RDA Table 2 (continued)

Age (years)	Trace Elements[b] *Chromium (mg)*	*Selenium (mg)*	*Molybdenum (mg)*	Electrolytes *Sodium (mg)*	*Potassium (mg)*	*Chloride (mg)*
0–0.5	0.01–0.04	0.01–0.04	0.03–0.06	115–350	350–925	275–700
0.5–1.0	0.02–0.06	0.02–0.06	0.04–0.08	250–750	425–1275	400–1200
1–3	0.02–0.08	0.02–0.08	0.05–0.10	325–975	550–1650	500–1500
4–6	0.03–0.12	0.03–0.12	0.06–0.15	450–1350	775–2325	700–2100
7–10	0.05–0.20	0.05–0.20	0.10–0.30	600–1800	1000–3000	925–2775
11+	0.05–0.20	0.05–0.20	0.15–0.50	900–2700	1525–4575	1400–4200
Adults	0.05–0.20	0.05–0.20	0.15–0.50	1100–3300	1875–5625	1700–5100

[a]Because there is less information on which to base allowances, these figures are not given in the main table of the RDA and are provided here in the form of ranges of recommended intakes.

[b]Since the toxic levels for many trace elements may be only several times usual intakes, the upper levels for the trace elements given in this table should not habitually be exceeded.

RDA Table 3

Recommended Energy Intakes for Individuals of Average Height, Weight, and Activity Levels

Age *(years)*	Weight *(kg)*	*(lb)*	Height *(cm)*	*(inches)*	Energy Needs[a] *(cal)*	*(MJ)*[b]
Infants						
0–0.5	6	13	60	24	kg × 115(95–145)	kg × 0.48
0.5–1.0	9	20	71	28	kg × 105(80–135)	kg × 0.44
Children						
1–3	13	29	90	35	1300 (900–1800)	5.5
4–6	20	44	112	44	1700 (1300–2300)	7.1
7–10	28	62	132	52	2400 (1650–3300)	10.1
Males						
11–14	45	99	157	62	2700 (2000–3700)	11.3
15–18	66	145	176	69	2800 (2100–3900)	11.8
19–22	70	154	177	70	2900 (2500–3300)	12.2
23–50	70	154	178	70	2700 (2300–3100)	11.3
51–75	70	154	178	70	2400 (2000–2800)	10.1
76+	70	154	178	70	2050 (1650–2450)	8.6
Females						
11–14	46	101	157	62	2200 (1500–3000)	9.2
15–18	55	120	163	64	2100 (1200–3000)	8.8
19–22	55	120	163	64	2100 (1700–2500)	8.8
23–50	55	120	163	64	2000 (1600–2400)	8.4
51–75	55	120	163	64	1800 (1400–2200)	7.6
76+	55	120	163	64	1600 (1200–2000)	6.7
Pregnant					+300	
Lactating					+500	

[a]The energy allowances for the young adults are for men and women doing light work. The allowances for the two older age groups represent mean energy needs over these age spans, allowing for a 2% decrease in basal (resting) metabolic rate per decade and a reduction in activity of 200 cal/day for men and women between 51 and 75 years, 500 cal for men over 75, and 400 cal for women over 75. The customary range of daily energy output, shown in parentheses, is based on a variation in energy needs of ±400 cal at any one age, emphasizing the wide range of energy intakes appropriate for any group of people. Energy allowances for children through age 18 are based on median energy intakes of children of these ages followed in longitudinal growth studies. The values in parentheses are 10th and 90th percentiles of energy intake, to indicate the range of consumption among children of these ages.

[b]MJ stands for megajoules (1 MJ = 1000 kJ).

Fourth Edition

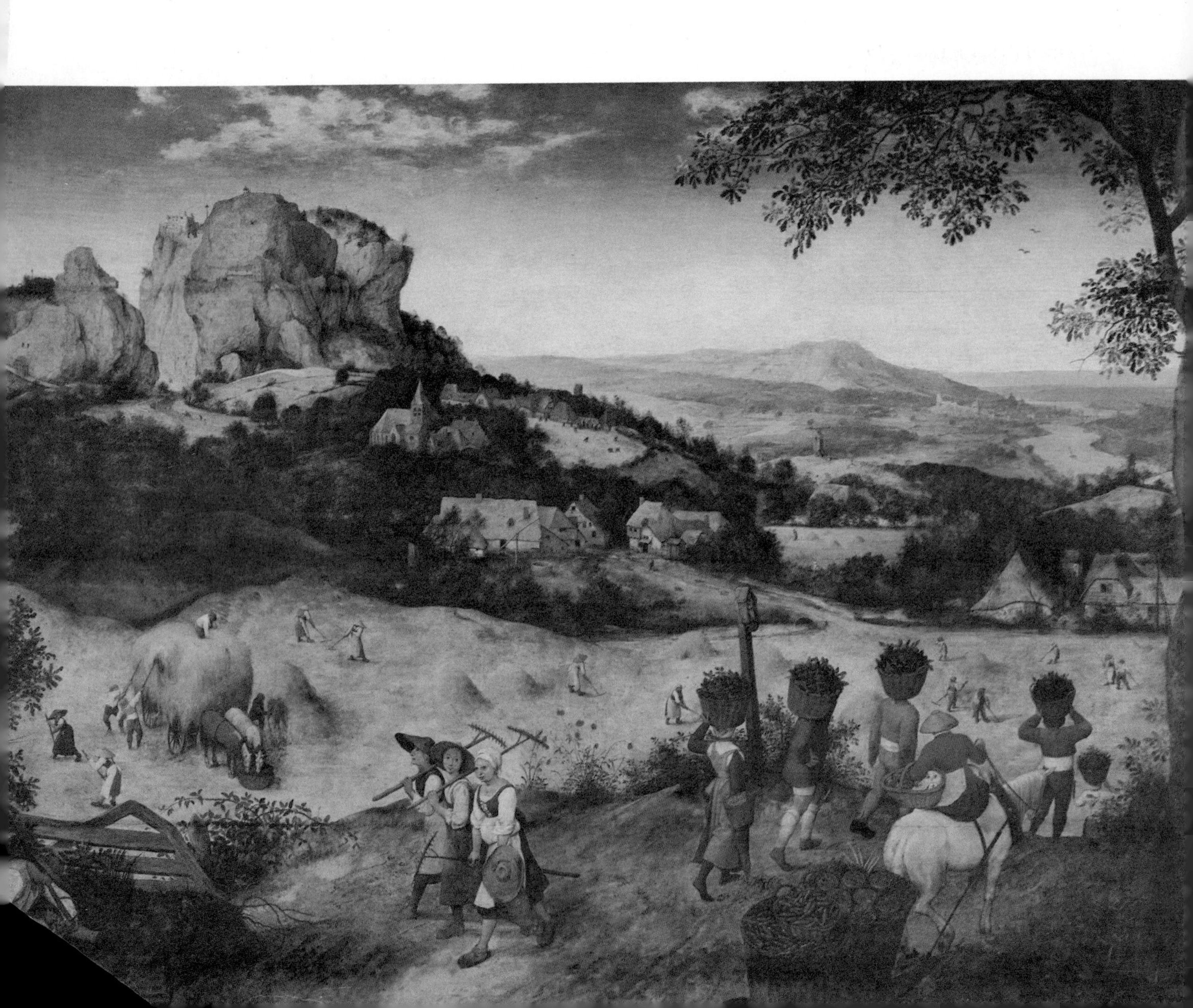

Nutrition: Concepts and Controversies

Eva May Nunnelley Hamilton

Eleanor Noss Whitney

Frances Sienkiewicz Sizer

Fourth Edition Prepared by

Eleanor Noss Whitney
Frances Sienkiewicz Sizer

West Publishing Company
St. Paul New York Los Angeles San Francisco

Production Credits

Cover Design: David Farr, Imagesmythe, Inc.
Text Design: Janet Bollow
Text Illustration: Asterisk Group; Brenda Booth
Cartoons: Kim Pickering, Barbara Clark
Copyediting: Mary Berry, Naples Editing Service
Index: Jo-Anne Naples, Naples Editing Service
Composition: Carlisle Communications

50 W. Kellogg Boulevard
P.O. Box 64526
St. Paul, MN 55164-1003

Printed in the United States of America

Library of Congress Cataloging-in-Publication Data

Hamilton, Eva May Nunnelley.
Nutrition : concepts and controversies / Eva May Nunnelley Hamilton, Eleanor Noss Whitney, Frances Sienkiewicz Sizer.—4th ed.

p. cm.
Includes bibliographies and index.
ISBN 0-314-59743-3
1. Nutrition. 2. Food. I. Whitney, Eleanor Noss. II. Sizer, Frances Sienkiewicz. III. Title.
QP141.H34 1988
613.2—dc19 87—34164
CIP

Photo Credits

p. 9 Sharon King; **17** Ray Stanyard; **19** Musee de l'Homme Paris; **41 (top)** Ray Stanyard; **41 (margin), 42** Courtesy of U.S. Department of Agriculture; **46, 47, 52, 56** Ray Stanyard; **59** PhotoEdit© Tony Freeman; **77, 87, 90** Ray Stanyard; **92** Anthony Vannelli; **95** PhotoEdit© Tony Freeman; **98** Ray Stanyard; **105** PhotoEdit© Tony Freeman; **109, 121, 122, 123, 126** Ray Stanyard; **131 (top)** Anthony Vannelli; **131 (bottom)** Reproduced by permission of ICI Pharmaceuticals Division, Cheshire, England; **147** Human hemoglobin model constructed by Dr. Makio Murayama, NIH, Bethesda, Maryland (scaled to ½ inch to angstrom). Atomic coordinates were supplied for the model by Dr. Max F. Perutz, Cambridge, England; **156, 164, 166** Ray Stanyard; **170** ©Jeffry W. Myers, Stock, Boston; **176** Ray Stanyard; **184** David Farr; **185** ©*Nutrition Today,* H. Sandstead, J. Carter, and W. Darby, Nutritional Deficiencies, Nutrition Today Teaching Aid Number 5 (Nutrition Today: Annapolis, MD); **186** Ray Stanyard; **187** Courtesy of Parke-Davis and Company; **195 (top)** ©*Nutrition Today,* C. Butterworth and G. Blackburn, Hospital Nutrition and How to Assess the Nutritional Status of a Patient. Nutrition Today Teaching Aid Number 18 (Nutrition Today: Annapolis, MD); **202** ©*Nutrition Today,* H. Sandstead, J. Carter, and W. Darby, Nutritional Deficiencies, Nutrition Today Teaching Aid Number 5 (Nutrition Today: Annapolis, MD), 1975; **204, 214** Ray Stanyard; **216** Anthony Vannelli; **227** Photo copyright ©Camera M.D. Studios, Inc.; **248** Ray Stanyard; **251** Reproduced with permission of *Nutrition Today* magazine, P.O. Box 1829, Annapolis, MD 21404, March, 1968; **252** Ray Stanyard; **253** Courtesy of H. Kaplan and V.P. Rabbach; **258** Ray Stanyard; **264** ©Ellis Herwig, Stock, Boston; **301, 302, 307** Ray Stanyard; **311** PhotoEdit© Tony Freeman; **340** A. Tannenbaum, Sygma; **350, 354** Ray Stanyard; **355** Courtesy of Andreas Cahling; **358** Ray Stanyard; **362** Anthony Vannelli; **371** Peter Menzel, Stock, Boston; **391, 401** Ray Stanyard; **405** PhotoEdit© Alan Oddie; **407** Ray Stanyard; **425, 431** Woodfin Camp and Associates© William Hubbell; **447** Anthony Vannelli; **449** Courtesy of H. Kaplan and V.P. Rabbach; **453** Anthony Vannelli; **454** Photos courtesy of Ann Pytkowicz Streissguth, University of Washington. Reprinted by permission of CIBA Foundation; **459, 462** Anthony Vannelli; **464** PhotoEdit© Richard Hutchings; **466** Anthony Vannelli; **483** ©Donald Dietz, Stock, Boston; **485, 489** Anthony Vannelli; **511** PhotoEdit, ©Mark Richards; **521** ©Jeff Dunn, Stock, Boston; **523** Anthony Vannelli; **524** ©Gabor Demjen, Stock, Boston; **527** PhotoEdit ©Myrleen Ferguson; **540 (left)** UNICEF photo by Arild Vollan; **540 (right)** World Health Organization/Pan American Health Organization; **541 (top)** David Wee and Karen Herseth Wee, St. Olaf College, Northfield, MN 55057; **541 (bottom)** Ray Stanyard; **552 (text)** Agency for International Development; **552, 553 (margin)** David Wee and Karen Herseth Wee, St. Olaf College, Northfield, MN 55057; **556** Agency for International Development; ©Bob Daemmrich, Stock, Boston; **573 (top)** PhotoEdit ©Tony Freeman; **573 (bottom)** PhotoEdit ©Alan Oddie

To the Quakers at Monteverde who showed me the rainforest.

Ellie Whitney

To the people whose work changes the world, Ellie, Gordie, Sharon, Linda, Marie and all the others.

Fran Sizer

About the Authors

Eleanor Noss Whitney, PhD, RD, received her BA in biology from Radcliffe College in 1960 and her PhD in biology with an emphasis on genetics from Washington University, St. Louis, in 1970. Formerly an associate professor at the Florida State University, she now devotes full time to research, writing, and consulting in nutrition and health. Her publications include articles in *Science*, the *Journal of Nutrition, Genetics,* and other journals, and the textbooks *Understanding Normal and Clinical Nutrition, Understanding Nutrition, Nutrition and Diet Therapy,* and *Life Choices: Health Concepts and Strategies.* She is president of Nutrition and Health Associates, an information resource center in Tallahassee, Florida.

Frances Sienkiewicz Sizer attended Florida State University where, in 1980, she received her BS, and in 1982, her MS in nutrition. As a founding member of Nutrition and Health Associates, Fran writes monographs for nutrition and health professionals on current topics in nutrition, and has published in *Shape* magazine, in the health newsletter *Healthline*, and in the *Journal of Chemical Senses.* In addition to *Nutrition: Concepts and Controversies*, she and Ellie Whitney have written *Life Choices: Health Concepts and Strategies*, a college health textbook.

Contents in Brief

Contents

Chapter Five

The Proteins and Amino Acids 145

Chapter Six

The Vitamins 181

Chapter Seven

Minerals and Water 225

Chapter Eight

Energy Balance and Weight Control 273

Preface

This edition of *Nutrition Concepts and Controversies* has come about in response to the requests and suggestions of users. The writing allowed us to enjoy discovering the new findings in research areas we first explored years ago, in the early editions. We see, too, that the research stories do not end, that seeming endings turn out to be beginnings, and that the field of nutrition continues to change. It is our hope that you will enjoy the new information and the new features of this text, and that beneath the new full-color format, you will recognize the old tradition of accurate and thorough information presented in a personally inviting style.

The order of the chapters has changed. Chapter 1 describes the body's basic needs for nutrients and gives the details of many of the body systems as they relate to nutrition. Chapter 2 brings together the concept of diet planning through food grouping systems, the nutrient density concept, and exchange systems. Chapters 3 through 5 are devoted to the energy-yielding nutrients—carbohydrates, lipids, and proteins. Chapters 6 and 7 present the vitamins, minerals, and water. Chapter 8 relates energy balance to the problems of overweight, obesity, and underweight. Chapter 9 is new to this edition, and presents the relationships between fitness, exercise, and nutrition, with specific suggestions for both the casual exerciser and the serious athlete. Chapter 10 delves into topics related to food (food processing, the safety of the food supply, how to avoid foodborne illness, and reading labels). Chapters 11, 12, and 13 develop nutrition themes important throughout life, from conception to old age. Chapter 14 describes the enormity of world food problems, with a focus on personal action.

The optional reading sections, the "Controversies" of this book's title, are printed on colored paper. Many are new to this edition, others are newly revised. These topics tantalize us with new research struggles appearing everywhere we look. We hope you enjoy those we selected for inclusion. Several deserve special mention here. Controversy 1 asks the question of whether modern people should strive to eat as their ancient ancestors did, and tells just what that diet might have been. Controversy 2 gives emphasis to a traditional topic of this book, how to become a sophisticated consumer of nutrition information. It defines explicitly how to tell the wheat from the chaff, the experts from the charlatans. Controversy 10 explores the fascinating contributions *non*nutrients make to the diet. Controversy 14 touches on a topic so vast that it may well shape the future of the world.

The Food Feature sections of Chapters 1 through 10 are much updated and offer new bridges between theory and practice; they are personal applications of the concepts in the chapters. The Self-Study sections at the ends of the chapters offer you a means of inspecting your own diet, to maximize your benefits from the study of nutrition. A new feature, repeated in every chapter, is the boxes for consumers on supplements and other nutrition-related products, including amino acids, vitamin-mineral supplements, calcium supplements, diet pills, supplements for the athlete, and more.

Glossary definitions of terms now appear on the pages where the terms are used in the text. This new format should ease learning new or major terms. Each new term appears in **boldface type** in the text, to call attention to its importance.

The appendixes are for your reference. Notice especially Appendix A, which presents the nutrient contents of over 1000 foods, including many fast foods not included earlier, and Appendix C, which offers help with nutrition calculations. Appendix I presents details of digestion and absorption beyond those given in the chapters.

Excitement leads us to want to write more about everything, but space constrains us (perhaps fortunately for the reader with limited time). To save space, we have included footnotes only where new information is presented. Anyone with an older edition of the book can find earlier notes, or you can request any reference from us through the publisher.

Thank you for your many good ideas that helped to shape this edition of *Nutrition: Concepts and Controversies*. We hope you enjoy it.

Eleanor N. Whitney
Frances S. Sizer
February, 1988.

Acknowledgments

We are grateful to our associates for their assistance in the preparation of this edition. Marie Boyle contributed much of Controversy 7, Nutrition and Hypertension, and Chapter 14, Nutrition Status: Domestic and World. Linda DeBruyne wrote Chapter 11, Mother and Newborn Infant. Sharon Rolfes wrote Chapter 12, Child and Teen. Linda Patton provided skilled and efficient help with library research and references. Our associates also supported us in other ways too numerous to mention.

We are also grateful to our editors and their staff Pete Marshall, Becky Tollerson, Sharon Walrath, and Jane Bacon whose efforts have greatly enhanced the quality of this book. We also thank Lorri Fishman, the preparer of the *Instructor's Manual,* Jana Kicklighter, preparer of the *Test Bank* and *Student Study Guide,* and Betty and Bob Geltz, creators of the food composition table (Appendix A), and the computerized diet analysis program that goes with this book.

The production staff have provided massive support, for which we cannot thank them enough. We especially appreciate the efforts of Joan Weber.

Our reviewers have supplied many helpful comments and suggestions. Finally, we wish to thank May Hamilton, from whose original work on this book we still draw inspiration.

Reviewers of *Nutrition: Concepts and Controversies*

(Fourth Edition) Reviewers

Carolyn Barnes
University of West Florida
Pensacola, FL

Hector Balcazar
University of Maine
Orono, ME

Dorothy Cope
Phoenix College
Phoenix, AZ

Nancy Green
Florida State University
Tallahassee, FL

Marsha Herrin
Dartmouth College
Hanover, NH

Susan Houston
San Francisco City College
San Francisco, CA

Nelda Loper
Seminole Community College
Sanford, FL

Judy Matheisz
Erie Community College-North Campus
Williamsville, NY

Pat Mogan
Orange Coast College
Santa Ana, CA

Dorice Czajka Narins
Northern Illinois University
DeKalb, IL

William Scheider
SUNY-Buffalo
Buffalo, NY

Sam Smith
University of New Hampshire
Durham, NH

Betty Jo Sullivan
Ohio University
Athens, OH

Sheron Sumner
University of North Carolina
Greensboro, NC

Susan Strahs
California State University
Long Beach, CA

Suzanne Tennis
College of San Mateo
San Mateo, CA

Cathleen Throssell
Loma Linda University
Loma Linda, CA

Linda Vaughan
Arizona State University
Tempe, AZ

Stan Winter
Golden West College
Huntington Beach, CA

Elizabeth Wirrick
University of Northern Colorado
Greeley, CO

June Wolgemuth
Florida International University
Miami, FL

(Third Edition) Revision Review

Nancy Betts
University of Nebraska
Lincoln, NE

Nancy Burzminski
University of Evansville
Evansville, IN

Effie Creamer
Eastern Kentucky University
Richmond, KY

Jane Garvin
University of Cincinnati
Cincinnati, OH

Margaret Harden
University of Guelph
Guelph, Ontario

Rosemary Richardson
Bellevue Community College
Bellevue, WA

Betty Jo Sullivan
Ohio University
Athens, OH

Sheron Sumner
University of North Carolina-Greensboro
Greensboro, NC

Suzanne Tennis
College of San Mateo
San Mateo, CA

Linda Vaughan
Arizona State University
Tempe, AZ

Lauretta Wasserstein
California State University-Northridge
Northridge, CA

Elizabeth Wirrick
University of Northern Colorado
Greeley, CO

Billie Wood
Daytona Beach Community College
Daytona Beach, FL

Chapter One

Contents

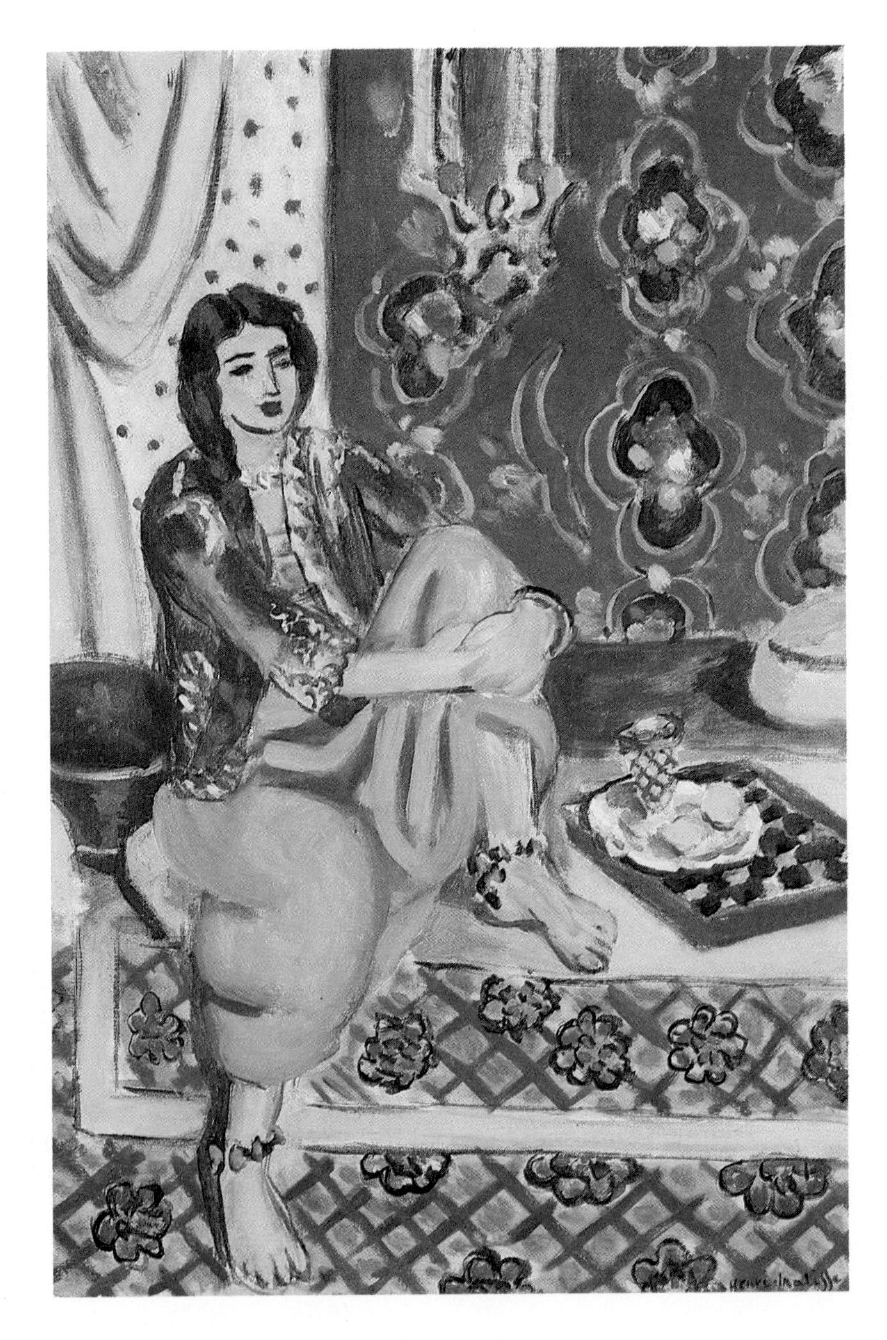

Seated Odalisque, Left Knee Bent, Ornamental Background and Checkerboard by Henri Matisse. The Baltimore Museum of Art: The Cone Collection, formed by Dr. Claribel Cone and Miss Etta Cone of Baltimore, Maryland (Photograph by Tennant). BMA 1950.255.

The Remarkable Body

You may be clothed in the latest fashions, and your car may be this year's model, but the body you live in is like that of your prehistoric ancestors. You have come a long way from the Stone Age in many ways: in language skills, in the arts, in medicine, and especially in the use of machinery. But in the ways your body handles food, bacteria, environmental pollutants, and other stresses, there have been few changes. You now have much the same body and brain your ancestors had 20,000 years ago.

Although the body has remained the same, the world has changed vastly, especially in the last hundred years. It is far more crowded than it used to be. In 1900, the world's population was 1 billion, now it is over 5 billion. Hunger and starvation today are for some a greater threat than ever before, especially in the developing countries, and some 15 million infants and children die each year from malnutrition and related causes.[1]

At the same time, abundance is also extreme, especially in the developed countries, for the technological era has brought great advantages. In much of the United States and Canada, for example, the food supply is abundant and relatively low in cost. The luxuries of convenience foods and high-speed cooking equipment, massive transportation and communication networks, and widespread economic security have made food so easily available that they have created problems of a different kind for people's health. People's diets are often much higher in fat, salt, and sugar and lower in fiber, vitamins, and minerals than those of the best-nourished people of the past. Most people's lifestyles offer much less physical activity than did the lives of their ancestors. Many people face, in their environments, new technological byproducts: smog, water pollution, and other forms of contamination. Your Stone Age body is stressed, contending with these new problems.

Whether you are poor or rich, hungry or overfed, all these differences from the past are relevant to you, for they are human problems of today. This book begins with the question how best to nourish yourself, individually, in a world in which foods are available. It assumes that, the better you understand and take care of yourself, the better you will be able to contribute to solving the problems of others.

Thanks to modern technology, you have far greater freedom to choose foods from a far greater variety in the local stores than people ever have had before. But with freedom comes both risk and responsibility; you have to make choices. This chapter describes the human body's needs and lays the groundwork for making wise food choices. The Controversy that follows asks the question whether we should actually try to eat as our ancestors did.

The brief anatomy lessons that follow are selected for their significance to nutrition. They review the body systems and terminology you need to understand in order to appreciate the points made in this book. The body is adapted to meet the life needs of its cells, so this discussion begins with them.

The Cells and Their Inheritance

The body is composed of millions of **cells**. Each is a self-contained, living entity (see Figure 1–1). Not one of them knows anything about food. You may get hungry for meat, milk, or bread, but each cell of your body needs **nutrients**—the vital components of foods. Each cell keeps itself alive just as its single-celled ancestors did, living alone in the ocean 3 billion years ago—by taking up the substances it needs from the surrounding fluid and releasing the wastes it produces into that fluid.

The cells' most basic need, always, is for **energy** fuel and the oxygen with which to burn it. Next, cells need water, the environment in which they live. Then they need building blocks to maintain themselves, especially the materials they can't make for themselves—the **essential nutrients**—which must be supplied preformed from food. The first principle of diet planning is that whatever foods we choose, they must provide energy, water, and the essential nutrients. If energy or nutrients are undersupplied or oversupplied, the result is **malnutrition,** a disease condition.

cells: the smallest units in which independent life can exist. All living things are single cells or organisms made of cells.

nutrients: components of food that help to nourish the body—that is, to provide energy, to serve as building material, or to help maintain or repair body parts. The nutrients include carbohydrate, fat, protein, vitamins, minerals, and water (see Chapter 2).

energy: the capacity to do work. The energy in food is chemical energy; it can be converted to mechanical, electrical, heat, or other forms of energy in the body. Food energy can be measured in *calories* (see Chapter 2).

essential nutrients: nutrients that can't be synthesized by the body in amounts sufficient to meet physiological needs. Chapter 2 presents a table of them.

malnutrition: any condition caused by excess or deficient food energy or nutrient intake, or by an imbalance of nutrients. Nutrient or energy deficiencies are classified as forms of *undernutrition*; nutrient or energy excesses are forms of *overnutrition*.

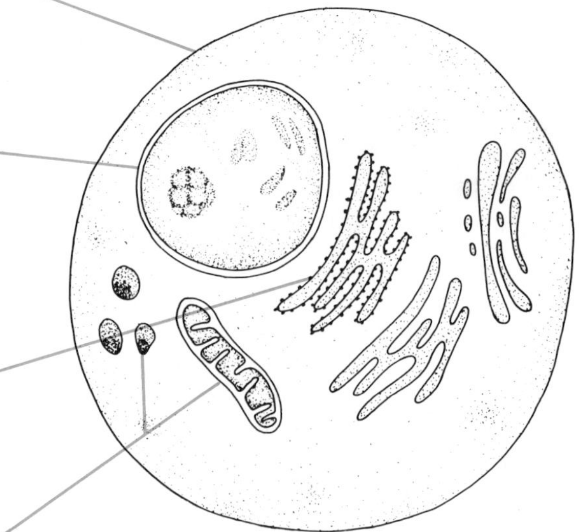

Figure 1–1 A Typical Cell (simplified diagram).

For most cells, death is not the natural end of life. A cell may grow until it has doubled its size and duplicated all its parts, at which point it may divide to form two daughter cells. These will grow and divide to form four, the four will become eight, and after only ten generations, if all survive, there will be almost 10,000 cells. The original cell has produced thousands of replicas of itself. Death comes to a cell only when its needs are not met—when its oxygen, water, or nutrient supply fails, the temperature becomes extreme, or its structure is somehow destroyed. The fact that you are alive today means that your cells' ancient ancestors successfully obtained these vital supplies in amounts sufficient to meet their needs, so that they could reproduce in an unbroken chain of generations for some 3 billion years.

In the human body, every cell works in cooperation with every other to support the whole. The cell's **genes** determine the nature of that work. Each gene is a blueprint that directs the making of a piece of protein machinery—most often an **enzyme**—that helps to do the cell's work. Each cell contains a complete set of genes, but different ones are active in different types of cells. For example, in the intestinal cells, the genes for making digestive enzymes are active; in the bone marrow cells, the genes for making the oxygen-carrying protein hemoglobin are active. Millions of cells group together to make the organs of the body. The organs promote the ultimate accomplishment—survival of the whole organism to reproductive age.

Genes are copied so accurately from one generation to the next that a mistake is made only once every 100 million times. Once made, however, the mistake will be as faithfully copied as the original gene was. Usually, such a mistake (a **mutation**) is a severe disadvantage, and the organism dies without reproducing the mistake. But one time in a thousand the mutation turns out to confer some advantage on its possessor. Mutations provide the variety of genes that give organisms different characteristics, so that **natural selection** can act.

If a gene or gene combination confers an advantage (for example, longer legs or stronger wings to better pursue prey), the organism that possesses them will eat well, survive to breeding age, and pass those genes on to successive generations. Ultimately, the descendants with those characteristics (and genes) take over the area, and the ones that are not so well adapted die out, leaving no descendents. The selected genes are then passed on to all succeeding generations.

Human evolution has been extremely slow. The time span of human generations is long—on the order of 20 to 30 years. New mutations appear infrequently, and beneficial ones are especially rare. Natural selection requires many generations to alter even slightly the gene frequencies in a population. The demands the environment placed on our ancestors, generation after generation, were powerful in determining which members of each generation survived to reproduce and pass on their physical characteristics to us. The natural selection process has made our species, humankind, highly successful under the conditions in which we evolved. But it has not solved all our problems for us. It is important to be aware that the way we are today is the result of natural selection during the Stone Age. It is life in that time, not life in modern industrial society, to which our bodies are adapted.

The Stone Age people ate foods in their natural state; many people today eat processed foods. The Stone Age people exercised vigorously all day long; many people today drive cars and sit all day. Ancient people had no purified

genes: units of a cell's inheritance, made of a chemical, DNA, that is copied faithfully so that every time the cell divides, both its daughters get identical copies. Genes direct the cells' machinery to make the proteins that form each cell's structures and that do its work.

enzyme: a protein catalyst. A catalyst facilitates a chemical reaction without itself being altered in the process. (Proteins are described fully in Chapter 5 and digestive enzymes in Appendix I.)

mutation: an event caused by chemicals, radiation, viruses, or unknown factors that alters a gene. A mutated gene codes for a slightly or greatly altered protein.

natural selection: the means by which evolution takes place. Among the varied offspring in a generation, those that are best adapted survive to reproduce and pass on the genes that gave them the adaptive advantage, so that the next generation has a different distribution of genes in its gene pool.

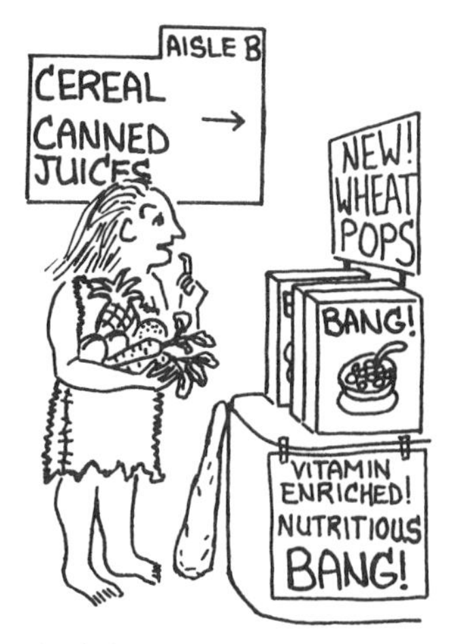

What foods best meet the needs of your Stone Age body?

blood: the fluid of the circulatory system—composed of water, red and white blood cells, other formed parricles, nutrients, oxygen, and other constituents.

lymph (LIMF): the fluid that bathes the cells, derived from the blood by being pressed through the capillary walls. Lymph is similar to the blood in composition but without red blood cells.

arteries: see Figure 1–3.

veins: see Figure 1–3.

capillaries: see Figure 1–3.

lungs: the organs of gas exchange. Blood circulating through the lungs releases its carbon dioxide and picks up fresh oxygen to carry to the tissues.

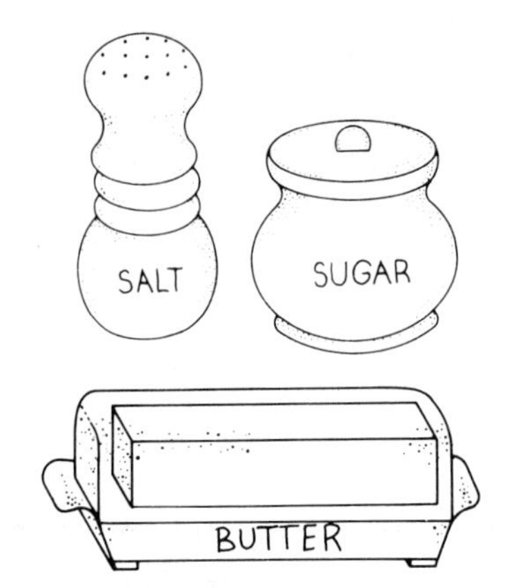

Familiar to us, new to the body.

fat, salt, or sugar; today, people use them liberally. The twentieth century food-ways and lifestyle impact the primitive body in ways that do not necessarily benefit health. To make choices of foods and activities that benefit our health, we need to learn how our bodies work and what they need. The body is designed to meet the needs of its cells for energy fuel, water, and nutrients. The body evolved in the natural world, but must meet its needs in today's changed world.

The Body Fluids and the Circulatory System

Every cell of the body needs a continuous supply of oxygen, energy, water, and building materials. The body fluids supply these necessities, bathing the outsides of all the cells much as the water of the ancient ocean bathed their one-celled ancestors. Every cell continuously uses up oxygen and nutrients (producing carbon dioxide and other waste products). The body fluids must circulate to pick up fresh supplies and deliver the wastes to points of disposal.

The fluids that bathe the cells and circulate around the body are the extra-cellular fluids, the **blood** and **lymph**. Blood travels within the **arteries, veins,** and **capillaries,** as well as the heart's chambers. (Figure 1–2). Lymph exits from the blood in the capillaries, circulates around the cells permitting exchange of materials, and returns to the blood farther along the capillaries or by way of its own vessels that return it to the veins.

As the blood travels through the circulatory system, it picks up wastes and delivers needed materials. Figure 1–3 shows its route, which ensures that all cells will be served. The blood picks up oxygen in the **lungs** and releases carbon dioxide there. All the blood circulates to the lungs, then returns to the heart, where it receives powerful impetus from the pumping heartbeats that push it out to all the other body tissues. Thus all tissues receive oxygenated blood fresh from the lungs.

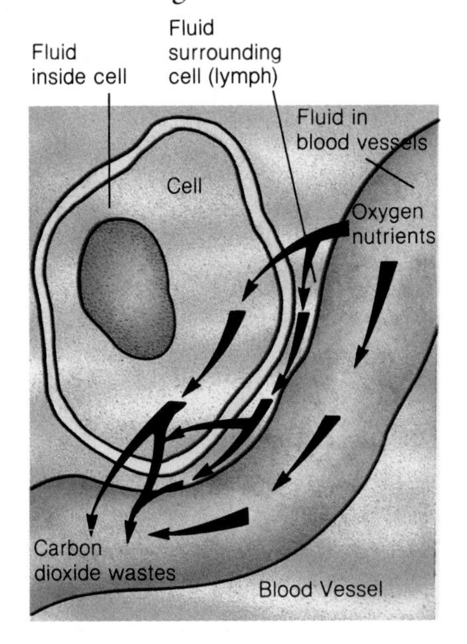

One cell and the surrounding fluids.

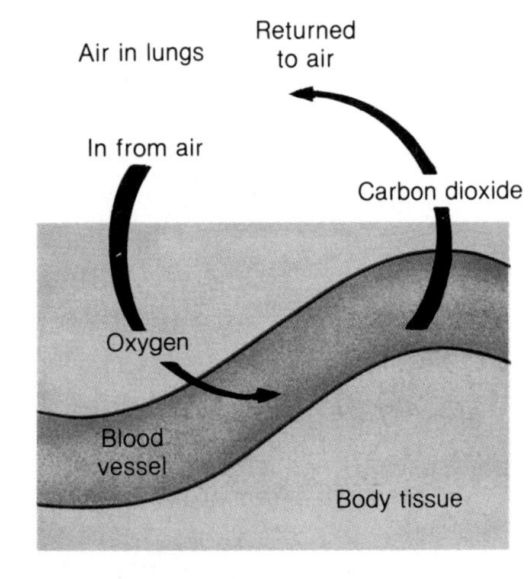

The lungs.

As it passes the digestive system, the blood delivers oxygen to the cells there and picks up nutrients for distribution elsewhere. All blood leaving the digestive system must go next to the **liver,** which has the special task of chemically altering the compounds it carries to make them better suited for use by other tissues. Then, in passing through the **kidneys,** the blood is cleansed of its wastes.

As it flows through the skin, the blood helps regulate the body temperature in two ways. First, heat generated by the internal organs is carried by blood to the skin, where it radiates into the surroundings. Second, fluid from lymph is used to make sweat, as explained later ("Temperature Regulation"). After being cooled, the blood returns to the deep body core, where it siphons off additional excess heat.

In summary, the blood is routed as shown in Figure 1–3:

- Heart to body to heart to lungs to heart (repeat).

The portion of the blood that flows by the digestive tract travels from:

- Heart to digestive tract to liver to heart.

To ensure the continued functioning of all your cells, clearly you need to ensure efficient circulation of fluid to them. This means drinking sufficient water to replace the water you necessarily lose every day—and also maintaining your cardiovascular fitness, a project that requires combined attention to nutrition and physical activity, as later chapters will show. You also need healthy red blood cells, because these carry oxygen to all the other cells, enabling them to burn their fuels for energy. Since red blood cells are born, live, and die within six weeks, you need to replace them constantly, a manufacturing process that requires many essential nutrients from food. Many kinds of blood disorders are caused by dietary deficiencies of vitamins or minerals; the blood is very sensitive to malnutrition.

liver: a large, many-lobed organ that lies under the ribs. It filters the blood, removing and processing nutrients, manufacturing materials for export to other parts of the body, and destroying toxins or storing them out of circulation.

kidneys: the organs that filter the blood to remove waste material and forward it to the bladder for excretion out of the body.

Another name for the circulatory system is the cardiovascular system.

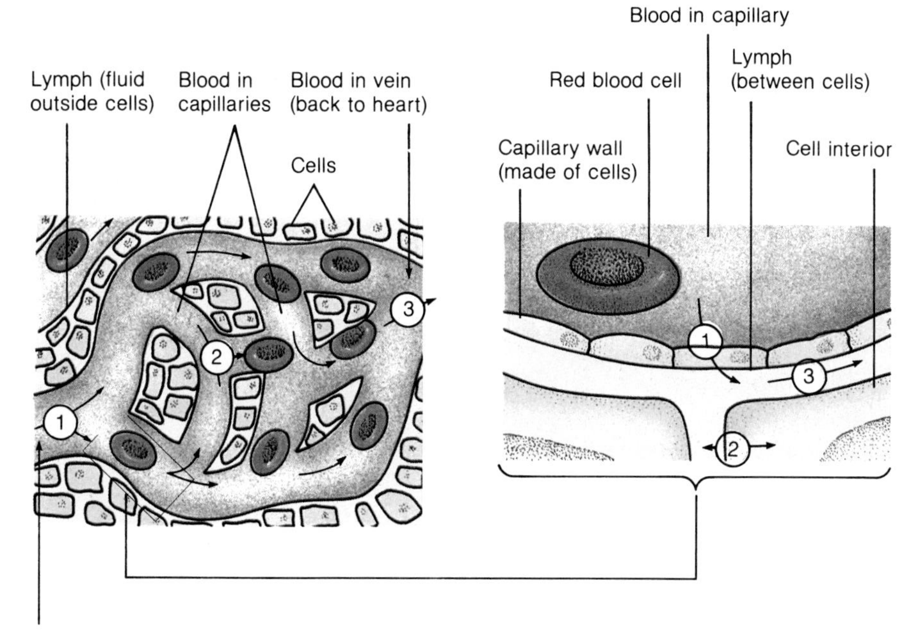

Figure 1–2 How the Body Fluids Circulate Around Cells.
A. Portion of body tissue.
1. Blood enters tissues by way of an artery.
2. Blood circulates among cells by way of capillaries.
3. Blood collects into veins for return to heart.

B. Detail of A.
1. Lymph filters out of capillary.
2. Exchange of materials takes place between cell fluid and lymph.
3. Lymph circulates away, later reentering bloodstream in a vein.

Figure 1–3 The Circulatory System.

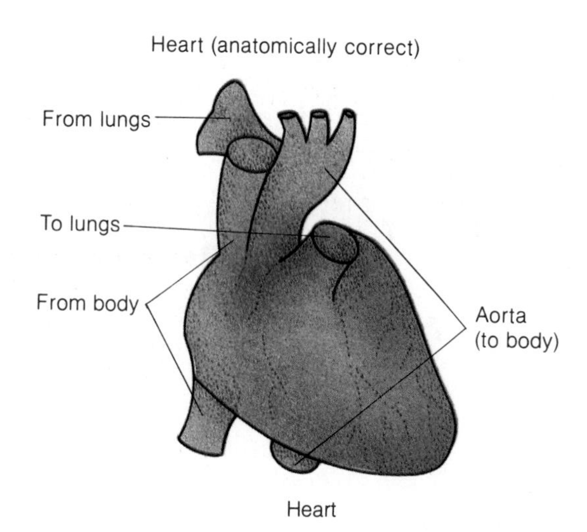

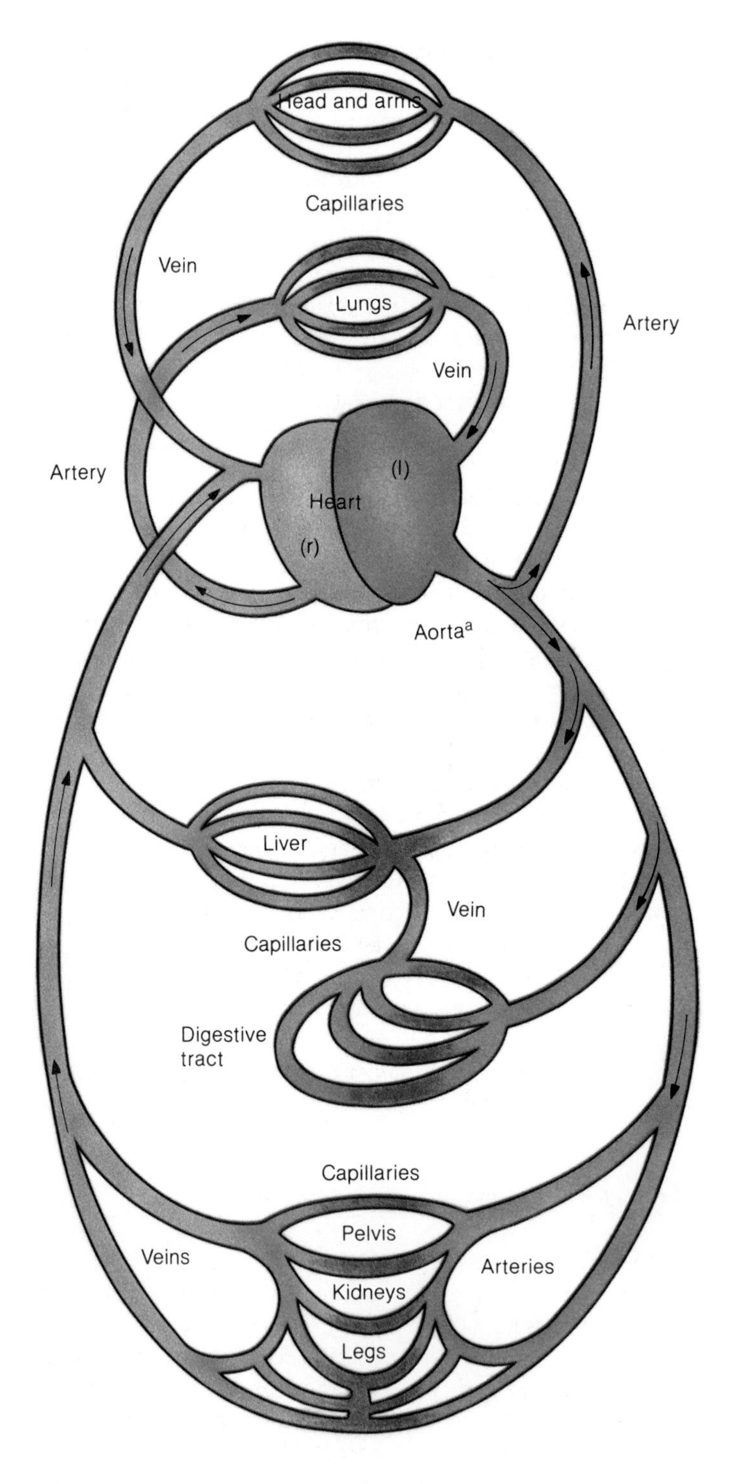

Blood leaves right side of heart, picks up oxygen in lungs, and returns to left side of heart. Blood leaves left side of heart, goes to head or digestive tract and then to liver or lower body, and then returns to right side of heart.

[a]The aorta is the main artery that launches blood on its course through the body. The picture is not anatomically correct but is drawn this way for clarity. The aorta actually arises behind the left side of the heart and arcs upwards, then divides. See detail of heart.

Blood and lymph deliver oxygen and nutrients to all the body's cells and carry waste materials away from them. The circulatory system ensures that these fluids circulate among all the organs, enabling each organ to contribute and remove materials.

The Immune System

Many of the body's cells cooperate to maintain its defenses against infection. The skin presents a physical barrier, and the body's cavities (lungs, digestive tract, and others) are lined with membranes that resist penetration by invading **microbes** or unwanted substances. The body's linings are sensitive to nutrient deficiencies, and clinicians inspect both the skin and the inside of the mouth to detect signs of malnutrition. (The chapters on protein, vitamins, minerals, and energy present details of the signs of deficiencies.)

Should these first lines of defense be breached, the lymph and blood present internal defenses: chemicals, enzymes, and cells that can inactivate, remove, or destroy microbes and foreign substances. Special cells are able to recognize minute aspects of the chemical structure of foreign materials and to store the memory of them for long times, so that they can quickly mobilize defenses when they see them again. This ability confers **immunity** against any disease that you have previously fought and conquered. Among the cells responsible for this immunity are some that produce ammunition (**antibodies**) designed to destroy specific targets (**antigens**), and still other cells that can gobble up and digest the injured invaders—to clean up the battlefield, so to speak.

Immune system components reside in compartments all over the body—inside the bones, along the linings of the blood vessels, in the lymph glands, and in glands of their own. They are in constant flux, being made and dismantled rapidly, and their maintenance requires a continuous supply of nutrients. A deficiency or an overdose of any nutrient is likely to affect the immune system adversely, and a deficiency of nutrients early in an infant's development can weaken that individual's immune defenses against infection for years.[2]

The immune system confers ability to resist disease. Its successful functioning depends on an adequate nutrient supply.

microbes: bacteria, viruses, or other organisms invisible to the naked eye; some cause disease.

immunity: the ability to successfully resist a disease, conferred on the body by way of the immune system's memory of previous exposure to that disease and its ability to mount a specific defense promptly and swiftly.

antibodies: proteins (see Chapter 5), made by the immune system, designed specifically to combine with and inactivate specific antigens.

antigens: microbes or substances that are foreign to the body.

hormones: chemical messages that are secreted by glands in response to conditions in the body that require a response, and that act on other organs to change those conditions.

endocrine (EN-doh-crin): a term to describe a gland or hormone: secreting or being secreted into the blood (*endo* means "into").

pancreas: an organ with two main functions. One is an endocrine function—the making of hormones, such as insulin, which it releases directly into the blood to assist in regulating the blood glucose level. The other is an *exocrine* function—the manufacture of digestive enzymes, which it releases through a duct into the small intestine to assist in digestion (*exo* means "out" into a body cavity).

insulin: a hormone from the pancreas that helps glucose get into cells (more in Chapter 3).

The Hormonal and Nervous Systems

The blood also carries messages, chemical signals from one system of cells to another, that communicate changing conditions that demand responses. These chemical messages, or **hormones,** are secreted and released into the blood by organs known as **endocrine** glands. For example, when the **pancreas** (a gland) experiences a too-high concentration of the blood's sugar, glucose, it releases **insulin** (a hormone). Insulin stimulates the liver, muscles, and fat cells to remove glucose from the blood and store it. When the blood glucose level falls too low, the pancreas secretes another hormone, glucagon. The liver responds by releasing glucose into the blood once again. (Chapter 3, whose subject is carbohydrates, describes this regulatory system in greater detail.)

Glands and hormones abound in the body. Each gland monitors a condition that needs regulation and produces one or more hormones to regulate it. Each

hunger: the physiological need to eat, experienced as an unpleasant sensation that demands relief.

appetite: the psychological desire to eat, experienced as a pleasant sensation that acccompanies the sight, smell, or thought of certain foods. Hunger and appetite usually occur together, but either may occur without the other (more in Chapter 8).

bladder: the sac that holds urine until time for elimination.

hormone is a message that stimulates certain organs to take appropriate action. Examples of the working of these hormones appear throughout this book.

Nutrition affects the hormonal system. Fasting, feeding, and exercise alter hormonal balances. People who become very thin have an altered hormonal balance that makes them unable to maintain their bones (see Chapter 9). People who eat high-fat diets have hormone levels that make them susceptible to certain cancers (details in Controversy 5).

Hormones also affect nutrition. They help to regulate **hunger,** and an abnormal hormonal state is probably at least partly responsible for the loss of **appetite** that sick people experience. Hormones also regulate the menstrual cycle in women, and they affect appetite—especially the appetite for carbohydrates—at different times in the cycle (see Chapter 12). They regulate the body's reaction to stress, too, suppressing hunger and the digestion and absorption of nutrients. Whenever questions about a person's nutrition are asked, the state of that person's hormonal system is always part of the answer.

The body's other major communication system is, of course, the nervous system. With the brain and spine as central controller, the system receives and integrates messages from receptors all over the body and returns instructions to the muscles and glands telling them what to do. The senses of sight, hearing, touch, smell, and taste all communicate to the brain the state of both the outer and inner worlds, including the availability of food and the need for it. The sensations of hunger and appetite are regulated by both nervous and hormonal systems—hunger communicating the physiological need for food, and appetite signifying the psychological willingness to eat it. Instructions then fly along the nerves to the voluntary muscles, saying "eat," and to the involuntary muscles and glands of the digestive tract, saying "make ready to digest food."

The hormonal and nervous systems facilitate regulation of body processes through communication among all the organs. They respond to the need for food and convey information about its availability. They mediate the willingness to eat it, govern the act of eating, and regulate digestion.

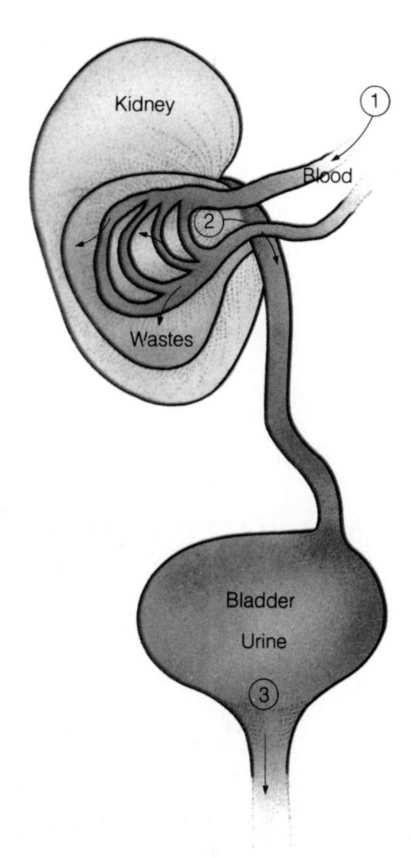

The excretory system.

1. Blood enters kidney by way of arteries, and splits into capillaries.
2. Kidney filters waste from blood and sends it as urine to the bladder.
3. Bladder periodically eliminates urine.

The Excretory System

To dispose of waste, the kidneys straddle the circulatory system and filter the passing blood. Waste materials removed with water are collected as urine in tubes that deliver them to the urinary **bladder,** which is periodically emptied. Thus the blood is purified continuously throughout the day, and dissolved materials are excreted as necessary (including sodium, to help keep blood pressure from rising too high). As you might expect, the kidneys' work is regulated by hormones secreted by glands that respond to conditions in the blood (such as the sodium concentration).

Whatever supports the health of the kidneys supports the health of the whole body, because the kidneys cleanse the blood. A strong cardiovascular system is important to keep blood flushing swiftly through the kidneys. An abundant water supply is also needed. In addition, the kidneys need sufficient energy to do their complex sifting and sorting job, and many vitamins and minerals serve as the cogs in their machinery. Exercise and nutrition are vital to healthy kidney function.

The kidneys adjust the blood's composition in response to the body's needs. Nutrients, including water, and exercise help keep them healthy.

metabolism (meh-TAB-o-lism): the sum total of all the chemical reactions that go on in living cells.

hypothalamus (high-poh-THAL-uh-mus): a part of the brain that senses a variety of conditions in the blood, such as temperature, glucose content, salt content, and others. It signals other parts of the brain or body to change those conditions when necessary.

cortex: the outermost layer of something. The brain's cortex is that part of the brain in which conscious thought takes place.

Temperature Regulation

All the body's cells obtain energy by breaking down the energy nutrients from food. Some of this energy they use to do work, some they store, and some they release as heat. The heat keeps the whole body warm, and excess heat radiates from the body surface whenever the surroundings are cooler than the skin. Temperature regulation involves speeding up or slowing down the cells' heat production (**metabolism**) and increasing or reducing heat loss through the skin. Specialized nerve cells in an area of the brain called the **hypothalamus** serve as a thermostat, measuring the temperature of the blood. These cells signal other cells, near the body surface, to respond appropriately. When the body is too hot, blood vessels immediately under the skin dilate, allowing warm blood to flow near the surface, where its heat can radiate away. In addition to this tactic, the sweat glands secrete fluid onto the skin surface, where its evaporation causes cooling—creating another need for the vital nutrient, water. When the body is cold, these mechanisms shut down. Blood is routed away from the skin, deeper into the tissues, and shivering and "goose bumps" are triggered, two muscular activities that generate heat.

The body's ability to maintain its temperature is especially sensitive to undernutrition. The fat under the skin provides insulation; when it is depleted, the circulating blood loses heat too rapidly. Not only fat loss, though, but also hormones account for the failure of temperature maintenance in starvation victims; they can't keep warm. Since some weight-loss diets are forms of starvation, they, too, alter hormone balances in a way that can cause a dieter to feel cold all the time, a sign that the dieter has gone to an unhealthy extreme (more about extreme diets in Chapter 8 and Controversy 12).

The body's heat production depends on the rate of cellular metabolism, which is regulated by the hypothalamus and by hormones. Undernutrition impairs the body's ability to keep warm.

The Digestive System

You may eat meals only two or three times a day, but your body's cells need their nutrients 24 hours a day. Providing the needed nutrients requires the cooperation of millions of specialized cells. When the body's cells are deprived of fuel, the hypothalamus (already mentioned) detects this condition and generates signals that travel to the conscious part of the brain, the **cortex,** signifying hunger. They also stimulate the stomach to intensify its contractions and secretions, creating hunger pangs and gurgling sounds. Becoming conscious of hunger, then, you eat, delivering a complex mixture of chewed and swallowed food to the digestive tract.

Many of the cells lining the digestive tract secrete powerful juices and enzymes to disintegrate nutrients into their component parts. Two organs outside the digestive tract also contribute digestive juices through a common duct into the

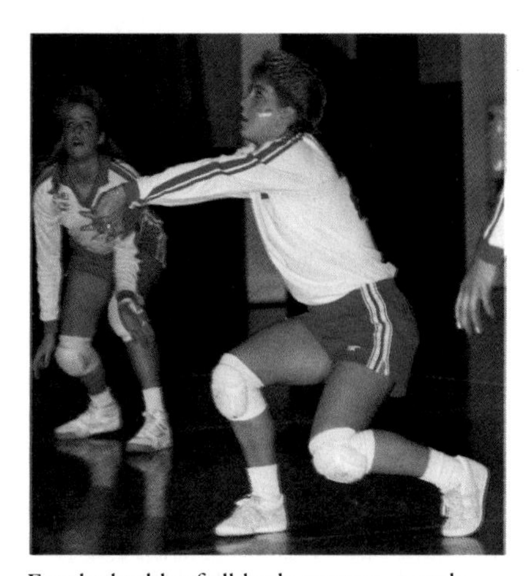

For the health of all body systems, people need exercise.

Figure 1–4 The Digestive System.

Mouth:
- Chews and mixes food with saliva

Esophagus:
- Passes food to stomach

Stomach:
- Adds acid and fluid
- Achieves some digestion
- Churns food to a liquid mass

Small intestine:
- Digests all components to nutrients
- Cells of wall absorb nutrients into blood and lymph

Liver:[a]
- Manufactures bile to emulsify fats

Gallbladder:[b]
- Stores bile until needed

Bile duct:
- Conducts bile into small intestine

Pancreas:[c]
- Manufactures enzymes to digest food and bicarbonate to neutralize stomach acid

Pancreatic duct:[d]
- Conducts pancreatic juice into small intestine

Large intestine (colon):
- Reabsorbs water
- Passes undigested waste (fiber, bacteria, and some water) to rectum

Rectum:
- Stores waste prior to elimination

Anus:
- Holds rectum closed
- Opens to allow elimination

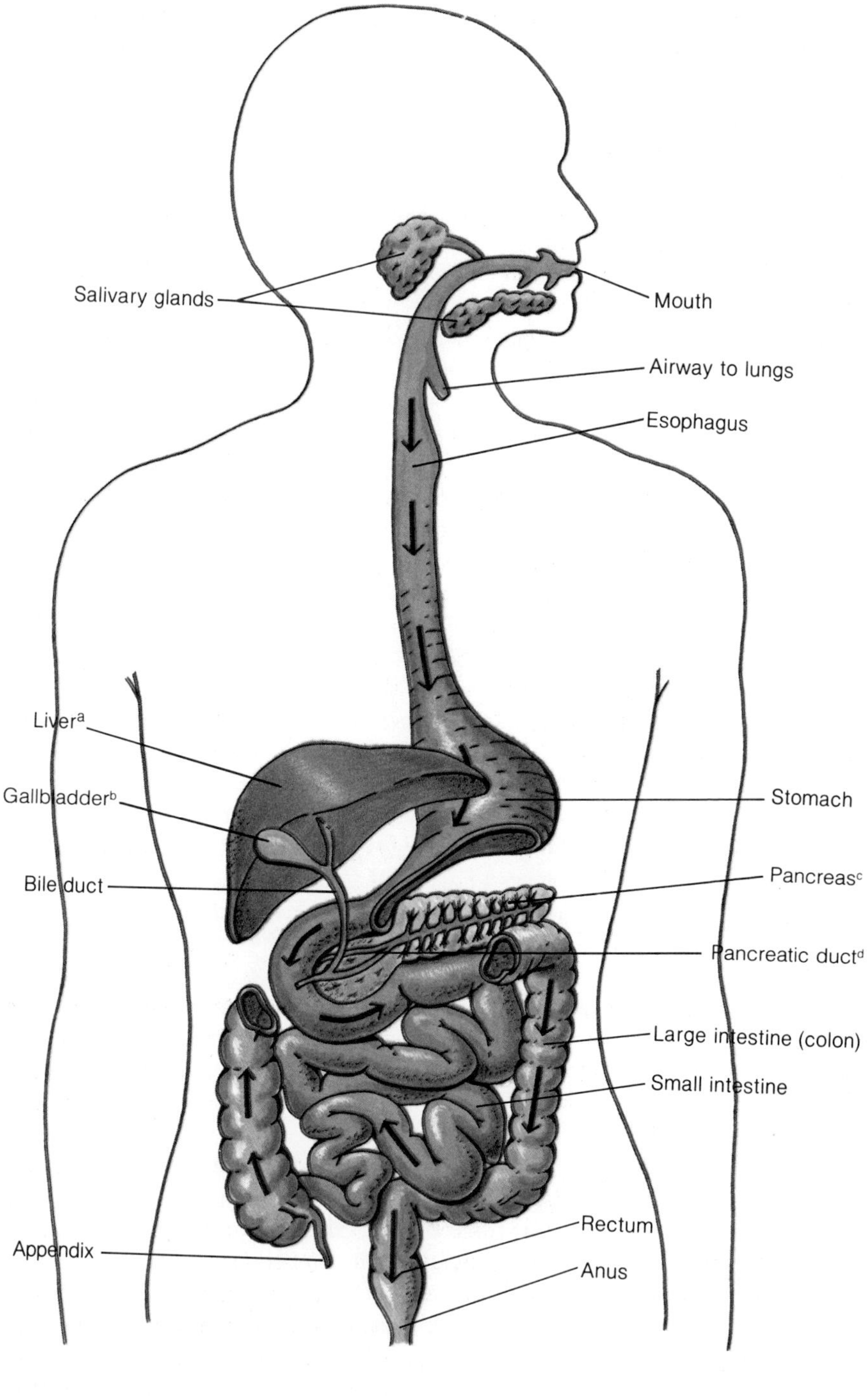

[a]The liver also serves other body systems. For example, it makes and stores glycogen (the storage form of glucose described in Chapter 3), it makes fat, and it adjusts the nutrient contents of the blood passing through it.

[b]The gallbladder is a sac embedded in the liver that stores a detergent-like substance, bile, to aid in the digestion of fat. The gallbladder releases bile through a duct into the small intestine whenever fat is present there.

[c]The pancreas also produces hormones that regulate the blood glucose level.

[d]In some people, the pancreatic duct merges with the bile duct before they open into the small intestine. The common portion is called the *common bile duct.*

small intestine. (One is the liver, already mentioned as a blood-adjusting organ; the other is the pancreas, already mentioned as an organ that produces insulin and digestive enzymes.) The cells of the intestinal lining then absorb nutrients from the digested mixture within the intestine and deposit them in the blood and lymph. Every nutrient must traverse a cell of the intestinal lining in order to enter the body fluids.

The small intestine's lining is wrinkled into thousands of folds, and each cell of its surface is also coated with tiny hairs, so that its absorbing surface is enormous. If that surface were spread out flat, it would occupy a third of a football field in area. The intestinal cells, weighing perhaps 4 to 5 pounds, absorb enough nutrients in a few hours a day to nourish the other 150 or so pounds of cells in the body.

The process of digestion can best be appreciated after learning about the constituents of food. The organs of the digestive tract are shown here, in Figure 1–4, but the steps they perform in digestion of the various nutrients are described later, in the chapters on those nutrients. The whole process is summarized in Appendix I, "Summary of Digestion and Absorption."

The digestive system is sensitive to an undersupply of energy, nutrients, dietary **fiber,** or exercise. In cases of severe undernutrition, the absorptive surface of the small intestine shrinks and may be reduced to a tenth of its normal area, making it impossible to obtain what few nutrients the limited food supply may make available. Without sufficient fiber, the digestive tract muscles have too little bulk to push against and so get too little exercise, becoming weak. Types of malnutrition that impair digestion are self-perpetuating, because impaired digestion makes malnutrition worse.

The digestive system feeds the rest of the body and is, itself, sensitive to malnutrition.

fiber: a nonnutrient constituent of foods, indigestible to the body and therefore useful in digestion because it adds bulk to the intestine's contents, giving the muscles something to push against. (Fiber is discussed in Chapter 3.)

glycogen: a storage form of carbohydrate energy (glucose), described more fully in Chapter 3.

fat: a storage form of energy, described more fully in Chapter 4.

fat cells: cells that specialize in the storage of fat.

Storage Systems

A meal may be eaten in half an hour, and the nutrients it provides reach the body fluids over a span of about four hours. However, as already mentioned, the cells of the body need their nutrients around the clock. Providing a constant supply requires that there be systems of storage and release to meet the cells' needs between meals.

Nutrients leave the digestive system by way of both branches of the circulatory system—the blood and the lymph. The blood carries some of the products of digestion, the lymph carries others, but all nutrients sooner or later find their way into the blood, and all sooner or later pass through the liver.

Nutrients collected from the digestive system move through a vast network of capillaries that weave among the liver cells, giving liver tissues access to the newly arriving nutrients. The liver cells process these nutrients. Later chapters provide the details, but it is important to know, now, that the liver converts excess energy-containing nutrients into two forms. It makes some into **glycogen,** and some into **fat.** It stores the glycogen to use for the body's short-term energy needs, and given the hormonal signal, the liver cells release this glycogen into the blood as glucose. The liver ships out fat in packages (see Chapter 4) via blood to other cells of the body. All body cells may withdraw fat from these packages; the excess fat winds up being stored in the **fat cells,** which hold it to meet longer-term energy needs.

The liver's glycogen provides a reserve supply of glucose, and thus can sustain cell activities if the intervals between meals become so long that glucose absorbed from ingested food is used up. But without food to replenish it, the liver's glycogen supply is used up within three to six hours. Similarly, the fat cells store reserves of fat, the body's other principal energy nutrient, but unlike the liver, the fat cells have virtually infinite storage capacity. They can continue to supply fat for days, weeks, or even months when no food is eaten. (Chapter 8 describes what happens during fasting, and Chapter 9 describes how the muscles also store glycogen—but for their own use, not for the body as a whole.)

These storage systems for glucose and fat ensure that the cells will not go without energy nutrients even if the body is hungry for food, except under extreme conditions. Body stores also exist for many other nutrients, each with a characteristic capacity. For example, the liver and fat cells store many vitamins, and the bones provide reserves of calcium, sodium, and other minerals that can be drawn on to keep the blood levels constant and to meet cellular demands.

Some nutrients are stored in the body in much larger quantities than are others. Some that are stored can become toxic, if too-large quantities are eaten. Others, the ones that are stored in only small amounts, can readily be depleted. As this book discusses the body's handling of various nutrients, it pays particular attention to how they are stored, so that you can know your tolerance limits. For example, you needn't eat fat at every meal, since fat is stored in virtually unlimited quantities in your body. On the other hand, you normally do need to have a source of carbohydrate at intervals throughout the day, because the liver can make glycogen available for only about three to six hours before becoming depleted.

The body stores large quantities of some nutrients, small quantities of others. Its energy stores are of two principal kinds: fat in the fat cells (in potentially large quantities) and glycogen in the liver cells (in smaller quantities).

Other Systems

In addition to the systems described above, the body has many more: the bones, the muscles, the brain and nerves, the reproductive organs, and others. All of these cooperate so that each cell can carry on its own life. Each system assures, through hormonal or nerve-mediated messages, that its needs will be met by the others, and each contributes to the welfare of the whole by doing its own specialized work. Each needs a continuous supply of many specific nutrients to maintain itself and carry out its work: calcium for the bones, for example; iron for the muscles; glucose for the brain. Each system is impaired by an undersupply or oversupply of nutrients. And each responds to exercise—the bones and muscles by becoming stronger, the brain and reproductive organs by remaining healthier.

Of the millions of cells in the body, only a small percentage make up the cortex of the brain, in which the conscious mind resides. These cells receive messages from other cells when they require you to "become conscious" of a need for decision and action. In modern life the need may be as complex as, for example, to notice that you feel anxious and to decide to consult an advisor, or it may be such a "simple" need as "I'm tired; I think I'll go to bed," or "I'm hungry; I guess I'd better eat."

Most of the body's work is done automatically by the other, unconscious portions of the brain and nervous system, and this work is finely regulated to achieve a state of well-being. But when your cortex does become involved, you would do well to cultivate an understanding and appreciation of your body's needs. Then your decisions will manifest themselves in health-promoting actions. Remember that your body is an "ancient" body, and that the life it is adapted to lead is the life of early human beings.

To achieve optimal function, the body's systems require nutrients from outside, and these have to be supplied through a human being's conscious food choices.

Human Food Behavior

If you live 65 years or longer, your remarkable body will consume and dispose of a hundred thousand pounds of food. It will extract energy from that food—and if you eat an amount of food energy that equals the energy you expend in physical activity, you will maintain desirable weight throughout your life. Your body will extract 40-plus nutrients from that food every day, and if you have eaten foods that supply neither too little nor too much of any nutrient, your body will carry out all of its vital functions efficiently, maintaining optimal nutritional health to the end of life. Your body will dispose of the unwanted constituents in all those foods to the extent that it is able to do so; and provided that you don't consume overwhelming quantities of cancer-causing or other toxic substances, the chances are good that you will remain relatively free of their effects.

Now, what is the probability that you will, over the 65-plus years of your life, select the right foods to just meet your body's needs for energy and all essential nutrients without consuming anything to excess? A look at the nation's older people helps to provide the answer. The chances of optimal health in later life are slim, unless you learn and begin to apply sound nutrition principles now. Many older people suffer from debilitating conditions that could have been largely prevented, had they known and applied the nutrition and fitness principles we know today throughout their lives.

We should hasten to say that not all of the so-called diseases of old age can be prevented by choice. The tendencies to develop heart disease, diabetes, many kinds of cancer, dental disease, and others differ among people, depending on their genetic constitutions. However, within the range set by your inheritance, the likelihood that you will develop certain diseases is strongly influenced by the life-style choices you make—such as whether to smoke; to consume alcohol; to exercise regularly; or to eat a nutritious, balanced diet. Figure 1–5 shows that many different diseases are responsive to nutrition to a greater or lesser extent, and Table 1–1 lists the nutrition measures you can take to help prevent these diseases.

With such information available, you might think that as soon as people knew how to obtain nutritional health, they would immediately set about eating the most beneficial diet possible. Such is not the case, however, because people's

Figure 1–5 Nutrition and Disease. Not all diseases are equally influenced by diet. Some are purely hereditary, like sickle-cell anemia. Some may be inherited (or the tendency to develop them may be inherited) but may be influenced by diet, like some forms of diabetes. Some are purely dietary, like the vitamin and mineral deficiency diseases. Some authorities are concerned that the offering of dietary advice to the public may seem to exaggerate the power of nutrition in preventing disease. Nutrition alone is certainly not enough to prevent many diseases, but it helps.
Source: Inspired by R. E. Olson, Are professionals jumping the gun in the fight against chronic diseases? *Journal of the American Dietetic Association* 74 (1979): 543–550, Figure 2.

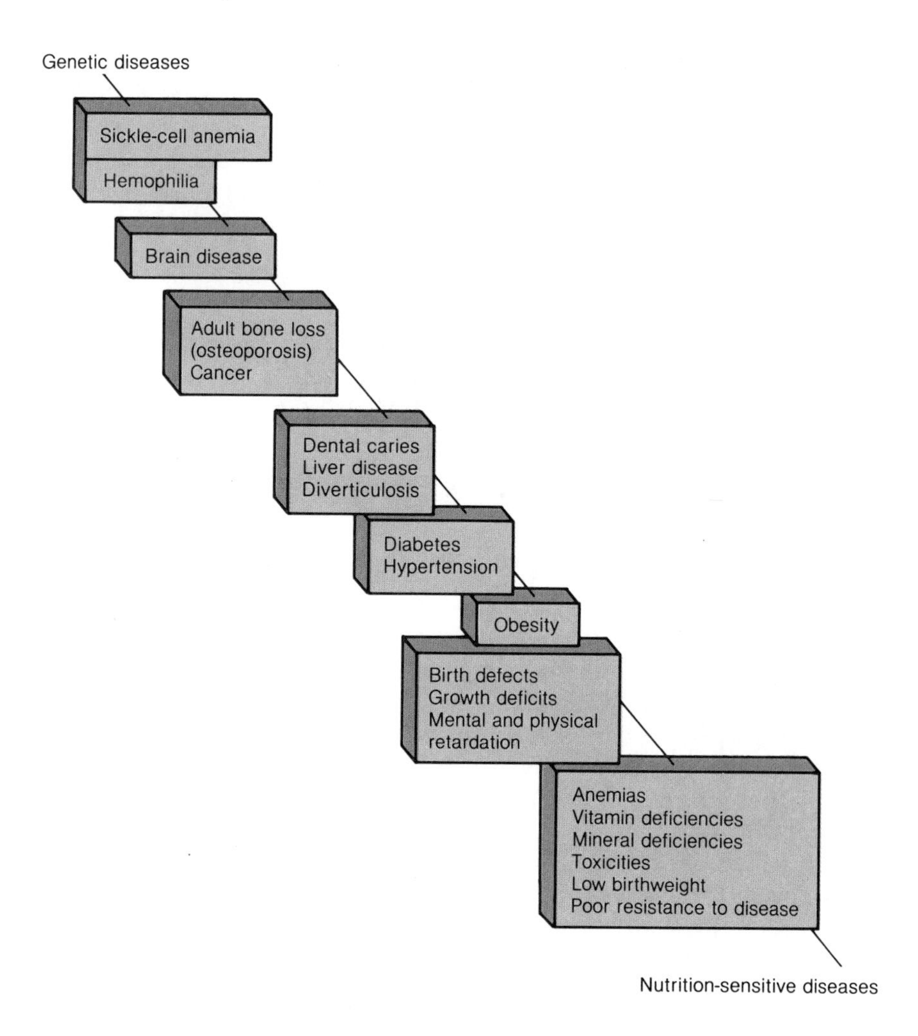

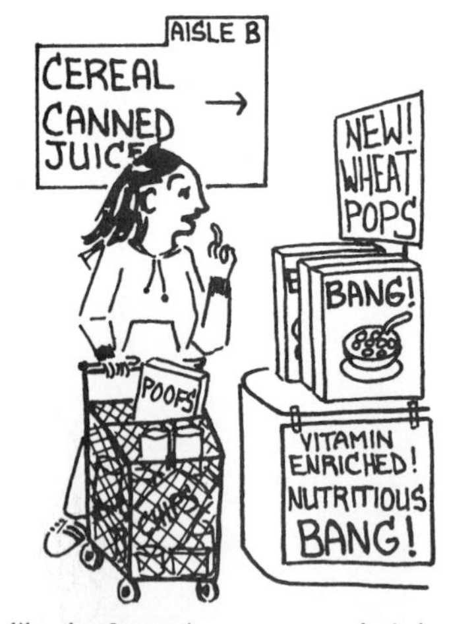

Unlike the Stone Age person, today's buyer faces many bewildering nutrition claims.

food choices are influenced by many factors other than the knowledge of what is best for their health, and most of these factors are irrational.

Among the reasons you choose the foods you eat today may be any of the following:

- Personal preference (you like them).
- Habit or tradition (they are familiar; you always eat them).
- Social pressure (they are offered; you feel you can't refuse them).
- Availability (there are no others to choose from).
- Convenience (you are too rushed to prepare anything else).
- Economy (they are within your means).
- Nutritional value (you think they are good for you).

Of these seven possible reasons people choose foods, only one has to do with nutrition directly. Even people who pride themselves on eating nutritious foods will admit that the other six factors also influence their food choices.

Although these factors influence everyone's food choices, the nutritional value of food has become a more important consideration for many consumers today

Table 1–1

Nutrition Measures to Prevent Diseases

Adequate intake of protein, food energy, or essential nutrients helps prevent:
- In pregnancy:
  - Birth defects
  - Mental/physical retardation
  - Low birthweight
  - Poor resistance to disease
- In infancy and childhood:
  - Growth deficits
  - Poor resistance to disease
- In adulthood and old age:
  - Malnutrition
  - Poor resistance to infectious and degenerative diseases

Moderation in food energy intake helps prevent:
- Obesity and related diseases, such as diabetes and hypertension

Adequate intake of any essential nutrient prevents:
- Deficiency diseases such as cretinism, scurvy, and folacin-deficiency anemia

Adequate calcium intake helps prevent:
- Adult bone loss

Adequate iron intake helps prevent:
- Anemia

Adequate fluoride intake helps prevent:
- Dental caries

Moderation in sodium intake helps prevent:
- Hypertension and related diseases of the heart and kidney

Adequate fiber intake helps prevent:
- Digestive malfunctions such as constipation and diverticulosis, and possibly colon or other cancers

Adequate vitamin A intake helps prevent:
- Susceptibility to certain cancers

Moderation in fat intake helps prevent:
- Susceptibility to some cancers and atherosclerosis

Moderation in sugar intake helps prevent:
- Dental caries

Moderation in alcohol intake helps prevent:
- Liver disease
- Malnutrition

Moderation in intake of essential nutrients prevents:
- Toxicity states

than ever before. As accumulating evidence continues to reveal nutrition's profound effects on human health, consumers are highly motivated to select foods that will provide the best possible nutrition.

Food producers and advertisers make use of all these motivations. They make their food as attractive to the senses of taste, smell, and sight as they can. If this means adding sugar, salt, and excess fat, they do so. They process their foods to be attractive or convenient to use, sometimes incurring serious nutrient losses. Some producers appeal to buyers who fear additives by selling foods with only "natural" ingredients (see Controversy 1). Some produce "light" snack foods and alcoholic beverages with slightly fewer calories per serving to entice weight-

Figure 1–6 Tags Identifying Questionable Nutrition Claims.

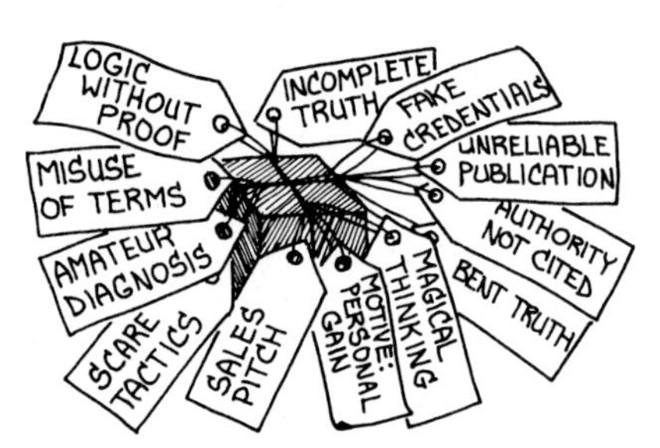

The more of these tags you can tie on a package of nutrition information, the less likely it is to be valid.

conscious people to imagine that these foods have a place in weight-reduction diets. And now that consumers have become sophisticated enough to begin selecting foods for their nutritional value, the food industry has responded by advertising its products as "nutritious." Further, as evidence that nutrition can help prevent some diseases has accumulated, advertisers have found legal ways to make claims to the effect on food labels. And some companies have gone to the extreme of producing products that are not foods at all, but claim to offer nutrients that will prevent disease by themselves—namely, supplements. This puts you, the consumer, in the position of being bombarded from all sides with claims that "our" foods are good for you, and that "their" foods are bad for you, or that "our" supplements are all you need. You therefore have still another problem in choosing what products to buy and not to buy: deciding whom to believe in the realm of nutrition information.

The consumer who cares about nutrition thus has at least a twofold task:

- To learn what nutrients the body needs and what kinds and combinations of foods and supplements supply them.
- To learn what kinds of claims are made by people who sell or write about foods and nutrients and how to tell whether the claims are valid.

The first task can be simplified by remembering that the three most basic needs of the body's cells, always, are for:

1. Energy fuel (along with the oxygen to burn it).
2. Water (the environment in which they live).
3. Building blocks (to maintain themselves).

Basic nutrition needs:

- Energy fuel.
- Water.
- Essential nutrients.

They especially need the building blocks they can't make for themselves—the essential nutrients, which must be supplied preformed from food. These needs are the basis for diet planning, and the chapters to come are devoted to them.

As for the second task, help with consumer problems will be offered throughout this book, wherever they come up. Special sections in almost every chapter deal with the claims made for supplements. To become skillful at recognizing false, misleading, or unproven nutrition information, consumers must learn the kinds of tricks that are used to mislead them. One way to do this is to have a collection of "tags" to identify these tricks, as shown in Figure 1–6.

Another way is to learn what qualifies a person to speak reliably about nutrition. Nutrition experts can be identified on the basis of their credentials. They have college and graduate degrees *in nutrition* (M.S., Ph.D.) from recognized universities, and they often have R.D. (registered dietitian) credentials. Controversy 2, "Who Speaks on Nutrition?" gives details. Appendix F provides a list of reliable nutrition resources.

A person must develop savvy to recognize valid nutrition information.

Food Feature

Managing It All

It is all very well to *talk* nutrition principles, but principles are no more nutritious than hot air. You have to take action before you will benefit from nutrition knowledge, and the action is no small thing. Putting nutrition principles into practice takes time, skill, energy, and personal commitment.

Many people are unable to perform the tasks associated with shopping, cooking, storing, and cleaning up. Children and the handicapped must depend on others for some or all of these services. Moreover, some mature and able-bodied people can't perform these tasks because they don't know how. This is where nutrition knowledge meets health in the real world; the following story illustrates this point. A man who had never prepared food for himself became a widower and suddenly became responsible for planning and preparing his own meals. During the year following his wife's death, he subsisted on a diet of black coffee, hamburgers, martinis, and steaks. He developed symptoms, and his health care providers treated him for many ailments. Finally, he was seen by a registered dietitian, who made the correct diagnosis: scurvy, the vitamin C deficiency disease. Even an occasional baked potato with his steak would have improved his vitamin C status, but without knowledge he was at a loss to select it, and baking it was beyond his skill.

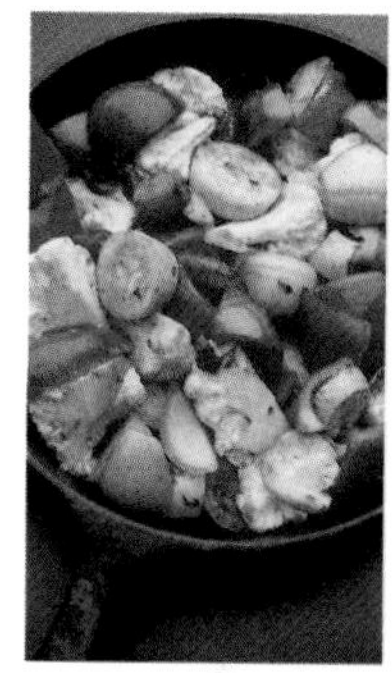

Would it take more time to prepare this dish than to prepare a pot of fudge? No, less time, and less cleanup, too.

Food planning, preparation, and cleanup require time and energy, as every worthwhile thing does. In our society, we have delegated the tasks of raising, harvesting, and transporting food to a few individuals, and we may even leave to others the task of preparing and serving our food. Still, we cannot delegate the responsibility for ensuring the adequacy of our diets; that responsibility falls squarely on our own shoulders.

Only if we arm ourselves with knowledge and commitment, can we obtain from our food the nutrients we need. For example, two people might spend exactly the same amount of time and money planning, shopping, cooking, and cleaning up. Whereas one may spend most of those resources on a fancy, high-fat and high-sugar dessert that dominates the meal, the other may use the money and time to buy, peel, and slice vegetables for a stir fry. The people who consumed the latter treat were much better nourished.

To maximize the return on your investment of time, money, and energy, you must plan menus, shop, and cook and handle food with care to conserve nutrients. The Food Features to come can help you do this. Each will provide a shopping list, like the one included here, suggesting some items to enhance the quality of your meals. By the time you read the last Food Feature, you will be aware of many staple items to keep in mind while you shop.

shopping list:

- paper and pencil, for planning and making shopping list
- nails and string, to hang them in a prominent place

Self-Study

Record What You Eat

Our purpose in providing these Self-Study exercises is to encourage you to study your own diet. Your reaction to them may be mixed. They will slow you down, and filling out all the forms is tedious. Like your checkbook, they have to be done carefully, with frequent checking of arithmetic and tidy handwriting, so that they will be accurate and meaningful.

The benefits, however, may well outweigh the drawbacks. Most students who do these activities with thoughtful attention report that unlike your checkbook, they are intriguing, informative, and often reassuring. They are also rewarding—in direct proportion to your accuracy.

In this first exercise you are to make a record of your typical food intake; in the next ones, you will analyze it for the nutrients it contains. You are undertaking this analysis before you have learned very much about the nutrients, but there's an advantage in that: having the results in front of you as you read will make the reading more meaningful. As you learn about each nutrient and ask yourself how much of it you consume, you will already have the answer in front of you, ready for interpretation and action.

Use three copies of Form 1 (Appendix H), and record on them all the foods you eat for a three-day period. If, like most people, you eat differently on weekdays than on weekends, then to get a true average you should probably record for two weekdays and one weekend day. Better still, make seven copies of Form 1, and record your food intakes for a week. Fill in only columns 1 and 2 for the moment. The Self-Study at the end of Chapter 2 will instruct you to look up the nutrients in the foods.

As you record each food, make careful note of the amount. Estimate the amount to the nearest ounce, quarter cup, tablespoon, or other common measure. (Appendix C provides help with conversion factors.) In guessing at the sizes of meat portions, it helps to know that a piece of meat the size of the palm of your hand weighs about 3 or 4 ounces. If you are unable to estimate serving sizes, measure out servings the size of a cup, tablespoon, and teaspoon onto a plate or into a bowl to see how they look. It also helps to know that a slice of cheese (such as sliced American cheese) or a 1½-inch cube of cheese weighs about 1 ounce.

You may have to break down mixed dishes to their ingredients. However, many mixed dishes, including fast foods, are listed in Appendix A, where you will look the foods up. Other mixtures are simple to analyze. A ham and cheese sandwich, for example, can be listed as 2 slices of bread, 1 tablespoon of mayonnaise, 2 ounces of ham, 1 ounce of cheese, and so on. If you can't discover all the ingredients, estimate the amounts of only the major ones, like the beef, tomatoes, carrots, and potatoes in a beef-vegetable soup.

You will, of course, make errors in estimating amounts. In calculations of this kind, errors of up to 20 percent are expected and tolerated. Still, you will have a rough approximation that will enable you to compare your nutrient intakes with the recommended ones.

Do not record any nutrient supplements you take. It will be interesting to discover whether your food choices alone deliver the nutrients you need. If they don't, you'll know better after analyzing your diet what supplement to choose.

You have now filled in columns 1 and 2 of Form 1 in Appendix H. The next Self-Study will guide you in filling in the remainder of the form.

Notes

1. D. R. Gwatkin, How many die? A set of demographic estimates of the annual number of infant and child deaths in the world, *American Journal of Public Health* 70 (1980): 1286–1289.

2. R. K. Chandra, Nutrition and immunity—practical applications, *Contemporary Nutrition* 11:12, 1986.

Our Ancestors' Diet: Is It Best for Us?

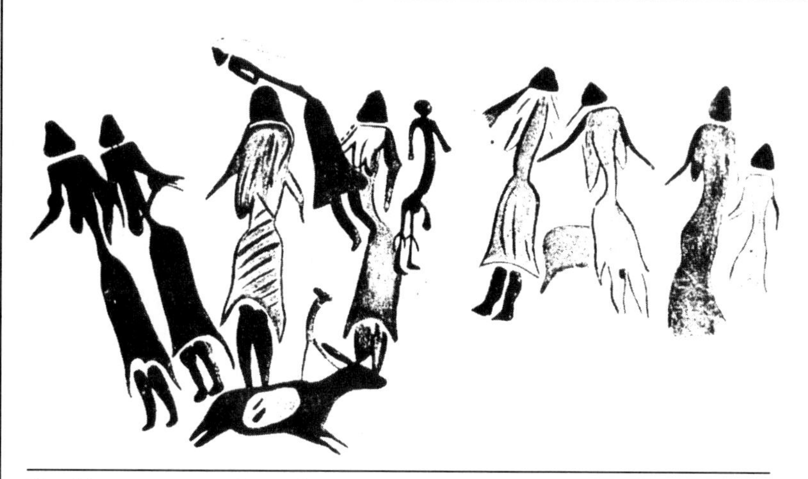

Should we eat as our Stone-Age ancestors did?

Should we eat as our ancestors did? Some people think we should. They say that the diet of the typical, prosperous, middle-class North American consumer today is not suited to the body's needs. It is too high in fat, sugar, and salt; and it is too low in fiber, vitamins, and minerals. It is unnatural, because the foods we eat are domesticated, refined, and processed to the point where they resemble very little the wild, natural, whole foods of earlier times. Some foods, they say, are even fabricated entirely from synthetic ingredients.

Others favor the ways we eat today. They say that our foods can be combined into one of the most healthful, nutritious diets people have ever consumed. Our ancestors died young of a host of diseases, including food poisoning and malnutrition, without knowing how to prevent them. We know how to keep foods safe, and we know our nutrient needs, so we can meet them—if not with foods alone, then with foods and appropriate supplementation. There is no reason why we should go back to the unpalatable, primitive foods of the past, when we can enjoy all the benefits of modern technology and eat delicious foods besides.

Who is right? Before arriving at any conclusions, it is necessary to know what our ancestors ate and how healthy they were. We have to begin by deciding which ancestors to study—our farmer forebears of 100 years ago, the early agricultural people who preceded them, or the hunter-gatherer people who lived still longer ago.

The people we should study are probably the earliest ones, the hunter-gatherers. They were the people of the Stone Age, the **paleolithic period.**[1] Their way of life and diet persisted for close to half a million years, vastly longer than the mere 10,000 years since the dawn of agriculture. It is hard to conceive of how long half a million years are, next to the times we are accustomed to thinking of, but two comparisons may help to dramatize the magnitude of the difference. Compared with the time since the beginning of the industrial era (about 1800), human beings have practiced agriculture since 10,000 years ago or more—five times longer. Ten thousand years may seem long, but try a second comparison. Imagine all of human existence on earth to have occurred within the last 24 hours. Then the agricultural era would have begun only 3½ minutes ago—and the industrial era would have begun 4 *seconds* ago. People who grew their own food have thus occupied the earth for "only" a few hundred generations, while people who hunted for their food roamed the earth for thousands of generations. Figure C1–1 depicts the magnitude of the differences between the earlier people's times on earth and our time.

Enough time elapsed during hunter-gatherer times to permit selection of genes that favored survival, generation after generation. The genes selected, naturally, tended to be those that adapted their owners' bodies to the hunter-gatherers' way of life and diet. Many of the genes that persist in our inheritance today are thousands of years old—the same ones favored by natural selection then, because in the few generations that have passed since then, not much more evolutionary change has taken place.[2]

The more we know about the Stone Age people, then, the better we can understand our needs today. The discussion that follows focuses on their food and physical activity, but many other aspects of their lives are worth studying. The publication of several popular novels in the

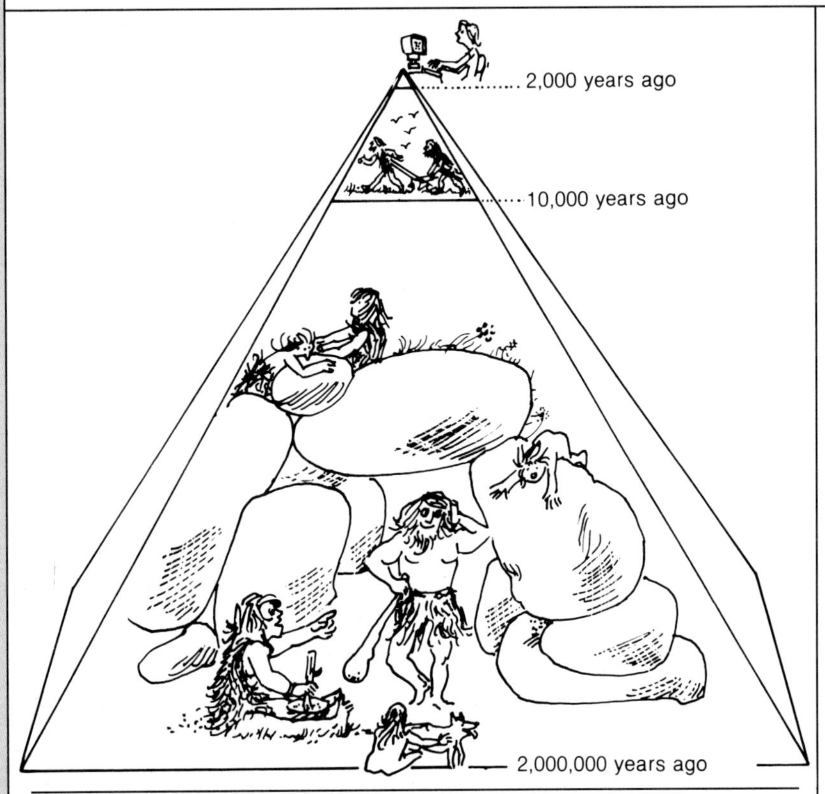

Figure C1–1
A perspective on modern human beings' time on earth. The space occupied in the pyramid is proportional to the time spent on earth.

Source: Inspired by A. Leaf and P. C. Weber, A new era for science in nutrition, *American Journal of Clinical Nutrition* 45 (1987): 1048–1053.

Earth's Children series by Jean Auel* has made it possible for people to enjoy informally learning about what the culture, traditions, and daily experiences of those people may have been like.

Life and Activities in the Stone Age

Food was not available all the time for the Stone-Age people. Times of plenty alternated with times of famine. The human body was well adapted to this state of affairs. It was the body of an **omnivore**—a creature able to digest and use the nutrients from both plants and animals. This made wide food choices possible and presented the least likelihood of starvation in the face of a food supply that depended on the geographical location and season. The body could also store excess energy-yielding nutrients when food was plentiful, and then draw on these nutrients when threatened by starvation from famine or debilitating illness.

The Clan of the Cave Bear, The Valley of Horses, and *The Mammoth Hunters* had been published at the time of this writing.

Our bodies still have those capabilities today. We can eat and derive nourishment from any of many different kinds of food, and we can store surplus energy in body fat—but now our stores often contribute to obesity, because for many people now, the food supply is quite reliable, and the times of famine never come. The storage of surplus energy in body fat that served the Stone Age person so well now produces conditions that may shorten life. Obesity is responsible for many of today's ills. It precipitates diabetes in susceptible people, it aggravates high blood pressure, it increases the likelihood of certain kinds of cancers, it worsens arthritis, and it harms health in many other ways.

The body feels hungry at approximately four to six-hour intervals, even though it may have sufficient fat stores to last for many days. This adaptation also served the Stone Age people well, for it drove them to continue stocking fuel within their bodies as often as their digestive systems could perform the task, even when they had sufficient reserves for temporary needs. Thus they never had to dip deeply into those stores until the food supply ran out. Furthermore, their appetites were stimulated whenever they encountered foods that were likely to be especially important for them to consume when available. Among these foods were those that were rich in food energy—those with the taste of energy-rich fat or the sweetness of concentrated sugar. Other foods that appealed to their taste buds were those that tasted of salt, for pure salt was rarely available in early times, and the essential nutrient sodium was harder to come by then than now. Novel foods also appealed to them. For long periods, their diets might be monotonous; their curiosity and willingness to try new foods probably helped to ensure that they would obtain the nutrients their regular diet might lack.

We have the same traits today. We feel hunger keenly every four to six hours during the day, whether we need to eat or not. We experience appetite on seeing, smelling, or tasting certain foods, even when we are not hungry—especially if the foods presented to us are rich in fat, sugar, or salt, or are foods that we don't often get the chance to eat. These traits still benefit people in many parts of the world where starvation and malnutrition are ever-present threats, but in food-abundant societies they contribute to vast overeating on the part of people who are already overfat.

Another adaptation of early human beings was the ability to call forth stored fuel instantaneously when physical danger threatened. The surge of energy this gave them helped them in overcoming or outrunning enemies and was frequently needed for these purposes. The reaction to physical danger, known as the **fight or flight reaction** or the **stress reaction,** is a magnificent adaptation for a creature confronted with the need to put forth maximum physical exertion in an emergency. The moment danger is detected, nerves and glands pour forth the stress hormones and every organ of the body responds. The pupils of the eyes widen so that you can see better; the muscles tense up so that you can jump, run, or struggle with maximum strength; breathing quickens to bring more oxygen to the lungs. The heart races to rush oxygen to the muscles, and the blood pressure rises to deliver efficiently the fuel the muscles need for energy. The liver pours forth glucose from its stored supply, while the fat cells release fat, another fuel. The digestive system shuts down, to permit all the body's systems to serve the muscles and nerves. With all its action systems at peak efficiency, the body can respond with amazing speed and strength to whatever threatens it.

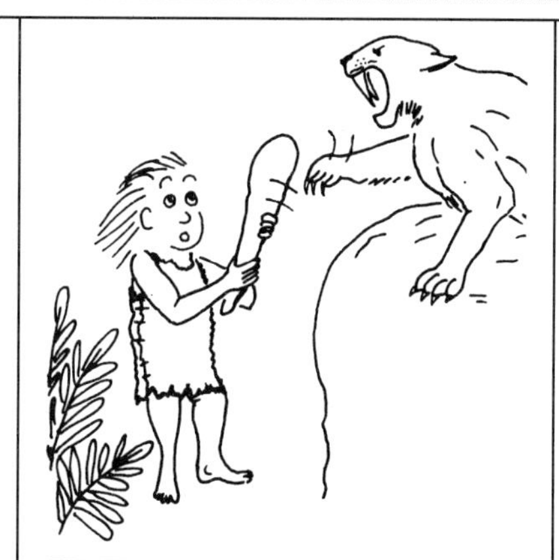

The fight-or-flight reaction.

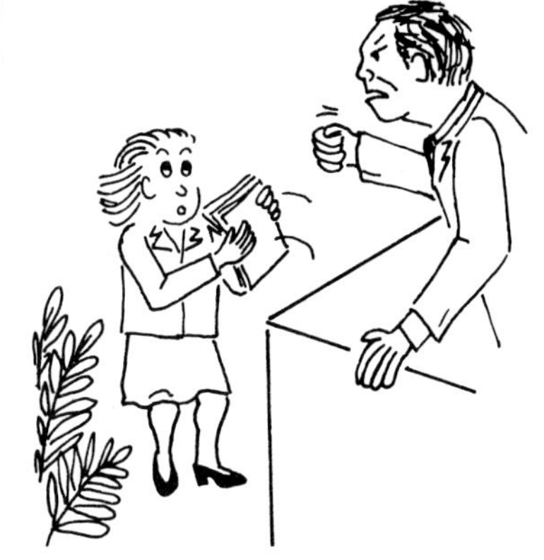

The stress reaction.

This adaptation, too, serves people well in modern times—but only in war or in sport, when the stresses they face are physical. However the stress reaction is called forth whenever any danger is perceived—even if it is an intangible, psychological or economic threat. What stresses you today may be a boss who threatens to fire you or a teacher who gives you an undeserved low grade. You can't eliminate these threats by fighting or running, as your early ancestors did; in fact, you may have to smile at the enemy and suppress your fear. But your heart still races, you feel it pounding, and hormones still flood your bloodstream with glucose and fat to support muscular action. At such a time, if you don't engage in vigorous exercise, eventually your body gets the message that these fuels are not needed, and it packs them away, to be stored as fat. Your blood pressure stays high for a long time after the event, and your digestion is upset. Stress today, because it is often psychological rather than physical, can cause or aggravate high blood pressure, ulcers, and other ills. People today have to learn to manage stress to avoid these ills, by learning to perceive the events as not so alarming, and by learning to work off their accumulated tension physically.

In other ways, too, the body is adapted to an earlier time. Heredity has given each human being a body that can respond to intense hard work by becoming stronger. The body can develop to run after prey, to fight enemies, or to carry heavy burdens long distances, and the more it is called upon to do these things, the stronger and swifter it becomes. Among the muscles that become stronger in response to exercise is the heart muscle, and it also (like all muscles) becomes weaker without it. In ancient times, there was little likelihood that anyone would sit around for months at a time, but today, people have to make special efforts to plan exercise into their daily routines if their muscles, including their heart muscles, are not to become weak.

Lack of opportunity for physical activity is a very new problem in human history. Even our farmer ancestors of 100 years ago had to work hard physically to milk the cows and bring in the harvest, but today, much of their work and that of many other people is done by machines. People drive to work and ride up and down in elevators rather than using their legs. They sit at desks or stand behind counters rather than moving about. Only a generation ago, children played games outdoors for hours every day with other neighborhood children, but now many sit passively in front of the television set watching others perform. Even when people spend many hours performing the work of house and child care, much of that time is spent sitting down. The sedentary life that many people lead has serious implications for their health.

Still another difference between the world our bodies are adapted for and the one they actually live in is the new chemicals present in our environments. The body has always had to defend itself against harmful substances ingested by mistake. The sense of taste is part of this defense; you refuse foods that do not taste right. A second part is the stomach's rejection response; you vomit up or wash out via diarrhea whatever "disagrees" with the digestive system. A third defense is the liver's filtering and detoxifying systems; toxins that get into the bloodstream are removed from it by the liver cells, which put them away in permanent storage or render them harmless and then release them for excretion in the urine or bile.

For example, protection against the harmful effects of one ancient and familiar substance—alcohol—is built into your genes. Two of those genes code for two enzymes that, in the liver, convert alcohol into substances the body can use or excrete (Controversy 12 provides details). So long as the liver is not overwhelmed by alcohol, the system works efficiently. But alcohol has been around ever since the first fruit ripened and fermented, so there have been thousands of generations for natural selection to mold a detoxifying system for it.

On the other hand, many of the present-day pollutants and toxins in our environment, including those that get into food by mistake, are new to the body. If it cannot efficiently excrete them, it may accumulate them in harmful quantities or convert them to odd, familiar substances that can interfere with metabolism or cause cancer or birth defects. It may not even recognize them: for example, it possesses no sense to detect radioactivity.

All of these differences add up to a set of circumstances that challenge your body and mind to maintain health against many odds. You are living with the food, the luxuries, the medical miracles, the smog, the contaminants, and all the other pleasures and problems of the twentieth century. However, you are housed in a body adapted to another world, in which the weak died before they could reproduce and strong men and women survived on simple foods obtained through hard physical labor. You now have the freedom to choose many different kinds of foods, to eat often or seldom, to eat a lot or a little. But the instincts you have inherited may tell you to eat foods whose tastes no longer signify the presence of beneficial nutrients, and to eat too much of them too often. You have not inherited any instincts for choosing correctly from among the foods available today, and in this country's melting pot of cultures and traditions, you may not have learned any time-tested and proven way of patterning your food intake, either. There is no guarantee that your diet, haphazardly chosen, will meet the needs of your Stone Age body.

Only with your brain can you compensate for these disadvantages of modern life. The Stone Age people used their brains to discover ways to obtain food; you must use yours, sometimes, to refuse delicious food and battle the ancient instincts that cry out for you to eat. They used their ingenuity to spare their energy when they could; you may have to use yours to find ways to increase your energy expenditure so that you can maintain appropriate weight and keep your heart and muscles fit. You have an advantage, though: you have access to more knowledge. Unlike your ancestors, you have the opportunity to learn how your body works and what it needs from food. For these reasons, researchers have turned to asking the question what the Stone Age people actually ate—what differences existed between the diet they ate long ago and the diets we eat today, and what significance those differences might have for us.

The Stone Age Diet

The probable diet of the Stone Age people has been analyzed to see what foods they ate and how much of each nutrient they received from it. Although the figures are undoubtedly not exact, it is interesting to compare them with those of today. These people probably consumed 3000 calories per day and were never obese. (Today, we consume fewer than 2000 calories a day and still, many are obese because they get so little exercise.)

Within their large energy allowances, the Stone Age people were able to meet all of their nutrient needs well. For example, their intakes of calcium were probably close to 1500 milligrams a day. Today, we fall short of 800 milligrams, although experts agree that we all (and especially women) need upwards of 1000 milligrams to preserve the integrity of our bones. They probably consumed close to 400 milligrams a day of vitamin C, whereas we take in less than 100 milligrams. They ingested much more fiber than we do today—45 grams or so, as compared with our 20 grams or less. They did this, using only two of the four groups of foods we think of as important: meat and fruits/vegetables. Their intakes of meat, and therefore of protein, were two to five times higher than ours are today. They apparently consumed cereal grains rarely if at all, and they had no dairy foods whatsoever.[3]

Although their total energy intakes were higher than ours, the people of the Stone Age had lower intakes of two no-no's that plague modern eaters: excess saturated fat, and sodium. Their cholesterol intakes were similar to ours, however, for the lean part of meat contains as much cholesterol as does the fat part. Also, their diet seldom contained concentrated sweets such as honey, and there was no such thing as purified, refined sugar.

Was this diet healthier for them than ours is for us? Stone Age people died younger than we do, but from causes we no longer face today. Judging from the evidence available on primitive people living today (tribes in Africa and other places, whose diets and ways of life resemble those of the Stone Age people), their way of life and diet can enable them to attain the age of 60 relatively free of the degenerative diseases that beset people in modern industrialized societies.[4] The differences between their diets and ours are those that most concern medical experts today. The heart associations, cancer societies, diabetes associations, and even political governing bodies of the United States, Canada, Sweden, Britain, and many other developed nations have recommended that, to remain healthy into old age, people should eat less fat, cholesterol, sugar, and salt, and more whole foods rich in fiber, vitamins, and minerals than they do (see Chapter 2).

What does all this mean in practice? Does it mean we should abandon the use of grains and dairy products and eat only meat and fruits/vegetables? Unfortunately, it is not all that simple, for our meats and fruits/vegetables are not the same as those the Stone Age people ate. Our meats are high in fat, theirs were lean. The fat in our meats is more saturated, that in theirs was more polyunsaturated. The polyunsaturated fats in our meats are primarily of the omega-6 kind; more of theirs were of the omega-3 kind—and we need more of those (Chapter 4 explains the fine points). As for the fruits and vegetables in our diets, none are the same as those the Stone Age people used to eat. It would be difficult for us to obtain enough calcium using the plant sources we have available today; we probably need dairy products for that reason.[5] The question whether we should eat as they did is, in any case, a moot question, for the foods the Stone Age people ate are no longer available today. The environment they experienced no longer exists for us.

For these reasons, it seems that even if it were desirable to return to the diet of our ancestors, it would not be possible in today's world. Still, even if we cannot eat the exact same foods as they did, we can attempt to duplicate their activity and nutrient intake levels using the foods available to us. Clearly, we should emulate them in incorporating more physical activity into our days. Chapter 9 is devoted entirely to nutrition and fitness, so suffice it here to offer just one observation. If you exercise more, you can eat more; if you eat more, you can obtain more nutrients; and if you obtain more nutrients, you are better protected against deficiencies.

Now about foods: how can we choose the ones that best will meet our needs? Should we try to eat foods that are as *natural* as possible? Should we take supplements, to increase our nutrient intakes?

Natural Foods

The word *natural,* with respect to foods, is widely abused. The common meaning is often stretched by food companies who produce a myriad of highly processed foods that bear the word on their labels. Common examples are beer and wine claiming to be natural, even though no brand of beer or wine ever grew in the woods or on a farm. Another example is natural candy bars. Because these candy bars are made from sources like fruit sugar, honey, and carob beans rather than from cane sugar and chocolate, they are advertised as natural. But they are not made of whole plants; they are made of concentrated ingredients derived from those plants. Only the sugar from the fruits has been used (leaving out the vitamins, minerals, and fiber), only the fat from the beans (again, leaving out the nutrients and fiber). Hence they are high in calories, low in nutrients, and hardly natural at all. Had the Stone Age people tasted them, they would have been amazed and delighted; had they had frequent access to them, they might have been able to replenish their energy stores more easily, but they would have obtained fewer nutrients in the process.

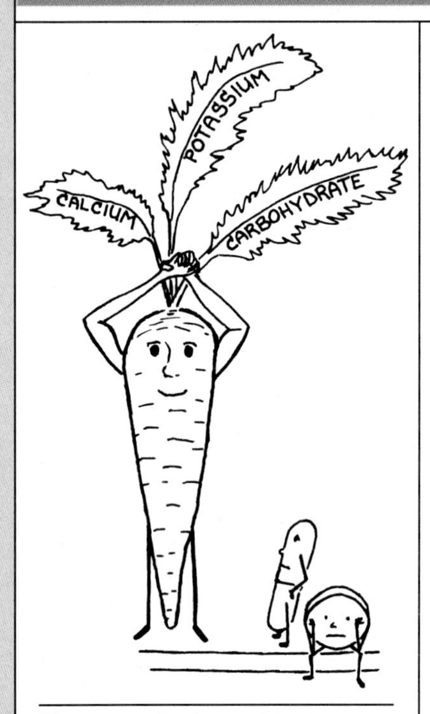

The more a food resembles the original, farm-grown product, the more nutritious it is likely to be.

It is too bad the term *natural* has been misused this way. We would have liked to use it in this book. But because of its widespread misuse in food advertising and on labels, we are choosing to use a different term instead: **whole foods**. With one exception, in general, the less a food has been taken apart, and the parts served separately, the more likely it is to have the characteristics experts agree are desirable: a high nutrient and fiber content relative to its calories, and a low saturated fat and sodium content. When this book speaks of whole foods, it means foods as similar as possible to the original, farm-grown product—and it often recommends them.

The one exception is foods from which the fat has been removed. For adults who lead inactive lives and who cannot afford to eat much of the meats and dairy products available today with their naturally high fat contents, defatted products are desirable. They should seek lean meats and nonfat milk products.

Many of the foods available today are *not* whole foods, but **partitioned foods.** Partitioning refers to the use of only parts of foods—sugars from beets or cane, refined flour from whole grains, butter from whole milk. Partitioning almost invariably yields products virtually empty of nutrients although usually high in calories. The food supply, which once consisted solely of whole foods, now offers two-thirds of its calories as partitioned foods: purified sugars, fats and oils, milled grains (primarily white flour), and alcohol.[6] These items should probably not be allowed to exceed about 20 percent of calories for people who eat a varied diet; they should occupy even less space in the diets of people whose energy intakes are low for reasons of dieting, illness, or aging.[7]

Notice that nothing has been said about processed foods. Processing is not the issue here; the nutritive value of foods is the issue. The term **processed foods** refers to foods that have been subjected to any procedure during preparation—freezing, canning, dehydration, addition of additives, or even simply cooking. Processing may not affect the nutrient content of a food, may affect it only minimally, or may improve it. A totally unprocessed food like honey from a wild bee tree is less nutritious than a package of frozen spinach or a can of salmon, because the honey is almost pure sugar, while the other foods named come from a plant and a fish, respectively, and are little altered from their original nutrient content. On the other hand, processing may seriously diminish a food's quality, rendering it nearly nutrient-free and high in unwanted constituents such as saturated fat and sodium. The question to ask is not whether a food has been processed or not, but how it has been processed, and how wholesome and nutritious it is now. Chapter 2 lays the groundwork for making the selection of whole foods according to patterns that will guarantee nutritional balance and adequacy.

Supplements

If what we are after from foods is simply nutrients and fiber without calories and fat, why wouldn't it make sense to take supplements of nutrients and fiber and not bother with food except to meet our energy needs? This represents an extreme argument that anyone could easily shoot down, but gives us the opportunity to present some introductory remarks about supplements—which are an issue of interest in every chapter in this book. One question of importance is whether we know all the nutrients people need.

We do know all the nutrients human beings need to *survive,* at least for a limited time. The 1970s and 1980s have seen an explosion of interest and skill in the making of **elemental diets**—diets that are totally chemically defined, used for people in the hospital who cannot eat ordinary food. These formulas can be administered to severely ill people in amounts up to 3000 calories a day. They support not only continued life but recovery from malnutrition and infection and the healing of wounds.

However, these diets are not sufficient to enable people to *thrive.* Used experimentally in laboratory animals, they support life but not optimal growth and health.[8] Often, people on all-synthetic diets develop nutrient deficiencies, as indicated by more than 100 separate reports.[9] Although each time this happens, the nutrient deficiency can be detected and corrected, it makes clear that the definition of these diets is not yet perfectly worked out in all the settings in which they are used.

Even if all the basic nutrient needs were perfectly understood, there might be something else foods offered that nutrients do not. The story of a girl who could not eat illustrates this possibility. This girl could not obtain nourishment from food, because she had a severe intestinal disorder that had rendered her digestive tract almost completely nonfunctional. She had to be fed nutrient mixtures through a vein. Deficiencies did develop, and were recognized and remedied, but still, something was missing: she wanted to eat food. Her health care providers therefore let her eat—whatever she wanted, even though everything she ate had to be collected into a bag through an opening in her abdominal wall after only a few minutes in her intestines. Clearly she gained something important from real food: "Her psychological outlook was completely changed. She was happy. The tastes, sounds, sights and smells of the food gave her great gratification. But, most especially, it was interesting to note the condition of her skin and hair improved and the pink on her cheeks and the look of 'wellness' returned." Whether the effect was physical or psychological remains unknown: "it was just something in food that gave this girl benefit, which we were not able to give through a needle."[10] The person reporting this was a physician with abundant knowledge and years of experience, not likely to ascribe mysterious powers to food without justification.

Some ingredient or characteristic of the food, other than its nutrients, may have been responsible for this health-promoting effect. This would not be surprising, for foods are composed of hundreds of chemicals, and we have much to learn about the effects of many of them on the body. Controversy 10 looks into the question of what else besides nutrients is present in foods that affects our reactions to them.

Another explanation is possible. Human beings are complex, and their reactions to foods may be different than to supplements for reasons rooted in the nervous system. We have, after all, needs for pleasure—which food gives in ways that supplements do not. We have needs for love—and the taking of nourishment is almost invariably associated with love from the first moment after birth when the baby is cradled and fed in loving arms. We have needs for stimulation and use of our nerves and muscles—and food stimulates the taste buds and requires chewing, as supplements do not. We have needs for social stimulation—and the taking of food is traditionally a social occasion among human beings.

For reasons like these, even if we don't understand them fully, it seems desirable to continue to rely as fully as possible on real foods, and as little as possible on supplements, to meet our nutrient needs. Later chapters offer much more information on supplements, but for the moment, let us suggest the following strategy: For the most part, choose *whole* foods. Never mind whether a food is *labeled* natural—just try to make sure that it

Miniglossary

elemental diets: diet composed of purified ingredients of known chemical composition such as amino acids, purified fats and sugars, vitamins, and minerals.

fight-or-flight reaction: the body's instinctive, hormone- and nerve-mediated reaction to danger, also known as the *stress reaction*.

natural food: a term that has no legal definition. Turn here to the definition of a *whole food,* which this book uses instead.

omnivore: an animal that eats both plant foods and the flesh of animals—for example, a human being. (Plant-eaters are *herbivores*; flesh eaters are *carnivores*.)

paleolithic period: the Stone Age, the period from 10,000 to about 500,000 years ago, before agriculture, when human beings were hunter-gatherers and used stone tools (*paleo* means "ancient"; *lith* means "stone").

partitioned food: a food composed of part of a natural food, such as butter (from milk), sugar (from beets or cane), or corn oil (from corn).

processed food: a food subjected to any process, such as enrichment, milling, alteration of texture, addition of additives, or cooking.

staple food: a food used frequently or daily—for example, potatoes (in Ireland) or rice (in the Far East).

stress reaction: see *fight-or-flight reaction*.

whole food: a food that has not been partitioned. Examples: a potato, an apple, a cut of meat, or a bowl of unpolished rice.

is natural, in the original, uncorrupted sense of the word. As for processed versus unprocessed foods, choose foods that processing has improved—by adding needed nutrients, rendering them safer to store and eat, or removing unwanted constituents such as fat and sodium. Avoid foods that processing has disimproved by adding fat, sugar, and salt or destroying or removing nutrients.

If this strategy forces you to look at one of your favorite treats with newly disapproving eyes, wait before you give it up. Ask yourself how much space the food occupies in your diet. There is no harm in indulging in any food as an occasional treat, but **staple food** items in your diet should be wholesome. For example, not every potato product you use must be recognizably potato, but if potatoes are one of your staple foods, then whole potatoes with their skins are a better choice than potato chips.

In conclusion, no one can go back to the days of the Stone Age people and really live as they did. We can learn from them, though—to get more exercise and to eat wholesome foods that will support our health as well as, or even better than, theirs did.

Notes

1. S. B. Eaton and M. Konner, Paleolithic nutrition, a consideration of its nature and current implications, *New England Journal of Medicine* 312 (1985): 283–289.
2. Eaton and Konner, 1985.
3. Eaton and Konner, 1985.
4. Eaton and Konner, 1985.
5. The 'caveman diet'? *Nutrition and the MD,* December 1985.
6. D. R. Davis, Nutrition in the United States: Much room for improvement, *Journal of Applied Nutrition* 35 (1983): 17–29.
7. A. E. Harper, U.S. dietary goals: Against, *Journal of Nutrition Education* 9 (1977): 154–156.
8. R. L. Koretz and J. H. Meyer, Elemental diets—facts and fantasies, *Gastroenterology* 78 (1980): 393–410.
9. D. Rudman and P. J. Williams, Nutrient deficiencies during total parenteral nutrition, *Nutrition Reviews* 43 (1985): 1–13.
10. F. D. Moore, Current thoughts on malabsorption: Parenteral, enteral, and oral feeding (commentary), *Journal of the American Dietetic Association* 86 (1986): 1169–1170.

Chapter Two

Contents

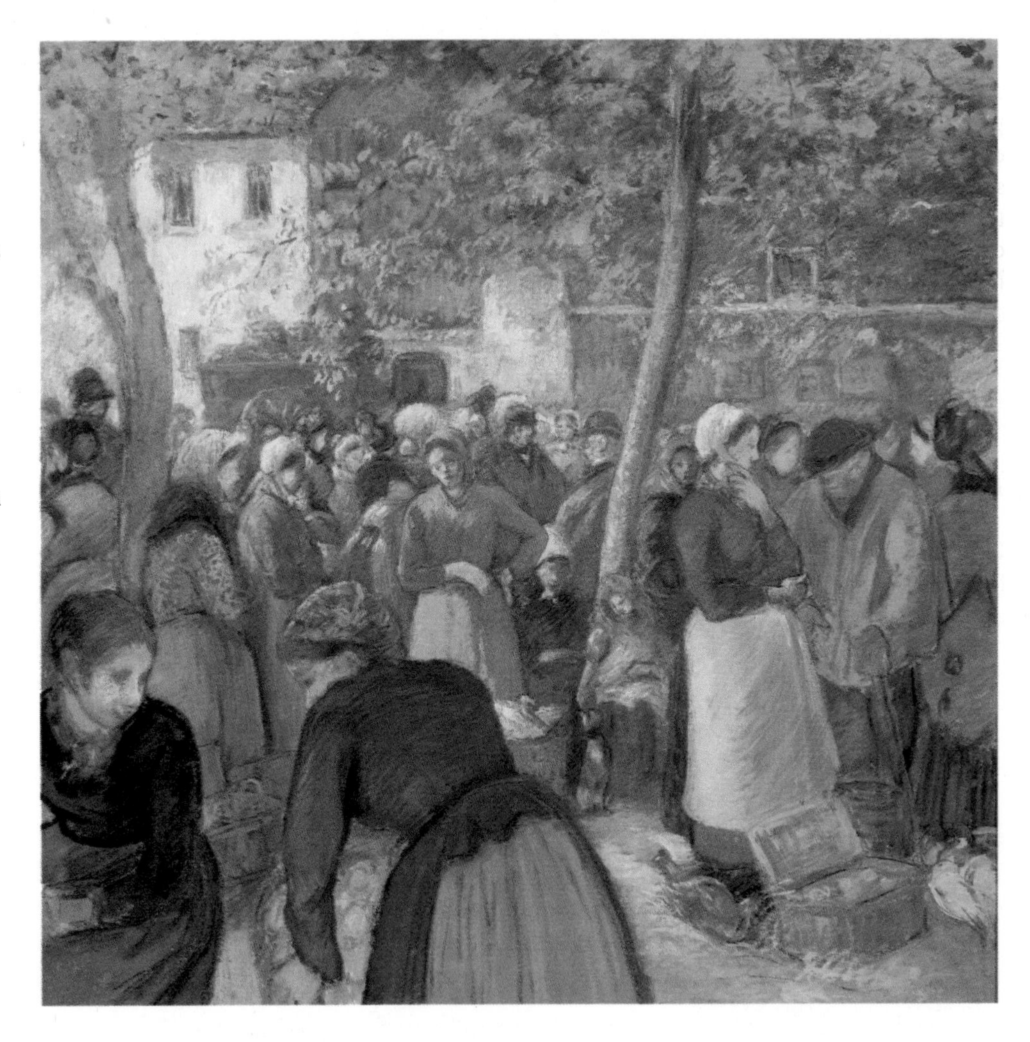

The Poultry Market at Gisors, 1885. By Camille Jacob Pissarro. Gouache and pastel on mounted paper 32¼ × 32½ inch (82 × 82 cm.) Bequest of John T. Spaulding.

Nutrients, Requirements, Foods, and Diet Planning

Eating well is easy, in principle. All you need to do is choose a selection of foods that supplies appropriate amounts of the essential nutrients, fiber, and energy. This is a simple enough assignment, but to master it and put it into practice requires that you know the answers to several questions. What are the essential nutrients? How much of each do you need? Which types of foods supply which nutrients and fiber? How much of each type of food do you have to eat, to get enough? And how can you eat all these foods without getting fat, or getting excess intakes of unwanted substances such as fat and salt? This chapter begins by identifying some dietary ideals, and ends with a Food Feature that shows how to achieve them.

adequacy: the description of a diet that provides all of the essential nutrients, fiber, and energy in amounts sufficient to maintain health.

balance: the description of a diet that provides foods of a number of types in balance with each other, such that foods rich in one nutrient do not crowd out of the diet foods that are rich in another nutrient.

calorie control: control of energy intake, a feature of a sound diet plan.

moderation: the description of a diet that provides no unwanted constituent in excess.

variety: the description of a diet in which different foods are used for the same purposes on different occasions—the opposite of *monotony.*

Dietary Ideals

If you succeed in planning an excellent diet for yourself, it will have all of the following characteristics: **adequacy** (it will provide enough of each essential nutrient, fiber, and energy), **balance** (it will not overemphasize any one food type or nutrient at the expense of another), **calorie control** (it will provide the amount of energy you need to maintain appropriate weight—not more, not less), **moderation** (it will not provide excess intakes of fat, salt, sugar, or other unwanted constituents), and **variety** (it will use different foods to provide the needed nutrients, rather than the same food day after day). Importantly, too, it will suit you—that is, it will consist of foods you realistically can obtain and enjoy eating—foods that fit your personality, family and cultural traditions, lifestyle, and budget. At its best, a well-planned diet is one of the chief sources of pleasure, as well as good health, in a person's life.

Any nutrient could be used to demonstrate the importance of dietary *adequacy.* Iron provides a familiar example. It is an essential nutrient; you lose some very day, so you have to keep replacing it, and you can only get it into your body by eating foods that contain it. If you eat too few of these foods, you can develop iron-deficiency anemia; you feel weak, tired, and unenthusiastic, may have frequent headaches, and can do very little muscular work without disabling fatigue. If you make the needed correction and add iron-rich foods to your diet, you soon feel more energetic.

Some foods are rich in iron; others are notoriously poor. Meat, fish, poultry, and legumes are in the iron-rich category, and an easy way to obtain the needed iron is to include these foods in your diet regularly.

nutrient density: a measure of nutrients provided per calorie of food.

To appreciate the importance of dietary balance, consider a second essential nutrient, calcium. Foods that are rich in iron are poor in calcium. Calcium's best food sources are milk and milk products, which happen to be extraordinarily poor iron sources. A diet lacking calcium causes poor bone development during the growing years and a gradual bone loss in adults that can totally cripple a person in later life. Adults are advised to use at least two, and preferably more, cups of milk or milk products a day to meet their calcium needs—but not so many as to crowd iron-rich foods out of the diet.

Clearly, to obtain enough of both nutrients, which don't appear together in foods, one has to balance the two. Balancing the whole diet is a juggling act that, if successful, provides enough but not too much of every one of the 40-odd nutrients the body needs for health. As you will see, food group plans address the problems of achieving dietary adequacy and balance, because they recommend specific amounts of foods of each type.

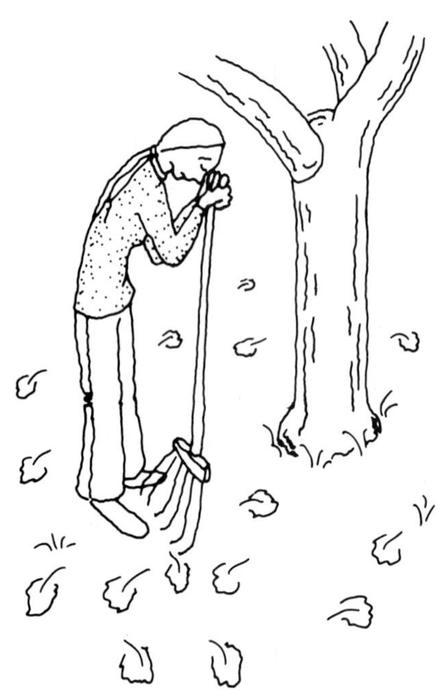

An iron deficiency makes a person feel tired.

Not all foods that supply iron or calcium have the same energy value, and this has further implications for food choices. Consider calcium sources, for example. A cup and a half of ice cream has about the same amount of calcium as does milk, but the ice cream may have over 500 calories, while the milk may have as few as 90. Or take iron: a 3-ounce serving of beef pot roast offers the same amount of iron as a 3-ounce serving of sardines, but the beef supplies 325 calories, the sardines 175. Most people cannot choose foods without regard to their energy content. To help with calorie control, the planner can use list of foods within each group that are similar in their calorie amounts per portion.

Foods that are rich in nutrients relative to their energy content are said to be foods with high **nutrient density.** The concept of nutrient density is especially useful for the person choosing foods within a limited energy allowance.

Other forms of moderation are useful in diet planning. The two substances people are most often advised to avoid today are fat and sodium. It helps if lists of foods to choose are provided that make clear which foods are low or high in these two substances.

As for variety, it is generally agreed that people should not eat the same foods day after day, for two reasons. One reason is that some lesser-known nutrients and some nonnutrient food components could be important to health; some foods may be better sources of these than others. Another reason is that a monotonous diet may deliver unwanted amounts of undesirable food constituents, such as plant toxins or chemical contaminants. Each undesirable component is diluted by all the other foods eaten with it and even further diluted if several days are skipped before it is eaten again. This is another reason why lists of interchangeable foods are useful—you can choose one today, and a different one tomorrow, to meet the same nutrient needs.

A well-planned diet is adequate and balanced, controls calories, contains only moderate amounts of unwanted constituents, and offers variety.

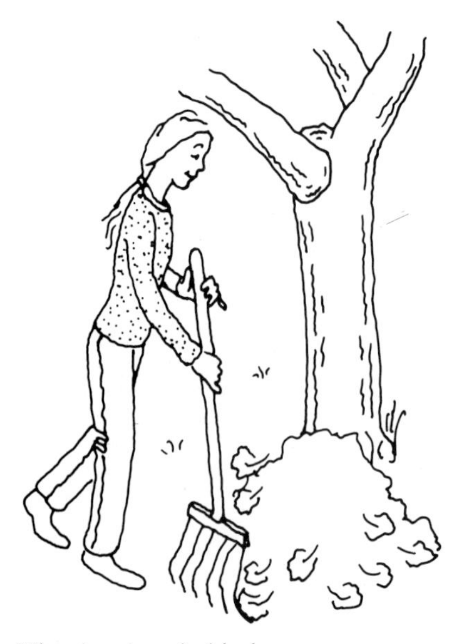

When iron is replenished, energy returns.

The Nutrients

The nutrients fall into six classes, and all six are found in most foods. Water usually predominates; carbohydrate (including fiber), fat, and protein are next in abundance. Last come the vitamins and minerals in smaller yet significant amounts.

The human body is made of similar materials, in roughly the same order of predominance. If you weigh 150 pounds, your body contains about 90 pounds of water and (if 150 pounds is the proper weight for you) about 30 pounds of fat. The other 30 pounds are mostly protein, carbohydrate compounds, and the major minerals of your bones—calcium and phosphorus. Vitamins, other minerals, and incidental extras constitute a fraction of a pound. Figure 2–1 compares the composition of the human body with that of two foods, corn and beef.

All of the six nutrients are composed of atoms of elements, bonded together by energy; all except the minerals contain hydrogen and oxygen, the elements of which water is made. Four nutrients also contain atoms of carbon and are therefore **organic** (carbon containing)—carbohydrate, fat, protein, and vitamins. This means that they can undergo **oxidation** or be burned (to carbon dioxide and water) and that energy will be released. But only three of these four—carbohydrate, fat, and protein—can be oxidized in the body to yield energy the body can use. The role of some vitamins is to help in the oxidation process, but one of the most common misconceptions people have is that the vitamins in some way yield energy for human use. They do not, although taking vitamin pills for energy is a common mistake. The only significance to us of vitamins' being organic is that they are easily destroyed by chemical and physical agents such as heat and light. Therefore, we have to be careful in cooking foods that contain vitamins (find out how in the Chapter 6 Food Feature).

Plants and animals that we use for food, as well as our own bodies, are made up primarily of six nutrients—water, carbohydrate, fat, protein, vitamins, and minerals. Of the four classes of organic nutrients, only three—carbohydrate, fat, and protein—yield energy that the body can use.

The Energy-Yielding Nutrients

The energy contained in carbohydrate, fat, and protein can be measured in **calories,** familiar to everyone as the constituent in foods that makes them fattening. (Properly speaking, however, they are kilocalories, and you will often see them referred to as **kcalories** or **kcal.*** This book uses the popular term

organic: carbon containing. The four organic nutrients are carbohydrate, fat, protein, and vitamins.

oxidation: with respect to nutrients in the body, breakdown of a nutrient and combination of its parts with oxygen—a process that releases energy.

calories: kilocalories **(kcalories, kcal),** or Calories. A calorie is the amount of heat necessary to raise the temperature of a kilogram (a liter) of water 1° C.

Elements in the Six Classes of Nutrients

	Hydrogen	Oxygen	Carbon	Nitrogen	Minerals
Carbohydrate	x	x	x		
Fat	x	x	x		
Protein	x	x	x	x	
Vitamins	x	x	x		
Minerals					x
Water	x	x			

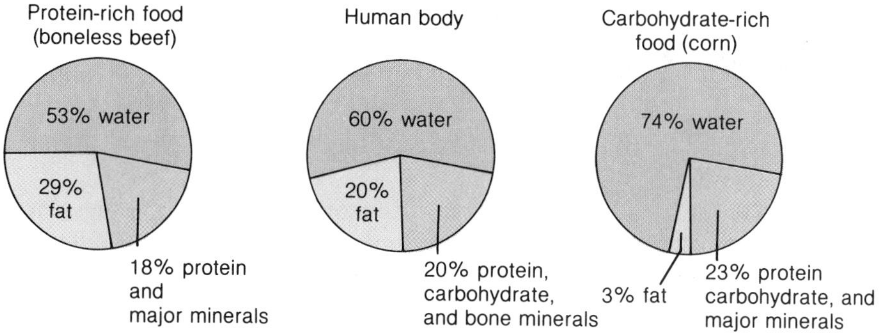

Protein-rich food (boneless beef): 53% water; 29% fat; 18% protein and major minerals

Human body: 60% water; 20% fat; 20% protein, carbohydrate, and bone minerals

Carbohydrate-rich food (corn): 74% water; 3% fat; 23% protein carbohydrate, and major minerals

Figure 2–1 Foods and the Human Body: Similarities in Composition.
(Vitamins are not shown, because the amounts are too small to be seen on a diagram this size.) Beef and the human body appear similar in composition, but corn offers carbohydrate, the body's ideal fuel, from which the body can make fat as needed.

*Food energy can also be measured in *joules, kilojoules,* or *megajoules.* A kilojoule is the amount of energy expended when a kilogram is moved 1 meter by a force of 1 newton. The kilojoule is now the international unit of energy and will become the unit of food energy for any country that shifts to the metric system. Conversions from calories to joules are on the inside back cover.

calorie, as most people do. The energy values of these nutrients appear in the margin. Note that they are measured in **grams (g)**.

grams: units in which weight is measured. A gram (g) is the weight of a cubic centimeter (cc) or milliliter (ml) of water under defined conditions of temperature and pressure. A note about grams appears in Figure 2–6, page 41.

The energy nutrients:
- Carbohydrate.
- Fat.
- Protein.

- 1 g carbohydrate = 4 cal.
- 1 g fat = 9 cal.
- 1 g protein = 4 cal.

Energy from food may be used by the body in several ways: to produce heat, to built its structure, to move its parts, or to be stored in body fat or other compounds for later use. Many people do not realize that even protein can be converted to body fat. Carbohydrate and fat are well known as calorie-laden villains against which the overweight wage constant war, but protein is not innocent in this respect. Protein does much more than simply contribute food energy, but an excess of any of the three energy-yielding nutrients can pad the body with an unwanted blanket of fat.

It is important not to forget one other organic compound—alcohol. Alcohol is not a nutrient, because it cannot be used in the body to promote growth, maintenance, or repair. It is a toxin that can be broken down and converted to fat. When alcohol contributes a substantial portion of the energy in a person's diet, its effects are damaging.

1 g alcohol = 7 cal. More about alcohol—Controversy 12.

Practically all foods contain mixtures of the three energy-yielding nutrients, although they are sometimes classed by the predominant nutrient. Thus it is incorrect to say that you are eating a protein when you eat meat; you are eating a protein-rich food. A protein-rich food like beef actually contains a lot of fat as well as protein. A carbohydrate-rich food like corn also contains fat (corn oil) and protein. Only a few refined foods are exceptions to this rule, the common ones being sugar (which is almost pure carbohydrate) and oil (which is almost pure fat). The nutrients in several hundred foods are shown in Appendix A, and the Self-Studies at the ends of the chapters direct you to look them up there.

Protein, carbohydrate, and fat contribute usable energy to the body, as does alcohol. Most foods contain mixtures of carbohydrate, fat, and protein.

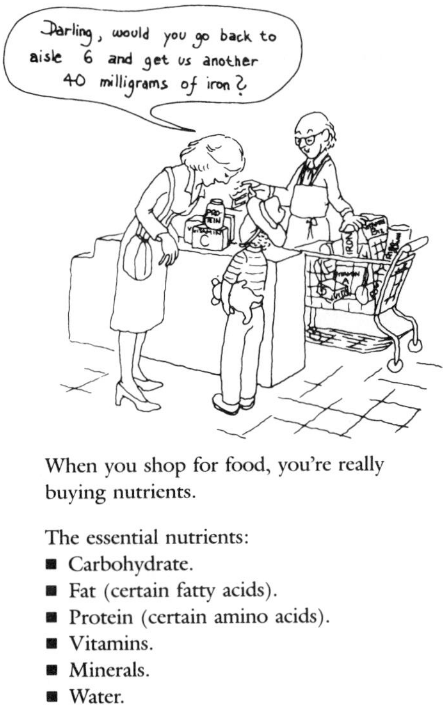

When you shop for food, you're really buying nutrients.

The Essential Nutrients

In nutrition, the word *essential* is used to distinguish between the nutrients that the body can manufacture from raw materials and those that must be obtained ready-made from food. For example, the body can convert some of the amino acids (parts of protein) into carbohydrate, if need be. It can manufacture one of the vitamins—niacin—from a certain amino acid. It can make most of its fats and oils from any of several different raw materials. These are nonessential nutrients. But the body cannot make for itself certain compounds absolutely indispensable to life processes, and these are termed the *essential nutrients* (p. 2). When used this way, the word *essential* means more than just "necessary." Many compounds the body makes for itself are necessary for good health, but *essential nutrient* means a necessary nutrient that can be obtained only from the diet.

The essential nutrients:
- Carbohydrate.
- Fat (certain fatty acids).
- Protein (certain amino acids).
- Vitamins.
- Minerals.
- Water.

About 40 nutrients are now known to be essential for human beings. How can you obtain all these nutrients? After all, you don't buy and cook nutrients; you usually think in terms of foods. This chapter will show you how to design a diet that meets all your nutrient needs, but it is important, first, to understand nutrient intake standards.

The essential nutrients are necessary nutrients that the body cannot make for itself.

Recommended Nutrient Intakes

The following section introduces the Recommended Dietary Allowances (RDA), used in the United States, as an example of recommended intakes. The Canadian equivalent is the Recommended Nutrient Intakes for Canadians (RNI), presented in Appendix 2. (The U.S. RDA used on food labels is different from the RDA and is described later.)

Recommended Dietary Allowances (RDA): nutrient intakes suggested by the Food and Nutrition Board (FNB) of the National Academy of Sciences/ National Research Council (NAS/NRC) for the maintenance of health in people in the United States. (The term *minimum daily requirement,* which some people confuse with the RDA, is no longer in use.)

The RDA

A committee of scientists funded by the U.S. government publishes recommendations concerning appropriate nutrient intakes for the people in this country.* These are the **Recommended Dietary Allowances (RDA),** and they are used and referred to so often that they are presented on the inside front cover of this book. As you can see, the main RDA table includes recommendations for protein, ten vitamins, and six minerals, while the additional tables include three more vitamins and nine more minerals, as well as energy (calories). About every five years, the Committee on RDA meets to re-examine and revise these recommendations on the basis of new research regarding people's nutrient needs. It then publishes an updated set of RDA.[1]

The RDA have been much misunderstood. One young woman, on first learning of their existence, was outraged: "You mean Uncle Sam tells me that I must eat exactly 45 grams of protein every day?" This is not the committee's intention, and the RDA are not commandments. The following facts will help put the RDA in perspective:

- The committee that makes them is funded by the government, but is composed of scientists representing a variety of specialties.
- They are based on reviews of available scientific research to the greatest extent possible and are revised about every five years to keep them up to date.
- They are recommendations, not requirements, and certainly not minimum requirements. The RDA include a substantial margin of safety.
- They are based on the concept that most healthy persons' intakes of nutrients probably should fall within a range. Individual needs differ.
- They are for healthy persons only. Medical problems alter nutrient needs.

Separate recommendations are made for different sets of people. Children aged 4 to 6 are distinguished from men aged 19 to 22, for example. Each individual can look up the recommendations for his or her own age and sex group.

No RDA is set for carbohydrate or fat. The assumption is that you will use a certain number of calories meeting your protein RDA and then will distribute the remaining calories among carbohydrate and fat and possibly alcohol, ac-

RDA are set for:

- Energy—a range.
- Protein.
- Vitamins:
  A, D, E, C, thiamin, riboflavin, niacin, B_6, B_{12}, folacin.
- Minerals:
  Calcium, phosphorus, magnesium, iron, zinc, iodine.

"Estimated safe and adequate intakes" are given in ranges for:
Vitamin K, biotin, pantothenic acid.

- Minerals (trace elements):
  Copper, manganese, fluoride, chromium, selenium, molybdenum, sodium, potassium, chloride.

See inside front cover.

*This is a committee of the Food and Nutrition Board (FNB) of the National Academy of Sciences/ National Research Council (NAS/NRC).

cording to your personal preference, to meet your energy RDA. (This chapter later shows how to balance energy sources to best support health; see "Food Groups and Exchange Lists.")

In 1985, the committee submitted the tenth edition of the RDA. These recommendations were, by and large, the same as those published in 1980, but the recommended levels of vitamins A and C had been reduced. These two new recommendations sparked a controversy that has delayed publication of the tenth edition of the RDA.

The critics of the revision pointed to recent findings that suggested that ample vitamins A and C in the diet might be protective against some types of cancer. In light of these findings, the critics believed the RDA for these vitamins should be raised or at least stay the same to best support national health objectives for disease prevention.

The RDA committee, however, argued that the main intent of the RDA was to establish levels of nutrient intakes that were adequate for populations. As such, they are widely used as standards for food labeling; for planning diets for schools, the armed services, and hospitals; and for administering public assistance programs.[2] To change the objective of the RDA to accommodate tentative research news about disease prevention would be to inflate the standard too much for its original purposes. As the philosophical debate continues, the ninth edition of the RDA is still in use.*

The next section describes the process the committee goes through in selecting the RDA values. It also makes clear that the RDA are tools best suited to evaluating the nutrient intakes of populations, and that they are less useful, but still often used, to guess at individual nutrition status.

The RDA and the RNI represent suggested daily nutrient intakes for healthy people in the United States and Canada.

The RDA for Nutrients

If you use the RDA to estimate the adequacy of your own diet, you need to be aware that individuals' nutrient needs vary, and that the allowances are designed only for use for whole groups of people. A theoretical discussion based on the way the Committee on RDA made its recommendation for protein will illustrate these points.

Suppose we were the Committee on RDA, and we had the task of setting an RDA for nutrient X (any nutrient). Ideally, our first step would be to try to find out how much of that nutrient individual persons need. We would review studies of deficiency states, of nutrient stores and their depletion, and of the factors influencing them. We would select the most valid data for use in our work. Among the experiments we might review or conduct might be measures

*Members of the RDA committee have published nutrient amounts they consider sufficient to maintain tissue saturation in human beings. They refer to these as RDI, Recommended Dietary Intakes. The RDI of folacin is 3 μg/kg body weight; of vitamin B_{12}, 2 μg; of vitamin K, 45 μg (men) and 35 μg (women); of vitamin C, 40 mg (men) and 30 mg (women); of vitamin A, 700 RE (men) and 600 RE (women); and of iron, lower than the RDA, depending on age and sex. See articles by V. Herbert, J. A. Olson, and R. E. Hodges in *American Journal of Clinical Nutrition* 45 (1987).

of the body's intake and excretion (in the case of nutrients that aren't changed before they are excreted) to find out how much of an intake is required for balance (this is called a **balance study**). For each individual subject, we could determine a **requirement** for nutrient X. Below the requirement, that person would slip into negative balance or experience declining stores that could, over time, lead to deficiency of the nutrient.

We would find that different individuals have different requirements. Mr. A might need 40 units of the nutrient each day to maintain balance; Ms. B might need 35; Mr. C, 65. If we looked at enough individuals, we might find that their requirements were distributed as shown in Figure 2–2—most near the midpoint, and only a few at the extremes.

Then we would have to decide what intake to recommend for everybody in order to set the RDA. Should we set it at the mean (shown in Figure 2–2 at 45 units)? This is the average requirement for nutrient X; it is probably the closest to everyone's need, assuming the distribution shown in Figure 2–2. (Actually, the committee usually doesn't have enough data to be sure that the distribution is so symmetrical.) But if people took us literally and consumed exactly this amount of nutrient X each day, half of the population would develop deficiencies, Mr. C among them.

Perhaps we should set the RDA for nutrient X at or above the extreme—say, at 70 units a day—so that everyone would be covered. (Actually, we didn't study everyone, so some individual we didn't happen to test might have a still higher requirement.) This might be a good idea in theory, but what about a person like Ms. B, who needs only 35 units a day? She would be forced to consume twice her need, and to do so, she might spend money needlessly on foods containing nutrient X to the exclusion of foods containing other nutrients she needs.

The choice we would finally make, with some reservations, would be to set the RDA at a reasonably high point so that the bulk of the population would be covered. In this example, a reasonable choice might be to set it at 63 units a day. By moving the RDA further toward the extreme, we would pick up few additional people but inflate the recommendation for most people (including Mr. A and Ms. B).

The committee makes choices of this kind when setting the RDA for nutrients. They set it well above the mean requirement as best they can determine it from the available information. In theory, relatively few people's requirements, then, are not covered by the RDA.

balance study: a laboratory study in which a person is fed a controlled diet and the intake and excretion of a nutrient are measured. Balance studies are valid only for nutrients like calcium (chemical elements) that don't change while they are in the body.

requirement: that amount of a nutrient that will just prevent the development of specific deficiency signs; distinguished from the RDA, which is a recommended and generous allowance.

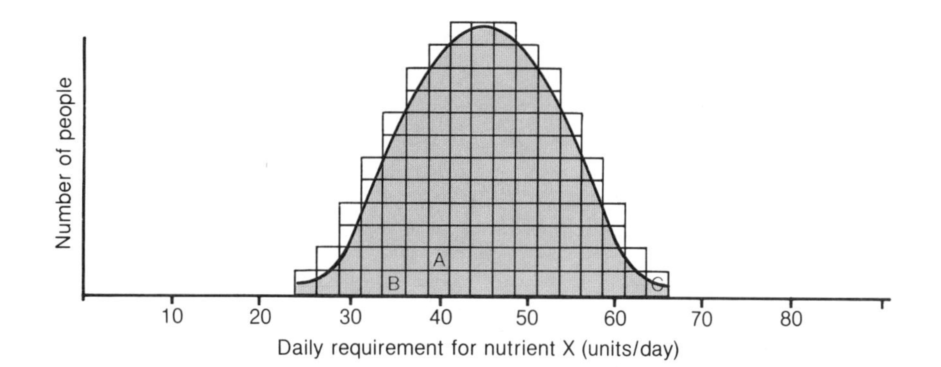

Figure 2–2 Individuality of Nutrient Requirements.
Each square represents a person. A, B, and C are Mr. A, Ms. B, and Mr. C.

reference man and woman: theoretical "average" figures used by the Food and Nutrition Board for calculating nutrient and energy needs. He is 5 feet 10 inches tall and weighs 154 pounds (70 kg); she is 5 feet 4 inches tall and weighs 120 pounds (55 kg). They are both aged 23 to 50 and lightly active.

For these reasons, the RDA cannot be taken literally by any individual; that is, you can't know exactly what your own personal requirement may be. The Committee on RDA makes several assumptions that may not apply to you at all. For example, they assume that you are eating a diet that includes protein, energy, and all the other nutrients. They assume, also, that you cook your foods with reasonable care and that nutrients are not lost in preparation. This may describe you exactly; then again, it may not. On the other hand, the RDA are not minimum requirements. *R* stands for "recommended," not for "required." The RDA are allowances, and they are generous. Even so, they do not necessarily cover every individual for every nutrient. It is probably necessary to aim at getting 100 percent of the RDA for every nutrient to ensure adequate intake.[3*]

Beyond a certain point, though, it is unwise to consume large amounts of any nutrient. It is naive to think of the RDA simply as a cutoff point. A more accurate view is to see your nutrient needs as falling within a range, with danger zones both below and above it. Figure 2–3 illustrates this point. The RDA reflect this consideration especially clearly in the tables for the trace minerals (inside front cover), which are stated in terms of "safe and adequate" ranges of intakes.

Figure 2–3 The Naive View versus the Accurate View of Optimal Nutrient Intakes.

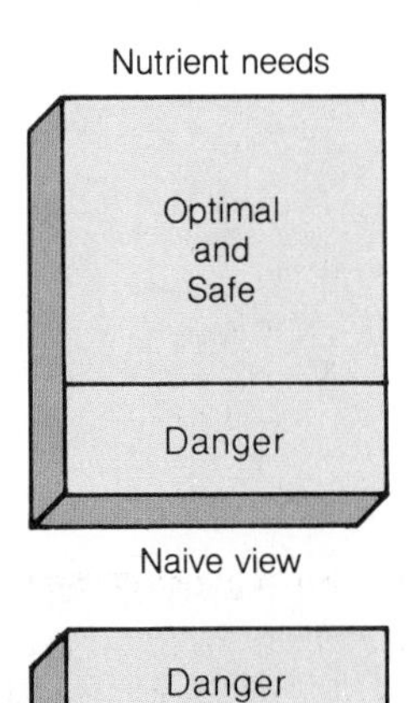

Remember, too, that the RDA and other such recommendations are for the maintenance, not the restoration, of health. Under the stress of serious illness or malnutrition, a person may require a much higher intake of certain nutrients. Separate recommendations are made for therapeutic diets; for use after surgery, burns, or fractures; and during recovery from illness or addictions.

With the understanding that they are approximate, flexible, and generous, we can use the RDA as a set of yardsticks to measure the adequacy of diets in whole populations, like that of the United States. Such standards have been applied in a number of surveys to determine people's nutrition status. (Chapter 14 presents more information about surveys and how well nourished today's people really are.)

The RDA are a set of yardsticks for measuring the adequacy of nutrient intakes of groups of people and can be used as a guide for planning group diets.

The RDA for Energy

In setting allowances for food energy intakes, the Committee on RDA took a different approach than for the nutrients. The committee had set generous allowances for protein, vitamins, and minerals, believing that a little bit extra, for a *nutrient,* would provide insurance against deficiencies. However, extra *energy,* even a little bit extra, would be harmful, because it would lead to obesity. The Committee on RDA therefore created a range of energy RDA centered around the mean. Figure 2–4 illustrates the difference between the nutrient and energy RDA set by the committee.

The energy RDA are thus recommendations for imaginary persons. The female is 23 to 50 years old, 5 feet 4 inches tall, and weights 120 pounds (55 kilograms). This **reference woman** requires (on the average) 2000 calories a

*It used to be thought that if a person consumed just two-thirds of the RDA, that person would be adequately nourished; now, though, a new interpretation of the data they are based on shows that two-thirds is inadequate.

day to maintain her weight. The **reference man** is the same age, 5 feet 10 inches tall, weighs 154 pounds (70 kilograms), and requires about 2700 calories. Both sleep or lie down for eight hours a day, sit for seven hours, stand for five, walk for two, and spend two hours a day in light physical activity. Very few people fit these descriptions exactly; but as Figure 2–4 shows, most people fall close to the mean. The best way to ensure that your food energy intake actually fits your own particular requirement is to monitor your weight over a period of time. Chapter 8 revisits the energy RDA and shows how to control your energy intake to meet your needs.

U.S. RDA: the RDA figures used on labels—the United States Recommended Dietary (or Daily) Allowances. In most instances, they are the highest RDA suggested in the RDA tables for any age and sex group for each nutrient (see inside back cover).

As mentioned previously, no RDA is set for carbohydrate or fat. The committee expects that you will use the energy RDA as a guide for deciding how much carbohydrate and fat to include in your diet.

The energy RDA was set at the mean, so as to discourage overconsumption of food energy.

The U.S. RDA

The term **U.S. RDA** appears on food labels and so deserves an explanation. The U.S. RDA were developed by selecting from the RDA tables a single set of recommendations for a reference adult human being. For each recommendation, a high value was chosen. Whereas a woman's RDA for vitamin A is 700 retinol equivalents (RE), a man's is 1000 RE, so the U.S. RDA is a single value, the higher of these. The amount of vitamin A in a food is expressed as a percentage of that standard on the label. Thus, instead of reading that a serving of the food contains "700 RE" of vitamin A, you read that it contains "70 percent of the U.S. RDA" for vitamin A. The advantage is that the consumer who wants information from a food label does not have to memorize all the different RDA, which are expressed in many different units (RE, milligrams, IU, and others). If you read on a label that a serving of cereal provides 25 percent of the U.S. RDA for a nutrient, you can be sure that it will also provide at least 25 percent of *your* RDA. Your need, if it is different from the U.S. RDA, is almost surely lower. The table on the inside back cover shows the U.S RDA. Chapter 10 explains more about food labels, and Figure 10–1 shows how to read them.

U.S. RDA—inside back cover.

The U.S. RDA are a single set of nutrient values drawn from the RDA tables. Nutrient contents of packaged foods are stated on food labels as percentages of the U.S. RDA.

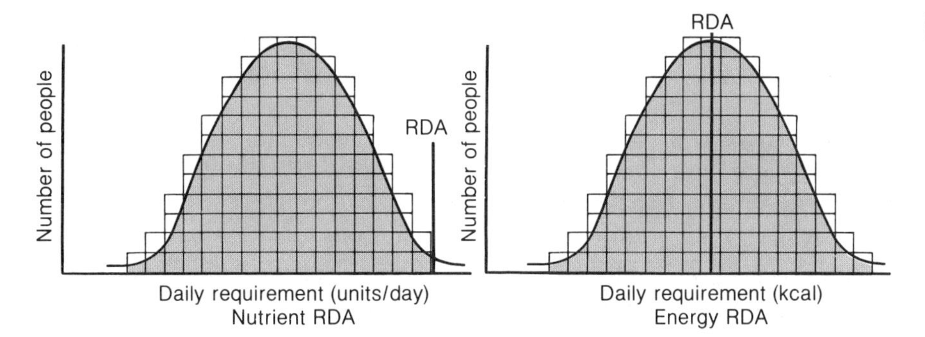

Figure 2–4 The Differences between the Nutrient RDA and the Energy RDA. The nutrient RDA are set so that nearly all people's requirements will be met by them. The energy RDA are set so that half the population's requirements will fall below and half above them.

Other Recommendations

Different nations and international groups have published different sets of standards similar to the RDA. The Canadian recommendations differ from the RDA in some respects, partly because of differences in interpretation of the data they were derived from and partly because conditions in Canada differ somewhat from those in the United States.

Among the most widely used sets of recommendations are those of two international groups: the Food and Agriculture Organization (FAO) and the World Health Organization (WHO). The FAO/WHO recommendations are considered sufficient for the maintenance of health in nearly all people. They differ from the RDA because they are based on slightly different judgment factors and serve different purposes. The FAO/WHO recommendations, for example, assume a protein quality lower than that commonly consumed in the United States and so recommend a higher intake. They also take into consideration that worldwide, people are generally smaller and more physically active than the population of the United States. The United States sets its calcium recommendation higher to keep it in balance with the higher protein intakes of its people. Nevertheless, the recommendations of different nations all fall within the same range.

Chapter 7 explains the impact of dietary protein on calcium balance. Appendix 6 provides addresses for FAO, WHO, and other agencies.

Dietary Goals and Guidelines

While the RDA and RNI make specific recommendations for protein, vitamins, and mineral intakes, they only make general statements about energy intakes, and they do little to protect people from excess intakes of fat, salt, sugar, cholesterol, and alcohol. The governments of many of the developed countries have published separate sets of recommendations in favor of moderation.

Among them have been the *Nutrition Recommendations for Canadians*, the *Dietary Goals for the United States,* and the *Dietary Guidelines for Americans*. These sets of guidelines are shown in Figure 2–5 and Tables 2–1 and 2–2. They speak in terms of foods: if you were to implement them, you would choose abundant fruits, vegetables, and whole grains, few foods high in sugar or fat, and few animal products.

Figure 2–5 The Current U.S. Diet and the Recommended Diet, According to the *Dietary Goals*.

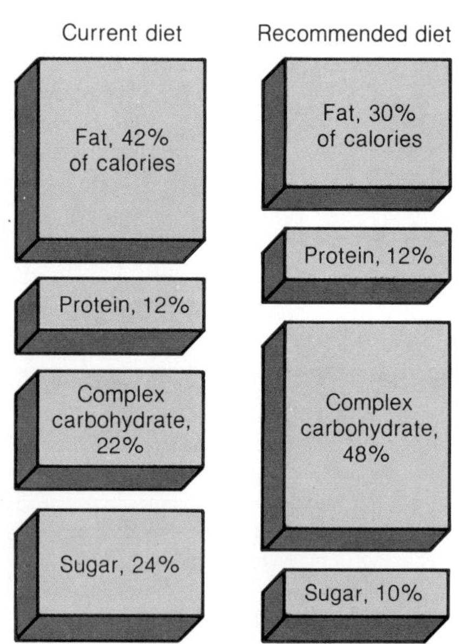

The dietary goals and guidelines are important to you as an individual, because they encourage health. They may also be the only human food consumption pattern that the earth can sustain into the future. The land areas used to feed meat animals are vast, especially if they are grain fed, as the majority of grocery store meat is. Some experts believe that to continue raising meat animals at today's rate is to threaten the world's agricultural future.[4] They point out that it takes many tens of thousands of calories of grain to produce a few hundred calories of beef. Thus it is more economical in terms of resources for people to eat the grain directly and benefit from its calories and nutrients.

Cattle also lay the land open to erosion. Grazing land is often obtained by destroying irreplaceable tropical rain forests upon which a stable world climate

Table 2–1

Dietary Guidelines for Americans/Suggestions for Food Choices

1. *Eat a variety of foods daily.* Include these foods every day: fruits and vegetables; whole-grain and enriched breads and cereals and other products made from grains; milk and milk products; meats, fish, poultry, and eggs; and dried peas and beans.
2. *Maintain desirable weight.* Increase physical activity; control overeating by eating slowly, taking smaller portions, and avoiding "seconds"; eat fewer fatty foods and sweets and less sugar, drink fewer alcoholic beverages, and eat more foods that are low in calories and high in nutrients.
3. *Avoid too much fat, saturated fat, and cholesterol.* Choose low-fat protein sources such as lean meats, fish, poultry, and dry peas and beans; use eggs and organ meats in moderation; limit intake of fats on and in foods; trim fats from meats; broil, bake, or boil—don't fry; limit breaded and deep-fried foods; read food labels for fat contents.
4. *Eat foods with adequate starch and fiber.* Substitute starchy foods for foods high in fats and sugars; select whole-grain breads and cereal, fruits and vegetables, and dried beans and peas, to increase fiber and starch intake.
5. *Avoid too much sugar.* Use less sugar, syrup, and honey; reduce concentrated sweets like candy, soft drinks, cookies, and the like; select fresh fruits or fruits canned in light syrup or their own juices; read food labels— sucrose, glucose, dextrose, maltose, lactose, fructose, syrups, and honey are all sugars; eat sugar less often to reduce dental caries.
6. *Avoid too much sodium.* Learn to enjoy the flavors of unsalted foods; flavor foods with herbs, spices, and lemon juice; reduce salt in cooking; add little or no salt at the table; limit salty foods like potato chips, pretzels, salted nuts, popcorn, condiments (soy sauce, steak sauce, and garlic salt), some cheeses, pickled foods and cured meats, and some canned vegetables and soups; read food labels for sodium or salt contents, especially in processed and snack foods; use lower-sodium products when available.
7. *If you drink alcoholic beverages, do so in moderation.* For individuals who drink, limit all alcoholic beverages (including wine, beer, liquors, and so on) to one or two drinks per day. "One drink" means 12 oz of beer, 3 oz of wine, or 1 1/2 oz of distilled spirits. Pregnant women should refrain from the use of alcohol. If you drink, do not drive.

Source: U.S. Department of Agriculture, U.S. Department of Health and Human Services, *Nutrition and Your Health: Dietary Guidelines for Americans,* 2d ed. (Washington, D.C.: Government Printing Office, 1985).

depends. Once converted from such forests to pastures and fields, the land is limited—topsoil is soon washed irretrievably into the oceans. Chapter 14 explores the relationships between people, their food and the planet's well-being.

Some people are already following the *Goals and Guidelines* like those shown here, but a person accustomed to the typical North American high-meat diet must make changes—especially to increase consumption of complex carbohydrate. Notice that all three sets of recommendations state not only what we should eat, but also what we should avoid, and that they make reference to weight maintenance and exercise.*

*Seven booklets have been made available to assist people in implementing the *Dietary Guidelines. Dietary Guidelines and Your Diet* is available from the Consumer Information Service, Dept. 187P, Pueblo CO 81009.

food group plan: a diet planning tool that sorts foods of similar origin and nutrient content into groups and then specifies that a person eat a certain number of foods from each group.

serving: an informal term that describes the amount of food a person might eat, similar to *helping*.

portion: a defined serving, such as a half cup or a cup.

exchange lists: lists of foods with portion sizes specified; the foods on a single list are similar with respect to energy-yielding nutrients and calorie amounts and so can be used interchangeably.

Table 2–2

Nutrition Recommendations for Canadians

1. Consume a nutritionally adequate diet, as outlined in Canada's Food Guide (see Table 2–4).
2. Reduce calories from fat to 35% of total calories. Include a source of polyunsaturated fatty acid (linoleic acid) in the diet.
3. Consume a diet that emphasizes whole-grain products and fruits and vegetables and minimizes alcohol, salt, and refined sugars.
4. Prevent and control obesity through reducing excess consumption of calories and increasing physical activity. Take precautions that no deficiency of vitamins and minerals occurs when total calories are reduced.

Source: Derived from the Report of the Committee on Diet and Cardiovascular Disease, 1976, by J. L. Beare-Rogers, Dietary goals and recommendations in Canada, *Journal of the Canadian Dietetic Association* 41 (1984): 325–329.

The U.S. Dietary Goals, *the* Dietary Guidelines for Americans, *and the* Nutrition Recommendations for Canadians *address the problems of overnutrition, recommending calorie control; reduced consumption of fat, salt, and sugar; and increased consumption of grains, fruits, and vegetables.*

Diet Planning with Food Groups and Other Tools

Diet planning is the bridge between nutrition theory and the food on the table. Standards such as the RDA and RNI, and guidelines such as those just described, can benefit you only if your diet meets them. To help with planning, two tools are commonly used—food group plans, and lists of foods to go with them.

A **food group plan** can tell you what types of foods to eat, and how much of each type. It helps to make the diet adequate and balanced. Many different food group plans are available, including some suited for people of different ethnic groups or religious persuasions.

A set of lists is useful along with a food group plan. The plan may tell you to use a **serving** of food from a certain group at each meal; you can then turn to the list to find out exactly what foods are in each group, and what **portion** sizes will offer the intended amounts of nutrients and calories. Figure 2–6 provides some help with recognizing portion sizes.

The lists most often used with food group plans are called **exchange lists**, because their members are interchangeable. Finding an apple and a pear on the same list, for example, you can trade one for the other without significantly altering the nutrient content or calorie count of your meal. Exchange lists help with calorie control, and permit you to vary your diet by making different choices on different days. The ones presented in this chapter also point out which foods are high in fat and sodium, so that you can avoid them if you wish,

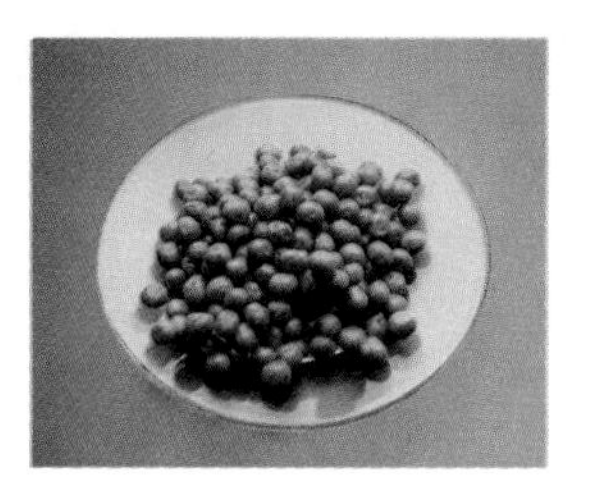

100 grams peas (about ½ cup).

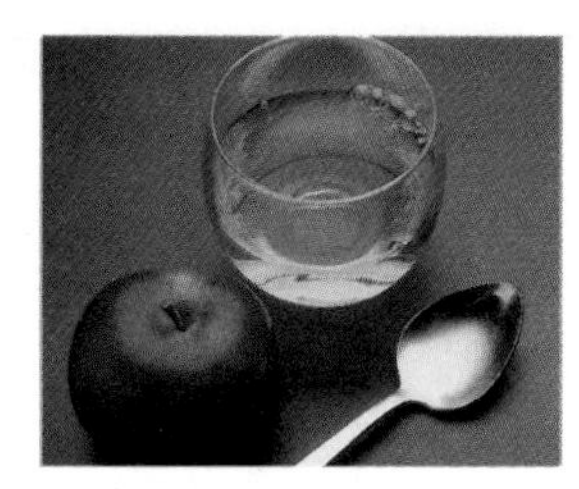

100 ml juice (about ½ cup).

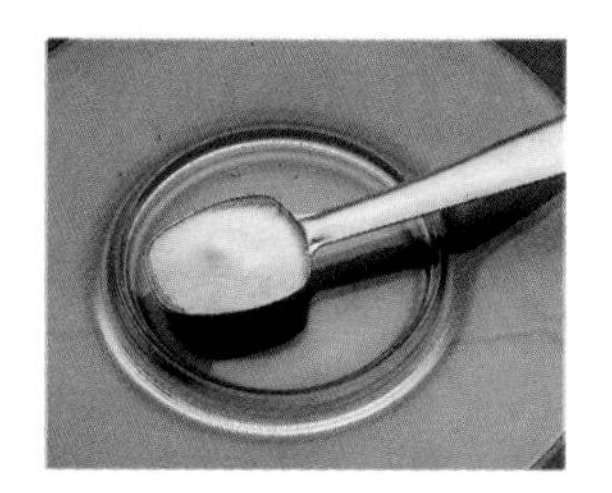

5 grams salt (about 1 teaspoon).

Figure 2–6 Portion Sizes.
A serving of a food can be any amount you like; portions are more specific. Shown here are three typical portions: 100 grams of a food (which is about the same as ½ cup), 100 milliliters of a juice (which is also about the same as ½ cup), and 5 grams of a powder, salt (which is about the same as a teaspoon). Cooks who like to switch back and forth between the British and metric systems have learned to use these values interchangeably.

and which are high in fiber, so that you can seek them out—thus helping with moderation.

Food Group Plans

One of the most familiar food group plans fits all foods into four groups and a miscellaneous category, as shown in Table 2–3 (next page). Each of the four groups contains foods that are similar in origin and that supply a characteristic array of nutrients. They are *whole foods* that form the foundation of a healthy diet: milks and milk products, fruits and vegetables, starches and grains, and meats and meat alternates. The plan suggests for adults a two, four, four, two pattern of servings from each group (see Table 2–3), although other patterns are possible and desirable for individuals.

The miscellaneous category contains *partitioned foods* (see p. 25) that do not fit into the four food groups. Among them are butter, margarine, cream, salad dressing, ketchup, jam and jelly, coffee and tea, herbs, soft drinks, alcoholic beverages, and others. These items may contain a few nutrients, but they are so greatly diluted with fat, sugar, or water, or used in such small quantities, that they make little contribution to nutrition.

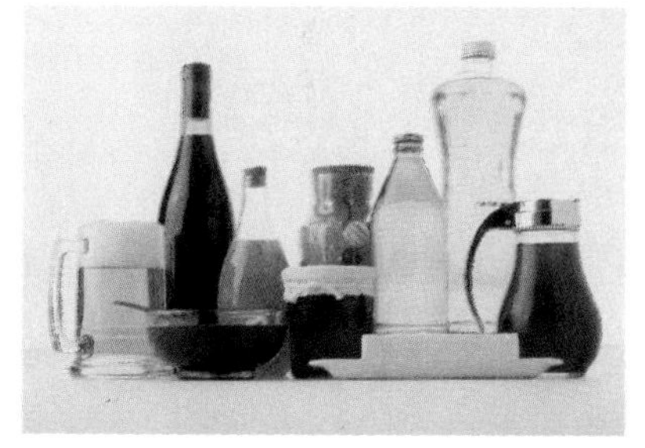

These are not whole foods, and so are grouped into a miscellaneous category.

Other food group plans are available. Canada has one of its own—Canada's Food Guide, shown in part A of Table 2–4. A plan specifically for vegetarians is shown in part B of the table. A person who spends many calories in vigorous physical activity might use the modified four food group plan shown in part C.

Food group plans alone don't provide as much detail as some people need. They give a framework, but don't specify exactly what to put in it. It helps to have lists of specific foods and serving sizes to fill in the frame.

Exchange Lists

Exchange lists are popular among careful diet planners—particularly people who wish to control calories as well as to obtain an adequate, balanced diet. Whether you use them or not, you may find them interesting, because they can help give you a "feel" for what is in the foods you choose to eat, and a sense of which foods are similar to each other. The system of lists used here is the same as that used to plan diets for people with diabetes—for they need to control the same dietary factors as most other people do—food energy, fat, other nutrients, fiber, and salt.

Table 2–3

The Four Food Group Plan

Food Group	Servings/Day (Adult)	Sample Foods and Serving Sizes	Main Nutrients
Milk and milk products	2[a]	(A)Nonfat milk, buttermilk, low-fat milk, plain yogurt;(B) whole milk, cheese, fruit-flavored yogurt, cottage cheese; (C) custard, milkshake, pudding, ice cream	Protein, riboflavin, vitamin B_{12},[b] calcium, magnesium
Fruits and vegetables	4[c]	(A)Apricot, bean sprouts, broccoli, Brussels sprouts, cabbage, cantaloupe, carrots, cauliflower, cucumber, grapefruit, green beans, green peas, leafy greens (spinach, mustard, and collard greens), lettuce, mushrooms, orange, orange juice, peach, strawberries, tomato, winter squash; (B) apple, banana, canned fruit, corn, pear, potato; (C) avocado, dried fruit, sweet potato	Vitamins A and C,[d] folacin, fiber
Grains (whole-grain and enriched bread and cereal products)	4[e]	(A)Whole grain and enriched breads, rolls, tortillas; (B) rice, cereals, pastas (macaroni, spaghetti), bagel; (C) pancake, muffin, cornbread, biscuit, presweetened cereals	Thiamin,[f] niacin, iron, zinc, fiber
Meat and meat alternates	2	(A)Poultry, fish, lean meat (beef, lamb, pork), dried peas and beans, eggs; (B) beef, lamb, pork, luncheon meats, refried beans; (C) hot dogs, peanut butter, nuts	Protein, thiamin, riboflavin, niacin, vitamins B_6 and B_{12},[b] folacin, magnesium, zinc

Note: Foods labeled (A) are lowest in calories, (C) highest, (B) in between. A miscellaneous category includes foods that tend to be high in fat, salt, sugar, alcohol, and, in most cases, calories. Foods high in fat include margarine, salad dressing, oils, mayonnaise, cream, cream cheese, butter, gravy, and sauces. Foods high in salt include potato chips, corn chips, pretzels, pickles, olives, bouillon, prepared mustard, soy sauce, steak sauce, salt, and seasoned salt. Foods high in sugar include cake, pie, cookies, doughnuts, sweet rolls, candy, soft drinks, fruit drinks, jelly, syrup, gelatin desserts, sugar, and honey. Alcoholic beverages include wine, beer, and liquor. Other miscellaneous foods, not high in calories, include spices, herbs, coffee, tea, and diet soft drinks.

[a]For children up to 9, 2–3 c; for children 9–12, 3–4 c; for teenagers and pregnant women, 3–4 c; for nursing mothers, 4 c or more; for women past 50, 3–5 c.

[b]Vitamin B_{12} is contributed only by foods that come from animals.

[c]One should be rich in vitamin C; at least one every other day should be rich in vitamin A.

[d]Dark green and deep orange vegetables are especially reliable vitamin A sources; other fruits and vegetables are not. For vitamin C, citrus fruits, green leafy vegetables, and selected other fruits and vegetables are superior sources. See Chapter 6 for more details.

[e]Enriched or, preferably, whole-grain products only. Whole grains include wheat, oats, rice, barley, millet, rye, and bulgur.

[f]If the recommended four or more servings are eaten, these foods contribute significant nutrients to the diet. They also contribute most of the complex carbohydrate of the diet. Whole-grain products are preferred over refined enriched products. For more details, see Chapter 3.

Sources: Adapted from *Building a Better Diet,* Food and Nutrition Service, USDA Program Aid No. 1241, 1979; and Food Group Chart, © Dairy Council of California (0020N, 1983, distributed by National Dairy Council).

Table 2–4

Alternative Food Group Plans

A. Canada's Food Guide	B. Four Food Group Plan for the Vegetarian	C. Modified Four Food Group Plan
Milk and milk products—2 servings[a] Meat, fish, poultry, and alternates—2 servings[b] Fruits and vegetables—4 to 5 servings, [b,c] Breads and cereals—3 to 5 servings[b]	Milk and milk products—2 servings[d] Protein-rich foods—2 servings[e] Legumes—2 servings[f] Fruits/vegetables—4 servings[g] Breads/cereals (whole-grain only)—4 servings	Milk and milk products—2 servings Meat, fish, or poultry—2 servings[h] Legumes—2 servings[i] Fruits/vegetables—4 servings Grains—4 servings[j]
[a]A serving is 250 ml, or about 1 c. See Appendix E for equivalents in the Canadian exchange system. Milk group servings differ for children up to age 11—2 to 3 servings; adolescents—3 to 4 servings; pregnant and nursing women—3 to 4 servings. [b]See Appendix E for equivalents in the Canadian exchange system. [c]Include at least two vegetables.	[d]If not using milk or milk products, use soy milk fortified with calcium and vitamin B_{12}. [e]Examples of protein-rich foods: cheeses, tofu (see meat alternates in Appendix E). [f]Legumes (2 c daily) should be eaten in addition to protein-rich foods, to help women meet iron requirements. [g]Include 1 c dark greens daily to help women meet iron requirements.	[h]Serving size is 3 ounces, not 2 to 3 ounces as in the Four Food Group Plan. [i]Serving size is 3/4 c. [j]Whole-grain products only, not enriched.
Source: Canada's Food Guide Handbook, revised (Health and Welfare Canada, 1985).	*Source:* Adapted from *Vegetarian Food Choices* (Gainesville: Shands Teaching Hospital and Clinics, Food and Nutrition Service, University of Florida, 1976).	*Source:* Designed to increase intakes of needed nutrients, especially iron, vitamin B_6, zinc, magnesium, and vitamin E, within about 2200 cal/day, by J. C. King and coauthors, Evaluation and modification of the basic four food guide, *Journal of Nutrition Education* 10(1978): 27-29.

There are six exchange lists, shown in their entirety in Appendix E. They go with the four food groups as follows:

Food groups	Exchange lists
Milk group: Milk and milk products Cheese	Milk list: Milk and milk products
Vegetable/fruit group: Low-calorie vegetables Starchy vegetables Legumes Fruits	Vegetable list: Low-calorie vegetables Fruit list: Fruits
Grains: Breads and cereals	Starches/grains list: Breads and cereals Starchy vegetables
Meat group: Meat, fish, poultry, eggs	Meat/meat alternate list: Meat, fish, poultry, eggs Cheese Legumes
Miscellaneous category: High-sugar foods High-fat foods Alcohol	Fat list: High-fat foods Alcohol Not on exchange lists: High-sugar foods

The Four Food Group Plan states that cheese can be substituted for milk, and so it can, but cheese is listed with the meats in the exchange lists. The truth is that cheese really doesn't fit very well in either system. It is like milk in being a significant calcium (and not iron) source, but like meat in its protein and fat contents. Except for very strict diet planning, such as may be necessary for people with severe diabetes, an informal instruction with respect to cheese should suffice: use it in place of milk sometimes (say, 1 to 2 ounces per cup of milk), and use it in place of meat sometimes (trading ounce for ounce).

The Four Food Group Plan groups together as vegetables all foods that a farmer would define as vegetables, but they appear on three different exchange lists. The starchy vegetables are listed with the grains, because of their high starch content, and the legumes are listed with the meats, because of their protein and iron contents. These differences illustrate the point that each food is unique—another argument for mixing and matching different ways on different days.

Sugar and high-sugar foods, which contribute calories but not significant nutrients, are often treated as simply adding calories without being assigned to any group. Besides pure fats, high-fat foods and alcohol, which also contribute nutrient-empty calories, are often included as members of the fat list.

Appendix E contains both the U.S. and Canadian exchange lists.

For each item on a list, a portion size is specified; that makes it possible to specify a calorie amount, too. Each list can be remembered by one of its typical members:

- *Milk*—1 cup nonfat milk—90 calories.
- *Vegetable*—½ cup green beans—25 calories.
- *Fruit*—½ small banana—60 calories.
- *Starches/grain*—1 slice bread—80 calories.
- *Meat*—1 ounce lean meat or low-fat cheese—55 calories.
- *Fat*—1 teaspoon butter—45 calories.

Table 2–5 shows the protein, fat, and carbohydrate values for the members of each list, and Table 2–6 (pages 46–47) shows some typical foods of each list.

Each list helps the user distinguish between the items of highest nutrient density and those that have significant added fat (and therefore calories). The milk list contains three categories of milk products: nonfat and very-low-fat, low-fat, and whole milk. The vegetable list includes only low-calorie vegetables, so that ½ cup of any of them will provide about 25 calories. The fruit list specifies "no added sugar or sugar syrup"—not to keep users from eating fruits with sugar but to make them aware when they do, and to help them keep track of sugar consumption. Portion sizes are adjusted so that fruit portions are equal in calories. One small banana is treated as "two fruits." A piece of cherry pie is not considered a fruit at all—it includes a fruit if it contains ten large cherries, but it also includes bread exchanges, fat exchanges, and sugar.

The starches/grains list also specifies portion sizes and makes clear which products contain added fat. Corn, lima beans, and other starchy vegetables are listed with the breads because they are similar to them in food energy and carbohydrate content. Meats and cheeses are, like the milks, separated into three categories—lean, medium-fat, and high-fat. Finally, the fat list includes unexpected items like bacon and olives, revealing their true character to the user.

The exchange lists point out fiber and sodium wherever they appear in significant quantities. Foods high in fiber can be picked out by the symbol (a stalk

Table 2–5

The Six Exchange Lists

Exchange List	Carbohydrate (g)	Protein (g)	Fat (g)	Calories
Milks				
Nonfat	12	8	Trace	90
Low fat	12	8	5	120
Whole	12	8	8	150
Vegetables[a]	5	2	—	25
Fruits	15	—	—	60
Starches/ breads[b]	15	3	Trace	80
Meats				
Lean	—	7	3	55
Medium fat	—	7	5	75
High fat	—	7	8	100
Fats	—	—	5	45

[a]This list includes low-calorie vegetables only.

[b]This list includes starchy vegetables such as lima beans and corn, as well as cereal, bread, pasta, and other grain products. For portion sizes see Appendix 5.

Note: This is the U.S. exchange system. The complete details, and those of the Canadian system, are shown in Appendix 5.

of grain) they bear (use them often). Another symbol (a salt-shaker) identifies those foods high in sodium so people can avoid them if they choose.

A refinement on diet planning is to create your own individualized pattern to follow, based on the number of calories you need and on the types of foods you particularly like to eat. A person eating 3000 calories a day, for example, could use considerably more bread portions than the person eating only 1500 calories a day. Table 2–7 shows sample patterns for different energy intakes.

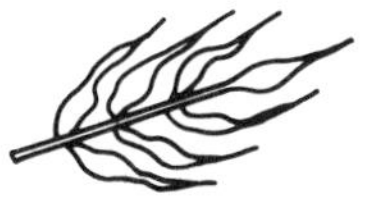

Fiber symbol. Sodium symbol.

The exchange system booklets available from the American Dietetic Association (ADA) identify foods high in fiber and sodium with these symbols, so that users can choose foods wisely. In Appendix E, the same foods are identified with superscripts a and b. To obtain the original booklet, write to the ADA at the address given in Appendix F.

Diet Planning

Table 2–8 provides an example of diet planning using the Four Food Group plan as a pattern. It shows that the plan's minimum specifications can be fulfilled within a total of about 1000 calories—leaving, for most people, many calories to spare. Even a moderately active adult woman could afford to eat at least 500 additional calories. A wise choice would be to invest many of those calories in additional vegetables, milk products, possibly legumes, and some fat. Some could be spent on luxury items—occasional sweet desserts or alcoholic beverages. Adequacy and balance should be achieved within the day, but need not characterize every single meal. The final plan might be like that outlined in column 3 of the table—one of many possible examples. The planner could then achieve variety by selecting different foods each day from each exchange list.

Food group plans and exchange lists, used together, ease diet planning. Food group plans provide the framework that ensures adequacy and balance; exchange lists supply the items to go in the frame, permitting calorie control, moderation, and variety.

Table 2–6

Exchange Lists: Typical Foods

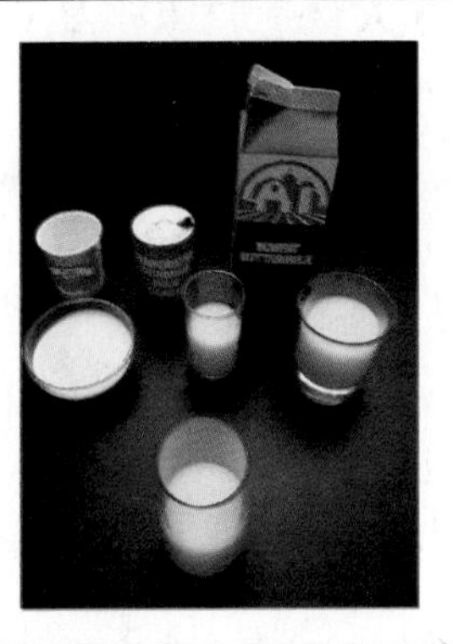

1. Milks
1 c nonfat milk is like:
1 c nonfat yogurt, plain
1 c nonfat buttermilk
½ c evaporated nonfat milk
(1 milk = 12 g carbohydrate, 8 g protein, trace of fat, and 90 cal.)

2. Vegetables
½ c carrots is like:
½ c greens
½ c brussels sprouts
½ c beets
(1 vegetable = 5 g carbohydrate, 2 g protein, and 25 cal.)

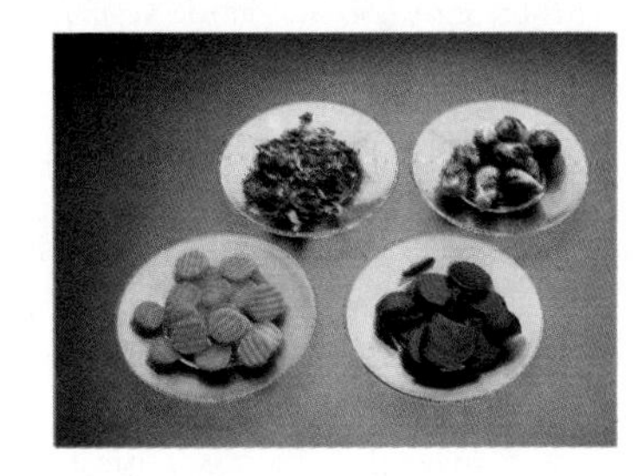

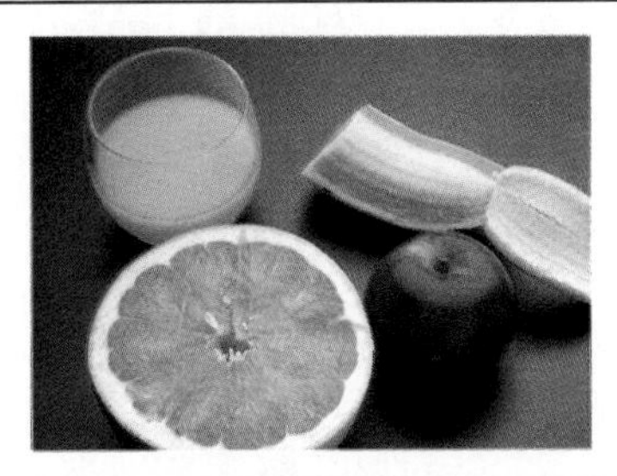

3. Fruits
½ small banana is like:
1 small apple
½ grapefruit
½ c orange juice
(1 fruit = 15 g carbohydrate and 60 cal.)

4. Starches/Grains
1 slice bread is like:
¾ c ready-to-eat cereal
⅓ c cooked beans
½ c corn
1 small (3-oz) potato
(1 bread = 15 g carbohydrate, 3 g protein, trace of fat, and 80 cal.)

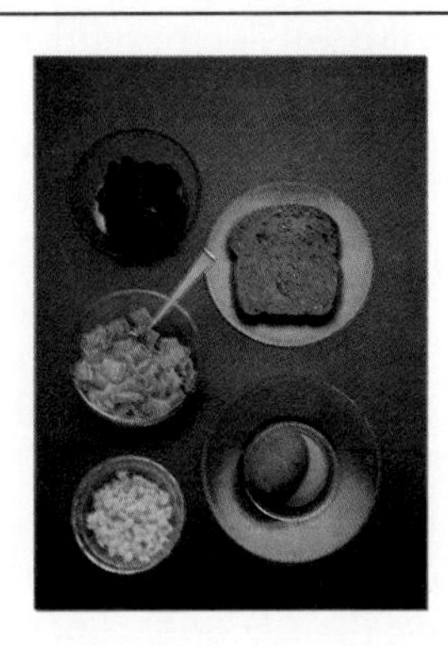

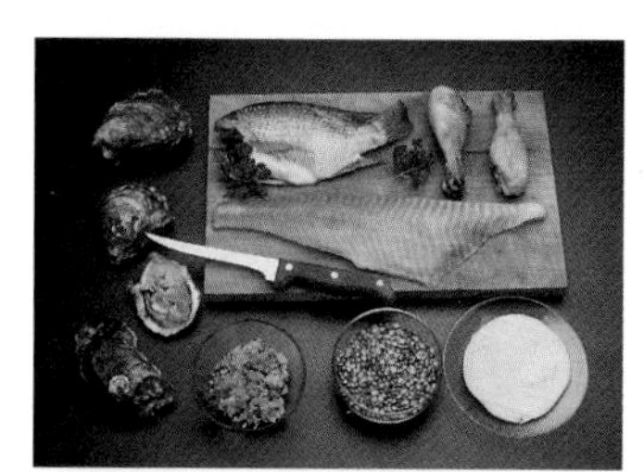

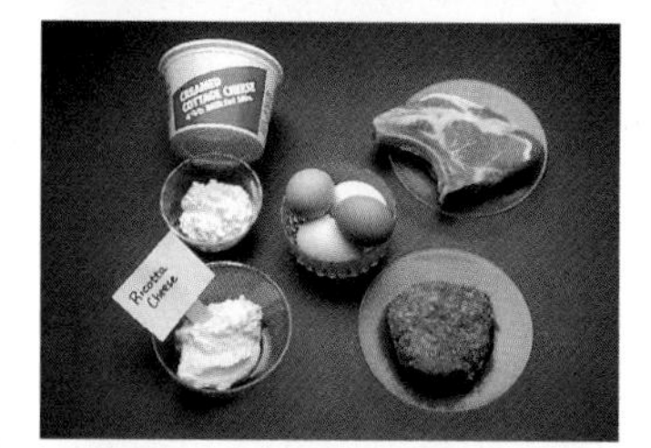

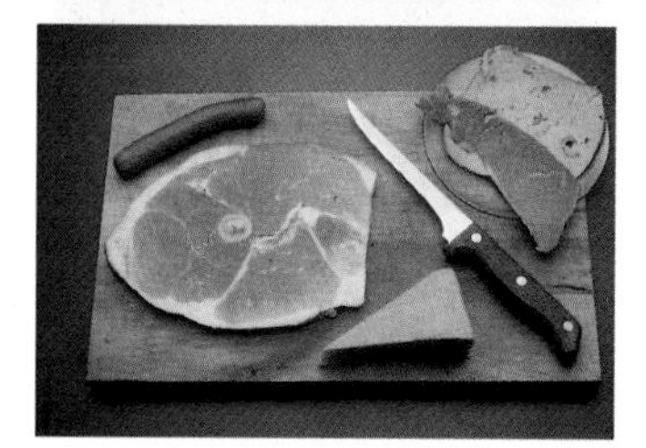

5A. Meats (lean)

1 oz lean meat is like:
1 oz chicken meat without the skin
1 oz any fish
¼ c canned tuna
1 oz low-fat cheese[a]
(1 lean meat = 7 g protein, 3 g fat, and 55 cal.) (One 3-oz portion of meat (such as a hamburger patty) = 3 meat exchanges. One meat exchange = ⅓ of a 3-oz hamburger patty.)

[a]Cheeses are grouped with milk in food group plans because of their calcium content but with meats in this system because, like meat, they contribute calories from protein and fat and have negligible carbohydrate content.

5B. Meats (medium fat)

1 oz medium-fat meat is like 1 oz lean meat in protein content but has 5 g fat (2 g more fat than lean meat). Examples:
1 oz pork loin
1 egg
¼ c creamed cottage cheese[a]
(1 medium-fat meat = 7 g protein, 5 g fat, and about 75 cal.)

5C. Meats (high fat)

1 oz high-fat meat is like 1 oz lean meat in protein content but is estimated to have an **extra "1 fat"**— that is, to have the 3 g fat of a lean meat and 5 g additional fat. Examples:
1 oz country-style ham
1 oz cheddar cheese[a]
1 small hotdog (frankfurter)[b]
(1 high-fat meat = 7 g protein, 8 g fat, and 100 cal.)

[b]The hotdog counts as 1 high-fat meat exchange plus 1 fat exchange.

5D. Legumes

Legumes are like meats because they are rich in protein and iron, but many are lower in fat than meat. They contain a lot of starch. They can be treated as:
1 c legumes = 1 lean meat + 2 starch.
(1 c legumes = 30 g carbohydrate, 13 g protein, 3+ g fat, and 215 cal.)

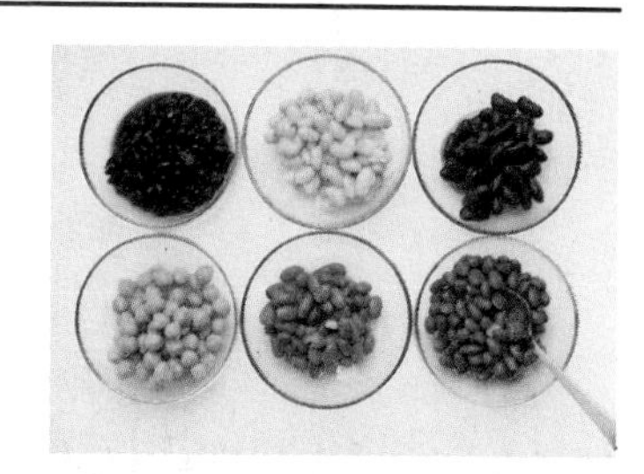

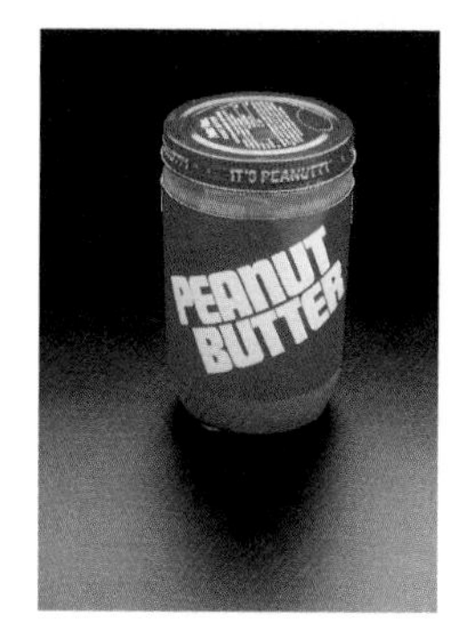

5E. Peanut butter

Peanut butter is like a meat in terms of its protein content. It is estimated as:
1 tbsp peanut butter = 1 high-fat meat (1 tbsp peanut butter = 7 g protein, 8 g fat, and 100 cal.)
Don't swear off peanut butter, necessarily. You'll need to appreciate the polyunsaturated character of its fat (see Chapter 4) and the B-vitamin contributions it makes (see Chapter 6), before deciding how much of a place it should have in your diet.

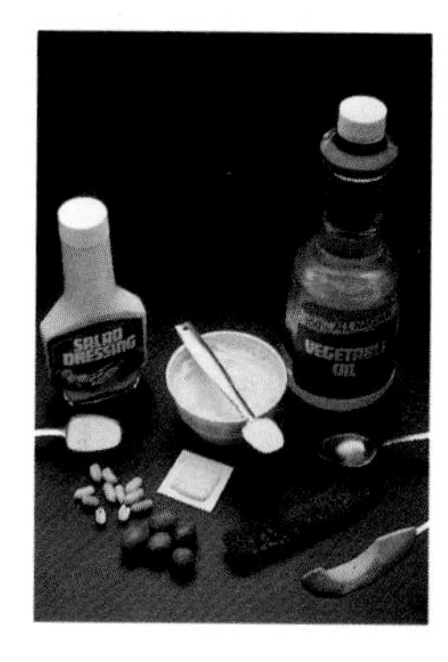

6. Fats

1 tsp butter is like:
1 tsp margarine
1 tsp any oil
1 tbsp salad dressing
1 strip crisp bacon
5 large olives
10 whole Virginia peanuts
(1 fat = 5 g fat and 45 cal.)

ethnic diets: diets associated with particular national origins, races, cultural heritages, or geographic locations.

vegetarian diets: diets that omit meat, or all animal flesh, or all animal products.

Table 2–7

Diet Plans for Different Energy Intakes

	Energy Level (cal)					
Exchanges	*1000*	*1200*	*1500*	*1800*	*2000*	*2200*
Milks	2	2	2	2	2	2
Vegetables	2	3	4	4	4	6
Fruits	3	3	4	5	5	5
Starches/grains	3	4	6	8	10	11
Meats	4	5	5	5	6	6
Fats	3	4	5	7	7	8

[a]These patterns of exchanges supply about 30% of the calories as fat, in accordance with the view that a moderate fat intake is desirable.

Ethnic and Vegetarian Diets

Every country, and in fact every region of a country, has its own typical foods and ways of combining them into meals. Immigrants to North America have brought those ways with them, and they have evolved here into patterns that we call—for lack of a better term—**ethnic diets** or cuisines. As generations have passed and people have migrated from one region of North America to another, these cuisines have melded together, and people have evolved their own styles that combine characteristics of many different original diets.

The mosaic of eating styles in North America evolved in a background of original North American foods, such as corn, sweet potatoes, pumpkins, fowl, and seafood, which were handed down by the first inhabitants, the Native American Indians. To those foods were added white potatoes, rice, barley, and others too numerous to name, brought by the original immigrants and those that followed over the years. Each ethnic group has molded the North American diet in its own way, by blending traditional seasonings and recipes with the abundant local foods. Today, when you think of southern Louisiana, you think of Cajun food: Cajuns are the Louisiana descendants of the Acadian French, famous for their cookery. The cuisine of southern Texas is TexMex, Texas food with a Mexican flavor. New England may bring to mind baked beans and brown bread; Wisconsin, German sausages and beer; the South, fried chicken and grits. Now that so many people travel from region to region, whatever people eat as their regular fare, they choose to enjoy what they call ethnic meals now and then—meaning whatever some *other* group typically eats—pizza, tacos, or chow mein. Many of these foods are not the same as what the original immigrants ate in the old country, but are Americanized versions of traditional foods.

Among the most highly evolved and least recognizable as coming from any particular place are the many meatless styles of eating people call **vegetarian diets.** The foods in these diets may be East Indian, Chinese, Middle Eastern, or other, but most of the diets have distinctly American—and modern—characteristics. They are very varied. People who call themselves vegetarians may eat

Table 2–8

Use of Diet-Planning Tools

Pattern from Four Food Group Plan	Selections Made from the Exchange Lists	Example	Energy Cost (cal)
Milk—2 c	Milk list—select 2 exchanges	2 c nonfat milk	180
Meat—2 servings (2 to 3 oz each)	Meat list—select 6 exchanges[a]	6 oz lean meat	330
Fruits and vegetables—4 servings	Fruit and vegetable lists—select 4 exchanges	2 vegetable exchanges; 2 fruit exchanges	50 120
Grains—4 servings	Starches/grains—select 4 exchanges[b]	2 bread exchanges; 2 starchy vegetable exchanges	320
		Total:	1000

[a]In the Four Food Group Plan, 1 serving is 2 to 3 oz. on the exchange lists, 1 exchange is 1 oz.
[b]Because the starchy vegetables are on the same list with the grains, some of them can be substituted for grains.

vegan (VAY-gun or VEDGE-un): a vegetarian who eats nothing but plant foods.

lacto-ovo vegetarian: a vegetarian who eats products from animals such as milk and eggs, but no animal flesh.

no foods of animal origin at all **(vegan),** may eat foods that come from animals such as milk and eggs but not meat **(lacto-ovo vegetarians),** or may abide by other rules, such as eating fish, or fish and poultry, but not red meat.

Table 2–9 shows some of the foods that are typical of some ethnic diets. It is a mistake, however, to assume that any particular individual eats the diet described for the group. Just as some New Englanders detest baked beans, and some Southerners never eat grits, preferences and practices of people within groups vary. Especially, as children of immigrants grow up, they modify old traditions. For example, in Puerto Rico, folklore classifies foods as "hot" or "cold," and for the local people, this property dictates when and in what combinations foods are used. Few people of Puerto Rican descent, born, raised, and educated here, hold such beliefs.

The kaleidoscopic mixture of traditional foodways that is available offers an opportunity to design diets to meet many ideals besides mere adequacy or economy. Diets can be colorful, tasty, exciting. They can even be designed idealistically, to be good for the earth. The two examples that follow are presented to reveal some of the potentials in diet planning for the thinking person.

People of the world have many foodways. Ethnic diets in America evolved from immigrants' traditional foodways that were modified by exposure to local customs and foods. Vegetarian diets, no longer recognizable as to origin, are among them.

The Chinese Diet

The Chinese diet makes a dramatic contrast with the typical United States diet (as described in the *Dietary Goals* and graphed in Figure 2–5). Tried and true, it has supported health without excess fatness in China for thousands of years.

Table 2–9

Traditional Diets of Ethnic Groups in the United States

Group and Place of Origin	Staple Foods	Foods Excluded	Strengths and Weaknesses of the Diet
Hispanic Americans from Cuba, Haiti, Puerto Rico	Steamed white rice; many varieties of beans; wheat breads; starchy vegetables such as cassavas, yuccas, yams, breadfruit, plantains, and green bananas; green peppers; tomatoes; garlic; dried, salted fish; chicken; pork; lard; olive oil; sugar; jams and jellies; sweet pastries; sugared fruit juices; coffee	Green leafy vegetables; milk as a beverage for adults; fish other than dried and salted	Provides adequate protein, many other nutrients, and fiber; may provide too much fat, especially animal fat; may lack calcium
Hispanic Americans from Mexico, Central America	Many varieties of beans; steamed rice; corn products such as tortillas made from lime-soaked cornmeal; chili peppers; tomatoes; mangoes; prickly pear fruit; potatoes; meat and sausages; fish; poultry; eggs; milk cheeses; milk custards and bread puddings; lard; sweet chocolate and coffee drinks; cakes; cookies; pastries	Green leafy vegetables; yellow vegetables; milk as a beverage for adults	Is high in calories and fat, especially saturated fat, and high in sugar; most nutrients can be obtained, but with many calories
Black Americans from West Indies, Africa, Central or South America	Dumplings or gruel made from millet, corn, wheat, rice, or barley; starchy roots such as cassavas, yams, plantains, and bananas; coconuts; peanuts; fresh fruits; hot peppers; tomatoes; onions; okra; palm oil; fruit wine; tea; coffee; honey; molasses	Milk and milk products (meat and fish limited use)	Is low in calcium, iron, and vitamin B_{12}; is potentially low in protein, depending on availability of foods; is low in fat and salt; is high in fiber
Southern black Americans from Africa (many generations in United States)	Hominy grits; biscuits; cornmeal and corn bread; rice; legumes; potatoes; green leafy vegetables; sweet potatoes; squashes; corn; cabbage; melons; peaches; pecans; smoked pork; fresh meats and poultry; fish; butter, shortening, and lard; sugar; bread puddings; pies and sweets	Milk and milk products; yeast breads	Provides ample fiber and many other nutrients; provides excess protein; is high in calories; provides excess fat, especially saturated fat; is high in salt; is low in calcium
Chinese Americans from China (diets vary sometimes with region)	Rice and rice gruel; wheat noodles; corn; green vegetables, especially from the cabbage family; squashes; cucumbers; eggplant; leafy vegetables; various shoots, including bamboo, mung, and soy; sweet potatoes; radishes; onions; peas and pods; mushrooms; roots; many local, seasonal vegetables; pickled vegetables; sea vegetables; plums; peaches; tangerines; kumquats and other citrus fruits; litchis; longans; mangoes; papayas; pomegranates; soybean products such as tofu (soybean curd), soy sauces, bean noodles, and soy milk; tiny portions of meat, fish with bones, or poultry; seafood; soup or tea as beverage; sugar as seasoning	Milk and most milk products	Depending on availability of protein-rich foods, protein and iron may be low; is low in fat; is high in fiber and many nutrients; see text for further discussion of the Chinese diet
Japanese Americans from Japan	Rice; vegetables; pickled vegetables; soy as miso (soup), tofu, bean paste, and soy sauce; fruits; salads; fish with bones; sugar as seasoning; sea vegetables; seafood; ginseng	Milk and milk products	Provides abundant nutrients with little fat; is high in salt

Group and Place of Origin	Staple Foods	Foods Excluded	Strengths and Weaknesses of the Diet
Korean Americans from South Korea	Rice; noodles; many leafy vegetables; kimchi (extremely hot pickled cabbage); sea vegetables; hot peppers; seasonal fruits; mushrooms; small fish with bones; large servings of grilled beef; chicken; fresh or dried squid, octopus, and lobster; fish with bones; mussels; eggs; lard and vegetable fat for frying; sesame oil; nuts and seeds; ginger; sugar as seasoning	Milk and milk products	Is high in fat and adequate in protein; is monotonous in winter (kimchi is served at each meal, to the exclusion of other vegetables); without the traditional small fish with bones, calcium can be lacking
Vietnamese Americans from Vietnam	Rice, rice noodles; french bread and croissants with butter; hot peppers; curries of asparagus and potatoes; salads; tropical fruits and vegetables; lemons and limes; small portions of poultry; eggs; fish pâtés; nuoc nam (a strong, fermented fish sauce); sweets, candies, sweetened drinks; coffee; tea	Milk and milk products	Can be low in iron or calcium
Seminole Indians, Natives of Southeastern United States	Corn; cornmeal; coontie (flour from a palmlike plant); swamp cabbage (now illegal to harvest); pumpkins; squashes; papayas; beef (largely replaces traditional meats such as alligator, snake, wild hog, duck, fish, and shellfish)	Milk and milk products	Is rich in protein and many nutrients; is high in calories and fat; calcium may be lacking

(There are, of course, many Chinese diets in that great country, but generalizations are still possible.)

Economy is essential for a country such as China, whose population is more than 1000 people per acre, and in which only 10 percent of the land can be used to grow food. China's population is estimated at about a billion people, with about 80 to 85 percent of that number involved in agriculture. There seems to be no malnutrition, and almost none of the Chinese people are fat.

Contrast the United States:
- Population density—113 per acre.
- Population—250 million.
- Farmers—1 to 2%.
- Land in farms—about 50%.

Chinese meals do not follow the separate meat/fish-vegetable-starch pattern of the West. The vegetables and meats are cooked together. The Chinese serve rice separately to each diner at almost every meal. They partake of soup or tea throughout each meal. Meat does not dominate any dish, but is used to add zest and variety to a meal. The total amount of meat, fish, or egg in a Chinese dish is very small by Western standards, but so much rice is eaten that the diet still supplies enough protein to meet the need. Diners have their own rice bowls, but the other dishes are served family style, and people reach for them with their chopsticks. Each person's meal thus centers on a staple starch food, and the person eats the other foods according to appetite.

Breakfast is usually light, consisting of rice, soft millet cereal, noodles, or steamed bread, with small dishes of salted fish or other well-seasoned food. Most Chinese eat three meals a day, but Western Chinese eat two main meals and three snacks, called "dot-the-heart" meals, consisting of fruit, meat or fish dumplings, or other special tidbits. This five-meal-a-day pattern meets nutrient needs equally well. There is no rule that says you must eat three meals a day, and there is no truth to the notion that snacks cannot be nutritious.

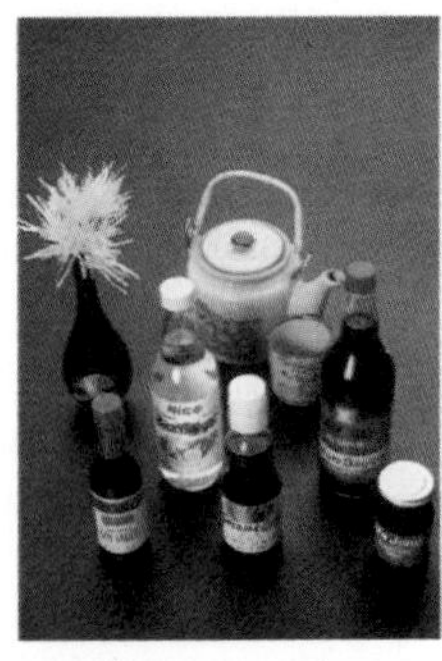

Sauces used in Chinese meals.

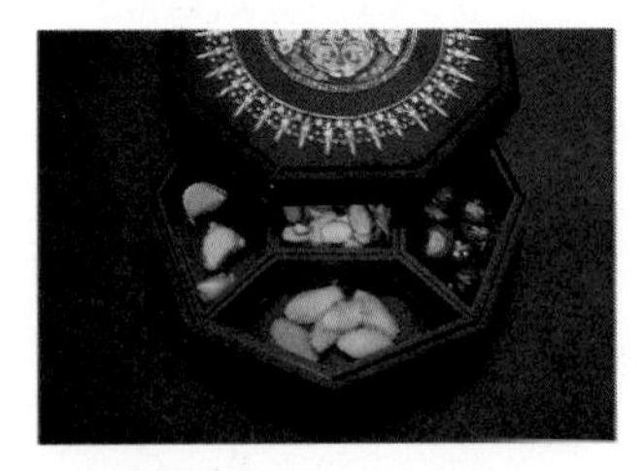

Seasonings used in Chinese meals.

The subtle flavors of Chinese dishes come partly from the foods themselves, and partly from the seasonings and sauces used in their preparation. Among the seasonings are ginger root, almonds, scallions, sesame seed oil, rice wine, and garlic. Sauces include dark and light soy sauce, hoisin sauce, oyster sauce, brown bean sauce, black bean sauce, and plum sauce. Chinese cooks use them in small quantities, only a tablespoon or so per dish. The sauces make no significant contribution of nutrients other than minerals; they add tasty flavors but no fat (unlike American gravies, butter, or sour cream); they are likely to be especially high in sodium.

The Chinese diet stands up well if measured against current dietary ideals. It is, or can be, *adequate* for all nutrients. Cooking foods the Chinese way tends to preserve nutrients. The water in which the rice is cooked soaks back into the rice rather than being thrown away. All food is cut into bite-sized pieces before cooking so that it will be easy to eat with chopsticks; cooking finely cut-up food requires only short times and so destroys few nutrients. No extra water is used, and none is thrown away, so nutrients are not lost.

As for *balance,* the diet emphasizes carbohydrate heavily, a point in its favor. Grains, together with sweet potatoes, are so extensively used that their carbohydrate provides more than 80 percent of the total calories. (Compare the typical American diet of Figure 2–5, which shows that it derives less than 50 percent of its calories from carbohydrate, and half of that from sugar.) Most of the remaining calories come from rice protein and other plant proteins. Fat calories are at a minimum, because the quantities of meat used are so small and the Chinese mode of cooking employs very little oil.

Vegetables and fruits provide tremendous *variety* in the Chinese diet, and its *nutrient density* is high. The nutrients in the foods are undiluted by fat and sugar; very seldom do the Chinese serve dessert, and seldom is it sweet. Nor do alcohol calories have a significant place, although the Chinese do make a wine and drink it on special occasions. The energy intakes of the Chinese man and woman are adequate but not excessive.

Chapter and Controversy 14 explore the links between world resources and people's foodwaste.

The Chinese diet and cooking techniques are also land efficient, as they must be in view of the scarcity of agricultural land and fuels. Nearly all of the calories come from plants rather than animals. A million calories in wheat or rice can be produced on less than an acre of land; a million calories in beef require 17 acres. In a world in which fuel and land are becoming increasingly scarce, the Chinese way of eating offers a model that industrialized nations might do well to adapt for their own use.

The staple food in the Chinese diet is rice; nearly all the remaining bulk comes from vegetables and fruits; and meats are sparingly used. Variety is characteristic of this time-tested, nutritious diet, and its cooking methods also conserve fuel and land.

Vegetarian Diets

Some ethnic diets are vegetarian, but many people from meat-eating cultures adopt vegetarian diets for reasons of their own—some for religious or ethical reasons; some because they feel it is ecologically sound; others because it costs less, because it supports health, or because they want to belong to a particular group. Vegetarianism does not require adopting any particular lifestyle; it implies no special mode of dress, set of political beliefs, or religious affiliation. It is simply a way of eating that anyone can adopt.

Vegetarianism has not been part of the mainstream of life in North America until the last few decades. People whose cultures have been vegetarian for centuries can look to tradition to be sure of dietary adequacy, but "new" vegetarians often build their diets from scratch. This can lead to nutrition problems.

There is no typical vegetarian diet, as there is a typical Chinese diet. Some vegetarian cuisines center on rice, vegetables, and fruits as do Asian diets; some on pasta, eggs, and cheese. Some vegetarians eat soybean curd (tofu; see Chapter 5) almost every day, others never use it. Some use whole foods only, others rely on modern, textured vegetable protein products that are formulated to look and taste like meat, fish, or poultry.

Provided that it is well planned, though, the vegetarian diet can be a model diet, nutritionally. Vegetarian protein sources are often higher than meats in fiber and richer in certain vitamins and minerals, and they are lower in fat. People practicing vegetarianism have been extensively studied, and are known to enjoy better health in several respects than comparable other people. They are more likely to be at the desirable weights for their heights, and to have lower blood cholesterol levels. They have less diabetes, fewer hernias, and better digestive function.[5] They experience fewer deaths from cardiovascular disease, even when compared with other people who are equally health conscious (see Controversy 4). They have less of certain kinds of cancer, too (Controversy 5). Often, vegetarianism goes with a clean-living lifestyle (no smoking, abstinence from alcohol, a supportive family life), so it is unlikely that the diet alone accounts for all the aspects of improved health. Clearly, however, it helps.

Vegetarian diets vary, some including eggs and cheese, some not. When practiced with care, vegetarian diets support health as well as, or better than, comparable diets that include abundant meat.

Problems with Ethnic and Vegetarian Diets

No diet is perfect simply by virtue of belonging to a particular ethnic group or by including or excluding a particular class of foods. In fact, each diet has problems typically associated with it—often, problems associated with the rapid changes that have taken place since the industrial era began, a hundred years ago. To rectify the likeliest problems in a diet, pay attention to two principles. First, look to your staple foods, to be sure they are as nutritious as those of your forebears were. Review your cultural traditions and recent changes in your eating pattern. Second, ask yourself how many whole foods you eat. Here are some examples.

If you are Chinese-American, you need to be warned that your staple food, polished rice, loses nutrients such as iron and B vitamins in this country's refining process. Therefore, although the rice-based diet in China may be adequate, your rice-based diet may not be. You are advised to use enriched or brown rice routinely. If you are Hispanic-American, you may have come from a homeland where the oil most often used in cooking was palm oil, rich in vitamin A, and practically the sole source of the vitamin in the diet. Here, you may be using a locally available commercial cooking oil (these contain no vitamin A), and this may leave you without a vitamin A source. There is a high incidence of deficiencies of this vitamin among Hispanic-Americans, whose traditional foods other than oil do not supply it. Find alternative sources such as dark green vegetables or fortified milk or cheese to make up for the deficit.

The Korean and Vietnamese traditional diets do not include dairy products. People in Korea use, as a staple food, small fishes with tender bones in them that provide abundant dietary calcium. Without these fish, Korean-Americans may have no significant dietary sources of calcium at all.[6] Similarly, people in Vietnam drink no milk but have a calcium-rich staple food—a stock made by soaking leftover pork and chicken bones in vinegar, then boiling and straining them.[7]* If you are of Korean or Vietnamese descent, learn to use small fish with the bones daily (learn about calcium in Chapter 7 to see how much you need), or learn to make and use a calcium-rich stock as described here. Alternatively, learn to drink milk as your neighbors of other ethnic groups do, to replace your lost supply of calcium. You might start by adding it to grain, to get used to the flavor. Then try it as a beverage. Native Americans of the Seminole Tribe face a similar problem. Their traditional calcium source, alligator meat, has been largely replaced by calcium-poor beef; they, too, traditionally use no dairy products; and they, too, need to find a reliable calcium source.

Certain problems are associated with vegetarian diets, too. For the lacto-ovo vegetarian, the Four Food Group Plan can be adapted by making a change in the meat group (see Table 2–4A). The strict vegetarian should find alternative sources of calcium and take a vitamin B_{12} supplement or use calcium- and vitamin B_{12}-fortified soy milk. Vegetarian diets are widely used, so many of the chapters to come address problems associated with them. Chapter 5 shows how vegetarians can meet protein needs. Chapters 6 and 7 provide more details on meeting needs for vitamins and minerals that vegetarian diets tend to lack.

No matter who you are, you should review your diet to see how much of it consists of whole rather than partitioned foods. As Controversy 1 mentioned, about two-thirds of the calories many people consume are taken from the non-nutritious parts of whole foods—purified sugars, fats and oils, milled grains, and alcohol. The more of these you eat, the lower the nutrient density of your diet is likely to be. Even vegetarian meals, reputed to be of high nutrient density, can be sabotaged by additions of too many high-fat foods such as butter, cream cheese, sour cream, olives, and nuts. The Food Feature that follows illustrates this problem and models a strategy to deal with it.

Finally, vary your diet creatively. Some people take this advice to the extreme by eating Jewish food one day, Greek the next, and grilled hotdogs with potato chips the next. This is fine, but such wide swings are not necessary. You need to loosen up only if you eat a limited number of different foods to the point of monotony or exclusion of whole classes of foods. To add variety, you might try one new food each week. Nobody is perfect, and nobody eats a perfect diet; in fact, it can't be determined what the perfect diet might be. If changes are needed, the goal to adopt is improvement, not perfection. Time spent improving your diet may, however, pay off in both pleasure and health.

While traditional foodways may have provided adequate nutrition, they may have changed recently so that they no longer do so. To solve problems associated with each diet requires comparison of traditional staple foods with modern ones, and review of the diet's proportion of whole to partitioned foods.

---

*One tablespoon of such stock may contain over 100 mg calcium.

Food Feature

Choosing Foods with High Nutrient Density

Figure 2–7 illustrates a playful contrast between two days' meals. One, labeled "High-fat choices," is an exaggerated version of the "typical American" way of eating—it emphasizes meat, eggs, and fats, and includes a fast-food lunch. The second, labeled "High-nutrient-density choices," shows the result of following some of the goals and guidelines cited in this chapter—it contains abundant plant foods, nonfat milk, modest amounts of fish and cheese, and no commercially prepared or processed foods.

The two sets of meals were made similar in energy and protein amounts, so that the other differences would stand out. Both add up to beween 1800 and 1860 calories, and both derive 18 percent of their calories from protein. To make them equivalent in these ways required altering both in ways real people probably would not have done. The high-fat eater had to be deprived of the milkshake such a person would probably have for lunch; this would have added too many calories. The high-nutrient-density eater had to be given 4 pats of butter and 2 packets of sugar, to raise the energy level without increasing the protein. Even so, the high-nutrient-density choices offer more than twice the bulk of the high-fat choices with only 24 percent of the calories from fat. The high-fat choices supply a whopping 48 percent of the calories from fat.

Real people eat both ways. Those who eat the abundant vegetable way are astonished that others can eat so much meat and fat. Those who eat the meat-and-potatoes way wonder how anyone could consume such a large bulk of food. A compromise between the two styles might be the reasonable alternative for many people, or at least a good starting point. In any case, the contrast illustrates clearly several things.

For one thing, by including abundant vegetables among your food choices, you can eat large amounts of food without having to consume too much food energy. Conversely, by choosing mostly animal products, with their abundant intrinsic fat, you can eat many calories without consuming much bulk of food. This means that, for most people who are struggling to keep their weight down, choosing vegetables most often will help—and will not reduce their protein intakes, as they might expect. For the minority, who have trouble consuming enough calories to keep their weight up, animal products can be eaten for extra calories and nutrients, and vegetables, for their vitamins and minerals.

For another thing, it is clear that anyone who eats a basically nutritious diet can afford a sweet treat now and then, or an occasional fast-food meal. Much of the art of balancing the diet, as the later chapters will continue to demonstrate, is a matter of learning appropriate frequencies with which to eat various foods.

The contrast between the two sets of meals illustrates another point. The high-nutrient-density eater chose the recommended number of servings from each food group and then some, obtaining 2 ½ portions of milk, 6 of vegetables, 4 of fruits, 6 of starches/grains, and 2 servings (5 ounces) of meats and cheeses. The high-fat eater included only 1 fruit and 1 vegetable in a day, and had no milk. As a result, the high-fat eater's nutrient intakes fell short of the RDA in many instances. The iron and zinc intakes, however, were higher than the high-

Figure 2–7 Two Days' Meals Compared.

High-nutrient-density choices
1809 cal

18% of calories from protein
24% of calories from fat
57% of calories from carbohydrate

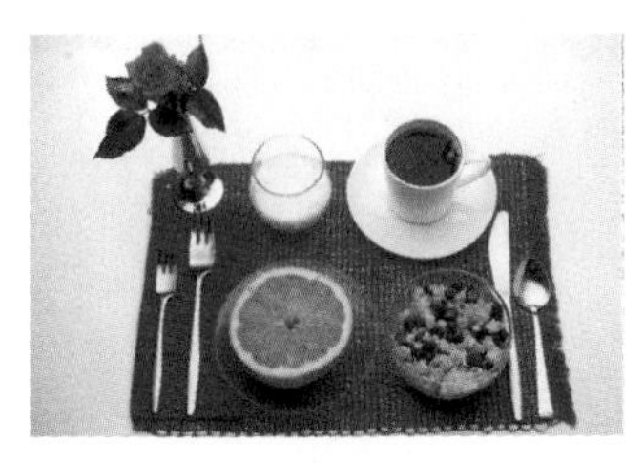

1 c coffee
1 c oatmeal
¼ c raisins
½ c nonfat milk
½ grapefruit

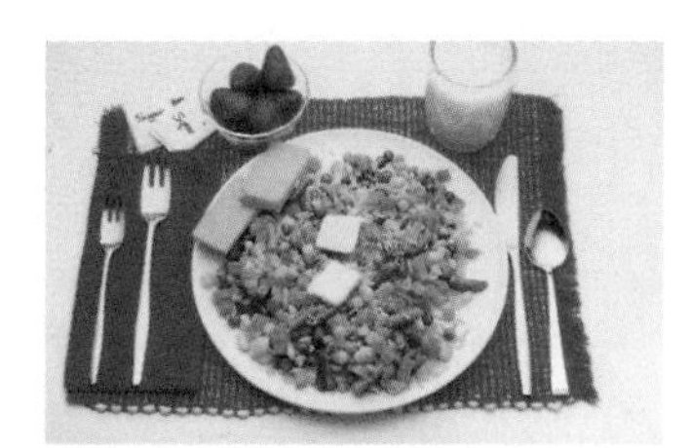

1 c cooked brown rice
2 c mixed vegetables
2 oz cheddar cheese
2 pats butter
⅔ c strawberries
1 c nonfat milk
2 packets sugar

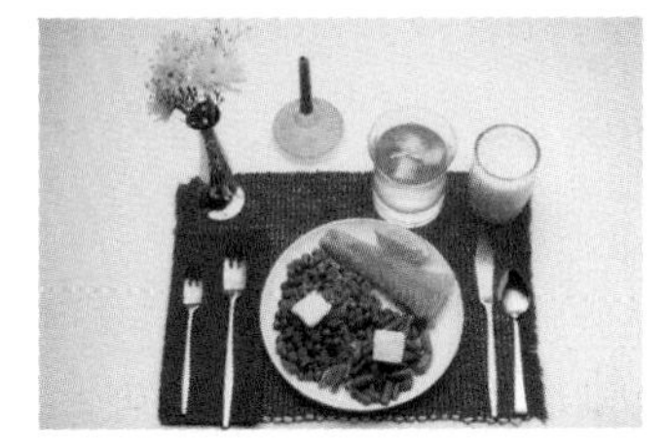

3 oz broiled fish
½ c green beans
½ c carrots
2 pats butter
½ c peas
1 c nonfat milk

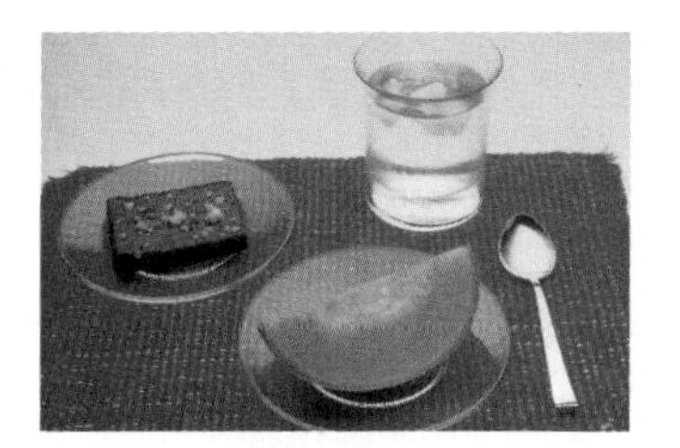

¼ cantaloupe
1 brownie

High-fat choices
1860 cal

18% of calories from protein
48% of calories from fat
34% of calories from carbohydrate

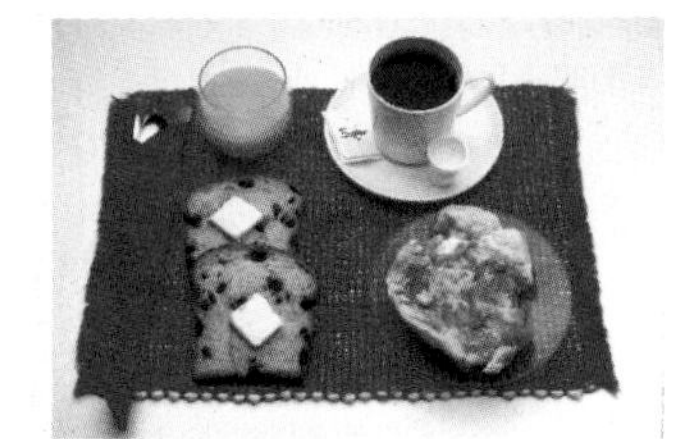

½ c orange juice
2 scrambled eggs
2 slices raisin bread
2 pats butter
1 c coffee
1 packet sugar
1 tbsp cream

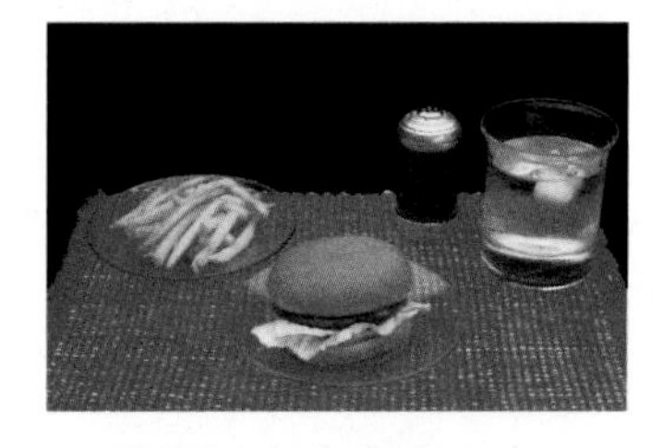

1 fast food hamburger
1 fast food small french fries

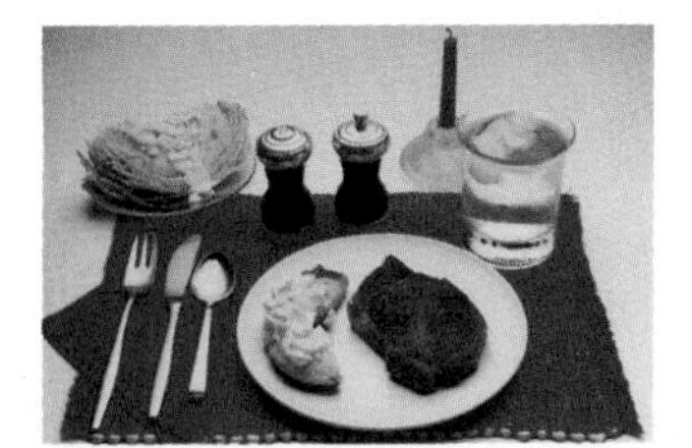

6 oz steak
½ baked potato
¼ head lettuce
1 tbsp blue cheese dressing
1 tbsp sour cream
2 pats butter

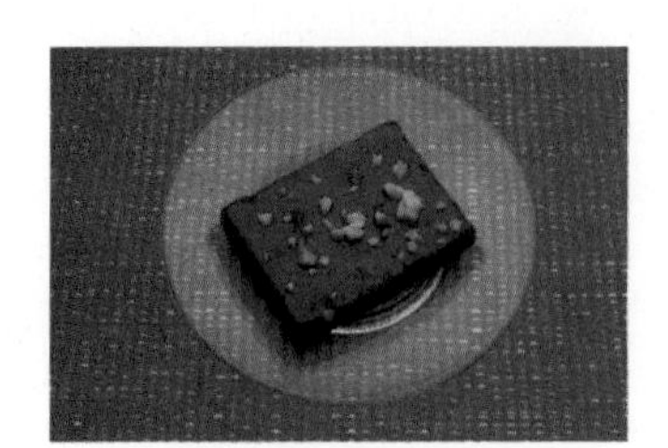

1 brownie

Table 2–10

Analysis of High-Fat versus High-Nutrient-Density Meals

	High-Fat Meals (Meat-Centered Meals)	High-Nutrient-Density Meals (Four Food Group plus added Vegetables)	Standard for Comparison (U.S. RDA)[a]
Thiamin	1.1 mg	1.5 mg	1.5 mg
Riboflavin	1.6 mg	2.1 mg	1.7 mg
Niacin	18.4 mg	18.1 mg	20 mg
Vitamin B_6	1.6 mg	1.7 mg	2.0 mg
Folacin	253 μg	294 μg	400 μg
Vitamin A	520 RE	4295 RE	1000 RE
Vitamin C	93 mg	195 mg	60 mg
Calcium	357 mg	1459 mg	1000 mg
Iron	15 mg	11 mg	18 mg[a]
Magnesium	384 mg	411 mg	400 mg
Potassium	2652 mg	3785 mg	1875–5625[b]
Zinc	15 mg	11 mg	15 mg
Fiber	10 g	48 g	20–30 g[b]
Cholesterol	761 mg	191 mg	<300 mg[b]

Meals were those described and illustrated in Figure 2–7.

[a]The menstruating woman's RDA is 18 mg, the man's is 10 mg. Thus, this person, if a man, has ample iron; if a woman, may need to take iron supplements or exercise more to earn more calories and then spend them on more good iron sources.

[b]Standard for comparison in the case of potassium is the recommended safe and adequate daily dietary intake. In the case of fiber, it is a suggested intake. In the case of cholesterol, it is a *Dietary Guideline*.

nutrient-density person's intakes, thanks to the steak and hamburger. Table 2–10 shows the complete analysis of the two day's meals.

The person who wants to apply these learnings could do no better than to begin by stocking up on the basic foods around which a nutritious diet is designed. If you have selected the Basic Four Food Group Plan to follow, for example, then you can make a list based on that. (You might resolve to purchase only the foods you have chosen, leaving nonessential items at the store.) After a while, you will be able to do less paper and pencil planning, except for a shopping list; you will automatically keep a mental tally of the groups and the number of portions you need from each. Now and then, return to pencil and paper to see if you really are on target, and to correct any tendency to stray. An example is shown on the shopping list; yours might be different.

shopping list:

(For each day:)
milk group selections, 2 portions
fruits and vegetables, 4 portions
starchy vegetables and whole-grain products, 4 portions
lean meats, 6 ounces

Notes

1. Food and Nutrition Board, Committee on Recommended Allowances, *Recommended Dietary Allowances,* 9th ed. (Washington, D.C.: National Academy of Sciences, 1980).
2. A. E. Harper and E. V. McCollum, Recommended Dietary Allowances in perspective, *Food and Nutrition News,* March/April 1986.
3. S. R. Rolfes and E. W. Whitney, A side note: RDA interpretation, *Instructor's Manual with Test Bank to Accompany Understanding Nutrition 4E* (St. Paul: West, 1987), pp. 22–23.
4. J. D. Gussow and K. L. Clancy, Dietary guidelines for sustainability, *Journal of Nutrition Education* 18 (1986): 1–5.

Self-Study

Calculate Your Nutrient Intakes

This Self-Study takes up where the last one left off, and directs you to calculate your nutrient intakes for the period in which you wrote down what foods you ate. Refer to Appendix C if you need help with the calculations.

1. Pick up Form 1 again (you filled out the first two columns in Self-Study 1). Using Appendix A, enter in the remaining columns of the form the amounts of nutrients each food contributed. If the foods you have eaten are not included in Appendix A, read the label on the package or use your ingenuity to guess their composition, using the most similar food you can find as a guide.

Be careful in recording the nutrient amounts in odd-sized portions. For example, if you used a quarter cup of milk, then you will have to record a fourth of the amount of every nutrient listed for a cup of milk. (Again, refer to Appendix C if you need help.) And note the units in which the nutrients are measured:

- Energy is measured in calories (cal), as explained on p. 31.
- Protein, carbohydrate, fiber, fat, and fatty acid breakdown are measured in grams (g).
- Cholesterol, calcium, iron, zinc, thiamin, riboflavin, niacin, vitamin B_6, and vitamin C (ascorbic acid) are measured in milligrams (mg)—thousandths of a gram (0.001 gram). Folacin is measured in micrograms (mcg or μg)—thousandths of a milligram or millionths of a gram (0.001 milligram or 0.000001 gram). Thus "800 milligrams calcium" is the same as "0.8 grams calcium," and "400 micrograms folacin" is the same as "0.4 milligrams folacin." Be sure to convert all calcium amounts to milligrams and all folacin amounts to micrograms before calculating.
- Vitamin A is sometimes measured in international units (IU) and sometimes in retinol equivalents (RE); 1 RE equals 3 IU of vitamin A from animal foods, 10 IU of vitamin A from plant foods,* or, on the average, 5 IU (for mixed dishes). Appendix A lists vitamin A in RE to ease comparison with the RDA, which is also in RE. (For more details, see Chapter 6.) If you eat a packaged food whose label lists vitamin A in IU, be sure to convert to RE before calculating.

If you eat a packaged food whose label lists nutrient amounts as "percent of U.S. RDA," use the table on the inside back cover to convert to grams, milligrams, micrograms, or RE. Suppose a food portion contains "25 percent of the U.S. RDA of iron," for example. The table shows that the U.S. RDA for iron is 18 milligrams. The food portion therefore contributes a fourth of 18 milligrams, or 4.5 milligrams of iron. Now, still using Form 1, total the amount of each nutrient you've consumed for each day.

2. Now transfer your totals from Form 1 to Form 2 in Appendix H. Form 2 provides a convenient means of deriving an average intake for each nutrient.

*One IU of vitamin A is equal to 0.344 microgram of crystalline vitamin A acetate or 0.6 microgram of all-*trans* beta-carotene.

3. As a final step, transfer your average intakes to Form 3 in Appendix H for future reference. For comparison, enter the intakes recommended for a person of your age and sex, using either the RDA (on the inside front cover) or the Canadian Recommended Nutrient Intakes (RNI; see Appendix B)—whichever you prefer. Note that no recommendations are made for intakes of fat or carbohydrate. Guidelines for these nutrients will be presented and discussed later, and tentative standards for fiber and cholesterol are provided on the form. Succeeding Self-Studies will guide you in focusing on each of the nutrients provided by your diet.

Suspend judgment about the adequacy of your diet for the moment. You have much to learn about your individuality, the nutrients, and the recommendations before you can reach any reasonable conclusions.

4. What percentage of the calories you consumed comes from protein, fat, and carbohydrate? (Use Form 4 in Appendix H to calculate, and Appendix C if you need help doing the calculation.) Is your diet in line with current recommendations in this respect? The suggested balance is about 10 to 15 percent of the calories from protein, about 30 percent (not more) from fat, and the remainder from carbohydrate.

5. You can get an indication of whether your diet is balanced on any particular day by using the Food Selection Scorecard (Form 5 in Appendix H—one copy for each day). How does your diet score by these criteria?

5. J. W. T. Dickerson, G. J. Davies, and M. Crowder, Disease patterns in individuals with different eating patterns, *Journal of the Royal Society of Health*, December 1985, pp. 191-194.

6. K. K. Kim and coauthors, Dietary calcium of elderly Korean American, *Journal of the American Dietetic Association* 84 (1984): 164–169.

7. A. Rosanoff and D. H. Calloway, Calcium source in Indochinese immigrants (correspondence), *New England Journal of Medicine* 306 (1982): 239–240.

Who Speaks on Nutrition?

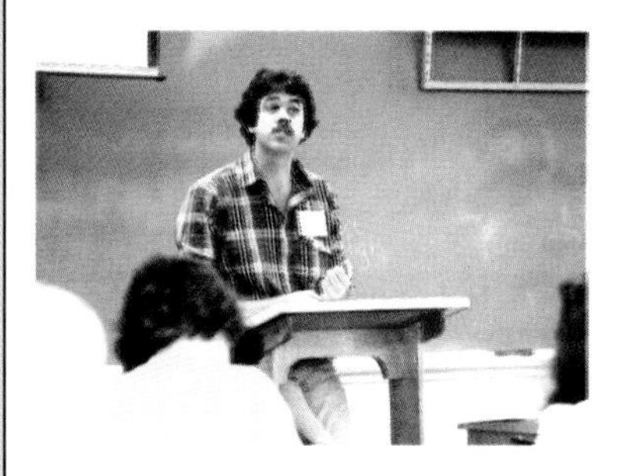

The quality of nutrition information depends on the credentials of the information provider.

When you need nutrition advice, whom can you ask? Many people automatically say, Ask the **doctor,** for "the doctor" is supposed to be an expert on everything related to health. But can you rely on your doctor to give you accurate information on nutrition? And if not, on whom can you rely? Do you have to go to a nutritionist? A dietitian? (What's the difference between those two?) Are people who sell nutrition products (health-food store owners, for example) qualified to teach nutrition to their customers? How can you tell?

The answer, as you will see, is that doctors may not be the best-qualified experts on nutrition; registered dietitians are. However, because so many people rely solely on physicians to deliver nutrition information, this Controversy begins with "the doctor."

Physicians' Nutrition Know-how

For the past two decades, the reputations of physicians as nutrition experts have suffered blow after blow. A big one came in 1974, when Dr. Charles E. Butterworth published a shocking article in *Nutrition Today* titled "The Skeleton in the Hospital Closet."[1] In it, he reported a high incidence of severe malnutrition in the hospital, which he called "physician-induced." He published pictures of emaciated patients, patients with bleeding gums and with sores on their skins, all caused by **iatrogenic malnutrition**—that is, malnutrition that had developed under physicians' care, and could have been prevented by physicians' actions. He cited some of the causes: physicians often deprived their patients of food for days at a time so that they could give them medical tests; they seldom ordered vitamin and mineral supplements for them; and they often administered inadequate solutions (bottles of glucose and salts without protein, vitamins, or minerals) for long periods. Under these circumstances, patients developed protein-energy malnutrition and iron-deficiency anemia, conditions that severely weakened them, delayed their recovery, prolonged their hospital stays, and increased the cost of their treatment. Reasons for the neglect of their nutrition care, Butterworth reported, included failure to notice low weight and weight loss, frequent staff rotations, diffusion of responsibility, and lack of communication between physicians and dietitians.[2]

The situation Butterworth was describing turned out to be typical of hospitals all across the country. His report was promptly followed by a report by two hospital physicians revealing that close to half of the patients in their hospitals showed evidence of protein-energy malnutrition—often caused not by the conditions that had brought them to the hospital, but by neglect of their nutrient needs while they were in the hospital.[3] These findings were later confirmed and extended by many other investigators.

Health Care Providers and Their Clients

In the past, the terms *doctor* and *patient* have been most often used to describe the pair of partners that attempted to make a sick person well. Today, other terms are displacing those—**physician** and **client.** The term *physician* is preferred, because it is more respectful, and because people with degrees other than the M.D. degree, and even quacks, can call themselves doctors. As for the term *client,* it implies characteristics altogether different from those of a patient. A patient is, literally, a passive person, one who waits, who is dependent on someone else for the solution to a medical problem. A client is an active person, one who is in charge of his or her own health, who pays for services rendered, and who has the right to expect quality service.

In this book, sometimes one pair of terms, sometimes the other, is used, depending on the historical period and situation. We reserve the terms *physician* and *client* for a cooperative relationship in which the responsibility for healing is shared. We also use the term **health care provider**—because today, physicians are not the only appropriate providers of health care. Depending on the client's need, the appropriate provider to see might be a physician, a physician's assistant, a nurse, a nurse practitioner, a pharmacist, or a dietitian.

Part of the blame for this deplorable situation was laid at the feet of the medical schools that educated the physicians. One physician remarked that, "often doctors are trained in nutrition by doctors who heard it from another doctor who made it up."[4] Another commented, "I would guess 90 percent of the graduates of our medical schools couldn't describe an adequate, nutritious diet."[5] Still another said, "The state of nutrition education in this country as it relates to health is in complete chaos. . . . One cause of that chaos is the medical profession's failure to take responsibility for this area."[6] Physicians were being taught how to give drugs and perform surgery, but not how to support people's health while they underwent these treatments. For all their knowledge of physiology, biochemistry, pharmacology, and the rest, most medical school graduates were blind to the signs of malnutrition in their patients.

Since then, the medical schools have responded to these accusations by evaluating the situation, identifying deficits, and attempting to remedy them. At first, a survey of 42 medical schools showed that seven of them offered no nutrition instruction of any kind and that thirteen more offered fewer than eleven hours in their four-year curriculum. Only three offered more than twenty hours, and only one had a nutrition department.[7] The schools immediately began scrambling to remedy the situation, however, and nutrition training of physicians-to-be began increasing,[8] a trend that resembled "a ground swell."[9] A medical journal reported that, "like sex, nutrition is increasingly discussed among physicians."[10]

Today, the situation has improved somewhat. Some physicians specialize in nutrition—50 medical centers provide postgraduate training.[11] But in the medical schools, regretfully, the situation is not fully remedied. A study that looked into nutrition education in U.S. medical schools in the mid-1980's concluded that it was still inadequate. The schools teach nutrition as an academic subject, but they still don't teach medical students how to apply it to cases in real practice (see Table C2–1). Many students graduate without even fully appreciating nutrition's role in supporting the work of medicine, much less realizing nutrition's "potential for prevention of diet-related diseases and overall maintenance of good health."[12]

The National Academy Board made several recommendations—among them, the following:

- That nutrition be a required science course.
- That 25 or more classroom hours be allocated to teaching its core concepts.
- That M.D.s and Ph.D.s be employed to teach nutrition, and that nutrition researchers be involved in teaching.
- That nutrition be a distinct department with at least one full faculty position devoted entirely to it.
- That the medical board examination cover all nutrition areas in proportion to their importance.

In relation to the last item, a recent review of the board exam showed that there were no questions on many important areas, including the relationships between nutrition and cancer, osteoporosis, and nutrient needs of the elderly.[13] These topics occupy large sections of this book in Controversy 5, Chapter 7 and Chapter 13.

Medical students themselves are dissatisfied with the nutrition education they are receiving in some medical schools. Of 236 students surveyed in 1986, 85 percent were dissatisfied with the quantity, and 60 percent with the quality, of the nutrition instruction they were receiving.[14] Meanwhile, in the hospital, physicians still are not using nutrition in their practices, they seldom if ever refer to the RDA tables to

Table C2–1

Core Concepts in Nutrition That Physicians Need to Learn
Energy balance
Role of specific nutrients
Nutrition in the life cycle
Nutrition assessment
Protein-energy malnutrition
Nutrition's role in preventing disease
Nutrition's role in treating disease
Risks of poor dietary practices

Source: Executive summary, *Nutrition Education in U.S. Medical Schools* (Washington, D.C.: National Academy of Sciences, 1986), as cited in S. Palmer and S. Berkow, Nutrition education in American medical schools, a commentary by the director of the Food and Nutrition Board and her staff scientist, *Nutrition Today*, January/February 1986, pp. 5–7. Copyright 1986 by Williams and Wilkins.

estimate their patients' needs, and they hardly ever ask how food is prepared, estimate food energy intakes, ask how much food is eaten, prescribe diets, advise on supplements, or consider the effects of prescription medicines on nutrition.[15]

All of this seems to mean that the consumer of medical care today still cannot rely on the physician to deliver competent nutrition advice and care. However, this disappointing conclusion does not apply to all physicians—not by a long shot. Some, after all, have received adequate nutrition training; some have sought it out on their own. Some are nationally recognized experts in nutrition. And some, recognizing that they cannot know everything about nutrition themselves, make use of properly credentialed nutrition experts as partners, consultants, or referrals.

Nutrition Support in the Hospitals

As of today, nutrition care in hospitals is still uneven—excellent in some, poor to nonexistent in others. A 1986 33-hospital screening study attempted to screen over 3000 clients' nutrition status, but could not complete the job for 60 percent of them because critical nutrition screening data had not been recorded at admission. The most important and simplest measures to record were height and weight, but many had not done even that. Of the other 40 percent, more than half had below-normal values for one or more of the indicators studied.[16]

On the positive side, though, many hospitals have worked out ways to deliver excellent nutrition care. A hospital entity called the **nutrition support team** has been defined—a team of selected physicians, nurses, dietitians, and pharmacists who work together to evaluate a client's nutrition status and develop an individualized nutrition care plan.[17] Books have been published to guide nutrition support teams in the delivery of nutrition services,[18] and the computer is being recruited for the task of identifying the clients most in need of attention.[19] In short, it is now clear what hospitals should be doing to meet the need adequately, and some are doing it. Table C2–2 presents a checklist for what a hospital ought to do to ensure that clients are well-nourished.

Outside the hospital, people wish to *maintain* their health, so that they will not have to *enter* the hospital. Such people are wise to seek nutrition counsel. But whom to ask? Physicians are disease treatment specialists, not health maintenance specialists, and are not often qualified to offer nutrition advice. For people who are obese or too thin, who are living with heart disease or cancer or diabetes, who have food allergies or digestive disorders, or who simply want to ensure that their nutrition status is optimal, the dietitian is the person to see.

Dietitians' Credentials

The **dietitian** is educated specifically to understand nutrition needs and deliver counsel and care. A dietitian who is the genuine article has an undergraduate degree requiring some 70 or so hours in nutrition and food science, has completed a year's clinical internship or the equivalent, has passed a national examination administered over six competency areas

Table C2–2

Checklist for Hospital Nutrition Care of Clients

Develop, and operate according to, a plan for meeting people's nutrition needs.

Follow a procedure at admission that is sure to evaluate people's nutrition status and allocate appropriate nutrition care to them from the beginning of their hospital stays. Include routine recording of height and weight as part of the admissions procedure.

Prepare people nutritionally for surgery; continue providing nutrition support afterward.

Monitor people's nutrition status while they are in the hospital, by periodic assessment, and by observing and recording food intake.

Make sure meals withheld for tests or procedures are provided later; make sure people given glucose/salt solutions for long times also receive supplements of essential nutrients.

Give antibiotics for infection only in conjunction with rehabilitative nutrition support; do not rely solely on antibiotics.

Assign specific responsibilities for parts of the plan to the physician, nurse, dietitian, and pharmacist.

Follow a procedure to be sure that the responsibility for nutrition support is passed on from one specific person to the next at the time of changes of staff.

Keep up with research findings; evaluate procedures in their light; apply them when appropriate.

by the American or Canadian Dietetic Association, and maintains up-to-date knowledge obtained through required continuing education (taking courses or writing professional papers). The dietitian can consult as an equal with the physician, both being knowledgeable in their specialties. And, importantly, dietitians almost invariably display the credentials **R.D.,** indicating **registration** with the American Dietetic Association, should a consumer want to check on their credentials. Dietitians come in several varieties: clinical, administrative, consultant, public health, food service, generalist, research, and teaching. An example of the competencies of a clinical dietitian is provided in Table C2–3.

Why, in talking about the dietitian, did we specify that the person had to be "the genuine article," when we did not say the same about the physician? For reasons no one quite understands, of all fields, nutrition is the most riddled with quack practitioners. During the past 50 years, perhaps 50 people have faked credentials as M.D.s and gotten away with it for a time. No one seems to fake dentistry, optometry, or chiropractic. But there are literally thousands of people with fake nutrition degrees. A well-known quack fighter says, "I am aware of no other field in which this phenomenon has ever taken place."[20]

The documents many of these people display indicate that they are dietitians, but without the R.D.; or nutritionists; or dietists; or other such. These titles are promoted as if they were equivalent in meaning to established credentials, but they are not.[21] That being the case, if we are to turn to dietitians for our diet advice, we have two tasks on our hands: first, to tell the real ones from the fake ones, and second, to tell the good ones from the poor ones—for, as with other health care providers, the possession of even a legitimate credential does not make a person a high-quality professional, or even an honest human being.

A person who wants to visit a dietitian and obtain nutrition advice needs to know that in many states the title ***dietitian*** is no guarantee of professionalism. Many states allow use of the title by anyone who wants to use it, just as anyone can call himself a counselor. Some states have passed laws to restrict use of the term—for example, as of 1982, California allows only qualified individuals to call themselves dietitians and R.D.s. Louisiana and Montana have similar laws. Many states are now considering a further guarantee: the **license to practice.**[22]* Licensing does not offer complete protection against nutrition quackery, but it makes it difficult for unqualified people to advertise widely that they are experts.

Some states are also regulating use of the title **nutritionist**—a welcome development, for that title has enticed thousands of consumers into scams where they have lost their health—and their shirts. If the term is to be meaningful, it should apply only to people who have an **M.S. (master of science) degree** or a **Ph.D. (doctor of philosophy) degree** in nutrition or related fields, not other forms of education. An M.S. or Ph.D. in nutrition requires five to seven years of training in an accredited graduate school. A course

Table C2–3

Competencies of the Clinical Dietitian

Competencies of the Clinical Dietitian
Assesses nutrition status
Develops individualized care plans
Implements, monitors, and evaluates care plans
Educates clients and families
Develops policies
Communicates effectively with physicians, nurses, and pharmacists regarding clients' nutrition status, needs, and treatment
Interfaces with food service personnel
Supervises dietetic staff
Participates in professional activities to enhance knowledge and skill
Serves the profession politically
Educates dietetics students and interns

Source: Adapted from P. M. Kris-Etherton and coauthors, A profile of clinical dietetics practice in Pennsylvania, *Journal of the American Dietetic Association* 83 (1983): 654–660. Material developed as part of the Continuing Professional Education Development Project, The Pennsylvania St. Univ. Funding provided by the W. W. Kellogg Foundation.

*As of 1983, Texas protects the titles *licensed dietitian* and *licensed registered dietitian* from fraudulent use. Georgia and Oklahoma have voluntary licensure laws. As of 1984, seven states had passed such laws. M. Mathieu, Licensure of nutrition professionals, *Journal of the American Dietetic Association* 84 (1984): 1228.

of (for example) six to nine months at a **correspondence school** is simply not the same. Some schools are not even legitimate correspondence schools, but **diploma mills**—places that, essentially, sell certificates of competency to anyone who pays their fees.

Some states are recognizing this distinction.* People who are not dietitians or R.D.s are allowed to call themselves nutritionists only if they have advanced degrees in nutrition from accredited colleges or universities.**

Evidence of **accreditation** is important in the description of the institution from which the education comes. (You have to be really, really careful in approaching a nutritionist.) The most rampant abuse of credentials is in the display of master's and doctoral degrees. According to the *New York Times,* doctorates are available for around $2300, master's degrees for $1250, and bachelor's for $800, with discounts for all three together. To obtain them, a candidate need not read any books or pass any tests. They are available from "accredited" schools, too, for there are 30 phony accrediting agencies.[23]

To dramatize the situation, one writer enrolled for $82 in a nutrition diploma mill that billed itself as a correspondence school offering nutrition degrees. She made every attempt to fail the course, even answering all the examination questions wrong on purpose. Even so, she received a "Nutritionist" certificate at the end of the course, together with a letter explaining that they were sure she must have just misread the test.[24]

In a similar stunt, Ms. Sassafras Herbert has been named a "professional member" of a professional association. Sassafras has a wallet card and is listed in a sort of fake who's who in nutrition that is distributed at health fairs and trade shows nationwide. Sassafras is a poodle; her master, Victor Herbert, M.D., paid $50 to prove that she could win these honors merely by sending in her name. Mr. Charlie Herbert also is a professional member of such an organization; Charlie is a cat.[25]

To check recommended providers' credentials, first look for the degrees listed by their titles in the Miniglossary. Then call and ask the state's health licensing agency if they are licensed to practice. Then find out what you can about the reputations of the institutions where they obtained their degrees. One of the best sources of information as to whether a school or other institution is legitimate or not is The National Council Against Health Fraud, whose address is in Appendix F.

If you set about researching whether an institution is a genuine graduate school, you may find yourself pursuing a fascinating detective story:

- The university should have an address, some buildings, and a faculty consisting of people with bona fide degrees. If you ask to speak to the dean of graduate studies, such a person should exist.

A post office box number without a street address is practically a guarantee that the degree-granting institution is a fraud.

- The university should show evidence of accreditation by the appropriate professional associations, membership in which constitutes a seal of approval to practice—for example, the AMA for a medical school, the ADA for a program in dietetics. (Read about the associations in the library's *Encyclopedia of Associations.*)
- The accrediting agency itself should be recognized by the U.S. Department of Education. (Look up the department under "United States" in the telephone book.)

Once you have found a *true* nutritionist (or preferably, registered dietitian), you still need to find a competent one. You may have to shop around and try appointments with more than one before you are satisfied on all counts.

Who Speaks on Nutrition

Dietitians may be the ideal professionals for serving people's nutrition education and care needs, but until recently, they have been so inconspicuous that many people have not known they were there. Dietitians themselves have been debating why this is, have identified some of the reasons, and have proposed some solutions.

The leaders in the professional organization of dietitians, the American Dietetic Association, have

---

*In Georgia, for example, the title *nutritionist,* as well as *dietitian* and *R.D.,* is forbidden except to such qualified individuals. Alabama also regulates the use of all three titles.

**One proposed wording of a law to protect consumers: "No person offering [services] who has received a degree from an institution [that] had no accreditation . . . by a national accrediting agency recognized by the U.S. Department of Education or the Council on Postsecondary Accreditation shall be entitled to use the title or degree . . . or [claim to be practicing the occupation] conferred by the degree or to represent that the degree holder possesses the skills, knowledge and educational background usually associated with such a title or degree." The proposed penalties range from $100 for the first offense to $1000 for the third, plus a jail term. *California Council Against Health Fraud Newsletter,* May/June 1984, p. 2.

phrased the problem as one of image: "qualities that make an excellent supportive professional have been nurtured at the expense of qualities that make a good leader. If dietetics is to flourish today, dietitians must learn leadership skills and . . . develop political savvy."[26] An observer who interviewed dietitians found that they were "naive about political power and organizational decision-making processes." They tended to be technically competent, but this focus indirectly reinforced their "political and organizational naivete."[27]

Miniglossary

accreditation: approval; in the case of hospitals or university departments, approval by a professional organization qualified to judge the quality of the service or educational program offered. There are phony accrediting agencies; the genuine ones are listed with the U.S. Department of Education.

client: the purchaser of health care, a term used in this book, wherever appropriate, in place of *patient*.

correspondence school: a school from which courses can be taken, and degrees granted, by mail. Those that are accredited offer respectable courses and degrees. See also *diploma mills*.

dietitian: a person trained in nutrition, food science, and diet planning. A **registered dietitian (R.D.)** is a dietitian who has graduated from a state-approved program of dietetics, has passed the professional American Dietetic Association registration examination, and has served in an internship program to practice the necessary skills. Some states require licensing for dietitians; others do not.

diploma mills: institutions that offer meaningless courses and degrees by mail.

doctor: see *physician*.

health care provider: a term used in this book to refer to a physician, physician's assistant, nurse, nurse practitioner, pharmacist, or dietitian.

iatrogenic malnutrition: malnutrition caused by inadequate physician care (*iatro* means "doctor").

license to practice: permission under state or federal law to use a certain title (such as *medical doctor, osteopath, attorney,* etc.) and to offer certain services. The procedure by which a license is granted involves passing a state-administered examination.

M.D.: see *physician*.

M.S. (master of science) degree: a degree granted by an institution of higher learning (graduade school). Only college graduates may study for the master's degree, which typically requires two to three years of course work in a specialty area, a research project, and the passing of a comprehensive set of examinations.

nutrition support team: a team of selected physicians, nurses, dietitians, and pharmacists who are experts in nutrition, and who, together, can evaluate a client's nutrition status and develop an appropriate nutrition care plan.

nutritionist: a person who specializes in the study of nutrition. Some nutritionists are registered dietitians, whereas others are self-described experts whose training may be minimal or nonexistent. If the term is to be meaningful, it should apply only to people who have M.S. or Ph.D. degrees from institutions accredited to offer such degrees in nutrition or related fields, not other forms of education.

Ph.D. (doctor of philosophy) degree: a degree granted by an institution of higher learning (graduate school). The doctoral degree typically requires four to seven years of course work in a specialty area, a research thesis or dissertation, and the passing of a comprehensive set of examinations. A person with a Ph.D. in any subject area can be addressed as "doctor."

physician: a medical practitioner with an M.D. (medical doctor) or D.O. (doctor of osteopathy) degree from an accredited medical school.

R.D.: see *dietitian*.

registration: listing; specifically with respect to health professionals, a listing with a professional organization signifying that the professional has satisfied certain requirements, such as course work, experience, and the passing of an examination, and so may use the title and practice the profession.

Today, dietitians are realizing that their specialty is precisely what is needed by a clientele interested in health rather than in disease, and in prevention of disease rather than attempts at cure after the fact. Recognizing their own special qualifications to offer nutrition education and care, dietitians have been becoming more vocal and more visible in the 1980s than ever before. They have been realizing they need to be assertive, to make their qualifications known in the face of the rampant nutrition quackery with which they have to compete. To fight quackery, as well as to gain the recognition to which they are entitled, they have identified several needs:

- They need to keep abreast of current issues, so that others claiming to know the latest will not get the jump on them.
- They need to be skilled at distinguishing valid from invalid information, so that they can win a reputation for knowing the facts.
- They need to develop sensitivity and tact in dealing with people, so as not to alienate their potential colleagues and clientele.[28]

Tact is especially important. In attempting to assume their rightful place as nutrition experts among a peer group of other experts, including physicians, dietitians do themselves a disservice when they openly criticize other professionals. It is not tactful to broadcast the statement that "doctors don't know beans about nutrition." Besides, it isn't true. In place of viewing physicians as their competitors, dietitians should accept them as their partners in a common enterprise—that of making and keeping people well. Instead of criticizing others for what they don't know, dietitians should step forward and display what they themselves

DR. SAM SMITH SAYS, "AND SO YOU MUST EAT BLAH BLAH BLAH..."
WHO IS DR. SAM SMITH?
FAKE CREDENTIALS

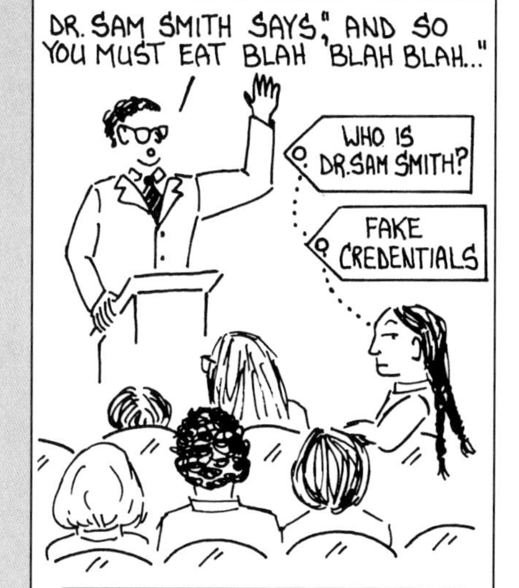

The title *doctor* should—but doesn't always—identify a reliable authority.

Miniglossary of Other Health Care Practitioners

These people's titles do not appear in this Controversy, but are included here for those who might be curious about them. Their qualifications to practice their professions are not as clearly defined as those of the people discussed in this Controversy. Their knowledge of nutrition may be extensive or nonexistent, or anything in between.

acupuncturist: a health practitioner who punctures the body with needles to relieve pain and achieve other physiological effects. Needles inserted at nerve synapses can alter the transmission of pain sensations. Acupuncture is an ancient art in China; depending on the practitioner, it has been found to be of some usefulness in the United States in relation to pain management.

chiropractor: a person who is trained to treat people with pain said to be caused by misalignment of the skeleton. Chiropractic treatments involve "adjustments"—that is, manipulations of the joints that can, in the best of cases, relieve pressure on nerves, and in the worst of cases, cause permanent disability. Chiropractors need have no more than two years of college, two of training, and two of supervised practice.

clinical ecologist: a practitioner who claims to be able to cure people's illnesses by diagnosing and treating allergies they have developed to substances and materials in their environments.

homeopath: a practitioner who uses small doses of poisons to prevent or relieve harm caused by those poisons (*homeo* means "same").

iridologist: a person who claims to be able to diagnose illnesses by studying the patterns of color in the iris of the eye. Training involves payment of $400 to purchase a chart of the iris and a list of diseases that various color patterns indicate.

naprapath: a person who treats connective tissue and ligament disorders by manipulation and massage (*napra* means "connective").

naturopath: a person who uses "natural" products such as foods and herbs to treat people's illnesses. Naturopaths distinguish themselves from traditional medical practitioners, whom they call *allopaths*—people who use medicine, surgery, x-ray examinations, and other "unnatural" tools to treat illnesses (*allo* means "other").

orthomolecular psychiatrist: a psychiatrist who uses "natural" treatments, especially vitamins and minerals, to rectify mental illnesses, assuming they are caused by wrong amounts of nutrient molecules in the system (*ortho* means "right amount").

know and can contribute to medical knowledge and practice. Similarly, with their clients, they need to learn how to facilitate behavior change effectively—by way of encouragement and example, not "telling what to do." They need to understand the emotional basis of food fads and practices, and take care to honor people's cultural beliefs even while molding their food behavior to better enhance their health. New curricula in dietetics are offering courses in assertiveness, communication, and counseling, as well as in the chemistry and biology.

Dietitians today can take their rightful places among their peers—on nutrition support teams, on the staffs of wellness centers, in home health agencies, in long-term care institutions, in private practice, and in sports training centers, as well as in the hospital. The needs are there, and dietitians are the professionals who can meet them.

Notes

1. C. E. Butterworth, The skeleton in the hospital closet, *Nutrition Today*, March/April 1974, pp. 4–8.
2. Butterworth, 1974.
3. A. Fonaroff, Undernutrition (letter to the editor), *Journal of the American Medical Association* 237 (1977): 1825–1826.
4. J. B. Schorr, as quoted by L. Hofmann, ed., *The Great American Nutrition Hassle* (Palo Alto, Calif.: Mayfield, 1978), p. 399.
5. P. R. Lee, as quoted by Hofmann, 1978, p. 321.
6. M. Winick, as quoted by R. Kotulak, Many doctors ignorant of nutrition, *Chicago Tribune*, May 1977.
7. E. S. Nelson, Nutrition instruction in medical schools—1976, *Journal of the American Medical Association* 236 (1976): 2534.
8. C. K. Cyborski, Nutrition content in medical curricula, *Journal of Nutrition Education* 9 (1977): 17–18.
9. W. J. Darby, The renaissance of nutrition education, *Nutrition Reviews* 35 (1977): 33–38.
10. Nutrition: No longer a stepchild in medicine (Medical News), *Journal of the American Medical Association* 238 (1977): 2245.
11. S. B. Heymsfield and coauthors, Biennial survey of physician clinical nutrition training programs, *American Journal of Clinical Nutrition* 42 (1985): 152–165.
12. Committee on Nutrition in Medical Education, Food and Nutrition Board, Commission on Life Sciences, National Research Council, *Nutrition Education in U.S. Medical Schools* (Washington, D.C.: National Academy Press, 1985), as reported in *American Journal of Clinical Nutrition* 43 (1986): 643–644.
13. Committee on Nutrition in Medical Education, 1985.
14. R. L. Weinsier and coauthors, Nutrition knowledge of senior medical students; A collaborative study of southeastern medical schools, *American Journal of Clinical Nutrition* 43 (1986): 959–968.
15. B. S. Levine and R. Tannenbaum, Frequency of nutritional considerations by practicing physicians (abstract), *American Journal of Clinical Nutrition* 43 (1986): 66.
16. S. K. Kamath and coauthors, Hospital malnutrition: A 33-hospital screening study, *Journal of the American Dietetic Association* 86 (1986): 203–206.
17. C. J. Krazit and W. W. Turner, The nutrition support advisory committee: A council of hospital services for nutrition support, *Journal of the American Dietetic Association* 86 (1986): 1067–1068.
18. S. H. Krey and R. L. Murray, eds., *Dynamics of Nutrition Support: Assessment, Implementation, Evaluation* (Norwalk, Conn.: Appleton-Century-Crofts, 1986), reviewed in *Journal of the American Dietetic Association* 86 (1986): 1642; M. A. Bernard, D. O. Jacobs, and J. L. Rombeau, *Nutritional and Metabolic Support of Hospitalized Patients* (Philadelphia: Saunders, 1985), reviewed in *Journal of the American Dietetic Association* 86 (1986): 1318; D. B. A. Silk, *Nutritional Support in Hospital Practice* (Boston: Blackwell Scientific Publications, 1983), reviewed by M. J. Hall in *American Journal of Clinical Nutrition* 40 (1984): 1309–1310.
19. P. W. Bunton, Using the computer as a referral source to find the patient at nutritional risk, *Journal of the American Dietetic Association* 86 (1986): 1232–1233.
20. S. Barrett, Why licensing of "nutritionists" is needed, *Nutrition Forum*, May 1985, p. 40.
21. Barrett, 1985.
22. M. B. Haschke, Licensure for dietitians: The issue in context (President's Page), *Journal of the American Dietetic Association* 84 (1984): 454–457.
23. New York Times Service story in the *San Bernardino* (California) *Times*, 6 August 1985, as cited by *National Council against Health Fraud Newsletter*, August 1985, p. 1.
24. V. Aronson, Bernardean University: A nutrition diploma mill, *ACSH News and Views*, March/April 1983, pp. 7, 11.
25. Meet Sassafras Herbert, professional nutritionist, *ACSH News and Views*, September/October 1983, p. 3.
26. S. C. Finn and J. D. Gussler, Women's issues and dietetics: Implications for professional development, *Dietetic Currents, Ross Timesaver*, January/February 1984.
27. V. Blanke, Political power and hospital dietitians, *Dietetic Currents, Ross Timesaver*, September/October 1982.
28. M. R. Polk, The dietitian vs. food faddism: An educational challenge, *Journal of the American Dietetic Association* 85 (1985): 1335–1337.

Chapter Three

Contents

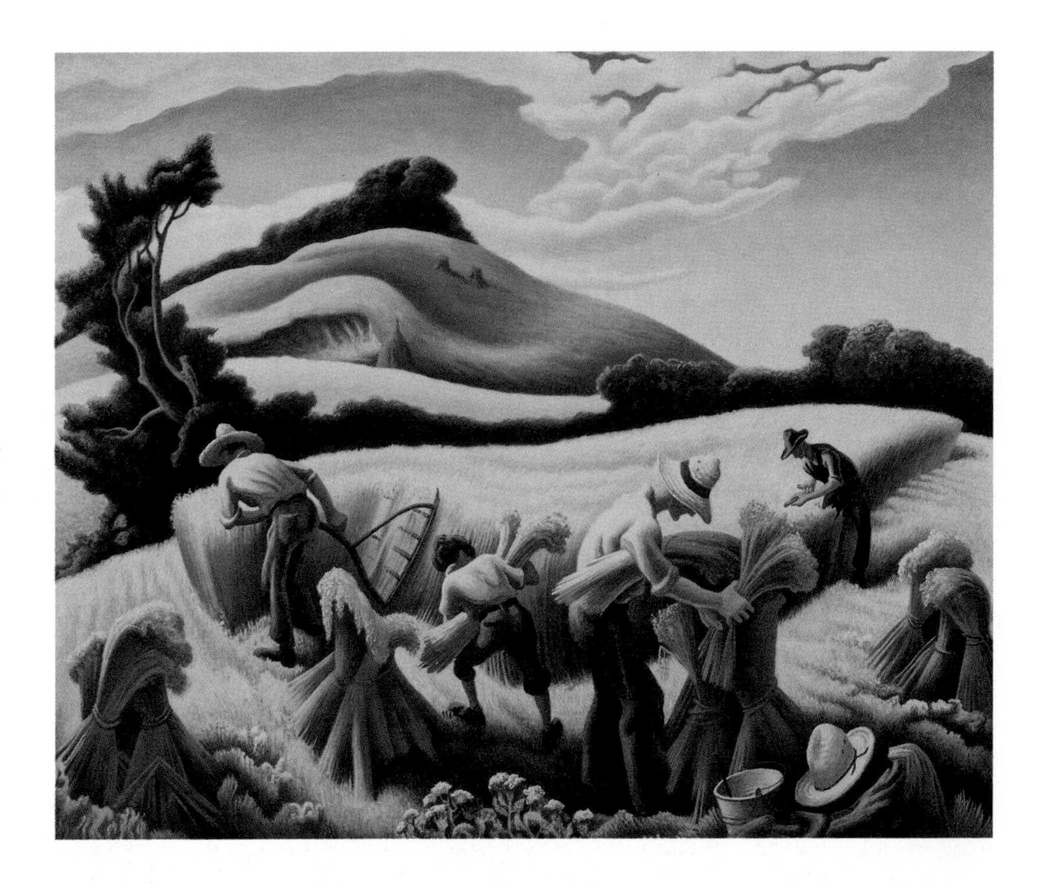

Cradling Wheat by Thomas Hart Benton, 1938. American, 1889–1975. The Saint Louis Art Museum Purchase.

The Carbohydrates: Sugar, Starch, and Fiber

It is impossible to point to the most important nutrient; the nutrients work together in harmony, each affecting the functions of many others. It is necessary, though, for the purpose of learning, to turn attention to each group, one at a time. This chapter is the first of a series of three on the energy-yielding nutrients: **carbohydrates,** fat, and protein. Those nutrients, together with fiber, give bulk to foods. The next chapters feature the vitamins and minerals.

This chapter invites you to learn to distinguish between the **complex carbohydrates**—such as starch and fiber—that are put to good use in the body and others—such as some of the **simple carbohydrates**—whose value is questioned. The Food Feature presents information about how to include enough of the right kinds of carbohydrate-rich foods in your diet. Appendix A displays the carbohydrate contents of foods.

carbohydrates: compounds composed of single sugars or multiples of them.

complex carbohydrates: long chains of sugars arranged as starch or fiber.

simple carbohydrates: sugars, both the single sugars and the double sugars.

chlorophyll: the green pigment of plants, which traps energy from sunlight and transfers this energy to other molecules, initiating photosynthesis.

glucose (GLOO-koce): a single sugar used in both plant and animal tissues as quick-energy currency; sometimes known as grape sugar, sometimes as blood sugar; also called **dextrose.**

photosynthesis: the synthesis of carbohydrates by green plants from carbon dioxide and water using the green pigment chlorophyll to trap the sun's energy (*photo* means "light"; *synthesis* means "making").

A Close Look at Carbohydrates

Carbohydrates support all life on earth. They are the first link in the food chain; they contain the sun's energy, captured in a form that living things can use to drive the processes of life. Carbohydrate-rich foods are obtained almost exclusively from plants; milk is the only animal-derived food that contains significant amounts of carbohydrate.

Carbohydrates:

- Sugars.
- Starch.
- Fiber.

When the sun beats down on the leaves of a plant, the energy of its rays, with the help of the green pigment **chlorophyll,** causes the carbon dioxide that the leaves take from the air and the water that the roots bring up from the soil to combine into the simple sugar called **glucose.** This complex reaction, **photosynthesis,** has been analyzed, and scientists know in minutest detail most of the steps in the total chemical reaction, yet it has never been reproduced from scratch; it requires the help of a green plant (see Figure 3–1).

Some of the energy that the sun gives to the reaction is used to make it happen, and some is lost as heat, but some—and this is the part that is important to our survival—is trapped in the chemical bonds that hold atoms of carbon in the special configuration that is glucose. The energy so caught and held will remain there until some agent (perhaps an enzyme) breaks the bonds, freeing the energy. The next few sections describe the forms that carbohydrates take, with their treasures of stored energy awaiting use in the human body.

Carbohydrate is made of carbon, hydrogen, and oxygen: carbo *means "carbon," C;* hydrate *means "water,"* H_2O.

Sugars and Starch

sugars: *simple carbohydrates*—that is, substances containing one or two sugar units.

fructose (FROOK-toce): a monosaccharide, sometimes known as fruit sugar (*fruct* means "fruit"; *ose* means "sugar").

Simple carbohydrates:
- Sugars.

Complex carbohydrates:
- Starch.
- Fiber.

The complex carbohydrates are also called the **polysaccharides.** *Poly* means "many," and *saccharide* means "sugar unit."

Glucose is a member of the chemical family, known as **sugars** or simple carbohydrates. These simple carbohydrates, made in the leaves of the green plant, provide energy for the work of all the plant's cells—those of the stem, roots, flowers, and fruits. For example, in the roots, far from the energy-giving rays of the sun, each cell takes some of the glucose, breaks it down (to carbon dioxide and water), and uses the energy thus released to fuel its own growth and water-gathering activities.

The plant makes other molecules from glucose—for example, **fructose,** the sweet sugar of fruit—by rearranging the atoms in glucose molecules. Fructose occurs mostly in fruits; in honey; and as part of another sugar, table sugar, to be described in a moment. Glucose and fructose are the most common single sugars, or **monosaccharides,** in nature. Another, **galactose,** has the same numbers and kinds of atoms, but they are arranged differently. Galactose, a monosaccharide that is part of the sugar in milk, does not occur free in nature; it is always bonded to something else until it is freed during digestion.

Some sugars are double sugars (**disaccharides**), made by bonding two single sugars together. When fructose and glucose are bonded together, they form **sucrose,** or table sugar, the product most people think of when they use the term *sugar.* This sugar is usually obtained by refining the juice from sugar beets or sugar cane, but it occurs naturally in many vegetables and fruits. It is of such major importance in human nutrition that most of controversy is devoted to it. Another disaccharide, **maltose,** appears wherever starch is being broken down. It occurs in germinating seeds and arises during the digestion of starch in the human body. Maltose consists of two glucose units. Finally, there is **lactose,** the sugar of milk, a disaccharide made by mammals from a galactose unit and a glucose unit. Table 3–1 summarizes the six sugars just named.

When you eat a food containing sugars, enzymes in your intestine first split the disaccharides into single sugars so that they can enter your bloodstream (see Figure 3–2). Your liver then quickly converts those other than glucose to glucose or to smaller pieces that can serve as building blocks of either glucose or fat. Monosaccharides other than glucose are not important inside the body.

Glucose may also be strung together in long strands to form compounds known as the **complex carbohydrates.** Starch is one of these; some of the fibers are others.

Figure 3–1 Carbohydrate—Mainly Glucose—Is Made by Photosynthesis. The sun's energy becomes part of the glucose molecule—its calories, in a sense. In the molecule of glucose here, dots represent the carbon atoms; bars represent the chemical bonds that contain energy.

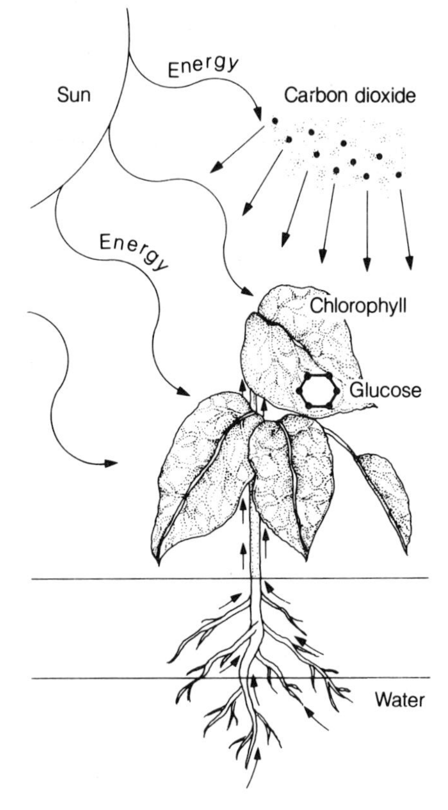

Table 3–1

The Sugars (Simple Carbohydrates)

Monosaccharides:		
Glucose	⬡	
Galactose[a]	GAL	
Fructose	FRU	
Disaccharides:		
Sucrose (fructose + glucose)		⬡-FRU
Maltose (glucose + glucose)		⬡-⬡
Lactose (glucose + galactose)		⬡-GAL

[a]Galactose never occurs free in nature; it is part of lactose.

As a plant matures, it provides not only energy for its own needs, but also food for the next generation. For example, after a corn plant reaches it full growth and has many leaves manufacturing glucose, it begins to store surplus energy for the growth of new plants from seeds next season. It can't store the glucose itself, because glucose is soluble in water and would be washed away by the winter rains. Instead, it must form an insoluble substance that will stay with the seed and nourish it until it puts out shoots with leaves to catch the sun's rays. This storage form of glucose is **starch,** and corn is really a package of seeds embedded in this nutritive material.

Starch is made up of many tiny glucose units bonded together—3,000 or so in each molecule. When you eat a starchy food, enzymes in your saliva break the bonds of the starch molecules, freeing maltose units (pairs of glucoses). Enzymes in your intestine follow through by breaking the maltoses apart, freeing glucose units, which are absorbed into the blood (see Figure 3–2). One to four hours after a meal, all the starch has been digested and absorbed, and is circulating to the cells as glucose.

Through photosynthesis, plants combine carbon dioxide, water, and the sun's energy to form glucose. Glucose is the most important monosaccharide in the human body. The liver converts monosaccharides and disaccharides other than glucose to units that can be converted to glucose or serve as building blocks for fat. Starch is a storage form of glucose. Enzymes in the saliva and in the intestine free the glucose units to be absorbed into the blood.

monosaccharides: a single sugar unit (*mono* means "one").

galactose (ga-LACK-toce): a monosaccharide; part of the disaccharide lactose.

disaccharides: two-sugar units (*di* means "two").

sucrose (SOO-crose): a disaccharide composed of glucose and fructose—table, beet, or cane sugar (*sucr* means "sugar").

maltose: a disaccharide composed of two glucose units—malt sugar.

lactose: a disaccharide composed of glucose and galactose—milk sugar (*lact* means "milk"; *ose* means "sugar").

starch: a plant polysaccharide composed of glucose, digestible by humans.

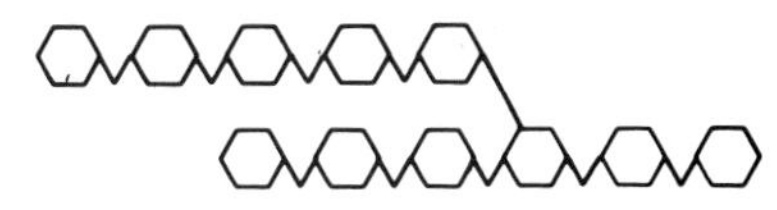

Starch. Glucose units are linked in long, occasionally branched chains to make starch. Human digestive enzymes can digest these bonds, retrieving glucose. Real glucose units are so tiny that you can't see them, even with the highest-power light microscope.

Fiber

The **fibers** of a plant contribute the supporting structures of its leaves, stems, and seeds. Most fibers are polysaccharides made of glucose, just as starch is, but

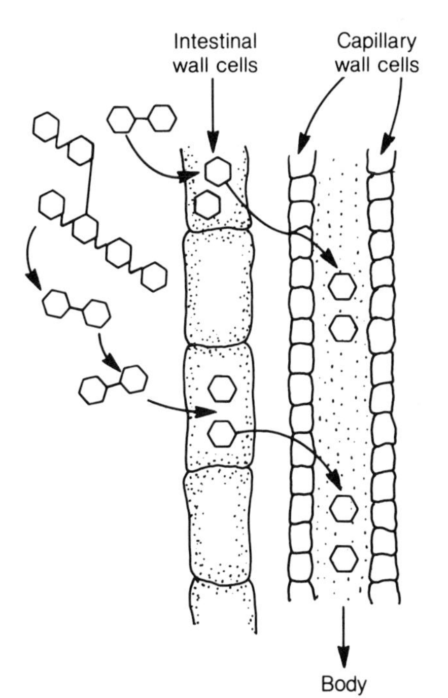

Figure 3–2 Digestion of Disaccharides and Starch.
Chapter 1 introduced the digestive system. Appendix I summarizes the whole process of digestion.

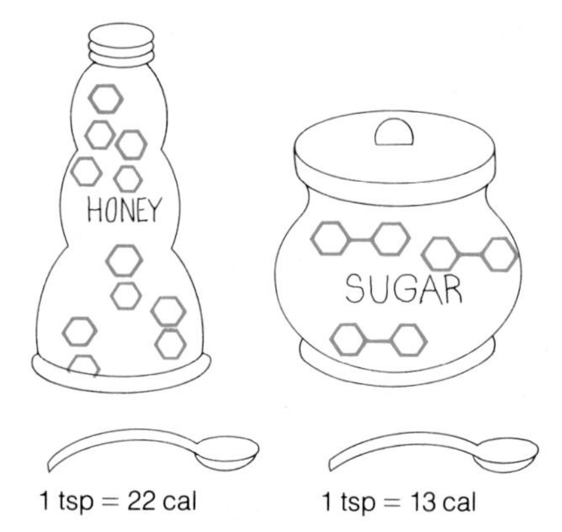

Honey and sucrose contain the same monosaccharides, but in sucrose they are linked together.

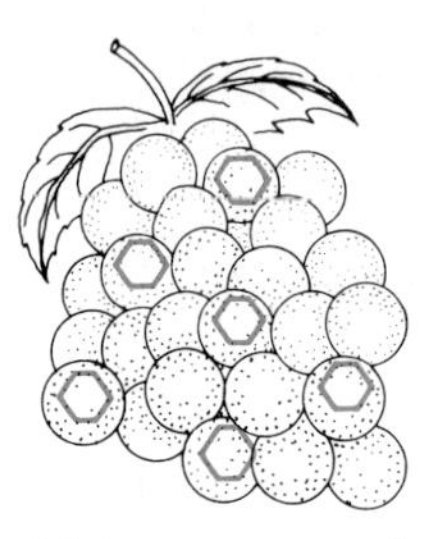

Compared with honey or sugar, fruit is truly nutritious.

White Sugar versus Purified Fructose versus Honey

The monosaccharide fructose is sold in purified, crystalline form, billed as a "natural" sugar that—unlike the nasty unnatural sugar sucrose—"won't cause ugly weight gain." This is just a sales pitch. What's natural about *any* purified, concentrated sugar? The calories in fructose are used for energy just as those in ordinary table sugar are—and too much of either can make you fat.

There has been some serious discussion to the effect that fructose may be a desirable sugar substitute for use in diabetes because it is sweeter (so people with diabetes might use less) and because it does not raise the blood glucose level as much as glucose does or require such an insulin response. However, early hopes that this might be true have been dampened. Fructose is not that much sweeter than sucrose; further, some of it becomes glucose after it enters the body, requiring insulin to be used. Anyway—and perhaps most importantly—most people with diabetes need to control their weight and fructose not only supplies nutrient-empty calories, but also requires less energy for its metabolism than does glucose, making it even more fattening.[1]

Some people believe that honey is better than white sugar, because it is "natural." As a matter of fact, chemically they are almost indistinguishable. Honey contains the two monosaccharides glucose and fructose in approximately equal amounts. Sugar contains the same monosaccharides, but joined together in the disaccharide sucrose. In the body, after digestion, sugar and honey are identical. Spoon for spoon, however, sugar contains *fewer* calories than honey, because the dry crystals of sugar take up more space than the sugars of honey dissolved in its water.

When people learn that fruit's energy comes from sugars, they may think that eating fruit is the same as eating concentrated sweets such as candy or cola beverages. However, fruits differ from concentrated sweets in important ways. The sugars of fruits are diluted in large volumes of water, packaged in fiber, and mixed with many vitamins and minerals needed by the body.

From these examples, you may see that the most significant difference between sugar sources is not between "natural" and "purified" sugar but between concentrated sweets and the dilute sugars of fruits and vegetables.

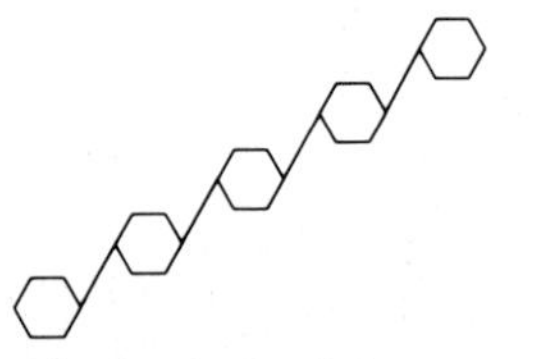

Cellulose. The bonds that link glucose units together are different from the bonds in starch and glycogen. Human enzymes cannot digest them.

with different bonds between the glucose units—bonds that cannot be broken by human digestive enzymes. The best known of these polysaccharides are **cellulose, hemicellulose,** and **pectin.** They are familiar as the "strings" of celery, the skins of corn kernels, and the membranes separating the segments in citrus fruits. Isolated from plants, they may be used to thicken jelly (citrus pectin), to keep salad dressing from separating (guar gum), to provide **roughage** (wheat bran, oat bran, and other brans), and to achieve other effects on texture and consistency.

A noncarbohydrate component of plants that has been included in the fiber family in the past is **lignin,** the woody material of heavy stems and bark. Foods are usually harvested before much lignin has formed, though, and a recent definition of fiber discounts it as a constituent. Thus fibers are "the nonstarch polysaccharides in foods."[2]

The bonds that hold the units of fiber together cannot be broken by human digestive enzymes, but some can be broken by the bacteria that reside in the human digestive tract. Therefore, we obtain a little glucose, some related products, and a barely detectable bit of energy from fiber molecules. Some animals, such as cattle, depend heavily on their intestinal bacteria to make available the energy of glucose derived from fiber. (When we eat beef, we receive indirectly some of the sun's energy that was originally stored in the fiber of the plants they ate. Beef, of course, contains no fiber itself.) Fibers exert important effects on people's health, and these are described in a later section.

Fiber is not digested by people for energy. Some fiber is changed by the intestinal bacteria into products that are absorbed; some fiber passes through the digestive tract unchanged.

fiber: the indigestible residue of food, composed mostly of the polysaccharides **cellulose, hemicellulose, pectin,** and **gums.**

The term **dietary fiber** refers to nutritionally significant fiber in food—that is, the fiber that resists human digestive enzymes. (A chemist might digest food, in a test tube, by a harsher procedure than the human intestine does, and so might find only one-third or one-half as much undigested material remaining; this fiber is termed *crude fiber.*)

A term not used here is **residue:** whatever material still remains solid when the intestinal contents reach the colon, such as undigested bits of protein, all the fibers, and other materials. Milk forms residue, for example, but contains no fiber.

roughage (RUFF-idge): the rough parts of food, an imprecise term that has been largely replaced by the term *fiber.*

lignin: the woody material of stems and bark, a noncarbohydrate classed by some as a fiber.

The Need for Starch and Fiber

Carbohydrate is the most efficient fuel for most body functions. There are only three other energy sources available to the body—protein, fat, and alcohol. Protein-rich foods are usually expensive and provide no advantage over carbohydrates when used to make fuel for the body. (The disadvantages of their overconsumption are explained in Chapter 5.) Fat cannot be used efficiently as fuel by the brain and central nervous system, and diets high in fat are associated with many disease states. Alcohol has the same disadvantage as fat, to say nothing of its well-known undesirable side effects. Thus, of all the possible alternatives, carbohydrate is the preferred energy source.

Carbohydrate has always been a major fuel source for plant-eating animals, and food starch has always been an important source of human energy. In fact, starchy plants made it possible for mammals and people to come into being. The first green plants contained no starch and could only support creatures like the ponderous dinosaurs of a hundred million years ago. Some of these great beasts were herbivores (plant eaters), and they had to eat enormous quantities of leaves and stems to supply the energy they needed.

Then came the flowering plants. The earlier plants had reproduced by means of spores carried by wind and water, but the flowering plants grew fruits packed with sugars and seeds filled with starch and oils. Thus they wrapped each of their offspring in a case with enough energy food inside to sustain it until it could make a foothold in the earth. This advantage enabled the seed-bearing plants to replace the earlier plants as the earth's main form of vegetation.

The seeds and fruits of the flowering plants contained enough concentrated energy food to support animals whose expenditures of energy were greater than those of the slow-moving herbivorous dinosaurs. As the ages passed, the mammals replaced the dinosaurs as the dominant animal life form. These animals made significant advances in their use of plant carbohydrate. They developed the ability to store small supplies of carbohydrate to keep their blood glucose

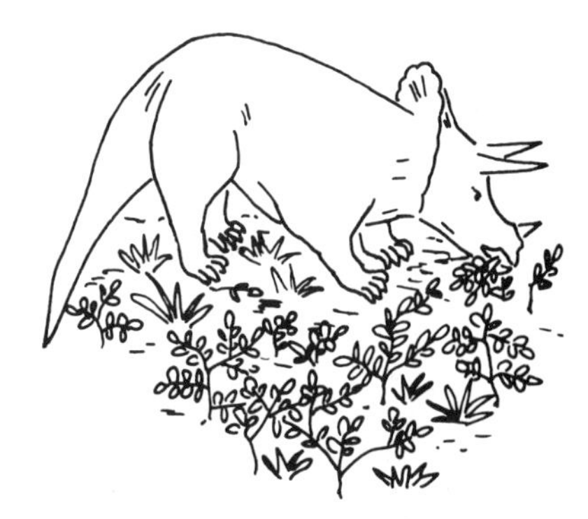

Dinosaurs had to eat masses of leaves and stems to obtain enough carbohydrate.

constipation: hardness and dryness of bowel movements, associated with discomfort in passing them.

appendicitis: inflammation and/or infection of the appendix, a sac protruding from the large intestine.

hemorrhoids (HEM-or-oids): swollen, hardened (varicose) veins in the rectum, usually caused by the pressure resulting from constipation.

diverticulosis (dye-ver-tic-you-LOH-sis): outpocketing of weakened areas of the intestinal wall, like blowouts in a tire (*divertir* means "to turn"; *osis* means "too much").

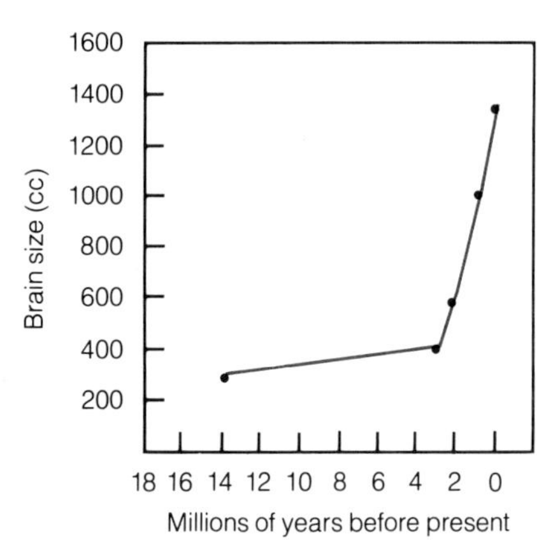

The graph shows that mammalian brain size "suddenly" increased during evolution. The increase coincided with the development of flowering plants.

Source: Adapted from D. Pilbeam, *The Ascent of Man* (New York: Macmillan, 1972), as adapted by E. O. Wilson, *Sociobiology: The New Synthesis* (Cambridge, Mass.: Belknap Press, Harvard University Press, 1975), p. 548, with the permission of both publishers.

levels constant between meals, to help burn other fuels, and to keep their bodies warm. A mammal doesn't need to eat constantly in order to think. A human being's large brain, supplied with constant warmth and fuel, doesn't have to turn off. Guaranteed energy even between meals, the brain can occupy itself with thoughts on a higher plane than that of gathering food. Thus the ultimate evolution of human beings and the explosion of their civilization and technology are partly a result of the development of seed-bearing plants.

The human brain still depends exclusively on carbohydrate for its energy whenever that fuel is available. And because the mind resides in the brain, to some extent your attitude toward life, the world, and other people is affected by the brain's glucose supply.

Carbohydrate has for years been wrongly accused of being "the" fattening ingredient of foods. If you have been exposed to as much anticarbohydrate propaganda as most people have been, the statement that we need to consume more carbohydrate, rather than less, may be startling. Yet much evidence supports it. The Senate committee that produced the *Dietary Goals for the United States* (see Chapter 2) made the observation that a young man's weight-reducing diet could include as many as 12 slices of bread in a day and still allow him to lose more than a pound a week.[3] The report urges consumption of all kinds of foods rich in complex carbohydrates, such as potatoes, pasta, and rice. Even people with diabetes, who used to be thought unable to handle carbohydrates, were exhorted to eat liberal amounts of certain kinds of starch. On the other hand, the Senate committee recommended that we reduce our intakes of sugar. Later, the *Dietary Guidelines for Americans* echoed these recommendations. The Canadian government made similar recommendations to its people, as have the governments of several other countries.

Starch and fiber come together in foods, and fiber affects health, too. Fiber comes in many forms. Not all have the same effects, but here are some of the things that different fibers do:

- Promote feelings of fullness, thereby reducing energy consumption, because high-fiber foods absorb water while donating little energy. Displacement of calorie-dense concentrated fats and sweets from the diet can help in weight control. Some fibers delay the emptying of the stomach so that you feel fuller longer.
- Possibly prevent **constipation** and bacterial infection of the appendix (**appendicitis**), by keeping the contents of the intestine moving along.
- Are associated with reduced incidence of colon cancer (see Controversy 5).
- Stimulate the muscles of the digestive tract so that they retain their health and tone; this prevents **hemorrhoids** (in which veins in the rectum swell, bulge out, become brittle, and bleed) and **diverticulosis** (in which the intestinal walls become weak and bulge out in places).
- Reduce the risks of heart and artery disease in several ways. Insoluble fiber binds fatty compounds (sterols) and carries them out of the body with the feces so that the whole body content of cholesterol is lowered. The substances produced from soluble fiber are absorbed and may inhibit the body's production of cholesterol, and enhance its clearance from the blood.[4]
- Also improve the body's handling of glucose, even in people with diabetes, perhaps by slowing the digestion or absorption rate of carbohydrate.[5] A high-fiber meal eaten for breakfast still exerts regulatory effects on people's blood glucose and insulin responses to lunch.[6]

When people choose high-fiber foods in hopes of receiving some of these benefits, they must choose with care. Wheat bran, which is composed mostly of cellulose, has no cholesterol-lowering effect, whereas oat bran and the fibers of legumes, apples, and carrots do lower blood cholesterol. On the other hand, wheat bran is one of the most effective stool- softening fibers. Table 3–2 shows the diversity of effects of different fibers, but its last item (food sources) reveals that they are only of academic interest. If a single practical conclusion were to be drawn from the table, it would have to be that all whole plant foods seem to contain many kinds of fibers and so can be expected to have the whole range of effects mentioned in the table.

Undoubtedly, including fiber in a daily meal plan has benefits—but how much is enough? Even fiber has potential for harm if taken in excess. Fiber carries water out of the body and can cause dehydration. Iron is mainly absorbed early during digestion, and excess fiber may limit its absorption by speeding up the transit of foods through the digestive system. Binders in some fibers link chemically with the minerals calcium, zinc, and others and carry them out of the body. Some fibers interfere with the body's use of carotene to make vitamin

Table 3–2

Health Effects of Fibers

Health Effect	Do Cellulose, Hemicellulose (insoluble fiber) Have Effect ?	Do Pectins, Gums (soluble fiber) Have Effect?
Obesity—displaces calories	Yes	Yes
Constipation/ hemorrhoids—reduces pressure, softens stools	Yes	No
Cancer—Increases bile acid excretion[a]	No	Yes
Speeds up transit time[b]	Yes	No
Diabetes—improves glucose tolerance	Yes, wheat bran does	Yes, some do
Cardiovascular disease—lowers blood cholesterol[c]	No[c]	Yes
Interferes with mineral absorption	Yes	No
Interferes with vitamin A supply from carotene	Not known	Yes, pectin does
Food sources	Fruits, vegetables, legumes, brans, nuts, seeds, popcorn, whole-grain flours, rice	Fruits, vegetables, seeds, legumes, oats, barley, rye

[a]Bile acids not excreted can be converted to cancer-causing substances and absorbed.

[b]Any cancer-causing substance has less chance to do its dirty work if it passes rapidly out of the system.

[c]Notably, wheat bran, which is largely composed of cellulose, does not lower blood cholesterol. Oat bran *does* lower blood cholesterol, and one of its soluble fiber constituents is probably responsible for the effect.

refined: refers to the process by which the coarse parts of food products are removed. For example, the refining of wheat into flour involves removing three of the four parts of the kernel—the chaff, the bran, and the germ—leaving only the endosperm (starch, with only a little protein).

enriched: refers to a process by which the nutrients thiamin, riboflavin, niacin, and iron are added to refined grains and grain products at levels specified by law. After enrichment, a grain product has approximately the same amount of thiamin, niacin, and iron, and about twice as much riboflavin, as the original whole-grain product had.

whole grain: refers to a grain milled in its entirety (all but the husk), not refined.

germ: the nutrient-rich inner part of a grain.

endosperm: the bulk of the edible part of a grain, the starchy part.

bran: the chief fiber-donator of a grain.

husk: the outer, inedible part of a grain.

gluten (GLOOT-en): an elastic protein formed in certain grain products by the mechanical action of kneading that confers structure and cohesiveness on them.

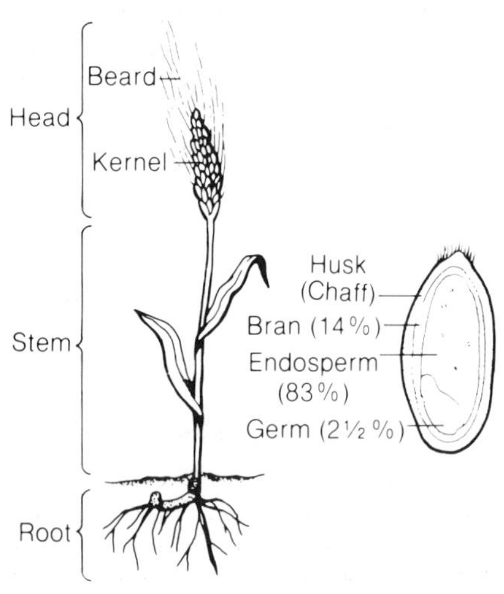

A wheat plant. A kernel of wheat.

Refined, Enriched, and Whole-Grain Bread

For many people, bread supplies most of the carbohydrate, or at least most of the starch, in a day's meals. Any food used in such abundance in the diet should be scrutinized closely, and if it doesn't measure up to high nutrition standards, it should be replaced with a food that does. For people who eat bread, the meanings of the words associated with the wheat flour that makes up the bread—**refined, enriched,** and **whole grain**—hold the key to understanding this product in which they invest many calories per day.

The part of the wheat plant that is made into flour and then into bread and other baked goods is the kernel. About 50 kernels cluster in the grain head, where they stick tightly until fully ripe. These kernels are first separated from the stem and then further broken apart by the milling process.

The wheat kernel (a whole grain) has four main parts: the **germ,** the **endosperm,** the **bran,** and the **husk.** The germ is the part that grows into a wheat plant, and so it contains concentrated food to support the new life. It is especially rich in vitamins and minerals. The endosperm is the soft, white inside portion of the kernel containing starch and proteins. The bran, a protective coating around the kernel similar in function to the shell of a nut, is also rich in nutrients and fiber. The husk, commonly called chaff, is unusable for most purposes except for animal feed. When made into white flour and mixed with liquid, the endosperm forms a stretchy protein called **gluten.** Gluten allows a lacy network of air bubbles to be baked in, making white-flour bread appealingly light and soft.

In earlier times, people milled wheat by grinding it between two stones, then blowing or sifting out the inedible chaff, but retaining the nutrient-rich bran and germ as well as the endosperm. Improved milling machinery made it possible to remove the dark, heavy germ and bran as well, leaving a whiter, smoother-textured flour. People came to look on this flour as more desirable than the crunchy, dark brown, "old-fashioned" flour, but were unaware of the nutrition implications at first.

Bread eaters suffered a tragic loss of needed nutrients in turning to white bread. A survey that took place in the United States in 1936 revealed that many people were suffering from deficiencies of the nutrients iron, thiamin, riboflavin, and niacin, which they had formerly received from bread. The Enrichment Act of 1942 standardized the return of these lost nutrients to commercial flour. Thus, in enriched bread, iron and niacin have been restored to the levels found in whole wheat; thiamin, and especially riboflavin, are added to higher levels. This doesn't make a single slice of bread "rich" in these nutrients, but people who eat several or many slices of bread a day obtain significantly more of them than they would from unenriched white bread.

To a great extent, the enrichment of white flour eliminated these known deficiency problems in the eaters of refined white bread, but many other deficiencies went undetected for years more. Today, you can almost take it for granted that all breads, grains like rice, wheat products like macaroni and spaghetti, and cereals, both cooked and ready-to-eat types, have been enriched. The law requires that all grain products that cross state lines must be enriched. Table 3–3 shows the trouble with enrichment: it makes refined bread comparable to whole-grain bread with respect to these four nutrients, but not with respect to others.

Enrichment does not compensate for many nutrient losses. When a grain is refined, many nutrients not replenished by enrichment, are also lost. The same losses are simultaneously occurring in other foods that are being refined and processed. Fiber needs are not being met, as fiber is refined out of many foods, not just bread and cereal. Some experts have attributed a few cases of diabetes to deficiency of a mineral that is refined out of processed foods—chromium, essential for insulin to act. Therefore, although the enrichment of wheat and other cereal products does improve them, it doesn't improve them enough. As Table 3–3 shows, whole-grain items are preferable to enriched products because they contain more magnesium, zinc, folacin, vitamin B_6, fiber, vitamin E, chromium, and many other nutrients than enriched bread and cereals. If bread is a staple food in your diet—that is, if you eat it every day—you would be well advised to learn to like the hearty flavor of whole-grain bread.

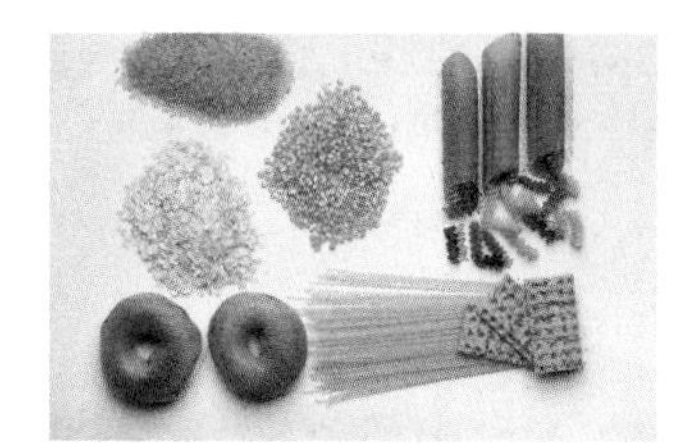

Learn to like the hearty flavor of whole grain.

A (the conversion is described in Chapter 6).[7] Too much bulk in the diet could limit the total amount of food consumed and cause deficiencies of both nutrients and energy. The malnourished, the elderly, and strict vegetarian children are especially vulnerable to this chain of events.

The average fiber intake in the United States is lower than has previously been thought. On any given day, about half the population reports an intake of less than 10 g per day. Women eat more fiber than do men, and most adults eat more as they grow older, but most do not consume as much as they need for their health.[8] There is no RDA for fiber, and not everyone agrees on just how to measure a food's fiber content. Still, with all the uncertainties, it is probably true to say that about 20 to 30 grams of dietary fiber daily is a desirable intake. The diet can supply that amount, given ample choices of whole foods,

Table 3–3

Nutrients in One-Pound Loaves of Bread

	Iron (mg)	Magnesium (mg)	Zinc (mg)	Thiamin (mg)	Riboflavin (mg)	Niacin (mg)	Vitamin B_6 (mg)	Folacin (mg)	Fiber (g)
Whole-grain bread	15.5 (100%)	422 (100%)	7.63 (100%)	1.59 (100%)	0.95 (100%)	17.4 (100%)	0.85 (100%)	250 (100%)	51.4 (100%)
		↑	↑				↑	↑	↑
Enriched white bread	83%	23%	36%	>100%	>100%	98%	18%	64%	24%
	↑			↑	↑	↑			
Unenriched white bread	21%	23%	36%	26%	28%	2%	18%	64%	24%

Note: The four "up" arrows in the bottom half of the table show that if you choose enriched over unenriched bread, you obtain significantly more iron, thiamin, riboflavin, and niacin, about the same as in whole-grain bread. The five "up" arrows in the top half of the table show that if you choose whole-grain over enriched bread, you obtain significantly more of *other* nutrients—magnesium, zinc, vitamin B_6, and folacin, as well as fiber. The same would be true of vitamin E, chromium, and other nutrients (not shown).

Table 3–4

Foods to Provide 25 Grams Dietary Fiber per Day

Fruits (with skins): about 2 g of fiber per portion; use four or more per day.	
apple, 1 small	cantaloupe, ½ melon
banana, 1 small	peach, 1
strawberries, ¾ c	pear, ½ small
cherries, 16 large	prunes, 2
Grains and cereals: about 2 g of fiber per portion; use four or more per day.	
whole-wheat bread, 1 slice	Cornbran, ¼ c
Rye Crisp, 2 crackers	oatmeal, cooked, 1 c
cracked-wheat bread, 2 slices	wheat bran, 1 tsp
Shredded Wheat, ½ biscuit	oat bran, 2 tsp
Grape-Nuts, ⅓ c	Puffed Wheat, 1½ c
barley, ½ c	popcorn, popped, 1½ c
All Bran, 1 tbsp	
Vegetables: about 2 g of fiber per portion; use four or more per day. These values are for cooked portions.	
broccoli, ½ c	lettuce, raw, 2 c
brussels sprouts, ½ c	green beans, ⅔ c
carrots, ½ c	potato, 1 small
celery, 1 c	tomato, 1 large
corn, ⅓ c	
Legumes (cooked): about 8 g of fiber per portion.	
garbanzo beans, ½ c	baked beans, canned, ½ c
kidney beans, ½ c	lentils, 1 c
dried peas, 1 c	lima beans, 1 c
Miscellaneous: about 1 g of fiber per portion.	
peanut butter, 2½ tsp	pickle, 1 large
peanuts, 7 nuts	strawberry jam, 5 tbsp
walnuts, ¼ c	

Source: Values for barley, puffed wheat, celery, lettuce, garbanzo beans, walnuts, pickles, and jam from Recommendations for a high-fiber diet, *Nutrition and the MD,* July 1981, in turn adapted from D. A. T. Southgate and coauthors, A guide to calculating intakes of dietary fiber, *Journal of Human Nutrition* 30 (1976): 303–313; Value for popcorn from Appendix 1; all others from: E. Lanza and R. R. Butrum, A critical review of food fiber analysis and data, *Journal of the American Dietetic Association* 86 (1986): 732–743.

as Table 3–4 demonstrates. The diet does have to be high in fruits, vegetables, and grains and relatively low in meats, fats, and concentrated sugar—the same recommendations put forth by the *Dietary Guidelines* and *Dietary Goals.*

The wholesale addition of purified fiber (for example, bran) to foods is probably ill advised, because it is so easily taken to extreme and because fiber types are mixed in foods. Taking only one isolated type deprives the taker of the benefits the other types of fiber provide, and a purified fiber, such as cellulose, may not have the same effect in the body as the celulose in whole grains.[9] Besides, in food, the fiber you need is found together with a package of benefits—water, minerals, vitamins, and the energy nutrients. Refined fiber could be compared in one way to refined sugar: the nutrients that normally accompany it have been lost. More information on obtaining fiber through food choices appears in the Food Feature at the end of this chapter.

Carbohydrate is the preferred energy source of the body; the brain and nerves prefer glucose as fuel. Fiber helps maintain the health of the digestive tract, and helps prevent or control certain diseases.

glycogen (GLY-co-gen): a polysaccharide composed of glucose, manufactured in the animal body and stored in liver and muscle. Glycogen is not a significant food source of carbohydrate and is not counted as one of the complex carbohydrates in foods.

The Body's Use of Glucose

Just as glucose is the original unit from which the wide variety of carbohydrate foods are made, so also is glucose the basic carbohydrate unit that each cell of the body uses. Cells cannot use whole molecules of lactose, sucrose, or starch; they require glucose. The task of the various body systems, then, is to make glucose available to the cells. The digestive system disassembles the disaccharides and polysaccharides to monosaccharides and absorbs them into the blood. The liver converts fructose and galactose to glucose or derivatives of glucose (such as fat), and the circulatory system transports the glucose and fat to the cells. Cells may store circulating glucose as glycogen or split it for energy. Similarly, they may store circulating fat or use it for energy.

This section refers to many body organs. If you want to review them, turn to Chapter 1.

The task of the various body systems is to break down carbohydrate into glucose to fuel the cells' work.

Storing Glucose as Glycogen

If the blood delivers more glucose than the cells need, the liver and muscles take up the surplus. From some of it, they build the polysaccharide **glycogen.** The muscles hoard two-thirds of the body's total store of this carbohydrate and use it themselves during intensive exercise. (Chapter 9 explores this relationship between glycogen and exercise and gives tips on how to make the most of glycogen stores.) The liver stores the other one-third, making it available when the brain or other organs need to draw on the supply.

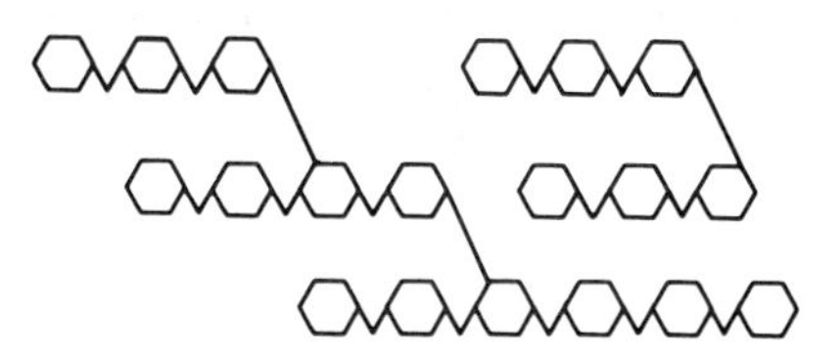

Glycogen. The bonds between glucose units are the same as in starch, but the chains are longer and more highly branched.

Glycogen is wondrously designed for its task of releasing glucose on demand. Instead of having long chains with occasional branches, like starch, which is cleaved one unit after the other during digestion, glycogen is highly branched, so that hundreds of ends stick out at its surface. On the tip of each chain is a glucose, whose attachment to the next glucose is easily accessible to the glycogen-splitting enzymes. When quick energy (glucose) is needed by the cells, a hormone (epinephrine, or what used to be called adrenaline) floods the bloodstream. Thousands of enzymes within the liver cells respond by attacking a multitude of ends simultaneously, and they release an abundance of glucose into the blood for use by all the other body cells. This response is part of the body's defense mechanism in times of danger.

For more about hormones, see Chapter 1.

The advantage to the Stone Age person of having an internal source of quick energy is obvious. Life was fraught with physical peril. The person who stopped and ate before running from the man-eating tiger did not survive to produce our ancestors. The quick-energy response in a stress situation works to our advantage today as well. (One example: It accounts for the energy you suddenly

protein-sparing action: the action of carbohydrate and fat in providing energy that allows protein to be used for other purposes.

ketosis (kee-TOE-sis): an undesirably high concentration of ketone bodies, such as acetone, in the blood and urine (*osis* means "too much in the blood"). **Ketone** (kee-tone) **bodies** are the product of the incomplete breakdown of fat when carbohydrate is not available.

have to clean up your room when you learn that a special person is coming to visit.) To meet such emergencies, we are well advised to eat and store carbohydrate every four to six hours when we are awake.

You might rightly ask, "What kind of carbohydrate?" Knowing only that energy is needed, you might conclude that the best source of energy is a concentrated sugar food, such as a candy bar or a sugary beverage. These do supply sugar energy quickly, but they are not the best choices. Advertisements of quick-energy foods use a logic based on partial truth; the whole truth is that starchy food will provide you with glucose just as well, and with a more nutritious assortment of other ingredients.

Mindful of this warning, when you encounter a sales pitch for an "energy food," you may ask, "What does the speaker stand to gain from having me believe this statement?" The answer is obvious: the speaker stands to gain whatever money you choose to spend.

NEED ENERGY?
EAT THE OLYMPIC CANDYBAR!
SALES PITCH
LOGIC WITHOUT PROOF
INCOMPLETE TRUTH

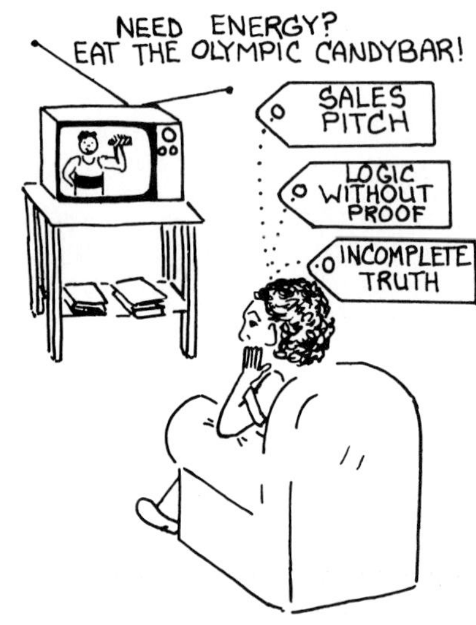

The implication that any kind of carbohydrate is a good energy food is often used to sell candy. Candy contains sucrose, but it's *starch* that makes the best fuel.

Glycogen is the body's form of stored glucose; the liver stores it for use by the whole body. Muscles have their own private glycogen stock for muscle use only.

Splitting Glucose for Energy

Glucose fuels the work of most of the body's cells. When a cell splits glucose for energy, it performs an intricate sequence of maneuvers that are of great interest to the chemist—and of no interest whatever to most people who eat bread and potatoes. There is only one fact that everybody needs to understand about the process, and it may help to give the punch line before telling the story: there is no good substitute for carbohydrate. There is a point at which glucose is forever lost in the body, and this can have serious consequences. The following details are given only for the purpose of making this point clear.

Inside the cell, glucose breaks in half, releasing some energy. These halves have two pathways open to them. They can be put back together to make glucose, or they can be further broken apart into smaller fragments. If they are broken into smaller fragments, they can never again be used to form glucose. They can yield still more energy, and in the process break down completely to carbon dioxide and water; or they can be hitched together into units of body fat. Figure 3–3 shows how glucose is broken down to yield energy and carbon dioxide.

Body fat can never regenerate enough glucose to feed the brain adequately. This is one reason why fasting and low-carbohydrate diets are dangerous. When there is a severe carbohydrate deficit, the body has two problems. Having no glucose, it has to turn to protein to make some (it has this ability), thus diverting protein from vitally important functions of its own. Protein's importance to the body is so great that carbohydrate should be kept available precisely to prevent this use of protein for energy. This is called the **protein-sparing action** of carbohydrate. For another thing, without sufficient carbohydrate, the body can't use its fat in the normal way. (Carbohydrate is needed to combine with the fat fragments so that they can be used for energy.) So the body has to go into **ketosis** (using fat without the help of carbohydrate), a condition in which unusual products of fat breakdown (**ketone bodies**) accumulate in the blood. Ketosis during pregnancy can cause brain damage and irreversible mental retardation in the infant, but even in nonpregnant adults it is a condition to avoid, because it disturbs the body's normal acid-base balance.

More about the hazards of fasting and low-carbohydrate diets—Chapter 8.

The amount of carbohydrate needed to ensure complete sparing of body protein and avoidance of ketosis is around 100 grams a day in an average-sized person. This has to be digestible carbohydrate, and considerably more than this minimum is recommended.[10]

Without glucose, the body is forced to use protein and fat differently. The body breaks down its own muscles and other protein tissues to make glucose, and converts its fat into ketone bodies, incurring ketosis.

insulin: a hormone secreted by the pancreas in response to high blood glucose levels; it assists cells in drawing glucose from the blood.

glycemic (gligh-SEEM-ic) **effect:** a measure of the extent to which a food raises the blood glucose level as compared with pure glucose.

Maintaining the Blood Glucose Level

The maintenance of a normal blood glucose level depends on two safeguards. When the level gets too low, it can be replenished by drawing on liver glycogen stores. When it gets too high, it can be corrected by siphoning off the excess into the liver, to be converted to glycogen or fat, and into muscle, to be converted to glycogen.

The correction of a too-low level has already been mentioned. The hormone epinephrine is involved in bringing about the release of glucose from liver glycogen. Other hormones also act in this manner, including some that promote the conversion of protein into glucose. However, the liver can store only half a day's worth of glycogen; then the available supply is depleted. As for protein, there is none that can be spared without cost. When body protein is used, it has to be taken from muscle, organ, or blood proteins—no surplus of protein is stored for emergencies. As for fat, you have already seen that it can't regenerate glucose.

Chapter 4 offers details of fat storage.

Obviously, when the blood glucose level falls and stores are depleted, a meal or a snack must be eaten to replenish the supply. The meal or snack you chose may require the body to protect itself against too *high* a blood glucose level.

When the blood glucose level rises, the body adjusts by storing the excess. The first organ to detect the excess glucose is the pancreas, which releases the hormone **insulin** in response. Most of the body's cells respond to insulin by taking up glucose from the blood. It has already been shown how they dispose of it—they make glycogen or fat. Thus the blood glucose level is quickly brought back down to normal as the body stores the excess.

If you eat a meal or snack that is unusually high in concentrated sugar and low in fiber, fat, or protein, your blood glucose concentration may rise too high, so that the pancreas oversecretes insulin and drives glucose into the cells too fast. Then the blood glucose level may fall too low or too fast. The effect of food on a person's blood glucose and insulin response is called the **glycemic effect**—how fast and how high the blood glucose rises, and how quickly the body responds by bringing it back to normal. Most people can quickly readjust, but people with abnormal carbohydrate metabolism should avoid foods with a strong glycemic effect.

It has long been thought that starch elicits a weaker glycemic effect than does simple sugar, but the old axiom "avoid sugar and eat starch" oversimplifies the case. The effects of different foods on blood glucose apparently depend on many factors:

- The digestibility of the starch in the food, depending partly on the form of the food (dry, paste, or liquid; coarsely or finely ground; cooked or raw).

Figure 3–3 The Breakdown of Glucose Yields Energy and Carbon Dioxide. The bonds between the carbon atoms in glucose are split apart by human-cell enzymes, liberating the energy stored there for the cell's use. The carbon atoms are combined with oxygen and released into the air, via the lungs, as carbon dioxide. Although not shown here, water is also produced at each step.

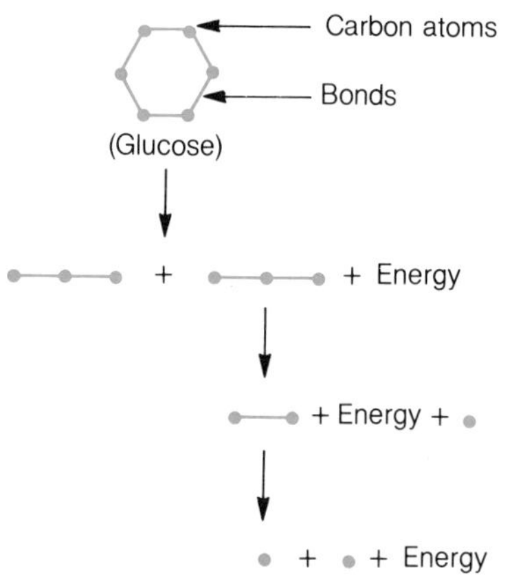

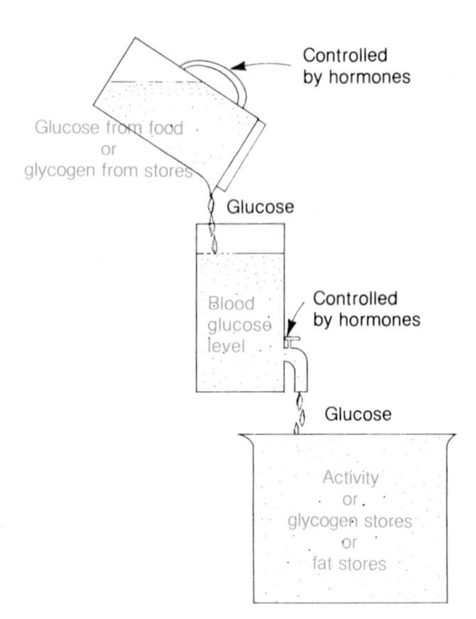

The close regulation of the blood glucose level shows how important a constant supply of glucose is to the body.

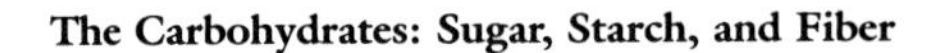

- Interactions of the starch with the protein, fat, sugar, and fiber in the food.
- The presence of other constituents, such as molecules that bind starch.

These factors work together, along with individual differences in metabolism, to determine the glycemic effect of individual foods and of whole meals, and the result is not always what a person might expect. Ice cream, for example, produces less of a response than potatoes; legumes are exceptional for slow release of glucose and have been associated with more controlled glycemic response.[11] In general, legumes produce the most even blood glucose response, dairy products next, fruits and cereals next, and pure sugar produces the greatest rise in blood glucose.

These findings might prompt you to switch to your favorite sweet goodies for lunch, but they don't really mean you should eat ice cream instead of potatoes. The glycemic effect is not the only factor to consider; ice cream is an appropriate occasional treat only for those who can handle the fat and afford the calories. More nutrient-dense choices are better for most of us, and even though most people suffer no acute effects from high-sugar foods, they may suffer long-term effects. For example, high-sugar diets may damage the lens of the eye over the years.[12]

The blood glucose level depends on hormones for its regulation. Certain carbohydrate foods are absorbed more quickly than others, producing a sudden rise in blood glucose. Eating well-spaced, carefully chosen meals can prevent rapid falls in blood glucose levels.

Converting Glucose to Fat

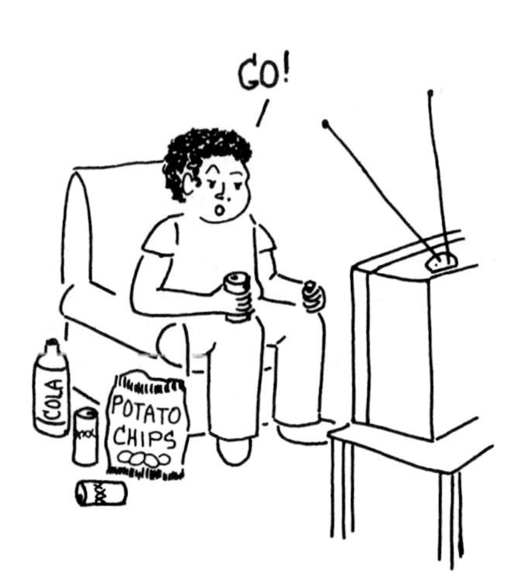

You had better play the game if you are going to eat the food.

After the glycogen stores are full and the cells' immediate energy needs are met, the body takes a third path for using carbohydrate. Say you have eaten. Now you are only sitting and watching a ball game on television, but you are eating pretzels and drinking beer. If your digestive tract is delivering glucose from the pretzels and alcohol from the beer to the liver, the liver will break the extra energy compounds into small fragments and put them together into the more permanent energy-storage compound—fat. The fat is then released, carried to the fatty tissues of the body, and deposited there. Unlike the liver cells, which can store only about half a day's worth of glycogen, the fat cells can store unlimited quantities of fat. Moral: you had better play the game if you are going to eat the food.

The story of carbohydrate turns out to be a cycle, as Figure 3–4 shows. Carbon dioxide, water, and energy are combined in plants to form glucose; the glucose may be stored in the polysaccharide starch. Then, in the body, the starch becomes glucose again, and this may be stored as the polysaccharide glycogen. Ultimately, the glucose delivers the sun's energy to fuel the body's activities; the waste products, carbon dioxide and water, are excreted to be used again by a plant.

The liver converts extra energy compounds into fat, a more permanent and less limited energy-storage compound than glycogen.

Abnormal Use of Carbohydrate

Some people have physical conditions that cause abnormal handling of carbohydrates in their bodies. Three such conditions are described here. Two are common: lactose intolerance and diabetes. The third, hypoglycemia, is rare as a true disease condition, but many people experience passing symptoms at times.

lactase: the intestinal enzyme that splits the disaccharide lactose to monosaccharides during digestion.

lactose intolerance: inability to digest lactose, due to a lack of the necessary enzyme; often sets in at age four in children of nonwhite races and makes them unable to drink milk.

Lactose Intolerance

A person can lose the ability to produce the enzyme (**lactase**) to digest lactose, the sugar of milk, during childhood or later. Thereafter, the person will experience nausea, pain, diarrhea, and excessive gas on drinking milk or eating lactose-containing products, because the intestinal bacteria will use the lactose for energy, producing gas and products that irritate the intestine. This condition, **lactose intolerance,** appears in many cases to be a racial trait, inherited by about 80 percent of the world's people—including most Africans, Greeks, and Asians. It also can develop temporarily in anyone who is malnourished or sick, making avoidance of milk and milk products temporarily necessary.

Because milk is an almost indispensable source of calcium for growth, a milk substitute must be found for a child who becomes lactose intolerant. Sometimes yogurt or cheese makes an acceptable substitute: these products contain less lactose, because the sugar is used as fuel by the bacteria that make them.

Sometimes, sensitivity to milk is due not to lactose intolerance, but to an allergic reaction to the protein in the milk. Children and adults with this problem often cannot tolerate cheese or yogurt, either, and they have to find nondairy

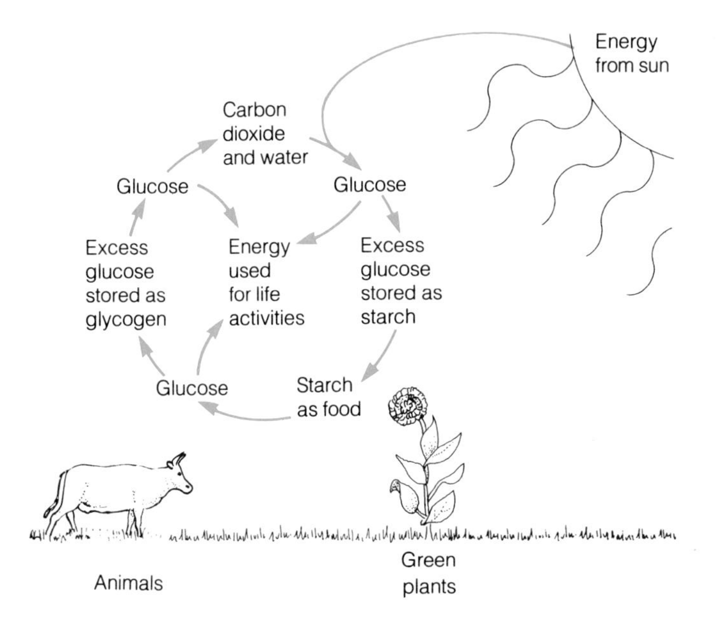

Figure 3–4 The Carbohydrate Cycle. The sun's energy is trapped by green plants and combined with carbon dioxide to make carbohydrates. Animals consume the plants, break down the carbohydrate to release the sun's energy for their use, and return the carbon, as carbon dioxide, to the air.

hypoglycemia (HIGH-po-gligh-SEEM-ee-uh): an abnormally low blood glucose concentration—below about 60 to 70 mg/100 ml (*hypo* means "too little"; *glyce* means glucose; *emia* means "in the blood"). **Reactive hypoglycemia** is a temporary symptom that may be experienced by any normal person. **Spontaneous** or **fasting hypoglycemia** is the symptom of any of several serious conditions and requires diagnosis, medical treatment, and sometimes a special diet.

calcium sources such as calcium-fortified soy milk, oysters, sardines, and legumes to compensate. Chapter 7 examines the value of milk in adult diets and discusses in more detail the problem of finding milk substitutes.

A common condition in which the body uses carbohydrate abnormally is lactose intolerance. People with lactose intolerance lack the enzyme lactase, and so are unable to properly digest the sugar in milk, leaving it available for bacterial use.

Hypoglycemia

The problem of **hypoglycemia** is not one of absorption, as is lactose intolerance, but a problem in blood glucose regulation, as the following example shows. Suppose the blood glucose falls, the glycogen reserves are exhausted, and you do *not* eat. Gradually, your body will shift into ketosis, breaking down its muscle and other proteins to feed glucose to the brain and its fat to fuel its other cells. Most times, the transition is smooth and not noticeable, but at other times, the blood glucose level may fall rapidly or below what is normal for you, and you may experience symptoms of glucose deprivation to the brain: anxiety, hunger, and dizziness. Your muscles become weak, shaky, and trembling, and your heart races in an attempt to speed more fuel to your brain. These, the symptoms of low blood glucose, sometimes called **reactive hypoglycemia,** signify that your system is out of balance. Reactive hypoglycemia is usually no cause for concern. All of us experience too-low blood glucose levels at times; and if the diagnosis of reactive hypoglycemia is correct, the treatment consists of learning to eat promptly and *properly.*

There is another type of hypoglycemia, however—**spontaneous hypoglycemia**—that requires treatment. True spontaneous hypoglycemia is a rare and often serious condition in which abnormal amounts of hormones are secreted, perhaps because of hidden tumors or other causes. As a result, the person's blood glucose is constantly too low. Also called **fasting hypoglycemia,** this condition causes symptoms of headache, confusion, fatigue, amnesia, seizures, or unconsciousness, after as little as 8 to 14 hours without food (for example, overnight). A person with spontaneous hypoglycemia urgently needs diagnosis and medical treatment.

Not only does spontaneous hypoglycemia have many possible causes, some of which are serious, but the same symptoms can arise from a multitude of other causes. For example, anything that reduces the flow of blood to the brain feels the same as glucose deprivation, because it cuts off the brain's energy supply. Poor circulation, as from heart and artery disease; poor lung function; dehydration, which lowers the blood volume; depression, which slows the metabolism; and other conditions have the same effect. Eating a large meal makes you sleepy, partly because the brain synthesizes compounds that favor sleep, and partly because the blood is routed temporarily to the digestive tract to pick up nutrients, so that less blood flows to the brain. Neither has anything to do with hypoglycemia. Some people can even bring on symptoms by simply eating a large dose of sugar. The sugar attracts large volumes of water from the bloodstream into the intestine, lowering the blood volume and causing a temporary reduction in the blood supply to the brain.

Hypoglycemia has been a popular buzz word for many decades. It is not a single entity; it is a symptom, not a disease. It may be simple and easy to avoid, or it may be a serious matter; diagnosis is properly left to a qualified health care provider, if symptoms are persistent or severe. But for anyone who has a hard time making it from one meal to the next, there can be no harm in eating balanced, sustaining meals of a kind most likely to blunt the glycemic effect—those containing adequate protein; a bit of fat; ample fluid; and abundant carbohydrate, including fiber, from vegetables, grains, fruits, and especially legumes.[13]

Everyone can experience symptoms from low blood sugar. Spontaneous hypoglycemia is a rare medical condition, brought on by disease, in which the blood glucose level is constantly too low.

diabetes (dye-uh-BEET-eez): a hereditary disease (technically, termed **diabetes mellitus**), characterized by inadequate or ineffective insulin, which renders a person unable to regulate the blood glucose level normally.

hyperglycemia (HIGH-per-gligh-SEEM-ee-uh): an abnormally high blood glucose concentration—above about 170 mg/100 ml (*hyper* means "too much"; *glyce* means "glucose"; *emia* means "in the blood").

Diabetes

Knowing how the blood glucose level is maintained, you can appreciate the problem of the person with **diabetes,** whose insulin fails to deposit blood glucose successfully into cells. Most adults with diabetes have the hereditary type, known as type II. They secrete insulin, but it is ineffective; the cells resist responding to it. Because of this characteristic, type II diabetes is named non-insulin-dependent diabetes. Often the diet of the person with type II diabetes can be adjusted to enable the body's own insulin, slow as it is, to do its work so that no insulin shots or drugs need be taken. The rarer type of diabetes—type I, or insulin-dependent diabetes—occurs in fewer than 20 percent of all cases. It involves a total lack of insulin, caused by an autoimmune response or viral infection, and it requires insulin shots.

The person with the common type of diabetes, who makes insulin but resists responding to it, tends to become obese, storing more fat than normal and being constantly hungry. This is because the liver takes up from the blood the glucose that the cells cannot take up, then converts it to fat and ships it out to the fat cells for storage. The fat cells respond—slowly, to be sure, but ultimately they store all the fat that is sent to them. Being slow to get the message that energy fuels are coming in from food, the person with diabetes is constantly hungry. Being slow to detect the presence of glucose in the blood, the person is hungry for sweets. Unfortunately, the larger the fat cells become, the more resistant they are to insulin, thus making the diabetes worse. People with diabetes in their families are urged not to get started gaining weight, for it is likely to precipitate the onset of the disease, and that will, in turn, greatly aggravate the weight gain.

The person with type I diabetes, who secretes no insulin, is likely to experience a sudden onset of the disease. Such a person may lose weight rapidly, because without insulin, the cells cannot store glucose or fat. Thus the two types of diabetes have opposite effects on body weight, one making the person fat; the other, thin.

In the person with diabetes, even if the blood glucose level rises too high (**hyperglycemia**), glucose still fails to get into cells and so stays at too high a level in the blood for an abnormally long time. The kidneys may respond by allowing some glucose to be lost in the urine—hence the myth that the person with diabetes can't handle carbohydrate. The person must only be careful to avoid concentrated sugar and eat balanced meals—providing a constant, steady, moderate flow of glucose to the bloodstream so that the body's slow responding ability will not be overwhelmed. Recent research indicates that people with

Table 3–5
The Warning Signs of Diabetes
Excessive urination and thirst
Weight loss with nausea, easy tiring, weakness, or irritability.
Craving for food, especially sweets.
Frequent infections of the skin, gums, or urinary tract.
Vision disturbances; blurred vision.
Pain in the legs, feet, or fingers.
Slow healing of cuts and bruises.
Itching.
Drowsiness.

Source: Adapted from J. M. Couric, Diabetes is a controllable disease with a growth factor, *FDA Consumer,* November 1982, pp. 21–23.

diabetes actually do best on a diet that is high in complex carbohydrate foods, especially those with plenty of fiber—as high as that recommended for any healthy person. The starch and protein in these foods help to regulate the blood glucose level, as already described.

Although the symptoms are controllable for the most part, diabetes is not to be taken lightly. The effects of the disease can be severe: disease of the feet and legs, sometimes necessitating amputation; kidney disease, sometimes requiring intensive hospital care or kidney transplant; cataracts in the eye, leading to blindness; and nerve damage. The root cause of all these conditions is the same. Diabetes causes destruction and blockage of the small arteries that feed the tissues—with effects like those of the artery disease atherosclerosis.[14] The tissues of the feet, kidneys, corneas, and other body parts die from lack of nourishment when the arteries that feed them become diseased. Diabetes is also a powerful predictor of the development of heart disease or stroke, and of conditions associated with them.[15]

Diabetes can be diagnosed by means of a glucose tolerance test, in which the body is challenged to handle a sudden large amount of glucose. After fasting overnight, the subject is fed a large, sugary drink. Four or six hours later, when blood glucose should be normal, the person with diabetes will show a blood glucose level that is still elevated. People should suspect diabetes and seek evaluation from their health care providers if they experience any of the symptoms listed in Table 3–5. For people with type II (obese type) diabetes, treatment consists of adopting eating habits and exercise to favor weight control or weight loss. Exercise also heightens tissue sensitivity to insulin. Some people must also supplement their own insulin production with insulin shots or with drugs that stimulate their own production of the hormone.

Diabetes is an example of the abnormal handling of glucose. Inadequate or ineffective insulin leaves blood glucose levels high and cells undersupplied with glucose energy, and causes blood vessel and tissue damage. Weight control is the most effective prevention for diabetes and the ills that accompany it.

Food Feature

Meeting Carbohydrate Needs

This Food Feature illustrates something the exchange system can do for you—to show you where the carbohydrates are in your meals, and how much you are getting. You can use it the same way to find fat and protein in meals by following this example.

Breads, cereals, fruits, vegetables, and milk—these are the foods noted for their contributions of valuable energy yielding carbohydrates: starches and dilute sugars. To learn how much starch and sugars these foods offer, consult the exchange lists. Carbohydrate-containing foods appear in four of the six lists; Figure 3–5 provides details.

More about the exchange lists—Chapter 2 and Appendix E.

The Milk List. A cup of milk or the equivalent is a generous contributor of carbohydrate, donating 12 grams. It also contributes high-quality protein (a point in its favor), as well as several important vitamins and minerals. (Milk products vary in fat content, an important consideration in choosing among them; Chapter 4 provides the details.) Similar to milk in these respects are the other items on the milk list:

- 1 cup buttermilk.
- 1 cup yogurt (plain).
- 1/3 cup dry milk powder.
- 1/2 cup canned evaporated milk, undiluted.

Cream and butter, although dairy products, are *not* on the milk list, because they contain little or no carbohydrate and insignificant amounts of the other nutrients important in milk. They are found on the fat list instead.

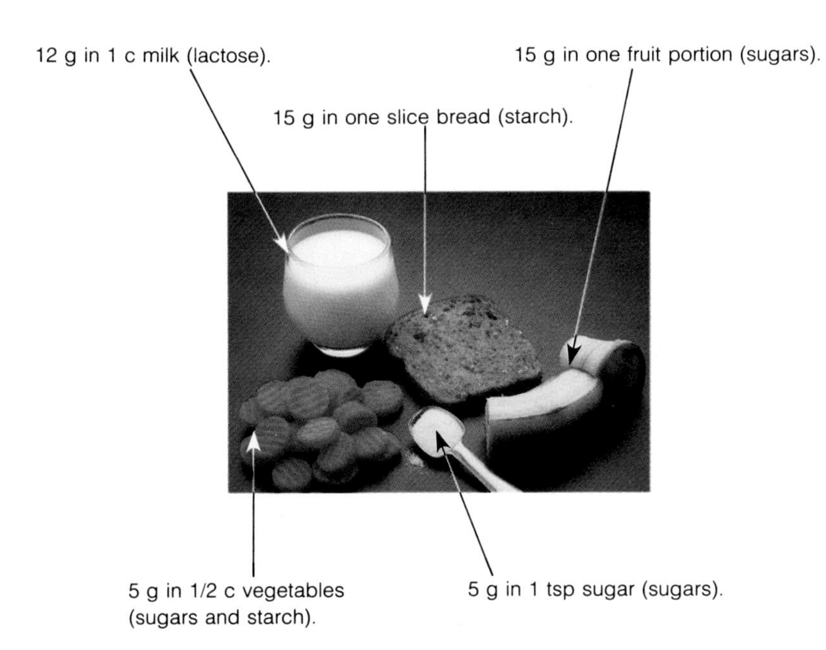

Figure 3–5 Carbohydrate in Foods. Four of the six exchange lists contain carbohydrate, so you need only know four values and learn a value for concentrated sugar (which is not on the exchange lists). The lists identify a few items that are especially high in fiber with a logo, but all whole plant foods are valuable fiber contributors if you eat enough of them.

One Exchange	Carbohydrate (g)
Milk	12
Vegetable	5
Fruit	15
Bread and starchy vegetable	15
Sugar	5
Meat	0
Fat	0

The Vegetable List. The exchange list portions of vegetables are small—only a half cup, a vestige from the days when people thought that meat should be the center of a meal and that vegetables should only decorate the plate. The opposite now seems a healthier strategy, so you are encouraged to double your servings to 1-cup portions of vegetables.

A half-cup portion of green beans or any other vegetable on this list contains 5 grams of carbohydrate as a mixture of starch and sugars. Such a portion is called a vegetable exchange. The vegetable exchanges include tomatoes, greens, okra, onions, beets, carrots, and others. Each of these foods also contributes a little protein and no fat. Some vegetables are so low in carbohydrate and calories that dieters call them "free foods." Among these are lettuce, parsley, and radishes.

For the lists of vegetable exchanges and "free foods," see Appendix E.

The Fruit List. A typical fruit portion, such as a half cup of orange juice, contains 15 grams of carbohydrate, mostly as simple sugars, including the fruit sugar, fructose. Fruits vary greatly in their water and fiber content, and therefore their sugar concentrations vary also. The portion sizes of different fruits are adjusted so that each contains 15 grams of carbohydrate. Thus you can "exchange" any fruit portion for any other without altering the amount of carbohydrate you eat. Among the fruit exchanges are one-third cup pineapple juice, one-half cup applesauce, and half of a small banana. The fruits contain insignificant amounts of fat and protein.

The Starch/Grain List. A slice of whole-wheat bread contains 15 grams of carbohydrate as starch. Equivalent foods are other breads, cereals, potatoes, rice, pasta, corn, peas, limas and other beans (legumes), and many other foods that are predominantly complex carbohydrate. Be aware that starchy vegetables such as corn and green peas actually resemble breads more closely than vegetables in their starch content. People who like breads and starchy vegetables are happy to learn that it is considered desirable to use them freely. They know that if calories are a problem, they should cut out fat, not complex carbohydrate foods. However, some foods in this group, especially baked goods such as biscuits, muffins, and snack crackers, do contain fat. Chapter 4 gives more information about the fats in foods.

For the lists of fruit exchanges and bread exchanges, see Appendix E.

Sugar. The exchange lists do not include concentrated sugar (not surprisingly, since the exchange system was originally designed for use by people with diabetes). But since we know that sweets supply carbohydrate, we need a portion size and calorie amount for them:

- 1 teaspoon brown sugar.
- 1 teaspoon molasses.
- 1 teaspoon corn syrup.
- 1 teaspoon honey.
- 1 teaspoon jam.
- 1 teaspoon jelly.
- 1 teaspoon any candy.
- 1 teaspoon maple syrup.

Each of the these teaspoons is equivalent in sugar content to a teaspoon of white sugar and can be assumed to supply about 20 calories. Most contribute less, actually, but in the case of concentrated sweets, it is better to overestimate, than to underestimate, their energy contributions, to encourage moderation in their use. (We repeated *1 teaspoon* with each item to reemphasize that each is like white sugar, in spite of many people's belief that some are different or "better.")

For a person who uses ketchup liberally, it may help to remember that a tablespoon of it contains a teaspoon of sugar. And for the soft-drink user, a 12-ounce can of a sugar-sweetened cola contains about 9 teaspoons of sugar. Controversy 3 offers more information on the sugar contents of foods.

wheat germ: the germ (see p. 76) of the wheat grain.

Carbohydrates in a Day's Meals. Chapter 2 introduced the basic tools to ensure that your diet provided at least the RDA for nutrients. There is, however, no RDA for carbohydrate, nor is there one for fiber. It is left to you to make sure that you plan to get enough.

According to dietary guidelines, people would do well to obtain about 60 percent of their daily energy from complex carbohydrate, an amount close to that in the sample diet plan of Figure 3–6 (p. 90). But the diet plan covers only 1000 of the day's total calories, and choices must be made concerning the other 600 or so calories without shortchanging the percentage from carbohydrate. Happily, fiber follows other carbohydrates into the diet. So long as the choices are made of whole foods, such as whole grains, potatoes with skins, or apples with peels, no special effort need be spent on obtaining fiber.

Does this mean that you can never eat white bread, rolls, or pancakes? Must you always choose the whole-grain types? The answer is no; you don't have to give up a favorite food, so long as the majority of such items are whole grain. An occasional white bread serving, like an occasional candy bar, will not ruin your plan for adequacy. The diet can easily supply 15 to 30 grams of dietary fiber daily. One slice of whole-grain bread, a cup of vegetables (raw or cooked), and two portions of fruit (fresh or dried) will provide 15 to 30 grams of fiber. Using the foods recommended in Table 3–4, you can plan to receive about 25 grams a day of dietary fiber. Appendix 1 lists the amounts of fiber in each of over 1000 foods.

If whole grains are new to you, start slowly. Choose breads made with a mixture of white and whole-grain flours (these appear as light tan breads with flecks of brown). Try whole-wheat crackers, breads sticks, or puffed grain cakes, which are especially easy to like. Experiment with several whole-grain breakfast cereals (the kind to which *you* add the sugar) to find one that appeals to you. One trick to add fiber and the nutrients of whole grain to your day's foods, especially if you are having trouble adjusting to whole-grain products, is to use **wheat germ** liberally in toppings, coatings, and mixed dishes, as well as on cereal. Wheat germ is rich in fiber and nutrients, but it also contains oil and so is high in calories; you might use it as a stepping stone to whole grains rather than as a permanent substitute.

Additional selections among the breads, fruits and fats will bring the total calorie level up to about 1500 with no significant change in the ratio between carbohydrate and other energy-yielding nutrients. If a person chose more meats instead (as is typical of the diet of developed nations), the fat and protein that those foods contain could easily overwhelm the carbohydrate, limiting the diet's total content of fiber and other constituents of the carbohydrate-rich foods.

Figure 3–6 displays the carbohydrate contents of the meals designated as high-nutrient density choices in Chapter 2. These foods are preferred partly because they contain abundant carbohydrate and fiber. Use the exchange system to estimate the carbohydrate content of each meal. You would estimate the cup of oatmeal as 2 breads, because one portion is a half cup of any cooked cereal.

shopping list:

- milk and milk products
- brown rice
- barley
- bulgur
- peas, carrots
- potatoes, corn
- other fresh vegetables
- dry beans
- whole-grain bread, crackers, bread sticks
- whole-grain cereal (unsweetened)
- wheat germ
- fresh fruit

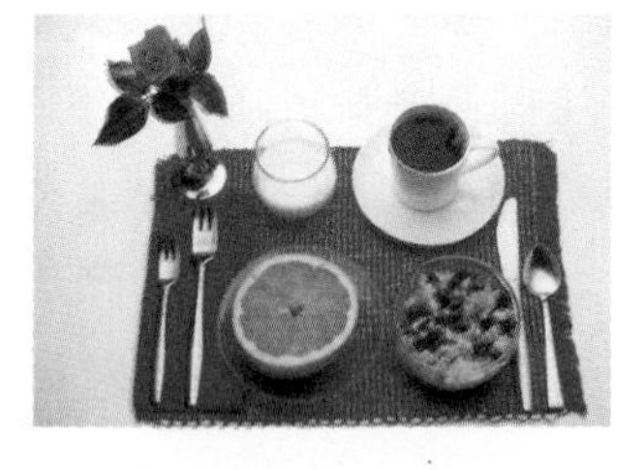

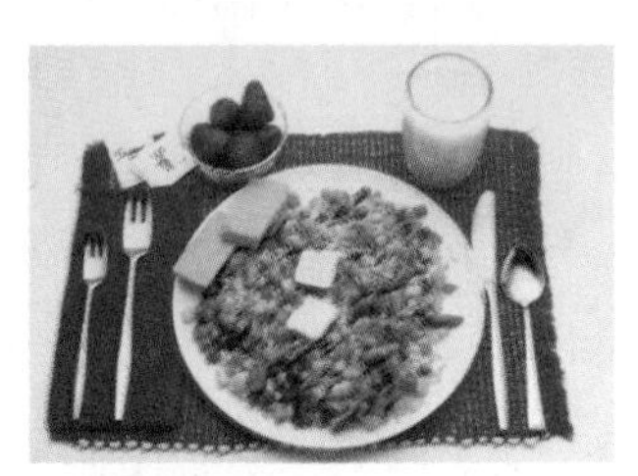

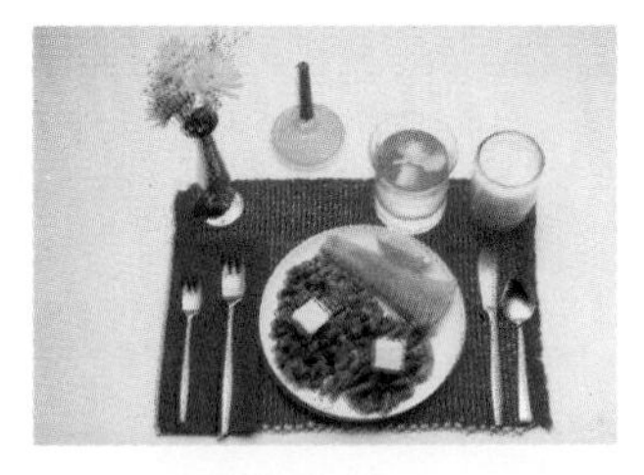

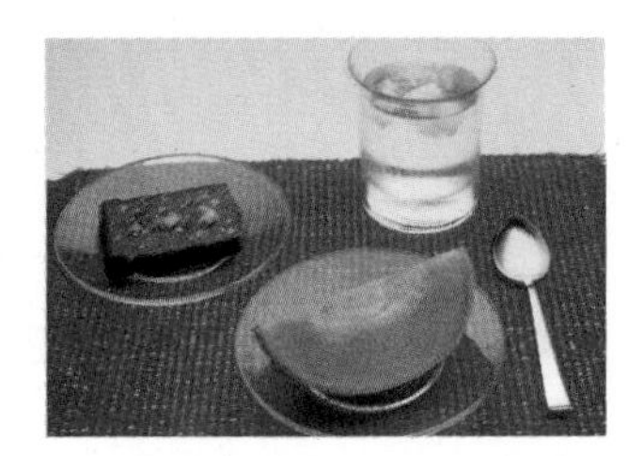

Figure 3–6

Carbohydrate and Fiber In the High-Nutrient-Density Meal Choices

		Carbohydrate (g)	Fiber (g)
Breakfast			
1 c oatmeal = 2 grain portions	=	30	9
¼ c raisins = 2 fruit portions	=	30	2
½ c nonfat milk = ½ milk portion	=	6	0
½ grapefruit = 1 fruit portion	=	15	2
		81	13
Lunch			
1 c cooked rice = 2 grain portions	=	30	3
2 c mixed vegetables might be figured as follows:			
1 c vegetables = 2 vegetable portions and	=	10	2
1 c starchy vegetables (lima beans, peas, and corn) = 2 starchy vegetables	=	30	7
2 oz cheddar cheese = 2 meat portions	=	0	0
⅔ c fresh strawberries = about 1 fruit portion	=	15	2
1 c nonfat milk = 1 milk portion	=	12	0
2 pats butter = 2 fat portions	=	0	0
2 packets sugar	=	10	0
		107	14
Dinner			
3 oz broiled fish = 3 meat portions	=	0	0
½ c green beans = 1 vegetable portion	=	5	2
½ c cooked carrots = 1 vegetable portion	=	5	2
½ c cooked peas = a starchy vegetable	=	15	8
2 pats butter = 2 fat portions	=	0	0
1 c nonfat milk = 1 milk portion	=	12	0
		37	12
Snack			
¼ cantaloupe = 1 fruit portion	=	15	1
1 brownie = 1 grain portion	=	15	0
		30	1
Day's total:	=	255	35

The quarter cup of raisins is 2 fruits, because 2 tablespoons of raisins is a fruit exchange. You have to become familiar with the exchange system before this technique saves time, but a few practice sessions are enough to make it easy to estimate carbohydrate grams. To estimate the fiber, remember that all vegetable list items donate between 2 and 3 grams per serving; Appendix A lists the specific amounts of fiber in these foods.

Carbohydrate is important, but it is only a part of the story. The next two Food Features will provide information on limiting fat and on obtaining enough, but not too much, protein.

Self-Study

Examine Your Carbohydrate Intake

Having read Chapter 3, you are in a position to study your carbohydrate intake. From the forms you filled out earlier, answer the following questions; if you need help with calculations, turn to Appendix C.

1. How many grams of carbohydrate do you consume in a day?
2. How many calories does this represent? (Remember, 1 gram of carbohydrate contributes 4 calories.)
3. It is estimated that you should have 125 grams or more of carbohydrate in a day. How does your intake compare with this minimum?
4. What percentage of your total calories is contributed by carbohydrate? You calculated this earlier, using Form 4.
5. How does this figure compare with the dietary goal that states that about 60 percent of the calories in your diet should come from carbohydrate? (Note: If you are on a diet to lose weight, then this goal does not apply to you. See the exercises in Self-Study 8, "Practice Diet Planning.")
6. Another dietary goal is that no more than 10 percent of total calories should come from refined and other processed sugars and foods high in such sugars. To assess your intake against this standard, sort the carbohydrate-containing food items you ate into three groups:

- Foods containing complex carbohydrate (foods found on the bread/starchy vegetable exchange lists).
- Nutritious foods containing simple carbohydrate (foods on the milk and fruit lists).
- Foods containing mostly concentrated simple carbohydrate (sugar, honey, molasses, syrup, jam, jelly, candy, cakes, doughnuts, sweet rolls, cola beverages, and so on).

How many grams of carbohydrate did you consume in each of these three categories? How many calories (grams times 4)? What percentage of your total calories comes from concentrated sugars? From other simple carbohydrates? Does your concentrated sugar intake fall within the recommended maximum of 10 percent of total calories?
7. Estimate how many pounds of sugar (concentrated simple carbohydrate) you eat in a year (1 pound = 454 grams). How does your yearly sugar intake compare with the estimated U.S. average of about 70 pounds per person per year?
8. You may be interested in evaluating your fiber intake as well. Compare your fiber intake with the recommendation of 25 grams of dietary fiber per day.

Notes

1. R. Levine, Monosaccharides in health and disease, *Annual Reviews of Nutrition* 6 (1986): 211–224.
2. D. A. T. Southgate, The relation between composition and properties of dietary fiber and physiological effects, in *Dietary Fiber: Basic and Clinical Aspects,* eds. G. V. Vahouny and D. Kritchevsky (New York: Plenum Press, 1986), pp. 35–48.
3. U.S. Senate, Select Committee on Nutrition and Human Needs, *Dietary Goals for the United States,* 2d ed. (Washington, D.C.: Government Printing Office, 1977).
4. W. J. L. Chen and W. J. Anderson, Hypocholesterolemic effects of soluble fiber, in *Dietary Fiber: Basic and Clinical Aspects,* eds. G. V. Vahouny and D. Kritchevsky (New York: Plenum Press, 1986), pp. 275–286.
5. J. W. Anderson, Dietary fiber in nutrition management of diabetes, in *Dietary Fiber: Basic and Clinical Aspects,* eds. G. V. Vahouny and D. Kritchevsky (New York: Plenum Press, 1986), pp. 343–360.
6. S. M. Shaheen and S. E. Fleming, High-fiber foods at breakfast: Influence on plasma glucose and insulin responses to lunch, *American Journal of Clinical Nutrition* 46 (1987): 804–811.
7. Dietary fiber reduces B-carotene utilization, *Nutrition Reviews* 45 (1987): 350–352.
8. E. Lanza and coauthors, Dietary fiber intake in the U.S. population, *American Journal of Clinical Nutrition* 46 (1987): 790–797.
9. J. L. Slavin, Dietary fiber: classification, chemical analyses, and food sources, *Journal of the American Dietetic Association* 87 (1987): 1164–1171; D. M. Klurfeld, The role of dietary fiber in gastrointestinal disease, *Journal of the American Dietetic Association* 87 (1987): 1172–1177.
10. Food and Nutrition Board, Committee on Recommended Allowances, *Recommended Dietary Allowances,* 9th ed. (Washington, D.C.: National Academy of Sciences, 1980).
11. D. J. A. Jenkins and coauthors, Simple and complex carbohydrates, *Nutrition Reviews* 44 (1986): 44–49.
12. Levine, 1986.
13. Hypoglycemia: Evolving concepts, *Nutrition and the MD,* November 1986.
14. W. H. Herman, S. M. Teutsch, and L. S. Geiss, Closing the gap: The problem of diabetes mellitus in the United States, *Diabetes Care* 8 (1985): 391–406.
15. G. L. Burke, L. S. Webber, and S. R. Srinivasan, Fasting and plasma glucose and insulin levels and their relationship to cardiovascular risk factors in children: Bogalusa heart study, *Metabolism* 35 (1986): 441–446.

Sugar and Sugar Substitutes

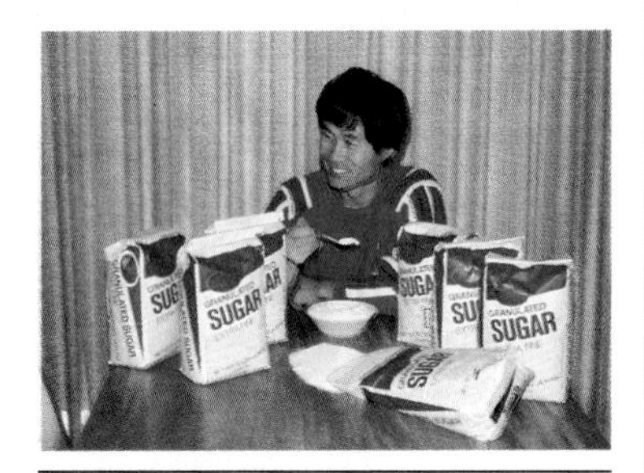

The average adult in the United States today eats 76 pounds of sugar a year.

People today are said to be eating about 70 pounds of purified sugar a year—amounting to almost a quarter of all the calories they consume (see Figure 2–5). Half of this sugar enters the diet in two major forms—as refined white sugar (sucrose) added to foods by consumers or during food processing, and as fructose in corn syrup, which is widely used by the food industry to sweeten and preserve foods.[1]* A century ago, people's intakes of sugars amounted to only 20 pounds per year, all from whole-food sources, and purified sugar was almost unknown.

Does sugar's large place in the diet harm people's health? Some people think so. In fact, sugar stands accused of causing several diseases. When they are scientifically investigated, how valid do these accusations prove to be? And if any are valid, are sugar substitutes a better choice? This Controversy addresses these questions.

*The total daily sugar intake is 95 g/day, or 21 percent of total daily calories. The total minus lactose is 80 g/day, or 18 percent of calories. This total minus naturally occurring sugars is 53 g/day, or 11 percent of calories, as calculated by The Sugars Task Force, from the 1977–1978 USDA National Road Consumption Survey data, which consisted of 3-day dietary intakes for about 30,000 individuals.

Evidence on Sugar

Sugar is thought, among other things, to (1) promote and maintain obesity, (2) cause and aggravate diabetes, (3) increase the risk of heart disease, (4) disrupt behavior in children and adults, and (5) cause dental decay and gum disease. In what respects is it guilty as charged? In what respects is it innocent?

1. Does sugar cause obesity? That is, do people who consume large amounts of sugar tend to be obese more than other people? Evidence from population studies shows that in many countries obesity rises as sugar consumption increases. But this evidence does not all point to sugar as the sole cause. Wherever sugar intake has increased, usually fat and total calorie intakes have also risen. Simultaneously, physical activity has decreased. Obesity also occurs where sugar intake is low, and fat people in many instances eat less sugar than thin people. Studies of populations do not, by themselves, make it possible to separate the effects of eating sugar from those of eating excess calories, or of exercising too little.

Concentrated sweets do make it easy for people to consume large amounts of calories fast, however, and that is why most diet plans recommend avoiding them. Some people believe that eating small amounts of sugar triggers binges; for them, conscientious sugar avoidance is an important part of weight-loss dieting.[2] For others, the inclusion of small amounts of sugar in a weight-loss plan makes the plan easier to follow.[3] In short, the effect of sugar on a person's weight depends on the user. It can be abused and lead to weight gain, or it can be used with discretion and not interfere with weight control.

2. Does sugar cause or contribute to diabetes? Recall from the chapter that diabetes is a disease (actually, several diseases) in which insulin secretion or responsivity becomes abnormal, and this, of course, affects the body's ability to manage sugar. At one time it was thought that eating sugar caused diabetes by "overstraining the pancreas," but this is now known not to be the case. Insulin-dependent (type I) diabetes, which afflicts about 20 percent of all persons with diabetes, appears to be caused or brought on by an autoimmune reaction (an attack on healthy body tissue by one's own immune system) or by a virus. Non-insulin-dependent (type II) diabetes, which is the predominant type, is clearly hereditary, and the most significant contributing factor to its onset is the development of obesity. High rates of diabetes have not been reported in any society where obesity is rare.[4] Still, it can be asked whether people with the genetic tendency to develop this type of diabetes should avoid eating sugar. The evidence on this point is conflicting and interesting.

In a number of populations around the world, as the diet has changed in the direction of increased sugar consumption, a profound increase—by as much as tenfold—in the incidence of diabetes has occurred. This has been true for the Japanese, Israelis,

Africans, Native Americans, Eskimos, Polynesians, and Micronesians. Yet in other populations, no relation has been found between sugar intake and diabetes. Wherever starch, rather than sugar, is the major carbohydrate in the diet, diabetes is rare, but this does not prove that sugar causes diabetes or that starch prevents it. The apparent protective effect of starch might be due to the chromium or fiber that comes with it, for example.

Animal experiments have also yielded conflicting evidence. Diabetes can be induced in experimental animals by feeding them diets high in fat, protein, *or* sugar, and its incidence can be reduced by lowering total food intake. From these facts, it is tempting to conclude that excess energy intake—obesity—causes diabetes; however, in some studies, diets very high in sugar bring on the disease even if the animals do not become obese.[5] One extensive and well-designed study on rats clearly implicated sugar as the cause of diabetes. In this study, one set of animals was fed a starch-based diet and the other, a similar, but sugar-based, diet. Those fed starch did not develop symptoms; those fed the sugar-based diet did.[6] The fairest conclusion that can be drawn is that obesity is a major causal factor, but that sugar has not been proven innocent as a contributor to diabetes.

One of the earliest symptoms of diabetes is excessive hunger. In the most common form of diabetes (the non-insulin-dependent type), the person typically first becomes obese. Obesity then causes resistance to insulin, and then the diabetes appears. In fact, in this type of diabetes there may be too much, rather than too little, insulin, but the tissues fail to respond to it. Both weight control and sugar avoidance have traditionally been recommended for the person who may be susceptible to diabetes.

Once a person has diabetes, is it all right to use moderate amounts of sugar? As recently as 1983, it was thought so, because sucrose-containing foods seemed to elicit no more of a glycemic response (see p. 81) in many instances than did starchy foods. The American Diabetes Association published a statement that "consumption of a modest amount of sucrose is acceptable, contingent on maintenance of metabolic control."[7] However, *other* body responses had not been looked at. Since then, researchers have shown that people with diabetes, eating a diet that contains a moderate amount of sucrose, experience many undesirable metabolic effects, among them raised blood lipid levels suggesting an increased risk of heart disease. The amount of sucrose was similar to that eaten by most U.S. citizens today, and the researchers concluded that for people with diabetes, this was too much.[8] Not all researchers agree; perhaps if the diet is low enough in fat and high enough in fiber, some sugar will do no harm.[9] The jury is still out on this question.

3. Does eating sugar raise the risk of heart disease? Logic says that sugar, turned to fat and transported through the bloodstream, might cause the sort of fat deposits in the arteries that are known to lead to heart disease. (More about heart disease appears in Controversy 4.) There is a hereditary condition, in 10 to 20 percent of the population, characterized by carbohydrate sensitivity. People with this condition tend to develop raised blood lipid levels in response to carbohydrate and alcohol in their diets, and the blood lipid pattern is associated with heart disease. If the risk seems high, they are told to restrict their intakes of carbohydrate and alcohol.[10] Some research has appeared to indicate that the blood lipid response is especially marked after these people eat the sugar fructose—or sucrose, which contains it.[11] However, this sensitivity may apply to complex, as well as to simple, carbohydrate. The foods to avoid are those that elicit the greatest glycemic response, and they are sometimes sugary, sometimes starchy, foods.[12]

Sugar may also have a relationship to high blood pressure, which contributes to heart disease. From studies of rats and monkeys, it appears that animals retain sodium when they are fed sucrose, and that this raises their blood pressure. From studies of people, it is known that human beings excrete large amounts of sodium and water at first, if they fast or restrict their carbohydrate intakes. When they resume eating carbohydrate (glucose, sucrose, or especially fructose), it causes them to regain both sodium and water.[13] However, the hormonal regulation of our fluid balances quickly adjusts to different carbohydrate intakes, and within a few days, the effect on blood pressure is gone. Such transient fluctuations in blood pressure are different from the dangerous, sustained hypertension associated with heart disease. A high-sugar diet does not cause a significant sustained increase in blood pressure in healthy subjects.[14]

Heart and artery disease generally correlates much more closely with obesity and fat intake than with sugar intake (see Controversy 4). High blood pressure in particular responds to sodium, several other minerals, and obesity more sensitively than to sugar (see Controversy 7). Animal experiments implicating sugar in heart and artery disease have used diets so high in sugar that the results may not reflect effects of people's real sugar intakes. No one has shown conclusively, throughout many years of research, that moderate amounts of sugar (10 to 20 percent of total calories) affect the disease process in human beings.

4. What about sugar and behavior? In the 1970s and early 1980s, many claims appeared that eating sugary foods caused children to become unruly and adolescents and adults to exhibit antisocial and even criminal behavior.[15] Sugar has been called a toxin and an addictive drug, and people have been warned that their lives would be destroyed if they allowed themselves or their children to consume it. A nationally publicized criminal defense was even won on the argument that the defendant was in the habit of eating junk food, notably Twinkies. It was argued that, under the influence of sugar, the accused had become hypoglycemic, and therefore not responsible for his actions. Is there any truth this or other claims that sugar can adversely affect behavior?

The idea that nutrition influences behavior is a popular one. There are many ways in which it might do so—by altering the levels of chemicals in the brain that affect mood, by delivering substances to which people are allergic, by way of nutrient deficiencies, and others. The relationships of nutrition, including carbohydrate nutrition, with behavior and mood are reviewed in Controversy 13, but the specific relationship of sugar to behavior is dealt with here. It has been proposed, specifically, that sugar adversely affects behavior by altering brain function. The brain is dependent on blood glucose for its energy, and according to the logic used by proponents of the sugar-behavior idea, eating sucrose causes wide fluctuations in blood glucose level, with frequent hypoglycemia and resultant irrational and violent behavior.

These ideas have generated a proliferation of research, all of which has yielded negative, or at most inconclusive, results. Some reports have simply not been based on valid researchtechniques (using hair analysis, for example, to diagnose hypoglycemia). One study claimed to show that abnormal glucose tolerance occurred at a higher-than-normal frequency among violent offenders, but it failed to take into account the probability that many of them were long-term alcohol abusers, a factor known to produce abnormal glucose tolerance test results.[16]

One careful study compared the seven-day spontaneous sugar intakes and behavior of 26 normal children with those of 28 hyperactive children. It was widely misinterpreted to show that sugar caused children to be hyperactive and aggressive, but it did not. Both groups of children, given free choice of how much sugar to consume, chose intakes in the same range. Among the normal children, the more active ones ate more sugar. Among the hyperactive children, a difference in overall activity level between low and high sugar consumers was not seen, but the higher sugar consumers were more aggressive. It was impossible to show whether the sugar intake was a cause or a result of the behavior. In the normal children, two conclusions were equally possible: either "the more active children tended to eat more sugar" or "the more sugar they ate, the more active they were." Similarly, in the hyperactive children, either "the more aggressive children tended to demand and receive more sugar" or "the more sugar they ate, the more aggressive they were."[17]

In another study using 13 children hospitalized for psychiatric disorders, researchers gave the children either orange juice or juice sweetened with pure sucrose or fructose. The children given the sugar-added drinks became more active and exhibited more inappropriate behavior, but the researchers critiqued their own study, saying that it showed only that added calories permit children to exert more energy, not that sugar, specifically, has a negative effect on behavior.[18] They made a follow-up attempt to demonstrate that a high sucrose intake tended to make children distractible, but they again critiqued their own study, showing other possible reasons for the weak, but apparently real, relationship they found.[19]

Clearly, though, sugary food, like any energy-containing food, will enable children to do more of whatever they do, including misbehave. The "Halloween effect" is an example: tired children, overstimulated by the excitement of costumery and late-night gallivanting, may act up afterward. Sugar has been accused of making them do so, but this has not been proven. It is more likely and more reasonable to suppose that sugar simply gives them the energy to do so.

In contrast to these inconclusive studies, one well-controlled study has shown that sugar calms children down, a finding consistent with convincing biochemical evidence. The subjects used were 21 boys whose parents described them as behaving badly after eating sugar. The study was designed to keep the parents' and the boys' expectations from influencing the results; none of them were told whether the boys were receiving glucose, sucrose, or a substitute (saccharin). The behavioral and physiological tests performed during the five hours following showed clearly that the boys were significantly *less* active after receiving the sugar than the substitute.[20] A follow-up study, using glucose, sucrose, saccharin, and aspartame in preschool children, showed no differences in activity, school performance, or emotional state in response to the four substances.[21]

Other studies have similarly failed to demonstrate any effects of sucrose on behavior, either in normal or hyperactive children.[22] One analysis showed a difference between sugar and a substitute in only one of 37 different measures, with children performing *better* on the sugar day.[23]

In the midst of all these inconclusive reports, one case stands out, in which a hyperactive boy was found to become irritable, hyperactive, and headachy when he received a sugary drink, but not when he received the same drink artificially sweetened. The physician tested in the same way the next 50 hyperactive children he saw but found no other cases in which this sensitivity to sucrose showed up.[24] In conclusion, very occasional behavioral reactions to sugar are not unheard of, but that sugar directly affects behavior adversely in most children or adults has been ruled out. That it has an effect indirectly, by displacing needed nutrients and contributing to malnutrition, is a real possibility (see Chapter 12).

5. Does sugar cause **dental caries**? Caries are a serious public health problem, afflicting nearly everyone in the country, half of them by the time they are two years old. One of the most successful measures taken to reduce the incidence of dental decay is fluoridation of community water (see Chapter 7), but sugar has something to do with dental caries, too.

Caries are actually caused by the acid by-product of bacterial growth in the mouth. Bacteria establish colonies known as **plaque** whenever they can get a foothold on tooth surfaces, and they multiply and affix themselves more and more firmly unless they are brushed, flossed, or scraped away. The acid they release as they grow erodes tooth surfaces, creating pits that deepen into cavities. Below the gum line, plaque works its way down until it erodes the roots of teeth and the jawbone they are embedded in, loosening the teeth and infecting the gums. Gum disease severe enough to threaten tooth loss afflicts 95 percent of our population by their later years.[25]

Bacteria thrive on food particles, especially if they contain carbohydrate, and so it is logical to implicate sugar as the cause of cavities. However, any carbohydrate, including starch, can support bacterial growth if the bacteria are allowed sufficient time to work on it.[26] Of prime importance is the length of time the food stays in your mouth, and this depends both on how sticky the food is and on whether you brush your teeth after eating it. Thus an "all-day" taffy bar, constantly bathing the teeth in sticky carbohydrate, sets the stage for cavity formation, while the same amount of sugar in a different form, say a cereal that is quickly swallowed and removed from contact with the bacteria of the mouth. Milk or water drunk with a meal will help wash the carbohydrate off the teeth. One large and well-controlled two-year study (979 children) showed that presweetened cereals eaten for breakfast did not increase cavities, probably because they were eaten at mealtimes and with milk.[27] Mechanically disturbing bacteria by flossing every 24 hours may effectively prevent formation of cavities, regardless of the carbohydrate content of the diet. And some people may *never* get cavities because they have inherited resistance to them. Thus in this matter, as in the others, sugar may not be the extreme villain that some have made it out to be. Still, it is clear that sugar is the best energy source for the bacteria that cause tooth decay, and that when eaten continuously over several hours or in a sticky form, it is guilty as charged.[28]

A personal strategy with respect to sugar might well involve substituting **artificial sweeteners** for it. However, before deciding whether to do so, the consumer must examine the evidence on their health effects.

Evidence on Artificial Sweeteners

The big three synthetic sweeteners are **saccharin, cyclamate,** and **aspartame** (see *Miniglossary of Artificial Sweeteners*). Saccharin has been around since before 1900, and it dominated the market except for a brief two decades, the 1950s and 1960s, when cyclamate was in wide

Miniglossary of Artificial Sweeteners

aspartame: a dipeptide with a methyl group attached, that is 200 times sweeter than sucrose. Being composed of amino acids, it has 4 cal/g, as does protein, but because so little is used as a sweetener, it is virtually calorie-free. In tabletop form it is mixed with lactose, however, so a 1-g packet contains 4 cal. Used in both the United States and Canada.

cyclamate: a 0-cal sweetener used in Canada but banned in the United States.

saccharin: a 0-cal sweetener used in the United States but banned in Canada.

use. Aspartame was approved by the FDA in 1981 and rapidly gained ascendancy over saccharin.[29]

Saccharin, used for nearly 100 years in the United States, is used primarily in soft drinks and secondarily as a tabletop sweetener. From the start, its safety has been questioned. The controversy over its use came to a head in 1977, when experiments showed that at high doses, saccharin caused bladder tumors in rats. As a result of those studies, the FDA proposed banning it. The public outcry in favor of retaining saccharin was so loud, however, that Congress placed a moratorium on any action, and the moratorium has since been repeatedly renewed. Products containing saccharin are required to carry the warning label, now familiar to all consumers of diet beverages; "use of this product may be hazardous to your health. This product contains saccharin which has been determined to cause cancer in laboratory animals."

Does saccharin really cause cancer? The evidence that it does so in animals is as follows. When male and female rats are fed diets containing saccharin from the time of weaning to adulthood and then mated, and their offspring are also fed saccharin throughout life, the offspring have a higher incidence of bladder tumors than comparable animals not fed saccharin. The question was raised for a while whether an impurity present in the commercial saccharin used in the tests might be causing the tumors, but it was clearly shown that the saccharin itself was responsible.[30] On the basis of these findings and in the face of public outcry as loud as that in the United States, Canada banned all uses of saccharin except as a tabletop sweetener to be sold in pharmacies, and it permits those sales only with a warning label.

Saccharin has not been shown conclusively to cause cancer in human beings. Three large-scale population studies were completed in 1980. One, involving 9000 people, showed a distinctly greater risk of cancers in some groups, such as women who drank two or more diet sodas a day and people who both smoked heavily and used artificial sweeteners habitually. Another study involving over 1000 people showed little or no excess risk of bladder tumors, but of course it could not conclude that there was no risk at all. Two alternative conclusions seemed possible:

1. Saccharin causes tumors in rats but not in people.
2. Saccharin is a weak carcinogen in people, and its effects will take more years of exposure, or perhaps several generations, to become apparent.

A 1985 review of all the evidence from experiments and population studies indicated that the first alternative was the more likely, and that saccharin was not associated with an increased risk of bladder cancer in human beings.[31]

Cyclamate has had a shorter life than saccharin, dominating the artificial sweetener market for only 20 years. The 1970 U.S. ban on its use, although repeatedly appealed, has been continued even though, like saccharin, cyclamate has never been conclusively proven guilty of causing cancer in human beings. In Canada, on the other hand, where saccharin is banned, cyclamate is still in legal use.

As for aspartame, within only a few years of receiving the FDA's final approval, it has appeared in dozens of familiar food products and in some totally new ones as well. Worldwide, people have gratefully accepted aspartame as NutraSweet in diet drinks, chewing gum, presweetened cereal, pudding, children's medications, and other commercial products, and as Equal, a powder to use at home in place of sugar. As of 1984, aspartame sales had already surpassed the sales of saccharin and were also encroaching on sugar sales in some markets.

This amazing popularity is mostly due to aspartame's flavor, which is almost identical to that of sugar. Another lure is the hope that aspartame may be completely harmless, unlike the other sweeteners whose laboratory records are tarnished. Too, aspartame is touted as safe for children, so families wishing to limit sugar are turning to it. Finally, as a sweet-toothed, overweight population, we perceive sugar substitutes as our only way to cheat the scales.

Aspartame is a simple chemical compound: two amino acids, phenylalanine and aspartic acid, joined together (see *dipeptide* in Chapter 5). One of the two carries an extra chemical detail, a methyl group. In the digestive tract, the two amino acids are split apart, absorbed, and used to build protein or burned for energy, just as they would be if they had come from protein in food. The methyl group becomes methanol, an alcohol. The flavors of the components give no clue to the combined effect; one of the amino acids tastes bitter, and the other is tasteless. But aspartame is incredibly sweet—200 times sweeter than sucrose.

Many safety concerns about aspartame have been raised, studied, and resolved to the satisfaction of the FDA. Among them: phenylalanine enters the brain and participates in the transmission of nerve impulses (see *neurotransmitter* in Controversy 13). Might the amounts of phenylalanine contributed by aspartame alter brain balances in subtle ways—especially in the long-term user?

Some people report headaches after using aspartame, although research has found no association.[32] Another question: methanol is produced as metabolism of aspartame proceeds: is there enough to cause harm? Another question: some people, without knowing it, carry one gene for the hereditary disease **PKU (phenylketonuria)**. People with two genes have the disease and cannot metabolize the phenylalanine part of aspartame; it can build up to possibly toxic levels in their bodies. Might people with one PKU gene be subtly harmed by aspartame? These questions have been answered no: the amount of aspartame consumed is below the threshold at which any of these effects would occur.

The FDA has approved aspartame based on the assumption that no one will consume more than 50 milligrams per kilogram of their body weight in a day.[33] People with both genes for PKU have a special warning to limit their intakes. Table C3–1 presents the aspartame contents of some frequently-used foods.

The maximum intake of 50 milligrams per kilogram of body weight, assumed by the FDA, is a lot. For a 132-pound person, it adds up to about 80 packets of Equal, or about 15 soft drinks, sweetened with aspartame only. The company that produces aspartame estimates that if all the sugar and saccharin in the U.S. diet were replaced with aspartame, 1 percent of the population would be consuming the FDA maximum. Some people actually do consume this amount, however. A child who drinks a quart of aspartame-sweetened beverage on a hot day and who has pudding, chewing gum, cereal, and other products with aspartame that day, too, might pack in more than the FDA maximum level. In practice, it is currently impossible for consumers to know for sure how much aspartame they or their children are taking in because labeling laws do not require quantities of aspartame to be specified. They require only that the label lists aspartame among its ingredients.

The newsletter for physicians *Nutrition and the MD* states that it is not known whether aspartame is safe for children under two years old, and it points out that there are "very few if any reasons to use a sugar substitute in infants and young children."[34] Until aspartame has been around for a longer time, it would be best not to let infants be unwitting testers of aspartame's safety. But for adults, it seems that a daily intake of several packets of aspartame or several servings of food or beverages sweetened with it is acceptable. This would take part of the burden of providing sweetness off sugar, and part of the

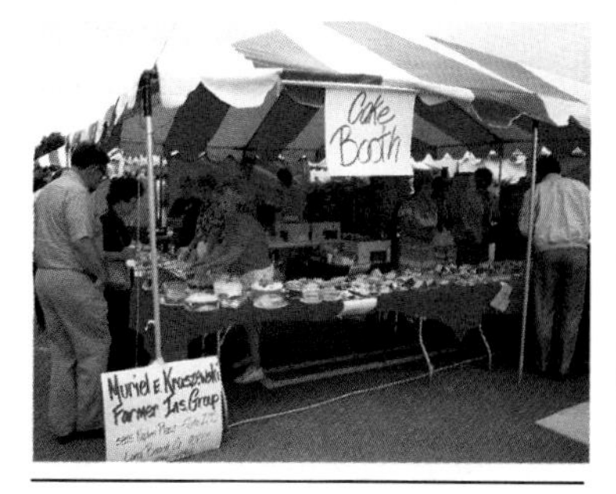

People love sugar, and if it is used appropriately, it can be a delightful addition to the diet.

Table C3–1

Approximate Aspartame Content in Food and Drug Administration Approved Categories

Product Category	Serving Size	Aspartame (mg)
Equal® Low-Calorie Sweetner	1 packet	35
Equal® Low-Calorie Sweetner	1 tablet	19
Carbonated beverage	12 oz	180
Gelatin dessert	4 oz	95
Powdered soft drink	8 oz	120
Hot chocolate	6 oz	50
Pudding dessert	4 oz	25
Cereal	1 c	55
Frozen confection/novelty	2½ oz bar	50
Fruit-flavored drink, 10% fruit juice	6 oz	70
Fruit juice drink, 60% fruit juice	6 oz	23
Tea	8 oz	80
Breath mint	1 mint	1.5
Vitamin	1 vitamin	4

Note: For specific information regarding individual products, contact the manufacturer. Exact formulation differ with each manufacturer and are proprietary.

Source: The NutraSweet Company, 1987, with permission. NutraSweet and The NutraSweet symbol are registered trademarks of the NutraSweet Company for its brand of sweetening ingredient. These data are not to be reprinted or distributed unless permission is granted by the NutraSweet Company. Equal® is a registered trademark of NutraSweet Consumer Products, Inc. for its brand of sweetener.

burden of consuming calories off the consumer, as well.

Evidence on Sugar Alcohols

Another alternative to using sugar and its relatives is to use alternative caloric sweetener—**sugar alcohols** such as **mannitol, sorbitol, xylitol,** or **maltitol.** These carbohydrates are either absorbed more slowly or metabolized differently than the sugars and so may be used by people who wish to limit their intake of ordinary sugars. Products made with sugar alcohols are labeled "sugar-free," but the sugar alcohols contain calories, just as many per gram as sucrose. Thus, for the person who is counting calories, they count. Also, the sugar alcohols can, by their prolonged presence in the digestive system, bring on diarrhea in some people. They do offer an advantage, though: they are considerably less supportive of oral bacterial growth, and they may even suppress it. Xylitol, in particular, has been reported to help *prevent* caries formation. It not only does not support cavity-producing bacteria; it actually inhibits their growth.[35]

Personal Strategy

Concentrated sugar is new in the human environment, and we are not biologically adapted to cope with it. It has been estimated that over a third of the calories in our diet now come from sugars and visible fats, and sugar is our number one additive today. Our consumption of it is not entirely voluntary; two-thirds of the sugar we eat comes already added to foods during processing.[36] To reduce such a high intake to half or less of the present level would surely do no harm and might well do some good.

Sugar does have its uses, however, so it makes no sense to try to omit it entirely. By tying up water, it serves as a preservative in foods such as jams and jellies. It provides tenderness and bulk in baked goods; artificial sweeteners cannot substitute for it in this role. It provides the fuel for fermentation processes used in creating the special flavors of many foods.[37] Al-

Miniglossary of Sugars and Sugar Alcohols

Note: These are terms that indicate the presence of simple sugars or sugar alcohols. All of these are about the same in energy value: 4 cal/g.

brown sugar: white sugar to which molasses has been added, about 95% pure sucrose.

confectioner's sugar: finely powdered sucrose, 99.9% pure.

corn sweeteners: corn syrup and sugar solutions derived from corn.

corn syrup: a syrup, mostly glucose, partly maltose, produced by the action of enzymes on cornstarch. **High-fructose corn syrup** (**HFCS**) may contain as little as 42% or as much as 90% fructose; dextrose and maltose make up the balance of the carbohydrates.

dextrose: an older name for glucose.

fructose, galactose, glucose: the monosaccharides (see Chapter 3).

granulated sugar: common table sugar, crystalline sucrose, 99.9% pure.

honey: a concentrated solution primarily composed of glucose and fructose produced by enzymatic digestion, by bees, of the sucrose in nectar.

invert sugar: a mixture of glucose and fructose formed by the splitting of sucrose in an industrial process. Sold only in liquid form, sweeter than sucrose, invert sugar forms during certain cooking procedures and works to prevent crystallization of sucrose in soft candies and sweets.

lactose, maltose, sucrose: the disaccharides (see Chapter 3).

levulose: an older name for fructose.

maltitol, mannitol, sorbitol, xylitol: sugar alcohols, chemical relatives of the sugars, which can be derived from fruits or produced from glucose; absorbed and metabolized differently from sugar in the human body, and not utilized by ordinary mouth bacteria.

maple sugar: a concentrated solution of sucrose derived from the sap of the sugar maple tree—mostly sucrose. Although once a common sweetener, this sugar is rarely added to foods and is commonly replaced by sucrose and artificial maple flavoring.

molasses: a syrup left over from the refining of sucrose from sugar cane; a thick, brown syrup. The major nutrient in molasses is iron, a contaminant from the machinery used in processing it.

natural sweeteners: a term used freely, without legal definition, to refer to any sugar or sweetener except refined sucrose.

raw sugar: crystals that form from concentrated sugar cane juice during the first evaporation; the first crop of crystals harvested during sugar processing, tan or brown because it contains impurities, including small amounts of vitamins and minerals. (White sugar—sucrose—is produced by redissolving these crystals, concentrating the solution, and letting purer crystals form.)

sugar: on a food label, this term means sucrose. See also p. 70.

though sugar is not an essential nutrient, it is certainly not a poison, as some hysterical headline makers have made it out to be.

Sugar is valuable to some people precisely because it is a delicious, concentrated source of calories. After all, although many people in our society need to lose weight, some need to gain, and sugary treats can be useful in a weight-gain effort. Sugar is also an acceptable source of some of the energy an athlete needs for an endurance event, although starch seems to enable the athlete to store more glycogen in muscle than a comparable amount of sugar.[38] Sugar is also, sometimes, the most suitable carbohydrate for use in sparing protein. For example, nutritionists recommend feeding Popsicles and hard candy to children with kidney disease to ensure that they don't waste protein by using it for needed energy.[39]

Sugar does, however, displace nutrients from the diet. Purified, refined white sugar—sucrose—contains no other nutrients—protein, vitamins, or minerals—and so can be termed an empty-calorie food. As Table C3–2 shows, if you choose 400 calories of sugar in place of 400 calories of starchy food like potatoes, you lose not only the starch, but also the vitamins, minerals, and fiber of the potatoes. You can afford to do this only if you have already met your nutrient needs for the day and still have calories to spend.

The point is that sugar can contribute to malnutrition by displacing nutrients from the diet. This is especially likely in the person who eats very large quantities of sugar, and in the person who eats too few calories to have room to spare for sugar. It is theoretically possible, with judicious food selection, to obtain all the needed nutrients within an allowance of about 1500 calories. A teenage boy can use up to 4000 calories a day, and if he eats some very nutritious foods first, then even the "empty calories" of sweets are useful to him. But many teenage girls or older people can eat only 1200 calories or even less without gaining weight, so they need nutrient-dense foods. Many teenage girls and other members of our population obtain too few nutrients, and to the extent that they use high-sugar (or other empty-calorie) foods to meet their energy needs, those foods can be said

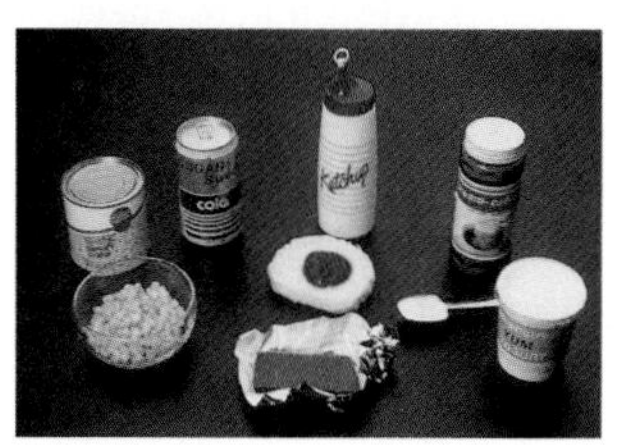

5 oz canned corn = 3 tsp sugar.
12 oz cola = 9 tsp sugar.
1 tbsp ketchup = 1 tsp sugar.
1 tbsp creamer = 2 tsp sugar.
8 oz yogurt = 7 tsp sugar.
2 oz chocolate = 8 tsp sugar.

Processed foods contain surprisingly large amounts of sugar.

Table C3–2

The Empty Calories of Sugar

Food	Energy (cal)	Protein (g)	Fiber (g)	Calcium (mg)	Iron (mg)	Magnesium (mg)	Potassium (mg)	Zinc (mg)	Vitamin A (RE)	Thiamin (mg)	Riboflavin (mg)	Niacin (mg)	Vitamin B_6 (mg)	Folacin (mg)	Vitamin C (mg)
Sugar (1 tbsp)	45	0	0	0	0	0	0	0	0	0	0	0	0	0	0
Honey (1 tbsp)	65	0	0	1	0.1	0	11	0.0	0	0	0	0.1	0	2	0
Toasted wheat germ (1 tbsp)	27	2	0.2	3	0.5	22	39	1	0	0.1	0.1	0.4	0.1	29	0
Potato (5 oz)	119	3	3.2	7	0.4	30	515	0.4	0	0.1	0	2.0	0.4	14	18
Cola beverage (12 fl oz)	151	0	0	9	0.1	3	4	0.1	0	0	0	0	0	0	0
% U.S. RDA	—	56	—	1	18.0	400	—	15	1000	1.5	1.7	20	2.0	400	60

At first glance, honey looks more nutritious than sugar, but when compared with a person's nutrient needs, neither contributes anything to speak of. The cola beverage is clearly an empty-calorie item, too. Wheat germ, though, offers some nutrients in a reasonable number of calories, and the potato is a nutritious food. Data from Appendix A, insignificant amounts rounded to zero.

to be contributing to their malnutrition. The solution is not to focus on the negative and say "Don't eat sugar!" but to focus on the positive: "Eat these nutritious foods, exercise more so that you can eat more food, and use sugar only to decorate your diet."

What about using a product such as blackstrap molasses in place of white sugar? Blackstrap molasses contains over 3 milligrams of iron per tablespoon and so, if used frequently, can make a major contribution of this important and, for women, hard-to-get nutrient. It is less sweet than the other sweeteners, however, and so does not satisfy the sweet tooth of people who like sugar. Also, its iron comes from the iron machinery in which the molasses is made: it is a salt not easily absorbed by the body. Most iron supplements would be at least equally absorbable, and could give more iron without the calories.

What about substituting raw or brown sugar or honey for white sugar? These sugars are virtually empty of nutrients. It would be absurd to rely on any of them for nutrient contributions, because one would have to eat so much to obtain significant amounts. Rather than go to the extreme of eating large quantities of any sweetener, it makes sense to ensure that the diet is otherwise adequate and then use sugar in moderation, if at all, for its taste appeal. You might then choose molasses, brown sugar, or honey correctly, not for its nutrient contributions but for the pleasure it gives. Other tricks to get the most sweetness for the calories:

- Serve sweet food warm (heat augments the perception of sweet taste).
- Add sweet spices such as cinnamon, nutmeg, allspice, or cloves.
- Add a tiny pinch of salt; it will enhance a food's sweetness.
- Try reducing the sugar added to recipes by one-third; this amount usually has little or no effect on the finished product except to diminish calorie content.

For the sake of our dental health, it seems sensible to partially substitute artificial and alternative sweeteners for sugar. Combining the recommendations of the *Dietary Guidelines for Americans* with those of authorities concerned about reducing the incidence of dental caries, we find that these suggestions best meet all needs:

- Learn to enjoy the natural sweetness of whole foods—fruits, melons, and berries. You'll be eating sugars, but in smaller quantities, and you'll get more nutrients with them.
- Use all concentrated sugars in small quantities, including white sugar, brown sugar, raw sugar, honey, and syrups.
- Eat limited amounts of foods containing added sugars—foods such as candy, soft drinks, ice cream, cakes, and cookies.
- Select fresh fruits, or fruits canned without sugar or in light syrup rather than heavy syrup.
- Use sugar substitutes that don't cause dental caries in place of sucrose and glucose in some foods, especially in snacks.
- Read food labels for clues on sugar content—if the names *sucrose, glucose, maltose, dextrose, fructose,* or *syrups* appear first, or if several appear anywhere on the ingredient list, then the food probably contains a large amount of sugar.
- For snacks between meals, use sugar-free foods and beverages. Remember, how frequently you eat sugar is as important as, and perhaps more important than, how much sugar you eat.

Miniglossary

artificial sweeteners: sugar substitutes such as saccharin, cyclamate, and aspartame (see Miniglossary of Artificial Sweeteners). Most people understand the term to refer to *noncaloric* or *nonnutritive* sweeteners, and that is how it is used in this book.

dental caries: decay of the teeth (*caries* means "rottenness").

plaque (PLACK): a mass of microorganisms and their resultant deposits on the crowns and roots of the teeth, a forerunner of dental caries and gum disease. (The term *plaque* is used in another connection—arterial plaque in atherosclerosis. See Chapter 4 and Controversy 4.)

PKU (phenylketonuria): the inherited inability to dispose of the amino acid phenylalanine when it is eaten in excess of the need for building proteins, a condition that can lead to severe brain damage and mental retardation, if not caught and treated early in infancy.

sugar alcohols: chemical relatives of the sugars (see Miniglossary of Sugars and Sugar Alcohols). They are *caloric,* or *nutritive,* sweeteners, as are the sugars; their energy content amounts to 4 cal per gram.

sugars: monosaccharides and disaccharides, as described in Chapter 3. See separate Miniglossary of Sugars and Sugar Alcohols.

■ To get children started right, omit sugar from baby foods.

■ Choose sweet foods that are not sticky or pasty, so that they will linger less long in the mouth. Buying these foods will encourage the food industry to modify the textures of sugar-containing foods to make them less likely to cause tooth decay.

Finally, enjoy whatever sugar you do eat. Sweetness is one of life's great sensations, and you need not forego it completely. The person who cares about nutrition and loves sweets can artfully combine the two by using moderate amounts of sugar with creative imagination to enhance the flavors of nutritious foods.

Notes

1. W. H. Glinsman, H. Irausquin, and Y. K. Park, *Evaluation of Health Aspects of Sugars Contained in Carbohydrate Sweeteners: Report of Sugars Task Force, 1986,* Divisions of Nutrition and Toxicology, Center for Food Safety and Applied Nutrition, Food and Drug Administration, 200 C Street, S.W., Washington, DC 20204.
2. M. A. Gannon and J. E. Mitchell, Subjective evaluation of treatment methods by patients treated for bulimia, *Journal of the American Dietetic Association* 86 (1986): 520–521.
3. D. K. Cowley and F. S. Sizer, *Fad Diets: Fact and Fiction?* (a 1987 monograph in the *Nutrition Clinics* series available from Stickley Publishing Co., 210 Washington Square, Philadelphia, PA 19106).
4. K. M. West, Prevention and therapy of diabetes mellitus, in *Nutrition Reviews' Present Knowledge in Nutrition,* 4th ed. (Washington, D.C.: Nutrition Foundation, 1976), pp. 356–364.
5. West, 1976.
6. A. M. Cohen, High sucrose intake as a factor in the development of diabetes and its vascular complications, in U.S. Senate, Select Committee on Nutrition and Human Needs, *Dietary Sugar and Disease* (hearings) (Washington, D.C.: Government Printing Office, 1973), pp. 167–198.
7. A. M. Coulston, How safe is sucrose for patients with NIDDM? *Nutrition and the M.D.,* January 1987, p. 1.
8. Coulston, 1987.
9. D. B. Peterson and coauthors, Sucrose in the diet of diabetic patients—Just another carbohydrate? *Diabetologia* 29 (1986): 216–220, as cited by *Modern Medicine,* October 1986, pp. 117, 120.
10. Nutritionists say reevaluation of sucrose "appears to be warranted," *Food Chemical News,* 21 February 1983, pp. 3–4.
11. J. Hallfrisch, S. Reiser, and E. S. Prather, Blood lipid distribution of hyperinsulinemic men consuming three levels of fructose, *American Journal of Clinical Nutrition* 37 (1983): 740–748.
12. D. J. A. Jenkins and coauthors, Low glycemic index carbohydrate foods in the management of hyperlipidemia, *American Journal of Clinical Nutrition* 42 (1985): 604–617.
13. T. Rebello, R. E. Hodges, and J. L. Smith, Short-term effects of various sugars on antinatriuresis and blood pressure changes in normotensive young men, *American Journal of Clinical Nutrition* 38 (1983): 84–94.
14. H. B. Affarah and coauthors, High-carbohydrate diet: Antinatriuretic and blood pressure response in normal men, *American Journal of Clinical Nutrition* 44 (1986): 341–348.
15. J. F. Wallace and M. J. Wallace, *The Effects of Excessive Consumption of Refined Sugar on Learning Skills, Behavior Attitudes and/or Physical Condition in School-Aged Children* (a 1978 booklet available from Parents for Better Nutrition, 33 North Central, Room 200, Medford, OR 97501); S. Buchanan, The most ubiquitous toxin, *American Psychologist,* November 1984, pp. 1327–1328, as cited by R. Milich, S. Lindgren, and M. Wolraich, The behavioral effects of sugar: A comment on Buchanan, *American Psychologist,* February 1986, pp. 218–220.
16. D. H. Morris, Diet and behavior: Sugar (sucrose) and criminal behavior, *Food and Nutrition News* 58, no. 1 (1986), pp. 5–6.
17. R. J. Prinz, W. A. Roberts, and E. Hantman, *Journal of Consulting and Clinical Psychology* 48 (1980): 760, as cited in Nutrition update: Sugar, *Dairy Council Digest,* July/August 1984.
18. C. K. Conners and A. G. Blouin, *Journal of Psychiatric Research* 17 (1982/83): 193, as cited in Nutrition update: Sugar, 1984.
19. R. J. Prinz and D. B. Riddle, Associations between nutrition and behavior in 5-year-old children, *Nutrition Reviews* (supplement), May 1986, pp. 151–158.
20. D. Behar and coauthors, *Nutrition and Behavior* 1 (1984): 277, as cited in Nutrition update: Sugar, 1984.
21. J. L. Rapoport, Diet and hyperactivity, *Nutrition Reviews* (supplement), May 1986, pp. 158–162.
22. H. B. Ferguson, C. Stoddart, and J. G. Simeon, Double-blind challenge studies of behavioral and cognitive effects of sucrose-aspartame ingestion in normal children, *Nutrition Reviews* (supplement), May 1986, pp. 144–150; M. L. Wolraich and coauthors, Dietary characteristics of hyperactive and control boys, *Journal of the American Dietetic Association* 86 (1986): 500–504.
23. Milich, Lindgren, and Wolraich, 1986.
24. M. G. Gross, Effect of sucrose on hyperkinetic children, *Pediatrics* 74 (1984): 876–878.
25. Gum disease largest threat to dental health, *Tallahassee Democrat,* 12 March 1987.
26. B. G. Bibby and coauthors, Oral food clearance and the pH of plaque and saliva, *Journal of the American Dental Association* 112 (1986): 333–337.
27. R. L. Glass and S. Fleisch, Diet and dental caries, *Journal of the American Dental Association* 88 (1974): 807–813.
28. S. M. Garn, M. A. Solomon, and A. Schaefer, Internal validation of sugar-food intakes in obese adolescents (letter to the editor), *American Journal of Clinical Nutrition* 33 (1980): 1890.
29. Aspartame was first approved in 1974, but approval was withdrawn. In 1981 it was again approved. C. Lecos, The sweet and sour history of saccharin, cyclamate, aspartame, *FDA Consumer,* September 1981, pp. 8–11.
30. Lecos, 1981.
31. Council on Scientific Affairs, Amer-

ican Medical Association, Saccharin: Review of safety issues, *Journal of the American Medical Association* 254 (1985): 2622–2624.

32. S. S. Schiffman and coauthors, Aspartame and susceptibility to headache, *New England Journal of Medicine* 317 (1987): 1181–1185.

33. *A Health Care Practitioner's Guide,* a pamphlet (1987) available from The NutraSweet Company, P.O. Box 111, Skokie, Illinois 60676.

34. Questions readers ask, *Nutrition and the MD,* January 1984.

35. K. K. Makinen and A. Scheinin, Xylitol and dental caries, *Annual Review of Nutrition* 2 (1982): 133–150.

36. Institute of Food Technologists' Expert Panel on Food Safety and Nutrition, Sugars and nutritive sweeteners in processed foods, *Food Technology* 33 (May 1979): 101–105.

37. R. A. Greenberg, Industrious ingredients, *ACSH News and Views,* March/April 1983, pp. 5–6.

38. D. L. Costill and coauthors, The role of dietary carbohydrates in muscle glycogen resynthesis after strenuous running, *American Journal of Clinical Nutrition* 34 (1981): 1831–1836; Dietary contributions to endurance athletics, *Nutrition and the MD,* September 1986; Sugar: Don't eat it to win, *Health,* June 1985, p. 12.

39. M. Berger, Dietary management of children with uremia, *Journal of the American Dietetic Association* 70 (1977): 498–505.

Chapter Four

Contents

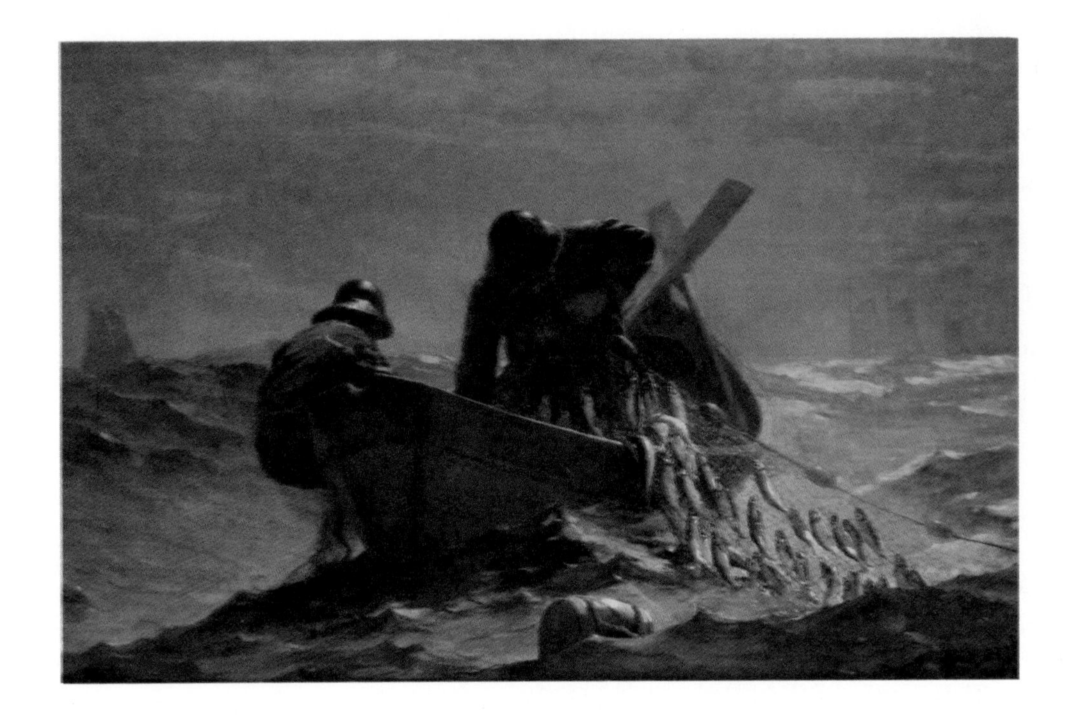

The Herring Net, by Winslow Homer, 1885 oil on canvas, 74.3 × 120.2 cm, Mr. and Mrs. Martin A. Ryerson Collection, 1937.1039.

The Lipids: Fats and Oils

A health care provider reports, "Your triglycerides are up." Your bill from a medical laboratory reads, "Blood **lipid** profile—$85." A health-food store advertisement recommends, "Use omega-fatty acids to lower your blood cholesterol." Triglycerides—blood lipid profile—omega-fatty acids—cholesterol. It is the mission of this chapter to provide an understanding of these and other terms related to **fats** and **oils**, and to make clear that they both contribute to health and detract from it.

lipid (LIP-id): a family of compounds soluble in organic solvents, which includes the triglycerides (fats and oils), phospholipids, and sterols.

fats: lipids that are solid at room temperature (70° F or 25° C).

oils: lipids that are liquid at room temperature (70° F or 25° C).

Usefulness of Fats

No doubt you have been expecting to hear that the fat in the diet has the potential to harm your health. It may be a surprise to hear that lipids are also valuable—more than valuable, they are absolutely necessary, and some lipids must be present in the diet for you to maintain good health. Luckily, at least a trace of fat is present in almost all foods, so you needn't make it a point to eat any extra. The next few paragraphs explore the usefulness of fat in the body and in foods.

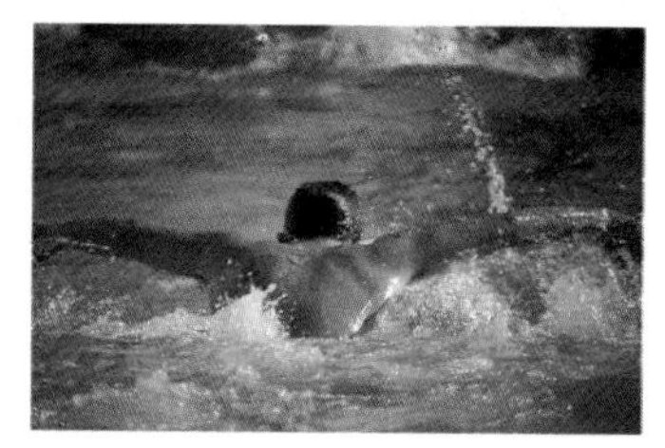

Body fat supplies much of the fuel these muscles need to do their work.

Fat is the body's chief storage form for the energy from food eaten in excess of need. The storage of fat is a valuable evolutionary mechanism for people who must live a feast-or-famine existence. It enables them to remain alive during the famine period. In addition, fats provide most of the energy needed to perform much of the body's work, and especially muscular work.

Most body cells can store only a limited amount of fat, but the fat cells seem able to expand almost indefinitely. The more fat they store, the larger they grow, until an obese person's fat cells may be a hundred times as large as a thin person's.

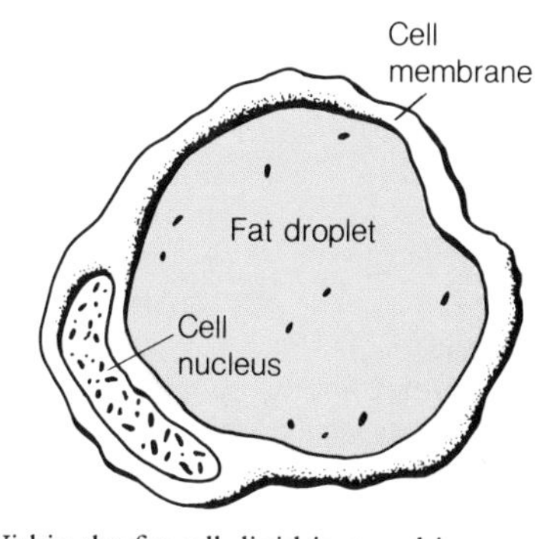

Within the fat cell, lipid is stored in a droplet. This droplet can enlarge indefinitely, and the fat cell membrane will grow to accommodate its swollen contents. More about fat cells and obesity—Chapter 8.

When a person's body starts to run out of fuel from food, it begins to use stored fat for energy. (It uses glycogen, too, as the last chapter showed.) Fat cells respond to the call for energy by breaking up stored triglycerides (see next section) and releasing the components into the blood. When energy-hungry cells receive them, they break them down in much the same way as they break down glucose (described in the last chapter). They first chop the fat components into fragments. Then they combine each fat fragment with another fragment made from glucose, and finish oxidizing them all the way to carbon dioxide and water.

Thus whenever you break down your body fat, you need carbohydrate to do so. Without carbohydrate, ketosis will occur; incomplete fat-breakdown

satiety (sat-EYE-uh-tee): the feeling of fullness or satisfaction after a meal. Fat provides more satiety than carbohydrate or protein, because it slows the stomach's motility.

products (ketone bodies) appear in the blood and urine. Because this process and its consequences are so important, Chapter 8 describes them in greater detail.

You may be wondering why glucose is not the body's major energy source. You will remember from Chapter 3 that the stored form of carbohydrate is glycogen. One characteristic of glycogen is that it holds a great deal of water, and as a result, it is quite bulky. The body cannot store enough glycogen to provide energy for very long. Fats, however, pack tightly together and can store many more calories of energy in a small space. The body fat found on a normal-weight, healthy person contains sufficient calories to fuel a marathon runner or a long-distance swimmer to the finish, or to give a sick person who cannot eat the energy to battle disease with minimum assistance from food.

1 g carbohydrate = 4 cal.
1 g fat = 9 cal.
1 g protein = 4 cal.

By the same token, foods rich in fat are valuable in many situations. A gram of fat or oil delivers over twice as many calories as a gram of carbohydrate. A hunter or hiker needs to consume a large number of calories to travel long distances or to survive in intensely cold weather. Such a person can carry more calories in fat-rich foods than in carbohydrate-rich foods. Also, fat slows digestion, lending **satiety** to meals.

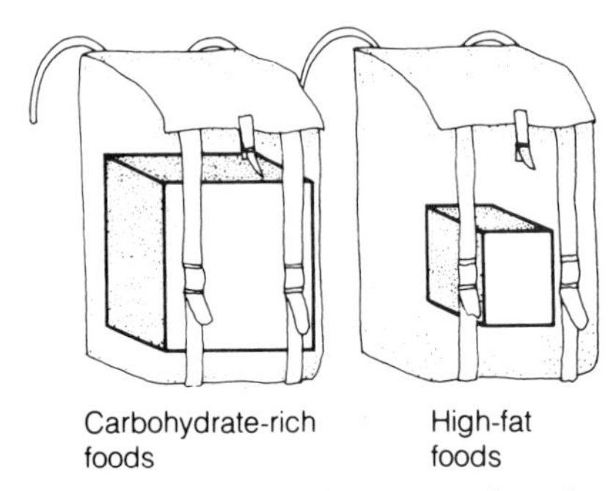

Both lunches contain the same number of calories, but the fat-rich lunch is lighter to carry.

On the other hand, high-fat foods may deliver many ***unneeded*** calories in only a few bites to the person who is not expending much energy in physical work. Overeating high-fat foods is especially likely because fat also carries with it many of the dissolved compounds that give food an enticing aroma and flavor, such as the aroma of frying bacon or french fries. In fact, when a person's appetite is poor, foods flavored with some fat may tempt that person to eat again.

It may be that fat is a more efficient fuel than is glucose.[1] Tests performed in the laboratory to judge how many calories a substance contains use the same reaction for all fuels—the fuels are completely burned, and the energy they release is measured in calories. But the body is different from a laboratory, in that it treats energy substances in various ways, depending on the substance and on body conditions. Glucose must undergo many chemical conversions in the body, each requiring energy to perform. Fat, on the other hand, requires fewer conversions. The body may spend less energy assimilating fat than assimilating carbohydrate. Thus it can store more calories when fat is eaten than it can store from the same number of calories (according to laboratory measurement) of carbohydrate. In short, you may get fatter on fat calories than on carbohydrate calories.

Fat in the body surrounds and cushions all the vital organs. It serves as a shock absorber, so that you can ride a horse or a motorcycle for many hours with no serious damage to internal organs. The fat blanket under the skin also insulates the body from extremes of temperature, thus assisting with internal climate control—and, in a pregnant woman, protecting her unborn baby.

Fats in the body:
- Store energy for life processes.
- Cushion the vital organs.
- Insulate the body.
- Transport some vitamins and essential fatty acids.
- Are part of cell membrane structures.
- Serve as raw materials for synthesis of other needed products.

Some essential nutrients are soluble in fat and therefore are found mainly in foods that contain fat. These nutrients are the essential fatty acids and the fat-soluble vitamins—A, D, E, and K.

Fat is important to all the body's cells as part of their surrounding envelopes—the cell membranes. Many dangerous household chemicals do their deadly work on the fat in cell membranes. Kerosene, gasoline, and paint thinners are a few of the substances that dissolve fat in human tissue when they come in contact with it. Such chemicals can injure the skin of the hands, or (if swallowed) the digestive tract membranes. This is why people must keep these substances out of the reach of small children. Harsh soaps have an excess of alkali, which combines chemically with the fat of the skin cells and washes away, leaving the hands dry and cracked. One must then apply an oily salve in an effort to return the lost fat and prevent further damage to the skin.

Lipids not only provide energy reserves but also protect the body from outside forces, help maintain body temperature, carry the fat-soluble nutrients, add flavor to foods, and provide the major material of which cell membranes are made.

Terminology

About 95 percent of the lipids in foods and in the human body are **triglycerides.** Other members of the lipid family are the **phospholipids** (of which **lecithin** is one) and the **sterols** (**cholesterol** is the best known of these). *Blood lipid profile* refers to a test conducted by a medical laboratory, which reveals the amounts of various lipids (especially triglycerides and cholesterol) found in the blood and the carriers in which they are found. The results of this test tell much about a person's risk of heart and artery disease, or **cardiovascular disease** (**CVD**). The blood cholesterol level is especially telling, and it bears on the question of whether people should avoid foods containing fat, those containing cholesterol, or both.

It is easy to become confused on first hearing that *blood* cholesterol, but not necessarily *dietary* cholesterol, is of concern relating to CVD.* Most important in this regard is *blood* cholesterol. A person's blood level of cholesterol is considered to be a predictor of that person's likelihood of suffering a fatal heart attack or stroke. Table 4–1 shows that blood cholesterol is one of the three major risk factors for CVD: the higher it is, the earlier in life a person may suffer from heart or vascular disease.

Food fats relate to blood cholesterol in the following way. Two kinds of lipids in foods are:

- Triglycerides in foods (commonly called fat).
- Cholesterol in foods.

Similarly, two kinds of lipids in the blood are:

- Blood triglycerides.
- Blood cholesterol.

triglycerides (try-GLISS-er-ides): the major class of dietary lipids. A triglyceride is made up of three units known as fatty acids and one unit called glycerol. More on fatty acids and glycerol later.

phospholipids (FOSS-foh-LIP-ids): one of the three main classes of lipids; lipids similar to triglycerides but having a phosphorus-containing acid in place of one of the fatty acids.

lecithin (LESS-ih-thin): a phospholipid, a major constituent of cell membranes, manufactured by the liver and also found in many foods.

sterols (STEER-alls): one of the three main classes of lipids; lipids with a structure similar to that of cholesterol.

cholesterol (koh-LESS-ter-all): one of the sterols, manufactured in the body for a variety of purposes and also found in animal-derived foods.

cardiovascular disease (CVD): disease of the heart and blood vessels. The two most common such diseases are *atherosclerosis* (Controversy 4) and *hypertension* (Controversy 7).

**Blood, plasma,* and *serum* cholesterol all refer to about the same thing; this book uses the term *blood* cholesterol. Plasma is simply blood with the cells removed; serum has the clotting factors also removed. The concentration of cholesterol is not much altered by these treatments.

Table 4–1

The Effect of Blood Cholesterol and Other Risk Factors on Age of Onset of CVD

The age listed is the hypothetical age of onset of the critical phase of CVD risk (60 percent coverage of artery surfaces by atherosclerosis).

Blood Cholesterol	200 mg/100 ml[a]	250 mg/100 ml	300 mg/100 ml
Age of nonsmoker	70	60	50
Age of smoker	60	50	40
Age of smoker with hypertension	50	40	30

The table shows that a nonsmoker with normal blood pressure and cholesterol of 200 would reach the critical phase at age 70. A smoker with high blood pressure and cholesterol of 300 would reach that phase at age 30.

[a]Milligrams cholesterol per 100 ml of blood.

Source: Data from S. M. Grundy, Cholesterol and coronary heart disease, *Journal of the American Medical Association* 256 (1986): 2849–2858.

Of the second pair, blood cholesterol is the major indicator of CVD risk (see Table C4–2, p. 133, for the risk associated with triglycerides). The question to ask, then, is, Which fat on the plate contributes more to blood cholesterol? The answer is not food cholesterol (that in eggs, liver, and the like). The important relationship is that food *fats* (triglycerides) raise blood cholesterol. People often fail to understand this point, and the question arises again and again: "Should I eat cholesterol?" When told, "It doesn't matter much," the questioner often jumps to the wrong conclusion—the conclusion that cholesterol doesn't matter. It does matter. High *blood* cholesterol is an indicator of risk for CVD, but the main food factor associated with it is a high *fat intake.** One more distinction must be made clear about fats on the plate: they come in two varieties, saturated and unsaturated, and the saturated type is most implicated in raising blood cholesterol. A later section describes the differences between saturated and unsaturated fats.

"Fat on the plate" includes visible fats and oils, such as butter, the oil in salad dressing, and the fat you trim from a steak. It also refers to some you can't see, such as the fat that marbles a steak or other meat or that is hidden in foods like nuts, cheese, biscuits, avocados, olives, and fried foods. The photos here show that when you remove the fat from foods, you remove something else: calories. A medium pork chop with a ½-inch border of fat contains 275 calories; the same chop with the visible fat trimmed off contains 165 calories. A baked potato with 1 tablespoon each butter and sour cream has double the calories of the plain potato. Choosing nonfat milk over whole milk provides a large saving of fat and calories; and so it goes. The single most effective step you can take to

*Heredity modifies everyone's ability to handle cholesterol somewhat, but a few individuals have inherited a total inability to clear from their blood the cholesterol they have eaten and absorbed. This condition is rare but well known, because the study of it led to the discovery of how cholesterol is transported in the body. People with hereditary high blood cholesterol must refrain from eating cholesterol in foods; perhaps this is where the general public's fear of dietary cholesterol has come from. The majority of people can eat eggs, shellfish, and other cholesterol-containing foods without fear of incurring high blood cholesterol.

fatty acids: organic acids composed of carbon chains with oxygens at the end and hydrogens attached all along their length.

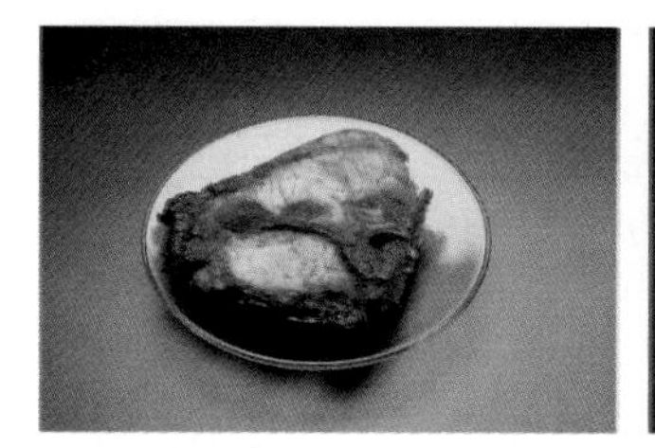

Pork chop with ½ inch of fat (275 calories).

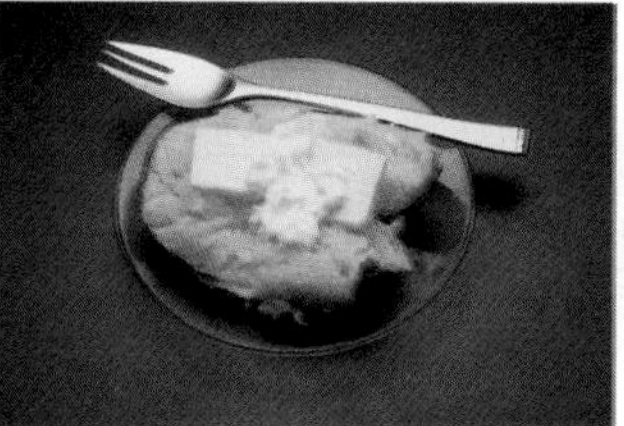

Potato with 1 tablespoon butter and 1 tablespoon sour cream (260 calories).

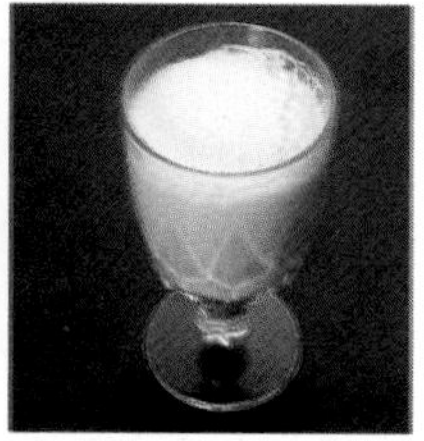

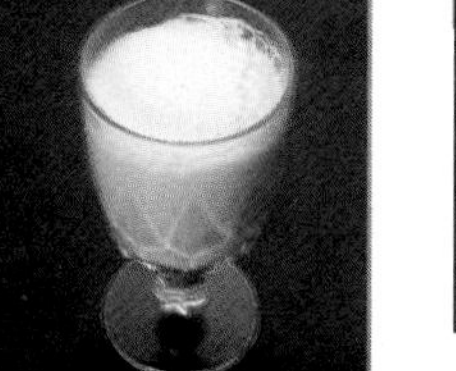

Whole milk, 1 cup (150 calories).

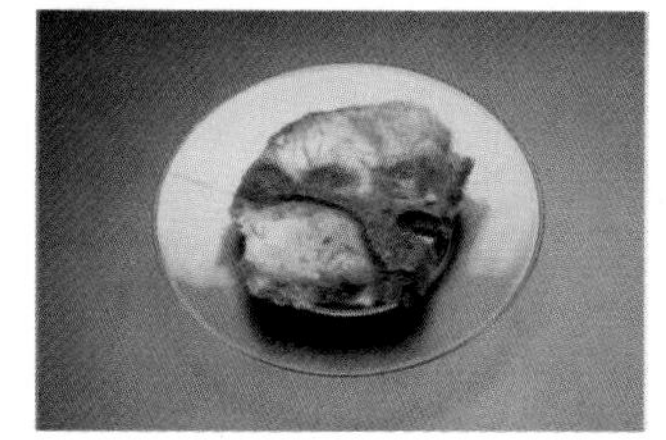

Pork chop with fat trimmed off (165 calories).

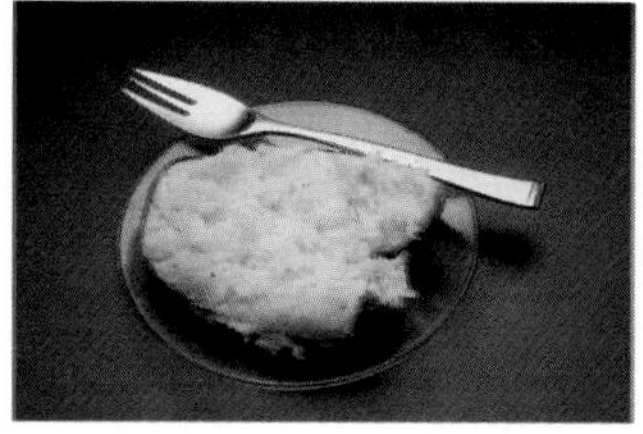

Plain potato (130 calories).

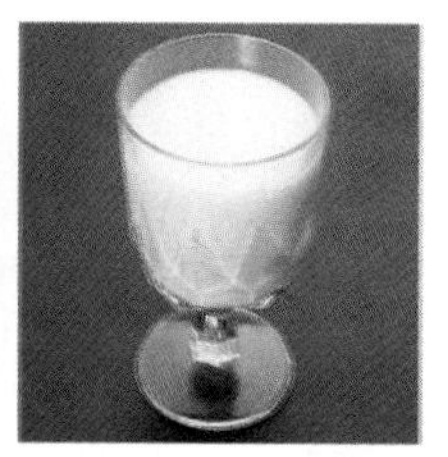

Nonfat milk, 1 cup (90 calories).

reduce the energy value of a food is to eat it without the fat. This step is also an effective dietary weapon against high blood cholesterol.

Triglycerides are the chief form of fat found in foods, and the next sections are mostly devoted to them. Later sections present information about lecithin and cholesterol; Controversy 4 asks the question of how diet is related to heart and artery disease, and Controversy 5 explores the relationships of dietary fat and other diet components to cancer risk.

An important distinction: total fat intake, and especially saturated fat intake (not dietary cholesterol intake), is the major dietary factor that raises blood cholesterol. Elevated blood cholesterol is a risk factor for cardiovascular disease.

A Chemist's View of Fats

The bulk of the fat in the human diet comes from animals. Animal fat, in turn, may have come from the fats and oils in plants; from the carbohydrates in plants, the last chapter showed; or from protein, which will be discussed later. When the energy of glucose is to be stored in fat, it is first broken into fragments—small molecules made of carbon, hydrogen, and oxygen. These fragments are then linked together into chains known as **fatty acids.** Fatty acids are the major constituent of triglycerides, the chief form of fat. The sections that follow show first the characteristics of fatty acids and then how they are put together into triglycerides.

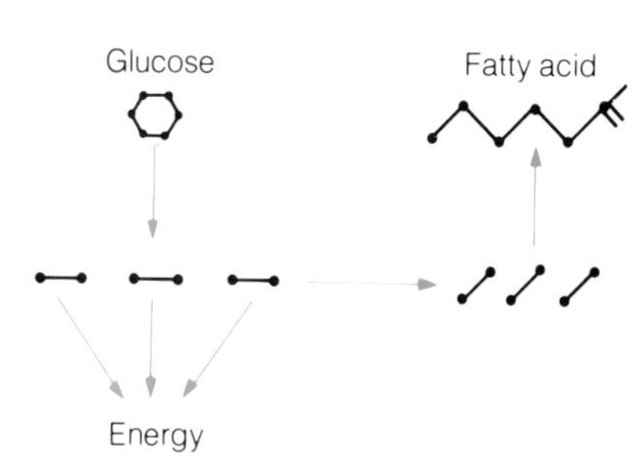

Glucose can be used for energy or changed into fat.

saturated fatty acid: a fatty acid carrying the maximum possible number of hydrogen atoms (having no points of unsaturation). A saturated fat is one that is made up of saturated fatty acids.

point of unsaturation: a site in a molecule where the bonding is such that additional hydrogen atoms can easily be added.

unsaturated fatty acid: a fatty acid in which one or more points of unsaturation occur. A lipid (triglyceride or phospholipid) in which one or more of the fatty acids is unsaturated is an unsaturated fat.

oleic (oh-LAY-ic) **acid:** a monounsaturated fatty acid found in animal and vegetable oils.

monounsaturated fatty acid: a fatty acid containing one point of unsaturation.

polyunsaturated fatty acid (**PUFA**): a fatty acid in which two or more points of unsaturation occur.

linoleic (lin-oh-LAY-ic) **acid, linolenic** (lin-oh-LEN-ic) **acid:** polyunsaturated fatty acids, essential for human beings.

essential fatty acids: fatty acids that cannot be synthesized in the body in amounts sufficient to meet physiological need.

omega: the last letter of the Greek alphabet (ω), used by chemists to refer to the position of the endmost double bond in a fatty acid. The **omega-6** fatty acids have their endmost double bond six carbons back along the chain; the **omega-3** acids, three carbons back. (The English alphabet letter *n* is sometimes used for ω.)

Fatty Acids

Fatty acids may differ from one another in two ways: in chain length and in degree of saturation. Chain length affects their solubility in water; the shorter chains are more water soluble. Saturation, a term that was mentioned earlier in relation to CVD, refers to the chemical structure—specifically, to the number of hydrogens the fatty acid chain is holding. If every available bond from the carbons is holding a hydrogen, the chain is a **saturated fatty acid**—filled to capacity with hydrogen.

Sometimes, especially in the fatty acids in plants and fish, there is a place in the chain where hydrogens are missing, an "empty spot," or **point of unsaturation.** A chain that possesses a point of unsaturation is an **unsaturated fatty acid**. (An example is **oleic acid.**) If there is one point of unsaturation (as in oleic acid), then it is a **monounsaturated fatty acid.** If there are two or more points of unsaturation, then it is a **polyunsaturated fatty acid.** (You sometimes see polyunsaturated fatty acids abbreviated on food labels as **PUFA.**)

The human body can synthesize all the fatty acids it needs from carbohydrate, fat, or protein, except two—**linoleic acid** and **linolenic acid.** These two cannot be made from other substances in the body or from each other, and they must be supplied by the diet; they are, therefore, **essential fatty acids.** These fatty acids are polyunsaturated fatty acids, widely distributed in plant and fish oils, and they are readily stored in the adult body. When *linoleic* acid is missing from the diet, the skin reddens and becomes irritated, infections and dehydration become likely, and the liver develops abnormalities. If the fatty acid is restored, the conditions reverse themselves. Infants are especially in need of linoleic acid for their growth, and it is no coincidence that human breast milk has a much higher percentage of it than cow's milk.

Linolenic acid (the other essential fatty acid) serves as a raw material from which the body makes hormonelike substances (see accompanying box) that regulate a wide range of body functions, including blood pressure. Research is currently exploring the possibility that adequate amounts in the diet protect against hypertension.[2]

Of the two essential fatty acids, linoleic acid is an **omega-6** fatty acid, related to a whole series of others. Linolenic acid is an **omega-3** fatty acid, with a similar family of its own.* Linoleic acid has long been known to be essential, but the essentiality of linolenic acid is only now becoming apparent. Its emerging importance, and that of the omega-3 fatty acid series of which it is a member, are discussed in the accompanying box, "Fish Oils and Omega-3 Fatty Acids."

Fatty acids are energy-rich chemical chains that can be saturated (filled with hydrogens), monounsaturated (with one point of unsaturation), or polyunsaturated (with more than one point of unsaturation). Two polyunsaturated fatty acids, linoleic acid (an omega-6 acid) and linolenic acid (omega-3), are essential nutrients.

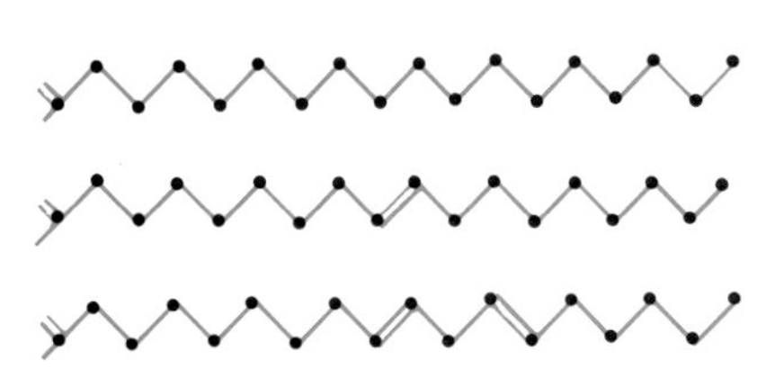

These are three fatty acids. The first is a saturated faty acid; the second one is a monounsaturated fatty acid (oleic acid); the third is a polyunsaturated fatty acid (linoleic acid).

*A fatty acid has two ends, designated the methyl end and the acid end. The carbons are usually numbered beginning at the acid end, but the numbering of these acids is an exception. When fatty acid chains are lengthened, the carbons are added at the acid end, not the methyl end, of the chain; when an ω3 acid is lengthened, the derivative is also an ω3 acid.

Fish Oils and Omega-3 Fatty Acids

It all began when someone thought to ask the question why the Eskimos of Greenland, who eat a diet very high in fat, have such a low death rate from heart disease. The trail led to the abundance of fish they eat, then to the oils in those fish, and finally to the ω3 (omega-3) fatty acids in the oils. Now, scientists are unraveling the mystery of what those fatty acids do. The essentiality of the ω6 (omega-6) fatty acids from plant oils such as corn and peanut oil had long been known—linoleic (18 carbons) and arachidonic (20 carbons) acids. However, the only ω3 thought to be important was linolenic acid (18 carbons), and it was thought to be dispensable. That is, as long as you had linoleic, you could do without linolenic:

Old Picture

Important: ω6	**Not so Important: ω3**
Linoleic acid (18 C)	Linolenic acid (18 C)
Arachidonic acid (20 C) (important, but can be made from linoleic acid)	(Linoleic acid can substitute for it)

The facts just stated are true: arachidonic can be made from linoleic, and linoleic can substitute for linolenic, but the importance of linolenic acid and its derivatives (described below) has been underrated. There are three ω3 fatty acids of interest:

New Picture

Important: ω6	**Also Important: ω3**
Linoleic acid (18 C)	Linolenic acid (18 C)
Arachidonic acid (20 C)	EPA[a] (20 C)
	DHA[a] (22 C)

The body cannot make any of the ω3 fatty acids from scratch, but furnished with the shortest one, linolenic acid, it can make the others.

The only one of these fatty acids that everyone has long agreed is essential (both necessary for growth and health and impossible to synthesize anew) is linoleic acid. Deficiency symptoms appear in the person deprived of this acid—a well-known skin rash and, in children, poor growth. However, linolenic acid is also beneficial—and it is also impossible to synthesize anew. Deficiency symptoms are not clear-cut, but subtle changes do appear in the person deprived of linolenic acid.

The reason the changes are subtle is that a lack of linolenic acid does not leave an unoccupied slot in the body; rather, a substitute fills its place—

[a]EPA is eicosapentaenoic (EYE-cossa-PENTA-ee-NO-ic) acid (*eicosa* means "20," referring to chain length; *penta* means "5," and *en* means "double bond," so there are 5 double bonds). DHA is docosahexaenoic (DOE-cosa-HEXA-ee-NO-ic) acid(*docosa* means "22" carbons long, and *hexa en* refers to the six double bonds).

(continued on following page)

eicosanoids (eye-COSS-uh-noyds): derivatives of a 20-carbon fatty acid, hormonelike compounds that regulate blood pressure, clotting, and other body functions.

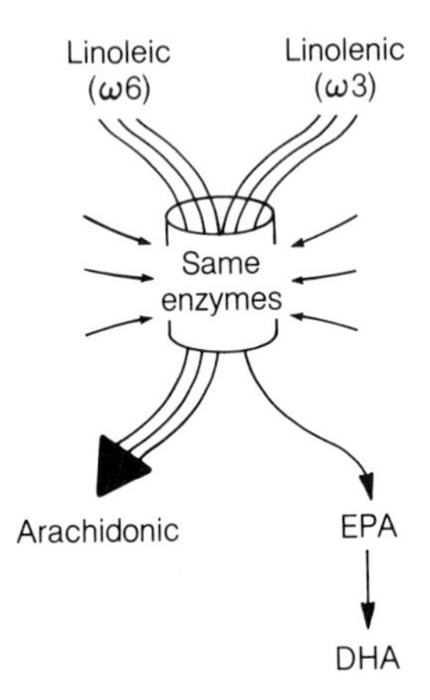

Competition between ω6 and ω3

linoleic acid. (The play goes on, but with an understudy who has not quite the talent of the original star.) The same is true of the longer-chain derivatives of these acids: if the ω3 acid is missing, the ω6 acid of the same length takes its place. The body is wise to make this substitution of one set of acids for the other, because the necessary jobs get done, but a price is paid: the jobs are not done as well.

Another connection between these two series of fatty acids is that they compete for the same chain-lengthening enzymes, and in that competition, the ω6 series seems to have the advantage. That is, given equal amounts of the ω6 and ω3 18-carbon starting materials, the enzymes will preferentially use linoleic acid and make its longer-chain derivative, and will use very little linolenic acid to make its longer-chain derivatives EPA and DHA (see margin). When the enzymes are given unequal amounts of ω3 and ω6 starting materials, though, the consequences are different. Thus, consider the consequences of taking supplements: if you took supplements of one but not the other, you might easily induce a deficiency of the other. In fact, the effect of taking linolenic acid without linoleic is known—eczema-like skin lesions and growth retardation. Now, people may be taking supplements of linoleic acid, and they may be inviting a deficit of the ω3 series and its consequences.

Even without supplements, our diets may be undesirably high in ω6 fatty acids. A comparison with the diet of the fish-eating Eskimos is illuminating. They eat more calories, and more of those calories come from ω3 acids. We eat fewer calories, and more of ours come from ω6 acids. Indeed, we eat about twice as much ω6 and half as much ω3 fatty acid as do the Eskimos. Researchers have speculated that that may be why we have so many more heart attacks than they do.

What, exactly, do the ω6 and ω3 fatty acids do in the body? The answer deals with the 20-carbon members of both series, arachidonic acid (ω6) and EPA (ω3).

Both arachidonic acid and EPA serve as starting materials for the synthesis of still other compounds in the body—compounds which as a class have been given the name **eicosanoids** (meaning 20-carbon compounds related to the 20-carbon fatty acids). The eicosanoids include groups with still more exotic sounding names,* and they play many regulatory roles in the body. They affect the formation of blood clots, the raising and lowering of blood pressure and blood lipid levels, the immune response, the inflammation response to injury and infection, and many other body functions.

Each eicosanoid comes in two forms (like words with two acceptable spellings)—one from the ω3 and the other from the ω6 fatty acid. A particular enzyme system makes the eicosanoids, and it is willing to work with either starting material. The final product will work the same way in either case—but with subtle differences. The eicosanoid made from an ω6

*Names of classes of eicosanoids: prostaglandins (PGs), thromboxanes (TXs), prostacyclins (PGIs), and leukotrienes (LTs).

fatty acid may produce a side effect that the one from the ω3 fatty acid does not produce. For example, an eicosanoid made from the ω6 fatty acid may cause blood clots to form and also constrict blood vessels; the same eicosanoid, if made from the ω3 fatty acid, will also cause clots to form, but will not constrict vessels. The eicosanoid made from the ω6 fatty acid may lower blood cholesterol by causing it to be degraded faster; the same eicosanoid, if made from the ω3 fatty acid, will also lower blood cholesterol, but by reducing the availability of carriers for it. (Yes, in this case it's the ω6 you need, not the ω3. But to counter this effect, the growth of certain tumors is slower in the presence of ω3 than in the presence of ω6 fatty acids.) These subtle differences, which might ordinarily have no impact on a person's health, may be crucial in the presence of certain factors leading to heart disease or cancer. Heart attacks and strokes are known to be caused by blood clots and narrowed blood vessels; cancer is known to advance by overwhelming the immune response. The types of eicosanoids made in the body may determine the degree of vulnerability to these diseases. In short, it may well matter which of the two types of polyunsaturated fatty acids you eat.

Two more questions come to mind. The first is, Aside from what we know about the Greenland Eskimos, what is the evidence that people who eat fish or fish oils have more or less heart disease or cancer than those who don't? More than 70 studies have now documented many connections. Diets high in ω3 fatty acids seem to bring about many desirable health effects. All are being investigated further: normalized blood pressure, reduced blood triglycerides, reduced LDL cholesterol, raised HDL cholesterol, a slowed clotting time, a slowed progression of atherosclerotic heart disease, enhanced defenses against cancer, reduced inflammation in arthritis and asthma sufferers. The Eskimos apparently had the right idea when they started fishing fish out of the sea to feed themselves. Clearly, we, too, could benefit from eating wild fish in abundance.

Notice that we didn't say "fish oil supplements." Many hazards may be associated with the taking of such supplements. (For one thing, they may upset the balance with the essential ω6 fatty acids, remember.) Too much fish oil might make a person susceptible to stroke, to the same degree as it reduced the risk of heart attack. Fish oils are notorious for accumulating toxins—not only the fat-soluble vitamins A and D, but also pesticides and other contaminants. Excesses of unsaturated oils can precipitate vitamin E deficiency. These and other risks do not accompany the eating of a variety of fish. Furthermore, fish contain other beneficial nutrients; the purified oils contain just oil. And oil is high in calories. If you tried to take enough fish oil to match the Eskimos' intake, you'd need 300 to 500 calories a day—enough to gain about 25 pounds a year. So don't. Substitute three to five fish meals a week for meals based on other protein-rich foods, and you'll accomplish a healthier thing more safely.

Source: Information from (among others) P. A. Anderson and H. W. Sprecher, Omega-3 fatty acids in nutrition and health, *Dietetic Currents* 14 (1987).

Fish especially high in EPA and DHA: Anchovies, herring, mackerel, sablefish, salmon, sardines, tuna (fresh), whitefish.
Fish moderately high in EPA and DHA: Bass, bluefish, hake, halibut, mullet, ocean perch, pollock, rainbow trout, rockfish, sea trout, smelt.
Shellfish moderately high in EPA and DHA: Oysters.

hydrogenation (high-droh-gen-AY-shun): the process of adding hydrogen to unsaturated fat to make it more solid and more resistant to chemical change.

antioxidant (anti-OX-ih-dant): a compound that protects other compounds from oxygen by itself reacting with oxygen (*anti* means "against"; *oxy* means "oxygen").

monounsaturated fats: triglycerides in which one or more of the fatty acids is monounsaturated.

polyunsaturated fats: triglycerides in which one or more of the fatty acids is polyunsaturated.

smoking point: the temperature at which fat gives off an acrid blue gas.

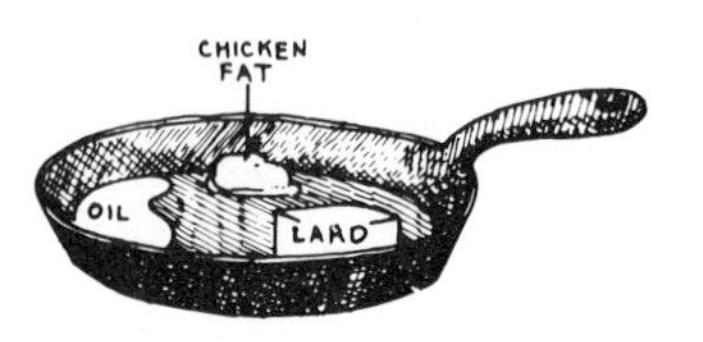

The more unsaturated a fat, the more liquid it is at room temperature.

Hydrogenation of Fats

Points of unsaturation in fatty acids are like weak spots, in that they are vulnerable to attack by oxygen. When the unsaturated points are oxidized, the oils become rancid. This is why oils should be stored in tightly covered containers. If stored for long periods, they need refrigeration to retard the oxidation reaction.

One way to prevent spoilage of oils containing unsaturated fatty acids is to change them chemically by **hydrogenation,** but this causes them to lose their unsaturated character and the health benefits that go with it. (This is often done to commercial fats.) A second alternative is to add a chemical that will compete for the oxygen and thus protect the oil. Such an additive is called an **antioxidant.** Examples are the well-known additives BHA and BHT listed on snack food labels and the natural antioxidants vitamin C and vitamin E. A third alternative, already mentioned, is to keep the product refrigerated.

When refrigerated, oils may become cloudy, because crystals of saturated fat form in them. This is no hazard to the user, but manufacturers of cooking oils sometimes prechill salad oils and remove the crystals that cause cloudiness before marketing them, a process called "winterizing."

The presence of unsaturated fatty acids in a fat affects the temperature at which the fat melts. The more unsaturated a fat, the more liquid it is at room temperature. In contrast, the more saturated a fat (the more hydrogens it has), the firmer it is. Thus, of three fats—lard, chicken fat, and safflower oil—lard is the most saturated and the hardest (it comes from pork); chicken fat is less saturated and somewhat soft (chicken is recommended over pork for people avoiding saturated fats); and safflower oil, which is the most unsaturated, is an oil at room temperature (and the only one of the three that comes from a plant). If your health care provider tells you to use **monounsaturated** or **polyunsaturated fats,** you can judge by the hardness of the fats which ones to choose. If you wish to see whether the oil you use contains saturated fats, place the oil in a clear container in the refrigerator and watch for cloudiness—winterized oils remain clear because the crystals of the most saturated fat have been removed.

Generally speaking, vegetable and fish oils are rich in polyunsaturates, olive oil is rich in monounsaturates, and the harder fats—animal fats—are more saturated. But not all vegetable oils are polyunsaturated. If you were looking for a substitute for cream, you might be inclined to choose a nondairy creamer, made from vegetable oil. Many nondairy creamers substitute coconut oil for cream (butterfat), however, and coconut oil is actually more saturated than cream. Palm oil, used frequently in food processing, is also highly saturated, but may not have the same effects on the body as other saturated fats. Olive oil may also be beneficial to heart health, if the people of the Mediterranean areas are any indication; they consume large quantities of olive oil and retain heart health.[3] You have to know your oils; it is not enough simply to prefer plant oils over animal fats.

When food producers want to use a polyunsaturated oil such as corn oil to make a spreadable margarine, they hydrogenate the oil. Hydrogen is forced into the oil, some of the unsaturated fatty acids accept the hydrogen, and the oil becomes harder. The spreadable margarine that results is more saturated than the original oil. If you, the consumer, were looking for polyunsaturated oils to include in your diet, these hydrogenated oils would not meet your need. A hydrogenated oil is easy to handle, stores well, has a high **smoking point,** and is a perfectly suitable product for some purposes, but it is more saturated than the oil it was made from. Margarines that list liquid oil as the first ingredient are usually the most polyunsaturated. Margarines that are sold in tubs and labeled "soft" are sometimes less saturated than the stick varieties.[4]

A chemical accident occurs when polyunsaturated oils are hydrogenated. They change in shape, creating unusual fatty acids that are not made by the body's cells and that occur only rarely in foods. These unfamiliar fatty acids, or ***trans*-fatty acids,** can be taken up into our cell membranes and may have the potential to alter cell functions. The issue is not clear, but some researchers believe that *trans*-fatty acids may make people prone to develop certain kinds of cancer. However, so many dietary factors are implicated in cancer causation that it is hard to sort them all out and decide which are significant. Undoubtedly, total fat consumption has much more bearing on susceptibility to cancer than does consumption of *trans*-fatty acids. Controversy 5 puts together the many factors that relate diet to cancer.

While the evidence on processed fats is still being collected, consumers can avoid them, if they wish. As an alternative to margarine, for example, you can mix warm butter and vegetable or olive oil in equal amounts. The result is a blend that is cheaper than butter, spreads well, is no more saturated than margarine, and contains more linoleic acid than margarine and fewer *trans*-fatty acids. As for peanut butter, you might choose the unhydrogenated "natural" varieties. The peanut mash and the oil may separate in these products, but you can stir them back together before using the product, or pour off the oil to use in cooking. If you pour off the oil, the remaining peanut butter will be lower in calories, although it's harder to spread. Ultimately, if *trans*-fatty acids are proven to contribute to disease, manufacturers can adopt manufacturing processes that, while more expensive, can produce solid fats without producing *trans*-fatty acids.

The degree of saturation of the fatty acids in a fat and the crystal size in a solid fat affect how the fat behaves. Vegetable margarines are partially hydrogenated oils that are more saturated than the oils they are made from.

***trans*-fatty acids:** fatty acids with unusual shapes that can arise when polyunsaturated oils are hydrogenated.

glycerol (GLISS-er-all): an organic compound, three carbons long, of interest here because it serves as the backbone for triglycerides.

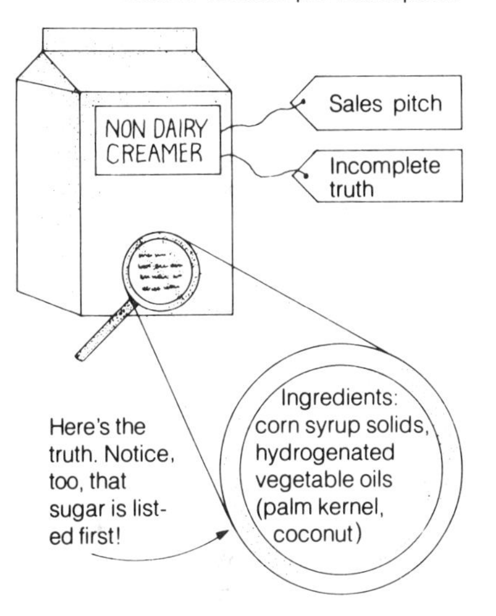

Triglycerides in the Body

Very few free fatty acids are found in the body or in foods. Usually, the fatty acids have been incorporated into large, complex compounds: triglycerides. The name almost explains itself: three fatty acids (*tri*) are attached to a molecule of **glycerol.** Figure 4–1 shows how glycerol and three fatty acids combine to make a triglyceride molecule.

Any combination of fatty acids can be incorporated into a triglyceride—long chain or short chain, saturated or polyunsaturated. Each species of animals (including people) has its own characteristic kinds of triglycerides, but within limits, fats in the diet can affect the types of triglycerides made. For example, animals raised for food can be fed diets with different fats in them in order to give them softer or harder fat, whichever is demanded by consumers.

When you eat food and do not put all of the stored energy in its energy-yielding nutrients (carbohydate, fat, and protein) to work right away, you can convert any of them to fat. To convert carbohydrate to fat, as already described,

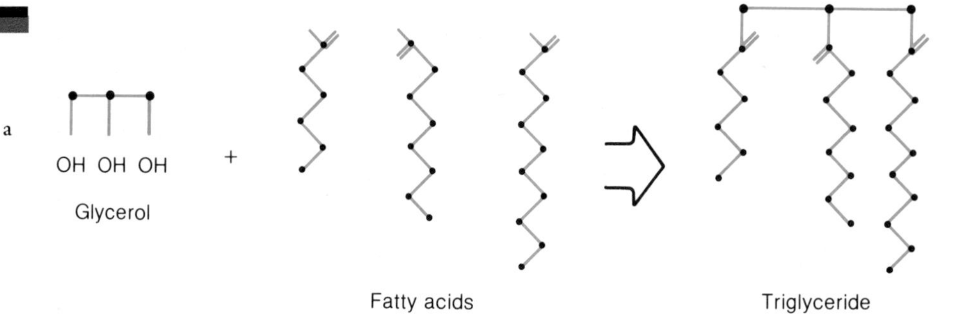

Figure 4–1
Triglyceride Formation.
Glycerol, a small, water-soluble carbohydrate, plus three fatty acids equals a triglyceride.

you first digest it, mostly to glucose. You may store some as glycogen, but you break down the rest to fragments. You may use some of these fragments for energy, but you join together the rest to make fatty acids. The fatty acids are attached to glycerol to make triglycerides. Finally, these are transported to the fat depots—muscles, breasts, the insulating fat layer under the skin, and others. Figure 4–2 shows the route glucose travels to become fat. Protein is converted to fat through similar intermediates, as described in the next chapter.

When you partake of animal flesh (meat, fish, poultry) or animal products (milk, cheese, eggs), you are eating fat and protein. Of the fat, 95 percent is triglyceride that has been made in the animal body, mostly from carbohydrate, the same way you make it. Animal fat can end up in fat stores in your own body, but first it has to be digested, absorbed, and transported to its cell destinations. Figure 4–3 (p. 118) shows how the body makes fat ready for absorption.

After digestion, most of the triglycerides that entered the body in food have been digested to their components—fatty acids, glycerol, and monoglycerides. They then move into the intestinal cells, where a difficulty must be overcome before they can be released into the body fluids, blood and lymph. Fats are insoluble in water, and lymph and blood are watery. The next section describes how the body solves this and other fat-transportation problems.

In the stomach, fats separate from other food components. In the small intestine, bile emulsifies them, enzymes digest them, and they pass into the intestinal cells.

Figure 4–2
How Glucose Becomes Fat.
Glucose must be broken down to fragments, the fragments assembled into fatty acids, and the fatty acids combined with glycerol in order to become the energy storage molecule, triglyceride.

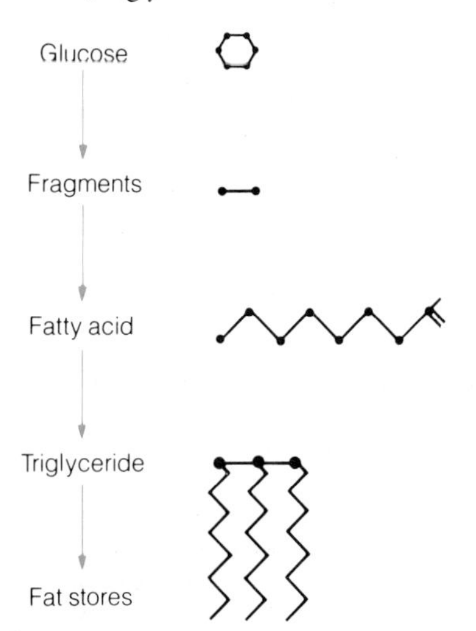

Lipid Transport within the Body

Within the body, fats always travel from place to place mixed with protein particles—that is, as **lipoproteins.** For example, monoglycerides and long-chain fatty acids liberated from food fat are too large to be released directly into the bloodstream—they would separate out and float in globules, disrupting the blood's normal functions. Instead, the intestinal cells allow them to cluster together, and before release, they combine them with protein, forming **chylomicrons,** a type of lipoprotein. The protein in the chylomicron is water soluble, and enables the fats to travel in the watery body fluids. That way, when the tissues of the body need energy from fat, they can extract what they need from these chylomicrons. What is left, the remnants, are picked up by the liver, which dismantles them and reuses their parts. Figure 4–4 (p. 119) shows the two routes that fat can travel from the digestive system—small fatty acids and glycerol travel freely in the blood, but monoglycerides and long-chain fatty acids must be combined to make triglycerides and travel as chylomicrons in the lymph and blood.

Lipoproteins are very much in the news these days. In fact, the health care provider who measures your blood lipid profile is interested not only in the types of fats in your blood (triglycerides and cholesterol), but also in the lipoproteins that carry them. One distinction among types of lipoproteins is of great importance because it has implications for the health of the heart and blood vessels; that is the distinction between **low-density lipoproteins (LDL)** and **high density lipoproteins (HDL).** The more protein in the lipoprotein molecule, the higher the density; a large percentage of lipids characterizes the lower-density molecules. Both LDL and HDL carry similar lipids around in the blood, but there is a functional difference between them. Raised LDL concentrations in the blood are a sign of high heart-attack risk. Raised HDL concentrations are associated with a low risk. A later section clarifies this relationship.

The characteristics of the four types of lipoproteins circulating in the blood are as follows:

- Chylomicrons—made by the intestine for transport of just-eaten fat to the body's cells. These carry mostly triglycerides.
- **VLDL (very-low-density lipoproteins)**—made by both intestine and liver for transport of fats around the body. These, too, carry mostly triglycerides.
- LDL (low-density lipoproteins)—made by the liver. These carry cholesterol (much of it synthesized in the liver) to the body's cells. A high blood cholesterol level usually reflects high LDL.
- HDL (high-density lipoproteins)—originally formed by fat cells to carry fats from storage to other tissues; HDL are remnants of unused cholesterol packages. It is believed that one of their functions is to return cholesterol to the liver for recycling or disposal.

Blood and other body fluids are watery, so non-water-soluble fats need a special transport system to travel around the body—the lipoproteins. Among the four types of lipoproteins, the HDL are unique, in that a high blood concentration indicates a reduced heart disease risk.

lipoproteins (LIP-oh-PRO-teens): clusters of lipids associated with protein; they serve as transport vehicles for lipids in blood and lymph. The four main types of lipoproteins are chylomicrons, VLDL, LDL, and HDL.

chylomicrons (KIGH-loh-MY-crons): a type of lipoprotein (very low in density) made by the cells of the intestinal wall; they serve as a means of transporting lipids from the intestine through lymph and blood. Chylomicrons donate lipids to all body cells, and the remnants are ultimately cleared from the blood by liver cells.

LDL (low-density lipoproteins): lipoproteins that transport lipids from liver to other (muscle, fat) tissues.

HDL (high-density lipoproteins): lipoproteins that return cholesterol from storage places to the liver for dismantling and disposal.

VLDL (very-low-density lipoproteins): lipoproteins made in the intestine and liver that transport lipids to other body organs.

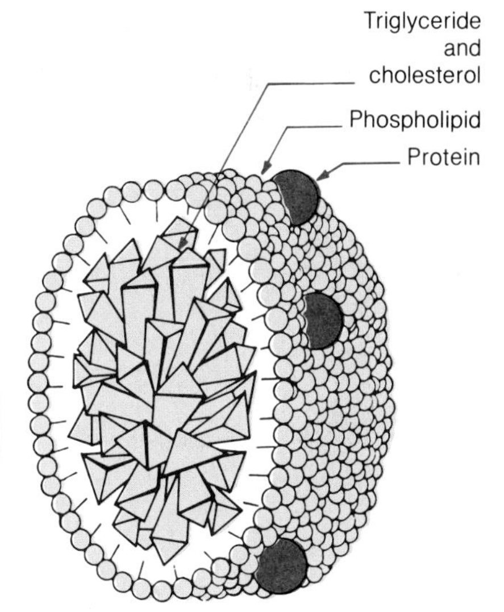

A lipoprotein. An LDL has a higher ratio of lipid to protein; an HDL has more protein relative to its lipid content.
Source: Adapted from D. Kritchevsky. An update on lipids, lipoproteins and fat metabolism, in *The Medicine Called Nutrition,* Medical Education (Meded) Programs, Ltd. (Englewood Cliffs, N.J.: Best Foods, 1979), p. 61.

Lecithin and Cholesterol

Lecithins and other phospholipids play key roles in the structure of cell membranes. Because of the way they are constructed, they have both water-loving and fat-loving characteristics, which enable them to help fats back and forth across the lipid-containing membranes of cells into the watery fluids on both sides. Almost magical health-promoting properties are sometimes attributed to the group of lipids called lecithin.

As for cholesterol, it is an important compound with many functions in the body. It is a part of bile, which is necessary in the digestion of fats. It is the starting material from which the sex hormones and other hormones are made.

bile: a mixture of compounds made from cholesterol by the liver, stored in the gallbladder, and secreted into the small intestine. It emulsifies lipids to ready them for enzymatic digestion and helps transport them into the intestinal wall cells. Bile works like a detergent (detergents, too, are emulsifiers; they remove grease spots from clothing—molecule by molecule they dissolve out the grease and hold it suspended in the water to be rinsed away).

emulsifier (ee-MULL-si-fire): a compound with both water-soluble and fat-soluble portions that can attract lipid into water solution.

monoglycerides (mon-oh-GLISS-er-ide): a product of the digestion of lipids; glycerol molecules with one fatty acid attached (*mono* means "one"; *glyceride* means "a compound of glycerol").

In the skin, it is made into vitamin D with the help of sunlight. It is an important lipid in the structure of brain and nerve cells. In fact, cholesterol is a part of every cell. Like lecithin, cholesterol can be made by the body, so it is not an essential nutrient. But while it is widespread in the body and necessary to its function, it also is the major part of the plaques that narrow the arteries in the killer disease atherosclerosis (see Controversy 4).

Although the cholesterol in foods does contribute somewhat to cholesterol in the blood, and it is prudent to avoid excesses, it is not as influential as total dietary fat in raising blood cholesterol—actually, LDL. It is LDL that forecasts heart and artery disease. The cholesterol of LDL comes mostly not from food cholesterol, but from food triglycerides—that is, plain old fat, and saturated fat in particular. As it turns out, the changes in diet that reduce serum cholesterol concentrations mostly do so by reducing LDL. HDL remain unaffected.

Among the most influential dietary factors that raise LDL are total fat intake, saturated fat, and high calories.[5] Among those that lower LDL are monounsaturated fats, including those of olive oil and rapeseed oil, and polyunsaturated fats, including those of other vegetable oils and fish oils. As for dietary cholesterol itself, it raises LDL slightly, depending on the amount being eaten and on the body's ability to compensate by making less. The American Heart Association offers recommendations for diet, based on these findings: eat no more than 30 percent of your calories as fat, with no more than a third of this fat as saturated fat; partially substitute polyunsaturated and monounsaturated fats for saturated fats; and reduce your cholesterol intake (see Table 4–2, p. 121).* This diet provides a total fat intake of 30 percent of calories, with 10 percent coming from each type of fat (saturated, monounsaturated, and polyunsaturated), and a cholesterol intake below 300 milligrams per day.

Figure 4–3
Digestion of Fats.

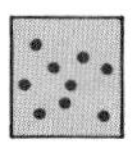
Water

Fat

Enzyme

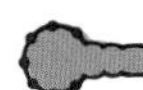
Emulsifier

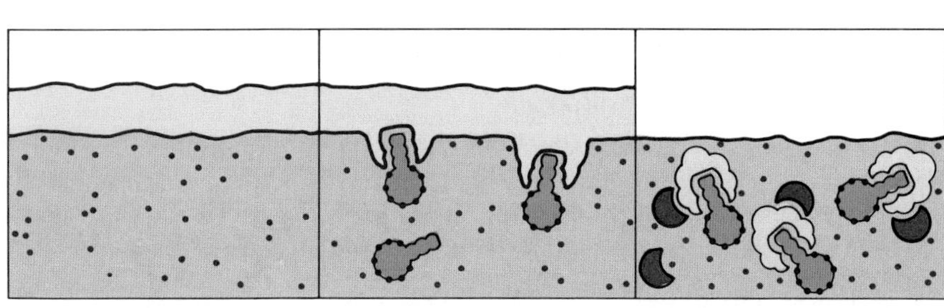

A. In the stomach, fats float to the top of the watery stomach fluid; fat slows digestion, lending satiety to the meal. Little digestion of fats takes place in the stomach.

B. Once in the small-intestine, fat encounters **bile,** an **emulsifier.** The gallbladder, a storage organ, squirts bile into the contents of the small intestine, to blend the fat with the watery digestive secretions.

C. Enzymes from the pancreas enter the small intestine. The enzymes can attack fat only after emulsification by bile. They break down the triglycerides to fatty acids, glycerol, and **monoglycerides** (a glycerol molecule with a fatty acid attached to the center carbon).

*The ratio between dietary polyunsaturated and saturated fat in the diet is called the P:S ratio. The significance of the P:S ratio to CVD development is altered by other dietary factors, including monounsaturated fats, fiber, and some sugars. To learn to calculate the P:S ratio of your diet, turn to Appendix C.

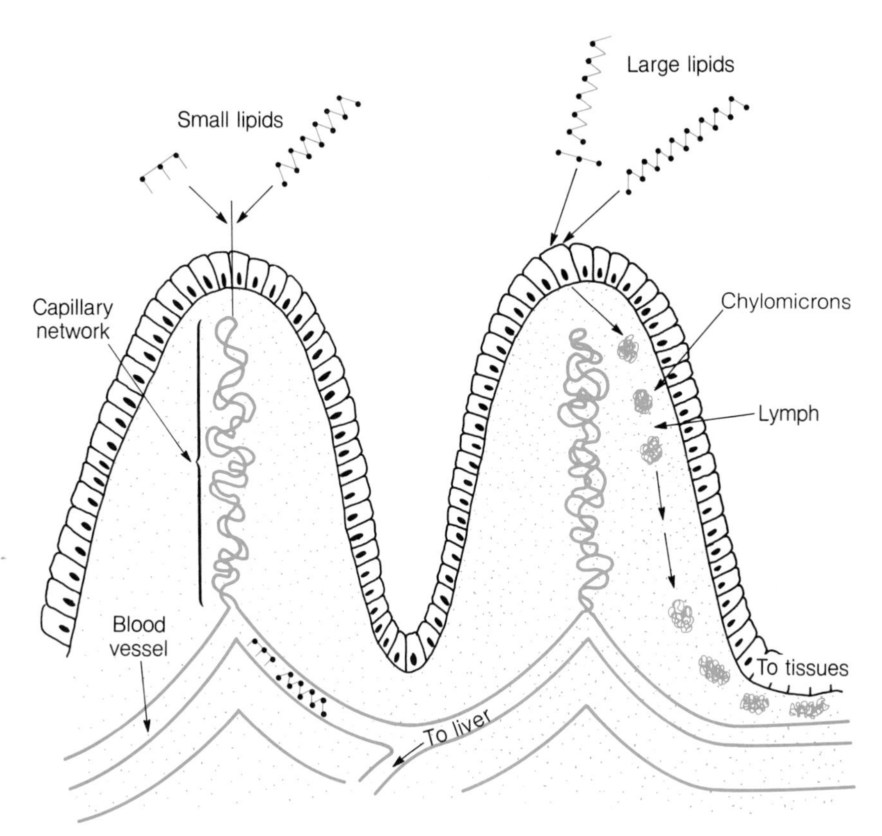

Figure 4–4
Two Routes Fat Takes from the Intestines to the Tissues.

A. The shortest free fatty acids pass by simple diffusion into the cells that line the intestine. Because these short-chain fatty acids are somewhat water soluble, they can, without any further processing, leave the cells on the other side and enter the body's capillaries. From these capillaries, the short-chain fatty acids are transported through collecting veins to the capillaries of the liver. The liver cells pick them up and convert them to other substances the body needs. The glycerol follows the same path as the short-chain fatty acids, because it too is water soluble.

B. The longer-chain fatty acids also pass into the intestinal cells, but there they reconnect with glycerol or with monoglycerides, forming *new* triglycerides. Now, triglycerides are insoluble in water, and the cells package them in chylomicrons for transport before releasing them into the lymph system. They, too, ultimately make their way into the bloodstream, because the lymph vessels ultimately pour into the bloodstream. Once the fats are in the blood, the tissues may pull them out of the packages for their use; if unused, the fats travel to the liver for dismantling.

While most blood cholesterol is carried in LDL and correlates *directly* with CVD risk, some is carried in HDL and correlates *inversely* with risk. In fact, for men over 50, the most potent single predictor of heart-attack risk may be the HDL level—the higher, the better for reducing risks.[6] While we must use the same caution here as formerly (since we don't know for sure whether it will have any beneficial effect), we can examine the question of how to raise HDL levels.

One way (although you can't do much about this) is to be female. Women have higher HDL than men. Another is not to smoke, or if you do, to stop. Nonsmokers have uniformly higher HDL than smokers. Still another is to be losing weight, but the most powerful influence on HDL is probably exercise, on a regular basis.

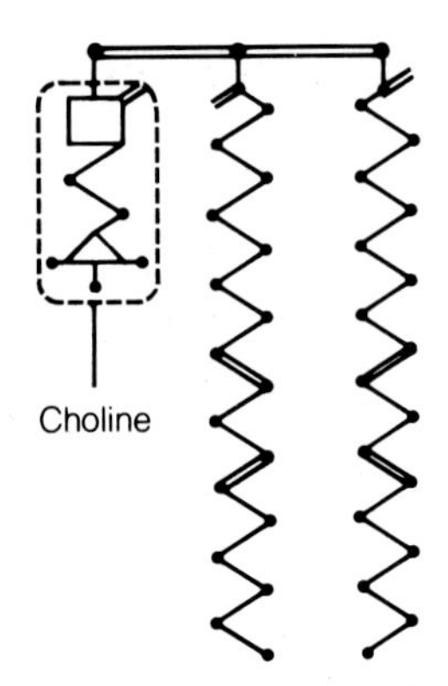

A molecule of lecithin is like a triglyceride but contains only two (polyunsaturated) fatty acids. The third position is occupied by choline, a B vitamin. The identity of the two fatty acids can vary, and all of the possible combinations are lecithins.

Lecithin

Lecithin periodically receives noisy attention in the popular press, being credited with great good deeds. You may hear that it is a major constituent of cell membranes (true), and that you must therefore purchase bottles of lecithin and give yourself daily doses (false). You might as well believe that in order to have healthy hair you must take supplements made from hair! One of the digestive enzymes takes most of the lecithin apart before it passes into the body fluids anyway, so not much of the lecithin you eat reaches the body tissues intact. All the lecithin you need for building cell membranes is made by your liver from scratch; in other words, lecithins are not essential nutrients. Furthermore, although once thought to be harmless, large doses of lecithin have now been seen to cause gastrointestinal upsets, sweating, salivation, and loss of appetite. These symptoms should serve to warn people to stop self-dosing with lecithin.

Another claim made for lecithin is that it helps improve people's memory. If only this were true, we could all benefit by eating lecithin; but if it is true at all, it seems to be so only for people with a specific kind of memory disorder. Even in those people, high doses are needed, suggesting that the effect is like that of a drug, not a nutrient. Lecithin probably works by contributing choline, which helps in several neurological disorders. But memory weakness is not a sign of lecithin deficiency. When you hear someone making claims for lecithin, especially someone recommending that you take it in order to escape deficiency, ask yourself, "Do I really need this? What is the evidence that my body is likely to be deficient?" In the case of lecithin, as with the overwhelming majority of other products that are hawked this way, such evidence is lacking.

Sources: J. L. Wood and R. G. Allison, Effects of consumption of choline and lecithin on neurological and cardiovascular systems, *Federation Proceedings* 41 (1982): 3015–3021; Choline and lecithin in the treatment of neurologic disorders, *Nutrition and the MD,* April 1980.

The discovery that exercise raises HDL has given great impetus to the physical fitness movement of the 1970s and 1980s, and especially to the popularity of running as a national pastime. The earliest reports of raised HDL were in long-distance runners, and continuing study of this elite group has repeatedly demonstrated that running does indeed elevate HDL.[7] Luckily, however, people do not have to become competitive athletes to raise their HDL—moderate or even light exercise such as walking may both lower LDL and raise HDL if the activity is consistently pursued.[8] Evidently, then, almost all people are capable of exercising enough to reap this and many other benefits. One more thing about athletes: some, under intense pressure to win, attempt to gain a competitive edge by abusing steroid drugs that increase muscle mass. These drugs negate any benefit against CVD that physical activity may impart—they promote CVD and reduce HDL in the blood of those who take them.[9]

Table 4–2

The American Heart Association Diet

Control the amount and kind of fat you eat:
- Limit your intake of meat, seafood, and poultry to no more than 5 to 7 oz/day.
- Use chicken or turkey (without skin) or fish in most of your main meals.
- Choose lean cuts of meat, trim all the fat you can see, and throw away the fat that cooks out of the meat.
- Substitute meatless or low-meat main dishes for regular entrees.
- Use no more than a total of 5 to 8 tsp of fats and oils per day for cooking, baking, and salads.
- Use low-fat dairy products.

Control your intake of cholesterol-rich foods to take in no more than 100 mg/1000 cal, or a maximum of 300 mg:
- Use no more than two egg yolks a week, including those used in cooking.
- Limit your use of shrimp, lobster, sardines, and organ meats.

Also control:
- Alcohol: use no more than 1.7 oz/day.
- Protein: consume no more than 15% of calories as protein.
- Sodium: use *no* more than 1 g/1000 cal, or a maximum of 3 g/day.
- Calories: eat just enough to maintain ideal weight.

Source: Adapted from *The American Heart Association Diet, An Eating Plan for Healthy Americans,* a booklet (1985) available from the American Heart Association National Center, 7320 Greenville Ave., Dallas, TX 75231; For a healthy heart, *Science News* 130 (1986): 135.

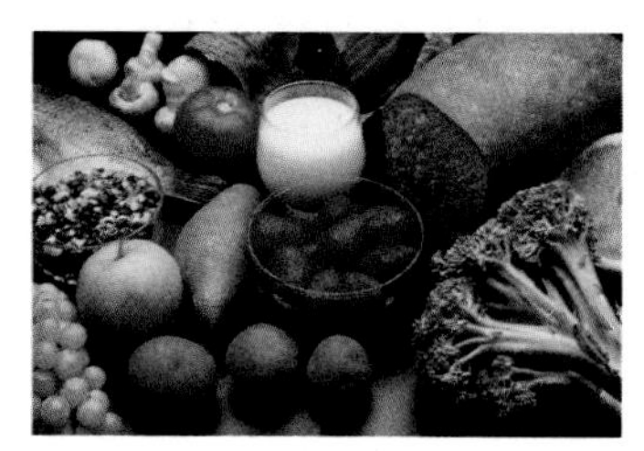

The AHA diet.

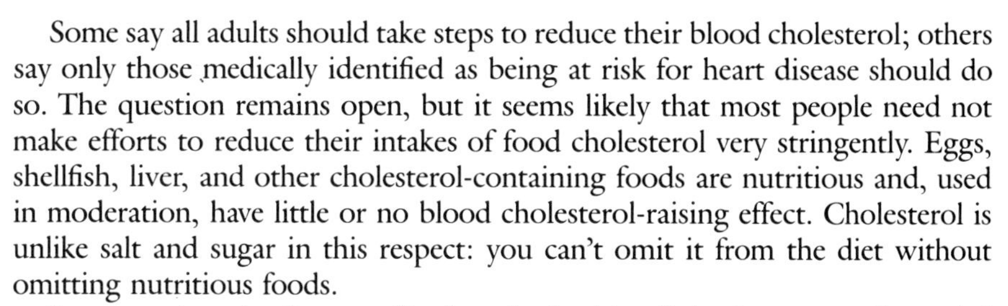

Some say all adults should take steps to reduce their blood cholesterol; others say only those medically identified as being at risk for heart disease should do so. The question remains open, but it seems likely that most people need not make efforts to reduce their intakes of food cholesterol very stringently. Eggs, shellfish, liver, and other cholesterol-containing foods are nutritious and, used in moderation, have little or no blood cholesterol-raising effect. Cholesterol is unlike salt and sugar in this respect: you can't omit it from the diet without omitting nutritious foods.

For more on diet changes to reduce blood cholesterol, read Controversy 4.

It seems that the factors affecting the health of the heart are all tangled together. The exact relationships among them have not yet been worked out; but although we don't know which causes what, all evidence points to the same general recommendations. For optimal wellness, and to avoid CVD, stop smoking; reduce blood pressure and weight if necessary; eat a balanced, adequate, and varied diet; use foods from animal sources sparingly and plant foods in abundance; reduce fat intake, especially saturated fat; exercise regularly; and—now that you have it all under control—enjoy life.

Dietary measures most effective in reducing the risk of heart disease are reducing total fat and saturated fats, and partially substituting monounsaturated and polyunsaturated fats. A third measure, perhaps effective to a lesser degree, is to reduce cholesterol intake. Don't omit cholesterol-containing foods altogether; they are nutritious. To lower LDL and raise HDL further, stop smoking and exercise regularly.

sucrose polyester (SPE): an artificial fat that can be substituted for oil, butter, margarine, and the like in meals. SPE is indigestible, so it does not contribute calories or raise blood cholesterol.

Fat in the Diet

The remainder of this chapter will help you to apply what you have learned about fats—that is, how to choose foods that supply enough, but not too much, of the right kinds of fat to support optimal health and provide pleasure in eating. To start, you must know where the fats are in the food groups.

Three food groups—fats and oils; meat, poultry, and fish; and dairy products—have traditionally accounted for about nine-tenths of the fat in the U.S. diet. However, recently there has been a shift from animal fats to fats of vegetable origin. The increasing consumption of vegetable fats and oils has come about because of three factors: their increased use by fast food chains serving fried foods like french fries and chicken, a shift away from the use of lard, and a shift from butter to margarine. A healthy trend is appearing: people are reducing their total fat intakes and increasing the proportion of unsaturated to saturated fat in their diets.[10]

Food chemists have developed and tested for safety an artificial fat that can substitute for the fat in foods but not be absorbed by the body. The artificial fat, **sucrose polyester (SPE),** was invented in the late 1960s and is just now earning a marketplace trial as the product Olestra. Tests with animals and people indicate that it looks, feels, and tastes like regular fats and that it is safe. SPE is made of sucrose molecules linked together in such a way that the digestive enzymes cannot break them apart, so it passes through the digestive tract undigested and unabsorbed. Some researchers suspect that it may carry with it some fat-soluble vitamins, causing deficiencies. It could also have the same effect in the digestive tract that mineral oil has—that of a laxative. Further tests will tell. But given that high blood cholesterol and obesity are so widespread, SPE is being viewed with hope as a possible help in the treatment of both.

The exchange lists show exactly where the fats are in foods. Two groups always contain fat (the fats and the meats) and two sometimes contain fat (the milks and the breads). The unprocessed vegetables and fruits are, for the most part, fat free. Figure 4–5 illustrates the fat values of foods.

Figure 4–5
Fat in Foods.

3 g in 1 oz lean meat.
8 g in 1 c whole milk.
5 g in 1 pat butter or margarine.

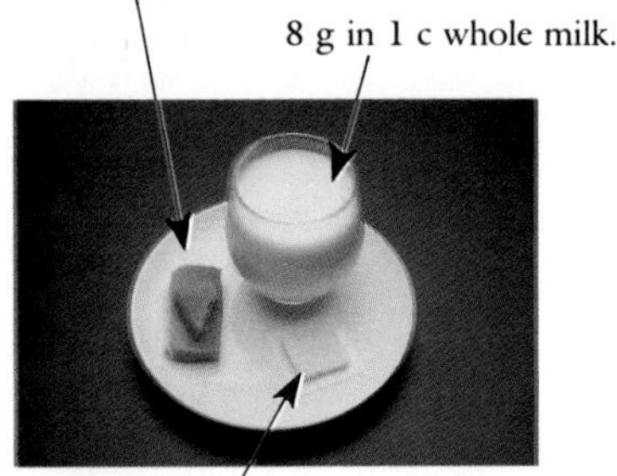

One Exchange	Fat (g)
Milk (1 c)	
Nonfat	Trace
2%	5
Whole	8
Meat (1 oz)	
Lean	3
Medium fat	5
High fat	8
1 tbsp peanut butter	8 (unsaturated)
Fat (1 tsp)	
Butter, margarine, or oil	5
Vegetables	0
Fruits	0
Breads and starchy vegetables	0
Sugar	0

The Fats

One portion of fat contains about 5 grams of fat, donating 45 calories and negligible protein and carbohydrate. Examples are:

- A teaspoon of butter or margarine.
- One-eighth of an avocado or five small olives.
- Two large whole pecans or 1 tablespoon of French dressing.
- Two tablespoons of sour cream or 1 tablespoon of heavy cream.
- A strip of crisp bacon.

Many are surprised to find bacon listed as a fat. They expect to find bacon fat included but think of crisp bacon as meat. It is classified as a fat, however, because its protein content is negligible, even if it is fried crisp and the melted fat is drained away.

The Meats

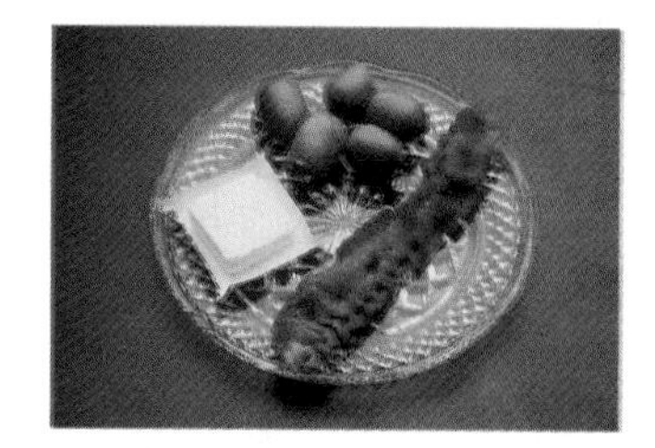

Fat exchanges. Each contributes 5 grams fat.

Meats probably conceal most of the fat that people unwittingly consume. Many people, when choosing a serving of meat, don't realize that they are electing to eat a large amount of fat. To help people "see" the fat in meats, the exchange lists present the meats in three categories according to their fat content. The three categories of meats contain about the same amount of protein per exchange, but the calorie amounts vary significantly among them. Table 4–3 lists some examples of lean, medium-fat and high-fat meats. The complete meat lists are in Appendix E.

A meat exchange is only 1 ounce of meat. This is a very small amount of meat and is not a serving size. A small fast-food hamburger, for example, weighs about 3 ounces (three exchanges), and 3 or 4 ounces of meat is thought of as a normal serving size for meal planning. Of course, your judgment of what is normal differs from other people's, and you might have to weigh your meat to discover the size of your servings.

People think of meat as protein food, but calculation of its nutrient content shows a surprising fact. A quarter-pound (4-ounce) hamburger contains 28 grams of protein and 23 grams of fat. Because protein offers 4 calories per gram and fat offers 9, the hamburger provides 112 calories from protein and a whopping 207 calories from fat. The total is over 300 calories. A hotdog is even higher in fat, which contributes 84 percent of its calories. From this, you might predict that overeaters of meat would tend to be overweight. This is because so much of the energy in a meat eater's diet is hidden from view—unrecognized.

Recently, some animal breeders have begun producing beef and pork that is lower in fat. This is a help to those people who choose lean cuts and eat small portions—they get less fat in the same quantity of meat. For the person choosing a hamburger, though, the change would not be significant—fat is ground together with the lean, negating any changes in the fat content of the lean. Chickens have also been bred to be leaner, but the nature of chicken meat remains mostly unchanged—chicken fat lies under the skin, not within the meat tissue. If you skin an ordinary chicken, you end up with a product that is much lower in fat than a lean-bred chicken with the skin left on.

Meat exchanges. Fat in these varies:

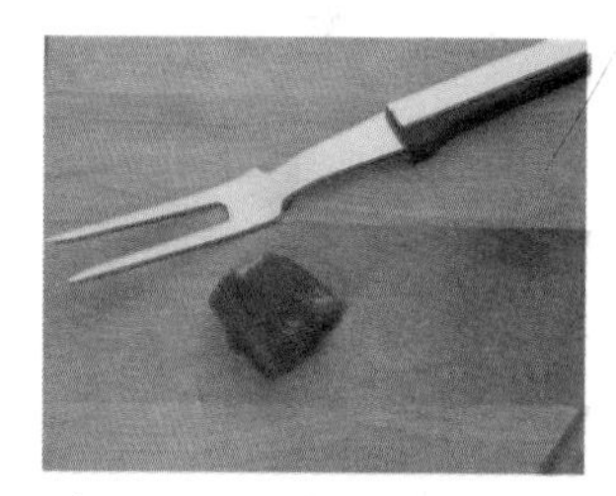

1 ounce lean meat = 3 grams fat.

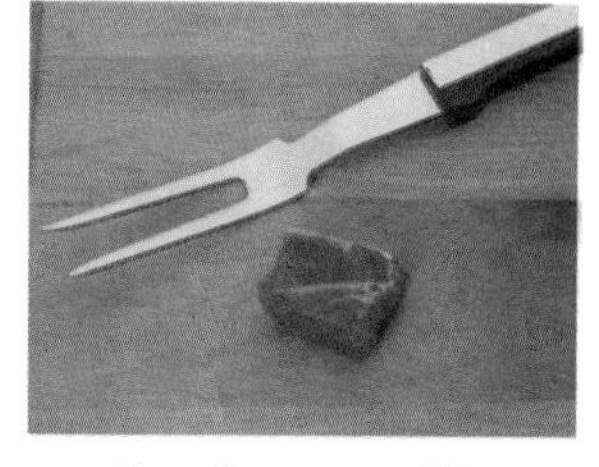

1 ounce medium-fat meat = 5½ grams fat.

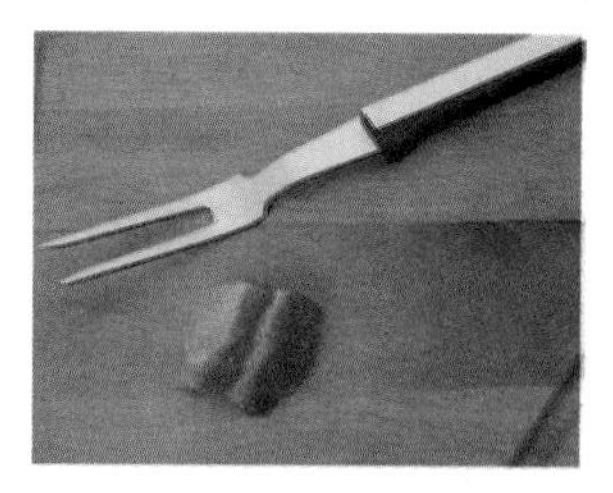

1 ounce high-fat meat = 8 grams fat.

Table 4–3

Some Examples of Lean, Medium-Fat, and High-Fat Meats

Lean Meat	Medium-Fat Meat	High-Fat Meat
Beef tenderloin, round steak	Corned beef, chuck	Hamburger; club or rib steaks
Chicken or turkey without skin	Ground round steak	Breast of lamb
Leg of lamb	Pork roast, liver, heart, kidney	Duck, goose
Fish	Eggs, creamed cottage cheese	Cold cuts
Dry cottage cheese		Hot dogs Cheddar cheese

1 oz = 28.4 g (dietitians often use "about 30 g" for an ounce).

1 oz meat = 28.4 g meat, containing about 7 g protein and from 3 to 15 g of fat.

Other Foods

Figure 4–5 showed that some milk exchanges contain fat. The exchange system views nonfat milk as milk and whole milk as milk with "added" fat. This is because, in homogenizing whole milk, milk processors blend in the cream, which otherwise would float and could be removed by skimming. The portion size is 1 cup; a cup of whole milk, then, contains the protein and carbohydrate of skim milk but, in addition, contains 8 grams (about 70 calories) of fat. (A cup of low-fat (2 percent) milk is halfway between whole and nonfat, with 5 grams of fat.) The fat occupies only a teaspoon of the volume but more than doubles the calories in the milk.

Milk and yogurt appear on the milk list, but cream and butter do not. Milk and yogurt are rich in calcium and protein, but cream and butter are not. Cream and butter are on the fat list, which also includes whipped cream, sour cream, and cream cheese.

Bread exchanges also sometimes contain fat. Notable are biscuits, corn bread, quick breads, french-fried potatoes, potato chips, snack and party crackers, pancakes, and waffles. People are often surprised to learn of the high fat content of these items.

A useful feature of the exchange lists is that they separate the polyunsaturated fat items from the saturated fat items. Of course, which of these you eat makes no difference in the total calories coming from fat, but it may make a difference in the unseen condition of your arteries.

People are eating more fat than they did 100 years ago. Fats, oils, meats, and dairy products contribute large amounts of fat to the diet. Reduce fat intake by using lean meats, nonfat milk products, and other foods containing little or no added fat.

Food Feature

Defensive Dining

Granola, "natural" cereals, breakfast bars, dinner rolls, snack crackers, biscuits, muffins—would you guess that these foods are high in fat? Although granola contains grain, check the ingredients on the label—fat is prominent, and sugar follows close behind. The fat of some foods is easy to see, and therefore to eliminate, but in foods like these, it is hidden. The purpose of this Food Feature is not to condemn familiar foods, but to enable you to choose or reject foods with a knowledge of their fat contents. It offers tips on using fats wisely to provide pleasure in eating and satiety to a meal, and on using restaurants to best advantage. The chief goal it addresses is to reduce fat, for that is the single most important dietary goal with respect to fat.

A place to begin is to read the labels on the foods you purchase in the grocery store. They can tell you much about their fat contents. The margin lists some words that can alert you to the presence of fat. Conveniently, the ingredients are listed in order of predominance in the product; if fat is one of the first ingredients listed, you know you are holding in your hands a high-fat product. Whether or not to choose it depends on how you intend to use it in your diet: as a staple item, as an occasional treat, or as a garnish for other foods.

You can find fat listed on a label as: Vegetable fat, lard, animal fat, shortening, oil, butter, margarine, cream.

Watch out also for mayonnaise, dressings, coconut, olives, cheese, nuts, and meats—they carry fat into foods, too.

Aside from labels, you can discern which foods may have hidden fat by studying the exchange lists in Appendix E. For example, yeast breads are listed with the bread, indicating that they contain negligible fat. On the other hand, biscuits and muffins are listed under a heading indicating that they were prepared with fat. The foods that are low in fat are the ones on all the regular and low-fat lists—cereals with no or little added fat (read the label), rice cakes and fatless wafers instead of snack crackers, nonfat milk and yogurt, lean meats, vegetables, and fruits.

If you want to limit fat in the foods you prepare at home, limit the fats that you add in preparation and at the table. Use an air popper for popcorn, and sprinkle the popcorn with butter flavoring. Spread a teaspoon of fruit butter on bread products instead of margarine. (Fruit butters contain only half the calories per teaspoon, and it's from sugar, not from fat.) Keep on hand low-fat substitute flavorings if you like them, such as imitation butter flavoring or diet margarine, low-fat salad dressings, and nonstick spray for frying in nonstick pans. Substitute low-fat ingredients in recipes where they will not affect the finished product detectably (see Table 4–4). By using such strategies, you can save hundreds of fat calories in a meal.

When you do add fats, be sure that they are detectable in the food and that you enjoy them. For example, if you use strongly flavored fat, a little goes a long way. Sesame oil, peanut butter, and the fats of strong cheeses are equal in calories to others, but they are so strongly flavored that you can use much less. Try small amounts of grated sapsago, romano, or other hard cheeses to replace larger amounts of less flavorful cheeses. Butter and regular margarine contain the same number of calories (35 per pat); diet margarine contains fewer calories, because water and fillers have been added. Imitation butter flavoring contains no fat and few calories.

Table 4–4

Substitutes for High-Fat Ingredients

Use	Instead of
Nonfat milk	Whole milk
Evaporated nonfat ("skim") milk (canned)	Cream
Yogurt[a]	Sour cream
Reduced-calorie margarine; butter replacers	Butter
Part-skim ricotta; low-fat cottage cheese	Whole-milk ricotta
Part-skim or low-fat cheeses	Regular cheeses
1 tbsp cornstarch (for thickening sauces)	1 egg yolk
Reduced-calorie mayonnaise	Regular mayonnaise
Low or reduced-calorie salad dressing	Regular salad dressing.

[a]If the recipe is to be boiled, the yogurt or cottage cheese must be stabilized with a small amount of cornstarch or flour.

If you use oil often, trade off, to obtain the benefits different oils offer. Peanut and sunflower oils are especially rich in vitamin E. Olive oil presents the heart health benefits associated with monounsaturates, mentioned earlier.

Here are some other tips to keep in mind while updating old high-fat recipes:

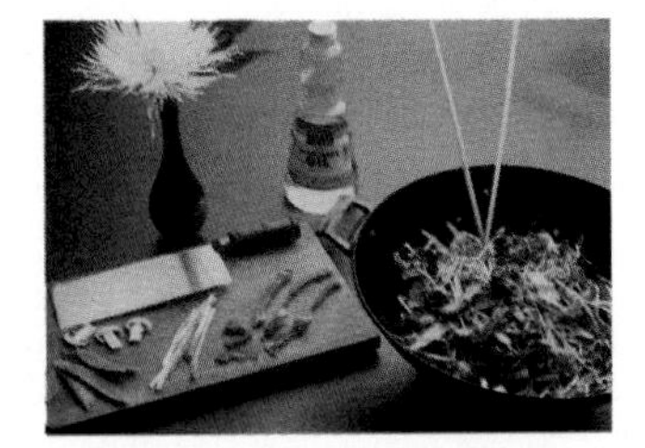

A little oil goes a long way in a pork and vegetable stirfry.

- Reduce the amounts of meats in recipes; substitute vegetables and starches.
- Trim all visible fat and skin from meat and poultry.
- Use the leanest meat you can find; pick a lean roast such as round, and have the butcher grind it without the fat. Then cut recipe amounts of the meat in half, and the meat price per recipe will be about the same as cheap, high-fat hamburger. Fill in the lost bulk with legumes, pasta, grains, or other low-fat items.
- Grill, roast, broil, boil, bake, stir-fry, microwave, or poach meats. Don't fry.
- Refrigerate pan drippings and broths, and lift off the fat when it solidifies. Then add the defatted broth to a recipe.
- Use water-packed canned tuna and chicken.
- If you use oil-packed tuna or chicken, place in a wire strainer and rinse with hot water to remove much of the fat.
- Use wine, lemon juice, or broth to replace butter.
- Use nonfat dairy products; replace cream with evaporated nonfat milk.
- Use low-fat yogurt instead of sour cream.
- Use reduced-calorie mayonnaise.
- When you use butter, margarine, or cream cheese, use the whipped variety—they contain half the calories of the regular types.
- Use commercial dry butter-flavored granules mixed with hot water as a substitute for melted butter.
- Use oil-free dressings for meat marinades.
- Add a little water to thick bottled salad dressings—they'll go farther this way.

Table 4–5 shows an example of a recipe modified to reduce the fat (and sodium, too—a need that Chapter 7 will explain fully).

All of these suggestions work well when a person carefully plans, selects, purchases, and prepares each meal with the loving attention it deserves. But in the real world, people fall behind schedule and don't have time to cook—they

Table 4–5

How to Modify A Recipe (Lasagne)

Original	Modified
⅓ c olive oil (to sauté vegetables)	[omit oil]
1½ c diced onions	1½ c onion, 1 green pepper, ½ lb mushrooms
2 cloves garlic	2 cloves garlic
1½ lb ground chuck	¾ lb ground round
2 t salt	[omit salt]
2 lb tomato sauce	use no-added-salt type
28 oz canned tomatoes	use no-added-salt type
6 oz canned tomato paste	use no-added-salt type
1 tbsp oregano	2 t oregano, 2 t basil, ¼ c fresh parsley
2 tsp onion salt	[omit salt]
1 lb lasagne noodles	1 lb whole wheat lasagne noodles
2 tbsp olive oil (to cook noodles)	[omit oil]
16 oz ricotta	16 oz low-fat cottage cheese, pureed
8 oz mozzarella	8 oz part skim mozzarella
10 oz parmesan	4 oz parmesan
oil to grease pan	spray to grease pan

Yield 16 servings (2 9″ × 12″ pans)

Analysis	Original	Modified
Energy (cal)	513	281
Protein (g)	35	21
Fat (g)	29 (6 t)	7 (1.4 t)
Sodium (mg)	1121	380
Cholesterol (mg)	73	32
Fat as % of calories	51	24

Source: Culinary Hearts Kitchen Course, Tallahassee, Fla., as taught by Sandi Woodruff, M.S., R.D., with permission.

eat fast food. Or they celebrate special occasions—they take a luxurious evening meal away from home. The next part of this Food Feature will show that you *can* eat in restaurants and dine nutritiously without being forced to accept high-fat foods you don't want.

To see how high the fast foods are in fat, look up a few in Appendix A.

What should you beware of in restaurant food? Let's begin with the foods typical of fast-paced, modern life: the fast foods. Fast foods can be extraordinarily high in fat because so many items are high in meat, are fried, or are made with whole milk, but they need not do you in.

The first question to ask about fast foods is, How often do I use them? If you visit a fast-food drive-in type restaurant only once a week, then the food consumed there accounts for only about 1 meal out of 20 and has little impact on your overall diet. The more often you visit fast-food places, the more important are the choices you make there. First, consider the choice of what place to visit. Places that sell tacos, hamburgers, pizza, or other foods offer meals with different characteristic nutrient arrays, and are rich in some nutrients. The old hamburger, french fries, and soft drink fast-food meal, for example, is *more* than adequate in protein, several of the B vitamins, and iron. Many fast-food

Figure 4–6
Calories in Fast-Food Choices.

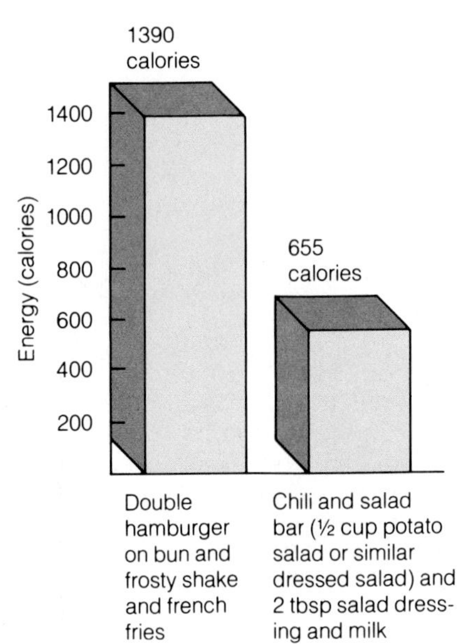

You have to choose carefully to limit calories in a fast-food meal.

places offer abundant vegetables and salads. If you have until now habitually chosen the old standby (hamburger, fries, and cola), here are some other possibilities you may want to consider:

- Except for pizza, fast-food meals are likely to be low in calcium. Choose milk or a milk shake for your beverage, or make sure to include milk or milk products in your other meals for the day.
- Hamburger/fries meals are low in vitamin A and folacin. The amount of lettuce and tomato provided in a typical hamburger, for example, doesn't make a dent on your need for these nutrients. Your next meal should be a large, raw salad or should include a generous serving of dark green vegetables.
- Fast foods are regrettably high in sodium—so high, in fact, that people on sodium-restricted diets have to stay away from them altogether.
- It is possible to vary your calorie intakes widely in a fast-food place. If your energy allowance is low, the salads are a good choice (use only about a quarter of the prepackaged dressing provided). Choose a small hamburger or fish sandwich to go with it if you are really hungry, or pick a salad that comes with meat, cheese, or egg. (People who need to lose weight can use fast foods as part of the diet plan, if they put their minds to it.) Figure 4–6 compares two fast-food meals.
- Finally, because fast foods are short on variety, let them be part of a lifestyle in which they complement the other parts. Eat differently, often, elsewhere.

Fast-food restaurants do not have a corner on the fatty meal market. This may be an even bigger problem for the eater in a traditional restaurant. Restaurant meals can be nutritious, but traditional restaurants seldom offer low-calorie choices or small servings, and an adult who asks for a "child's plate" is told the restaurant will serve them only to children. Nonfat milk is seldom available. Restaurants sometimes offer a "diet plate" of a 6-ounce patty of high-fat ground beef and a cupful of creamed cottage cheese, decorated with a sugar-packed peach half and gelatin dessert. Such a so-called diet plate can easily run up a fat total of more than that in the largest double burger, dripping with mayonnaise sauce and served with french fries. In fact, one hamburger chain noticed this and displayed placards claiming that its hamburger meals were lower in fat than a diet plate. The claim is true, but it only means that the diet plate is a hoax, not that hamburger meals are low in fat or calories.

Not all restaurants have these faults, and some people choose to avoid those that do. But in any restaurant, you can ask for changes that are to your benefit. For example, if the choices for potato are french fries, butter-soaked baked, or fat-carrying mashed, ask whether you can get a plain baked potato with butter on the side or double vegetable portions in place of the potato. (The latter is an especially useful strategy for the person with a small appetite.) You can also:

- Ask the person who is serving you how the dishes are prepared.
- Give an explicit order, so the chef knows exactly how to prepare the food.
- Order first so the other orders you hear won't sway you.
- Order all dressing, gravy, and butter on the side. Ask that the butter and other fats be placed on the far side of the table from you.
- Be creative with the menu; consider ordering from the appetizer list only—clear soup, salad, and a seafood cocktail can make a delicious low-fat meal.
- Don't read the menu at all; just ask for the foods you want.

Another strategy requires an effort that many consumers find mind-boggling:

- Leave some food on the plate.

It can be argued that the problem of overeating is caused not by restaurants but by overeaters themselves.

With practice, you can maximize the benefits of eating in restaurants. Here are a few more general strategies:

- Look for soup-and-salad restaurants.
- Order fruits, juices, vegetables, or salads whenever they are available. Ask for a vegetable plate even if it isn't on the menu as such.
- In a steak house, order the filet mignon. It is a smaller portion, and one of the only steaks on the menu that is truly a lean cut of meat (check Table 4–3).
- Ask for a "people bag" as soon as you get your food. Cut portions in half, eat half, and take the rest home to enjoy for lunch or supper the next day.
- If you are dining with a friend who's in the same boat you are, you can ask to share one large meal between you. There is usually a fee for the extra plate and sometimes they will split the food for you.
- Order fish and ask that it be broiled, not fried.
- If you must garnish your potato with fat, choose sour cream at 30 calories per tablespoon, rather than butter or margarine at 35 calories per teaspoon.

There is little question that eating out involves a trade-off. One loses in cost and control, but gains in convenience and in pleasure.

That covers the subject of reducing fat intake in meals, as far as the foods are concerned. But it hasn't focused long enough on the most important character in the picture: the diner. While it is possible to find nutritious *foods* in abundance in our fast-food places and restaurants, we do not find well-nourished *people* in such abundance. One survey of 600 people who eat in restaurants showed that a fourth of them had suboptimal intakes of one or more nutrients, that half of them were overweight, and that 20 percent of them were underweight. They had poor breakfast habits and tended to snack on nonnutritious foods, especially sweets and high-calorie foods. They suffered feelings of nausea, dizziness, and headaches before lunchtime and felt fatigued long before the day was over.[11]

Perhaps these people were trying to give to others the responsibility for seeing to their own needs. As pointed out in the first Food Feature of this book, nutrition is a personal matter; no one else can fully take the responsibility—not restaurant owners, not chefs, not even mothers or spouses. When the spotlight falls on the diner rather than on the foods served, it becomes clear where the responsibility lies.

shopping list:

- lean, lean meat
- water-pack tuna or chicken
- diet margarine or whipped margarine or butter
- commercial dry butter-flavored granules
- reduced-fat salad dressings
- oil-free dressing for meat marinades
- imitation butter flavor (liquid or granules)
- sesame or other strong-flavored oils, peanut butter
- fruit butters

- cooking spray
- nonstick pans
- nonfat milk products
- fresh and dried fruit, for dessert
- raw vegetables, for cooking and salads
- wine, lemon juice, or both, for cooking

Self-Study

Examine Your Fat Intake

These exercises make use of the information you recorded on Forms 1 to 4 in Appendix H.

1. How many grams of fat do you consume in a day?
2. How many calories does this represent? (Remember, 1 gram of fat contributes 9 calories.)
3. What percentage of your total energy is contributed by fat? You calculated this earlier, using Form 4.
4. A dietary guideline says fat should contribute not more than 30 percent of total energy. How does your fat intake compare with this recommendation? If it is higher, look over your food records: what specific foods could you cut down on or eliminate and what foods could you add to your diet to bring your total fat intake into line?
5. How much linoleic acid do you consume? (Refer to Form 1, polyunsaturated fatty acid column, and assume that most of this fatty acid is linoleic acid.) Remembering that linoleic acid is a lipid (energy value, 9 calories per gram), calculate the number of calories it gives you. What percentage of your total energy comes from linoleic acid? The guideline recommends 1 to 3 percentof *total* calories.
6. How much cholesterol do you consume daily? How does your cholesterol intake compare with the suggested limit of 300 milligrams a day? If your intake is high, you might want to read Controversy 4 before arriving at any conclusions regarding the importance of this limit.

Notes

1. S. W. Corbett, J. S. Stern, and R. E. Keesey, Energy expenditure in rats with diet-induced obesity, *American Journal of Clinical Nutrition* 44 (1986): 173–180.
2. E. M. Berry and J. Hirsch, Does dietary linolenic acid influence blood pressure? *American Journal of Clinical Nutrition* 44 (1986): 336–340.
3. Is it the olive oil? Cardiovascular benefits of the 'Mediterranean diet,' *Nutrition and the MD,* September 1987, p. 4.
4. M. Burros, Margarine choices: A guide for consumers, *New York Times,* 21 November 1984.
5. Consensus conference: Lowering blood cholesterol to prevent heart disease, *Journal of the American Medical Association* 253 (1985): 2080–2086.
6. Dozens of research articles now support this finding. A typical one: J. G. Brook and coauthors, High-density lipoprotein subfractions in normolipemic patients with coronary atherosclerosis, *Circulation* 66 (1982): 923–926.
7. P. D. Wood and coauthors, The distribution of plasma lipoproteins in middle-aged male runners, *Metabolism* 25 (1976): 1249–1257; R. H. Dressendorfer and coauthors, High-density lipoprotein-cholesterol in marathon runners during a 20-day road race, *Journal of the American Medical Association* 247 (1982): 1715–1717.
8. T. R. Thomas, Effects of interval and continuous running on HDL-cholesterol, apoproteins A-1 and B, and LCAT, *Canadian Journal of Applied Sports Sciences* 10 (1985): 52–59; A. Weltman, S. Matter, and B. A. Stamford, Caloric restriction and/or mild exercise: Effects on serum lipids and body composition, *American Journal of Clinical Nutrition* 33 (1980): 1002–1009; J. A. Cauley and coauthors, The epidemiology of high density lipoprotein cholesterol levels in postmenopausal women, *Journal of Gerontology* 37 (1982): 10–15.
9. M. Alen and coauthors, Reduced high-density lipoprotein-cholesterol in power athletes: Use of male sex hormone derivatives, an atherogenic factor, *International Journal of Sports Medicine* 5 (1984): 341–342; O. L. Webb and coauthors, Severe depression of high-density lipoprotein cholesterol levels in weight lifters and body builders by self-administered exogenous testosterone and anabolic steroids, *Metabolism, Clinical and Experimental* 33 (1984): 971–975.
10. R. Goor and coauthors, Nutrient intakes among selected North American populations in the Lipid Research Clinics Prevalence Study: Composition of fat intake, *American Journal of Clinical Nutrition* 41 (1985): 299–311.
11. R. B. Alfin-Slater and B. Gillis, Nutrition and work performance, *Nutrition and the MD,* August 1979.

Nutrition and Atherosclerosis

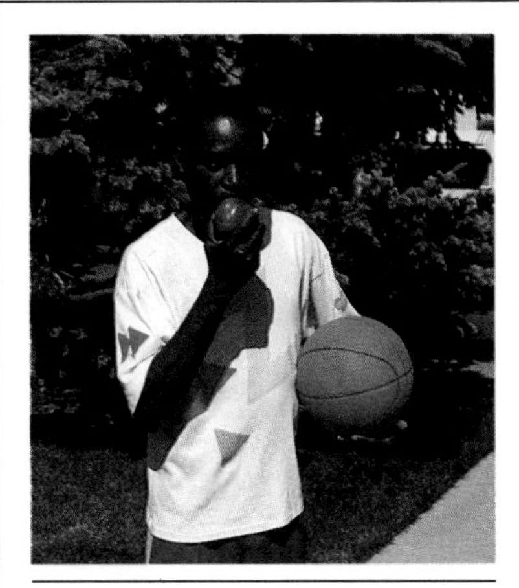

Is it because the fiber of apples lowers blood cholesterol that they keep the doctor away?

For decades, now, our major cause of death has been disease of the heart and blood vessels (cardiovascular disease, or CVD). CVD accounts for more than half of the nation's deaths each year, mostly by way of heart attacks and strokes.[1] Efforts to fight CVD have led to valuable discoveries and public education. We now know that smoking, high blood pressure, and high blood cholesterol are the three major risk factors for CVD, and many people have changed their lifestyles accordingly. Many have quit smoking, or refused to begin. Many who have hypertension have learned to control it. Many have been willing to change their diets, eating fewer calories and less fat, and are exercising more. The rate of CVD has fallen steadily since 1950, for some or all of these reasons; still, it is high. Can we lower it further? In particular, what are the factors we can control that will increase our chances of leading long and healthy lives?

The twin demons that lead to most CVD are **atherosclerosis** and **hypertension.** Atherosclerosis, the subject of this Controversy, is the common form of hardening of the arteries; hypertension (the subject of Controversy 7) is high blood pressure; and each makes the other worse.

How Atherosclerosis Develops

No one is free of atherosclerosis. The question is not whether you have it but how far advanced it is and what you can do to retard or reverse it. It usually begins with the accumulation of soft mounds of lipid, known as **plaques,** along the inner walls of the arteries, especially at branch points (see Figure C4–1). These plaques gradually enlarge, making the artery walls lose their elasticity and narrow-

Figure C4–1

The Formation of Plaques in Atherosclerosis.
When plaques have covered 60 percent of the coronary artery walls, the critical phase of heart disease begins.

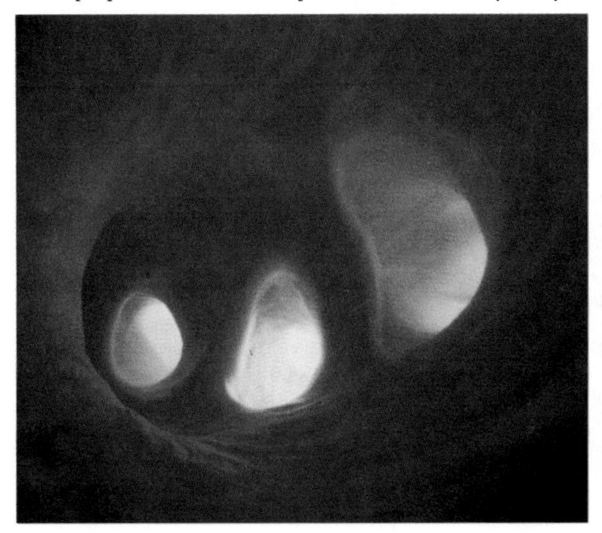

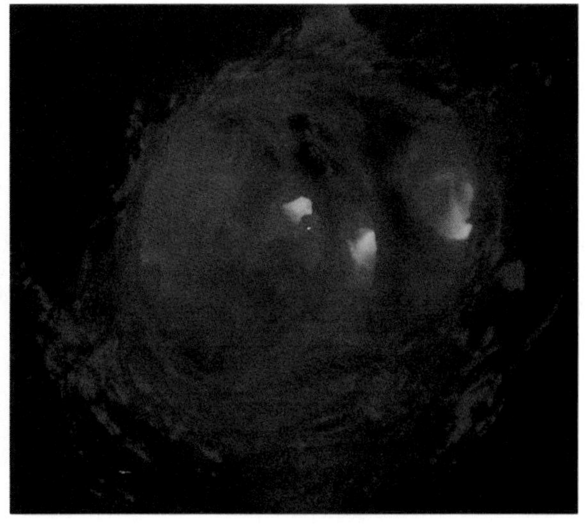

ing the passage through them. Most people have well-developed plaques by the time they are 30.

Normally, the arteries expand with each heartbeat to accommodate the pulses of blood that flow through them. Arteries hardened and narrowed by plaques cannot expand, and so the blood pressure rises. The increased pressure puts a strain on the heart and damages the artery walls further. At damaged points, plaques are especially likely to form; thus the development of atherosclerosis is a self-accelerating process.

As pressure builds up in an artery, the arterial wall may become weakened and balloon out, forming an **aneurysm.** An aneurysm can burst, and when this happens in a major artery such as the aorta, it leads to massive bleeding and death.

Abnormal blood clotting also contributes to life-threatening events. Clots form and dissolve in the blood all the time, and the balance between these processes ensures that they do no harm. That balance is disturbed in atherosclerosis. Small, cell-like bodies in the blood, known as **platelets,** are supposed to cause clots to form whenever they encounter injuries in blood vessels, but they respond in the same way to plaques and form clots when none are needed. Eicosanoids (see p. 112) control the action of the platelets, and an imbalance among these compounds may contribute to the formation of clots. Substances released by platelets also may aggravate the growth of plaques.

A clot, once formed, may remain attached to a plaque in an artery and gradually grow until it shuts off the blood supply of that portion of the tissue supplied by the artery. That tissue may die slowly and be replaced by scar tissue. The slow death of heart tissue caused by reduced blood flow is **ischemia,** and the stationary clot is called a **thrombus.** When it has grown large enough to close off a blood vessel, it is a **thrombosis.** A **coronary thrombosis** is the closing off of a vessel that feeds the heart muscle. A **cerebral thrombosis** is the closing off of a vessel that feeds the brain.

A clot can also break loose, becoming an **embolus,** and travel along the system until it reaches an artery too small to allow its passage. Then the tissues fed by this artery will be robbed of oxygen and nutrients and will die suddenly (**embolism**). Such a clot can lodge in an artery of the heart (Figure C4–2), causing sudden death of part of the heart muscle; we say that the person has had a **heart attack.** When the clot lodges in an artery of the brain, killing a portion of brain tissue, we call the event a **stroke.**

Figure C4–2
The Arteries That Feed the Heart Muscle.
The heart is a muscle, and like all muscles, it needs nutrients and oxygen. These are the **coronary arteries,** which bring nourishment to the heart muscle. If one of these arteries becomes blocked by plaque, the part of the heart muscle that it feeds will die.

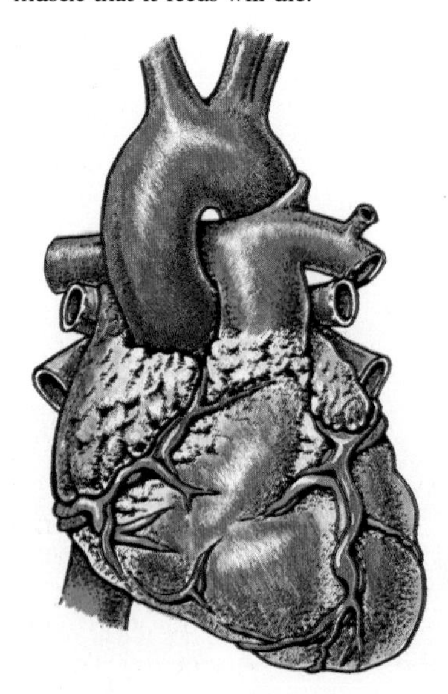

On many occasions, it is not clear what has caused a heart attack or stroke. An artery appears to go into spasms, and the blood supply to a portion of the heart muscle or brain is cut off, but examination reveals no visible cause.[2] Much research today is devoted to asking what causes plaques to form, what causes arteries to go into spasms, what governs the activities of platelets and the synthesis of eicosanoids, and why the body allows clots to form unopposed by clot-dissolving cleanup activity.

Hypertension makes atherosclerosis worse. A stiffened artery, already strained by each pulse of blood surging through it, is more greatly stressed if the internal pressure is high. Lesions (injured places) develop more frequently, and plaques grow faster.

Atherosclerosis also makes hypertension worse. By hardening the arteries, it makes them unable to expand with each beat of the heart, so the pressure rises, instead. This leads to further hardening of the arteries, as already explained. Hardened arteries also fail to let blood flow freely through the body's blood pressure–sensing organs, the kidneys; the kidneys respond as if the blood pressure were too low—and raise it further (see Controversy 7).

Risk Factors for CVD

The **risk factors** for atherosclerosis are listed in Table C4–1. It befits a nutrition book to focus on dietary strategies to reduce them. It should be noted, though, that diet is not the only, and perhaps not even the most important, factor in the causation of CVD. In fact, among the many con-

Table C4–1

Risk Factors for Atherosclerosis

Smoking
Hypertension
High blood cholesterol
Obesity
Glucose intolerance (diabetes)
Lack of exercise
Stress
Heredity
Gender (being male)

Table C4–2

Standards for Atherosclerosis Risk Factors

Hypertension	Obesity
Diastolic[a] pressure: 90–104 = mild 105–114 = moderate 115+ = severe	Body mass index greater than 27.2 for men or 26.9 for women (see Chapter 8, Figure 8–1)

	Blood Cholesterol[b]		Blood Triglycerides
Age	Moderate Risk (mg/100 ml)[c]	High Risk (mg/100 ml)[c]	Fasting levels: 250–500 mg/100 ml[d]
20–29	>200	>220	
30–39	>220	>240	
40+	>240	>260	

[a]When the blood pressure is taken, two measures are recorded: the systole first and diastole second (example: 105/70). Diastolic pressure is used in this table because it is the most sensitive indicator of hypertension. Adapted from Figure 17–10, How to interpret your blood pressure, F. S. Sizer and E. N. Whitney, Chapter 17, Heart and artery disease, in *Life Choices: Health Concepts and Strategies* (St. Paul, Minn.: West, 1988, in press).

[b]National Institutes of Health, *Cholesterol Counts: Cholesterol Management Principles from the Coronary Primary Prevention Trial,* NIH publication no. 85–2699, October 1985.

[c]100 ml is sometimes called a *deciliter (dl),* a term not used in this book. Values for blood cholesterol given in mg/100 ml are the same as those given in mg/dl. New values for blood cholesterol are also given in millimoles, another term not used in this book.

[d]High triglycerides are not normally indicative of direct risk, but possibly of risk by way of carbohydrate sensitivity, impaired glucose tolerance, or diabetes (see Controversy 3). Dietary management of patients with hypertriglyceridemia (clinical update), *Nutrition and the MD,* October 1986, pp. 4–5. High fasting triglycerides over many years may predict a probability of heart attack death, according to a follow-up heart disease risk factor study after more than ten years' elapsed time. L. A. Carlson and L. E. Bottinger, Risk factors for ischaemic heart disease in men and women: Results of the 19-year follow-up of The Stockholm Prospective Study, *Acta Medica Scandinavica* 218 (1985): 207–211, as cited in Plasma triglycerides: Fasting levels linked to risk for MI death, *Modern Medicine,* July 1986, p. 144.

troversies over diet and nutrition in recent years, one of the noisiest ones has been over the questions of whether diet is of any importance at all in heart disease; whether changes in diet can reduce the risk; and if so, whether such changes should be advocated for everyone, or just for selected high-risk individuals.

The big *diet-related* risk factors for CVD are hypertension, obesity, high blood cholesterol, and glucose intolerance. The standards by which each of these risk factors is labeled "high" are shown in Table C4–2. The rest of this discussion addresses the areas of disagreement among the experts on diet and atherosclerosis—the so-called **diet-heart controversy**—and attempts to arrive at suggestions for a personal strategy despite the confusion.

The Diet-Heart Controversy

No one disputes the fact that high blood cholesterol, particularly high blood LDL, predicts CVD, but people do dispute the hypothesis that links *diet* to CVD. The hypothesis is that high blood cholesterol (LDL) is at least partly caused by a diet high in saturated fat and cholesterol, among other things, and that reducing the amounts of saturated fat and cholesterol in the diet will lower blood cholesterol and reduce the rate of CVD. Both parts of this hypothesis have some strong support, but pieces are missing. With respect to the first part (whether or not a high-fat diet elevates blood cholesterol), blood cholesterol can be raised in both animals and people by raising the amounts of saturated fat and cholesterol in their diets—but whether the high blood cholesterol we see among so many people in the real world is *caused* by that aspect of their diets has been impossible to demonstrate. With respect to the second part (whether or not reducing fat intake will reduce blood cholesterol), it is possible to lower blood cholesterol in both animals and people by reducing the amounts of saturated fat and cholesterol in their diets—but whether this reduces their risks of heart disease has been impossible to demonstrate.

A strong voice against the diet-heart hypothesis is that of G. V. Mann, associate professor of medicine and biochemistry at Vanderbilt University School of Medicine, and a career investigator of CVD for the National Institutes of Health (NIH). In 1977, Mann presented several lines of evidence against the diet-heart hypothesis:

1. Two major studies showing no correlation between people's diets and their blood cholesterol levels.
2. A major decline in mortality from CVD that occurred between 1950 and 1980, a time during which people's saturated fat and cholesterol intakes were not changing.
3. Studies, in which people had been given diet changes to reduce blood cholesterol to prevent or treat heart disease, that had not proven any correlation.
4. Studies in which drugs had been used to reduce blood cholesterol—drugs that either succeeded in doing so without affecting the heart disease rate or caused excess deaths from other causes.

Mann argued that the high blood cholesterol seen in developed countries was not related to the saturated fat and cholesterol in the diet. He called for an investigation of other possibilities—abnormal oxidized forms of cholesterol that arise in foods when they are processed, *trans*-fatty acids that arise in oils when they are hydrogenated, an excess of vitamin D that is added to foods to "enrich" them, or excess carbon monoxide in the atmosphere that might interfere with the enzymes responsible for handling cholesterol. "Somewhere in the environment of Western man there is a noxious agent that causes trouble by inducing high blood cholesterol and, as a consequence, obstructive cardiovascular disease," but it is not dietary fat and cholesterol, Mann said. He suggested that regular vigorous exercise would be more effective than diet as a preventive strategy, although studies had not yet shown it to be so.[3]

The prevailing view was the opposite of Mann's, however. Many investigators and many organizations, including the American Heart Association, saw links between our high-fat, high-cholesterol diet and heart disease, and they held out the hope that continued research would confirm and clarify these relationships. The ferment of argument and research activity surrounding the issue continued, and by 1984, many more trials had been made. One of the most extensive was the Multiple Risk Factor Intervention Trial (MRFIT), involving a ten-year-long study of over 12,000 men who were persuaded to quit smoking, control their blood pressure, and make dietary changes to reduce their blood lipid levels. MRFIT was inconclusive: it did not demonstrate that diet changes would reduce the risk of CVD. In fact, it did not even demonstrate that controlling blood pressure would reduce mortality, partly because side effects of the drugs used to control high blood pressure confounded the results.

Another major trial was the Coronary Primary Prevention Trial (CPPT), involving about 4000 men for 7½ years. Initially, 48,000 men, aged 35 to 59, were screened. Those free of CVD, with the highest (top 5 percent) blood cholesterol levels, were chosen for the study—3,806 men altogether. All were given diet advice; half were given a cholesterol-lowering drug. The experiment was designed to lower blood cholesterol and measure any resulting changes in heart disease mortality, but it used drugs, not diet, to lower the blood cholesterol.

At the conclusion of the CPPT in 1984, the NIH stated that the reduction of blood cholesterol (using a drug) in the participants had successfully reduced heart attack risk. For each 1 percent reduction in blood cholesterol, a 2 percent reduction in heart attack risk was seen, they reported. The conclusion went on to say that for the men given the cholesterol-lowering drug in the study, an average 19 percent reduction in risk was seen; for those who had the full degree of cholesterol lowering, the reduction in risk was 49 percent.[4]

The reaction was instantaneous. The editor of the popular magazine *Nutrition Today* invited 27 experts to comment, and 20 responded, many with heavy criticism of the study and of the conclusions drawn from it. A sampling of the responses: "The trial proves nothing. There were 68 deaths out of 1906 men on the drug against 71 of 1900 on placebo."[5] "Only a small proportion of middle-aged men are prone to heart attacks and of those who are, only a fraction respond to cholesterol-lowering drugs."[6] "Several of the major clinical trials of reduction of raised serum cholesterol levels have shown an increase in non-cardiovascular mortality."[7] "Extrapolation of the . . . study data to the general population is far-fetched, [and] its projection into diet effects is illogical and indefensible. . . . The test may be said to demonstrate a *lack* of effect of diet."[8]

Disagreements on the meanings of the numbers of heart attacks and heart attack deaths were particularly troublesome. One critic reviewed the trial design from the start and found several flaws. For example, during the 7½ years of the study, 187 fatal and nonfatal heart attacks occurred in the untreated group and 155 in the treated group. The authors drew the erroneous conclusion that a 19 percent difference had been observed. The difference was actually only 1.6 percent—8.6 percent of the untreated men versus 7 percent of the treated men. The appropriate statistical test showed this difference to be insignificant. Based on this reevaluation of the data, "It is totally unreasonable to accept the statement . . . that these results have widespread implications for many millions of Americans." Only men with the highest blood cholesterol levels—265 and above—were studied. Therefore, any results apply only to males with elevated blood cholesterol and have hardly any significance even for them. "There is no evidence that reducing serum cholesterol in normal persons from 210 mg/100 ml will reduce the incidence of CVD in this group."[9]

The president of the American Heart Association (AHA) stated the exact opposite view: "The results of the CPPT clearly show the benefit of lowering plasma cholesterol. . . . The AHA has taken the position that a diet recommendation for the healthy U.S. population is warranted. . . . Americans . . . should consume a diet containing less total fat, saturated fat, and cholesterol."[10]

At the end of 1984, the NIH gathered together a panel of experts to attempt to arrive at a consensus on the question of whether lowering blood cholesterol would help prevent heart disease. They concluded that elevated blood cholesterol levels are clearly a major cause of artery disease, and that lowering them would reduce the risk of heart attack in men and probably in women. They agreed that the top 25 percent of blood cholesterol levels should receive top priority in treatment, but they also stated that the whole population has too-high levels, "in large part because of our high dietary intake of calories, saturated fat, and cholesterol." They went on to state that "there is no doubt that appropriate changes in our diet will reduce blood cholesterol levels [and] afford significant protection against coronary heart disease."[11]

The NIH Consensus Conference report went on to recommend that:

1. People at high risk (values in the top 10 percent) receive intensive dietary treatment and, if not successful, treatment with drugs.
2. People at moderate risk (the next 15 percent) receive intensive diet treatment (few should need drugs).
3. All U.S. citizens from age two up be advised to adopt a preventive diet with 30 percent of calories from fat (with 10 percent from polyunsaturated fat and 10 percent from monounsaturated fat) and a maximum of 300 milligrams a day of cholesterol (as described in Chapter 4).
4. All people with obesity reduce their weight by means of diet and exercise.
5. People with high blood cholesterol also be counseled to control hypertension and diabetes, abstain from smoking, and exercise regularly.

Additional recommendations addressed education of health professionals and the public, cooperation by the food industry, adoption of informative food labels, universal screening of adults' blood cholesterol levels, further research, and ongoing monitoring and evaluation of these efforts.

Even while the "consensus" was being broadcast to the public, the conferees disagreed. They had been unanimous only in agreeing that everyone should be screened for high cholesterol and that obese people should reduce. There were strong dissenting opinions on the notion that so many people should attempt to lower their cholesterol levels or should eat a low-fat diet after the age of two. According to the dissenters, it had not been proven that these measures would benefit people, nor even that they would do no harm.* The publication that emerged from the conference, in fact, was accused of being a "nonsensus," rather than a "consensus," document.[12]

While the nation mobilizes to reduce everyone's blood cholesterol, the arguments continue unabated. In fact, the squabble over diet and heart disease is one of the most prolonged and complicated in 20th century nutrition. The missing piece is still missing. The question of whether dietary fat and cholesterol have any effect on heart disease risk is still unanswered. It is agreed that high blood cholesterol is a major risk factor for atherosclerosis. It is agreed that stringent dietary control can alter blood cholesterol levels somewhat. But what if the blood cholesterol is only a symptom of some underlying problem? Then altering it would not get at the cause.

If dietary fat and cholesterol do have effects on heart disease risk, they

*A scare for a while that low blood cholesterol might be a risk factor for cancer has been cleared up. Low blood cholesterol is associated with cancer, but it is a consequence, not a cause. A. I. Neugut, C. M. Johnson, and D. J. Fink, Serum cholesterol levels in adenomatous polyps and cancer of the colon: A case-control study, *Journal of the American Medical Association* 255 (1986):365–367.

may be so small as not to be worth all the hullabaloo that surrounds them. One team of statisticians calculates from the available data that a lifelong program of blood cholesterol reduction by diet might increase life expectancy only 3 days to 3 months among people with normal blood pressure who do not smoke. For people at high risk, added life expectancy would range from 18 days to 12 months. Public health would be better served by reducing smoking and high blood pressure, rather than lowering cholesterol intake in the general public.[13] In the same vein, ten years after the first of his statements mentioned here, Mann is still voicing objections. He states that there are people in East Africa who eat twice as much saturated fat and cholesterol as Americans do, and their cholesterol levels are rarely above 150 milligrams per 100 milliliters. He urges that diet and cholesterol be downgraded in importance in treating people at risk for heart disease, and that measures to manage hypertension be emphasized more strongly: don't smoke; seek potassium and avoid sodium; seek seafood; and follow a regular, vigorous exercise program.[14]

Even among those who agree that dietary fat and cholesterol should be reduced, there are other questions. For example, the NIH conferees noted that the trials had mostly been on middle-aged men, but they believed that women and older men would benefit, too, from a general lowering of blood cholesterol. Two years later, reviews of statistics were leading to doubts about the broad applicability of the recommendations. Using data from the longest available, original diet-and-heart-disease study, the Framingham Study (5000 people, 30 years), it was clear only that CVD risk for men under 50 was increased at cholesterol levels above 180 milligrams per 100 milliliters. For women, and for men over 50, there was little or no association.[15]

If people over 50 and women are excluded from the recommendations, what about infants and children? Experts (you will not be surprised to learn) disagree on this point. The Mayo Clinic and the American Heart Association have stated that it is appropriate and safe for all members of the family older than 2 years to eat a diet in which 30 percent of the total calories are from fat and cholesterol is limited to 300 mg a day.[16] The American Academy of Pediatrics, however, has warned that such a diet has not been tested on people under 20, may not reduce their blood cholesterol levels, and may not adequately support growth. Its recommendation for children is to avoid extremes in their

Miniglossary

Note: Not all of the terms presented here are used in the text, but they are common in general reading about cardiovascular disease and seem worth defining here.

aneurysm (AN-you-rism): the ballooning out of an artery wall at a point where it has been weakened by deterioration.

angina (an-JYE-nuh; some people say ANN-juh-nuh) **pectoris** (peck-TORE-us): pain in the heart region caused by lack of oxygen (*angos* means "blood vessel"; *angere* means "to strangle"; *pectoris* means "of the chest").

atherosclerosis (ath-er-oh-scler-OH-sis): the most common form of artery disease, characterized by plaques along the inner walls of the arteries (*athero* means "porridge" or "soft"; *scleros* means "hard"; *osis* means "too much"). (The related term **arteriosclerosis** means *all* forms of hardening of the arteries and includes some rare diseases.)

CAD (coronary artery disease): atherosclerosis in the arteries feeding the heart muscle.

CHD (coronary heart disease): another term for CAD.

CVA (cerebrovascular accident): a stroke or aneurysm in the brain.

CVD (cardiovascular disease): a general term for all diseases of the heart and blood vessels. Atherosclerosis is the main form of CVD.

diet-heart controversy: the controversy over the questions of whether a high-fat, high-cholesterol diet causes atherosclerosis and whether a low-fat, low-cholesterol diet can prevent it.

embolus (EM-boh-luss): a thrombus that breaks loose. When it causes sudden closure of a blood vessel, it is an **embolism** (*embol* means "to insert").

heart attack: the event in which an embolus lodges in vessels that feed the heart muscle, causing sudden tissue death. Also called *myocardial infarct*.

high-risk approach: the approach (to prevention of CVD) that says that only those with blood cholesterol levels above 240 mg/100 ml should change their diets. (See also *population approach.*)

hypertension: high blood pressure (see Table C4–2 for quantitative definition and Controversy 5 for discussion).

IHD (ischemic heart disease): another term for atherosclerosis and its relatives.

diets except where careful screening of their family histories and blood cholesterol levels indicates unusual hereditary risk. Most children should eat a diet in which fat contributes 30 (not less) to 40 percent of the calories, an amount deemed moderate.[17] Low-cholesterol diets have not been tested on children and their effects during the growing years are not sufficiently well known to permit their use.[18] One thing seems clear to us: poor nutrition in early life seems to predispose children to CVD; so whatever else you do, feed them an ***adequate*** diet in infancy and early childhood.[19]

Although controversy sizzles around all the areas discussed above, health professionals are continuing to function, many of them by adopting a policy of screening every adult and selected children (the children of high-risk families) for high blood cholesterol. When high blood cholesterol is found, many agree that the first treatment should be diet.[20] If we agree thus far, we still have two more questions to address before attempting to put the lid back down on this controversy. The first is about blood cholesterol: how high is too high? The second is about diet: which diet?

How High Is Too High?

It is a much debated question, at what level of blood cholesterol to sound alarms. In our society, all people's blood cholesterol levels rise as they grow older. Should higher blood cholesterol levels in the later years therefore be considered acceptable? Some say yes, but the louder voices say no. Even moderately elevated cholesterol levels increase the odds of dying from CVD, and the danger is present even in people who do not smoke or do not have hypertension. According to one expert, who has worked with heart disease and public health for several decades, the optimal cholesterol level is 180 milligrams per 100 milliliters, and 80 percent of middle-aged men have levels higher than that.[21] Readings from 180 to 240 have been defined as "moderate" by some, but people with readings over 180 have elevated risks that rise higher, the higher they go.

According to the authors of the Whitehall Study, a study of over 15,000 middle-aged men whose mortality was followed over ten years, most deaths related to cholesterol occur among men with cholesterol levels in the *middle* three-fifths of the distribution. That means that if treatment were aimed only at those with the highest levels, it would miss an enormous number of people. The only way to save these lives, according to those who believe they *can* be saved by lowering their cholesterol

Miniglossary (continued)

ischemia (iss-SHE-me-uh): the deterioration and death of tissue (for example, of heart muscle), often caused by atherosclerosis (*is* means "to restrain"; *hem* means "blood").

multifactorial: having many causes.

myocardial infarct (MI) (my-oh-CARD-ee-ul IN-farct or in-FARKT): the sudden shutting off of the blood flow to the heart muscle by a thrombus or embolism; the same as a heart attack (*myo* means "muscle"; *cardial* means "of the heart"; *infarct* means "blocking off").

occlusion (ock-CLOO-zhun): shutting off of the blood flow in an artery (*ob* or *oc* means "in the way"; *clude* means "to shut").

plaques (PLACKS): mounds of lipid material, mixed with smooth muscle cells and calcium, which develop in the artery walls in atherosclerosis. The same word is also used to describe an entirely different kind of accumulation of material on teeth, which promotes dental caries (*placken* means "patch").

platelets: tiny, disk-shaped bodies in the blood, important in blood clot formation (*platelet* means "little plate").

population approach: the approach (to prevention of CVD) that argues that the whole population should change its diet. (see also *high-risk approach.*)

prostaglandins: hormonelike compounds (eicosanoids) related to and derived from polyunsaturated fatty acids (*prostagland* because the first such compound discovered was from the prostate gland).

risk factors: factors known to be related to (or correlated with) a disease but not proven to be causal.

stroke: the sudden shutting off of the blood flow to the brain by a thrombus or embolism.

thrombus: a stationary clot. When it has grown enough to close off a blood vessel, it is a **thrombosis.** A **coronary thrombosis** is the closing off of a vessel that feeds the heart muscle. A **cerebral thrombosis** is the closing off of a vessel that feeds the brain. (*Coronary* means "crowning" (the heart); *thrombo* means "clot"; *cerebrum* is part of the brain.)

levels, would be to lower cholesterol levels in the whole population.[22] Other researchers agree that it wouldn't help to treat only the high-risk people, because most heart attacks occur in people at moderate risk.[23] They therefore propound the **population approach.**

An exactly opposite view is put forth by the authors of a study involving over 10,000 middle-aged Israelis followed for 15 years. They found no association between elevated cholesterol and mortality until cholesterol levels rose above 240 milligrams per 100 milliliters, and they therefore viewed it as premature to support a policy of reducing mean cholesterol below 220 in the general population.[24] They therefore advocate the **high-risk approach.**

The president of the American Heart Association takes the position that cholesterol levels near the low end of the range should be considered risky, even though overt disease doesn't appear until levels are high. Figure C4–3 shows what may be going on. As he sees it, while a person's blood cholesterol steadily rises from the teen years onward, plaques are silently accumulating in that person's arteries. When 60 percent of the inner walls of the arteries are covered with accumulations of cholesterol, the CVD risk suddenly becomes apparent, but it has been developing for a long time. If this is the case, it can be argued that to minimize CVD risk, the process should be stopped near its beginning, not just shy of the danger point. Accordingly, the AHA president takes the preventive approach, recommending that:

- For people over 30, the line should be drawn at 200 milligrams per 100 milliliters. For people under 30, the line should be drawn at 180.
- If total serum cholesterol is above this line, then more sensitive indicators of risk should be measured: LDL and HDL cholesterol in particular.
- Triglycerides should be measured, too. They may or may not indicate risk for CVD, but they do indicate diabetes, kidney problems, and other conditions, and they should be treated.[25]

Another constructive suggestion has been made. Rather than argue over whether to target only those with the highest cholesterol levels or to educate everyone to control their blood cholesterol, why not do both? It has been pointed out that the two are complementary, not contradictory, strategies.[26]

Thus cholesterol screening goes on, in the hope of reducing this risk factor for atherosclerosis. Meanwhile, the reader may wonder what became of the loose ends mentioned earlier. What if the culprit responsible for high blood cholesterol and associated heart disease in the Western world is not fat and cholesterol, but some other factor—oxidized cholesterol, *trans*-fatty acids, vitamin D fortification, or something else? Investigations pursuing each of these

Figure C4–3

The Silent Progression of Plaque Formation.
As blood cholesterol rises from 100 to 300 mg/100 ml, plaques form in the arteries, first covering 25 percent, then 50, then 75, then 100 percent of their surfaces (straight line and numbers at left. The arteries here are coronary arteries, the ones that feed the heart muscle). However, heart disease symptoms remain at 0 until 60 percent of the artery walls are covered by plaques; then they rise steeply (curved line and numbers at right). Thus it appears that heart disease is nonexistent at cholesterol levels below 200 to 250 mg/100 ml. Actually, it is present but invisible—and progressing.

Most people with a cholesterol level of 200 and no other risk factors reach a critical degree of atherosclerosis at age 70. If their cholesterol level were 250 or 300, they would reach this critical point earlier—at age 60 or 50. Knowing the cholesterol level enables the health professional to predict the age of onset of CVD.

Source: Adapted from S. M. Grundy, Cholesterol and coronary heart disease: A new era: *Journal of the American Medical Association* 256 (1986): 2849–2858, Figure 6, p. 2851.

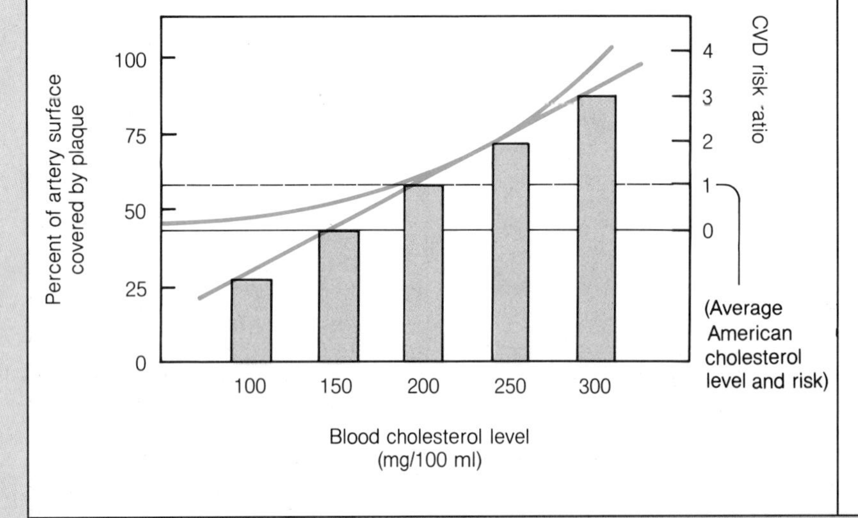

Table C4–3

Nutrients That Raise or Lower Blood Cholesterol[a]

Nutrients and Nutrient Variables That Raise Blood Cholesterol	Nutrients That Have No Effect	Nutrients That Lower Blood Cholesterol
	Carbohydrates	
Sucrose	Starch	Lactose
Fructose	Glucose	
	Fibers	
	Fine wheat bran	Coarse wheat bran
	Cellulose	Citrus pectin
	Soybean fiber	Oat bran
	Lignin	Guar gum
		Xanthan gum
		Other water-soluble fibers and gums from fruits, legumes, and vegetables
		Hemicellulose
	Lipids	
Total fat	Dietary cholesterol (in some individuals)	Polyunsaturated fat
Saturated fat		Monounsaturated fat
Trans-fatty acids[b]		Artificial fat (sucrose polyester)[c]
Dietary cholesterol (in some individuals)		
	Protein	
Animal protein, especially milk protein	Soybean protein (in some experiments)	Soybean protein (in some experiments)
		Plant protein
	Vitamins	
Vitamin C deficiency	Vitamin C; vitamin C megadoses	Vitamin C administered to correct deficiency
	Vitamin E	
	Vitamin B_6[d]	
	Minerals	
Fluoride deficiency		
Other mineral and trace mineral deficiencies or imbalances[e]		
	Water	
Soft water[f]		Hard water[f]
	Other Constituents of Foods	
		Plant sterols
		Flavones (from chick peas)
		Saponins (from alfalfa)

[a]References available on request; write the authors in care of the publisher.

[b]*Trans*-fatty acids raise blood cholesterol but do not cause atherosclerosis.

[c]Sucrose polyester doesn't actively lower blood cholesterol, but substitutes for saturated fat, which would otherwise raise it. See Chapter 4.

[d]Vitamin B_6 has no effect on blood cholesterol but does inhibit blood clotting. Inhibition of platelet aggregation and clotting by pyridoxal-5′-phosphate, *Nutrition Reviews* 40 (1982): 55–57.

[e]Optimal intakes of all of the following are necessary to keep cholesterol normal and prevent atherosclerosis: sodium, magnesium, calcium, chromium, copper, zinc, iodine, iron, and selenium. W. Mertz, Trace minerals and atherosclerosis, *Federation Proceedings* 41 (1982): 2807–2812. Magnesium deficiency also causes spasms of coronary arteries. P. D. M. V. Turlapaty and B. M. Alturn, Magnesium deficiency produces spasms of coronary arteries: Relationship to etiology of sudden death ischemic heart disease, *Science* 208 (1980): 198–200.

[f]Perhaps because soft water contains sodium and hard water, magnesium. R. Masironi and A. G. Shaper, Epidemiological studies of health effects of water from different sources, *Annual Reviews of Nutrition* 1 (1981): 375–400.

Table C4–4

Foods That Raise or Lower Blood Cholesterol[a]

Foods That Raise Blood Cholesterol	Foods That Have No Effect	Foods and Diet Variables That Lower Blood Cholesterol
	Meat, Fish, Poultry	
	Fatty fish (in some experiments) Shellfish	Fatty fish (in some experiments: salmon, sardines, mackerel, kippers, herring, pilchard, trout)
	Dairy Products	
Eggs (in some experiments)	Eggs (in some experiments)	Milk, nonfat milk, fermented milk and milk products
	Vegetables, Fruits	
		Fruits and vegetables Vegetarian diet Garlic[b]
	Legumes	
		Legumes[c] Soy milk[d] Textured soy protein
	Grains	
		Alfalfa, barley, oats, and other grains[e]
	Fats, Oils	
Butter Beef fat Other animal fats Hydrogenated fat products		Corn oil Soy oil Cod-liver oil Other fish oils Garlic oil Olive oil
	Other	
Refined sugar Coffee[g]	Hot peppers[f]	Ginseng Weight reduction in obese subjects

[a]References available on request; write the authors in care of the publisher.

[b]Garlic reduces blood cholesterol, slows the development of plaques, inhibits blood clotting, lowers LDL, and raises HDL (see also Controversy 10).

[c]Table C4–3 shows some of the constituents of legumes that may be responsible for their cholesterol-lowering effect.

[d]Soy milk lowered cholesterol "substantially" in subjects above the 50th percentile for North American cholesterol levels, but not in those with lower initial levels. W. A. Check, Switch to soy protein for boring but healthful diets (medical news), *Journal of the American Medical Association* 247 (1982): 3045–3046.

[e]Table C4–3 identifies some of the components of grains that lower blood cholesterol.

[f]Hot peppers (capsicum) don't lower blood cholesterol but do have an anticlotting effect. S. Visudhiphan and coauthors, The relationship between high fibrinolytic activity and daily capsicum ingestion in Thais, *American Journal of Clinical Nutrition* 35 (1982): 1452–1458.

[g]Although caffeine in animals lowers blood cholesterol, coffee (especially boiled coffee) raises it.

possibilities are under way but have, so far, yielded no findings suggesting that answers will lie there.[27] As mentioned, a piece is still missing from the heart disease puzzle.

If Diet, Which Diet?

Suppose that despite the conflicting evidence, a person wanted to adopt a diet consistent with the *possibility* that it might help avert cardiovascular disease. The next question is, what diet to choose? The conferees at the NIH Consensus Conference recommended the AHA Diet as the one of choice, but several dissenting opinions were voiced. Alternatives were a vegetarian diet with a high ratio of polyunsaturated to saturated fat, a diet rich in monounsaturated fats, and a diet rich in fish oils.[28] Extremists might propose the Pritikin diet—a diet with only 5 to 10 percent of its calories from fat, with negligible cholesterol, and with severely limited meats (Nathan Pritikin, who advocated this diet, died at 69 of causes unrelated to heart disease, with a blood cholesterol level of less than 100 milligrams per 100 milliliters and no plaques in his arteries at all.[29])

For interest's sake (and it may be purely academic interest), Tables C4–3 and C4–4 show the fruits of some fifty recent studies on individual diet components that influence blood cholesterol levels (higher or lower). They seem to point in the same direction as most other information so far presented. It seems to make sense to combine all reasonable possibilities: Why not? Eat a calorie-controlled, low-fat, low-cholesterol, high-fiber, high-complex-carbohydrate, adequate, balanced, varied diet. Abstain from too much coffee, alcohol, and sodium. Use olive oil among your oils; garlic, onions, and hot peppers among your vegetables. Include raw vegetables daily. Use whole grains (especially oats, and not especially wheat) and sprouts (especially alfalfa sprouts) often. Eat periodic meals of fish. Feel free to use shellfish; they are not as high in cholesterol as has been believed, and they do contain EPA and other fatty acids in the ω3 series. Use eggs and other animal protein foods in moderation.

Why do all this? Body weight has proven, in some studies, to be the most important single determinant of blood cholesterol level,[30] but even if weight control doesn't help ward off heart disease by reducing blood cholesterol, it will help by reducing blood pressure (see Controversy 7). So will eating a low-fat diet. Even if the high-fiber, high-complex-carbohydrate aspect doesn't help by way of cholesterol, it will help by improving glucose tolerance (diabetes, remember, is a major risk factor for CVD). Even if the monounsaturated oils and the ω3 oils from the fish don't help by way of cholesterol, they may help by favoring the right eicosanoid balance so that clot formation is unlikely. Even if the vegetable protein doesn't help by way of cholesterol, it may help in some other way. An adequate diet will protect the health of the heart muscle itself; mineral deficiencies precipitate disease of the heart muscle and arteries.[31] Also, stay with whole foods for the sake of every aspect of your health (not just the heart disease angle). While you are at it, exercise daily. Relax. Meditate or pray. Play. Happy people have lower blood cholesterol levels.[32]

Notes

1. *America's Health: A Century of Progress but a Time of Despair,* a booklet (1983) available from the American Council on Science and Health, 47 Maple St., Summit, NJ 07901.

2. H. Sheldon, *Boyd's Introduction to the Study of Disease,* 9th ed. (Philadelphia: Lea and Febiger, 1984), pp. 347–348.

3. G. V. Mann, Diet-heart: End of an era, *New England Journal of Medicine* 297 (1977): 644–650.

4. C. Lenfant and B. M. Rifkind, in Diet and heart disease: Responses to the LRC-CPPT findings, *Nutrition Today,* September/October 1984, pp. 22–29.

5. P. Elwood (director of the Medical Research Council Epidemiology Unit, Cardiff, Wales), in Diet and heart disease, September/October 1984.

6. A. E. Harper (professor of biochemistry and nutrition at the University of Wisconsin, Madison), in Diet and heart disease, September/October 1984.

7. M. F. Oliver (professor of cardiology at the Cardiovascular Research Unit, Department of Medicine, University of Edinburgh, Scotland, in Diet and heart disease, September/October 1984.

8. R. Reiser (professor emeritus, Department of Biochemistry and Biophysics at Texas A&M University, College Station, Texas), in Diet and heart disease, September/October 1984.

9. R. E. Olson (professor of medicine and pharmacology, State University of New York at Stony Brook), in Diet and heart disease: Responses to the LRC-CPPT findings, *Nutrition Today,* November/December 1984, pp. 22–25.

10. A. M. Gotto, Jr. (president of the American Heart Association; professor, Department of Medicine, Baylor College of Medicine and professor, Methodist Hospital, Baylor, Texas), in Diet and heart disease, November/December 1984.

11. Lowering blood cholesterol to prevent heart disease, NIH Consensus Conference, *Journal of the American Medical Association* 253 (1985): 2080–2086.

12. M. F. Oliver, Consensus or nonsensus conferences on coronary heart disease, *Lancet,* 11 May 1985, pp. 1087–1089.

13. W. C. Taylor and coauthors, Cholesterol reduction and life expectancy, *Annals of Internal Medicine* 106 (1987): 605–614; A. M. Epstein and G. Oster, Cholesterol reduction and health policy: Taking clinical science to patient care (editorial), *Annals of Internal Medicine* 106 (1987): 621–623; M. H. Becker, The cholesterol saga: Whither health promotion? *Annals of Internal Medicine* 106 (1987): 623–626.

14. G. Mann, interviewed in High cholesterol and heart disease: Experts disagree on the evidence, *Modern Medicine,* September 1985, pp. 229, 233–235.

15. K. M. Anderson, W. P. Castelli, and D. Levy, Cholesterol and mortality: 30 years of follow-up from the Framingham study, *Journal of the American Medical Association* 257 (1987): 2176–2180.

16. W. H. Weidman, Cardiovascular risk modification in childhood: Hyperlipidemia, *Mayo Clinic Proceedings* 61 (1986): 910–913.

17. Committee on Nutrition, American Academy of Pediatrics, Prudent life-style for children: Dietary fat and cholesterol, *Pediatrics* 78 (1986): 521–525.

18. R. E. Olson, Mass intervention vs screening and selective intervention for the prevention of coronary heart disease, *Journal of the American Medical Association* 255 (1986): 2204–2207.

19. D. J. P. Barker and C. Osmond, Infant mortality, childhood nutrition, and ischaemic heart disease in England and Wales, *Lancet,* 10 May 1986, pp. 1077–1081.

20. A. M. Gotto, Hypercholesterolemia: An assessment of screening and diagnostic techniques, *Modern Medicine,* April 1987, pp. 28–32.

21. J. Stamler, D. Wentworth, and J. D. Neaton, Is the relationship between serum cholesterol and risk of premature death from coronary heart disease continuous and graded? Findings in 356,222 primary screenees of the multiple risk factor intervention trial (MRFIT), *Journal of the American Medical Association* 256 (1986): 2823–2828.

22. G. Rose and M. Shipley, Plasma cholesterol concentration and death from coronary heart disease: 10 year results of the Whitehall study, *British Medical Journal* 293 (1986): 306–307.

23. D. M. Hegsted, Nutrition: The changing scene (1985 W. O. Atwater Memorial Lecture), *Nutrition Reviews* 43 (1985): 357–367.

24. U. Goldbourt, E. Holtzman, and H. N. Neufeld, Total and high density lipoprotein cholesterol in the serum and risk of mortality: Evidence of a threshold effect, *British Medical Journal* 290 (1985): 1239–1243, as cited in Cholesterol:

Mortality risk for CHD linked to a specific threshold, *Modern Medicine,* November 1985, pp. 147, 151.
25. Gotto, 1987.
26. M. F. Oliver, Strategies for preventing coronary heart disease, *Nutrition Reviews* 43 (1985): 257–262.
27. A. M. Pearson and coauthors, Safety implications of oxidized lipids in muscle foods, *Food Technology,* July 1983, pp. 121–129; M. Cleveland, Determination of oxidized cholesterol compounds in commercially processed cow's milk, Thesis (Ph.D.), Florida State University, 1986; J. E. Hunter and T. H. Applewhite, Isomeric fatty acids in the U.S. diet: Levels and health perspectives, *American Journal of Clinical Nutrition* 44 (1986): 707–717.
28. E. H. Ahrens, Jr., The diet-heart question in 1985: Has it really been settled? (editorial), *Lancet,* 11 May 1985, pp. 1085–1087.
29. J. D. Hubbard, S. Inkeles, and R. J. Barnard, Nathan Pritikin's heart, *New England Journal of Medicine* 313 (1985): 52.
30. Body weight and serum cholesterol, *Nutrition Reviews* 43 (1985): 43–44.
31. Diet, metals, and hidden heart disease, *Science News* 130 (1986): 201.
32. Try a little TLC, *Science 80,* January-February 1980, p. 15.

Chapter Five

Contents

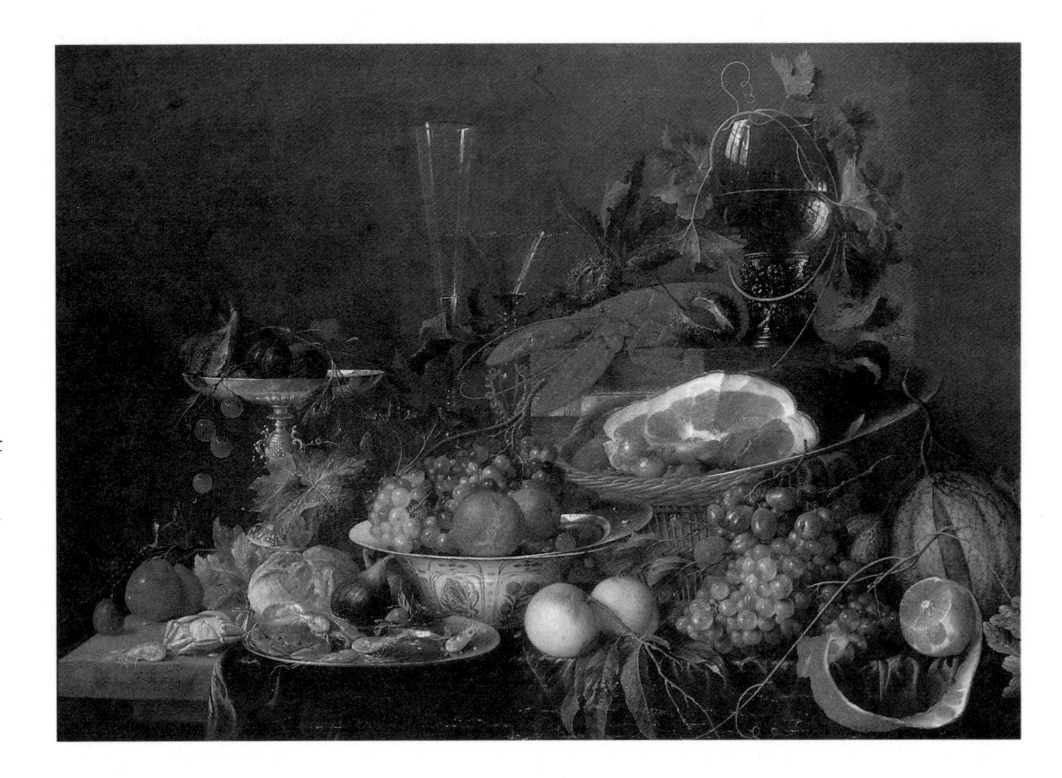

Still-life with Ham, Lobster, and Fruit by Jan Davidsz de Heem. Museum Boymans-van Beuninger, Rotterdam.

The Proteins and Amino Acids

The **proteins** are amazing, versatile, and vital cellular machines. Without them, life would not exist. First named 150 years ago after the Greek word *proteios* ("of prime importance"), proteins have revealed countless secrets of the ways living processes take place, and they account for many nutrition concerns. Why do we need to eat certain chemical substances (nutrients) and not others? How do we grow? How do our bodies replace the materials they lose? How does blood clot? What gives us immunity to diseases we have encountered? Understanding the nature of the proteins gives us many of the answers to these questions.

Protein machinery comes in many forms: enzymes, antibodies, transport vehicles, cellular "pumps," oxygen carriers, tendons and ligaments, scars, the cores of bones and teeth, the filaments of hair, the materials of nails, and more. But before describing the individual roles of protein, it is necessary to describe what all protein molecules have in common.

proteins: compounds—composed of carbon, hydrogen, oxygen, and nitrogen—arranged as strands of amino acids. Some amino acids also contain the element sulfur.

amino (a-MEEN-o) **acids:** building blocks of protein; each is a compound with an amine group at one end, an acid group at the other, and a distinctive side chain.

amine (a-MEEN) **group:** the nitrogen-containing portion of an amino acid.

The Structure of Proteins

To appreciate the many vital functions of proteins, we must understand their structure. One key difference from carbohydrate and fat, which contain only carbon, hydrogen, and oxygen atoms, is that protein contains nitrogen atoms. These nitrogen atoms give the name *amino* ("nitrogen-containing") to the **amino acids** of which protein is made. Another key difference is that in contrast to the carbohydrates, whose repeating units—glucose molecules—are identical, the amino acids in a strand of protein are different from one another. A protein is a strand of individual amino acids of 20 *different* kinds.

Amino Acids and Their Side Chains

All amino acids have a simple chemical backbone with an **amine group** (the nitrogen-containing part) at one end. At the other end is the acid group. This backbone is the same for all amino acids. The differences between them depend on a distinctive structure, the chemical side chain, that is attached to the backbone (see Figure 5–1). It is the nature of the side chain that gives identity and chemical nature to each amino acid. Twenty amino acids with 20 different side

Figure 5–1 An Amino Acid.
The "backbone" of the amino acid is the same as that of carbohydrates (p. 81) and fats (p. 109)—two carbon atoms joined together. *R* stands for the radical (as chemists call it), or side chain (as we call it), which differs from one amino acid to the next. The nitrogen is in the amine group. In later figures, amino acids will appear as rectangles and this structure will be understood.

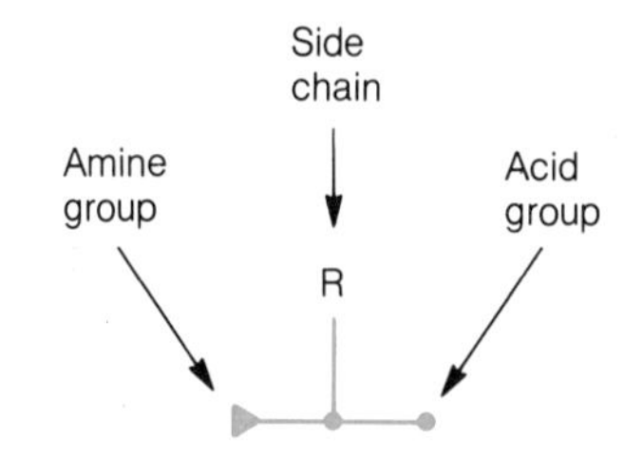

essential amino acids: amino acids that cannot be synthesized at all by the body or that cannot be synthesized in amounts sufficient to meet physiological need.

The amino acids:

- alanine
- arginine**
- aspartic acid
- cysteine**
- cystine
- glutamic acid
- glutamine
- glycine
- histidine*
- isoleucine*
- leucine*
- lysine*
- methionine*
- phenylalanine*
- proline
- serine
- threonine*
- tryptophan*
- tyrosine**
- valine*

*Essential amino acids for adults.
**Conditionally essential amino acids.

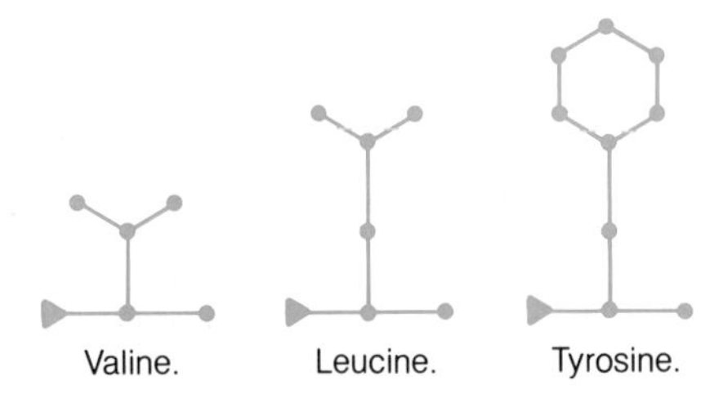

Examples of amino acids with different side chains.

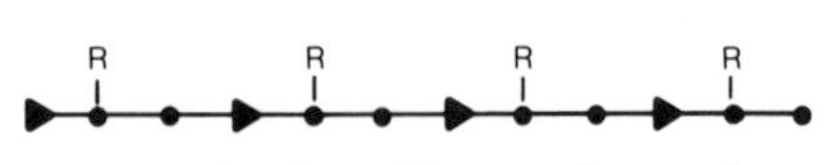

A strand of amino acids, part of a protein.

chains make up most of the proteins of living tissue. (Other rare amino acids appear in a few proteins.)

The side chains vary in complexity. This makes the amino acids differ in size, shape, and electrical charge. Some are negative, some are positive, and some have no charge. These side chains help to determine the character and functions of the larger protein molecules that the amino acids make up.

The body can make most of the amino acids for itself, given the needed parts: nitrogen to form the amine group, and backbone fragments derived from carbohydrate or fat. But there are some amino acids that the healthy adult body cannot make. These are the **essential amino acids.** If the diet does not supply them, the body cannot make the proteins it needs to do its work. The indispensability of the essential amino acids makes it necessary to eat food sources of protein every day.

The distinction between essential and nonessential amino acids is not quite as clear-cut as the list in the margin makes it appear. Histidine often appears not to be essential, perhaps because the diet supplies it in abundance; now, however, it has been added to the list of essential amino acids.[1] Arginine may, under some conditions, be synthesized too slowly to fully meet the human need.[2] Cysteine and tyrosine normally are not essential, because the body makes them from methionine and phenylalanine—but if there is not enough of these precursors to make them from, then they have to be supplied in the diet. Another amino acid, taurine, is not listed with the standard 20 because it is not used in protein strands. However, it is used to make materials important in brain and eye function and in the digestion of fat. Its concentration in human milk is high, and under special circumstances, human infants may require an external dietary source. States of illness can interfere with amino acid transformations in the body and so make other amino acids essential for individual human beings.

Proteins, unique among the energy nutrients because they possess nitrogen-containing amine groups, are composed of 20 different amino acid units. Some amino acids are essential or conditionally essential.

Proteins: Strands of Amino Acids

In the first step of making a protein, each amino acid is hooked to the next. A bond, called a peptide bond, is formed between the amino end of one and the acid end of the next. The side chains bristle out from the backbone of the structure, and these will give the protein molecule its unique character.

A strand of protein is not a straight chain. Proteins are made of many amino acid units, from several dozen to as many as 300. The amino acids at different places along the strand are attracted to each other, and in the second step of making a protein, this attraction causes the strand to coil into a shape reminiscent of a metal spring. A third step in forming a completed protein is achieved when side chains of the amino acids are attracted to, or repelled from, one another, causing the entire coil to fold back on itself this way and that, forming a globular structure. The amino acids whose side chains are electrically charged are attracted to water, and in the body fluids, they orient themselves on the outside of the structure. The amino acids whose side chains are neutral are repelled by water and are attracted to one another; these tuck themselves into the center, away from the body fluids. All these interactions among the amino acids and the surrounding fluid result in the unique architecture of each type of protein. One final step may be needed for the protein to become functional. Several strands may gather together and depend on one another to function, or a metal ion (mineral) or a vitamin may be needed to complete the unit and activate it.

The dramatically different shapes of proteins enable them to perform different tasks in the body. In proteins that give strength and elasticity to body parts, several springs of amino acids coil together and form ropelike fibers. Some are more than ten times as long as they are wide, forming stiff, rodlike structures that are somewhat insoluble in water and very strong. Other proteins, like those in the blood, don't have such structural strength, but they are water soluble, having globular shapes like balls of steel wool. Some are hollow balls, which can carry and store minerals in their interiors. Still others act like glue. Among the most fascinating are the **enzymes,** which act on other substances to change them chemically. The variety of proteins is endless. A photo of a model of a single large protein molecule, the one that carries oxygen in the red blood cells, is shown in Figure 5–2.

enzymes (EN-zimes): protein catalysts (as mentioned in Chapter 1). A catalyst is a compound that facilitates a chemical reaction without itself being altered in the process. (Additional details on digestive enzymes are in Appendix I.)

The great variety of proteins in the world is due to the infinite number of sequences of amino acids that is possible. If you consider the size of the dictionary, in which every word is constructed from just 26 letters, you can visualize the variety of proteins that are designed from 20 or so amino acids. The letters in a word must alternate between consonant and vowel sounds, but the amino acids in a protein need follow no such rules. Also, there is no restriction on the length of the chain of amino acids. Thus there are as many or more possible proteins as possible English sentences. There may be as many as 10,000 different proteins in a single human cell, each one present in thousands of copies.

The sequences of amino acids that make up a protein molecule are specified by heredity with exquisite order and precision. For each protein there is only

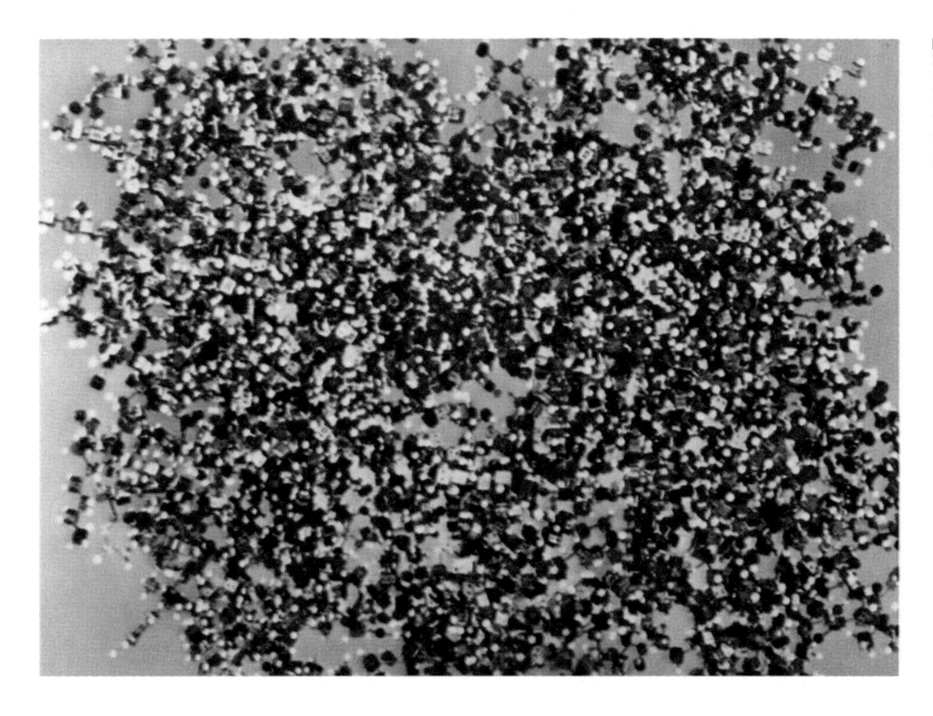

Figure 5–2 The Protein Hemoglobin. Each ball is an atom; the red cubes are iron atoms. This model represents one molecule of hemoglobin, magnified 27 million times.

denaturation: the change in shape of a protein brought about by heat, acid, base, alcohol, heavy metals, or other agents.

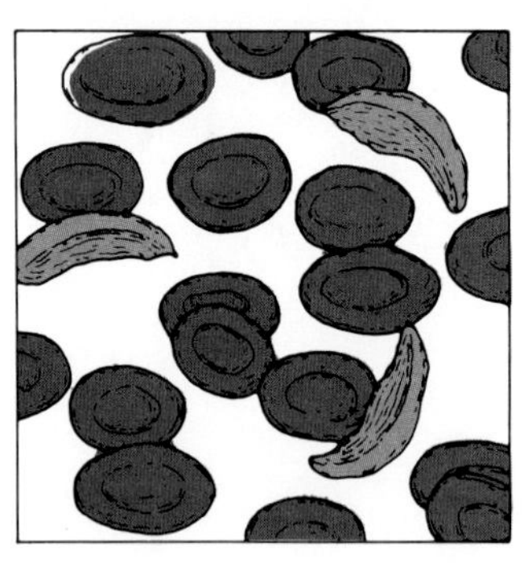

Normal cells (disk-shaped) and sickle cells (crescent-shaped).

one proper sequence. If the wrong amino acid is inserted or if one is out of place, the result may be disastrous.

Sickle-cell disease—in which hemoglobin, the oxygen-carrier protein of the red blood cells, is abnormal—is an example of an inherited mistake in the amino acid sequence. Normal hemoglobin contains two kinds of chains. One of the chains in sickle-cell hemoglobin is an exact copy of that in normal hemoglobin. But in the other chain, the sixth amino acid, which should be glutamine, is replaced by valine (see Table 5–1). The character and shape of the protein are so much affected by this difference that the protein is unable to carry and release oxygen. The red blood cells collapse into crescent shapes instead of remaining disk shaped as they normally do. If too many abnormal hemoglobins appear in the blood, the result is illness and death. One of the methods of detecting the disease is to observe under the microscope the altered shape of the red blood cells.

Each species of animal (including people) has proteins particularly designed for it. There may be great similarities; for example, the sequence of amino acids in the hormone insulin is nearly identical in most animals. But there are also some differences that make each insulin most suitable for the animal it belongs to. When an animal eats protein, the digestive and absorptive systems break it down and deliver the separated amino acids to the body cells. The cells then put them together in the order dictated by the animal's heredity to produce the particular proteins the animal needs. Figure 5–3 shows how the genes passed down to a cell from its parent cell dictate the sequences of the amino acids in its proteins, and Figure 5–4 shows the amino acid sequence of human insulin.

Amino acids link into long strands that fold or coil to make a wide variety of different proteins. Each type of protein has a distinctive sequence of amino acids and so has great specificity. Each type of animal builds species-typical proteins.

Denaturation of Proteins

Proteins can undergo **denaturation** (that is, distortion of shape) by heat, alcohol, acids, or the salts of heavy metals. Many reactions are harmful or useful because of their effects on protein. The denaturation of a protein is the first step in its destruction; thus excess acidity or alkalinity in the body is dangerous because it damages the body's proteins. However, the same reaction is useful to the body in digestion. During the digestion of a food protein, an early step is denaturation by the stomach acid, which opens up the protein's structure, permitting digestive enzymes to get at it. Cooking an egg denatures the proteins of the egg and makes it more appetizing. Perhaps more important, cooking denatures two raw-egg proteins that bind the B vitamin biotin and the mineral iron, as well as another protein that slows the digestion of other proteins. Cooking eggs liberates biotin and iron and aids in protein digestion.

Many well-known poisons are salts of heavy metals like mercury and silver; these alter the structure of proteins wherever they touch them. The common first-aid remedy for swallowing a heavy-metal poison is to drink milk. The poison then acts on the protein of the milk rather than on the protein tissues of the mouth, esophagus, and stomach. (Then vomiting is induced to expel the poison.)

Proteins can be denatured by heat, acid, alcohol, or the salts of heavy metals.

Table 5–1

The First Eight Amino Acids in One of the Chains of Human Hemoglobin

Normal		Sickle-Cell Disease
Valine	1	Valine
Histidine	2	Histidine
Leucine	3	Leucine
Threonine	4	Threonine
Proline	5	Proline
Glutamine	6	Valine
Glutamine	7	Glutamine
Lysine	8	Lysine

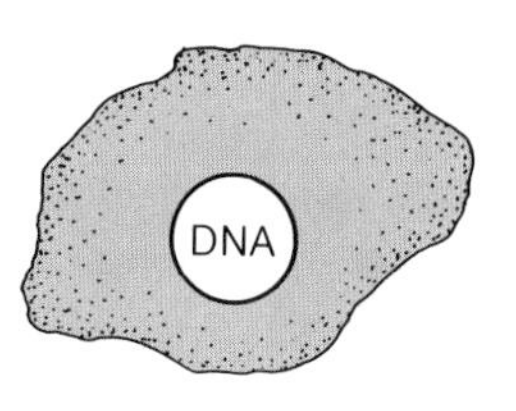

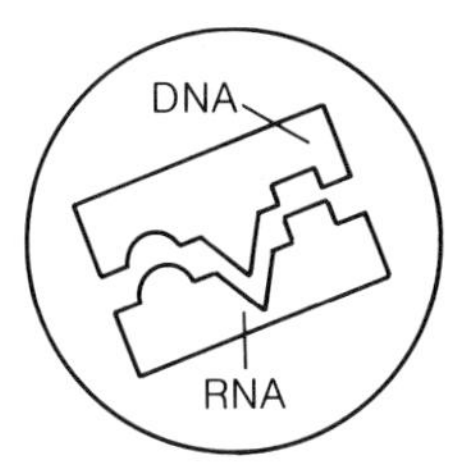

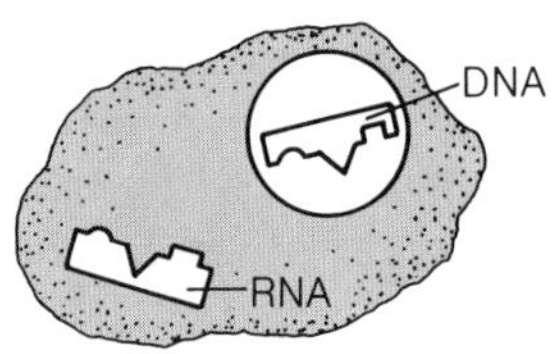

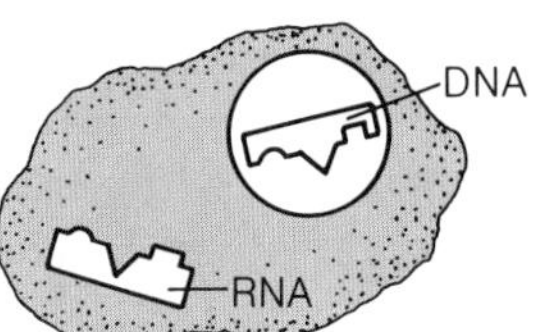

1. DNA is in the nucleus of each cell.

2. DNA makes a copy of that portion of itself that has the instructions for the protein the cell needs.

3. RNA leaves the nucleus.

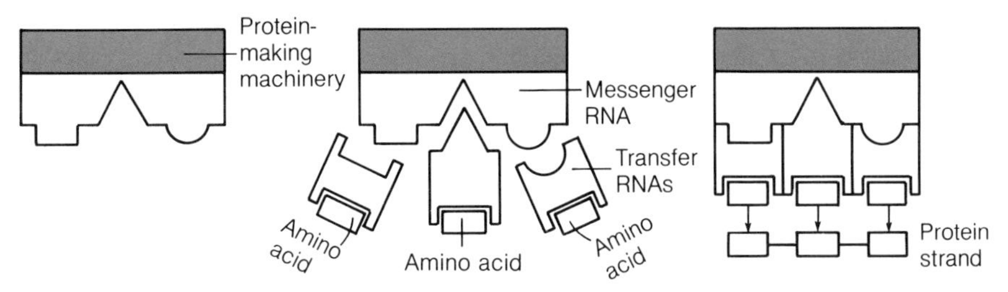

4. RNA attaches itself to the protein-making machinery of the cell.

5. Transfer RNAs carry their amino acids to the messenger RNA, where they are snapped into place.

6. The completed protein strand is released, and the messenger RNA is degraded.

Figure 5–3 Protein Synthesis.

The instructions for making every protein in a person's body are transmitted in the genetic information he or she receives at conception. This body of knowledge is filed away in a master file in the nucleus of every cell. The master file is the DNA (deoxyribonucleic acid), which never leaves the nucleus. The DNA is identical in every cell and is specific for each individual. Each specialized cell has access to the total inherited information but calls on only the instructions needed for its own functions.

In order to inform the cell of the proper sequence of amino acids for a needed protein, a "carbon copy" of the appropriate portion of DNA is made. This copy is messenger RNA (ribonucleic acid), which is able to escape through the nuclear membrane. In the cell fluid, it seeks out and attaches itself to one of the ribosomes (a protein-making machine, itself composed of RNA and protein). Thus situated, the messenger presents the specifications for the amino acids to be linked into a protein strand.

Meanwhile, other forms of RNA, called transfer RNAs, collect amino acids from the cell fluid and bring them to the messenger. For each amino acid there is a specific transfer RNA. Thousands of these transfer RNAs, with their loads of amino acids, cluster around the ribosomes, like vegetable-laden trucks around a farmer's market awaiting their turn to unload. When an amino acid is called for by the messenger, the transfer RNA carrying it snaps into position. Then the next and the next and the next loaded transfer RNAs move into place. Thus the amino acids are lined up in the right sequence. Then an enzyme bonds them together.

Finally, the completed protein strand is released, the messenger is degraded and the transfer RNAs are freed to return for another load. It takes many words to describe these events, but in the cell, 40 to 100 amino acids can be added to a growing protein strand in only a second.

The Roles of the Body's Proteins

Only a few of the great many roles of proteins will be described here, to give an appreciation of their versatility and importance. Primary among their functions is the support of growth.

hormones: as defined in Chapter 1, chemical messages that are secreted by a variety of body organs in response to conditions that require regulation. Each hormone affects a specific organ or organs and elicits a specific response.

Growth and Maintenance One function of protein in the diet is to ensure that amino acids are available to build the proteins of new tissue. The new tissue may be in an embryo; in a growing child; in the blood that replaces that which has been lost in burns, hemorrhage, or surgery; in the scar tissue that heals wounds; or in new hair and nails. Not so obvious is the protein that helps replace worn-out cells. The red cells of the blood are useful for about three or four months and then must be replaced by new cells that have been manufactured in the bone marrow. The cells that line the intestinal tract live for about three days and are constantly being shed and excreted. You have probably observed that the cells of your skin die and rub off and are replaced from underneath. Nearly all cells are constantly being replaced, and within each cell, too, proteins are constantly being made and broken down. For this new growth to take place, amino acids must be supplied constantly from food.

Figure 5–4 Amino Acid Sequence of Human Insulin.
This picture shows a refinement of protein structure not mentioned in the text. The amino acid cysteine (cys) has a sulfur-containing side group in it, and these groups on two cysteine molecules can bond together, creating a bridge between two protein strands or two parts of the same strand. Insulin contains three such bridges.

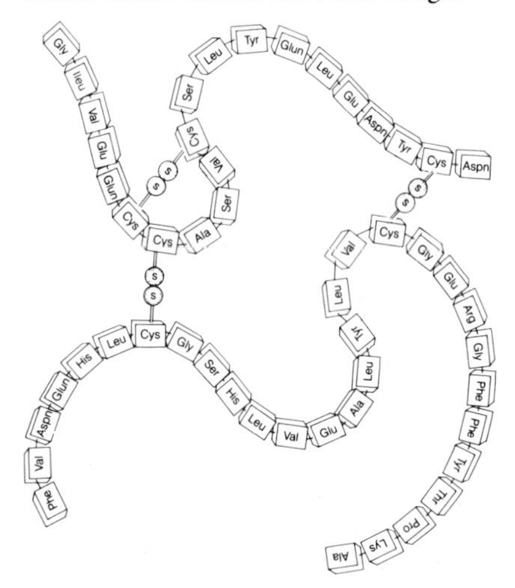

Enzymes and Hormones Enzymes are among the most important of the proteins formed in living cells. Enzymes are catalysts—they help chemical reactions take place. There are thousands of enzymes inside a single cell, each one facilitating a specific chemical reaction.

One of the mysteries that has been partially explained in recent years is how an enzyme can be specific for a particular reaction. The surface of the enzyme is contoured so that the enzyme can recognize the substances it works on and ignore others. The surface provides a site where two substances may become attached, first to the enzyme itself, then to each other. The newly formed product is then expelled by the enzyme into the fluid of the cell. Figure 5–5 shows compounds A and B parking for a moment on the enzyme, then leaving it as the new compound AB (a substance that is needed in some way). It could be that A and B, because they were both swimming around in the cell fluid, would have eventually discovered each other and combined without help. However, the enzyme attracted them and made them snap into the exact position for bonding. In this way, the enzyme speeded up the reaction time. A single enzyme can facilitate several hundred such reactions in a second. Enzymes are the "hands-on" workers in the production and processing of substances needed by the body.

Similar to the enzymes in the profoundness of their effects are the **hormones.** However, these molecules differ from the enzymes in that not all of them are made of protein and in that they don't catalyze chemical reactions directly.

Figure 5–5 Enzyme Action.
Each enzyme facilitates a specific chemical reaction.

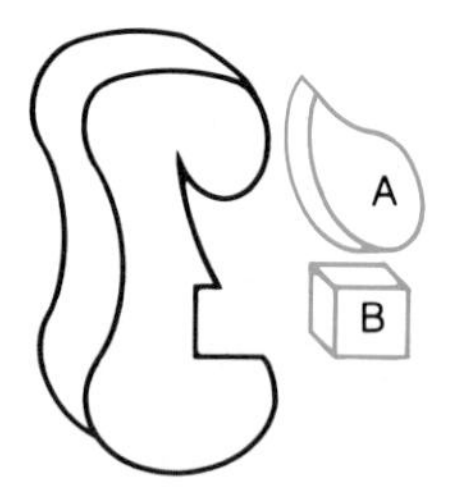

Enzyme plus two compounds, A and B

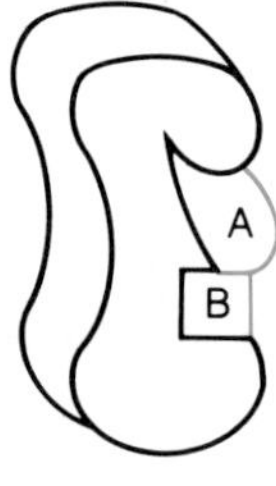

Enzyme complexed with A and B

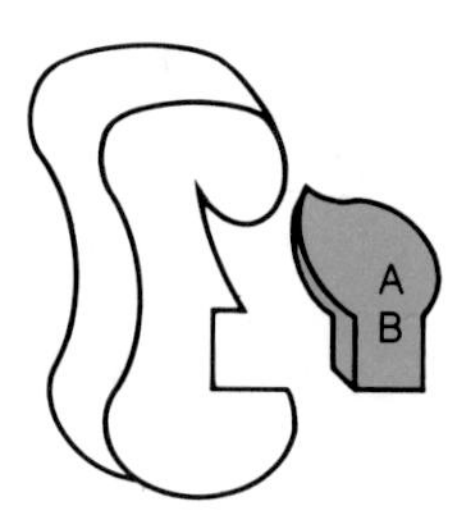

Enzyme plus new compound AB

Rather, they signal the appropriate enzymes to do what the body needs. Hormones regulate overall body conditions, such as the blood glucose level (insulin) and the metabolic rate (thyroxine), and they do it through the work of enzymes.

antibodies (introduced in Chapter 1): large proteins of the blood, produced by the immune system in response to invasion of the body by foreign substances (antigens); they combine with and inactivate them.

immunity (introduced in Chapter 1): specific disease resistance, derived from the immune system's memory of prior exposure to specific disease agents and its ability to mount a swift defense against them.

fluid and electrolyte balance: distribution of fluid and dissolved particles among body compartments (see also Chapter 7).

acids: compounds that release hydrogens in a watery solution.

bases: compounds that accept hydrogens from solutions.

Antibodies Of all the great variety of proteins in living organisms, the **antibodies** best demonstrate that proteins are specific for one organism. Antibodies are formed in response to the presence of foreign particles (usually proteins) that invade the body. The foreign protein may be part of a bacterium, a virus, or a toxin, or it may be present in a food that causes allergy. The body, after recognizing that it has been invaded, manufactures antibodies, and they inactivate the foreign protein.

One of the most fascinating aspects of this response is that each antibody is designed specifically to destroy one invader. An antibody that has been manufactured to combat one strain of influenza would be of no help in protecting a person against another strain. Once the body has learned to make a particular antibody, it never forgets; and the next time it encounters that same invader, it will be equipped to destroy it even more rapidly. In other words, it develops an **immunity.** This is the principle underlying the vaccinations and antitoxins that have almost eradicated childhood diseases in the Western world.

In some cases, the immune response can cause harm. If a transfusion should accidentally deliver the wrong blood type, the body would make antibodies to inactivate the foreign blood proteins. The first time this happened, the body might be able to tolerate or get rid of the gradual accumulation of inactivated foreign blood cells. But with a second transfusion of the wrong type, the body would be overwhelmed by an immediate, massive immune response, and death would result.

Fluid and Electrolyte Balance Proteins help regulate the quantity of fluids in the compartments of the body to maintain the **fluid and electrolyte balance.** To remain alive, a cell must contain a constant amount of fluid. Too much might cause it to rupture, and too little would make it unable to function. Although water can diffuse freely into and out of the cell, proteins cannot—and proteins attract water. By maintaining a store of internal proteins, the cell retains the fluid it needs (it also uses minerals this way). Similarly, the cells secrete proteins (and minerals) into the spaces between them to keep the fluid volume constant in those spaces. The proteins secreted into the blood can't cross the vessel walls, and thus they maintain the blood volume in the same way. (The control of water's location by particles is called *osmosis* and is discussed further in Chapter 7).

Not only the quantity, but also the composition, of the body fluids is vital to life. Transport proteins in the membranes of all the cells respond sensitively to small changes in the circulating fluids and work to maintain equilibrium by transferring substances into and out of cells. Thus, for example, sodium is concentrated outside the cells, and potassium is concentrated inside—a condition that is critical to the functioning of nerve and muscle cells. A disturbance of the fluid and electrolyte balance can impair the action of the indispensable heart, lungs, and brain, triggering a major medical emergency.

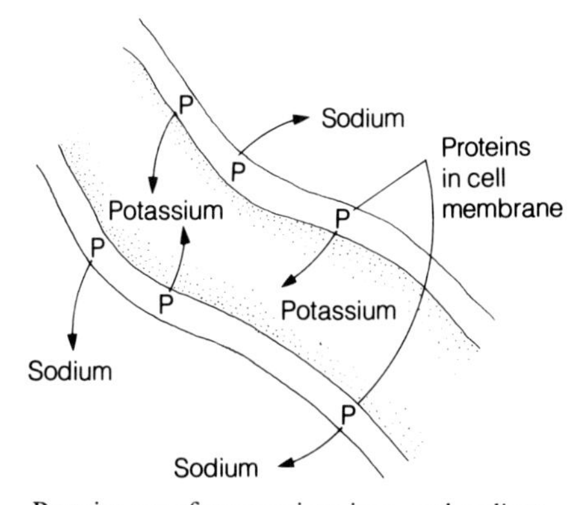

Proteins transfer potassium into, and sodium out of, nerve cells.

Acid-Base Balance Normal processes of the body continually produce **acids** and their opposite, **bases,** which must be carried by the blood to the organs of

acid-base balance: equilibrium between acid and base concentrations in the body fluids (see also Chapter 7).

acidosis (a-sih-DOSE-iss): blood acidity above normal, indicating excess acid (*osis* means "too much in the blood").

alkalosis (al-kah-LOH-sis): blood alkalinity above normal (*alka* means "base"; *osis* means "too much in the blood").

urea (yoo-REE-uh): the principal nitrogen-excretion product of metabolism, generated mostly by removal of amine groups from unneeded amino acids or from amino acids' being sacrificed to a need for energy.

excretion. The blood must do this without allowing its own **acid-base balance** to be affected. This magical feat is another trick of the proteins in the blood, which act as buffers. They pick up hydrogens (acid) when there are too many and release them again when there are too few. The secret is that the negatively charged side chains of the amino acids can accommodate additional hydrogens (which are positively charged) when necessary.

The acid-base balance of the blood is one of the most rigidly controlled conditions in the body. If it changes too much, the dangerous condition **acidosis** or the opposite, basic condition, **alkalosis,** can cause coma or death. The hazard of these conditions is due to their effect on proteins. When the proteins' buffering capacity is exceeded—when they have taken on board all the acid hydrogens they can accommodate—additional acid deranges their structure by pulling them out of shape; that is, it denatures them. Knowing how indispensable the structures of proteins are to their functions and how vital their functions are to life, you can imagine how many body processes would be halted by such a disturbance.

These are but a sampling of the major roles proteins play in the body, but should serve to illustrate their versatility, uniqueness, and importance. No wonder they are said to be the primary material of life.

Energy Only protein can perform all the functions described above, but it will be sacrificed to provide needed energy if insufficient fat and carbohydrate foods are eaten. The body's top priority need is for energy. All other needs have a lower priority.

When amino acids are degraded for energy, their amine groups are stripped off and used elsewhere or incorporated by the liver into **urea** and sent to the kidney for excretion in the urine. The fragments that remain are composed of carbon, hydrogen, and oxygen, as are carbohydrate and fat, and can be used to build those substances or be metabolized like them.

Not only can amino acids supply energy, but also about half of them can supply energy as glucose, as fat can never do. Thus, if need be, protein can help maintain a steady blood glucose level and so serve the brain.

A perspective on the three energy-yielding nutrients—their similarities and differences—now should be clear. Carbohydrate offers energy; fat offers concentrated energy; and protein, if needed, can offer energy plus nitrogen (see Figure 5–6).

Figure 5–6 Three Different Energy Sources.
Carbohydrate offers energy; fat offers concentrated energy; and protein, if necessary, can offer nitrogen plus energy.

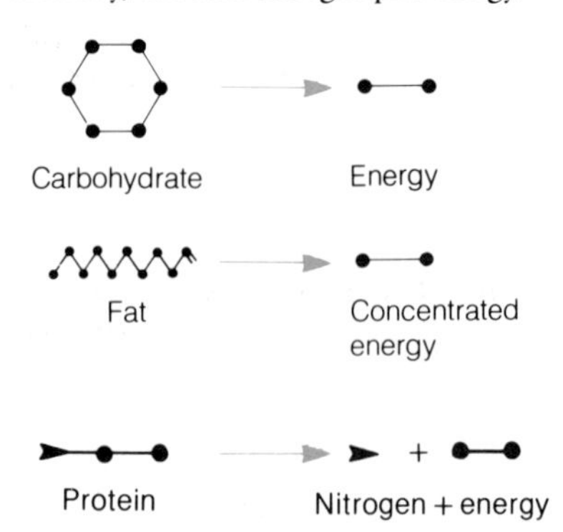

Only if the protein-sparing energy from carbohydrate and fat is sufficient to power the cells will the amino acids be used for the work only they can perform—making proteins. Thus energy deficiency (starvation) is always accompanied by the symptoms of protein deficiency.

If amino acids are oversupplied, the body has no place to store them. It will remove and excrete their amine groups and then convert the residues to glucose and glycogen or to fat for energy storage. Amino acids are not stored in the body, except in the sense that they are present in all the tissues. In case there is a great shortage of amino acids, tissue proteins, such as those of the blood, muscle, and skin, have to be degraded so that their amino acids can be used to maintain the heart, brain, and lungs.

Proteins serve many diverse functions, all of which are essential to life. When insufficient carbohydrate and fat are provided to meet the body's energy need, food protein and body protein are sacrificed to supply energy. The nitrogen part is removed from each amino acid, and the resulting fragment is oxidized for energy.

The Body's Handling of Protein

dipeptides (dye-PEP-tides): protein fragments two amino acids long. (A *peptide* is a strand of amino acids: *di* means "two.")

tripeptides (try-PEP-tides): protein fragments three amino acids long (*tri* means "three").

Each protein is designed for a special purpose in a particular tissue of a specific kind of animal or plant. When a person eats food proteins, whether from cereals, vegetables, beef, or cheese, the body must break them down into amino acids in order to rearrange them into its own unique sequences.

Digestion and Absorption in the Stomach and Small Intestine

Other than being crushed and mixed with saliva, nothing happens to protein until it reaches the very strong acid of the stomach. There, the acid helps to uncoil (denature) the protein's tangled strands so that the stomach enzymes can attack the bonds. You might expect that the stomach enzymes themselves, being proteins, would be attacked, but these are the only proteins in the body designed to resist strong acid and to become most active in it. Their job is to break apart the protein strands into smaller pieces. The stomach lining, which is also made partly of protein, is protected by a coat of mucus, secreted by its cells.

The whole process of digestion is an ingenious solution to a complex problem. Proteins (enzymes), when activated by acid, digest proteins (food) denatured by acid, and the mucous coating of the stomach wall protects *its* proteins from being affected by either acid or enzymes. The acid in the stomach is so strong (pH 2) that no food is acid enough to make it stronger. It is obvious from this that the stomach is supposed to be acid to do its job.

TV commercials sometimes promote antacids for relief of "acid indigestion," but antacids only put the burden on the stomach to produce even more acid to restore its normal balance. Antacids are useful to protect bleeding ulcers from stomach acid, but they are not appropriate for normal, healthy people. It is normal to have an acid stomach.

Sometimes the stomach acid backs up and burns the lining of the esophagus or throat, which are not as well protected by mucus as the stomach. When this happens, the person shouldn't take an antacid but should consult a doctor. The cause may simply be overeating, but it may be a condition that requires medical treatment—a hernia or obstruction. Self-diagnosis and treatment, even with over-the-counter medicines that are advertised to the general public, may not be a wise move.

By the time proteins slip into the small intestine, they are already broken into different-sized pieces. There are some single amino acids and many strands of two, three, or more amino acids **(dipeptides, tripeptides,** and longer chains). In the small intestine, the acid delivered by the stomach is neutralized by alkaline juice from the pancreas. The raising of the pH (to about 7) enables the next enzyme team to accomplish the final breakdown of the strands. Digestion continues until almost all pieces of protein are broken into small fragments and more free amino acids.

Absorption of amino acids takes place all along the small intestine. As for dipeptides and tripeptides, the cells that line the small intestine capture them on their surfaces, split them into amino acids, absorb them, and then release them into the bloodstream.

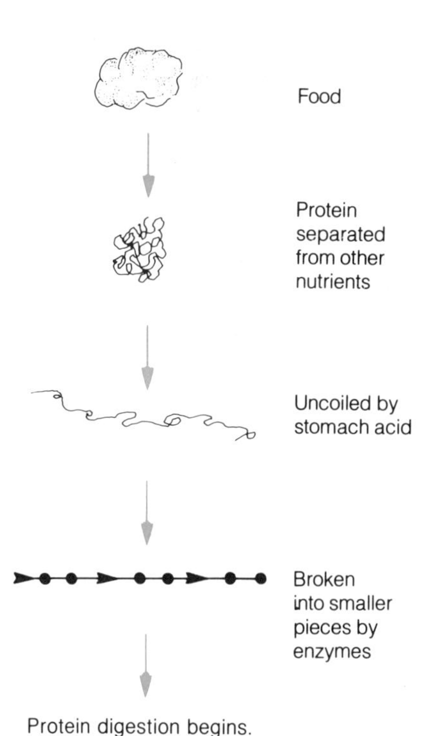

Protein digestion begins.

complete proteins: proteins containing all the essential amino acids in the right balance.

incomplete proteins: proteins lacking or low in one or more of the essential amino acids.

The cells of the small intestine possess different sites for the absorption of different classes of amino acids. A specific protein carrier helps the neutral amino acids across the cell membranes; another helps the acid ones; and another, the basic ones. Within each class, amino acids compete for the carriers. The presence of specific sites for the absorption of amino acids explains why we advise against supplementing the diet with specific amino acids, as is sometimes recommended (see the box entitled "Protein and Amino Acid Supplements" later in this chapter).

Digestion of protein involves denaturation by stomach acid, followed by enzymatic digestion by the stomach and small intestine to amino acids, dipeptides, and tripeptides. The cells of the small intestine complete digestion, absorb amino acids, and release them into the blood.

Use of Amino Acids inside Cells

Once they are circulating in the bloodstream, the amino acids are available to be taken up by any cell of the body. The cells can then make proteins, either for their own use or for secretion into lymph or blood for other uses.

If a *nonessential* amino acid (that is, one the cell *can* make) is unavailable for a growing protein strand, the cell will synthesize it and continue attaching amino acids to the strand. If an *essential* amino acid (one the cell *cannot* make) is missing, the building of the protein will be halted. Partially completed proteins are not held for later completion (for example, on the next day). Rather, the partial structures are dismantled, and the surplus amino acids are returned to the circulation to be made available to other cells. If they are not soon inserted into protein, their amine groups will be removed and excreted, and the residues will be used for other purposes. The need that prompted the calling for that particular protein will not be met.

It follows that all the essential amino acids must be eaten within the same time period, probably within about four hours.[3] This presents no problem to people who regularly eat **complete proteins**, such as those of meat, fish, poultry, cheese, eggs, or milk. The proteins of these foods contain ample amounts of all the essential amino acids. An equally sound choice is to eat two **incomplete protein** foods from plants, each of which supplies the amino acids missing in the other. This strategy is described in this chapter's Food Feature.

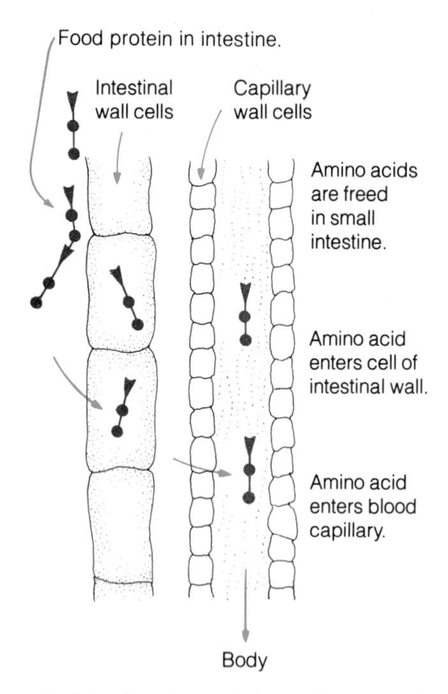

Protein digestion and absorption proceed.

The diet should supply all essential amino acids simultaneously. If an essential amino acid is missing at the time of protein synthesis, synthesis stops, and the amino acids present are degraded.

To review the body's handling of amino acids, let us follow the fate of an amino acid that was originally part of a protein-containing food. When the amino acid arrives in a cell, it may be used in several different ways, depending on the needs of the cell at the time.

The amino acid may be used as is and become part of a growing protein. Alternatively, the cell may dismantle it and use its amine group to build a different amino acid. The remainder may be used for fuel or, if not needed, stored as glycogen or fat.

Nearly the same fate awaits the amino acid if it arrives at a cell that is screaming for energy but has no fuel in the form of glucose or fatty acids. Even though this amino acid may be needed to build a vital protein, the energy need will be given top priority. Without energy, the cell dies. Therefore, this valuable amino acid will be stripped of its amine group, and the remainder of its structure will be used for energy. The amine group will be excreted from the cell and, finally, from the body in the urine.

Another circumstance in which amino acids are used for energy is when there is a surplus of amino acids and energy-yielding nutrients. In this case, the body does not waste this resource. It takes the amino acid apart, excretes the nitrogen as urea, converts the rest to fat, then stores it in the fat cells. In this way, valuable, expensive, protein-rich foods can contribute to obesity.

In summary, amino acids in the cell can be used to:

- Synthesize protein.
- Provide glucose (half of them can be converted to glucose).
- Provide nitrogen in the form of amine groups to build nonessential amino acids.
- Provide energy if there is a scarcity of energy nutrients.
- Increase the stores of fat.

Amino acids are wasted (not used to build protein) whenever there is:

- Not enough energy from carbohydrate and fat.
- An imbalance, with not enough essential amino acids (low-quality protein).
- Too much protein so that not all is needed.
- Too much of any amino acid from a supplement.

Factors that must be supplied in the diet for the body to be able to synthesize protein include:

- All essential amino acids simultaneously and in the proper amounts.
- An adequate total amount of protein (to supply amine groups to synthesize the nonessential amino acids).
- Adequate energy-yielding carbohydrate and fat (to spare the protein).

Amino acids can be metabolized to protein, glucose, nitrogen + energy, or fat. They will be metabolized to protein only if sufficient energy is present from other sources and if all of the essential amino acids are present simultaneously.

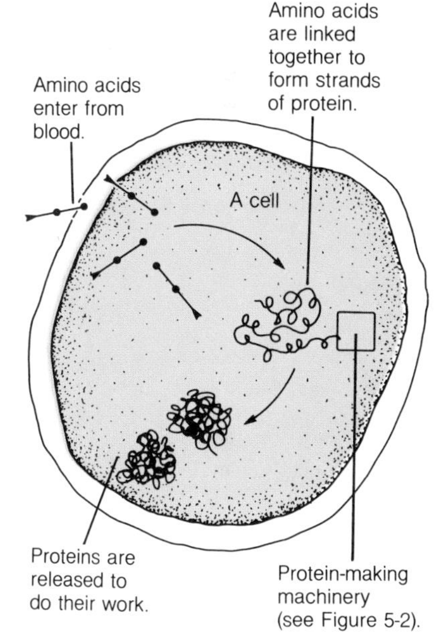

Cells absorb amino acids and build their own proteins.

Food Proteins: Quality and Use

The body responds to different proteins in different ways, depending on many factors: the body's state of health, as well as the food source of the protein, its digestibility, the other nutrients taken with it, and its amino acid assortment. Protein will be used most efficiently if accompanied by carbohydrate, fat, and the full array of vitamins and minerals. To know whether, say, 30 grams of a

biological value (BV): a measure of protein quality, assessed by determining how well a given food or food mixture supports nitrogen retention.

reference protein: egg protein, the standard with which other proteins are compared to determine biological value.

chemical scoring: a method of evaluating protein quality by comparing its chemically determined amino acid composition, on paper, with human amino acid requirements.

protein is enough to meet a person's daily needs, it is necessary to know how all these other factors affect the body's use of the protein.

A person in good health can be expected to use dietary protein efficiently. However, malnutrition or infection can seriously impair digestion (by reducing enzyme secretion), absorption (by causing degeneration of the absorptive surface of the small intestine or losses from diarrhea), and the cells' use of protein (by forcing amino acids to meet other needs). In addition, infections cause the stepped-up production of antibodies made of protein. Malnutrition or infection may greatly increase the needs while making it harder to meet them.

Concern about the quality of individual food proteins is of theoretical interest only, in settings where food is abundant. Most people in the United States and Canada would find it next to impossible *not* to meet their protein requirements, even if they ate no meat, fish, poultry, eggs, or cheese—provided only that they were meeting their energy needs from relatively nutritious foods; not, say, from cookies, potato chips, cola beverages, or alcoholic beverages. (They would still have to pay attention to other nutrients richly supplied by animal foods. Chapters 6 and 7 point these out.) Tradition has it that if you don't eat meat, you have to use milk, cheese, and eggs, and that if you don't eat any foods taken from animals, you have to mix and match plant products carefully, to obtain the numbers and balance of amino acids necessary to build body protein. This chapter's Food Feature offers many ways of meeting protein needs and shows that it is very easy to do, even for the "pure" vegetarian.

However, the situation is different when food energy intake is limited (where malnutrition is widespread), or when the selection of foods available is severely limited (where a single food such as potatoes, rice, or cassava provides 90 percent of the calories). Even then, protein intake may be adequate (it would be, on potatoes or rice), but it may not be (it would not be, on cassava). In these cases, the primary food source of protein must be checked, for its quality is of great importance. Thus scientists have studied many different individual foods as protein sources and have developed many different methods of evaluating their quality. The generalizations that follow come from such studies.

Amino acids from animal proteins are best absorbed (over 90 percent). Those from legumes follow (about 80 percent), and those from grains and other plant foods vary (from 60 to 90 percent). Cooking with moist heat generally improves protein digestibility, whereas dry heat methods may impair it.

All other things being equal, a protein that supplies all the essential amino acids in exactly the right ratio will be most completely used. If an essential amino acid is in short supply, it limits the use of all the others for building protein. A protein that almost entirely lacks an essential amino acid does not, by itself, support protein synthesis.

When amino acids are wasted, their nitrogen can't be stored. Therefore, the efficiency of a protein in maintaining body tissue can be assessed by measuring the net loss of nitrogen from the body when that protein is fed by itself. The more nitrogen is retained, the higher the quality of the protein. This is the basis for determination of the **biological value (BV)** of proteins.

A high-quality protein by this standard is egg protein. It has been designated the **reference protein** and given a score of 100; other proteins are scored against this standard. Three other ways of scoring protein quality are in common use. One is **chemical scoring**—a pencil-and-paper method of calculating which amino acid is in shortest supply relative to human physiological need. The second is

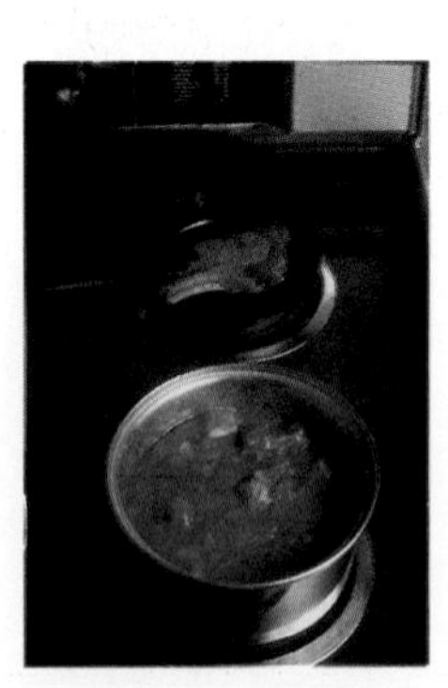

Cooking with moist heat improves protein digestibility.

net protein utilization (NPU)—a measure of the amount of protein retained from that ingested. The third is **protein efficiency ratio (PER)**—a method that involves feeding the protein to young, growing rats and measuring their weight gains per unit of time. These different methods of evaluating proteins give different results. The chemical scores and NPUs of several proteins are listed in Table 5–2 to illustrate this point.

The PER is used as a standard for food labeling. The U.S. RDA recommends two different daily intakes of protein, depending on the quality. If the protein is of as high quality as milk protein (casein) or higher, then 45 grams a day is considered sufficient for an adult; if the protein's quality is lower than that, then 65 grams a day is recommended. (See inside back cover for the U.S. RDA table.)

These methods and others have uses and disadvantages. For example, the PER is time-consuming to determine and is complicated by the problem that growing children have different amino acid needs from those of rats. Furthermore, its use in labeling products such as bread makes the protein appear less nutritious than it actually is. The World Health Organization (WHO) now believes that a protein's digestibility may be the most important feature determining its quality for human use. WHO has scored proteins for digestibility, using milk, eggs, and meat as the standard (given a score of 100). WHO recommends that if plant proteins are used instead, since their digestibility ranges from 80 to 100, their recommended intakes be adjusted accordingly.[4]

Protein scores help policy-makers deal with widespread malnutrition. For the average well-fed Westerner, however, perhaps their major message is that the scores of animal proteins and plant proteins overlap considerably. The best guarantee of amino acid adequacy is to eat mixtures of foods containing protein in the presence of adequate amounts of vitamins, minerals, and energy from carbohydrate and fat.

Protein use depends on the user's health, the protein's digestibility, the nutrients eaten with it, and its amino acid assortment. The quality of a protein is measured by how much of its nitrogen is retained by the body or by how well the protein supports growth.

net protein utilization (NPU): a method of evaluating protein quality by comparing the amount animals retain to the amount they ingest.

protein efficiency ratio (PER): a measure of protein quality assessed by determining how well a given protein supports weight gain in laboratory animals.

nitrogen balance: the amount of nitrogen consumed compared with the amount excreted in a given period of time.

The Protein RDA

Protein is at the heart of a good diet. Menu planners build their meals around the RDA for protein. The RDA is designed to cover the need to replace protein-containing tissue people lose and wear out every day. Therefore it depends on body size: larger people have a higher protein RDA. The protein RDA also is adjusted to cover additional needs for building new tissue and so is higher for growing children and pregnant and lactating women. The Canadian recommendation for protein is similar and is based on similar assumptions.

Underlying the protein RDA are **nitrogen balance** studies, which measure nitrogen lost by excretion compared with nitrogen eaten in food. Nitrogen-in must equal nitrogen-out. The laboratory scientist measures the body's daily nitrogen losses in urine, feces, sweat, and skin under controlled conditions and can then estimate the amount of protein needed to replace these losses. The

The RDA table is on the inside front cover.

Table 5–2

Chemical Scores and NPUs of Various Proteins

Protein	Chemical	NPU
Eggs	100	100
Milk	93	75
Rice	86	67
Beef	75	80
Fish	75	83
Corn	72	56

Source: Adapted from Assessment of proteins, *Nutrition and the M.D.*, June 1985, pp. 3–4.

average amino acid is 6.25 times as heavy as the nitrogen it contains, so as a rule of thumb, the scientist multiplies the nitrogen weight by 6.25 to estimate the protein's weight.

Under normal circumstances, healthy adults are in nitrogen equilibrium, or zero balance—that is, they have at all times the same amount of total protein in their bodies. When nitrogen-in exceeds nitrogen-out, they are said to be in positive nitrogen balance; this means that somewhere in their bodies more proteins are being built than are being broken down and lost. When nitrogen-in is less than nitrogen-out, they are said to be in negative nitrogen balance; they are losing protein.

Growing children add to their bodies new blood, bone, and muscle cells every day. These cells contain protein, so children must have in their bodies more protein (and therefore more nitrogen) at the end of each day than they had at the beginning. A growing child is therefore in positive nitrogen balance. Similarly, when a woman is pregnant she is, in essence, growing a new person; she too must be in positive nitrogen balance. When she is lactating, she may be in equilibrium again, but it is a sort of enhanced equilibrium. She is eating more protein than before to make her milk and is secreting it whenever the baby nurses.

Negative nitrogen balance occurs when muscle or other protein tissue is broken down and lost. Consider the situation when people have to rest in bed for a period of time. Their muscles degenerate, and they suffer a net loss of protein. One of several problems faced by the nutritionists responsible for the welfare of astronauts involves the negative nitrogen balance that occurs as astronauts are lying down for days in the space capsule. Their muscles fail to receive enough exercise to maintain themselves.

Protein RDA (adult) = 0.8 g/kg.
To figure your protein RDA:

1. Find your body weight.
2. Convert pounds to kilograms (pounds divided by 2.2 lb/kg equals kilograms).
3. Multiply by 0.8 g/kg to get your RDA in grams per day.

For example:

1. Weight = 110 lb.
2. 110 lb ÷ 2.2 lb/kg = 50 kg.
3. 50 kg × 0.8 g/kg = 40 g.

For healthy adults, the RDA for protein has been set, at present, at 0.8 grams for each kilogram (or 2.2 pounds) of body weight. Athletes need slightly more (see Chapter 9). For children who are growing, the RDA is higher per unit of body weight; for infants it is highest of all (see Table 5–3).

The protein RDA listed in the RDA table are intended for the mythical creatures of Chapter 2—the reference man and woman, who are "average" figures for our population. Real, live people may have a hard time discovering how the RDA apply to them. This is not surprising: recall that all the RDA are values for *populations,* not individuals. Still, they can yield a rough, ballpark estimate of protein needs for people of appropriate weight for height.

Table 5–3
The Protein RDA

Age (yr)	RDA (g/kg)[a]
0–½	2.2
½–1	2.0
1–3	1.8
4–10	1.1
11–14	1.0
15–18	0.9
19 and up	0.8

[a]The RDA increases by 30 g/day during pregnancy and by 20 g/day during lactation.

Very little attention has been paid to the protein needs of the obese person. Some people reason that because the excess fat is mostly metabolically dormant tissue, the person's protein needs are about the same as for a normal-weight person of the same height. Similarly, the underweight person lacks fat, but not lean tissue, so that person, too, probably needs the same amount of protein as the normal-weight person of the same height.

It would be easier to state people's protein needs if there were an easy way to measure lean tissue. There is an easy way to measure weight, but this doesn't reveal much about lean tissue. The very inactive fat person may have a severely underdeveloped lean body, and so need less protein than the person's weight seems to imply; the heavyweight football player may have a greatly overdeveloped lean body and so need much more than the inactive person of the same weight. In the absence of other guidelines, the best way to estimate protein needs seems to be to use the RDA and the person's *appropriate* weight—another frustratingly rough approximation (see Chapter 8).

In making its recommendations for protein intakes, the members of the Committee on RDA took into consideration that the protein in a normal diet would be mixed—that is, a combination of animal and plant protein. They also recognized that not all proteins are used with 100 percent efficiency and that individuals vary in the efficiency with which they use protein. In short, they made the RDA quite generous. Many normal people can consume less than the RDA for protein and still meet their bodies' needs. What this means in terms of food selections is presented in this chapter's Food Feature.

The RDA must be interpreted with caution. For the present, perhaps the most important point to be made is that the RDA are generous recommendations and that there is no need for the healthy person to exceed them. A look at food sources of protein will show that it is abundantly supplied in the foods people normally eat.

The amount of protein needed daily depends on size and stage of growth. The RDA for adults is 0.8 grams of protein per kilogram of body weight.

protein-energy malnutrition (PEM), also called **protein-calorie malnutrition (PCM):** the world's most widespread malnutrition problem, including both kwashiorkor and marasmus and states in which they overlap.

kwashiorkor (kwash-ee-OR-core, kwash-ee-or-CORE): the deficiency disease caused by inadequate protein in the presence of adequate energy.

marasmus (ma-RAZ-mus): the energy-deficiency disease; starvation.

Protein and Health

With all the attention that has been paid to the health effects of starch, sugars, fibers, fats, oils, and cholesterol, protein has been slighted. Protein deficiency effects are well known, because together with energy deficiency, they are the world's main form of malnutrition. But the effects of too much protein, and particularly the effects of proteins of different kinds, are far less well known. Let us consider each in turn: deficiency, excess, and type of protein.

Protein-Energy Malnutrition

Protein deficiency and energy deficiency go hand in hand so often that public health officials have given a nickname to the pair: **protein-energy malnutrition (PEM).** The two diseases and their symptoms overlap all along the spectrum, but the extremes have names of their own. Protein deficiency is **kwashiorkor,** and energy deficiency is **marasmus.**

Kwashiorkor is the Ghanaian name for "the evil spirit that infects the first child when the second child is born." In countries where kwashiorkor is prevalent, parents customarily give their newly weaned children watery cereal rather than the food eaten by the rest of the family. The child has been receiving from the mother breast milk containing high-quality protein designed beautifully to support growth. Suddenly the child receives only a weak drink with scant protein of very low quality. Small wonder the just-weaned child sickens when the new baby arrives.

The child who has been banished meets this threat to life by engaging in as little activity as possible. Apathy is one of the earliest signs of protein deprivation; the body is collecting all its forces to meet the crisis and so cuts down on any expenditure of protein not needed for the heart, lungs, and brain. As the apathy increases, the child doesn't even cry for food. All growth ceases; the child is no

edema (eh-DEEM-uh): the swelling of body tissue caused by leakage of fluid from the blood vessels, seen in (among other conditions) protein deficiency.

dysentery (DISS-en-terry): an infection of the digestive tract that causes diarrhea.

larger at four than at two. New hair grows without the protein pigment that gave it its color. The skin also loses its color, and when sores open, they fail to heal. Digestive enzymes are in short supply, the digestive tract lining deteriorates, and absorption fails. The child can't assimilate what little food is eaten. Proteins and hormones that previously kept the fluid correctly distributed among the compartments of the body now are diminished, so that fluid leaks out of the blood **(edema)** and accumulates in the belly and legs. Blood proteins, including hemoglobin, are not synthesized, so the child becomes anemic; this increases the weakness and apathy. The kwashiorkor victim often develops a fatty liver, caused by lack of the protein carriers that transport fat out of the liver. Antibodies to fight off invading bacteria are degraded to provide amino acids for other uses; the child becomes an easy target for any infection. Then **dysentery,** an infection of the digestive tract that causes diarrhea, further depletes the body of nutrients, especially minerals. Measles, which might make a healthy child sick for a week or two, kills the kwashiorkor child within two or three days.

If the child is taken into the hospital, this starved condition may not be obvious. Water in the tissues may cause the body to look almost fat. Only when the fluid balance is restored will it be seen that the child is just a skeleton thinly covered with skin.

If caught in time, a kwashiorkor child's life may be saved by careful nutrition therapy. The fluid balances are most critical. Diarrhea will have depleted the body's potassium stores and upset other salt balances. Careful remediation of these critical balances will prevent sudden death from heart failure about half the time. Only later can skim milk, containing protein and carbohydrate, be safely given; then comes fat, when body protein is sufficient to provide carriers.

Children with marasmus suffer symptoms similar to those of children with kwashiorkor, since both cause loss of body protein tissue, but there are also differences between the two. Kwashiorkor children retain some of their stores of body fat (because they are still consuming calories), accumulate fat in their livers (because they can't make protein to carry it away), and develop edema (from protein lack). Marasmus children experience ketosis to conserve body protein, while kwashiorkor children do not, because they are receiving some carbohydrate; so kwashiorkor is actually a less balanced state and a more fatal disease than marasmus for children at any given age.

A marasmic child looks like a wizened little old person—just skin and bones. The child is often sick, because resistance to disease is low. All the muscles are wasted, including the heart muscle, and the heart is weak. Metabolism is so slow that body temperature is subnormal. There is little or no fat under the skin to insulate against cold. The experience of hospital workers with victims of this disease is that their primary need is to be wrapped up and kept warm. They also need love, because they have often been deprived of maternal attention as well as food.

Unlike the kwashiorkor child, who is fed milk until weaning, the marasmic child may have been neglected from early infancy. The disease occurs most commonly in children from 6 to 18 months of age in all the overpopulated city slums of the world. Since the brain normally grows to almost its full adult size within the first two years of life, marasmus impairs brain development and may have a permanent effect on learning ability.

Kwashiorkor occurs not only in Ghana but in other African countries, Central America, South America, the Near East, and the Far East. Cases have also been reported on the Indian reservations and in the slums of the United States. Both marasmus and kwashiorkor also occur in adults in countries where PEM is prevalent. In recent years, PEM has also been recognized in many undernourished hospital patients and is the major threat to the person with anorexia nervosa (Controversy 9). The extent and severity of malnutrition worldwide is a political and economic problem and is discussed further in Chapter 14.

Protein deficiency symptoms are always observed when either protein or energy is deficient. Extreme protein deficiency with amply energy is kwashiorkor; extreme energy deficiency is marasmus. The two diseases overlap most of the time, and together are called PEM.

Protein Excess

Many of the world's people struggle to obtain enough food and enough protein to keep themselves alive, but in the developed countries protein is so abundant that the opposite problems are seen. There are no benefits, and there are risks, associated with the overconsumption of protein. For one thing, as we have said before, protein-rich foods are often high-fat foods that contribute to obesity and its accompanying health risks. In addition, infants and children do not adjust well to diets containing large amounts of protein; their body composition is altered.[5] Animals fed high-protein diets experience a "protein overload effect," seen in the enlargement of their livers and kidneys. In human beings, high-protein diets eaten over a lifetime may cause problems in kidney function.[6]

Animals experimentally fed high-protein diets of the same nature as those Americans typically eat also experience losses of zinc from their tissues as they age.[7] Such zinc excretion is also seen in pregnant women and infants on protein supplements. The use of such supplements during pregnancy may do more harm than good, even to undernourished women.[8] In infants, their use has been linked to deficits in cognitive development.[9]

YOU NEED PROTEIN.
TRUE.
YOU NEED MY PROTEIN POWDER
BENT TRUTH
SALES PITCH
MOTIVE: PERSONAL GAIN

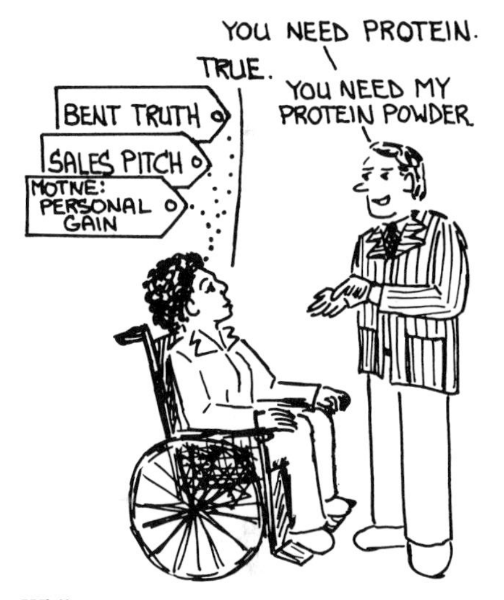

While protein is immensely important in nutrition, there is no need to take it in powder or liquid form. Most diets provide plenty.

Protein also creates a demand for certain vitamins for its metabolism; vitamin B_6 is an example. An overabundance of protein without accompanying vitamin B_6 can cause a deficiency of the vitamin, and such deficiencies are suspected of contributing to our population's high incidence of atherosclerosis.[10] High dietary protein also increases the tendency to obesity, a finding in direct contrast to the popular belief that such diets cause people to "burn off fat." Fed *low*-protein diets, even with ample calories from carbohydrate, obese subjects can lose weight.[11]

Diets high in protein also increase the body's excretion of calcium, depleting the bones of their chief mineral.[12] Overconsumption of protein can also cause dehydration, because water is needed to help excrete the wasted nitrogen—a problem the athlete should be warned about, because water balance is of such great importance to athletic performance (see Chapter 9). In a world where protein deficiency is such a threat to so many, it is ironic that some people in developed countries should be overconsuming protein.

While eating excess protein is clearly ill-advised, taking protein or amino acid supplements (except for abnormal conditions, on competent medical advice) is even more so. The accompanying box, "Protein and Amino Acid Supplements," tells why.

Health risks follow the overconsumption of protein foods.

Protein and Amino Acid Supplements

Why do people take protein supplements? Athletes take them to build muscle. Dieters take them to spare their bodies' protein while losing weight. Women take them to improve the strength of their fingernails. People take individual amino acids, too—to cure herpes, to make themselves sleep better, to relieve depression. Do protein and amino acid supplements really do any of these things? Almost never. Are they safe? No.

Muscle work builds muscle; protein supplements do not, and athletes do not need them. Food energy spares body protein; protein and carbohydrate serve this purpose equally well, and carbohydrate is safer (see Chapters 8 and 9 for details). Fingernails remain unaffected by protein supplements, provided the diet is otherwise adequate in protein, and if it is not, it must be sorely lacking in foods, altogether. The chapter has demonstrated that no decent diet fails to supply enough protein, so protein supplements never are needed by the normal, healthy person.

Furthermore, protein supplements are expensive and less well digested than protein-rich food; and when used as a replacement for such food, they are often downright dangerous. The "liquid protein" diet, advocated some years ago for weight loss, caused deaths in many users, and even the physician-supervised protein-sparing modified fast (also based on liquid protein) causes abnormal heart rhythms.

As for amino acid supplements, they, too, are unnecessary and can be dangerous. The body is designed to handle whole proteins best. It breaks them into manageable pieces (dipeptides and tripeptides), then splits these a few at a time, simultaneously absorbing them into the blood. When proteins are predigested in a laboratory and served up as mixtures of single amino acids, they are less well absorbed and digested, because they overwhelm the absorptive mechanism and not all can be accommodated. When amino acids are presented singly, severe imbalances and toxicities can occur. Groups of chemically similar amino acids compete for the carriers that absorb them into the blood, and an excess of one can create such demand for a carrier that it prevents the absorption of another. The result is a deficiency. Every amino acid is toxic when taken in excess. In some cases, "excess" means not very much above normal daily intake levels.

In two cases, recommendations for amino acids have led to widespread public use—lysine to prevent or relieve the infections that cause herpes cold sores and sexually transmitted diseases; and tryptophan to relieve pain, depression, and insomnia. In both cases, enthusiastic popular reports and careful scientific experiments are at odds. Lysine does not relieve or cure herpes infections, and if long-term use helps prevent them, it does so only in some individuals and with unknown associated risks. Tryptophan does have some interesting effects with respect to pain and sleep in responsive individuals as Controversy 13 explains further, but people taking large doses may be damaging their livers. It is safer to take amino acids in protein foods with a little carbohydrate to facilitate absorption—a turkey sandwich, for example.

This is the third chapter that has presented evidence on purified nutrients added to foods or taken singly. Chapter 3 showed that the enrichment of a nutritionally inferior food (refined bread) with four added nutrients left it still deficient in many others. It also debunked the notion that purified fructose is in any sense natural. Chapter 4 showed that supplements of one kind of fatty acid can impose on the taker a deficiency of the other kind. With amino acids, the same thing is true. Even with all we know about science, it is hard to improve on nature.

Source: R. A. Lantigua and coauthors, Cardiac arrhythmias associated with a liquid protein diet for the treatment of obesity, *New England Journal of Medicine* 303 (1980): 735–738; N. J. Benevenga and R. D. Steele, Adverse effects of excessive consumption of amino acids, *Annual Review of Nutrition* 4 (1984): 157–181; Myth of the month: Lysine for herpes, *Nutrition and the M.D.*, December 1984, p. 4; L. J. Fitten, J. Profita, and T. G. Bidder, L-tryptophan as a hypnotic in special patients, *Journal of the American Geriatrics Society* 33 (1985): 294–297; M. E. Trulson and H. W. Sampson, Ultrastructural changes of the liver following L-tryptophan ingestion, *Journal of Nutrition* 116 (1986): 1109–1115.

Animal versus Vegetable Protein

Protein from animals is invariably accompanied by fat; that from land animals, by saturated fat, mostly. Protein from plants is likely to have little lipid with it, and that lipid is mostly oil. Scientists studying heart disease and cancer have observed that people who ate large amounts of meat had higher disease rates than people who ate large amounts of vegetables, and the difference has usually been attributed to the lipids in those diets. When the lipids are factored out, though, it becomes apparent that the proteins from animals and plants differ in character. Independently of the accompanying lipids, animal and plant proteins may make a difference in risk factors and associated diseases.

One difference is that diets containing purified proteins from animal sources raise blood cholesterol higher than do similar diets containing purified vegetable proteins. Fed diets based on animal protein for a long time, experimental animals are more prone to develop atherosclerosis than their vegetable-protein–fed counterparts.[13] It is suggested that people with high blood cholesterol can bring it down by altering the ratio of the animal to vegetable protein in their diets. The typical ratio is 2 to 1; the suggested altered ratio, 1 to 1. In animals, the 1-to-1 ratio maintains blood cholesterol as low as a diet containing vegetable protein alone.[14] For people with blood cholesterol in the lower ranges, though, no effect is seen, and some investigators believe that the type of dietary protein is of little significance in this regard.[15]

The question of whether animal or vegetable proteins, by themselves, raise or lower blood cholesterol may not be directly applicable to people's food choices, for people eat foods, not purified proteins. The purified proteins most often used in experiments that involve dietary protein and raised blood cholesterol are milk protein (casein) and soy protein. If the whole foods are used instead of the isolated proteins, the contrast is not seen. Milk *lowers* blood cholesterol (see Controversy 4), just as soy does.

The use of diets high in animal protein may be associated with increased risks of heart disease and cancer.

Food Feature

Enough, But Not Too Much, Protein

People who learn of the dire consequences of protein deficiency may, understandably, become concerned about their own intakes. For people in developed nations, however, that concern may be misdirected, for such people usually eat ample protein. The protein RDA is generous: it more than adequately covers the estimated needs of most people, even those with unusually high requirements.

Overconsumption of protein is understandable in a country such as ours, because meat is a major part of the diet. A single ounce of meat donates 7 or 8 grams of protein, and where the RDA for an average-size individual is only about 50 grams per day. The meat list is one of two lists of foods in the exchange system that contribute an abundance of high-quality protein; the milk list is the other. Two others—the vegetable and grain lists—contribute smaller amounts of proteins, but they can add up to significant quantities, as you will see. The protein values assigned to each of the exchange lists permit you to estimate the protein content of foods (see Figure 5–7).

To illustrate how easy it is to overconsume protein, assume that *your* protein RDA is 50 grams per day. This would divide easily into three meals: 10 grams at breakfast, 20 grams at lunch, and 20 grams at dinner. An egg and a glass of milk at breakfast would add up to 15 grams, exceeding the allowance for that meal by half. At lunch, a chef's salad with an egg, an ounce of ham, and an ounce of cheese would deliver 21 grams—and the greens would be additional.

Figure 5–7 Protein in Foods.

One Exchange	Protein (g)
Milk (1 c)	8
Vegetable (½ c)	2
Fruit (1 portion)	0
Bread and starchy vegetable (1 slice or ½ c)	3
Sugar	0
Meat (1 oz)	7
Fat	0

8 g in 1 c milk.
3 g in 1 starch portion.
2 g in ½ c vegetables.
7 g in 1 oz meat.

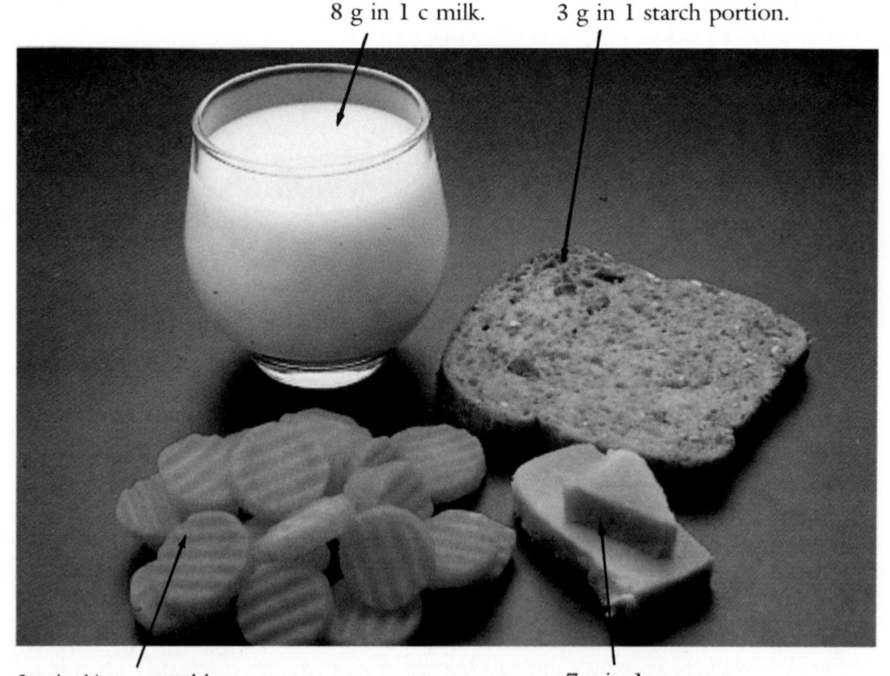

A 4-ounce piece of chicken for dinner would contribute 28 more. By the time you added the vegetables, the second milk serving, and the four bread/cereal servings suggested by the Four Food Group Plan, you would have added at least 20 grams more, exceeding your protein needs for the day by far. Finally, if you also included a cup of legumes, you would add over 10 grams more protein to your day's meals for a total of more than 94 grams. No wonder most people get more than twice the protein they need.

Protein is of prime importance, but overemphasis on protein-rich foods in the diet can easily lead to nutrient imbalances. Protein-rich foods carry with them a characteristic array of vitamins and minerals, including vitamin B_{12} and iron. By the same token, they are notoriously lacking in others—vitamin C and folacin, for example (more about these nutrients appears in the next two chapters). To overemphasize protein-rich foods, then, would be to ensure an overabundance of vitamin B_{12} and iron while shortchanging vitamin C and folacin. In addition, many protein-rich foods such as meat are high in calories, and to overconsume them is to invite obesity.

In Figure 2–7 of Chapter 2, two days' meals were compared. They both contained the same amount of protein, but the meat and potatoes meals delivered far fewer nutrients. The person eating such meals, which are typical of Western developed nations, cannot improve that diet by simply adding nutritious foods on top of it. If the person added milk, whole grains, or vegetables; the protein would far exceed the need. To keep from vastly overconsuming protein (and calories), the person must delete something, and the obvious "something" to delete is some of the meat.

Figure 5–8 repeats the high-nutrient-density meals from that comparison, and shows another point about the protein content of the high-nutrient-density meals. As you can see, even these meals provide almost double the average person's protein RDA, mostly from milk, vegetables, and grains. Only small amounts of cheese and fish are used. Plant foods, then, can contribute large amounts of protein, provided that you eat enough of them. Given the variety of foods chosen, the amino acid assortment is excellent. In fact, to bring the *calories* up to match those in the high-fat meals without adding more protein, we had to add pure fat and pure carbohydrate. That's why you see the butter pats and sugar packets on the plates. There is only half as much fat in the high-nutrient-density meals as in the high-fat meals, but almost all the fat is visible (and therefore optional). Removing it would leave a large volume of highly palatable, nutritious, low-calorie food to eat (a hint for the dieter who thinks that the way to cut calories is to eat *meat*).

Today, more people are turning to grains and vegetables instead of meat for the protein they need, and an old distinction is beginning to blur—that between meat eaters and vegetarians. People are tailoring their eating plans not to a rigid definition, but to their own preferences. For example, in addition to meat eaters and the traditional types of vegetarians described in Chapter 2, there are people who eat seafood but not other meats; those who include chicken and other poultry but not red meat; those who eat just fish, cheese, and plant foods; those who center their diets on legumes, pasta, or rice and use just tiny amounts of meats to season their meals; and others. These people are not at risk for protein deficiency, so long as they follow the diet-planning rules for variety and balance.

Is it at all possible, then, that a person may have trouble meeting protein needs? Yes, if adequate energy foods are not consumed or if nonnutritious energy

mutual supplementation: the strategy of combining two plant protein foods in a meal so that each provides the essential amino acid(s) lacking in the other.

complementary proteins: two or more proteins whose amino acid assortments complement each other in such a way that the essential amino acids missing from each are supplied by the other.

foods such as pure fats, sugars, and alcohol are overemphasized. Too, someone who overemphasizes one group of foods, especially the fruits or even certain vegetables (cassava root, for example), at the expense of others could conceivably create a protein deficiency. More often, though, people who eat too few protein-rich foods will suffer from *many* deficiencies—calcium, iron, and many of the vitamins as well as protein and food energy. In other words, the condition would be one of starvation.

Traditionally, people who have relied solely on vegetables, fruits, and grains have made a conscious effort to combine proteins from these sources in such a way as to guarantee that the whole array of essential amino acids would be present in each meal. The method, known as **mutual supplementation,** reassures the eater that meals composed of plant foods alone meet protein needs.

Figure 5–9 shows how mutual supplementation works. The two protein foods chosen are **complementary proteins.** Table 5–4 shows how to choose complementary proteins.

Some sincere vegetarians, when they first learn about mutual supplementation, are eager to know how much of each essential amino acid is required daily.

Figure 5–8 Protein in the High-nutrient-density Meals.
The values presented in Figure 5–8 provide a way to estimate the amount of protein eaten at a meal or in a day. Using those values, let's estimate the amounts of protein in the meals shown here. (These are the same meals used as examples in Figure 2–7 of Chapter 2.) The fruits and fats (butter) can be assumed to contain no protein, so the only foods to inspect are the meats, milks, grains/starchy vegetables, and vegetables. The exchange system slightly overestimates the protein in these meals. Peas and beans (members of the legume family) contain more protein than other vegeables do. Still, the estimate is higher than the actual amount of protein by only 8 percent.

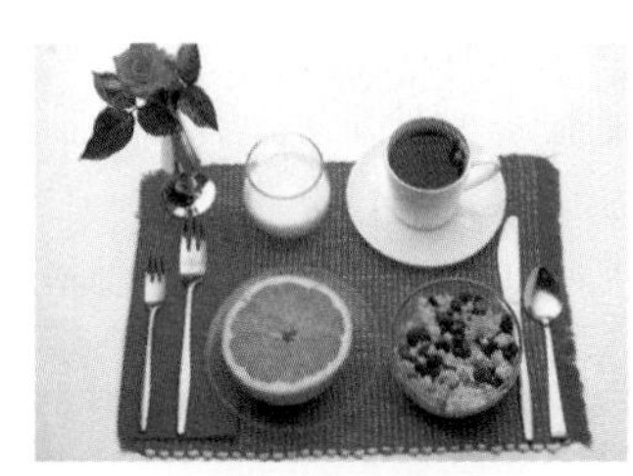

	Protein (g) (estimated)
Breakfast	
1 c oatmeal = 2 starch portions	6
½ c nonfat milk = ½ milk portion	4
	10

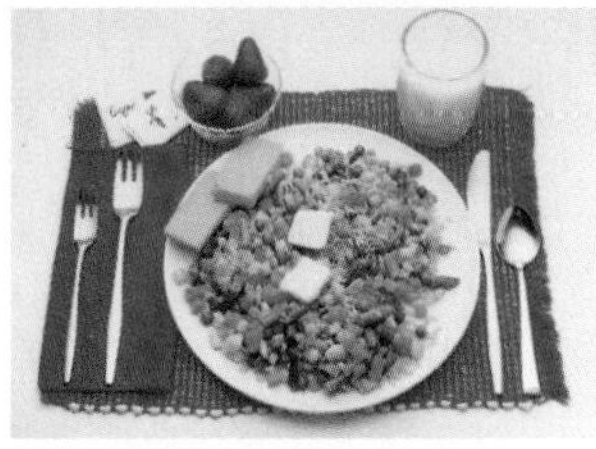

	Protein (g) (estimated)
Lunch	
1 c cooked rice = 3 starch portions	9
2 c mixed vegetables = 2 starchy vegetables + 2 vegetables	10
2 oz cheddar cheese = 2 meat portions	14
1 c nonfat milk = 1 milk portion	8
	41

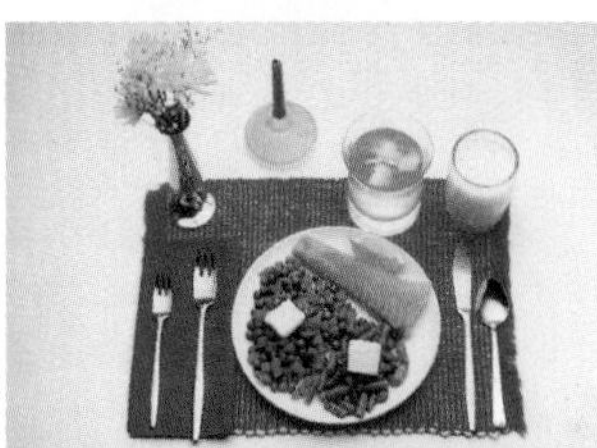

	Protein (g) (estimated)
Dinner	
3 oz broiled fish = 3 meat portions	21
½ c green beans = 1 vegetable portion	2
½ c cooked carrots = 1 vegetable portion	2
½ c cooked peas = 1 starchy vegetable	3
1 c nonfat milk = 1 milk portion	8
	36

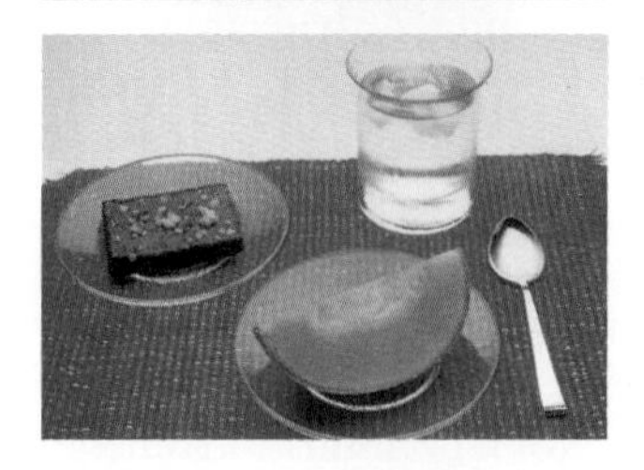

	Protein (g) (estimated)
Snack	
1 brownie = 1 starch portion	3
	3

Day's total 90

They also want to know exactly how much of each is contained in their favorite plant foods. This information is available. However, much time can be squandered calculating the amino acid contents of a meal. Instead of computing amino acid quantities from tables, the eater should adopt the strategy of using a wide variety of whole foods in generous servings. Meals planned this way not only meet a person's needs for nutrients without much fat, but also make the best use of the world's resources. (That fast-food hamburger could have much farther reaching effects than you might imagine. Controversy 14 tells the story.)

Once you have the confidence that you will not short yourself with respect to protein, planning meatless meals can become a pleasure. Many interesting, novel sources of protein are available. One class of protein-rich foods other than meats has already been mentioned many times: the plant family known as the **legumes** (see Figure 5–10).

The protein of legumes is of a quality almost comparable to that of meat. Legumes are also excellent sources of fiber, many B vitamins, iron, calcium and other minerals. A cup of cooked legumes contains 31 percent of the protein and 42 percent of the iron recommended daily for an adult male. Like meats, though, legumes do not offer every nutrient, and they do not make a complete meal by themselves. They contain no vitamin A, vitamin C, or vitamin B_{12}, and their balance of amino acids can be improved by using grains and other vegetables with them.

The heavy use of soy products in place of meat severely inhibits iron absorption. The effect can be alleviated, though, by using small amounts of meat and/or foods rich in vitamin C in the same meal with the soy products.[16]

legumes (leg-GYOOM, LEG-yoom): plants of the bean and pea family having roots with nodules that contain special bacteria. These bacteria can trap nitrogen from the air in the soil and make it into compounds that become part of the seed. The seeds are rich in high-quality protein compared with those of most other plant foods.

tofu (TOE-foo): a curd made from soybeans, rich in protein and calcium, used in many Asian and vegetarian dishes in place of meat.

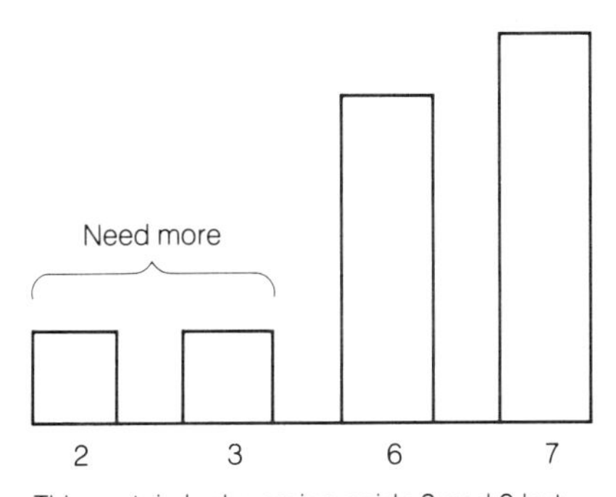

This protein lacks amino acids 2 and 3 but has plenty of 6 and 7.

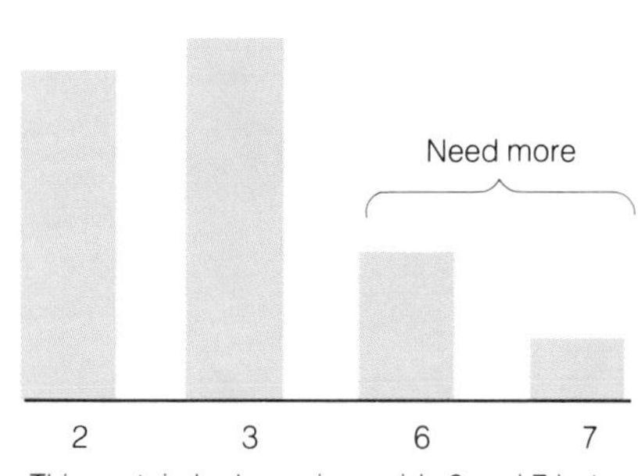

This protein lacks amino acids 6 and 7 but has plenty of 2 and 3.

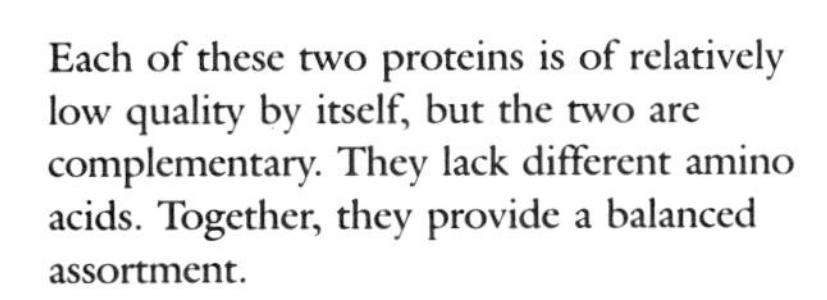
Each of these two proteins is of relatively low quality by itself, but the two are complementary. They lack different amino acids. Together, they provide a balanced assortment.

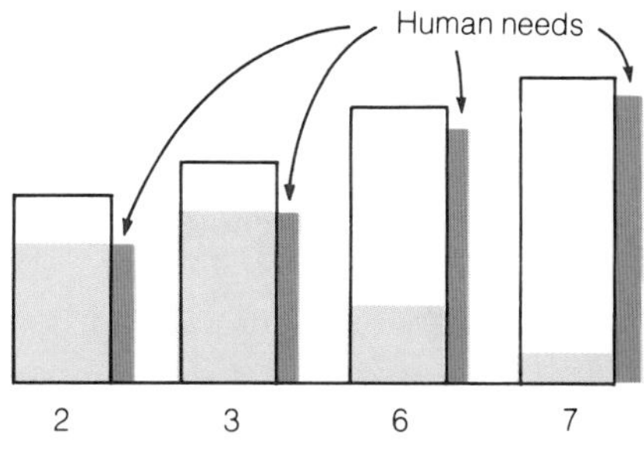

Put them together in a half-and half mixture, and the balance of amino acids meets human needs quite well.

Figure 5–9 Mutual Supplementation.

Figure 5–10 A Legume.

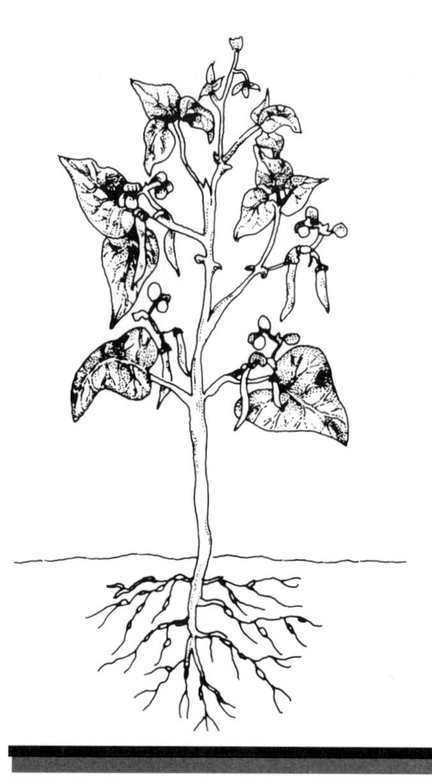

The legumes are the seeds of such plants as the kidney bean, soybean, garden pea, lentil, black-eyed pea, and lima bean. Bacteria in the root nodules can "fix" nitrogen, contributing it to the beans. Ultimately, thanks to these bacteria, the plant leaves in the soil more nitrogen than it takes out. So efficient at trapping nitrogen are the legumes that farmers often grow them in rotation with other crops to fertilize fields. For a variety of legumes used in cooking, see photographs in Table 2–6 of Chapter 2.

Table 5–4

Traditional Complementary Protein Combinations

Lentils	+	Wheat, rice
Legumes	+	Cereals (enriched or whole grain)
Sesame, or sunflower seeds	+	Leafy vegetables, whole grains
Brewer's yeast	+	Peanuts, legumes, seeds, nuts, whole grains, corn, leafy vegetables
Leafy vegetables	+	Seeds, whole grains, yeast
Soybeans	+	Rice (Indochina)
Peas	+	Wheat (middle East)
Beans	+	Corn (Central and South America)

shopping list:

- small meat portions
- ample dairy products
- whole grains
- a variety of legumes
- a legume-centered cookbook

Another form in which the nutrients of soybeans are available is as bean curd or **tofu,** a staple used in many Asian dishes. Thanks to the way tofu is made, it is high in calcium and can serve as a milk substitute for people who are allergic to milk or can't tolerate it.

The protein-rich, high-fiber, nutrient-dense foods from plants are most often lower in fat than animal-derived foods. People who eat mostly plant foods can therefore enjoy a nutritious diet that is low in fat, but only if other high-fat foods like nuts, olives, butter, cream cheese, and sour cream are limited, too.

The key to getting enough, but not too much, protein seems to be to use a variety of foods in ample quantities; to de-emphasize meats; and to emphasize vegetables, grains, legumes, and nonfat milk and milk products. If you have followed the Food Features so far, you may now see that the recommendations for the three energy-yielding nutrients go hand in hand—if you reduce fat and increase carbohydrate, protein totals automatically come more into line with the requirements.

Self-Study

Evaluate Your Protein Intake

These exercises make use of the information you recorded on Forms 1 to 4 in Appendix H.

1. How many grams of protein do you consume in a day?
2. How many calories does this represent? (Remember, 1 gram of protein contributes 4 calories.)
3. What percentage of your total energy is contributed by protein? You calculated this earlier, using Form 4.
4. The U.S. *Dietary Goals* suggest that protein should contribute about 10 to 15 percent of total energy. How does your protein intake compare with this recommendation? (Note: If you are on a calorie-restricted diet, then a higher percentage of your calories should come from protein. See the Self-Study for Chapter 8.) If your protein intake is out of line, what foods could you consume more of—or less of—to bring it into line?
5. Calculate your protein RDA (see p. 158). Is it similar to the RDA for an "average" person of your age and sex, as shown in the RDA tables (inside front cover)?
6. Compare your average daily protein intake with your RDA. On the average, about what percentage of your RDA for protein are you consuming each day? If you are healthy, the RDA is probably a generous recommendation for you, and yet you may be eating more than the recommendation. This means that you may be spending protein prices for an energy-yielding nutrient. What substitutions could you make in your day's food choices so that you would derive from carbohydrate, rather than from protein, the energy you need?
7. How many of your protein grams are from animal, and how many from plant, foods? Assuming that the animal protein is all of high quality, no more than 20 percent of your total protein need come from this source. Should you alter the ratio of plant to animal protein in your diet? If you did, what effect would this have on the total *fat* content of your diet?
8. How is your protein intake distributed throughout the day? (At what times do you eat? How many grams of protein each time?) Is the distribution even enough to sustain your blood glucose supply throughout the day and evening? (Remember from Chapter 3 that protein helps regulate blood glucose.)

Notes

1. S. A. Laidlaw, Indispensable amino acids, *Nutrition and the M.D.,* August 1986, pp. 1–3; K. C. Hayes, Taurine requirements in primates, *Nutrition Reviews* 43 (1985): 65–70.
2. W. J. Visek, Arginine needs, physiological state and usual diets: A reevaluation, *Journal of Nutrition* 116 (1986): 36–46.
3. A. A. Albanese and L. A. Orto, The proteins and amino acids, in *Modern Nutrition in Health and Disease,* 5th ed., eds. R. S. Goodhart and M. E. Shils (Philadelphia: Lea and Febiger, 1973), p. 59.
4. World Health Organization Technical Report no. 724, as cited in Energy and protein requirements, *Cereal Foods World* 31 (1986): 694–695.
5. Albanese and Orto, 1973, pp. 28–88; L. E. Holt, Jr., Protein economy in the growing child, *Postgraduate Medicine* 27 (1960): 783–798.
6. J. Klug, Overeating possible cause of renal disease, *Internal Medicine News,* December 1–14, 1982, pp. 1, 30–31.
7. A. R. Sherman, L. Helyar, and I. Wolinsky, Effects of dietary protein concentration on trace minerals in rat tissues at different ages, *Journal of Nutrition* 115 (1985): 607–614.
8. H. H. Sandstead, Zinc: Essentiality for brain development and function, *Nutrition Today,* November/December 1984, pp. 26–30; B. Worthington-Roberts, Nutrition and maternal health, *Nutrition Today,* November/December 1984, pp. 6–19; D. Rush, Z. Stein, and M. Susser in Diet in pregnancy: A randomized controlled trial of prenatal nutritional supplementation (New York: Alan Liss, 1979).
9. E. Pollitt and N. Lewis, Nutritional and educational achievement, *Food and Nutrition Bulletin* 2 (1980): 33–37, as cited by C. G. Neumann and E. F. P. Jelliffe, Effects of infant feeding, in *Adverse Effects of Foods,* eds. E. F. P. Jelliffe and D. B. Jelliffe (New York: Plenum Press, 1982), p. 549.
10. R. B. Alfin-Slater, Vitamin B_6 and coronary heart disease, *Nutrition and the M.D.,* March 1983, p. 4.
11. Dietary protein and body fat distribution, *Nutrition Reviews* 40 (1982): 89–90.
12. A. A. Licata, Acute effects of increased meat protein on urinary electrolytes and cyclic adenosine monophosphate and serum parathyroid hormone, *Americal Journal of Clinical Nutrition* 34 (1981): 1779–1784.
13. K. K. Carroll, Dietary protein and heart disease, *Nutrition and the M.D.,* June 1986, p. 1.
14. Carroll, 1986.
15. S. M. Grundy and J. J. Abrams, Comparison of actions of soy protein and casein on metabolism of plasma lipoproteins and cholesterol in humans, *American Journal of Clinical Nutrition* 38 (1983): 245–252; A. C. Beynen and coauthors, Dietary soybean protein and serum cholesterol, *American Journal of Clinical Nutrition* 39 (1984):840–841.
16. Soyfoods and iron bioavailability, *Nutrition and the M.D.,* March 1983, pp. 4–5.

Nutrition and Cancer

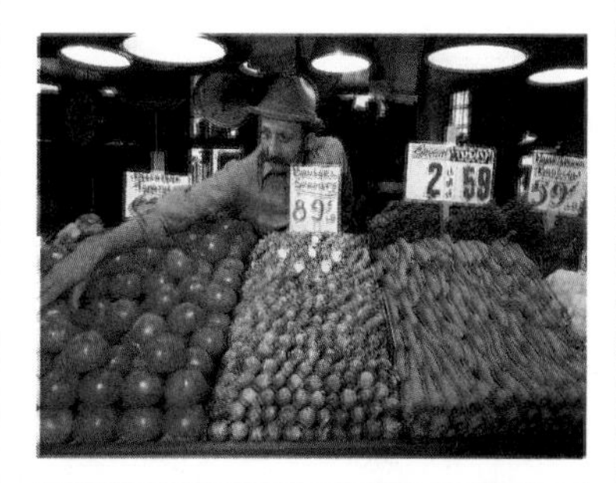

People who enjoy vegetables enjoy good health.

Almost everyone knows someone who has had cancer; according to present statistics, one in every four people in the United States will contract it.[1] Within the last 50 years, the outlook for recovery from most kinds of cancer has improved somewhat, and for a few kinds, it has improved dramatically. But still, after many years spent in the laboratory and untold millions of research dollars invested, no cures exist for many types of cancer, and virtually none for advanced cases. Some experts are beginning to say that resources should be used to support efforts to find causes, and that the hope of the future lies in preventing, not curing cancer.[2]

Cancer is a complex disease, and its causes are not easily discovered. Prevention is straightforward only when a culprit has been identified. Smoking and other tobacco use, for example, are known to cause cancer; quitting tobacco use helps to prevent it. Some cancers start when viruses attack the genes. Others involve other environmental factors—water and air pollution, for example.[3] The links between nutrition and cancer are not nearly so clear-cut, but research has revealed tantalizing connections—clues to where researchers might dig deeper for answers. This Controversy is about the intriguing, conflicting, and hopeful results of research in the field of cancer and diet.

Conclusions as to what to do would be premature. People urgently want to know about discoveries that will give them some degree of control over cancer, especially in areas of life that they themselves can manage, such as diet. The writers and publishers of books and articles offering such advice are merely responding to demand—people will buy promises of control over cancer. Do not think because you see such magazines and books boasting of anticancer diets, recipes, workouts, or other schemes, that a consensus has been reached among scientists who study cancer and diet. Not a single issue is settled in this regard.

Still, many connections exist between nutrition and cancer. Constituents in foods may be responsible for starting cancer or for speeding its development, or they may protect against cancer. Also, for the person who has cancer, diet can make a crucial difference to recovery.

The steps in cancer development are thought to be:

1. Exposure to a **carcinogen.**
2. Entry of the carcinogen into a cell.
3. A change inside the cell—**initiation,** probably by the carcinogen's altering the cell's genetic equipment.
4. Facilitation of the cancer's growth—**promotion,** probably involving several more steps before the cell multiplies out of control to form a tumor.

Most people think that the first step is the one that has the nutrition implications. That is, they think that they must learn to avoid eating foods that contain carcinogens. In particular, many people have learned to fear food additives, believing that they are responsible for diet-related cancer.

In reality, food additives probably have little to do with the causation of cancer. The law forbids the addition to food of any substances that have ever been shown to cause cancer in any animal (see box, "The Delaney Questions"). However, foods themselves contain substances that may influence whether or not people get cancer. These substances may promote or inhibit cancer after the initiating event—that is, after the cancer has been started by some other environmental influence.

The overall adequacy of the diet has far-reaching effects in preventing or promoting cancer. At each step, including the initiation process, the immune system plays a role in stopping cancer development. A diet that fails to provide the essential nutrients weakens the body's immune defenses, making cancer more likely. The reverse is also true—an adequate diet supports optimal defenses in every cell and system, to combat and overcome cancer at each stage of development.[4] Calorie control and dietary variety are important, too, and specific nutrients and nonnutrients have been singled out as allies against cancer (these are discussed later).

Several kinds of research have led to what we now know about diet and cancer. Studies of whole populations in different areas of the world—**epidemiological studies**—provide one source of information on diet and cancer. Another approach is to conduct **case-control studies**—studies of people who have cancer and of other people as closely matched to them as possible in age, occupation, and other key variables—to see what differences in their lifestyles may account for the differing cancer incidences. Still another approach is to test possible causes of cancer on animals under controlled laboratory conditions in which all other variables can be ruled out. The most powerful research tool, human **intervention trials**, are only now beginning to be employed to a limited degree in cancer research.[5] In these trials, human subjects agree to adopt a new behavior and continue it for years, so that any effect of the behavior on cancer can be discovered. Generally, researchers have a firm suspicion from animal research that the treatment is protective, and not harmful. Currently, for example, a number of physicians have agreed to take daily supplements of the vitamin A compound carotene for many years into the future, to determine if levels greater than those in food may protect against cancer development. Each type of study has its limitations and must be interpreted with an awareness of those limitations.

Four Types of Studies

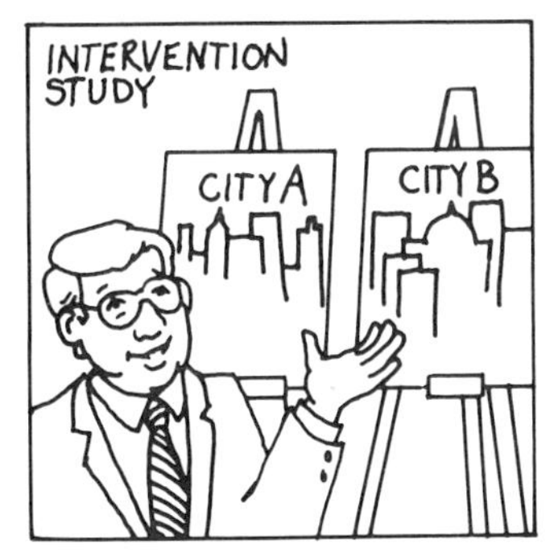

"Now let's see; what's different about the environment in these two places?"

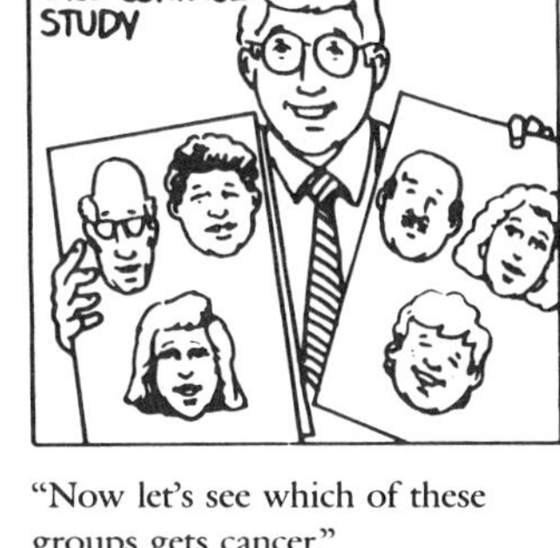

"Now let's see which of these groups gets cancer."

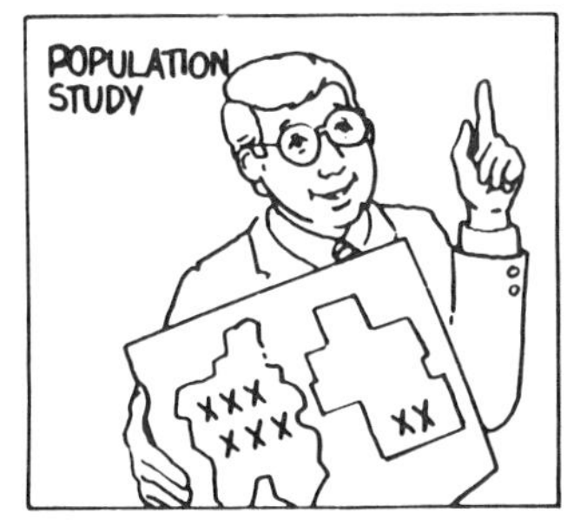

"Now let's see; what was different in these people's lifestyles?"

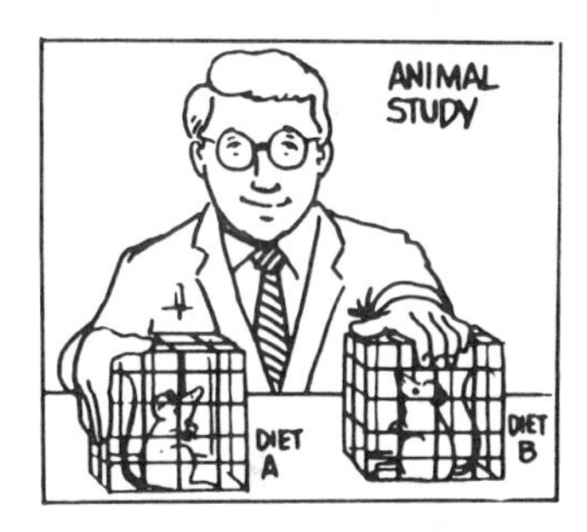

"Let's intervene in City A for ten years and compare its cancer incidence to that of City B."

Findings from Epidemiological Studies

A thought-provoking finding from studies of populations comes from the comparison of high-risk and low-risk areas. If only 10 people out of 1000 get a certain kind of cancer in location X, while 100 out of 1000 get that same kind of cancer in location Y, researchers are inclined to conclude that 90 percent of the cancers in location Y are caused by some environmental factor and are therefore, in theory, preventable. Comparison of high-risk and low-risk areas suggests that 80 to 90 percent of human cancers may indeed be preventable.[6] Hence the great challenge to nutrition researchers is to discover what dietary factors differ between people who do and do not get cancer, and to what extent such factors may influence the development of cancer.

Japanese immigration to the United States after World War I provided an especially interesting opportunity for cancer research. The Japanese living in Japan develop more stomach cancers and fewer colon cancers than people in the United States and other Western countries. However, when Japanese people have come to the United States, their children have developed both stomach and colon cancers at a rate like that of U.S. citizens. What changes the susceptibility of Japanese immigrants? It probably isn't pollution, because Japan and the United States are both industrial countries. However, something in the environment has changed, and an obvious candidate is diet.

Some other interesting questions arise from this comparison. Curiously, even though the incidence of colon cancer rises in the immigrants,

Japanese women of the second generation retain the same rate of breast cancer as women in Japan; a change in breast cancer rates doesn't show up until the third generation.[7] This contrasts with worldwide trends, where breast and colon cancer correlate, rising and falling together in the same population. Does the rate of breast cancer in adulthood reflect the food intakes of childhood, so that it takes more than one generation to bring about a change? Perhaps the women who become pregnant adopt the trusted traditional diet of the old country, thereby changing the uterine environment and also their offspring's predisposition to cancer. (We know that maternal diet affects the cancer rates of offspring of mice; the effect could possibly work in people, too.[8]) Answering one question raises many more questions.

Other epidemiological studies provide additional clues for the cancer detectives. For example, Seventh-day Adventists have rates of most forms of cancer lower than those of the general population. The difference can't be attributed entirely to their nutrition, because members of this religion also refrain from smoking and using alcohol. But when cancers linked to smoking and alcohol are taken into account, Seventh-day Adventists still have a mortality rate from cancer about one-half to two-thirds that of the rest of the population.

Seventh-day Adventists' foodways center on a lacto-ovo vegetarian diet (one that includes milk and eggs). While not all church members are vegetarians, those who eat meat do so sparingly and do not eat Biblical "unclean meat," such as pork and shellfish. Most church members also follow health recommendations to avoid caffeine and certain spices. Could their low cancer mortality be due to their low meat intakes, or to their high intakes of vegetables and cereal grains? Could some other dietary factor, such as coffee or egg avoidance, be responsible? Or could factors other than diet, still unidentified, be the keys to their good health? Seventh-day Adventists are of a higher-than-average socioeconomic level, and most are college educated. What influence might these factors have on their cancer rates?[9]

In an early study of dietary factors and cancers, one pair of investigators studied the diets of people in 37 countries. They documented the food available per person per day, as well as other indicators of lifestyle, such as possession of radios and motor vehicles. They found many correlations, but one of the most interesting showed both breast and colon cancer to be strongly associated "with indicators of affluence, such as a high-

The Delaney Questions

In 1958, a clause was added to the food safety laws, known as the Delaney Clause. It stated that "no substance that is known to cause cancer in animals or human beings at any dose level shall be added to foods." Its purpose was to protect the public, but its usefulness has been questioned.

One question is, Why focus on cancer? Is cancer different from other diseases that food additives might cause? Although serious, cancer is not the only disease that threatens from food—we face bacterial poisoning, lead and other poisoning, and nervous system damage from tainted foods, too. General laws govern the addition of dangerous substances to foods, and cancer-causing substances are already covered under those provisions.

Another question centers around how much of a carcinogen is a risk to the human body, and how much the body can safely dispose of. The Delaney Clause was written at a time when the technology available could detect only large quantities of substances in foods. With today's technology, scientists can detect just a few molecules of carcinogens in foods, and here lies the debate. Where should the line be drawn? Is there a threshold at which the risk from a carcinogen is negligible? One side says there is no safe amount—that ultimately, one molecule of carcinogen starts every cancer. The other says that although this is true, vast numbers of molecules must be present before the one *will* cause cancer.

To fully understand the arguments, you must consider how the first steps in cancer causation occur. Inside a single body cell, a single molecule alters the cell's genetic material, causing a mutation. A simple view of what happens next is that the altered genes create altered cell proteins, and a tumor begins to grow. So cancers do start from a single event, involving one cell and one molecule of carcinogen. But it is also true that the body repairs or replaces such damaged genes every day, and it is a normal function to do so. Not every altered string of genetic material results in cancer—not by a long shot.

Still, carcinogens are unique that way—no other toxic substance can affect the body unless present in amounts greater than a certain threshold. Does the unique nature of carcinogens warrant their being treated with special dread, as in the Delaney Clause? Some say no—that it is also true that there is a threshold below which the presence of a carcinogen presents a negligible threat. In other words, many thousands of carcinogenic molecules are present in every cell, and the intrusion of a single molecule would be lost against this background. Science supports this view in many ways—with studies of cancer itself, with population studies that show that there is a threshold below which carcinogens pose no significant threat, and with risk assessment techniques that would fat diet rich in animal protein."[10] Other researchers analyzed almost 100,000 medical records and found that high blood cholesterol (an indicator of a high-fat diet) predicted colon and rectal cancer.[11]

Such an attempt to link dietary components with disease must be approached with caution. An increase in one component of the diet causes increases or decreases in others. If a close correlation is shown between a disease and, say, the consumption of animal protein, it would not prove the critical factor to be the animal protein. It might be increased fat consumption; fat goes with animal protein in foods. Or the disease might occur because of what was crowded out: the vitamins, minerals, or fiber contained in the missing fruits, vegetables, and cereals. Remember, too, that owning radios and motor vehicles was also positively linked to the cancers studied. While it is improbable that the gadgets themselves cause cancer, they do foster a sedentary lifestyle, and evidence points to lack of exercise as a contributor to many diseases, including some forms of cancer.[12]

Another problem inherent in population studies is that they depend on dietary recall. People tend to have trouble remembering how much of each food they have eaten. Moreover, in the case of cancer studies, the need is not so much to know what the diet is like now as to know what it was like at an earlier time—say, 30 years ago—when the initiating event may have taken place. In this connection, study of the Seventh-day Adventist vegetarians offers hope of clarifying the relationship between animal protein and cancer. Most can recall exactly when they quit eating meat—they quit when they joined the church.

In general, studies of populations have suggested that low cancer rates correlate with low meat and high vegetable and grain intakes, but there are exceptions. For example, another religious group, the Mormons, do not limit meat; they consume it in amounts that are typical of most people living in the United States. Still,

The Delaney Questions (continued)

allow an accurate accounting of exactly what that threat level is for each substance considered. Such thinking leads to the conclusion that some additives with the potential to cause cancer would not have to be banned altogether; they could be tolerated at an acceptable risk level, perhaps with warning labels to the users.

The problems do not end there, though. For example, scientific testing to determine whether a compound is carcinogenic is itself problem-laden. It is unethical to test a potential carcinogen by feeding it to cancer-free adults and then watching to see if cancer develops. To get around this problem, researchers must test the substance on other species, usually bacteria and small mammals. Even if a substance receives a clean billing from these studies, it is uncertain how well results from animal studies apply to human beings. And another question: do tests of exposure to one isolated chemical hold true for real people in the real world, where they are exposed to many substances that may work synergistically to produce cancer? For example, alcohol, although not known to be a carcinogen in of itself, promotes cancer formation when it is present with other carcinogens. Still, animal testing is, to most people's way of thinking, the only way to evaluate the cancer risk associated with new additives.

In summary, the regulation of additives suspected of causing cancer is controversial. It is debatable whether they should be treated like other harmful food constitutes. If thresholds should be permitted, there is a question how to establish them. And the question how they should be identified also draws argument: bacterial screening and animal tests are useful, but their interpretation is difficult. The need to resolve these questions is becoming more pressing, as new analytical techniques allow lower and lower levels of carcinogenic materials to become detectable in foods.

At present, the Delaney Clause is still in force, although many wish to modify or abolish it. It prohibits the addition to foods of any substance that has been shown to cause cancer in animals at any dose level. No threshold is considered safe, and risk assessment is not permitted. It has been proposed that the law be changed to base safety decisions related to additives more on the assessment of theoretical risk to people, to allow the FDA more latitude in creating regulations, and to allow food companies more freedom of choice in their use of low-risk additives.

Source: Adapted from E. N. Whitney, C. B. Cataldo, and S. R. Rolfes, Highlight 13A, Questions about additives and cancer, in *Understanding Normal and Clinical Nutrition* (St. Paul: West, 1987), pp. 475–479.

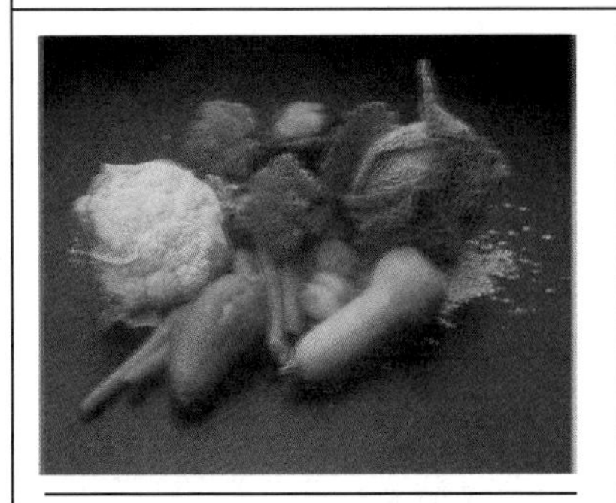

These foods contain nutrients and nonnutrients that are protective against cancer.

Mormons experience lower rates of breast and colon cancer than other U.S. citizens do.[13] Case-control studies, in which researchers can control some of the variables, can help to confirm or refute the meat-cancer relationship.

Findings from Case-control Studies

Case-control studies have generally implicated diet in cancer causation. When 179 Hawaiian Japanese people with colon cancer were carefully matched with 357 Hawaiian Japanese people without cancer, those with cancer were seen to have a strikingly higher consumption of meat, especially beef. An Israeli study showed fiber consumption to be lower in victims of colon cancer than in comparable people who did not have cancer. A study of U.S. blacks with colon cancer showed that they ate less fiber and more saturated fat than others without cancer. These studies and many others like them have led reviewers to the view that a diet "high in total fat, low in fiber, and high in beef [is] associated with an increased incidence of large-bowel cancer in man."[14] Others deny that these findings have established the existence of a strong association between fat consumption and colon cancer.[15]

Findings from Studies on Animals: Fat and Cancer

Once population and case-control studies have identified a possible dietary link to cancer, researchers often turn to experiments with laboratory animals. By using animals, researchers can control many variables while manipulating only the diet.

Laboratory studies using animals confirm suspicions that fat, of all dietary components, is most strongly correlated with cancer. For example, it is well known that the number of mammary tumors in rats increase with increased dietary fat, and especially if the fat is unsaturated.[16]

People are often surprised to learn that fat may be far more significant in cancer causation than food additives, which have long been suspected and feared. Fat is thought to act as a **promoter** that somehow enhances the process by which cancer becomes established in a cell or tissue. A high-fat diet may advance cancer:

- By altering body tissue responsiveness to certain hormones (for example, growth hormone), thus stimulating cell division and the advancement of certain cancers.
- By promoting the secretion of bile into the intestine; bile may then be converted by organisms in the colon into compounds that cause cancer.
- By supplying unsaturated fat, which can split into molecules that can initiate cancer.
- By inhibiting the production of molecules that modulate cell division (prostaglandins).
- By blocking the communications pathways cells use to signal their neighbors to stop dividing.
- By reducing the immune system's effectiveness in destroying cancerous cells.
- By contributing to obesity (a known cancer risk factor).
- By being incorporated into cell membranes and changing them so that they offer less defense against cancer-causing invaders.
- By delivering to tumors the concentrated energy they need to grow rapidly.

Fat in general is associated with increased cancer, but studies seem to point to polyunsaturated fat specifically. Could it be that polyunsaturated fat in the diet is responsible for some kinds of cancer? Some think so. Others criticize laboratory methods for falsely implying this association. The box on the omega fatty acids in Chapter 4 mentioned that diets high in certain polyunsaturated fatty acids, the ω3 series, seem to *enhance* defenses against cancer.

As an example of criticism against this line of research, consider the following problem. Laboratory chow fed to rats is made up of synthetic ingredients, and is tightly controlled in composition. Even ordinary grains have too much natural fat to include in the chow. When scientists make rat chow with only *saturated* fat, it lacks the essential fatty acids, no matter how much saturated fat they add. Hence, tumor growth will be slow. If the scientist should then try a chow with even small amounts of added unsaturated fat, the nutrient needs of the tumor would be supplied and cancer would advance uninhibited. Such a finding might make it look as if the unsaturated fat had promoted tumor growth. However, this situation was artificial, and would not have relevance to the human diet.

At this writing, the jury is still out on whether polyunsaturated fats promote cancer, whether some types may help prevent it, or whether they simply allow its advancement in the same way other nutrients do. What is clear is that diets relatively higher in total fat (20 percent or more), and in energy, enhance cancer development.[17] We can safely say that overnutrition, and overweight, are directly related to a high cancer risk.[18]

Scientifically, experimental findings about rats cannot be assumed to be true for people. At present, studies are in progress to determine if people who are at risk for certain cancers, or who already have them, can benefit from the same kind of diet that benefits the rats, one that is very low in fat.[19] There would appear to be no harm in reducing the fat intake of adults from the widespread 40 or so percent to 20 percent or less of total calories, and to bring energy intakes into line with energy needs. (For children, this may be too low. Fat supports growth.) For the average Westerner, accomplishing this would mean choosing low-fat alternative foods, drastically reducing the amount of fat used in food preparation, and refraining from adding fat, such as butter, margarine, or salad dressings to foods at the table.

Implications

In general, wherever the diet is high in fat-rich foods, it is simultaneously low in vegetable fiber. The association of fat with cancer is stronger than that of low fiber intake, but fiber may independently help to protect against some cancer—for example, by promoting the excretion of bile from the body, or by speeding up the transit of all materials through the colon so that the colon walls are not exposed for long to cancer-causing substances. That fiber does have an independent protective effect of some kind is supported by evidence from Finland. The Finns eat a high-fat diet, but unlike other such diets, theirs is very high in fiber as well. Their colon cancer rate is low, suggesting that fiber has a protective effect even in the presence of a high-fat diet.[20]

If fat and/or a meat-rich diet are implicated in the causation of certain cancers, and if fiber and/or a vegetable-rich diet are associated with prevention, then vegetarians should have a lower incidence of those cancers. They do. The Seventh-day Adventists have already been mentioned; other vegetarian women also have less breast cancer than do meat eaters. A study of people in Minnesota and Norway found less frequent use of vegetables in people with colon cancer; a New York study found, specifically, less use of the so-called **cruciferons vegetables**—such as cabbage, broccoli, and brussels sprouts—in colon cancer victims. Similarly, careful comparisons of stomach cancer victims' diets with those of case controls show less use of vegetables in the cancer group—in one case, vegetables in general; in another, fresh vegetables; in others, lettuce and other fresh greens; or vegetables containing vitamin C.[21]

One of the suspects for the causation of stomach cancer is nitrosamines, produced in the stomach from nitrites. The vegetables may help keep nitrosamines from forming by contributing vitamin C, which inhibits the conversion of nitrites to nitrosamines. Nitrites occur naturally in the environment. They are present in the water supply and are present in high concentrations in many vegetables. They are also made in the human body in quantities much larger than those found in food. We can't avoid nitrites, but perhaps we can help to prevent their conversion to nitrosamines (which cause cancer) by eating vitamin C-containing vegetables and fruits along with them. This approach to the prevention of stomach cancer has a strong theoretical basis, but as yet, no actual experiments on human beings have proven it effective. Among unanswered questions: Within what range of stomach acidities is vitamin C effective in preventing nitrosamine formation? How effective is it in the presence of other agents that promote nitrosamine formation? How much vitamin C has to be present for an effect to occur?[22] It makes sense, for other reasons, to eat foods containing plenty of vitamin C, so

Miniglossary

carcinogen (car-SIN-oh-jen): a cancer-causing substance. (*carcin* means "cancer"; *gen* means "gives rise to").

case-control studies: studies of individuals with a disease, matched as closely as possible to other individuals without the disease in the attempt to identify possible causes of the disease.

cruciferous vegetables: vegetables of the cabbage family (*cruci* means "cross-shaped," referring to the shape of the flowers).

epidemiological studies: studies of populations in which differing incidences of a disease are correlated with other factors in the attempt to identify possible causes of the disease.

initiation: an event, probably in the cell's genetic equipment, caused by a carcinogen or by radiation, that can give rise to cancer.

intervention trials: studies in which preventive measures are tried on half of a population to see if they will reduce the incidence of a disease.

promotion: assistance in the development of cancer.

promoter: a substance that does not initiate cancer, but that favors its development once the initiating event has taken place.

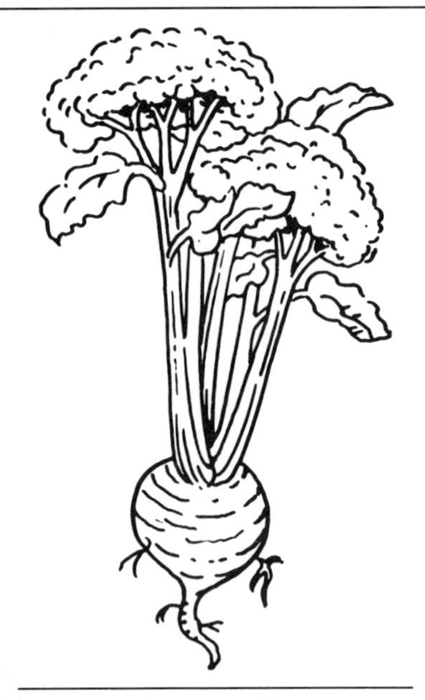

By combining vegetables, you can achieve all the vitamins you would receive in a supplement, in addition to other needed nutrients.

go ahead and do it. Drink orange juice with your breakfast bacon; eat broccoli with your ham; enjoy fresh fruits and vegetables with every meal. It may help and it can't hurt.

When environmental causes of another kind of cancer—that of the head and neck—have been sought, the major factor has appeared not to be diet but the combination of alcohol and tobacco consumption. Again, however, some dietary factors have turned up here and there, pointing to a low intake of fruits and raw vegetables in cancer cases. This time, intakes were low specifically of the fruits and vegetables that contribute carotene (the vitamin A precursor) and riboflavin. Carotene and its relatives the retinoids are also important in preventing cancers of epithelial origin, including skin cancer.[23]

Among the known actions of vitamin A are the important roles it plays in maintaining the immune function. A strong immune system may be able to prevent cancers from gaining control, even after they have gotten started in the body. Some studies suggest that this may be one place vitamin A makes its contribution. In Norway, a five-year study showed lung cancer incidence to be 60 to 80 percent lower in men with a high vitamin A intake than those with a low intake. In Japan, a study of 280,000 people showed lung cancer rates to be 20 to 30 percent lower in smokers who ate yellow or green vegetables daily than in those who did not. In ex-smokers who ingested yellow or green vegetables daily the reduction was much greater, as if something in the vegetables enhanced the *repair* of damage done by smoking after the initiation of cancer.[24] Other studies of the microscopic events that occur during cancer initiation indicate that vitamin A may also play a role in defending against the earliest cancerous changes.[25] Abundant evidence along these lines makes clear that anyone at risk for the development of cancer should obtain adequate vitamin A and its previtamin carotene. Whether *excess* carotene is extra beneficial against cancer remains for the group of physicians mentioned earlier to prove or disprove by taking their daily carotene supplements.

What other substances might vegetables contribute to help protect the body against cancer? Among other nutrients now known to be important in the functioning of the immune system are vitamin B_6, folacin, pantothenic acid, vitamin B_{12}, vitamin E, iron, and zinc. Doubtless there are others.

Cancer Prevention

In 1980, the Food and Nutrition Board of the National Academy of Sciences stated that not enough evidence was yet available to justify making any recommendations for the dietary prevention of cancer. Two years later, however, under heavy pressure from the public, the Academy did publish some provisional recommendations.[26] It was as if they were saying, "This is what we are tempted to recommend, but we don't think we can, yet." Among the provisional recommendations were these:

- Reduce the consumption of both saturated and unsaturated fats.
- Include fruits (especially citrus fruits), vegetables (particularly carotene-rich and cruciferous vegetables; see Table C5–1), and whole-grain products in the daily diet.
- Consume only moderate amounts of alcohol, if any.

In addition, they recommended minimizing consumption of cured and smoked foods on the supposition that the carcinogens they contained would increase the risk of cancer. They also endorsed protection of the food supply against contamination with carcinogens from any source and continued evaluation of food additives for carcinogenic activity. A summary of the evidence that backed these guidelines included these points:

- Attention should also be paid to nitrates and their relatives in foods.
- Toxic substances in drinking water are also of concern.

It bears repeating that additives legally permitted in foods do not contribute significantly to people's overall risk of cancer.[27]

Obviously, much remains to be learned about the connections between nutrition and cancer. Still, many people working in cancer research believe that we already know enough to take the tentative preventive steps provisionally recommended by the National Academy. One pair of reviewers says, "The public is looking for answers regarding this diet-cancer link and will look to anyone willing to provide answers, regardless of his/her qualifications. . . . The recommendations offered here constitute no risk and may help lower the incidence of . . . cancers." In other words, it can't hurt, and it may help. To the recommendations made in these guidelines, we would add only one other: Vary your choices. Don't let your diet become monotonous.

This last suggestion is based on the concept of dilution, first mentioned in Chapter 2 and taken up again later in Controversy 10. It is specific to the prevention of cancer initiation. Whenever you switch from food to food, you are diluting whatever is in one food with what is in the others. It is safe to eat *some* processed meats, but don't eat them all the time. Eat many kinds of green, yellow, and orange vegetables; they are all needed in the diet for many good reasons. If you include high-fiber foods, reduce your fat intake, and control your energy intake, you have every reason to feel confident that you are providing your body with the best nutrition at the lowest possible risk for cancer. A fringe benefit is that you are probably helping protect yourself against heart disease, diabetes, and many other diseases as well.

Table C5–1

Cruciferous Vegetables and Carotene-rich Fruits and Vegetables

Cruciferous vegetable	Carotene-rich fruits and vegetable
broccoli	apricots
brussels sprouts	asparagus
cabbage (all varieties)	broccoli
cauliflower	cantaloupe
greens (collards, mustards, turnips)	carrots
kale	green onions
kohlrabi	greens (all varieties)
rutabaga	lettuce (dark green)
turnip roots	mango
	oriental cabbages
	papaya
	parsley
	spinach
	squash (hard, winter)
	sweet potato

Notes

1. Parts of this Controversy are adapted from Highlight 4A: Nutrition and Cancer, in *Understanding Nutrition,* 4th ed., by E. N. Whitney, E. M. N. Hamilton and M. A. Boyle (St. Paul, Minn.: West, 1987).
2. J. C. Bailar and E. M. Smith, Progress against cancer? *New England Journal of Medicine* 314 (1986): 1226–1232.
3. A. E. Reif, The causes of cancer, *American Scientist* 69 (1981): 437–447.
4. L. A. Poirier, Stages in carcinogenesis: Alteration by diet, *American Journal of Clinical Nutrition* 45 (1987): 185–191.
5. S. Graham, Fats, calories, and calorie expenditure in the epidemiology of cancer, *American Journal of Clinical Nutrition* 45 (1987): 342–346.
6. B. S. Reddy and coauthors, Nutrition and its relationship to cancer, *Advances in Cancer Research* 32 (1980): 238–245.
7. Reddy and coauthors, 1980.
8. G. L. Wolff, Body weight and cancer, *American Journal of Clinical Nutrition* 45 (1987): 168–180.
9. R. L. Phillips and D. A. Snowdon, Dietary relationships with fatal colo-rectal cancer among Seventh-day Adventists, *Journal of the National Cancer Institute* 74 (1985): 307–317.
10. B. S. Drasar and D. Irving, Environmental factors and cancer of the colon and breast, *British Journal of Cancer* 27 (1973): 167–172.
11. S. A. Törnberg and coauthors, Risks of cancer of the colon and rectum in relation to serum cholesterol and β-lipoprotein, *New England Journal of Medicine* 315 (1986): 1629–1633, as reported in *Modern Medicine,* May 1987, pp. 136, 141.
12. J. E. Vena and coauthors, Occupational exercise and risk of cancer, *American Journal of Clinical Nutrition* 45 (1987): 318–327; R. E. Frisch and coauthors, Lower lifetime occurrence of breast cancer and cancers of the reproductive system among former college athletes, *American Journal of Clinical Nutrition* 45 (1987): 328–335.
13. R. Doll and R. Peto, The causes of cancer: Quantitative estimates of avoidable risks of cancer in the United States today, *Journal of the National Cancer Institute* 66 (1981): 1191–1308, as cited by M. W. Pariza, *Diet and Cancer* (Summit, N.J.: American Council on Science and Health, 1985), p. 12.
14. Reddy and coauthors, 1980.
15. L. N. Kolonel and coauthors, Role of diet in cancer incidence in Hawaii, *Cancer Research* 43 (1983 Supplement): 2297s–2402s; W. C. Willet and B. MacMahon, Diet and cancer: An overview, *New England Journal of Medicine* 310 (1984): 697–703.

16. C. W. Welsch, Enhancement of mammary tumorigenesis by dietary fat: Review of potential mechanisms, *American Journal of Clinical Nutrition* 45 (1987): 192–202.

17. I. Clement, Fat and essential fatty acid in mammary carcinogenesis, *American Journal of Clinical Nutrition* 45 (1987): 218–224.

18. M. W. Pariza and R. K. Boutwell, Historical perspective: Calories and energy expenditure in carcinogenesis, *American Journal of Clinical Nutrition* 45 (1987): 151–156.

19. P. Greenwald and coauthors, Feasibility studies of a low-fat diet to prevent or retard breast cancer, *American Journal of Clinical Nutrition* 45 (1987): 347–353.

20. E. L. Wynder, Dietary habits and cancer epidemiology, *Cancer* 43 (1979): 1955–1961, as cited by S. H. Brammer and R. L. DeFelice, Dietary advice in regard to risk for colon and breast cancer, *Preventive Medicine* 9 (1980): 544–549.

21. Reddy and coauthors, 1980.

22. S. A. Kyrtopoulos, Ascorbic acid and the formation of N-nitroso compounds: Possible role of ascorbic acid in cancer prevention. *American Journal of Clinical Nutrition* 45 (1987): 1344–1350.

23. J. L. Werther, Food and cancer, *New York State Journal of Medicine,* August 1980, pp. 1401–1408.

24. Werther, 1980.

25. L. M. Deluca and E. M. McDowell, Deletion of essential functions and tumorigenesis, *Journal of Nutrition* 116 (1986): 2064–2065.

26. Committee on Diet, Nutrition, and Cancer, National Research Council, *Executive Summary: Diet, Nutrition, and Cancer* (Washington, D.C.: National Academy Press, 1982).

27. Committee on Diet, Nutrition, and Cancer, 1982.

Chapter Six

Contents

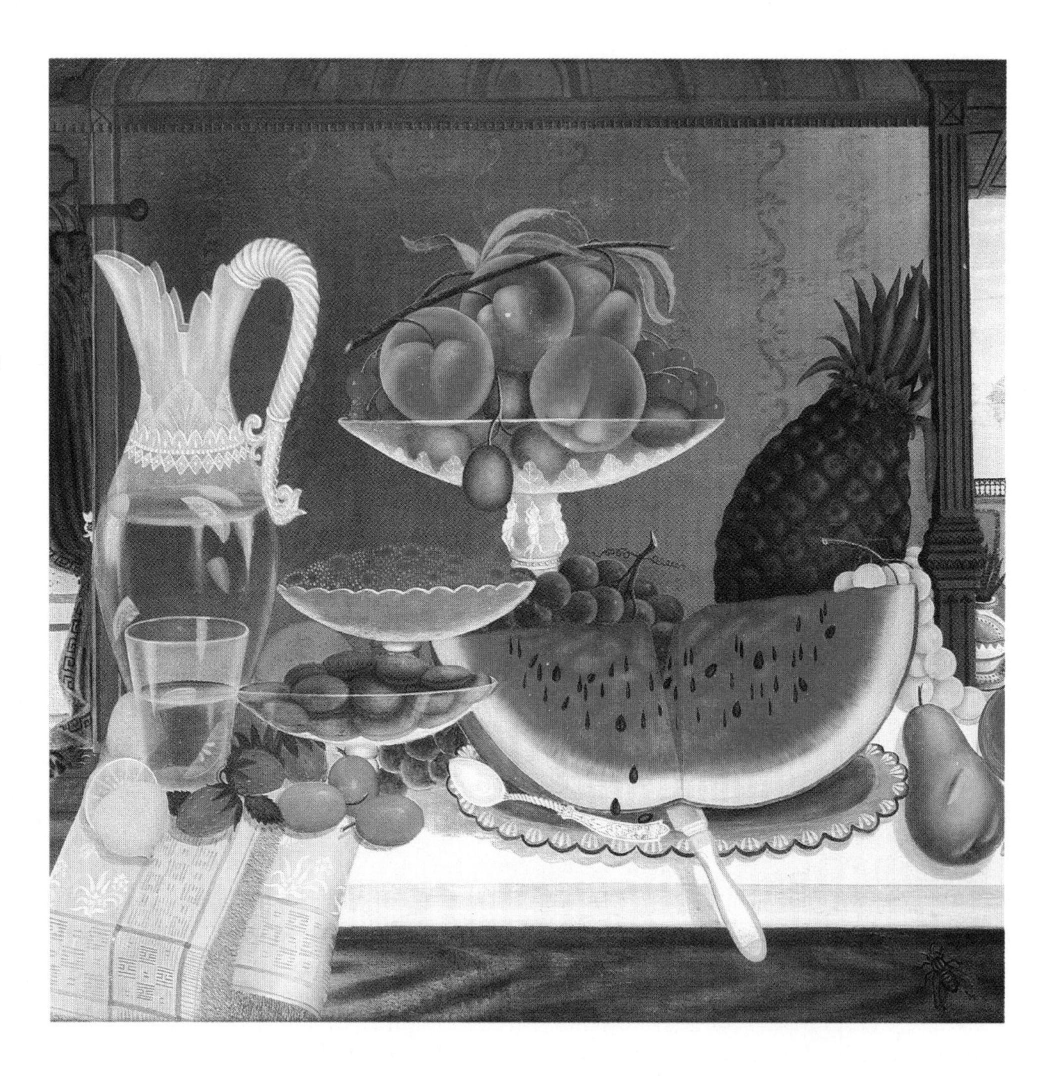

Still Life by Henry Church, © 1870s, oil on paper backed on cloth 26 × 28 inches. Collection of Mrs. Donald Stem.

The Vitamins

Since the turn of this century, the romance and thrill of the discoveries of the first **vitamins** have captured the world's heart. People love the vitamins. Catapulted from the shrouded mystery of folk cures to the high-tech era that brings us vitamin pills, they seem a perfect answer to people who are looking for an easy way to good health. Today, scientists are stepping back from their microscopes to appreciate the complexity of the interactions of vitamins in the body. The media bombard us with a never-ending stream of advertisements for "miracle vitamins," and the supplement business is a multi*billion* dollar industry.

vitamins: organic compounds, vital to life, indispensable to body function, needed in minute amounts; noncaloric essential nutrients.

From a review of the history of vitamin discoveries, it is easy to see why people are so impressed. The story line has been repeated over and over with the discovery of each new vitamin. Whole groups of people are unable to walk (or are going blind or bleeding profusely) until an alert scientist stumbles onto the substance missing in their diets. According to the plot, the scientist usually confirms the discovery by feeding vitamin-deficient feed to laboratory animals. The animals respond by becoming unable to walk (or going blind or bleeding profusely). Then, miraculously, they recover when the one missing ingredient is restored to their diet. Miraculous cures of people follow, as their vitamin deficiencies are remedied. On reading of dramatic events like these, people come to believe that vitamins will cure a host of ailments. But the truth is that the only disease a vitamin will cure is the one caused by a deficiency of that vitamin.

The only disease a vitamin will cure is the one caused by a deficiency of that vitamin.

At first, vitamins were given letters: vitamin A, vitamin B, vitamin C. Later, chemical analysis revealed that what had been thought to be one chemical was actually two or more, and sub-numerals were used to differentiate these: B_1, B_2, and so on. In addition, some vitamins received names. This led to confusion that still exists today. This chapter uses the current, officially correct names of the 13 known vitamins (see Table 6–1).*

It took a sophisticated knowledge of chemistry and biology to isolate the vitamins and to learn their chemical structures. Today, chemists can synthesize most of them, and people can therefore take them in supplement form.

Each of the previous chapters has included a box on supplements related to that chapter's subject. So many supplements of vitamins are available that this chapter's entire Controversy is devoted to them. Read it to learn when to take vitamin supplements.

IF YOU'RE TIRED, YOU NEED TO BUY SOME B_{12} PILLS.
LOGIC WITHOUT EVIDENCE
MOTIVE: PERSONAL GAIN
AMATEUR DIAGNOSIS

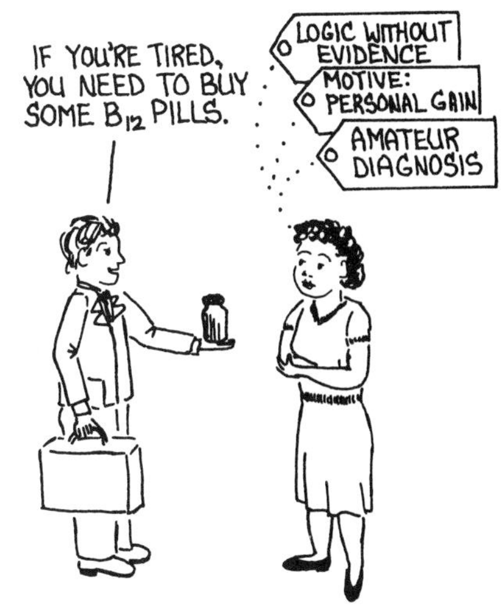

Vitamins are frequently offered as cures for people's symptoms.

*The vitamin names used here are those agreed on, and published by, the Committee on Nomenclature of the American Institute of Nutrition, in Nomenclature policy: Generic descriptors and trivial names for vitamins and related compounds, *Journal of Nutrition* 112 (1982): 7–14. Alternative names are given in Tables 6–2 and 6–3.

precursors: compounds that can be converted into active vitamins; also known as **provitamins**.

Definition and Classification of Vitamins

A child once defined a vitamin as "what, if you don't eat, you get sick." Although the grammar left something to be desired, the definition was accurate. Less imaginatively, a vitamin is defined as an essential, noncaloric organic nutrient needed in tiny amounts in the diet. The role of many vitamins is to help make possible the processes by which other nutrients are digested, absorbed, and metabolized, or built into body structures.

Some of the vitamins occur in foods in a form known as **precursors,** or **provitamins**. Once inside the body, these are changed chemically to one or more active forms. Thus, in measuring the amount of a vitamin found in food, it is often most accurate to count not only the amount of the true vitamin, but also the vitamin activity potentially available from its precursors. Tables 6–2 and 6–3 later in this chapter show which vitamins have precursors.

Fat-soluble vitamins:

- Vitamin A.
- Vitamin D.
- Vitamin E.
- Vitamin K.

Water-soluble vitamins:

- B vitamins.
- Vitamin C.

The vitamins fall naturally into two classes. The fat-soluble vitamins—A, D, E, and K—generally occur together in such foods as fish oils and plant oils. Like the lipids, once these vitamins have been absorbed from the intestinal tract, they are not easily excreted. Instead, they are stored in the liver and fatty tissues. Excesses, especially of vitamins A, D, and K, can reach toxic levels. As you read about each, you may want to refer to the table in Controversy 6 that lists safe doses for the vitamins. The fat-soluble vitamins *can* be inadvertently lost from the digestive tract with undigested fat; any disease that produces fat malabsorption (such as liver disease that prevents bile production) can bring about deficiencies of them. A person who uses mineral oil (which the body can't absorb) as a laxative risks losing the fat-soluble vitamins by excretion.

All of the other vitamins—the B vitamins and vitamin C—are water soluble. They can be leached out of foods easily by incorrect preparation. They are easily excreted in the urine, should a person ingest more than the needed amount. Under ordinary circumstances, you need not be concerned about small excesses. Some of the water-soluble vitamins can remain in the lean tissues for periods of a month or more; but these tissues are actively exchanging materials with the body fluids at all times, and so these vitamins are likely to be picked up by the extracellular fluids, carried away by the blood, and excreted in the urine. As a rule of thumb, it is recommended that you eat foods every day that are rich in the water-soluble vitamins; food sources never deliver toxic doses. The large doses provided by vitamin supplements can reach toxic levels, but the greatest hazard they usually present is that, as one person aptly noted, "If you take supplements of the water-soluble vitamins, you may have the most expensive urine in town."

Table 6–1

Vitamin Names
Fat-soluble vitamins
Vitamin A
Vitamin D
Vitamin E
Vitamin K
Water-soluble vitamins
B vitamins
Thiamin
Riboflavin
Niacin
Vitamin B_6
Folacin
Vitamin B_{12}
Pantothenic acid
Biotin
Vitamin C

It is common for drugs to act as antagonists to vitamins. For example, tuberculosis bacteria have very high needs for vitamin B_6. The drug INH (isonicotinamide hydrazide), by interfering with the action of that vitamin, kills the bacteria. Of course, human cells need the vitamin, too, but they are not as quickly affected by its lack as are the bacteria. (You'll read more about drug and nutrient interactions in Chapter 13).

Although small in quantity, the vitamins accomplish mighty tasks. In some instances, their exact functions are still unknown. Some of the most important facts will be discussed separately for each vitamin in the following sections;

Tables 6–2 and 6–3 at the end of the chapter sum up the basic facts about all of the vitamins.

Vitamins are essential, noncaloric nutrients, needed in tiny amounts in the diet, that serve as helpers in cell functions. The fat-soluble vitamins are vitamins A, D, E, and K; the water-soluble vitamins are the B vitamins and vitamin C.

The Fat-Soluble Vitamins

The fat-soluble vitamins are diverse, as you will see. Vitamin A is, among many other things, a visual pigment. Vitamin A and also D can act somewhat like hormones, directing cells to convert one substance to another, store this, or release that. Vitamin E swarms all over the body, preventing oxidative destruction of tissues. Vitamin K helps in blood clotting. Each is worth a book in itself, but each receives only a section here.

Vitamin A

Vitamin A has the distinction of being the first fat-soluble vitamin to be recognized. It is certainly one of the most versatile, with roles in such diverse functions as vision, maintenance of body linings and skin, bone growth, and reproduction. It is the most flashy, too; the active form **retinol** is yellow, and the precursor form **carotene** is bright orange, calling attention to its presence in foods. When carotene is converted to retinol in the body, losses occur, so rather than express the amount of carotene in foods, nutrition scientists use the **retinol equivalent (RE)**—the amount of retinol the body actually receives from a plant food after conversion. The body can make one unit of retinol from about three of carotene.

Perhaps the most familiar function of vitamin A is in eyesight. When you were a child, someone may have told you to "eat your carrots, because they're good for your eyes." While you may not have believed it at the time, that person may have known the two indispensable functions vitamin A plays in the eye—in the events of light perception at the **retina** and in the maintenance of a healthy, crystal-clear outer window, the **cornea**.

When light falls on the eye, it passes through the clear cornea and strikes the cells of the retina, bleaching many molecules of the pigment **rhodopsin** that lies within them. Vitamin A is a part of rhodopsin. The vitamin is broken off when bleaching occurs, initiating the signal that conveys the sensation of sight to the optic center in the brain. The vitamin then reunites with the pigment, but a little vitamin A is destroyed each time this reaction takes place, and fresh vitamin A arriving in the blood regenerates the supply. If the supply is low, a lag occurs before the eye can see again after a flash of bright light at night (see Figure 6–1). This lag in the recovery of night vision, termed **night blindness,** may indicate a vitamin A deficiency. (The diagnosis is not certain, though, because the mineral zinc is also needed to regenerate rhodopsin.)

retinol: one of the active forms of vitamin A.

carotene: a vitamin A precursor found in plants; an orange pigment.

RE (retinol equivalent): a measure of vitamin A activity; the amount of retinol that the body will derive from a food containing vitamin A (preformed retinol) or its precursor carotene.

retina (RET-in-uh): the layer of light-sensitive nerve cells lining the back of the inside of the eye.

cornea (KOR-nee-uh): the hard, transparent membrane covering the outside of the eye.

rhodopsin: the light-sensitive pigment of the cells in the retina; it contains vitamin A (*rhod* refers to the rod-shaped cells; *opsin* means "visual protein").

night blindness: slow recovery of vision after flashes of bright light at night; an early symptom of vitamin A deficiency.

keratin (KERR-uh-tin): a water-insoluble protein; the normal protein of hair and nails.

keratinization: accumulation of keratin in a tissue, a sign of vitamin A deficiency.

xerosis: a second stage of vitamin A deficiency in the cornea—drying.

xerophthalmia (ZEER-ahf-THALL-me-uh): hardening of the cornea of the eye in advanced vitamin A deficiency that can lead to blindness (*xero* means "dry"; *ophthalm* means "eye").

epithelial (ep-ih-THEE-lee-ull) **tissue:** the layers of the body that serve as selective barriers to the environment. Examples are the cornea, the skin, the respiratory lining, and the lining of the digestive tract.

A deficiency of vitamin A that has progressed well beyond the night blindness stage may be reflected in an accumulation of a protein, **keratin,** which clouds the eye's outer vitamin A–dependent part, the cornea. The condition is known as **keratinization,** and it can progress to **xerosis** (drying) and then to thickening and permanent blindness—**xerophthalmia**. Tragically, vitamin A–deprived children will often become blind because of this preventable condition. If the deficiency is discovered early, it can be reversed by vitamin A therapy. If allowed to progress too long, the disease causes children as young as two or three to lose their sight permanently.

Vitamin A is needed by all **epithelial tissue** (external skin and internal linings), not just the cornea. The skin and all of the protective linings of the lungs, intestines, vagina, urinary tract, and bladder serve as barriers to infection from bacteria, or to damage from other sources. If vitamin A is deficient, some of the cells in these areas are displaced by cells that secrete keratin, which is normally produced only in the hair and fingernails. Keratin makes the surfaces dry, hard, and vulnerable to infection (see Figure 6–2). The cells then cannot perform their jobs; they die, accumulate on the surface, and become hosts to bacterial infection. In the cornea, keratinization leads to xerophthalmia; in the lungs, the displacement of mucus-producing cells makes respiratory infections likely; in the vagina, the same process leads to vaginal infections.

Controversy 5 offers more on vitamin A and cancer.

Adequate vitamin A has been shown to be important in the prevention of certain cancers. Healthy skin and internal linings are able to interrupt the process by which cancers get started, but vitamin A deficiency handicaps this defense. Skin, lung, bladder, and larynx cancers become more likely when vitamin A or carotene is lacking.

Figure 6–1 Night Blindness.
This is one of the earliest signs of vitamin A deficiency.

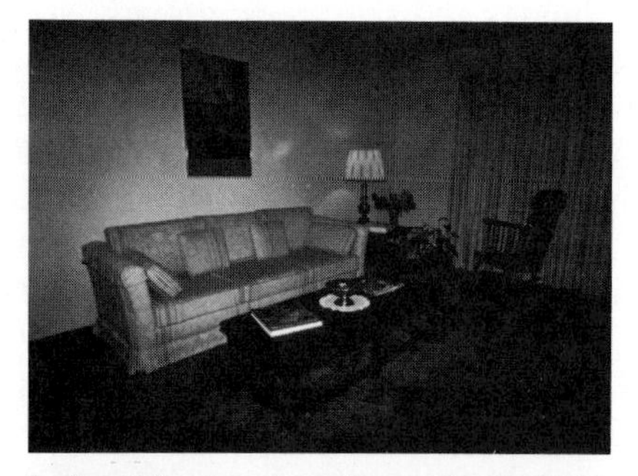
In dim light, you can make out the details in this room.

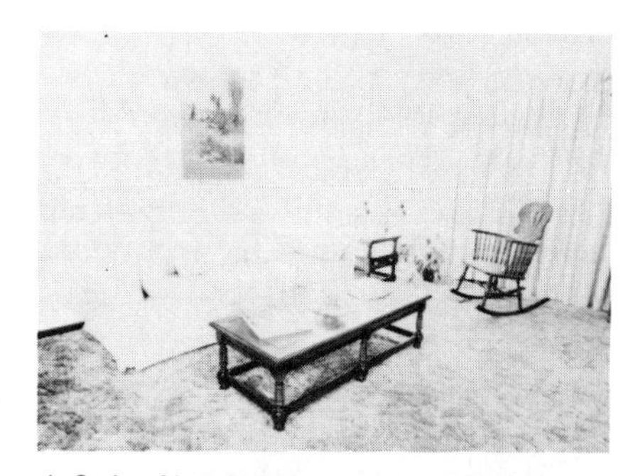
A flash of bright light momentarily blinds you as the pigment in the retina is bleached.

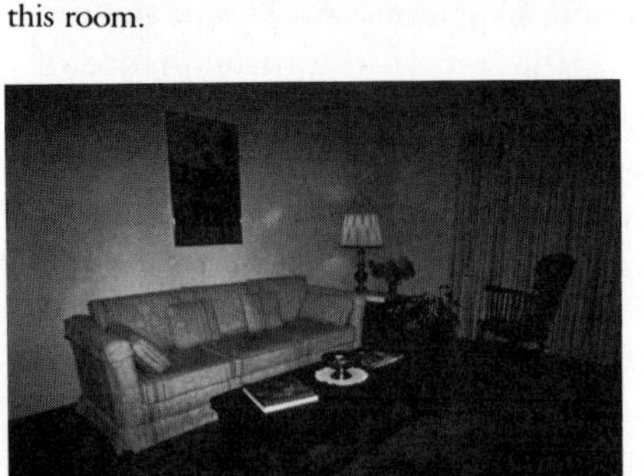
You quickly recover, and can see the details again in a few seconds.

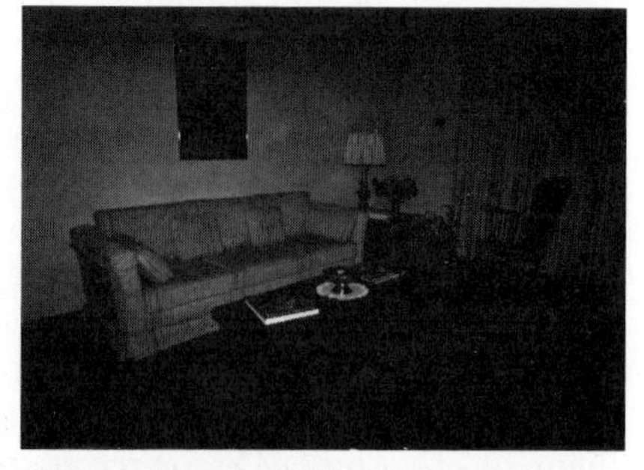
With inadequate vitamin A, you do not recover but remain blind for many seconds; this is night blindness.

Vitamin A also assists in bone growth. Normal children's bones grow longer, and the children grow taller, by remodeling of each old bone into a new, bigger version. In order to convert a small bone into a large bone, the body must dismantle parts and then rebuild. Vitamin A is needed in the dismantling step. Without it, bones cannot change shape. By helping reshape the jawbone as it grows, vitamin A permits normal tooth spacing. Crooked teeth and poor dental health can result from a deficiency in prenatal or early postnatal life. In children, failure to grow is one of the first signs of poor vitamin A status.

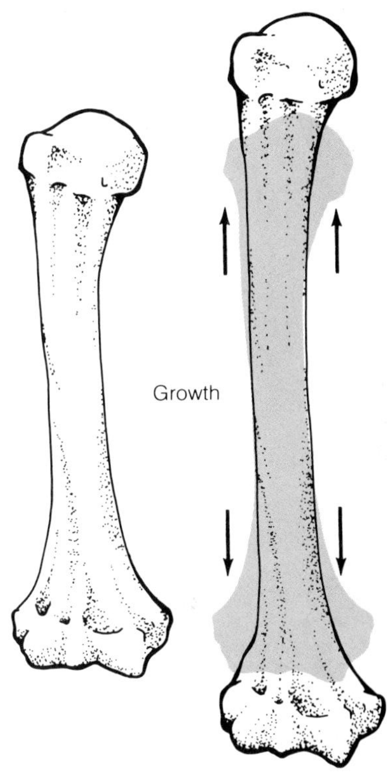

As bone lengthens, vitamin A helps remove old bone (arrows).

Vitamin A is also essential for normal reproduction, the stress response, metabolism, the nervous system, immunity, and the making of blood. In short, it is needed everywhere.

Vitamin A deficiency is a vast problem worldwide. It causes as many as 100,000 new cases of blindness a year, placing a heavy burden on society. Countless more children suffer from less obvious signs of vitamin A deficiency—stunted growth, poor appetite, and impaired immunity leading to infections, illness, and death. It is estimated that 20 to 35 percent of all childhood mortality may be related to vitamin A deficiency.[1] To prevent all this sickness and death would cost only a few pennies per child per year, for vitamin A capsules are inexpensive to make and each child would need only two or three a year.

Toxicity is an equally real danger for people who take excess vitamin A in capsule form. It can cause many symptoms, including hair loss, joint pain, stunted growth, bone and muscle soreness, cessation of menstruation, nausea, diarrhea, rashes, and enlargement of the liver and spleen. Taken during pregnancy, vitamin A megadoses can cause major birth defects; much smaller doses given to animals during pregnancy cause permanent learning disabilities in their offspring, implying that they may do so in human children, too.[2] Early symptoms of overdoses in children are loss of appetite, growth failure, and itching of the skin. Carotene from plant foods is not converted to the active form of vitamin A rapidly enough to be hazardous but has been known to turn people bright yellow if they eat too much. This happens because the brightly colored carotene is stored in the fat layer, directly below the skin surface. Foods containing vitamin A compounds can be eaten in large amounts without causing toxicity symptoms, with the possible exception of liver. Polar bears, because they eat fish whole (and thus fish livers), store very large amounts of the vitamin in *their* livers, which have therefore become notorious as a dangerous food source for the Inuit people and for arctic explorers.

Experts argue about how much vitamin A is too much. Some authorities think people take too much vitamin A in supplements and that "we may be on the verge of an epidemic of vitamin A toxicity."[3] Other authorities point to a relatively low supplemental dose (five to ten times the RDA) given over many years as a cause of toxicity in the long run. Still others cite evidence that it takes 40 to 120 times the RDA to achieve a toxic dose. A table in Controversy 6 lists a safe dose of vitamin A that will not be toxic even over a long period of time, but the best way to ensure a safe vitamin A intake is to steer clear of supplements and simply eat foods that contain it.

Figure 6–2 The Skin in Vitamin A Deficiency.
The hard lumps reflect accumulations of keratin in the epithelial cells.

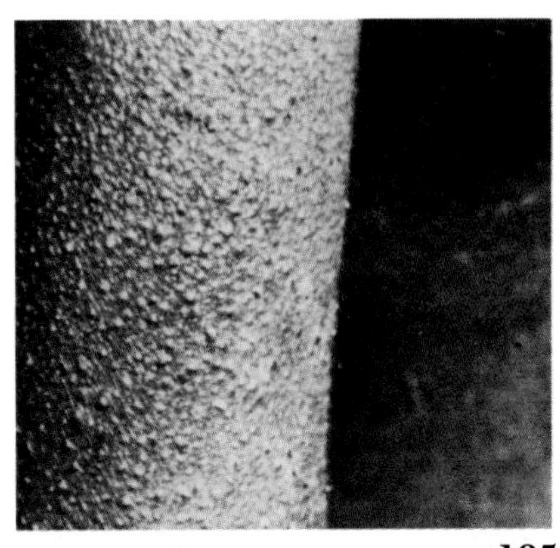

Foods from animal sources that include some fat contain the active vitamin retinol. Among the richest sources are liver, cod-liver oil, butter, egg yolks, whole or fortified milk, cream, and cheeses made from whole milk or cream.

Foods from plants contain carotene, the orange pigment that is a precursor to vitamin A. They are so brightly colored that they decorate the plate. Carrots, sweet potatoes, pumpkins, cantaloupe, apricots, and peaches are all rich sources.

IU (international unit): a measure of fat-soluble vitamin activity.

Another colorful group, such *dark* green vegetables as spinach, other greens, or broccoli, owe their color to chlorophyll and carotene: the two pigments together give a deep, murky, dark green color to the vegetables. Other green and yellow vegetables can fool you into thinking they contain carotene—yams, lettuce, and sweet corn—but these derive their color from other pigments and are poor sources of carotene, along with the "white" plant foods like grains and potatoes, which have none. Recommendations state that a person should eat *dark* green or *deep* orange vegetables and fruits at least every other day. Figure 6–3 shows a sampling of the richest food sources of vitamin A; this chapter's Food Feature discusses the best way to obtain sufficient vitamin A and all of the vitamins.

Studies of typical fast-food meals indicate that these foods are particularly lacking in vitamin A. Recently, however, even fast-food restaurants have been offering salad bars with raw spinach, shredded carrots, and other vitamin A–rich foods as alternatives to the plain burgers, fries, and cola meals of yesterday.

The RDA tables are on the inside front cover.

The amount of vitamin A a person needs is proportional to the body weight. Because it is stored, the vitamin does not need to be eaten every day, although the RDA for vitamin A is stated as a daily amount. Any excess eaten is stored, mostly in the liver, where it is available constantly to the bloodstream, and thereby to the cells of the body. According to the RDA, to be assured of adequacy, the average man needs about 1000 RE daily and the average woman, about 800 RE. According to the more recent tentative recommendations, the RDI, the need is lower (see note, p. 34). Needs increase during pregnancy; children need less.

1 RE = 5 IU vitamin A, on the average. More accurately, when you convert IU of vitamin A from a plant source, divide by 10 to get RE. When you convert IU from an animal source, divide by 3.3 to get RE.

Vitamin A recommendations are expressed in RE as of 1980, but food contents of vitamin A are sometimes still expressed using a different unit, the **IU (international unit)**. Until this discrepancy is corrected in food tables, if you want to compare your vitamin A intakes with recommendations, you have to convert from one to the other. A rule of thumb is that on the average, given foods that contain both retinol (from animal sources) and carotene (from plant sources), 1 RE equals 5 IU. For plant foods alone, 1 RE equals 10 IU; for foods taken from animals (which have already converted the carotene to retinol), 1 RE equals 3.3 IU. Not everything in nutrition is arranged for the consumer's convenience; people working with the amounts of vitamin A in foods have to remember to make sure that they are all expressed in the same units before making comparisons.

Broccoli 220 RE per cup
Sweet potato 2490 RE per potato
Asparagus 150 RE per cup
Carrots 3830 RE per cup
Fortified milk 250 RE per cup
Butternut squash 1435 RE per cup
Cantaloupe 861 RE per ½ melon
Apricots 280 RE per 3 apricots

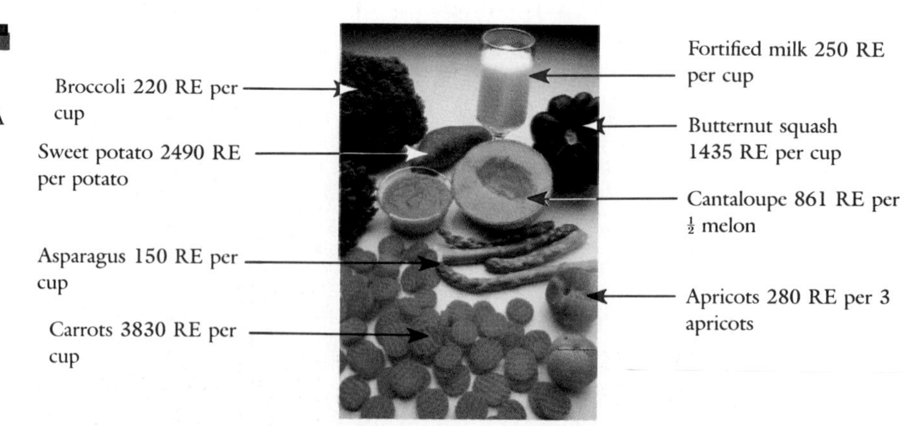

Figure 6–3 A Sampling of Rich Food Sources of Vitamin A.
The U.S. RDA for vitamin A is 1000 RE. A 3-ounce portion of beef liver (not shown) contains 9120 RE. See also this chapter's Food Feature and Appendix A.

Vitamin A is essential to vision, integrity of epithelial tissue, growth of bone, reproduction, and more. Vitamin A deficiency causes blindness, sickness, and death, and is a major problem worldwide. Overdoses are possible and cause a variety of symptoms. Brightly colored foods are richest in vitamin A.

rickets: the vitamin D deficiency disease in children, characterized by abnormal growth of bone, manifested in bowed legs or knock knees, outward-bowed chest, and knobs on the ribs.

Vitamin D

Vitamin D is one member of a large and interacting team of nutrients and hormones that continuously maintains bone. The vitamin's special role is to be sure that sufficient minerals are available in the blood that feeds the growing bone structure. (The major minerals of bone are calcium and phosphorus, and you'll read more about them in Chapter 7.) Vitamin D's role with respect to calcium is especially well known.

Calcium is indispensable to the proper functioning of all the cells of the body, and it arrives at the needed sites via the blood. The skeleton serves as a vast warehouse of stored calcium that can be tapped if the supply from food is low. Calcium to raise the blood level can be drawn from only two other places: from food in the digestive tract and from the kidney, which conserves it by retrieving it from the fluid destined to become urine. Vitamin D acts, when needed, at all three locations to raise the blood calcium level.

The most obvious sign of vitamin D deficiency is abnormality of the bones. The disease **rickets**, caused in children by vitamin D deficiency, has been recognized for several centuries, and it was even known in the 1700s that it could

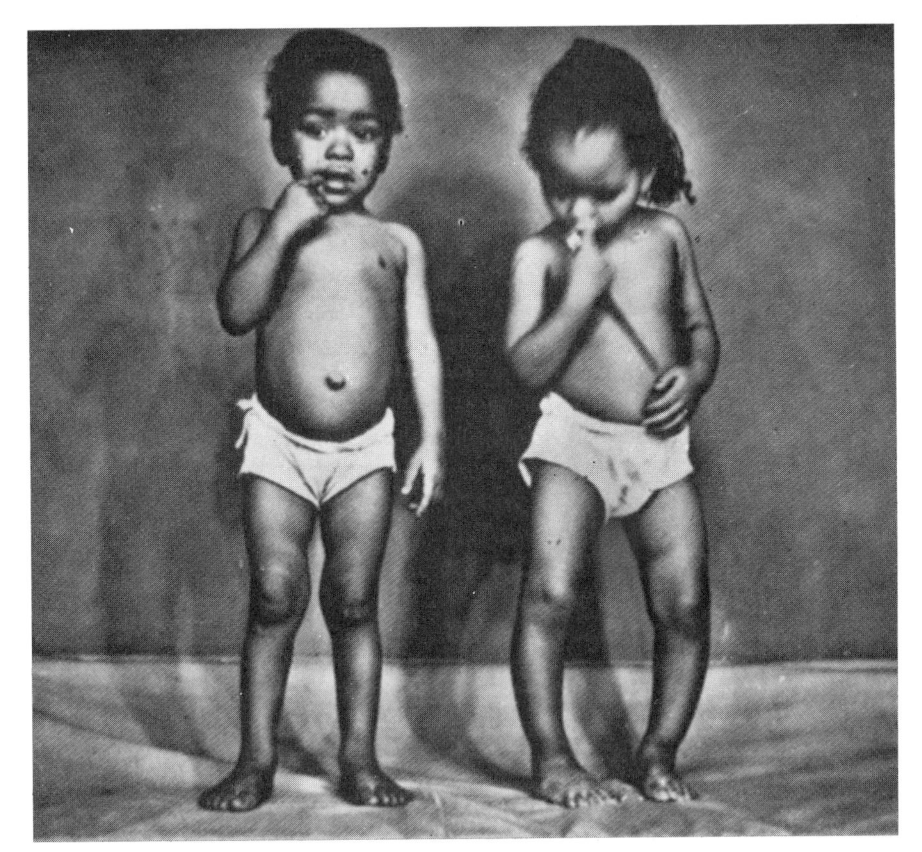

The child on the right has the vitamin D deficiency disease rickets.

osteomalacia (OS-tee-o-mal-AY-shuh): the vitamin D deficiency disease in adults (*osteo* means "bone"; *mal* means "bad"). Symptoms include bending of the spine and bowing of the legs with consequent loss of height.

be cured with cod-liver oil. However, not until the turn of this century was enough known about rickets to reproduce it in laboratory animals. When the condition was linked to the newly discovered vitamin, the tragedy of rickets was greatly reduced. The bowed legs, knock-knees, and pigeon breasts of children with rickets are no longer common sights.

In adults, the comparable deficiency disease is **osteomalacia,** in which calcium is withdrawn from the bones but not picked up efficiently from the intestine or saved by the kidney. The bones lose their minerals and protein understucture, becoming porous, weak, and easy to break. Deafness, too, can result from vitamin D deficiency, because sounds are transmitted to the brain along tiny ear bones, and these bones also degenerate when vitamin D is lacking.[4]

Vitamin D is the most toxic of all vitamins. As little as four to five times the recommended daily intake can create an overdose. Toxicity symptoms include diarrhea, headache, and nausea; if overdoses continue to occur, the vitamin will increase the blood mineral level to dangerous extremes, and there will be calcium deposits in the soft tissues like the heart and other vital organs. If calcium deposits form in the heart's major artery, the aorta, the consequence of overdosing can be death.

The likeliest victims of vitamin D poisoning are infants whose mothers have been misguided to think that if some is good, more is better. People who take supplements containing vitamin D, too, may easily overdose, not realizing that their tissues are building up a stockpile of the vitamin. Physicians don't always recognize the symptoms of vitamin D toxicity and have sometimes performed unnecessary surgery or therapy.[5] The pathological conditions can be reversed by withdrawal of the supplemental vitamin D. To protect people from toxic effects of vitamin D, the law permits its sale as a single supplement only in low doses.

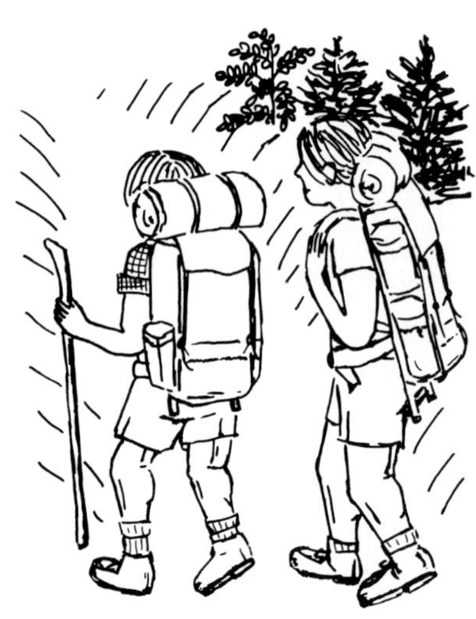
Sunlight promotes vitamin D formation in the skin.

People don't necessarily have to eat vitamin D to have enough in their bodies. They can make it from cholesterol whenever the sun shines on their skin, and they absorb it from there directly into the blood. Dark-skinned people require longer exposure to the sun (about three hours) than light-skinned people do (they need about 30 minutes) to get a full day's supply of vitamin D. The experiments that have revealed these findings also suggest that overexposure to the sun cannot produce a toxic amount of vitamin D, as supplements can, because the skin only allows a certain amount to be made, no matter how long the exposure. (Of course, long exposure to the sun can have some other negative effects, such as sunburn, wrinkling of the skin, and increased risk of skin cancer.) The ultraviolet rays of the sun, the rays that promote vitamin D formation in the skin, are filtered out by clouds, smoke, smog, clothing, window glass, and even window screens.

There was a time when rickets seemed to have been almost completely eliminated from the developed countries, but since the 1970s it has been creeping back, with cases being reported in inner-city children, especially blacks; in children breastfed for an exceptionally long time; and in vegetarian children.[6] The slower vitamin D production in dark-skinned people may account for most of today's cases of rickets. In the United States and Canada, almost all cases show up in dark-skinned people who live in smoggy northern cities. Worldwide, rickets is still a major health problem, especially in those societies that traditionally clothe themselves in concealing garments.

The few significant food sources of vitamin D are fish oils (like cod-liver oil), butter, cream, egg yolks, and liver. In the United States and Canada, milk, whether fluid, dried, or evaporated, is usually fortified with vitamin D, so that a quart or liter will supply the amount recommended for an adult daily. That way, the adult who drinks the recommended 2 cups a day receives half the daily need and has only half to get from other sources. Children who drink 2 cups or more will have a head start towards meeting their vitamin D needs for growth. Milk is not naturally a rich source of vitamin D, because it contains only 4 to 5 percent cream, but it is an ideal vehicle for fortification because it is a major source of calcium. Breakfast cereals may also be fortified with vitamin D, as their labels indicate. The natural food sources of vitamin D, such as milk and butter before fortification, vary with the seasons, with spring and summer contents being significantly higher.

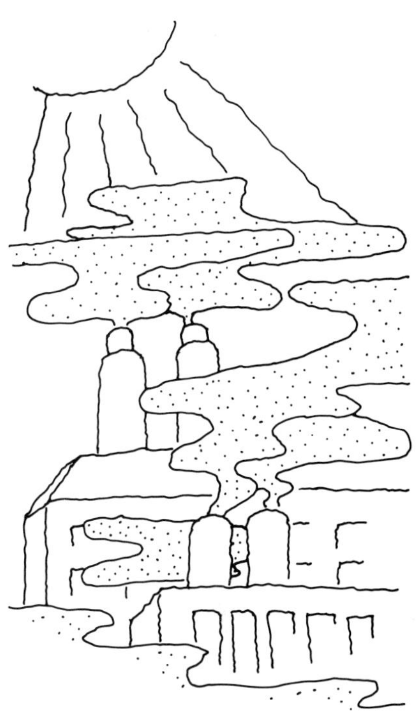

Smog filters out ultraviolet rays of the sun.

Strict vegetarians, if they do not receive sufficient sun exposure, need supplemental vitamin D. Children receive sufficient vitamin D if their parents supply them with vitamin D–fortified milk; otherwise, they are likely to develop rickets. Infants receiving formula receive sufficient vitamin D, because all formula is required by law to meet a standard (see Chapter 11). Infants being fed breast milk may need supplements prescribed by the pediatrician.

The RDA for vitamin D is 5 micrograms per day for adults, and is higher wherever growth is occurring—in pregnancy, lactation, childhood, and adolescence. Contrary to popular belief, people do need vitamin D in adulthood and can suffer from deficiencies, especially if they are housebound or institutionalized, or if they work at night. Prolonged deficiency (for years) of vitamin D in an adult leads to deficiency of calcium severe enough to cause its loss from bones and the deficiency disease osteomalacia. Milk is therefore a good food for adults as well as for children. Daily doses of vitamin D are not necessary, because the body stores surpluses in its fat.

Vitamin D increases the blood level of minerals, notably calcium and phosphorus, permitting bone formation and maintenance. A deficiency in childhood can cause rickets and in later life, osteomalacia. People exposed to the sun make vitamin D from cholesterol; fortified milk is an important food source. Vitamin D is the most toxic of all vitamins, and excesses are dangerous or deadly.

Vitamin E

Vitamin E, because it can be oxidized, is like a bodyguard for other substances; it serves as an antioxidant. By being destroyed itself, vitamin E protects the polyunsaturated fats and other fat-soluble substances such as vitamin A from destruction by oxygen. Vitamin E exerts an especially important antioxidant effect in the lungs, where the cells are exposed to high oxygen concentrations that can destroy their membranes. As the red blood cells carry oxygen from the lungs to other tissues, vitamin E protects their cell membranes, too. Vitamin E also protects the white blood cells that defend the body against disease. Indeed, deficiency of vitamin E suppresses the immune system, and large doses of the vitamin stimulate it in several species of animals. Normal nerve development also depends on vitamin E.

A deficiency of vitamin E produces a wide variety of symptoms in laboratory animals, but most of these symptoms have not been reproduced in human beings, despite many attempts. Two reasons have been given for this. First, the vitamin is so widespread in food that it is almost impossible to create a vitamin E–deficient diet. Second, the body stores so much vitamin E in its fatty tissues

tocopherol (tuh-KOFF-er-all): a kind of alcohol. The active form of vitamin E is *alpha*-tocopherol.

erythrocyte (eh-REETH-ro-sight) **hemolysis** (he-MOLL-ih-sis): rupture of the red blood cells, caused by vitamin E deficiency (*erythro* means "red"; *cyte* means "cell"; *hemo* means "blood"; *lysis* means "breaking").

fibrocystic breast disease: a harmless disease in which the breasts become lumpy and painful, caused sometimes by vitamin E deficiency and sometimes associated with caffeine toxicity (*fibro* means "fibrous tissue"; *cyst* means "closed sac").

intermittent claudication: pain on walking and nighttime cramps in the calves, caused sometimes by vitamin E deficiency (*claudicare* means "to limp").

that a person could not keep on eating a vitamin E–free diet for long enough to deplete these stores and produce a deficiency. It may be, however, that occasional vitamin E deficiencies are seen in people without diseases. People in whom they are most likely are those who, for years, eat diets extremely low in fat, who use fat substitutes such as diet margarines and salad dressings as their only sources of fat, or who consume low-fat diets composed largely of highly processed or "convenience" foods—for vitamin E is destroyed by extensive heating at high temperatures.

A number of disease conditions, however, do cause vitamin E deficiencies—notably, conditions that cause malabsorption of fat. These include disease or injury in the liver (which makes bile, the emulsifier that breaks up fat prior to digestion and absorption), the gallbladder (which stores bile and squirts it into the intestine when needed), and the pancreas (which makes fat-digesting enzymes), as well as a number of hereditary diseases. In children, supplements given in time can prevent damage to the developing nervous system, including the retina of the eye. In adults, vitamin E supplements also prevent neurological disorders caused by vitamin E deficiency due to disease.[7]

Although vitamin E deficiency is rare, many horror stories have been told about vitamin E deficiency diseases in human beings. Extravagant claims have been made that it cures all sorts of things, because it has effects on animals' hearts, muscles, and reproductive systems that it does not have in human beings. While research has revealed possible roles for vitamin E, it has also clearly discredited claims that vitamin E prolongs the life of the heart, improves athletic endurance and skill, enhances sexual performance, or cures sexual dysfunction in males. Some of this research gave vitamin E its name, **tocopherol.** *Tokos* is a Greek word meaning "offspring."

A cruelly false claim has been that vitamin E cures the hereditary and usually fatal disease muscular dystrophy in human children. This claim sprang from the observation that laboratory animals develop symptoms of muscular wasting and weakness when they are fed vitamin E–deficient diets and recover when the vitamin is reintroduced into their diets. However, this malnutrition-induced condition of animals has been scientifically shown to be unrelated to hereditary muscular dystrophy in human beings.

One proven vitamin E deficiency symptom in human beings is found in premature babies, because there is little transfer of the vitamin from the mother to the infant until the very last weeks of pregnancy. Without vitamin E, the red blood cells rupture (**erythrocyte hemolysis**), and the infant becomes anemic. Two other conditions are apparently caused sometimes by vitamin E deficiency in human beings. One is a painful, but nonmalignant disease characterized by lumps in the breasts (**fibrocystic breast disease**). This can also be worsened by caffeine toxicity, so it sometimes responds to vitamin E supplements and sometimes to abstinence from caffeine. The other is a disorder that involves pain on walking and cramps in the calves at night (**intermittent claudication**).

The RDA for vitamin E is based on body size—8 milligrams for women, 10 for men. The need for vitamin E rises as polyunsaturated oil intake rises. Conveniently, vitamin E occurs with most oils in foods, with the exception of cooking oils, which are usually poor vitamin E sources. People who need vitamin E supplements are, as mentioned, people with very low fat intakes, as well as people with diseases impairing fat absorption, which cause vitamin E deficiency.

Cases of vitamin E toxicity are rare. The medical literature contains isolated reports of adverse effects on laboratory animals and of nausea, intestinal distress, and other vague complaints in human beings. However, the impression remains that for most individuals, daily doses below 300 milligrams are harmless.

Most vitamin E is in plant oils, the richest being wheat germ oil. Whole grains, green plants, egg yolk, milk fat, butter, liver, nuts, and seeds are all good sources. Thus all four food groups provide generous amounts of vitamin E, so long as they are represented by whole, rather than highly processed, foods.

Vitamin E acts as an antioxidant in cell membranes, and is especially important for the integrity of cells that are constantly exposed to high levels of oxygen—the lungs and blood cells, both red and white. Vitamin E deficiency is rare in human beings, but it does occur in newborn premature infants. The vitamin is widely distributed among foods; toxicity is rare.

Vitamin K

Vitamin K is the fat-soluble vitamin necessary for the synthesis of at least two proteins involved in blood clotting. It also works with vitamin D in helping to regulate blood calcium levels (calcium is also needed for blood to clot). If blood cannot clot, then wounds may bleed for a dangerously long time; this is the reason why people's blood is drawn to measure clotting time before they go into surgery. Vitamin K is sometimes administered before operations to reduce bleeding in surgery, but is of value at this time only if a vitamin K deficiency has existed.

K stands for the Danish word ***koagulation*** (clotting).

In some heart problems, there is a need to *prevent* the formation of clots within the circulatory system. (This is popularly referred to as "thinning" the blood.) One of the best-known compounds for this purpose is dicumarol, which interferes with the action of vitamin K in permitting clotting. Vitamin K therapy is necessary in people taking dicumarol if hemorrhaging occurs.

Like vitamin D, vitamin K can be obtained from a nonfood source—in this case, the intestinal bactèria. Billions of bacteria normally reside in the intestines, and some of them synthesize vitamin K. People obtain about half of their daily needs from foods and about half through the courtesy of their intestinal inhabitants. Vitamin K is found in dark green leafy vegetables, and there is one rich animal food source—liver.

Newborn infants, whose intestinal tracts are not yet inhabited by bacteria, and people who have taken antibiotics that have killed the intestinal bacteria have vitamin K deficiencies, manifested in a delayed clotting time. Vitamin K supplements are needed in these cases.

Vitamin K is not toxic in the range of amounts commonly consumed from natural sources, but toxicity can result when supplements of a synthetic version of vitamin K are given, especially to infants or to pregnant women.* Toxicity symptoms include breakage of the red blood cells, releasing their pigment into the general circulation; a resultant yellowing of the skin; and brain damage.

---

*A toxic dose of a vitamin K compound such as ***menadione*** causes the liver to release a bile pigment into the blood (***hyperbilirubinemia***), and leads to jaundice of certain areas of the brain (***kernicterus***).

Because amounts of the vitamin contained in supplements can easily reach toxic levels, it is available as a single vitamin only by prescription.

Vitamin K is necessary for blood to clot; deficiency causes uncontrolled bleeding. Excesses are toxic. The bacterial inhabitants of the digestive tract produce vitamin K, and most people derive about half their requirement from them and half from foods.

coenzyme (co-EN-zime): a small molecule that works with an enzyme to promote the enzyme's activity. Many coenzymes have B vitamins as part of their structures (*co* means "with").

The B Vitamins and Their Relatives

The B vitamins and vitamin C are known together as the water-soluble vitamins. Because the B vitamins have much in common, they are treated as a group here; vitamin C has a separate section.

The B vitamins act as part of coenzymes. A **coenzyme** is a small molecule that can combine with an inactive protein to make it an active enzyme. Sometimes the vitamin part of the enzyme is the active site, where the chemical reaction takes place. The substance to be worked on is attracted to the active site and snaps into place, and the reaction proceeds instantaneously. The architecture of each enzyme is designed to accomplish just one kind of job. Without its coenzyme, however, the enzyme is as useless as a padlock without its key. Figure 6–4 shows how a coenzyme enables an enzyme to do its job.

Figure 6–4 Coenzyme Action.

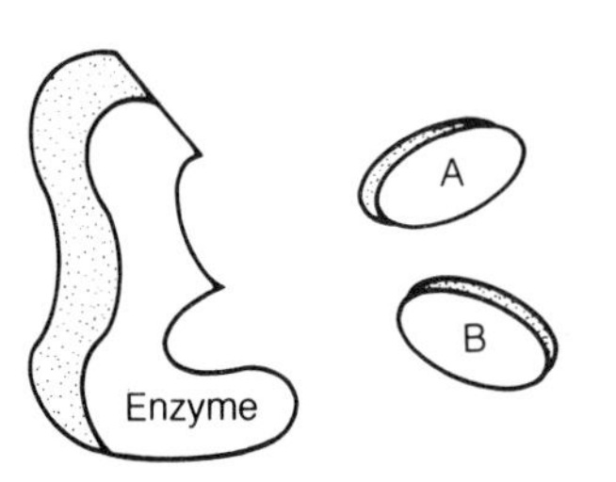

Without the coenzyme, compounds A and B don't respond to the enzyme.

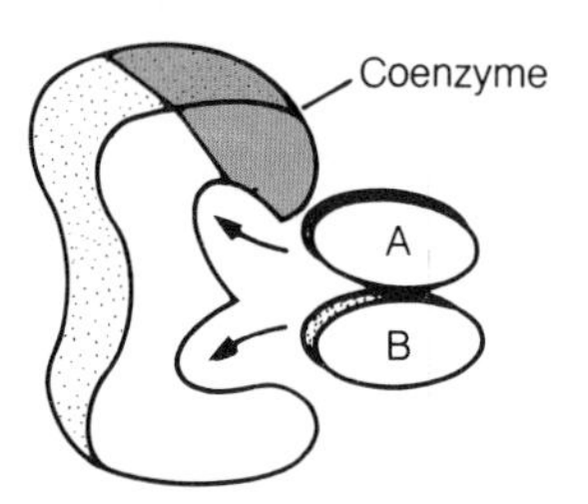

With the coenzyme in place, A and B are attracted to the active site on the enzyme, and they react.

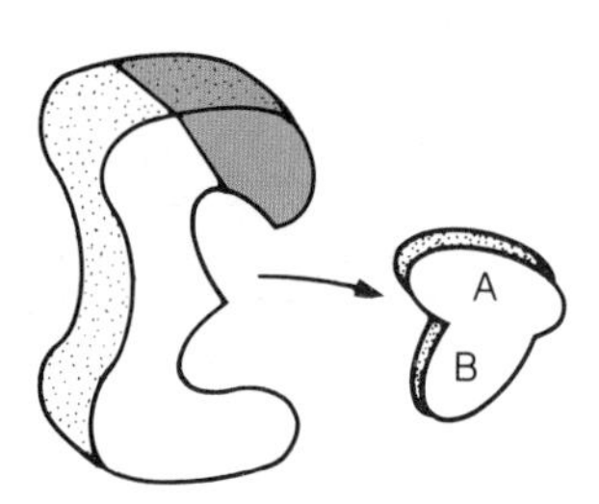

The reaction is completed.

Each B vitamin has its own special character, and the amount of detail known about each one is overwhelming. To simplify this introduction to them, this section describes some of the ways in which the B vitamins work together in the body, and emphasizes the consequences of deficiencies. The Food Feature at the end of this chapter shows how to select foods that will provide adequate amounts of all of the B vitamins.

B Vitamin Roles in Metabolism

Figure 6–5 shows some of the interconversions of carbohydrates, lipids, and amino acids in metabolism. It is not presented to teach many details; that is a subject for whole graduate courses in biochemistry. The purpose of the figure is to give an impression of how intimately involved the B vitamins are in the processes by which the body makes use of the energy nutrients, and also of how interdependent these vitamins are on one another. A few details are presented in the figure legend.

The amounts of B vitamins people need are determined differently for each vitamin. For three of the B vitamins, the amounts needed are proportional to energy expenditure. For vitamin B_6, which is tied closely to amino acid metabolism, the amount is proportional to protein intake. The recommended intakes are summarized in the RDA tables (inside front cover).

The B vitamins facilitate the work of every cell. Some help generate energy, and others help make DNA, RNA, protein, and new cells.

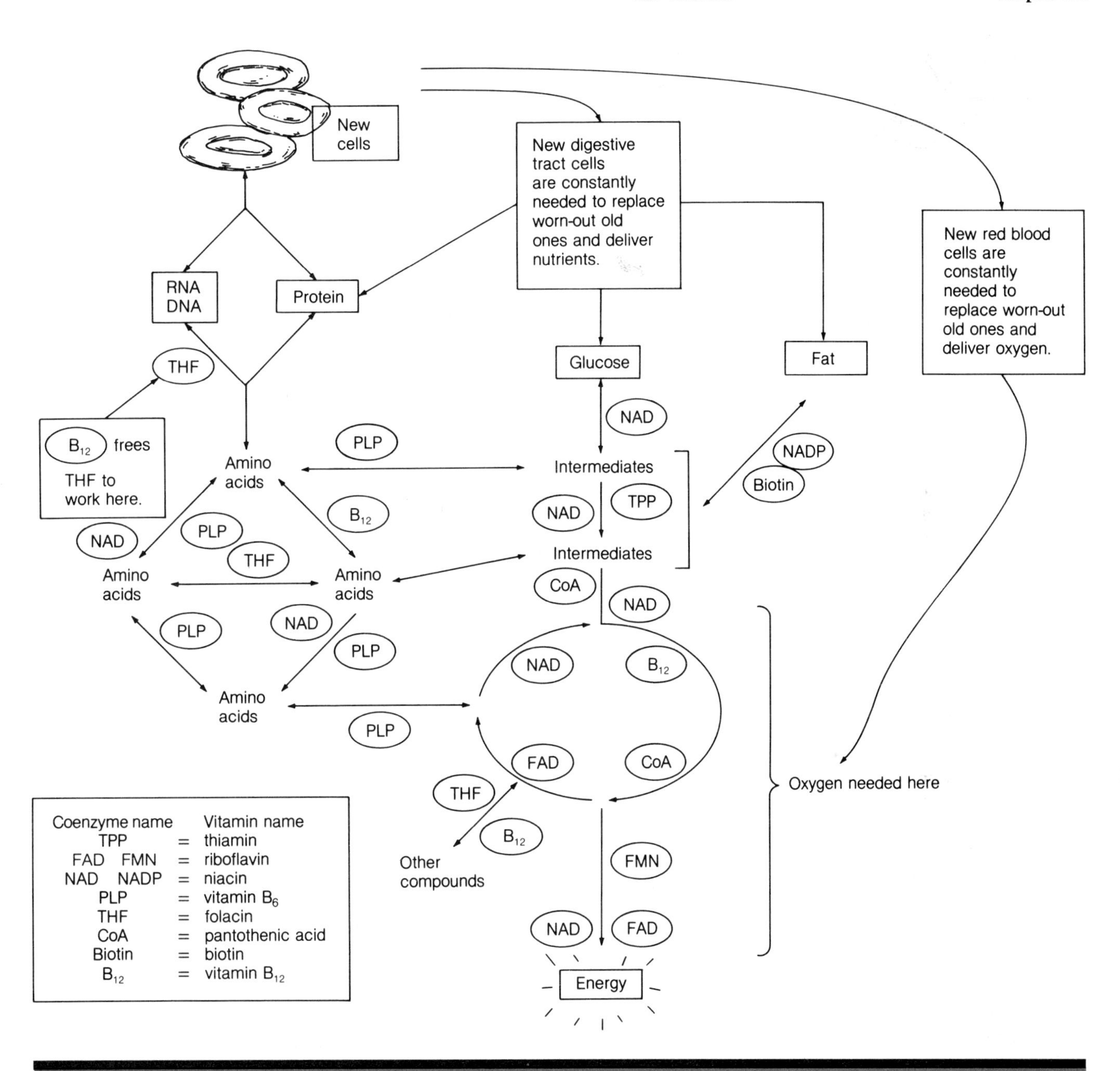

Figure 6–5 The B Vitamins in Metabolism.
The figure shows some starting and ending points of the pathways nutrients take in the body. For example, glucose can yield energy or fat. Protein can yield energy or can be used to build new cells. New cells in the digestive tract are needed to deliver glucose. New blood cells are needed to deliver oxygen, making possible the release of energy from glucose or fat. Each B vitamin is part of one or more coenzymes that make possible the body's chemical work. For example, the niacin coenzymes are necessary for most of the energy pathways. The folacin and vitamin B_{12} coenzymes are necessary for the making of RNA and DNA and thus, new cells. The vitamin B_6 coenzyme is necessary for the making of many amino acids and therefore, of protein. The riboflavin coenzymes are important in the pathways involving oxygen. Inspection of the figure will reveal other relationships.

thiamin (THIGH-uh-min): a B vitamin.

beriberi: the thiamin-deficiency disease, characterized by loss of sensation in the hands and feet, muscular weakness, advancing paralysis, and abnormal heart action that can cause death.

riboflavin (RIBE-o-flay-vin): a B vitamin.

niacin, nicotinic acid, niacinamide, nicotinamide: four names for the same B vitamin. Niacin can be eaten preformed or can be made in the body from tryptophan, one of the amino acids.

B Vitamin Deficiencies and Toxicities

So long as B vitamins are present, their presence is not felt. Only when they are missing does their absence manifest itself in a lack of energy and a multitude of other symptoms, as you can imagine after looking at Figure 6–5. The reactions in the central part of the figure (below glucose), by which energy is released, take place in every cell, and no cell can do its work without energy. Thus in a B vitamin deficiency, every cell is affected. Among the symptoms of B vitamin deficiencies are nausea, severe exhaustion, irritability, depression, forgetfulness, loss of appetite and weight, pain in muscles, impairment of the immune response, loss of control of the limbs, abnormal heart action, severe skin problems, teary or bloodshot eyes, and many more. Because cell renewal depends on energy, protein, and DNA/RNA availability, and because all these depend on the B vitamins, tissues in which the cells' life spans are shortest are readily damaged by B vitamin deficiency. Thus the digestive tract (whose cells replace themselves every three days) and the blood (whose cells live an average of six weeks) are invariably damaged. In children, full recovery may be impossible; in the case of a thiamin deficiency, for example, permanent brain damage can result.

In academic discussions of the vitamins, clearly different deficiency symptoms are given for each one. Actually, such clear-cut symptoms are found only in laboratory animals that have been fed contrived diets that lack just one ingredient. In real life, a deficiency of any one B vitamin seldom shows up by itself, because people don't eat nutrients singly; they eat foods that contain mixtures of nutrients. Still, the deficiency of one B vitamin may appear predominant in a cluster of deficiencies, and often, if it is corrected by giving wholesome food rather than single supplements, the subtler deficiencies will be corrected along with it. Table 6–3 at the end of the chapter summarizes the symptoms of B vitamin deficiencies and toxicities.

The **thiamin** deficiency disease, **beriberi**, was first observed in the Far East, where rice provided about 90 percent of the total calories most people consumed, and therefore was almost their sole source of thiamin. When the custom of polishing rice (removing its brown coat, which contained the thiamin) became widespread, beriberi swept through the population like an epidemic. Most other vitamins can be obtained by taking a helping of this or that (if you choose the right food), but thiamin is so evenly distributed in foods that its removal from such a major staple food effectively removes it from the diet altogether. Scientists wasted years of time and effort hunting for a microbial cause of beriberi before they realized that the cause of beriberi was not something present in the environment, but something absent from it.

Just before the year 1900, an observant physician in a prison in India discovered that beriberi could be cured with proper diet. The physician noticed that the chickens at the prison developed a stiffness and weakness similar to that of the prisoners who had beriberi. The chickens were being fed the rice left on the plates of prisoners. When the rice bran, which had been discarded in the kitchen, was given to the chickens, their paralysis was cured. As might be expected, the doctor met resistance when he tried to feed the rice bran—the "garbage"—to the prisoners. Later, extracts of rice bran were used to prevent infantile beriberi; still later, thiamin was synthesized.

When thiamin is deficient, **riboflavin** may be lacking, too, but the deficiency symptoms may be unseen because those of thiamin deficiency are more severe.

When foods remedy the thiamin deficiency, because they invariably also contain some riboflavin, both deficiencies clear up.

The **niacin**-deficiency disease, **pellagra,** appeared in Europe in the 1700s when corn from the New World came into wide acceptance as a staple food. At about the turn of this century in the United States, pellagra was wreaking havoc throughout the South and Midwest. Hundreds of thousands of pellagra victims were thought to be suffering from a contagious disease, until the dietary deficiencies were pinned down.

Early workers seeking to find the cause of pellagra observed that well-fed people *never* got it. From there, they defined a diet that reliably produced the disease—one of cornmeal, pork fat, and molasses. The disease still occurs in urban slums today where such a poor diet is eaten. Figure 6–6 shows the skin disorder associated with pellagra. For comparison, Figure 6–7 shows a skin disorder associated with vitamin B_6 deficiency—a reminder that any nutrient deficiency affects the skin and all other cells. The skin just happens to be the organ you can see.

The key nutrient that prevents pellagra is niacin—but any protein containing sufficient amounts of the amino acid tryptophan will serve in its place. Tryptophan, which is present in almost all proteins (but is absent from the protein of corn), is converted to niacin in the body. In fact, it is possible to cure pellagra by administering tryptophan alone. Thus a person eating adequate protein will not be deficient in niacin. The amount of niacin in a diet is therefore stated in terms of **niacin equivalents,** a measure that takes available tryptophan into account. Self-Study exercise 1, on p. 215, shows how to estimate niacin equivalents.

The vitamin **folacin** is required for making all new cells. If the RDA is correct, folacin deficiencies are common; the RDI for folacin is somewhat lower (see note, p. 34). In any case, deficiencies may result from an inadequate intake, impaired absorption, increased excretion, or increased metabolic need for the vitamin. Deficiencies cause anemia and abnormal digestive function (the blood cells and digestive tract cells divide most rapidly and so are most vulnerable to deficiency). A significant number of cases of folacin-deficiency anemia occur among the poor, and especially among people with alcoholism, and among pregnant women.

Folacin deficiency is also likely to be caused by the taking of medication. Ten major groups of drugs have been shown to interfere with the body's use of folacin, including aspirin and its relatives, anticonvulsants, and oral contraceptives.[8]

Folacin needs the help of **vitamin B_{12}** to manufacture red blood cells. Vitamin B_{12} also maintains the sheaths that surround and protect nerve fibers. One of the most obvious symptoms of a vitamin B_{12} deficiency is the anemia of folacin deficiency, because without vitamin B_{12}, folacin cannot get to its sites of action. Giving extra folacin will clear up this blood condition. The trouble is, though, that the deficiency of vitamin B_{12} can continue undetected, causing a creeping paralysis of the nerves and muscles, which begins at the extremities and works inward and up the spine. The name **pernicious anemia** comes from the hidden, sneaky, and frightening way in which vitamin B_{12} deficiency damages nerves, even after the blood symptom has normalized.

A deficiency of vitamin B_{12} must be detected early by the presence of very large, immature red blood cells in order to prevent the severe nerve damage that otherwise will develop. The vegetarian's high intake of folacin helps the red blood cells to develop (despite the lack of vitamin B_{12}) to normal size and

pellagra (pell-AY-gra): the niacin-deficiency disease (*pellis* means "skin"; *agra* means "seizure"). Symptoms include the "4 D's"—diarrhea, dermatitis, dementia, and ultimately, death.

niacin equivalents: the amount of niacin present in food, including the niacin that can theoretically be made from its precursor tryptophan present in the food.

folacin (FOLL-uh-sin), or **folic acid**: a B vitamin that acts as part of a coenzyme important in the manufacture of new cells.

vitamin B_{12}: a B vitamin that enables folacin to get into cells and also helps maintain the sheath around nerve cells.

pernicious (per-NISH-us) **anemia:** the vitamin B_{12} deficiency disease, characterized by large, immature red blood cells, and damage to the nervous system undetectable by blood test.

Figure 6–6 Pellagra.
The typical dermatitis of pellagra develops on skin that is exposed to light.

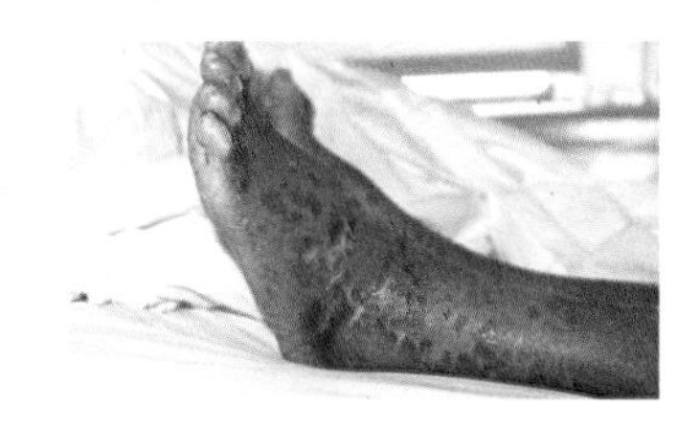

Figure 6–7 Vitamin B_6 Deficiency.
In this dermatitis, the skin is greasy and flaky, unlike the dermatitis of pellagra.

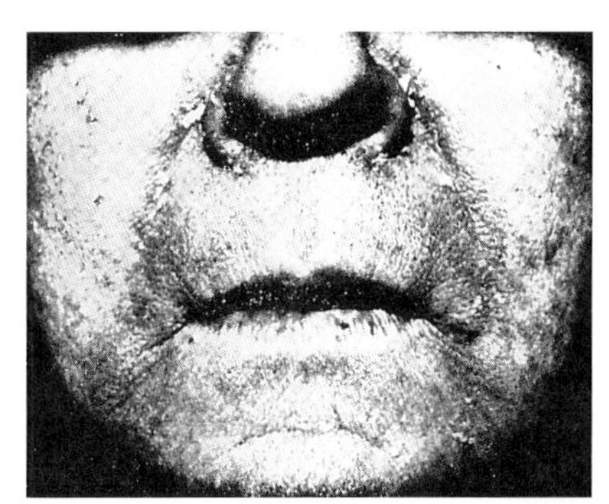

intrinsic factor: a factor found inside a system. The intrinsic factor necessary to prevent pernicious anemia is now known to be a compound made in the stomach that helps in the absorption of vitamin B_{12}.

maturity. This deceives the physician who examines a blood sample for signs of abnormality. However, the folacin can do nothing toward repairing the nerve damage caused by vitamin B_{12} deficiency, so this damage proceeds unchecked. Because of the danger of masking a lack of vitamin B_{12}, the amount of folacin in over-the-counter vitamin preparations is limited by law.[9]

Vitamin B_{12} deficiency takes a long time to develop after a person gives up animal foods, because up to five years' worth can be stored in the body, but when it does occur, it can irreversibly damage the brain and nerves. A pregnant or lactating woman who is eating a vegan diet should be aware that her infant can develop a vitamin B_{12} deficiency, even if the mother remains healthy. A deficiency of this vitamin can cause irreversible nervous system damage in the infant; all vegan mothers must be sure to use B_{12}–fortified products, or take the appropriate supplements.

The absorption of vitamin B_{12} requires an **intrinsic factor**—a compound made inside the body. The design for this factor is carried in the genes. The intrinsic factor is synthesized in the stomach, where it attaches to the vitamin; the complex then passes to the small intestine and is absorbed into the bloodstream.

A few people have in their genetic makeup a gene for the intrinsic factor that becomes defective, usually in midlife. Without the intrinsic factor, they can't absorb vitamin B_{12} even though they are taking enough in their diets, and so they develop deficiency symptoms. In such a case vitamin B_{12} must be supplied by injection to bypass the defective digestive system. The same problem arises when the stomach has been injured or partially removed by surgery and cannot produce enough of the intrinsic factor.

The tendency of a high intake of folacin to mask the anemia caused by vitamin B_{12} deficiency exposes the uninformed strict vegetarian to a special risk. Strict vegetarians are most apt to be deficient in vitamin B_{12}, because it is obtainable only from animal products. In addition, they are most likely to be well supplied with folacin, because, as its name—related to *foliage*—implies, folacin is abundant in vegetables and fruits. The amount of vitamin B_{12} that can be stored in the body is 1000 times the amount used each day, so it may take years to develop a deficiency in a new vegetarian, but when it does occur, it may be masked by a high folacin intake. Sometimes the nervous system damage of pernicious anemia is first seen in the breast-fed infant of the vegan mother. The Food Feature discusses vitamin B_{12} sources for the vegetarian.

The way folacin masks the anemia of vitamin B_{12} deficiency underlines a point already made several times. It takes a skilled professional to make a correct diagnosis, and the risk you take when you diagnose yourself or listen to would-be experts is clearly serious. A second point should also be underlined here. Since vitamin B_{12} deficiency in the body may be caused either by a lack of the vitamin in the diet or by a lack of intrinsic factor necessary to absorb it, a change in diet alone may not correct it—another reason for professional diagnosis of physical symptoms.

The history of the discovery of vitamin B_{12} makes an intriguing story. In the 1920s, researchers discovered that genetic pernicious anemia could be controlled but not cured by eating large amounts of calf liver. (Researchers concluded that liver contained a factor—the "extrinsic factor"—needed to prevent the disease, and later they identified the factor as vitamin B_{12}.) The concentration of vitamin B_{12} in liver was so great that people who ate liver absorbed some of the vitamin even without the help of the intrinsic factor. At one time people who suffered from pernicious anemia had no choice but to eat about a pound of liver a day, but now they can be cured by the injection of a few micrograms of the purified vitamin every three weeks.

Most of the B vitamins are toxic in excess. A particularly notable example—that of **vitamin B_6**—is described in the accompanying box, "Vitamin B_6 Supplements." Others are in the summary tables at the end of the chapter, and safe doses are listed in Controversy 6.

Two other B vitamins, **biotin** and **pantothenic acid**, are important in metabolism, and rare diseases may precipitate deficiencies. However, both vitamins are widespread in foods, and healthy people eating ordinary diets are not at risk for deficiencies.

vitamin B_6: a B vitamin. Its three active forms are *pyridoxine, pyridoxal, and pyridoxamine.*

biotin (BY-o-tin): a B vitamin; a coenzyme necessary for fat synthesis and other metabolic reactions.

pantothenic (PAN-to-THEN-ic) **acid:** a B vitamin.

inositol (in-OSS-ih-tall): a nonessential nutrient.

lipoic (lip-OH-ic) **acid:** a nonessential nutrient.

choline (KOH-leen): a nonessential nutrient.

acetylcholine (ASS-uh-teel-KOH-leen): a transmitter of nerve-to-nerve messages within the brain; a substance that can be made from dietary choline.

Historically famous vitamin B deficiency diseases are beriberi (thiamin), pellagra (niacin), and pernicious anemia (vitamin B_{12}), but folacin-deficiency anemia is probably the most common. Pellagra can be prevented by adequate protein, because the amino acid tryptophan can be converted to niacin in the body. A high intake of folacin can mask the blood symptom of pernicious anemia but will not prevent the associated nerve damage.

Non-B Vitamins

The section on the B vitamins has left a few compounds unrecognized that are sometimes *called* B vitamins. These are **inositol, lipoic acid,** and **choline**. These are not essential nutrients for human beings, although deficiencies can be induced in laboratory animals for experimental purposes. Like the B vitamins described above, they serve as coenzymes in metabolism. Even if they were essential in human nutrition, supplements would be unnecessary, because they are abundant in foods. Choline has an interesting role with respect to a special kind of memory defect in the elderly, however, that is worth a moment of attention.

The nerves that are responsible for the storage and retrieval of information in the brain rely on chemicals to transmit their signals. One of these transmitter chemicals is **acetylcholine,** which is made from choline. Normally, the brain has to make all such substances for itself, because it is shielded from the rest of the body by a protective barrier that won't allow changed concentrations of chemicals in the blood to affect the brain. There are only a few exceptions: among them, a few drugs such as alcohol, narcotics, and choline. High doses of choline given to animals raise the blood concentration, and this raises the brain concentration higher than normal—and the brain synthesizes more acetylcholine as a result. Other neurotransmitters that respond this way to diet are described in Controversy 13.

Some elderly people develop Alzheimer's disease, a progressive impairment of memory that can lead over several years' time to total incapacity to care for themselves. Some work suggests that the progress of this disease may be slowed or halted by large doses of choline. The researchers working with it emphasize that this is not a deficiency disease but that they are simply taking advantage of a curiosity of the brain to treat nonnutritional diseases. Poor memory from poor circulation, brain damage, social isolation, or other causes would not be helped by choline.

Another specific use of choline is for clients with mental disorders who have been treated for a long time with the major psychoactive drugs. In reaction to the drugs they develop bizarre movements of the facial muscles, and this side

Chinese restaurant syndrome: an intolerance reaction that may occur in one out of several hundred people, 20 minutes after the ingestion of the additive MSG (monosodium glutamate, or Accent). Symptoms include burning sensations, chest and facial flushing and pain, and throbbing headache.

carpal tunnel syndrome: tingling and numbness in part of the hand and wrist and shooting pains up the arm caused by swelling of tissue surrounding a nerve that passes through the wrist bones. Possible causes include fluid accumulation and hormone imbalances as well as vitamin B_6 deficiency. A *syndrome* is a cluster of symptoms.

Vitamin B_6 Supplements

Juanita gets sick in Chinese restaurants; Joann has pain in her left hand. Harriet is taking oral contraceptives, and James has had a heart attack and fears another. George has sores in his mouth, Angela is becoming senile, and Margie feels miserable before her menstrual period. What do all these people have in common? All are taking 1 g/day of vitamin B_6 supplements. Some of them are getting better, and some are beginning to get sicker than they were to begin with because they are beginning to suffer the toxic effects of an overdose.

Chinese restaurant syndrome is a sensitivity to the flavor enhancer monosodium glutamate (MSG) used in Asian cookery; Chapter 10 discusses it in detail. The symptoms are warmth, stiffness, weakness, and tingling in the limbs; chest and facial flushing; headaches; light-headedness; and stomachaches or sensations like heartburn. In 1981, a group of researchers, speculating that Chinese restaurant syndrome might be a manifestation of borderline vitamin B_6 deficiency, sought out 27 students who didn't take vitamin supplements and who, by a clinical test, were in poor vitamin B_6 status. They tested the students to see if they were sensitive to MSG; of the 27, 12 were and 15 were not. They then tested the 12 students further: they gave vitamin B_6 (50-mg doses each day for three months) to nine of them and an inert placebo (see p. 202) to the other three without telling them which was which. At the end of that time, eight of the nine who had received the vitamin were no longer sensitive to MSG, while all three of the untreated subjects still reacted adversely to it.

People have thought this indicated that Chinese restaurant syndrome was caused by vitamin B_6 deficiency, and it seems possible that some cases are, but the experimental design shows clearly that some also are not. The people in this experiment were selected *because* they were deficient in vitamin B_6. It showed that eight out of nine people with vitamin B_6 deficiencies who suffer from Chinese restaurant syndrome experience relief when their deficiencies are remedied. The one subject whose reaction didn't change proves that there are people with the syndrome who are nonresponders to B_6. Even after her vitamin B_6 status became entirely normal, she wasn't cured. The dose the researchers used was 50 mg a day, showing that when a deficiency does occur, this amount will relieve it. Juanita should not be taking a gram a day of vitamin B_6—that's 1000 mg, 20 times more than the therapeutic dose, and it isn't even clear that she has a deficiency. Any responsible clinician would test her directly, to see.

In **carpal tunnel syndrome,** a tendon in the wrist tightens on the nerves of the hand, causing excruciating pain. Often, a health care provider will consider surgery to relieve it. However, in 1978, a case was reported in which a 40-year-old man with carpal tunnel syndrome gained relief by taking supplements of 100 mg/day of vitamin B_6 for 10 to 11 weeks. At the same time, an enzyme in his red blood cells that was dependent on vitamin B_6 as a coenzyme went from abnormal to normal in its action. When he was given a placebo for nine weeks, both his physical state and the enzyme activity deteriorated; when he was given the real vitamin again, both were restored to normal. The man seemed to have been eating a vitamin B_6–deficient diet for ten years or more, and RDA levels of vitamin B_6 (2 mg a day) were not enough to correct his deficiency.

The researchers who reported this case also reviewed evidence that other people with carpal tunnel syndrome may have vitamin B_6 deficiencies. Anyone reading their report, which was published in a reputable journal, would be inclined to test any client with carpal tunnel syndrome for a possible vitamin B_6 deficiency.

However, there can be other causes of carpal tunnel syndrome not related to vitamin B_6 deficiency. Joann should not blindly self-prescribe the vitamin without first receiving a diagnosis.

The basis for Harriet's taking vitamin B_6 supplements is the belief that oral contraceptive users need more than the RDA. Perhaps some women have an exceptional reaction of this kind to the Pill. The hormones in oral contraceptives affect the way the body handles tryptophan (an amino acid) so that substances appear in the urine that would normally be metabolized in the body. Vitamin B_6 assists in the metabolism of tryptophan, and when women on the Pill take added vitamin B_6, the abnormality largely disappears (5 mg of vitamin B_6 is all that is needed). This suggests, but does not prove, that women on the Pill have a vitamin B_6 requirement greater than the RDA of 2 mg/day, although not greater than 5 mg. Larger doses might bring about undesirable alterations in amino acid metabolism and might even interfere with the effectiveness of the Pill's hormones. (The vitamin, in megadose amounts, interferes with the action of this class of hormones generally.) Like the other enthusiasts in this story, Harriet hasn't been tested to see if she has the abnormality that indicates a B_6 need, and she is way out on a limb in taking 1000, rather than 5, milligrams a day.

With respect to heart disease, vitamin B_6 deficiencies have been observed to cause injuries in the arteries of monkeys, dogs, rats, and rabbits. High doses of the vitamin (perhaps 40 mg/day) may modify a protein that affects platelet aggregation so that blood clots are less likely to form. The tests showing this effect were performed on blood samples in test tubes, however, not in human beings, and experiments will have to address many more research questions before they can assess the safety or effectiveness of vitamin B_6 supplements to prevent clotting or determine the appropriate dose. James needs a test to see if his vitamin B_6 status is normal. Only if he had blood enzyme levels consistent with a deficiency would he be justified in taking supplements—and then not megadoses, just therapeutic doses.

Oral lesions can also be a manifestation of vitamin B_6 deficiency. However, practically every vitamin and mineral deficiency and many other conditions also cause oral lesions of one kind or another. Their presence indicates George's need for a diagnosis, not a need for vitamin B_6.

Should people who are getting older take vitamin B_6 supplements to help ward off senility? Vitamin B_6 deficiency has been shown to cause alterations in the brain cells of rats suggesting premature aging of the brain, and it is known that older people in general have an increased likelihood of vitamin B_6 deficiency. But to demonstrate degenerative brain changes in animals, the researchers had to deprive them almost totally of

(continued on following page)

the vitamin; total absence of the vitamin is *not* seen in human populations and is surely not the case for Angela. (On the other hand, people live much longer than rats, so time is available for the effects of slight vitamin deficiency to accumulate.) Angela should certainly be checked for vitamin B_6 deficiency—but then, if she is concerned about the signs that she is aging prematurely, her entire nutrition profile should be studied, and she should also go through a standard diagnostic workup, including questions about chest infections, urinary tract infections, depression, use of medications, alcohol use, and other possibilities.

What about vitamin B_6 and PMS (premenstrual syndrome)? No one, as of this writing, knows what causes PMS. Vitamin B_6 seems related to it somehow, but many other nutrients are, too. Because PMS is a topic of great current interest, the chapter on teen nutrition (Chapter 12) devotes a section to it.

This narrative illustrates the point that people are unwise to dose themselves with supplements of vitamin B_6 (or, by implication, any other nutrient) without a competent diagnosis and sound professional advice. The point should be reinforced by a word about the consequences. The first major report of toxic effects of vitamin B_6 appeared in 1983. The doctors told the stories of seven different individuals who had been taking more than 2 g/day of vitamin B_6 for two months or more, most of them attempting to cure the edema of PMS. Three had simply self-prescribed it; two were following their gynecologists' advice; one had a prescription from an "orthomolecular psychiatrist"; and one was taking it after reading about it in a health magazine. All seven cases were similar with only minor variations. They started with numb feet, then lost sensation in their hands, then became unable to work. Later, in some cases, their mouths became numb. In all but two cases they had started with much lower doses, found they didn't work, and progressed to higher and higher doses seeking an effect. They may have suffered irreversible nerve damage. At the last report, although their symptoms had been clearing up after withdrawal of the supplements, they hadn't completely disappeared.

Since then, 16 more cases have been reported in which doses as low as 200 mg, taken for a long time, caused "pins and needles," numbness of the hands, difficulty walking, and other symptoms. When clients stopped taking the vitamin, they reported improvement, but not complete disappearance, of their symptoms. Then followed a report on 58 women who were taking 50 to 300 mg/day of vitamin B_6. In these women, other symptoms—in fact, those normally associated with PMS—improved or disappeared on *stopping* taking the vitamin: depression, headaches, tiredness, bloatedness, irritability, and nerve malfunction. The evidence seems to be mounting that high doses of this vitamin are ill-advised.

Vitamin B_6 is only one of many nutrients that work together, and there are some roles it can't play. It can cure its own deficiency symptoms, and possibly, in high doses, it can act as a drug, but it can't work miracles. Deficiencies of vitamin B_6 do exist in our population, but if you or anyone you know suspects a vitamin B_6 deficiency, consult an R.D. and an M.D. The R.D., if he is worth his salt, will check your diet history. The M.D., assuming she is enlightened, will check for clinical signs of vitamin B_6 deficiency. And both should review your medical and drug history for interactions of diseases and medications with the vitamin. If they have reason to believe you have a vitamin B_6 deficiency, *and once they have excluded other diagnoses,* they will recommend a therapeutic dose supplement for a finite period of time—probably 50 to 200 mg for not more than six to ten weeks. Meanwhile, they will counsel you on improving your diet so that supplementation will not continue to be necessary, and they will advise you to come back for follow-up and further diagnostic work if B_6 replacement proves ineffective.

Sources: Possible vitamin B_6 deficiency uncovered in persons with the "Chinese restaurant syndrome," *Nutrition Reviews* 40 (1982): 15–16; K. Folkers, Biochemical evidence for a deficiency of vitamin B_6 in the carpal tunnel syndrome based on a crossover clinical study, *Proceedings of the National Academy of Sciences USA* 75 (1978): 3410–3412; The vitamin B_6 requirement in oral contraceptive users, *Nutrition Reviews* 37 (1979): 344–345; Does pyridoxal phosphate have a non-coenzymatic role in steroid hormone action? *Nutrition Reviews* 38 (1980): 93–95; Inhibition of platelet aggregation and clotting by pyridoxal-5′-phosphate, *Nutrition Reviews* 40 (1982): 55–57; S. Bapurao, L. Raman, and P. G. Tulpule, Biochemical assessment of vitamin B_6 nutritional status in pregnant women with orolingual manifestations, *American Journal of Clinical Nutrition* 36 (1982): 581–586; E. J. Root and J. B. Longenecker, Brain cell alterations suggesting premature aging induced by dietary deficiency of vitamin B_6 and/or copper, *American Journal of Clinical Nutrition* 37 (1983): 540–552; S. C. Vir and A. H. G. Love, Vitamin B_6 status of the hospitalized aged, *American Journal of Clinical Nutrition* 31 (1978): 1383–1391; H. Schaumberg and coauthors, Sensory neuropathy from pyridoxine abuse, *New England Journal of Medicine* 309 (1983): 445–448; More B_6 toxicity reported, *Nutrition Forum,* November 1985, p. 84; K. Dalton, Pyridoxine overdose in premenstrual syndrome, *Lancet,* 18 May 1985, pp. 1168–1169.

effect seems to be countered by choline. Both of these uses of choline are instances of nonnutrition therapies developed out of the discovery that large doses of a normal substance may sometimes have unexpected, beneficial druglike effects. It is still too early to say, however, whether these treatments may also incur some risk.

In addition to choline, inositol, and lipoic acid, other substances have been mistaken for essential nutrients for people because they are needed for growth by bacteria or other life forms. These substances include PABA (para-aminobenzoic acid), bioflavonoids ("vitamin P" or hesperidin), and ubiquinone. Other names you may hear are "vitamin B_{15}" or pangamic acid (a hoax), "vitamin B_{17}" (laetrile or amygdalin, not a cancer cure and not a vitamin by any stretch of the imagination), "vitamin B_T" (carnitine, an important piece of cell machinery, but not a vitamin), and more.

Many substances people claim are B vitamins are not, although some may have nonnutrient effects or be useful as drugs. Among them are inositol, lipoic acid, and choline.

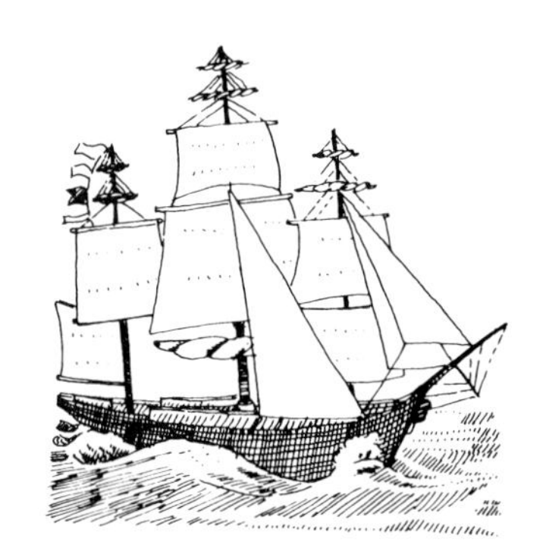

Vitamin C

Two hundred-odd years ago, any man who joined the crew of a seagoing ship knew he had only half a chance of returning alive—not because he might be slain by pirates or die in a storm, but because he might contract the dread disease

Long voyages without fresh fruits and vegetables spelled death by scurvy for the crew.

scurvy: the vitamin C deficiency disease.

ascorbic acid: one of the active forms of vitamin C (the other is dehydroascorbic acid). Many people consistently and incorrectly refer to all vitamin C by the name *ascorbic acid.*

collagen (COLL-a-jen): the chief protein of most connective tissues, including scars, ligaments, and tendons, and the underlying matrix on which bones and teeth are built.

placebos (plah-SEE-bows): inert, harmless substances that resemble medicine, used in research to distinguish the effects of faith and hope from the effects of the medicine.

placebo effect: the healing effect that faith in medicine, even inert medicine, often has.

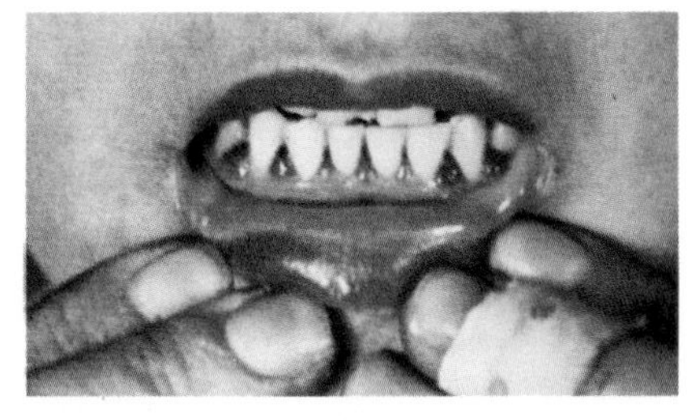

Scurvy. Vitamin C deficiency causes breakdown of collagen, which supports the teeth.

scurvy. As many as two-thirds of a ship's men might die of scurvy on a long voyage. Only ships that sailed on short voyages, especially around the Mediterranean Sea, were safe from this disease. It was not known at the time that the special hazard of long ocean voyages was that the ship's cook used up his fresh fruits and vegetables early and relied for the duration of the voyage on cereals and live animals.

The first nutrition experiment to be conducted on human beings was devised nearly 250 years ago to find a cure for scurvy. A British physician divided some sailors with scurvy into groups. Each group received a different test substance: vinegar, sulfuric acid, seawater, oranges, or lemons. The ones receiving the citrus fruits were cured within a short time. Sadly, it was 50 years before the British Navy made use of the information and required all its vessels to provide lime juice to every sailor daily. The term *limey* was applied to the British sailors in mockery because of this requirement. The name later given the vitamin, **ascorbic acid**, literally means "no scurvy."

Vitamin C is required for the production and maintenance of **collagen,** a protein substance that forms the base for all connective tissues in the body—bones, teeth, skin, and tendons. Collagen forms the scar tissue that heals wounds, the reinforcing structure that mends fractures, and the supporting material of capillaries that prevents bruises. Besides helping to produce and maintain collagen, vitamin C protects against infections and promotes the absorption of iron.

Many substances found in foods and important in the body can be destroyed by oxidation. Remember the role of vitamin E in protecting fat-soluble substances. Vitamin C works in much the same way with water-soluble substances, protecting them from oxidation by being oxidized itself instead. The vitamin is also important to the production of thyroxine, the hormone that regulates basal metabolic rate and body temperature.

In times of stress, the supply of vitamin C is depleted because it is involved in the release of the stress hormones from the adrenal gland. Vitamin makers have used this fact to sell supplements that are largely vitamin C with B vitamins added. In truth, the amount of extra vitamin C used up during stress is so small that it is well within the safety margin of the RDA. If you are under stress (and who isn't?), generous servings of vitamin C–rich fruits and vegetables will more than cover your needs.

Most of the symptoms of scurvy can be attributed to the breakdown of collagen in the absence of vitamin C: loss of appetite, growth cessation, tenderness to touch, weakness, bleeding gums, loose teeth, swollen ankles and wrists, and tiny hemorrhages in the skin. One symptom, anemia, reflects an important role that vitamin C plays in helping the body to absorb and use iron (see Chapter 7).

In the United States, scurvy is seldom seen today except in infants. Breast milk supplies enough vitamin C, but the formula-fed infant must receive vitamin C in formula or from an outside source early. Fruit juices fortified with vitamin C may be used for this purpose at first. By six months of age, a baby should be guaranteed enough vitamin C by also having some fruits and vegetables in the diet. ·

Researchers find evidence of subclinical vitamin C deficiency in some groups of people, particularly male teenagers and elderly men who do not eat fruits, vegetables, or salads. Smoking cigarettes seems to interfere with the use of vitamin C, but people's intakes are usually high enough to cover this extra need. Taking extra vitamin C does not protect against the damage caused by smoking.

The RDA for vitamin C is 60 milligrams per day for adults, with an extra 20 to 40 milligrams recommended for pregnant and lactating women; the RDI is somewhat lower (see note, p. 34). These amounts are midway between two extremes. At one extreme is the requirement, 10 milligrams per day, which is all you need to prevent the symptoms of scurvy from appearing. At the other extreme is the amount at which the body's pool of vitamin C is full to overflowing: about 100 milligrams per day. Other authorities have set different standards; for example, Canada recommends 30 milligrams per day and Germany, 75. The differences between these recommendations may seem large, but when you consider that vitamin C intakes from foods can easily vary from below 10 to over 1000 milligrams (1 gram) a day, you can see that the official recommendations are all within the same rather narrow range.

An advocate of the taking of large doses of vitamin C is Dr. Linus Pauling, whose first popular book, *Vitamin C and the Common Cold,* came out in 1970. According to Pauling, much larger quantities than the RDA are necessary to enable the vitamin to perform functions other than preventing scurvy, like protecting cells from attack by cold viruses. Pauling advocates taking 1 or 2 grams (1000 to 2000 milligrams) of vitamin C per day, about 20 to 40 times the RDA.

Many controlled, double-blind studies on vitamin C and colds have been performed since Pauling's controversial book first came out. Taken together, they show that the effects of vitamin C, if any, are statistically very small. This does not exclude the possibility that the effects on a few individuals might be considerable, especially if their vitamin C intake has been low. Research of this kind is difficult to perform, because people tend to be influenced by what they expect from their medicine. In one, now classic, study, a questionnaire given at the end revealed that the subjects who received **placebos** who thought they were receiving vitamin C had fewer colds than the group receiving vitamin C who thought they were receiving placebos.[10] The **placebo effect** can sometimes be more important to cure than any medicine.

Pauling and others have also suggested that vitamin C megadoses might be effective against cancer, but careful research using 10-gram-per-day doses of the vitamin on people with advanced cancer has shown no difference in either symptoms or survival time. The notion that vitamin C may cure cancer thus seems to be a false hope. However, no one questions the need for adequate amounts of vitamin C to defend the body against the onset of cancer.

The widespread use of megadoses of vitamin C has enabled researchers to study their toxic effects. Some effects are theoretically possible, but have not been seen with intakes as high as 3 grams a day. Among unconfirmed effects are formation of stones in the kidneys, upset of the acid-base balance, destruction of vitamin B_{12} resulting in a deficiency, and interference with the action of vitamin E.

Other toxic effects, however, have been seen often enough to warrant concern. Nausea, abdominal cramps, and diarrhea are often reported. Several instances of interference with medical regimens are known. The large amounts of vitamin C excreted in the urine can obscure the results of tests used to detect diabetes, giving a false-positive result in some instances and a false-negative result in others. People taking medications to prevent blood clotting may unwittingly abolish their effect if they also take massive doses of vitamin C.

People of certain racial groups are more likely to be harmed by vitamin C megadoses than others. Some black Americans, Sephardic Jews, Asians, and members of other groups have an inherited enzyme deficiency that makes them susceptible to high doses of vitamin C, which can make their red blood cells

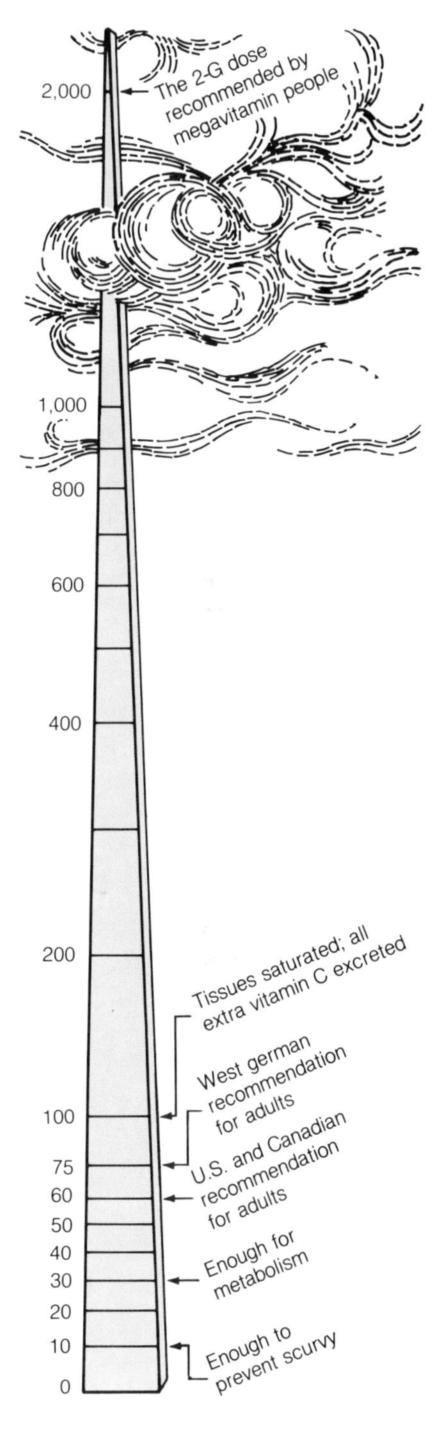

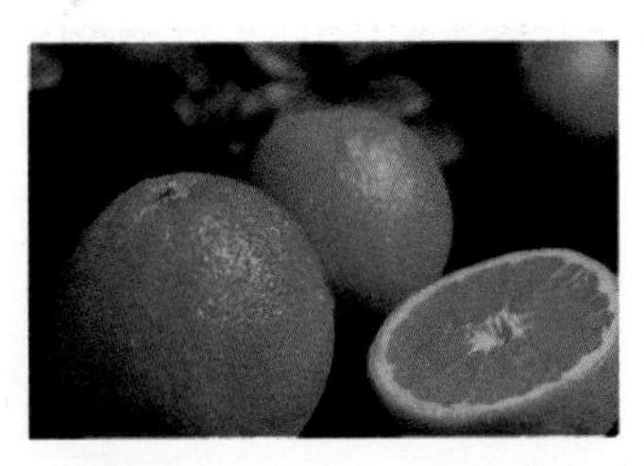

When nutritionists say "vitamin C," people think "oranges" . . .

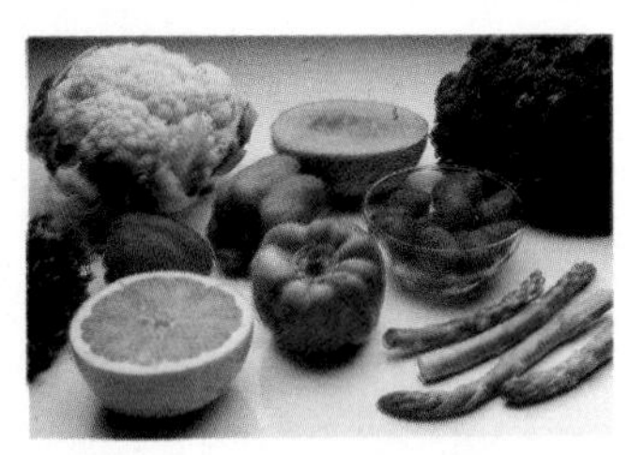

But these foods are actually richer in vitamin C for their calorie cost.

burst, causing hemolytic anemia. Those with sickle-cell anemia may also be more vulnerable to megadoses of vitamin C. In sickle-cell anemia, the hemoglobin protein is abnormal; it responds to a reducing agent by assuming a shape that distorts the red blood cells (see p. 148), making them clump and clog capillaries. Those who have a tendency toward gout and those who have a genetic abnormality that alters the way they break down vitamin C to its excretion products are more prone to forming stones if they take megadoses.

The published research on large doses of vitamin C reveals few instances in which taking more than 100 to 300 milligrams a day is beneficial. Adults may not be taking major risks if they dose themselves with 1 to 2 grams a day, but doses approaching 10 grams are clearly unsafe. In short, the range of safe vitamin C intakes seems to be broad. Between the absolute minimum of 10 milligrams a day and the reasonable maximum of 1000 milligrams, nearly everyone should be able to find a suitable intake. People who venture outside these limits do so at their own risk.

Citrus fruits are among the best and most popular sources of vitamin C, and these can be fresh, canned, or frozen. Other vitamin C–rich fruits are strawberries and cantaloupe. The best vegetable sources are broccoli and other members of the cabbage family and green leafy vegetables. Green peppers, okra, tomatoes, and potatoes are considered good sources, although a single serving will not by itself meet the vitamin C RDA. Milk, meat (except liver), and eggs are poor sources, as are breads and cereals. The Food Feature offers suggestions on making the diet rich in vitamin C.

This chapter has treated all 13 of the vitamins. Tables 6–2 and 6–3 sum up the basic facts about each one.

Vitamin C, an antioxidant, is needed for proper maintenance of the connective tissue protein collagen, protects against infection, and aids in iron absorption. The theory that vitamin C prevents or cures colds or cancer is not well supported by research. Vitamin C megadoses may be hazardous; ample vitamin C can be obtained from foods.

Table 6–2

The Fat-Soluble Vitamins—A Summary

Vitamin Names	Chief Functions in the Body	Deficiency Disease Name	Deficiency Symptoms	Toxicity Symptoms	Significant Sources
			Blood/Circulatory System		
Vitamin A (retinol, retinal, retinoic acid); precursor is provitamin A carotenoids such as beta carotene	Vision; maintenance of cornea, epithelial cells, mucous membranes, skin; bone and tooth growth; reproduction; hormone synthesis and regulation; immunity; cancer protection	Hypovitaminosis A	Anemia (small-cell type)[a]	Red blood cell breakage, nosebleeds	Retinal: fortified milk, cheese, cream, butter, fortified margarine, eggs, liver Beta carotene: Spinach and other dark leafy greens, broccoli, deep orange fruits (apricots, peaches, cantaloupe) and vegetables (squash, carrots, sweet potatoes, pumpkin)
			Digestive System		
			Diarrhea, general discomfort	Abdominal cramps and pain, nausea, vomiting, diarrhea, weight loss	
			Immune System		
			Depression; frequent respiratory, digestive bladder, vaginal, and other infections	Overreactivity	
			Mouth, Gums, Teeth		
			Abnormal tooth and jaw alignment		
			Nervous/Muscular Systems		
			Night blindness (retinal)	Blurred vision, pain in calves, fatigue, irritability, loss of appetite, bone pain	
			Skin and Cornea		
			Keratinization, corneal degeneration leading to blindness,[b] rashes	Dry skin, rashes, loss of hair	
			Other		
			Kidney stones, impaired growth	Cessation of menstruation, growth retardation, liver and spleen enlargement	
			Blood/Circulatory System		
Vitamin D (calciferol, cholecalciferol, dihydroxy-vitamin D); precursor is the body's own cholesterol	Mineralization of bones (raises calcium and phosphorus blood levels by increasing absorption from digestive tract, withdrawing calcium from bones, stimulating retention by kidneys)	Rickets osteomalacia		Raised blood calcium	Self-synthesis with sunlight; fortified milk, fortified margarine, eggs, liver, fish
			Digestive System		
				Constipation, weight loss	
			Nervous System		
				Excessive thirst, headaches, irritability, loss of appetite, weakness, nausea	
			Other		
			Abnormal growth, joint pain, soft bones	Kidney stones, stones in arteries, mental and physical retardation	

[a]Small-cell anemia is termed ***microcytic anemia.***

[b]Corneal degeneration progresses from ***keratinization*** (hardening) to ***xerosis*** (drying) to ***xerophthalomia*** (thickening, opacity, and irreversible blindness).

Table 6–2

(continued)

Vitamin Names	Chief Functions in the Body	Deficiency Disease Name	Deficiency Symptoms	Toxicity Symptoms	Significant Sources
E (alpha-tocopherol, tocopherol)	Antioxidant (detoxification of strong oxidants), stabilization of cell membranes, regulation of oxidation reactions, protection of PUFA and vitamin A	(No name)	*Blood/Circulatory System* Red blood cell breakage, anemia *Nervous/Muscular Systems* Degeneration, weakness, difficulty walking, intermittent claudication *Other* Fibrocystic breast disease	*Blood/Circulatory System* Interference with anticlotting medication *Digestive System* General discomfort	Plant oils (margarine, salad dressings, shortenings), green and leafy vegetables, wheat germ, whole grain products, butter, liver, egg yolk, milk fat, nuts, seeds
Vitamin K (phylloquinone, naphtho-quinone)	Synthesis of blood-clotting proteins and a blood protein that regulates blood calcium	(No name)	*Blood/Circulatory System* Hemorrhaging	*Blood/Circulatory System* Interference with anticlotting medication; vitamin K analogues may cause jaundice	Bacterial synthesis in the digestive tract; liver, green leafy vegetables, cabbage-type vegetables, milk

Table 6–3

The Water-Soluble Vitamins—A Summary

Vitamin Names	Chief Functions in the Body	Deficiency Disease Name	Deficiency Symptoms	Toxicity Symptoms	Significant Sources
Thiamin (vitamin B_1)	Part of a coenzyme used in energy metabolism, supports normal appetite and nervous system function	Beriberi	*Blood/Circulatory System* Edema, enlarged heart, abnormal heart rhythms, heart failure *Nervous/Muscular Systems* Degeneration, wasting, weakness, pain, low morale, difficulty walking, loss of reflexes, mental confusion, paralysis	*Blood/Circulatory System* Rapid pulse *Nervous/Muscular Systems* Weakness, headaches, insomnia, irritability	Occurs in all nutritious foods in moderate amounts; pork, ham, bacon, liver, whole grains, legumes, nuts

Table 6–3

(continued)

Vitamin Names	Chief Functions in the Body	Deficiency Disease Name	Deficiency Symptoms	Toxicity Symptoms	Significant Sources
			Mouth, Gums, Tongue		
Riboflavin (vitamin B_2)	Part of a coenzyme used in energy metabolism, supports normal vision and skin health	Ariboflavinosis	Cracks at corners of mouth,[a] magenta tongue	(No symptoms ordinarily reported)	Milk, yogurt, cottage cheese, meat, leafy green vegetables, whole-grain or enriched breads and cereals
			Nervous System and Eyes		
			Hypersensitivity to light,[b] reddening of cornea		
			Other		
			Skin rash	Interference with anticancer medication	
			Digestive System		
Niacin (nicotinic acid, nicotinamide, niacinamide, vitamin B_3, vitamin G); precursor is dietary tryptophan	Part of a coenzyme used in energy metabolism; supports health of skin, nervous system, and digestive system	Pellagra	Diarrhea	Diarrhea, heartburn, nausea, ulcer irritation, vomiting	Milk, eggs, meat, poultry, fish, whole grain and enriched breads and cereals, nuts, and all protein-containing foods
			Mouth, Gums, Tongue		
			Black, smooth tongue[c]		
			Nervous System		
			Irritability, loss of appetite, weakness, dizziness, mental confusion progressing to psychosis or delirium	Fainting	
			Skin		
			Skin rash on areas exposed to sun	Painful flush and rash	
			Other		
				Abnormal liver function, low blood pressure	
			Blood/Circulatory System		
Vitamin B_6 (pyridoxine, pyridoxal, pyridoxamine)	Part of a coenzyme used in amino acid and fatty acid metabolism, helps convert tryptophan to niacin, helps make red blood cells	(No name)	Anemia (small-cell type)[d]		Green and leafy vegetables, meats, fish, poultry, shellfish, legumes, fruits, whole grains
			Digestive System		
				Bloating	
			Mouth, Gums, Tongue		
			Smooth tongue[c]		
			Nervous/Muscular Systems		
			Abnormal brain wave pattern, irritability, muscle twitching, convulsions	Depression, fatigue, irritability, headaches, numbness, damage to nerves, difficulty walking	

[a]Cracks at the corners of the mouth are termed *cheilosis* (kee-LOH-SIS).
[b]Hypersensitivity to light is *photophobia*.
[c]Smoothness of the tongue is caused by loss of its surface structures and is termed *glossitis* (gloss-EYE-tis).
[d]Small-cell type anemia is *microcytic anemia*; large-cell type is *macrocytic* or *megaloblastic anemia*.

Table 6–3

(continued)

Vitamin Names	Chief Functions in the Body	Deficiency Disease Name	Deficiency Symptoms	Toxicity Symptoms	Significant Sources
			Skin		
Vitamin B_6 (continued)			Irritation of sweat glands, rashes		
			Other		
			Kidney stones		
Folacin (folic acid, folate, pteroylglutamic acid)	Part of a coenzyme used in new cell synthesis	(No name)	*Blood Circulatory System*		Leafy green vegetables, legumes, seeds, liver
			Anemia (large-cell type)[d]		
			Digestive system		
			Heartburn, diarrhea, constipation	Diarrhea	
			Immune System		
			Depression, frequent infections		
			Mouth, Gums, Tongue		
			Smooth red tongue[c]		
			Nervous System		
			Depression, mental confusion, fainting	Insomnia, irritability	
			Other		
				Masking of vitamin B_{12} deficiency symptoms	
			Blood/Circulatory System		
Vitamin B_{12} (cyanocobalamin)	Part of a coenzyme used in new cell synthesis, helps maintain nerve cells	(No name[e])	Anemia (large-cell type)[d]	(No toxicity symptoms known)	Animal products (meat, fish, poultry, shellfish, milk, cheese, eggs)
			Mouth, Gums, Tongue		
			Smooth tongue[c]		
			Nervous System		
			Fatigue, degeneration progressing to paralysis		
			Skin		
			Hypersensitivity		
			Digestive System		
Pantothenic acid	Part of a coenzyme used in energy metabolism	(No name)	Vomiting, intestinal distress	Occasional diarrhea	Widespread in foods
			Nervous System		
			Insomnia, fatigue		
			Other		
				Water retention (infrequent)	

[c]Smoothness of the tongue is caused by loss of its surface structures and is termed *glossitis* (gloss-EYE-tis).
[d]Small-cell type anemia is *microcytic anemia*; large-cell type is *macrocytic* or *megaloblastic anemia*.
[e]The name *pernicious anemia* refers to the vitamin$_{12}$ deficiency caused by lack of intrinsic factor, but not to that caused by inadequate dietary intake.

Vitamin Names	Chief Functions in the Body	Deficiency Disease Name	Deficiency Symptoms	Toxicity Symptoms	Significant Sources
			Blood/Circulatory System		
Biotin	Part of a coenzyme used in energy metabolism, fat synthesis, amino acid metabolism, and glycogen synthesis	(No name)	Abnormal heart action	(No toxicity symptoms reported)	Widespread in foods
			Digestive System		
			Loss of appetite, nausea		
			Nervous/Muscular Systems		
			Depression, muscle pain, weakness, fatigue		
			Skin		
			Drying, rash, loss of hair		
			Blood/Circulatory System		
Vitamin C (ascorbic acid)	Collagen synthesis (strengthens blood vessel walls, forms scar tissue, matrix for bone growth), antioxidant, thyroxine synthesis, amino acid metabolism, strengthens resistance to infection, helps in absorption of iron	Scurvy	Anemia (small-cell type),[d] atherosclerotic plaques, pinpoint hemorrhages	Blood cell breakage in certain racial groups[f]	Citrus fruits, cabbage-type vegetables, dark green vegetables, cantaloupe, strawberries, peppers, lettuce, tomatoes, potatoes, papayas, mangos
			Digestive System		
				Nausea, abdominal cramps, diarrhea	
			Immune System		
			Depression, frequent infections		
			Mouth, Gums, Tongue		
			Bleeding gums, loosened teeth		
			Muscular/Nervous Systems		
			Muscle degeneration and pain, hysteria, depression		
			Skeletal System		
			Bone fragility, joint pain		
			Skin		
			Rough skin, blotchy bruises		
			Other		
			Failure of wounds to heal	Interference with medical tests; aggravation of gout symptoms; deficiency symptoms may appear at first on withdrawal of high doses	

[d]Small-cell type anemia is *microcytic anemia*; large-cell type is *macrocytic* or *megaloblastic anemia*.
[f]Groups susceptible to vitamin C toxicity are Sephardic Jews, Africans, and Asians.

Food Feature

Making Meals Rich in Vitamins

This discussion reviews an old way of choosing foods rich in vitamins, and then introduces a new way. The old way is to compare typical food servings and ask how much of each vitamin is in them. The left side of Table 6–4 shows the result. Except for liver, the foods richest in vitamin A per serving are vegetables; those richest in thiamin appear to be meats and seeds. For riboflavin, the richest food sources appear to be meats and dairy products, while for vitamin B_6, too, meats are among the best sources. Highest on the list of folacin and vitamin C contributors are vegetables and fruits. Such a table seems to suggest that the best way to obtain ample amounts of all of the vitamins is to mix meats, milk products, legumes and other seeds, vegetables, and fruits in about equal amounts in your meal plans. (If a table of vitamin E were shown, it would indicate that these foods should include a little oil.) Indeed, this strategy works well, but another approach is worth considering, especially for the person who can afford to consume only a limited number of calories—especially if the person likes to eat large portions of food.

The other way of selecting foods for their vitamin contributions is to ask how much of the vitamins they contribute per calorie, or per 100 calories. When you compare foods on this basis, the vegetables suddenly assume considerably greater prominence as rich sources of all of the vitamins—again, especially if you like to consume large quantities of them. Comparisons of foods as sources of vitamins, on a per-100-calorie basis, are presented on the right side of Table 6–4.

The right side of the table is designed to reveal several things. It is also intended to make you laugh. It shows how ridiculous it is to try to use any one food to meet a nutrient need—with the notable exceptions of vitamins A, folacin, C, which are concentrated in a few foods. The column headed, "If you wanted 100% of your need of the nutrient from this food," is most useful for making comparisons.

Just for fun, then, the right side of the table shows how much of a serving of each food would deliver your entire need of the nutrient for the day—and for what calorie cost. Thus, for example, to get your vitamin A for the day, you could eat about a cup of almost any kind of dark green, leafy vegetables—but you could also eat half a carrot—or 1 bite of fried beef liver. Vitamin A is clearly a nutrient that is easy to get in adequate amounts. Notice, though, that all the apples in Washington can't meet your need for vitamin A. Poor food sources of every vitamin have been included in every table, to remind you to keep your diet balanced.

Thiamin presents a contrast. To meet your thiamin need for the day with any one food would be almost impossible; clearly, you have to do it by eating reasonable portions of several nutritious foods. A rule of thumb is that ten portions of nutritious foods will deliver a day's worth of thiamin. Inspection of the other tables will reveal other patterns of distribution of the vitamins in foods.

The riboflavin part of the table illustrates another point. On the left side, five of the top six items are meats and dairy products. On the right, five of the top six are vegetables. The point is that, while you *could* eat sirloin steak to meet your need for riboflavin, you would have to eat more than a pound to do so—together with more than 1000 calories. On the other hand, you could eat mushrooms (if you could wolf down four cups of them), and the accompanying calories would amount to only 155. Clearly, vegetables (especially dark green vegetables) are a richer source of riboflavin per calorie than meats are, and a day's meals that included generous servings of several vegetables would make the inclusion of so much meat unnecessary.

The vitamin B_6 part of the table illustrates the same point. Meats and legumes are near the top on a per-serving basis (the left side), but vegetables fly to the top on a per-calorie basis (the right side). As for folacin and vitamin C, any way you look at them, vegetables and fruits are the richest sources. Such analyses are enough to make even the most dedicated meat-eater resolve to eat more vegetables, and to reassure the meat-avoider that vegetables can deliver adequate quantities of almost any vitamin if you eat enough of them.

It is for this reason that the total amount of vegetables provided in the high-nutrient-density meals of Chapter 2 was 3 ½ cups for the day. It is more than many people have ever dreamed of eating, but from a nutrition standpoint, it makes sense. The calorie cost is nil; the nutrient contributions are highly significant; and the nutrients that are still needed can be obtained from economical portions of milk products, meats, and related foods. The pleasures of sweet or fat-containing foods can then be fitted in, within a reasonable calorie allowance, without incurring the price of obesity.

It also makes sense not to leave animal products out of the diet altogether. Vitamin B_{12} is unique among the nutrients in being found almost exclusively in meats and animal products. Anyone who eats meat is guaranteed an adequate intake, and lacto-ovo vegetarians (who use milk, cheese, and eggs) are also protected from deficiency. But vegans must use vitamin B_{12}-fortified soy milk, fermented foods, or other such products or take vitamin B_{12} supplements.

There is no limit to the amount that you can learn about the nutrient contents of foods from studying tables like Table 6–4. People who enjoy that sort of thing continue picking up new bits of information throughout their lives ("Oh, mushrooms are the richest in thiamin per 100 calories?"). The tables shown here can only whet your appetite for more information (and vegetables); Appendix A shows the complete nutrient contents of more than 1000 foods.

Once you have selected the most nutritious foods at the market and brought them home, you have the task of storing and preparing them so that they deliver the nutrients to you when you eat them. This requires some understanding of ways to conserve the vitamin value of foods in the kitchen. Vitamins are organic compounds synthesized and broken down by enzymes in the foods that contain them. The enzymes in fruits and vegetables work best at the temperatures at which the plants grow, normally about 70 degrees Fahrenheit (25 degrees Centigrade), which is also the room temperature in most homes. After a fruit has been picked, synthesis of vitamins largely stops; degradation continues. Chilling the fruit slows down this degradation. To protect the vitamin content, fruits and vegetables should be vine ripened (if possible), chilled immediately after picking, and kept cold until they are used.

Riboflavin is light sensitive; it can be destroyed by the ultraviolet rays of the sun or by fluorescent light. For this reason milk is not sold (and should not be stored) in transparent glass containers. Cardboard or plastic containers screen out light, protecting the riboflavin.

Table 6–4

Food Sources of Vitamins Selected to Show a Range of Values

If you eat this size serving of:	You will receive this % of your need[a] of VITAMIN A:	If you wanted 100% of your need[a] of VITAMIN A from this food:	You would have to eat this size serving:
Beef liver, fried (3 oz, 185 cal)	912%	Carrot, whole fresh	0.5 carrot (16 cal)
Sweet potato, baked (1, 118 cal)	249	Beef liver, fried	0.3 oz (19 cal)
Carrot, whole fresh (1, 31 cal)	203	Dandelion greens, cooked	0.8 c (28 cal)
Spinach, cooked (1 c, 41 cal)	147	Spinach, cooked	0.7 c (29 cal)
Butternut squash, baked (1 c, 83 cal)	144	Turnip greens, cooked	1.3 c (38 cal)
Dandelion greens, cooked (1 c, 35 cal)	123	Sweet potato, baked	0.4 potato (47 cal)
Cantaloupe melon (½, 94 cal)	86	Butternut squash, baked	0.7 c (58 cal)
Turnip greens, cooked (1 c, 29 cal)	79	Cantaloupe melon	0.6 melon (113 cal)
Oysters, raw (1 c, 160 cal)	22	Broccoli, cooked	4.5 c (207 cal)
Nonfat milk (1 c, 86 cal)	15	Nonfat milk	6.7 c (576 cal)
Broccoli, cooked (1 c, 46 cal)	22	Oysters, raw	4.5 c (720 cal)
Cheddar cheese (1 oz, 114 cal)	9	Cheddar cheese	11 oz (1254 cal)
Sole/flounder, baked (3 oz, 120 cal)	5	Apple, fresh medium	too much (too many cal)
Apple, fresh medium (1, 80 cal)	1	Sirloin steak, lean	too much (too many cal)
Sirloin steak, lean (8 oz, 480 cal)	<1	Sole/flounder, baked	too much (too many cal)
Whole wheat bread (1 sl, 70 cal)	<1	Whole wheat bread	too much (too many cal)

If you eat this size serving of:	You will receive this % of your need[a] of THIAMIN:	If you wanted 100% of your need[a] of THIAMIN from this food:	You would have to eat this size serving:
Pork chop (3.1 oz, 275 cal)	58%	Mushrooms, raw sliced	20 c (360 cal)
Sunflower seeds, dry (¼ c, 205 cal)	55	Green peas, cooked	3.2 c (403 cal)
Green peas, cooked (1 c, 126 cal)	31	Sunflower seeds, dry	0.5 c (410 cal)
Watermelon (1 sl, 152 cal)	26	Pork chop	5.3 oz (468 cal)
Sirloin steak, lean (8 oz, 480 cal)	19	Broccoli, cooked	11 c (506 cal)
Oysters, raw (1 c, 160 cal)	19	Watermelon	3.8 sl (578 cal)
Broccoli, cooked (1 c, 46 cal)	9	Turnip greens, cooked	20 c (580 cal)
Whole wheat bread (1 sl, 70 cal)	7	Oysters, raw	5.3 c (848 cal)
Nonfat milk (1 c, 86 cal)	6	Whole wheat bread	14 sl (980 cal)
Mushrooms, raw sliced (1 c, 18 cal)	5	Nonfat milk	17 c (1462 cal)
Turnip greens, cooked (1 c, 29 cal)	5	Sole/flounder, baked	100 oz (3960 cal)
Sole/flounder, baked (3 oz, 120 cal)	5	Sirloin steak, lean	42 oz (2544 cal)
Apple, fresh medium (1, 80 cal)	1	Apple, fresh medium	100 apples (8000 cal)
Cheddar cheese (1 oz, 114 cal)	0	Cheddar cheese	too much (too many cal)

If you eat this size serving of:	You will receive this % of your need[a] of RIBOFLAVIN:	If you wanted 100% of your need[a] of RIBOFLAVIN from this food:	You would have to eat this size serving:
Beef liver, fried (3 oz, 185 cal)	207%	Beef liver, fried	1.4 oz (93 cal)
Braunschweiger sausage (2 pcs, 205 cal)	51	Mushroom pieces, cooked	3.7 c (155 cal)
Sirloin steak, lean (8 oz, 480 cal)	41	Spinach, cooked	4 c (164 cal)
Mushroom pieces, cooked (1 c, 42 cal)	27	Broccoli, cooked	5.3 c (244 cal)
Ricotta cheese, part skim (1 c, 340 cal)	27	Dandelion greens, cooked	9 c (319 cal)
Oysters, raw (1 c, 160 cal)	25	Braunschweiger sausage	4 (410 cal)
Spinach, cooked (1 c, 41 cal)	25	Nonfat milk	5 c (430 cal)
Nonfat milk (1 c, 86 cal)	20	Oysters, raw	4 c (640 cal)
Broccoli, cooked (1 c, 46 cal)	19	Cheddar cheese	9 oz (1026 cal)
Dandelion greens, cooked (1 c, 35 cal)	11	Sirloin steak, lean	19.5 oz (1152 cal)
Cheddar cheese (1 oz, 114 cal)	6	Ricotta cheese, part skim	3.7 c (1258 cal)
Sole/flounder, baked (3 oz, 120 cal)	5	Whole wheat bread	25 sl (1750 cal)
Whole wheat bread (1 sl, 70 cal)	4	Sole/flounder, baked	60 oz (2400 cal)
Apple, fresh medium (1, 80 cal)	1	Apple, fresh medium	100 apples (8000 cal)

If you eat this size serving of:	You will receive this % of your need[a] of VITAMIN B_6:	If you wanted 100% of your need[a] of VITAMIN B_6 from this food:	You would have to eat this size serving:
Sirloin steak, lean (8 oz, 480 cal)	39%	Spinach, cooked	4.5 c (185 cal)
Navy beans, cooked dry (1 c, 225 cal)	36	Mustard greens, cooked	11 c (231 cal)
Baked potato, whole (1, 220 cal)	35	Cauliflower, cooked	8 c (240 cal)
Watermelon (1 sl, 152 cal)	35	Broccoli, cooked	6.3 c (290 cal)
Banana, peeled (1, 105 cal)	33	Banana, peeled	3 banana (315 cal)
Chicken breast, roasted (½, 142 cal)	26	Watermelon	2.9 sl (441 cal)
Sunflower seeds, dry (¼ c, 205 cal)	23	Chicken breast, roasted	4 halves (568 cal)
Spinach, cooked (1 c, 41 cal)	22	Navy beans, cooked dry	2.8 c (630 cal)
Tuna, canned (3 oz, 135 cal)	21	Tuna, canned	14 oz (635 cal)
Broccoli, cooked (1 c, 46 cal)	16	Baked potato, whole	2.9 potato (638 cal)
Sole/flounder, baked (3 oz, 120 cal)	14	Sunflower seeds, dry	1 c (820 cal)
Cauliflower, cooked (1 c, 30 cal)	12	Sole/flounder, baked	21 oz (840 cal)
Mustard greens, cooked (1 c, 21 cal)	9	Sirloin steak, lean	20.5 oz (1248 cal)
Nonfat milk (1 c, 86 cal)	5	Nonfat milk	20 c (1720 cal)
Apple, fresh medium (1, 80 cal)	4	Apple, fresh medium	25 apples (2000 cal)
Whole wheat bread (1 sl, 70 cal)	3	Whole wheat bread	33 sl (2310 cal)
Cheddar cheese (1 oz, 114 cal)	1	Cheddar cheese	100 oz (11,400 cal)

If you eat this size serving of:	You will receive this % of your need[a] of FOLACIN:	If you wanted 100% of your need[a] of FOLACIN from this food:	You would have to eat this size serving:
Spinach, cooked (1 c, 41 cal)	66%	Romaine lettuce, chopped	5.3 c (48 cal)
Asparagus, cooked (1 c, 44 cal)	44	Spinach, cooked	1.5 c (62 cal)
Turnip greens, cooked (1 c, 29 cal)	43	Turnip greens, cooked	2.3 c (67 cal)
Lima beans, cooked (1 c, 260 cal)	43	Parsley, chopped fresh	3.6 c (72 cal)
Beef liver, fried (3 oz, 185 cal)	38	Asparagus, cooked	2.3 c (101 cal)
Parsley, chopped fresh (1 c, 20 cal)	28	Broccoli, cooked	3.7 c (170 cal)
Broccoli, cooked (1 c, 46 cal)	27	Mushrooms, raw sliced	25 c (450 cal)
Romaine lettuce, chopped (1 c, 9 cal)	19	Beef liver, fried	7.9 oz (481 cal)
Oysters, raw (1 c, 160 cal)	6	Lima beans, cooked	2.3 c (598 cal)
Sirloin steak, lean (8 oz, 480 cal)	5	Whole wheat bread	25 sl (1750 cal)
Whole wheat bread (1 sl, 70 cal)	4	Nonfat milk	25 c (2150 cal)
Nonfat milk (1 c, 86 cal)	4	Oysters, raw	17 c (2720 cal)
Mushrooms, raw sliced (1 c, 18 cal)	4	Apple, fresh medium	100 apples (8000 cal)
Cheddar cheese (1 oz, 114 cal)	1	Sirloin steak, lean	10 lb (9600 cal)
Apple, fresh medium (1, 80 cal)	1	Cheddar cheese	100 oz (11,400 cal)

If you eat this size serving of:	You will receive this % of your need[a] of VITAMIN C:	If you wanted 100% of your need[a] of VITAMIN C from this food:	You would have to eat this size serving:
Papaya, whole fresh (1, 117 cal)	313%	Green peppers, whole	0.6 pepper (11 cal)
Cantaloupe melon (½, 94 cal)	190	Parsley, chopped fresh	1.2 c (24 cal)
Broccoli, cooked (1 c, 46 cal)	163	Cauliflower, cooked	0.9 c (27 cal)
Brussels sprouts, cooked (1 c, 60 cal)	161	Broccoli, cooked	0.6 c (28 cal)
Green peppers, whole (1, 18 cal)	160	Strawberries, fresh	0.7 c (32 cal)
Grapefruit juice, fresh (1 c, 96 cal)	160	Papaya, whole fresh	0.3 papaya (35 cal)
Strawberries, fresh (1 c, 45 cal)	142	Brussels sprouts, cooked	0.6 c (36 cal)
Oysters, raw (1 c, 160 cal)	120	Mustard greens, cooked	1.8 c (38 cal)
Orange, fresh medium (1, 60 cal)	116	Cantaloupe melon	¼ melon (47 cal)
Cauliflower, cooked (1 c, 30 cal)	115	Orange, fresh medium	0.9 orange (54 cal)
Parsley, chopped fresh (1 c, 20 cal)	90	Grapefruit juice, fresh	0.6 c (58 cal)
Mustard greens, cooked (1 c, 21 cal)	58	Oysters, raw	0.8 c (128 cal)
Apple, fresh medium (1, 80 cal)	13	Apple, fresh medium	7.7 apples (616 cal)
Nonfat milk (1 c, 86 cal)	3	Nonfat milk	33 c (2838 cal)
Sole/flounder, baked (3 oz, 120 cal)	2	Sole/flounder, baked	150 oz (6000 cal)
Cheddar cheese (1 oz, 114 cal)	0	Cheddar cheese	too much (too many cal)
Whole wheat bread (1 sl, 70 cal)	0	Whole wheat bread	too much (too many cal)

[a]The U.S. RDA is used as an approximation of "your need."

Some vitamins are acids or antioxidants, and so are most stable in an acid solution, away from air. Citrus fruits, tomatoes, and many juices are acid. As long as the skin is uncut or the can is unopened, their vitamins are protected from air. If you store a cut vegetable or fruit or an opened container of juice, cover it with an airtight wrapper and store it in the refrigerator.

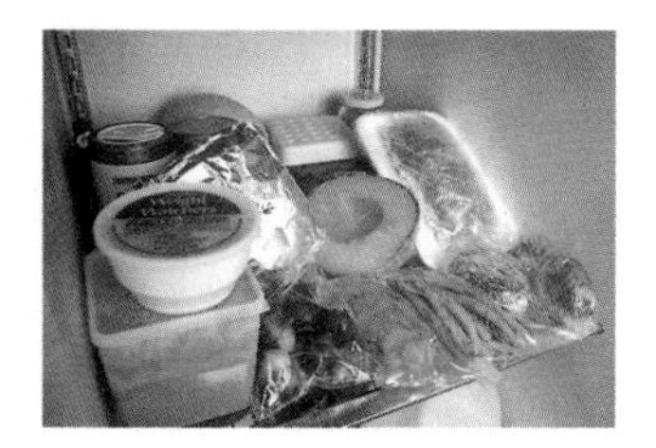

To preserve nutrients, refrigerate and wrap tightly.

You have seen labels on frozen foods that tell you "Do not refreeze." As food freezes, the cellular water expands into long, spiky ice crystals that puncture cell membranes and disrupt tissue structures, changing the texture of the food. People sometimes wonder if there is any danger in eating a twice-frozen food. Provided that they haven't let it spoil while it was thawed, the only problem is that the food may be less appealing.

Generally, chest-type freezers keep foods coldest, because they aren't opened as often as the refrigerator's freezing compartment. You might consider owning both types, and use the refrigerator's freezing compartment for ice and foods to be used quickly, while keeping things longer in the chest type. Be sure that the refrigerator keeps food at 40 degrees Fahrenheit and the freezer at 0 degrees Fahrenheit (use a freezer thermometer).

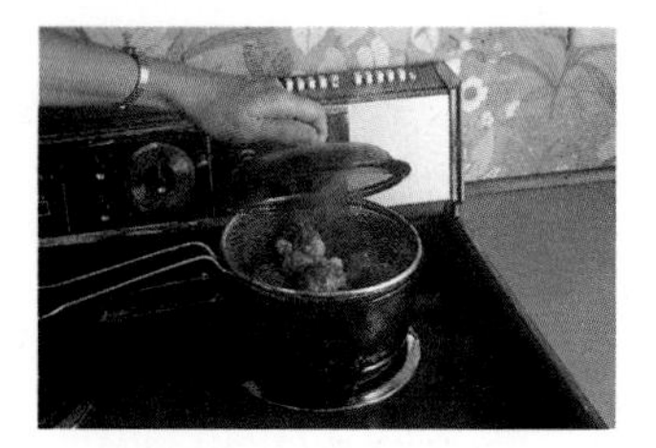

Steam vegetables.

The water-soluble vitamins readily dissolve into the water in which cut vegetables are washed, boiled, or canned. If the water is discarded, as much as half of the vitamin content of the food is poured down the drain with it. To minimize this kind of loss, steam vegetables over water rather than in it, or boil them in a volume of water small enough to be reabsorbed into them by the time they are cooked. Wash the food vigorously and briefly, don't soak it, and cut it later.

The nutrient contents of canned foods are usually shown as "solids and liquids." If you throw away the liquid from a canned food, you are throwing away all the nutrients that have leaked into that liquid—up to half the amount in the original product. A bit of southern folk wisdom is to serve the cooking liquid with the vegetable rather than throwing it away; this liquid is known as the "pot liquor." The user of canned vegetables who can think of a way to use the "liquor"—for example, by saving it to make soups, cook rice, or moisten casseroles—is displaying similar wisdom.

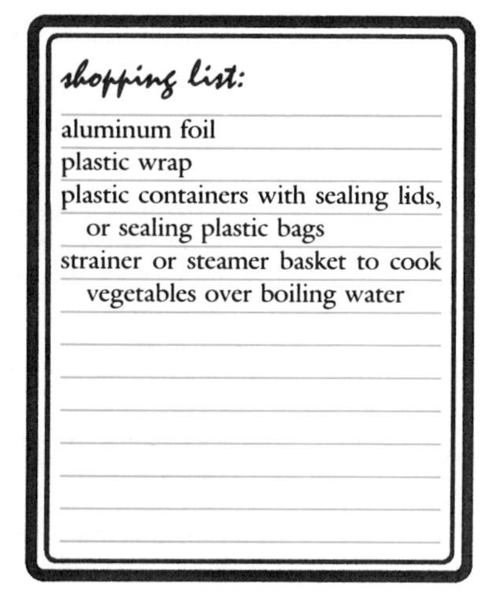

shopping list:

aluminum foil
plastic wrap
plastic containers with sealing lids, or sealing plastic bags
strainer or steamer basket to cook vegetables over boiling water

During cooking, minimize the destruction of vitamins by avoiding high temperatures and long cooking times. Iron destroys vitamin C, but perhaps the benefit of increasing the iron content of foods by cooking in iron utensils outweighs this disadvantage. Each of these tactics is small by itself, but saving a small percentage of the vitamins in foods daily can mean saving significant amounts in a year's time.

Meanwhile, however, a law of diminishing returns operates. Most vitamin losses under reasonable conditions are not catastrophic. (For example, frozen orange juice that has been reconstituted and refrigerated typically retains 80 percent of its original vitamin C activity after eight days of storage.) You need not fret over small vitamin losses that occur in your kitchen; you may waste time that is valuable to you in other ways. You can be assured that if you start with fresh, whole foods containing ample amounts of vitamins and you are reasonably careful in their preparation, you will receive a bounty of the nutrients that they contain.

Self-Study

Evaluate Your Vitamin Intakes

Several of these exercises make use of the information you recorded on Forms 1 to 3 in Appendix H.

1. Start with vitamin A. Compare your average intake with the standard (RDA or RNI); you recorded these earlier on Form 3. What percentage of your recommended intake did you consume? Was this enough? What foods contribute the greatest amount of vitamin A to your diet? If you consumed more than the recommendation, was this too much? Why or why not? In what ways would you change your diet to improve vitamin A intake? Answer these same questions for thiamin, riboflavin, niacin, vitamin B_6, folacin, and vitamin C.

Note on niacin: Remember that preformed dietary niacin is not the only source your body uses; it also uses the amino acid tryptophan, if there is extra available after protein needs are met. If your niacin intake seems low, perform the following calculation. Record the total protein you consumed (in grams). Subtract your recommended protein intake to obtain an estimate of "leftover" protein available to make niacin (in grams). Divide this number by 100 to obtain the total tryptophan you might have had available from which to make niacin (tryptophan represents about 1/100 of the weight of most dietary proteins). Multiply this number by 1000 to convert grams to milligrams.

Now, about 60 milligrams of tryptophan can be converted to about 1 milligram of niacin in the body, so divide by 60 to get "niacin equivalents." Finally, add the amount of niacin you obtained preformed in your diet, and compare this total with the recommended intake. This is only a rough estimate of the amount of niacin you might have derived from your diet, but perhaps better than none. If your niacin and protein intakes are both low, you should do something about it—probably increase your protein intake, for a start.

2. Appendix A does not show vitamins D, E, and K, but you can guess at the adequacy of your intakes. For vitamin D, answer the following questions. Do you drink fortified milk (read the label)? Eat eggs? Fortified breakfast cereal? Liver? Are you in the sun frequently? (Remember, though, that excessive exposure to sun increases the risk of skin cancer in susceptible individuals.)

3. For vitamin E, consider the foods you ate in 24 hours. Vitamin E often accompanies linoleic acid in foods. Did you consume enough linoleic acid? (See Self-Study 4.)

4. For vitamin K, does your diet include 2 cups of milk or the equivalent in milk products every day? Does it include leafy vegetables frequently (every other day)? Do you take antibiotics regularly (which inhibit the production of vitamin K by your intestinal bacteria)?

Notes

1. U.S. House of Representatives, Select Committee on Hunger, *Vitamin A: An Urgent Nutritional Need for the World's Children* (Washington, D.C.: Government Printing Office, 1985).
2. J. E. Olson, Vitamin A and cancer (a letter to the editor), *Journal of the American Dietetic Association* 86 (1986): 1730, 1732.
3. Masked hypervitaminosis A and liver injury, *Nutrition Reviews* 40 (1982): 303–305.
4. T. Ziporyn, Possible link probed: Deafness and vitamin D, *Journal of the American Medical Association* 250 (1983): 1951–1952.
5. Occult vitamin D intoxication . . . , *Nutrition and the MD,* October 1979.
6. M. Rudolf, K. Arulanantham, and R. M. Greenstein, Unsuspected nutritional rickets, *Pediatrics* 66 (1980): 72–76; Vitamin D deficiency rickets, revisited, *Nutrition Reviews* 38 (1980): 116–118.
7. M. A. Guggenheim, *Vitamin E Deficiency Diseases,* a booklet available from the Vitamin Nutrition Information Service, Hofmann-La Roche, Inc., Nutley, NJ 07110; D. P. R. Muller, J. K. Lloyd, and O. H. Wolff, Vitamin E and neurological function, *Lancet,* 29 January 1983, pp. 225–228.
8. D. A. Roe, *Drug-Induced Nutritional Deficiencies* (Westport, Conn.: AVI, 1976), pp. 3, 16–17.
9. Over-the-counter preparations in doses greater than 0.4 milligrams per day are marketed only for pregnant and lactating women. Federal Regulation 21, *Code of Federal Regulations,* Section 172, 345, cited by L. Alhadeff and coauthors (letter), *Nutrition Reviews* 42 (1984): 265–267.
10. T. C. Chalmers, Effects of ascorbic acid on the common cold, *American Journal of Medicine* 58 (1975): 532–536.

Controversy 6

Vitamin Supplements

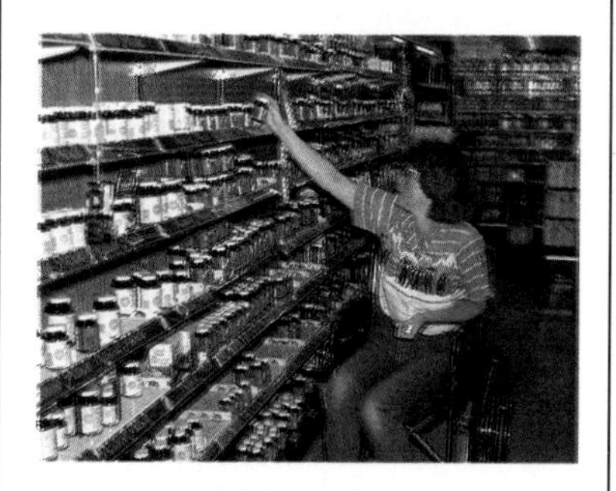

First of all, do you really need a supplement?

Many people are not sure that they meet their nutrient needs using foods alone. Fully half the population uses nutrient supplements regularly, collectively spending billions of dollars on them each year.[1] Many take a single daily pill; others take huge quantities of single nutrients. Many are self-prescribed, or taken on the advice of friends, relatives, or magazines that may or may not be reliable.

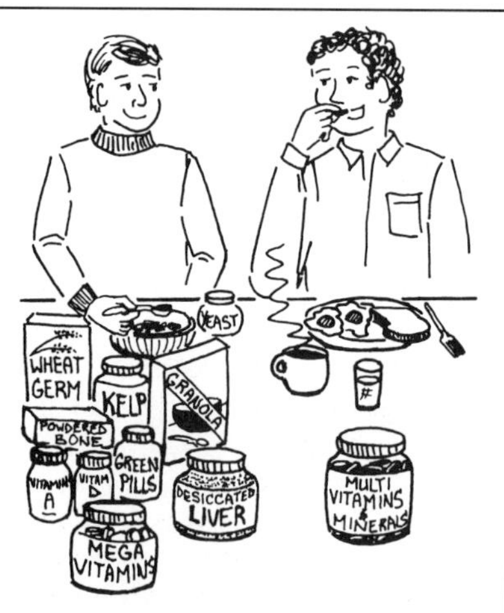

What do you need: an arsenal of supplements, a single daily pill, or just food?

This Controversy examines several questions related to supplement taking. What are the arguments for taking supplements? What are the arguments against taking them? Should a person choose to do so, how should the person go about choosing one?

Arguments for Supplements

Nutrition surveys of the U.S. and Canadian populations do detect deficiencies of protein, vitamins, and minerals (Chapter 14 provides details). The incidence of these deficiencies is low, but they do exist, and they provide the basis for the argument that ordinary people may need to take nutrient supplements. A favorite argument is that if deficiency symptoms are seen, then **marginal** or **subclinical deficiencies** must also exist, causing symptoms that have not been well characterized yet and are probably not always recognized even by skilled, experienced health care providers. Perhaps many individuals, although cloaked in fat, are more or less subtly impaired by nutrient deficiencies.

The newsletter *Nutrition and the MD* describes marginal deficiencies as states of unwellness shy of classical deficiencies:

- When people are becoming deficient in thiamin, classic signs of beriberi don't appear until the sixth week. But, as the deficiency develops, loss of appetite and weight, irritability, insomnia, and malaise appear within three to four weeks, together with a fall in a blood enzyme (transketolase, detectable only by laboratory test).
- No clinical signs of a developing riboflavin deficiency appear until the eighth week, but behavioral symptoms can be detected by the sixth week.
- As vitamin B_6 deficiency develops, clients complain of fatigue and headache; only later does one see the classic small red blood cells of anemia.

In other words, somewhere between the adequate intake of a nutrient and the development of a physically observable deficiency, there is an area in which people don't feel well and don't function well. Since physically observable deficiencies are seen in North America, even if they are not very common, there must be people—in fact, more people—in the in-between area, too.

In some cases there are predisposing conditions (the people aren't healthy, they are addicted to alcohol or other drugs, they have kidney diseases, or they use medications that interfere with nutrient action). But *Nutrition and the MD* adds: "There is probably a large additional group of people **at risk** of developing marginal vitamin deficiencies. These include young and older women consuming diets that are marginally adequate for energy, and those patients with chronic debilitative illness who are often anorexic and have poor food intake."[2]

To give one specific example, the authors of a hospital study on surgery clients observed that a slight thiamin deficit resulted in poor wound healing. They were impressed: "The data served to emphasize once more the invaluable benefits of **optimal nutrition** in preventive and post-operative medicine."[3]

For people who are at risk of marginal deficiencies, supplements may be a rational and beneficial choice. It has been suggested that all of the following adults are on that list:[4]

- People with low energy intakes, such as habitual dieters.*
- The elderly, especially if they are malnourished.
- People who eat bizarre or monotonous diets, such as some food faddists.
- People with illnesses that take away the appetite.*
- People with illnesses that impair absorption of nutrients—including diseases of the liver, gallbladder, pancreas, and digestive system.*
- People taking medications that interfere with the body's use of specific nutrients (such as INH, mentioned on p. 182).
- People who have diseases, infections, or injuries, or who have undergone surgery resulting in increased metabolic needs.
- Women who are pregnant or lactating, whose metabolic needs are therefore increased.*
- Strict vegetarians.*
- Women who bleed excessively during menstruation.*
- People whose calcium intakes are too low to forestall osteoporosis.

Most of those people would benefit from a multivitamin-mineral supplement that supplied approximately the RDA amount of every essential nutrient. Those taking drugs that interfered with specific nutrients would need individual advice. Pregnancy and lactation incur increased needs for iron, calcium, and folacin in particular; strict vegetarians need special provisions to meet their needs for calcium, iron, and zinc; and women who lose much blood during menstruation need iron supplements.

*The taking of supplements by groups tagged with an asterisk is endorsed by the societies mentioned in note 12 (p. 222).

Other special cases exist. For example, newborns are routinely given a single dose of vitamin K at birth,* and infants may need supplements depending on whether they are receiving formula or not, and on whether their water is fluoridated or not (see Chapter 11).

The special cases are discussed later. Calcium and iron supplements receive attention in Chapter 7; supplements for pregnancy, lactation, and infancy in Chapter 11, and for people taking medications in Chapter 13. The end of this Controversy comes back to the question of how to choose a general multivitamin-mineral supplement, but first, there are arguments against doing so.

Arguments Against Supplements

One argument is not so much against supplements in general as against high-dose supplements. High doses of almost every nutrient are dangerous. People's tolerances for high doses of nutrients vary, just as their thresholds for deficiencies vary. Thus amounts that some can tolerate may not be safe for others, and no one knows who falls into which category.

Toxic overdoses of vitamins and minerals may be more common than we realize. One physician, reporting several cases of harm from vitamin overdoses in his local community, warns that the cases we hear about are just the tip of the iceberg.[5] Sometimes even an alert health care provider who is on the lookout for such cases fails to spot them. Only a few recognize the signs of short-term acute toxic doses; and no doubt many cases of chronic nutrient toxicity, in which the effects develop more subtly and slowly, go unrecognized.[6] Because supplements are, under the law, classed as foods rather than as drugs, manufacturers are not required to prove their safety or effectiveness. In view of the hazards they present, many authorities believe they should be required to bear warning labels.

In hopes of learning the extent and severity of the problem of supplement toxicity, the FDA has been, as of 1987, collecting reports of adverse reactions to overdoses of nutrients from physicians and will report on them in due course. The project is titled the Adverse Reaction Monitoring System.[7] FDA is also developing a set of **safety indexes** for nutrients—indexes of the safety of doses higher than the RDA. The safety index for calcium is 10, for example (up to 10 times the U.S. RDA is a safe dose for an adult); that for selenium is only 5.[8]

In light of today's knowledge, it is impossible to say just how much of a nutrient is too much. Assuming, however, that is is best to err on the conservative side, Table C6–1 presents upper limits for vitamin and mineral doses to be obtained from supplements.

Another argument against the use of supplements is that no one knows exactly how to formulate the "ideal" supplement. What nutrients should be included? How much of each? On whose needs should the choices be based? And how should an individual choose a supplement, since no individual's needs are exactly like anyone else's?

Another argument against supplements is that they may lull the taker into a false sense of security. A person might eat irresponsibly, thinking, "My supplement will cover my needs." Or, experiencing the warning sign of a disease, a person might postpone seeking a diagnosis, thinking, "I probably need a nutrient supplement to make this go away." Such self-diagnosis is always dangerous.

Other invalid reasons why people may take supplements include:

- Their feelings of insecurity about the nutrient content of the food supply.
- Their desire for additional energy or strength.
- Their belief that extra vitamins and minerals will help them cope with stress.
- Their desire to prevent, treat, or cure symptoms or diseases from the common cold to cancer.

Ironically, though, one study found that supplement users actually eat more nutrient-dense diets than those who don't use supplements and therefore need the supplements the least.[9] In addition, little relationship exists between the nutrients individuals need and the ones they take in pills.[10]

Another problem is that of **bioavailability.** In general, nutrients are absorbed best from foods, in which they are diluted and dispersed among other ingredients that may facilitate their absorption. Taken in pure, concentrated form, they are more likely to interfere with each other's absorption or with the absorption of the nutrients in foods eaten simultaneously with them. Documentation of these effects is particularly extensive for minerals: zinc hinders copper and calcium absorption, iron hinders zinc absorption, calcium hinders magnesium and iron absorption, and magnesium hinders the absorption of calcium and iron. The same interference takes place when people use foods that are fortified with added minerals, leaving no recourse other than the use of ordinary whole foods to the consumer who wants the benefits of optimal absorption of nutrients.[11]

In view of all the negatives associated with supplement taking, several professional nutrition societies have joined to issue guidelines indicating that people should ordinarily *not* use them:

Healthy children and adults should obtain adequate nutrient intakes from dietary sources. Meeting nutrient needs by choosing a variety of

Table C6–1

Vitamin and Mineral Doses for Supplements

Substance	Safe Dose (FDA, RDA[b]) *Prevention*	*Treatment of Deficiency*
Vitamins		
Vitamin A (IU)	1250 to 2500	5 to 10,000
Vitamin D (IU)	400 (up to age 18) 200 (adults)	Do not use[a]
Vitamin E (mg)	50	300
Thiamin (mg)	1 to 2	5 to 25
Riboflavin (mg)	1 to 2	5 to 25
Niacin (as niacinamide, mg)	10 to 20	25 to 50
Vitamin B_6 (mg)	1.5 to 2.5	7.5 to 25
Folacin (mg)	0.1 to 0.4 1.0 (pregnancy, lactation)	Do not use[a]
Vitamin B_{12} (μg)	3 to 10	Do not use[a]
Pantothenic acid (mg)	Not recommended in supplement form	
Biotin (mg)	Not recommended in supplement form	
Vitamin C (mg)	50 to 100	300 to 500
Minerals		
Calcium (mg)	400 to 800	Do not use[a]
Phosphorus (mg)	No need to supplement	
Magnesium (mg)	No need to supplement	
Iron (mg)	10 to 30 (women) 30 to 60 (pregnancy, lactation)	Do not use[a]
Zinc (mg)	10 to 25 (adults) 25 (pregnancy, lactation)	Do not use[a]
Iodine (mg)	Iodized table salt is the accepted way to supplement dietary iodine in the United States	

[a]The FDA and the Committee on RDA do not recommend that these nutrients be used to attempt to correct deficiencies, because deficiencies often arise from nonnutritional causes such as disease or interference by drugs. In these cases, the underlying causes of the deficiencies must be correctly diagnosed and treated; supplements may mask, but will not correct, the problems.

Source: Parts adapted from A. Hecht, Vitamins over the counter: Take only when needed, *FDA Consumer,* April 1979, pp. 17–19; Food and Nutrition Board, *Recommended Dietary Allowances,* 9th ed. (Washington, D.C.: National Academy of Sciences, 1980).

foods in moderation, rather than by supplementation, reduces the potential risk for both nutrient deficiencies and nutrient excesses. Individual recommendations regarding supplements and diets should come from physicians and registered dietitians. . . .

The Recommended Dietary Allowances represent the best currently available assessment of safe and adequate intakes, and serve as the basis for the U.S. Recommended Daily Allowances shown on many product labels. There are no demonstrated benefits of self-supplementation beyond these allowances.[12]

The societies agree that supplement use may be warranted only in the instances marked with an asterisk in the list presented earlier. They urge that, whenever a person's diet is reviewed and found to be inadequate, the action to take is not to begin supplementation but to improve the person's food choices and eating patterns.[13]

From the perspective of the experts, then, it seems that supplementation is not the wisest course for most people. Still, when a supplement is needed, some pointers can assist in its selection.

Selection of Supplements

People often think in terms of "vitamin pills." However, when you go looking for an all-purpose supplement, it is important to remember that if vitamins are needed, minerals will be needed, too. A single, balanced vitamin-mineral supplement should do the job.[14]

If you decide to take a vitamin-mineral supplement, you may find yourself bewildered in front of a drugstore counter, reading the clever, and usually deceptive, ads on labels—"For vitality!" "Infants only!" "For those with active lives!" "What you need for stress!" or "Be more fun, sexier, smarter, and more healthy!"—the key to each quality to be found, of course, in *that* particular supplement. The first step in escaping the clutches of the health hustlers is to imagine that you have a bottle of white paint and can simply white out the picture of the sexy people on the beach and the meaningless, glittering generalities like "new and improved." No matter how lovely the container, you are shopping for a nutrient supplement. (If a pretty container is what you actually need, you can get one for less in housewares.) After you have whited out the label claims, all you have left is the list of ingredients, what form they are in, and the price. Here's where the truth lies, and from here you can make a rational decision based on facts.

You have two basic questions to answer. The first question: What form do you want—chewable, liquid, or pills? If you'd rather drink your vitamins and minerals than chew them, fine. (Remember, you whited out *infant* on the labels, so now those bottles are just liquid supplements.) The second question: Who are you? What vitamins and minerals do *you* need? The RDA table on the inside front cover and the table for Canadians (Appendix B) are the standards appropriate for virtually all reasonably healthy people (if you aren't healthy, see your health care provider).

Generally, most people who need a supplement should choose one that provides all the RDA nutrients in amounts smaller than, equal to, or very close to the RDA. Avoid any preparation that, in a daily dose, provides more than the RDA of vitamin A, D, or any mineral, or more than ten times the RDA for *any* nutrient. Other warnings:

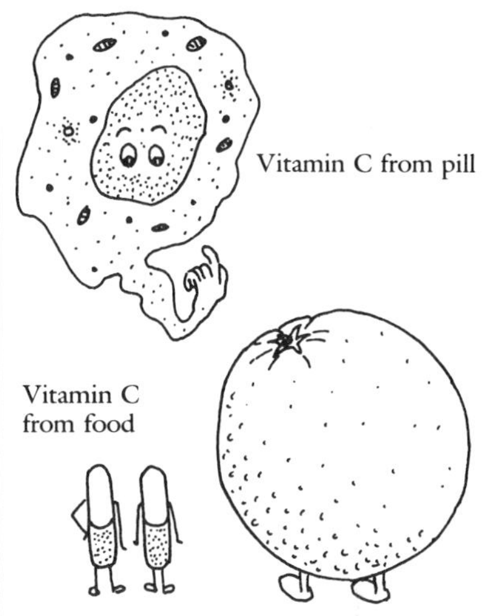

The cell can't tell which vitamins come from pills and which from foods.

- Avoid preparations with high iron concentrations (say, more than 10 milligrams per dose) except for menstruating women. People who menstruate need more iron, but people who don't, don't. Iron is hard to get rid of once it's in the body, so an excess of iron can cause problems, just as a deficiency can (Chapter 7).
- Avoid "organic" or "natural" preparations. They are no better than standard pharmacy types. The word *synthetic* may sound like "fake," but to synthesize just means to put together. The synthetic supplement is not a fake, but the real thing, identical in every way to the vitamins that are synthesized by plants and animals. Your body can't tell the difference, but your wallet can.
- Avoid products that make "high potency" claims. More is not better. If a supplement covers your RDA, it's more than enough. You're eating foods, too, after all, so you're getting well over RDA amounts of vitamins and minerals.

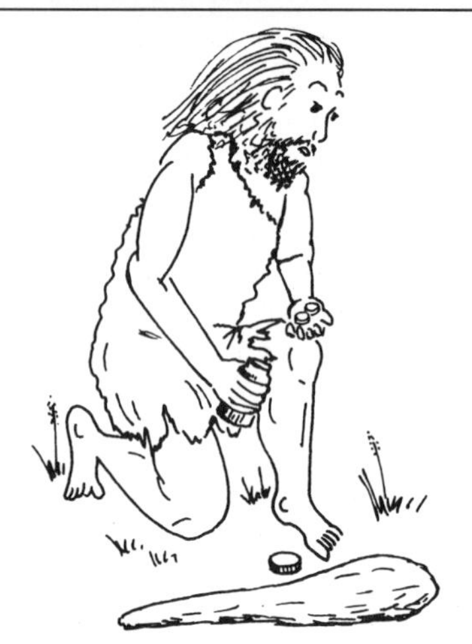

It really isn't natural to take any kind of pills.

■ Avoid megadoses unless they are prescribed by a physician. Nutrients can build up and cause unexpected problems. (For example, a man who takes vitamins and begins to lose his hair may think it means he needs *more* vitamins, when in fact hair loss may be an early sign of vitamin A overdose.)

■ Avoid preparations that contain items not needed in human nutrition, such as choline and inositol. It's not that those particular items will harm you, but they reveal a marketing strategy that makes the whole mix suspect. The manufacturer may want you to believe that its brand of pills contains the latest "new" nutrient that the takers of all other brands will miss out on, but in fact, for every valid discovery of this kind these days, there are 999,999 frauds.

■ Avoid pills containing ground parsley, alfalfa, and other vegetable components. They may deliver a few of the same nutrients as a plate of salad or broccoli, but salad and broccoli are much more nutritious—and cheaper.

■ Avoid geriatric "tonics." They are generally poor in vitamins and minerals, and yet so high in alcohol as to threaten inebriation. The liquids designed for infants are more complete.

The tables presented in Appendix D list the nutrient amounts in some nationally advertised supplements. Blank columns are provided for the addition of local brands you may wish to compare with the national brands shown. Local or store brands are just as good as the nationals. If they are less expensive, it is not because they are inferior, but because the price does not have to cover the cost of national advertising. (One full-page color ad in a national magazine costs upwards of $60,000.) The less expensive pills may well have come from the same batch as the higher-priced ones, but without the price tag associated with the brand name.

Steer clear of doses that are too high. Think of the original Stone-Age person, who had to depend only on foods for life and health. If the foods available to Stone-Age people *could* have supplied the amount of a nutrient being advocated, then perhaps it is not unsafe for us, their descendants, to ingest that amount ourselves.

By this standard, the doses some people take are clearly excessive. To obtain 840 milligrams of vitamin E

Miniglossary

at risk: a term used in nutrition to describe people on the verge of developing nutrient deficiencies.

bioavailability: absorbability, a term used to refer to the individual differences in nutrients' ease of absorption.

bone meal: a nutrient supplement made from bone, intended to supply calcium and other bone minerals.

desiccated liver: dehydrated liver, a powder sold in health-food stores and supposed to contain in concentrated form all the nutrients found in liver. Possibly not dangerous, this supplement has no particular nutritional merit, and grocery store liver is considerably less expensive (*desiccated* means "totally dried").

garlic oil: an extract of garlic.

granola: a cereal mixed from rolled oats and other grains.

green pills: pills containing dehydrated, crushed vegetable matter. One pill contains nutrients equal to those in one small forkful of fresh vegetables—minus losses incurred in processing. Sixty pills costing $15 deliver vegetable matter worth about $1.50.

kelp: a kind of seaweed used by the Japanese as a foodstuff. Kelp tablets are made from dehydrated kelp.

marginal deficiency: see *subclinical deficiency.*

nutritional yeast: a preparation of yeast cells, often praised for its high nutrient content. Yeast is a concentrated source of B vitamins, as are many other foods. The type of yeast used is brewer's, not baker's, yeast; see items 992 and 993 in Appendix A.

from its best food source, wheat germ, for example, you would have to eat 15 pounds of wheat germ—yet some people take supplements containing more than 840 milligrams of vitamin E every day. To obtain 5 grams of vitamin C, you would have to eat 19 pounds of oranges, yet some people consume more than that much vitamin C daily from supplements.

Our ancestors survived for centuries without nutrient supplements and arrived successfully at the point of producing us. On this basis alone, it can be argued that we must need no more vitamins or minerals than what *we* can obtain from food. That much, but not more, would be reasonable to look for in a supplement.

But, come to think of it, if all the nutrients we need can come from food, why not just get them from food? Foods have so much more to recommend them than do supplements. Nutrients in foods come in an infinite variety of combinations with a multitude of different carriers, absorption facilitators, antioxidation protectors, and other benefits. They come with water, fiber, and a host of beneficial and interesting nonnutrients (see Controversy 10). They come with calories (you have to eat some calories each day; why not ask nutritious foods to deliver them?) They offer pleasing mouth sensations, satiety, and opportunities for socializing while eating. In no way can nutrient supplements hold a candle to foods as a means of meeting human health needs.

Sharing Nutrition Knowledge

A problem that remains for the reader who is persuaded of the view presented here is, How do I tell my friends? Trying to convince a pill-popping friend not to take pills and powders can easily turn into the unfortunate experience of losing the friend. Dr. Alfred E. Harper, Ph.D., professor of nutritional sciences, University of Wisconsin, has put it like this: "Isn't it amazing how, when you explain to someone that what they have accepted as fact is not so, they become angry with *you* rather than with the person who gave them the inaccurate information in the first place."[15] Yes, it is amazing and painful. But the response is not surprising when you recall that the person who has paid his or her own money as the price for believing a bogus fact has a personal stake in having the fact be true.

To avoid alienating the people we try to reach with valid information, we can adopt several strategies. For one thing, we can always acknowledge the validity of the feelings and values that underlie these practices. Then, we can make ourselves responsible for learning the facts of the matter as thoroughly as we can, getting them all in perspective, and communicating them clearly. Finally, we can distinguish between practices that are dangerous and those that are merely neutral. We can ignore the neutral ones and confront only the dangerous ones.

To demonstrate this skill, let us rank some items selected by a friend who, with great enthusiasm for nutrition, takes huge stockpiles of nutrient supplements. Let's say that at breakfast, this person takes 500 milligrams of vitamin C, 1000 units of vitamin E, several tablespoons of **nutritional yeast,** some **kelp** tablets, several different pills containing vitamins A and D, a **spirulina** tablet, some **green pills,** and assorted other pills containing trace minerals. This

Miniglossary (continued)

optimal nutrition: the best possible nutrition; distinct from merely adequate nutrition, which characterizes the person who has no overt deficiency signs. This term describes people free of marginal deficiencies, imbalances, and toxicities, and who is not at risk for them.

powdered bone: a nutrient supplement made from bone, intended to supply calcium and other bone minerals.

safety index: a numerical statement of the safety of high doses of nutrients. A safety index of 5, for example, means that doses up to 5 times the U.S. RDA are safe.

spirulina: a kind of algae ("blue-green manna") said to contain large amounts of vitamin B_{12} and to suppress appetite. It does neither.

subclinical deficiency (also called a *marginal deficiency):* a nutrient deficiency that has no visible or otherwise detectable (clinical) symptoms. It is possible for such a deficiency to develop, but the term is often used as a scare tactic to persuade consumers to buy nutrient supplements they don't need.

supplement: a preparation (such as a pill, powder, or liquid) containing nutrients; not a food. Breakfast cereals that contain "100 percent of the U.S. RDA" for certain nutrients are defined by law as dietary supplements, not foods. See also Chapter 10.

wheat germ: the oily embryo of the wheat kernel, rich in nutrients.

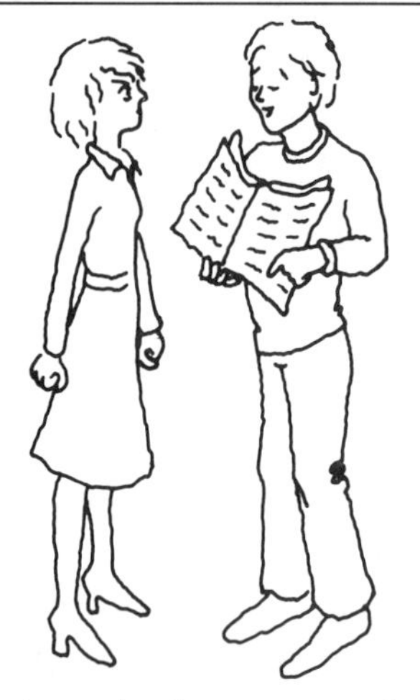

Isn't it amazing how angry people can become when you tell them the facts?

person sprinkles **dessicated liver, powdered bone, bone meal, garlic oil,** and **wheat germ** on a bowl of **granola,** then pours powdered nonfat milk over it all. Where would you begin?

- Most risky: the A and D capsule and the minerals, because overdoses are a real possibility and have serious ill effects.
- Next: the nutritional yeast (it is not needed, and may contribute to B vitamin overdose); the powdered bone (the calcium from such a source is very poorly absorbed, and some bone meal has been found to contain high levels of lead), and the kelp tablets (which may contain too much iodine and even arsenic, a poison and a possible cancer-causing agent[16]).
- Next: the vitamin C and the vitamin E. These are not the highest doses people take and get away with, but they are high enough to be toxic in some individuals. (See Chapter 6 for more about vitamin toxicity.)
- Next: the desiccated liver. Using it may be a neutral practice (although it is high in cholesterol, and the liver is an organ that concentrates toxins); it is easy to get the nutrients delivered in ordinary foods, but there may be no harm in this practice other than to the wallet.
- Last: the wheat germ, the granola, and the powdered nonfat milk. These are nutritious foods, they can be bought in the grocery store, and the nonfat milk in particular is an economical source of valuable nutrients.

In counseling the user of megasupplements, you might offer a caution about the use of the potent supplements listed first and keep your own counsel about the remaining ones unless you are asked. This way you may preserve your friendship, and you may provide a substantial boost to exactly what the person treasures most—good health.

Notes

1. $2.9 billion for vitamins, *FDA Consumer,* April 1987, p. 4.
2. Marginal vitamin deficiency, *Nutrition and the MD,* July 1983.
3. Thiamin and wound repair, *Nutrition Reviews* 40 (1982): 316–318.
4. D. Heber and W. Mertz, Food versus pills versus fortified foods, *Dairy Council Digest,* March-April 1987; A. E. Harper, "Nutrition insurance"—A skeptical view, *Nutrition Forum,* May 1987, pp. 33–37.
5. Santa Barbara physician warns of vitamin overdosing, *California Council against Health Fraud Newsletter,* March/April 1983, p. 2.
6. Nutrient toxicity: A special report, *Nutrition Reviews* 39 (1981): 249–256.
7. Heber and Mertz, 1987.
8. Heber and Mertz, 1987.
9. N. Kurinij, M. A. Klebanoff, and B. I. Graubard, Dietary supplement and food intake in women of childbearing age, *Journal of the American Dietetic Association* 86 (1986): 1536–1540.
10. S. J. A. Bowerman and I. Harrell, Nutrient consumption of individuals taking or not taking nutrient supplements, *Journal of the American Dietetic Association* 83 (1983): 298–305.
11. Heber and Mertz, 1987.
12. The societies that joined to make this statement were the American Dietetic Association, the American Society for Clinical Nutrition, and the American Institute of Nutrition. The American Medical Association reviewed it and endorsed it. Heber and Mertz, 1987.
13. Heber and Mertz, 1987.
14. This discussion is adapted with permission from L. K. DeBruyne and S. R. Rolfes, *Selection of Supplements* (a 1987 monograph in the *Nutrition Clinics* Series available from Stickley Publishing Co., 210 Washington Square, Philadelphia, PA 19106).
15. A. E. Harper, Science and the consumer, *Journal of Nutrition Education* 11 (1979): 171.
16. FDA request for lead warning rejected, *Nutrition Week,* 9 June 1983, p. 6; V. Herbert and G. Drivas, *Spirulina* and vitamin B_{12}, *Journal of the American Medical Association* 248 (1982): 3096–3097; Spirulina discounted (update), *FDA Consumer,* September 1981, p. 3.

Chapter Seven

Contents

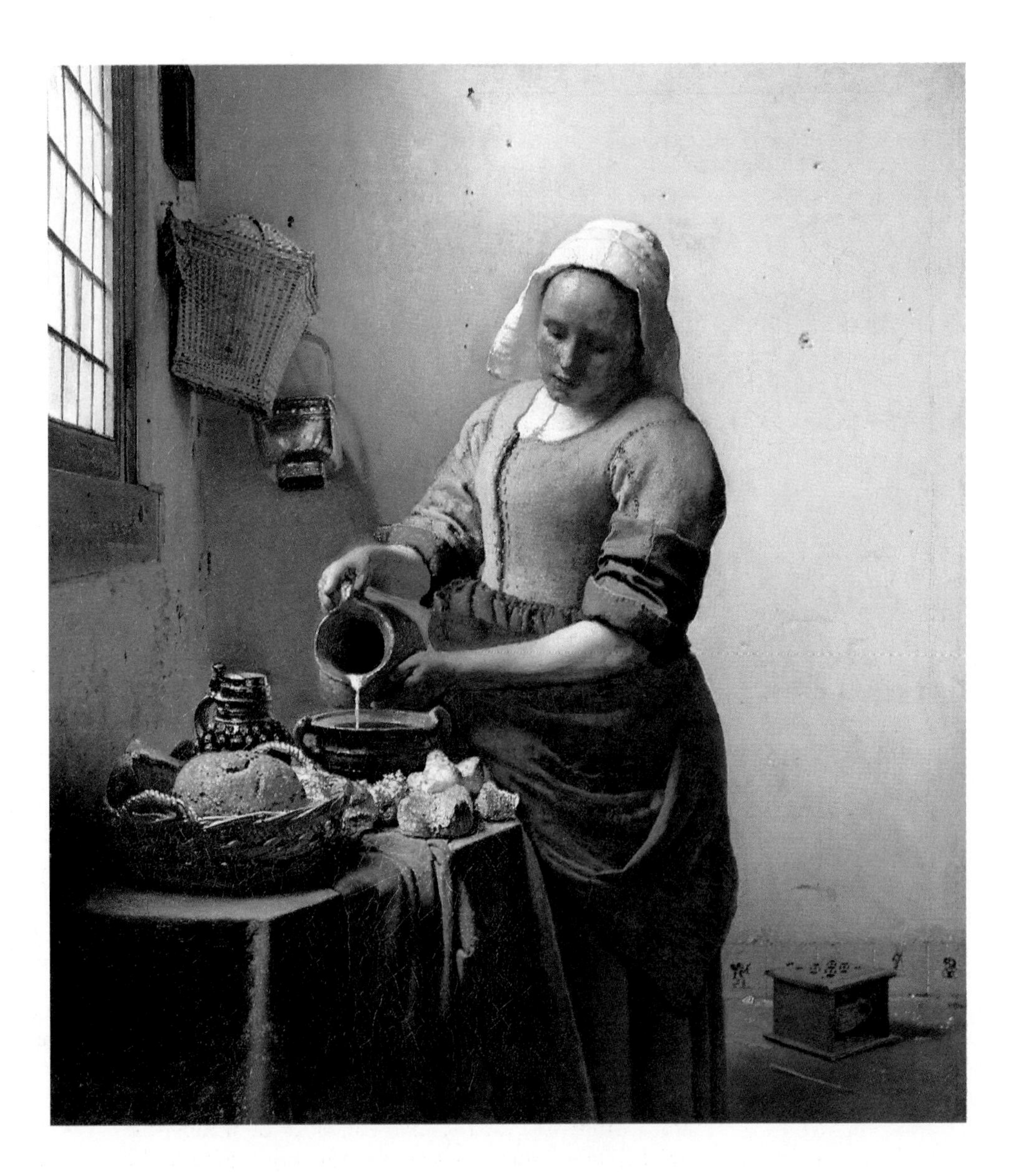

The Milkmaid by Johannes Vermeer. The Rijksmuseum, Amsterdam.

Minerals and Water

"Ashes to ashes and dust to dust." This familiar quotation is used often to remind us of our mortality. Perhaps we need this reminder to put our own importance into perspective, and it is true that when the life force leaves the body, what is left behind ultimately becomes nothing more than a small pile of ashes. Carbohydrates, proteins, fats, vitamins, and water are present at first, but they soon disappear.

The carbon atoms in all the carbohydrates, fats, proteins, and vitamins combine with oxygen to produce carbon dioxide, which vanishes into the air; the hydrogens and oxygens of those compounds unite to form water; and this water, along with the water that was a large part of the body weight, evaporates. The ashes that are left behind are the **minerals,** a small pile of only about 5 pounds. The pile is not impressive in size, but when you consider the tasks these minerals perform, you may realize their great importance in living tissue.

Consider calcium and phosphorus. If you could separate these two minerals from the rest of the pile, you would take away about three-fourths of the total. Crystals made of these two minerals, plus a few others, form the structure of the bones and so provide the architecture of the skeleton.

Run a magnet through the one-fourth of the pile that remains and pick up the iron. It would not fill a teaspoon, but it is billions of billions of iron atoms. As part of billions of protein molecules, these iron atoms have the special property of being able to attach to oxygen and make it available at the sites where metabolic work is taking place, deep inside the body.

If you were able to extract all the other minerals, leaving only copper and iodine in the pile of ashes, you would want to close the windows before you did it. A slight breeze would blow these remaining bits of dust away. Yet the copper in the dust is the catalyst necessary for iron to hold and release oxygen, and iodine is the critical mineral in the hormone thyroxine. Figure 7–1 shows the amounts of **major minerals** and a few of the **trace minerals** in the human body.

The distinction between the major and the trace minerals doesn't mean that one group is more important than the other. A deficiency of the few micrograms of iodine needed daily by the body is just as serious as a deficiency of the several hundred milligrams of calcium. However, the major minerals, because of their larger total quantities, influence the body fluids, and so affect the whole body in a general way as well as playing specific roles.

This chapter begins with a discussion of the characteristics of water—the most indispensable nutrient of all—and then goes on to show how some of the major minerals affect it. Then the chapter discusses the minerals that play specialized roles.

minerals: naturally occurring, inorganic, homogeneous substances; chemical elements

major minerals: essential mineral nutrients found in the human body in amounts larger than 5 g.

trace minerals: essential mineral nutrients found in the human body in amounts less than 5 g.

Only 25 chemical elements are essential to life:

- Carbon.
- Hydrogen.
- Oxygen.
- Nitrogen.
- Major minerals:
  - Calcium.
  - Chlorine.
  - Magnesium.
  - Phosphorus.
  - Potassium.
  - Sodium.
  - Sulfur.
- Trace minerals:
  - Chromium.
  - Cobalt.
  - Copper.
  - Fluorine.
  - Iodine.
  - Iron.
  - Manganese.
  - Molybdenum.
  - Nickel.
  - Selenium.
  - Silicon.
  - Tin.
  - Vanadium.
  - Zinc.

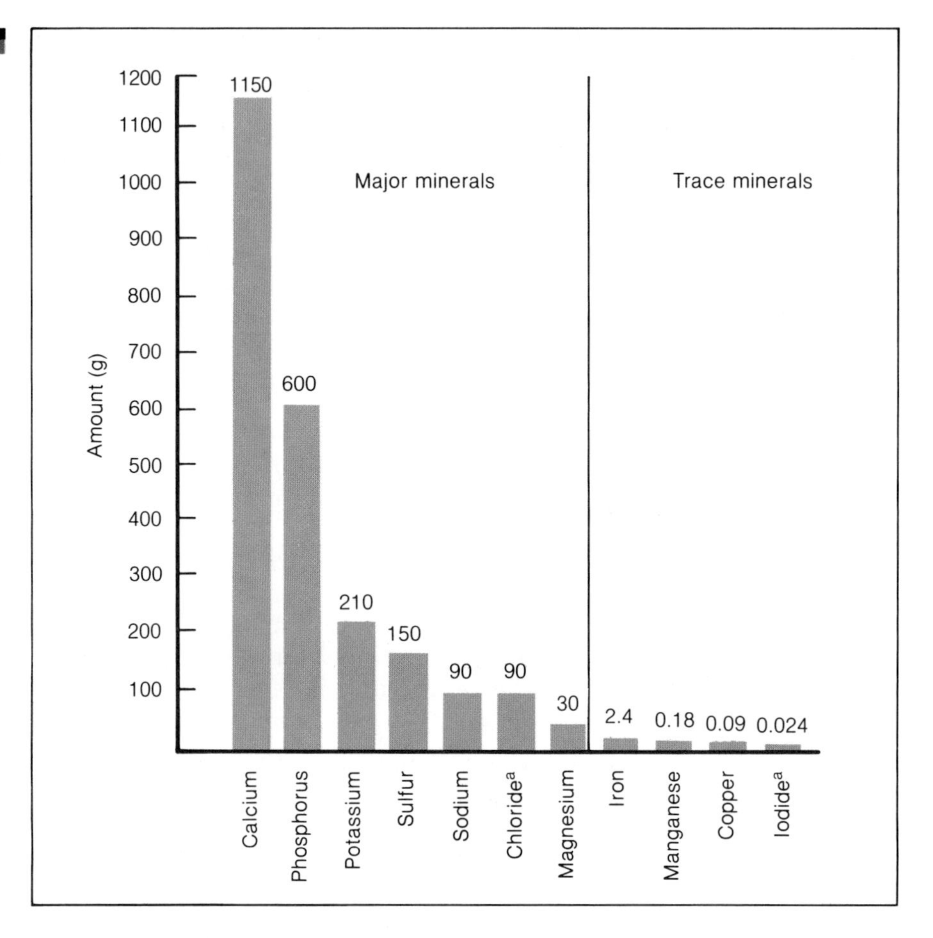

Figure 7–1 Minerals in a 60-kg Person. The major minerals are those present in amounts larger than 5 grams (a teaspoon). The trace minerals number a dozen or more; only four are shown. A pound is about 454 grams; thus only calcium and phosphorus appear in amounts larger than a pound.

[a]Chlorine and iodine appear in the body as the ions chloride and iodide, and hence are referred to as such.

Water

You began life as a single cell bathed in a nourishing fluid. Even after you became a beautifully organized, air-breathing body of billions of cells, each individual cell had to remain next to water to remain alive. That water brings to each cell the exact ingredients it requires and carries away the end products of the life-sustaining reactions that take place within its boundaries.

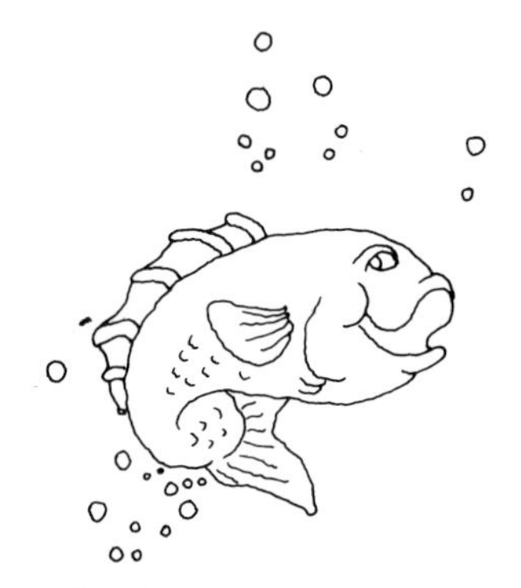

We, too, live in water.

Water in the body is not simply a river coursing through the arteries, capillaries, and veins. Some of the water is part of the chemical structure of compounds that form the cells, tissues, and organs of the body. For example, proteins hold water molecules within them. This water is locked in and is not readily available for any other use. Water also participates actively in many chemical reactions.

Boasting scientist: I'm working on discovering the universal solvent.

Skeptical backwoodsman: Is that so? Well, when you've got it, what are you going to keep it in?

As the medium for the body's traffic of nutrients and waste products, water is nearly a universal solvent. Luckily for our physical integrity, this is not quite the case, but water does dissolve amino acids, glucose, minerals, and many other substances needed by the cells. Fatty substances are specially packaged with water-soluble proteins so that they too can travel freely in the blood and lymph. Water is thus the transport vehicle for all the nutrients.

Another important characteristic of water is its incompressibility. Its molecules resist being crowded together. Thanks to this characteristic, water can act as a lubricant around joints. For the same reason, it can protect a sensitive tissue such as the spinal cord from shock. The fluid that fills the eye serves in a similar way to keep optimal pressure on the retina and lens. The unborn infant is cushioned against shock by the bag of amniotic fluid in which it develops. Water also lubricates the digestive tract and all tissues moistened with mucus.

Still another of water's special features is its heat-holding capacity. This characteristic of water is familiar to coastal dwellers, who know that land surrounded by water is protected from wide variations in temperature from day to night. Water itself changes temperature slowly; at night, when the land cools, the water gives up its heat gradually to the air, moderating the coolness of the night. In contrast, the desert has a wide variation in temperature from day to night because it is dry. Similarly, water helps to maintain body temperature. A great deal of heat is required to change water from a liquid to a gas, so when we sweat, the evaporated water carries off large quantities of body heat.

Life is possible on earth because of a fascinating characteristic of water. Although water contracts like other substances as it gets colder, it abandons this behavior at 4 degrees Centigrade and then expands as it cools down to 0 and freezes. Ice is therefore *lighter* than cold water, and so it floats. This protects the water beneath the ice from the coldness of the air. Thus living things in pond water below ice can survive through hard winters, even when the temperature of the air goes many degrees below freezing. If ice were to sink, instead of float, ponds and lakes would freeze from the bottom up, they would become solid and colder than freezing temperature, and all living things in them would die.

Water provides the medium for transportation, chemical reactions, protection, lubrication, and temperature regulation in the human body.

The Water Supply

When you draw water from the tap into a glass and drink it, it is not only water that you are drinking. Chlorine may have been added to it, to kill microorganisms that might otherwise convey disease. Fluoride may have been added to it, if your community has adopted fluoridation. In addition, it contains naturally occurring minerals, toxic heavy metals, live microorganisms, and a miscellany of organic compounds.

The distinction between **hard water** and **soft water,** which has some important health implications, is based on three minerals. Hard water has high concentrations of calcium and magnesium. Soft water's principal mineral is sodium. Most people distinguish between these two types of water in practical terms. Soft water makes more bubbles with less soap; hard water leaves a ring on the tub, a jumble of rocklike crystals in the teakettle, and a gray residue in the wash. Hence consumers often consider soft water to be the more desirable and may even purchase water-softening equipment, which removes magnesium and calcium and replaces them with sodium. However, soft water can add appreciable sodium to people's diets, and it appears to contribute to a higher incidence of hypertension and heart disease in areas where it is used. About half

hard water: water with a high calcium and magnesium concentration.

soft water: water containing a high sodium concentration.

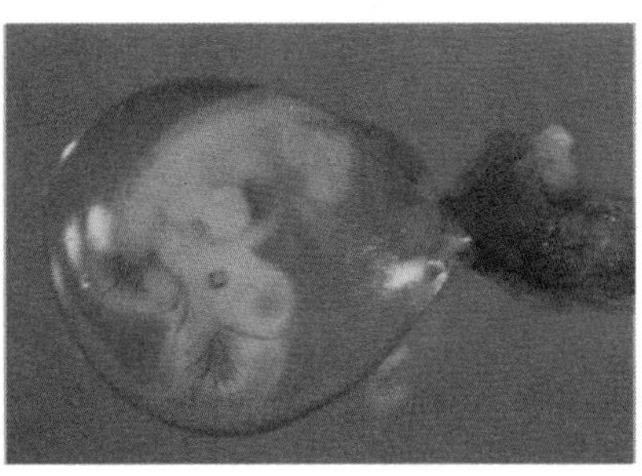

Life begins in water.

of the U.S. population drinks water containing more than 20 milligrams of sodium per liter—an amount small enough not to matter to healthy people, but enough to be significant to persons who must restrict their sodium intakes severely. (Controversy 7 takes up the issue of nutrition and hypertension.)

Soft water also dissolves certain metals, such as cadmium and lead, from pipes. Cadmium is not an essential nutrient. In fact, it can harm the body, affecting at least some enzymes by displacing zinc from its normal sites of action. Cadmium is also suspected of promoting hypertension. Lead is another toxic metal, and the body seems to absorb it more readily from soft than from hard water—possibly because the calcium in hard water protects against its absorption.

The examples just given show that the choice to install a water softener in your home may be unwise, especially if your family is prone to heart disease. One family we know solves the problem by connecting the water softener only to the hot-water line, then using hot water for washing and bathing, and only cold water for cooking and drinking.

Ordinary groundwater does not normally contain toxic heavy metals. In the wilderness, water cycles rapidly through living systems, undergoing a natural purifying process in every cycle. Animal waste excreted onto the earth is filtered out by the soil and never arrives in underground water. Pollutants entering rivers quickly disappear back into the earth as the rivers flow along, leaving the water pure. But neither the earth nor its rivers can purify completely the heavily polluted water expelled as city sewage or industrial waste. Water leaving a factory may contain concentrations of toxic metals so high that some are still present when it is recycled to become drinking water. And if the water is cycled through the same factory again, it will contain still higher concentrations the next time around.

Human technology bears the burden of purifying water contaminated by human technology. The Public Health Service sets drinking water standards (upper limits for the amounts of toxic substances permitted in water), and public law distributes the responsibility for adhering to these standards among the industries and the water-processing plants.

The metals of greatest concern are mercury, cadmium, and lead. These metals may be absorbed into the body, where they change cell membrane structure, alter enzyme or coenzyme functions, or even change the structure of the genetic material DNA, causing cancer or birth defects. If they happen to alter the DNA in the eggs or sperm, the changes (mutations) will become hereditary. When combined with organic compounds, these metals may be absorbed especially rapidly and may damage body tissue even more.

In contrast to heavy metals, bacteria are an expected and natural constituent of the water supply. Many harmless, even beneficial, bacteria dwell in the human digestive tract and are excreted into sewage. If these were the only inhabitants of sewage, there would be no concern about their presence in drinking water. But disease organisms are also excreted into sewage, and others are introduced into it by flies and other carriers. Before a sewage treatment plant releases water into the public water supply, it must reduce the bacterial count enough so that the further dilution that follows will make recycled water safe for drinking.

High standards for sewage treatment in the developed countries ensure that most people's drinking water is safe, but for the rest of the world, microbial contamination remains the primary cause of human diseases and epidemics. Two of the most basic public health needs of the world's people are safe drinking water and an acceptable standard of waste disposal.

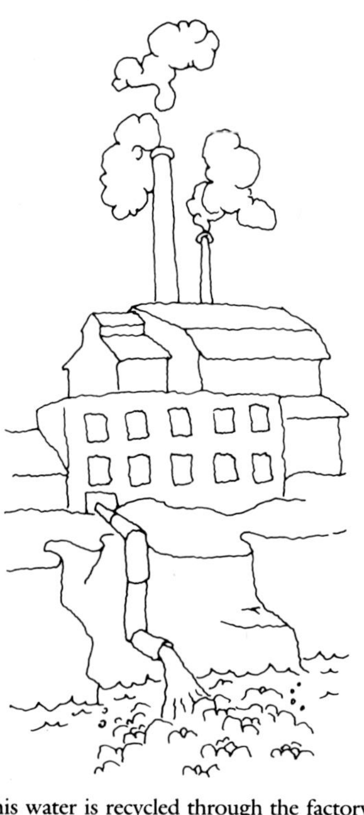

If this water is recycled through the factory, it will be more polluted the next time.

The fourth class of substances that may occur in water is organic compounds from sewage, insecticides, petroleum-based industries, and elsewhere. Research on these substances is less than 25 years old, and few of them have been identified, but many are known to be toxic. Some cause birth defects; some cause cancer; some cause mutations of the genes. Many contain chlorine, and some may be formed during the chlorination of water. No information is available on the risks now presented by water containing these compounds; standards are only now being established, and if public water exceeds them, new filtering systems may be called for.

In some regions, people have become alarmed about their local water supplies and have turned to buying bottled water. The choice is an individual matter. However, in buying water, as in buying any other product, the consumer needs to be alert to fraudulent claims. Mineral waters from "famous spas" offer no known health advantages and may be undesirably high in sodium. Manufacturers use scare tactics to try to convince people to spend money on useless water-purifying tablets or machines. On the other hand, bottled water sold in the United States must be tested by the producers once a year to be sure that its purity at least equals that required of all public water supplies.

The quality of drinking water can be affected by the minerals, heavy metals, micro-organisms, and organic compounds it contains. Hard water is high in calcium and magnesium; soft water is high in sodium and dissolves cadmium and lead from pipes. Industry pollutes water with toxic metals. Human diseases can be transmitted through water supplies. Pollutants from industry can cause cancer or birth defects. Strict quality regulations are necessary to prevent hazards.

dehydration: loss of water. The symptoms progress rapidly from thirst through weakness to exhaustion and delirium, and end in death.

water intoxication: the condition in which body water content is too high. Symptoms are headache, muscular weakness, lack of concentration, poor memory, and loss of appetite.

water balance: the balance between water intake and water excretion, which keeps the body's water content constant.

solutes (SOLL-yutes): dissolved substances.

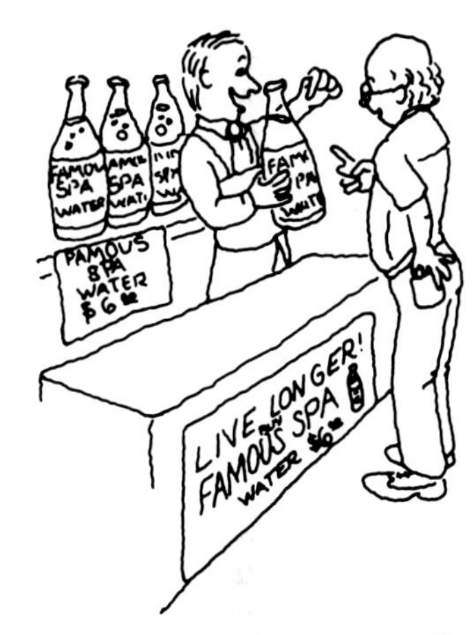

Mineral waters from "famous spas" offer no health advantage and may be undesirably high in sodium.

The Body Fluids

Water makes up about 60 percent of the body's weight. It is such an integral part of us that people seldom are conscious of its importance—unless they are deprived of it. You can survive a deficiency of any of the other nutrients for long times, some of them even for months or years, but you can survive only a few days without water. Since the body's self-purification process requires that it excrete at least a quart of water a day, a person must drink that much each day to avoid life-threatening losses.

The total amount of fluid in the body is kept constant by delicate balancing mechanisms. Imbalances can occur—**dehydration** and **water intoxication**—but they are restored to normal as promptly as the body can manage it. Both intake and excretion are controlled to maintain **water balance.**

Nearly all foods contain some water, and some are over 90 percent water. The energy-yielding nutrients in them give rise to additional water as they are oxidized during the breakdown process. The remainder of the water that you need comes from beverages.

Thirst and satiety govern water intake. When the blood is too concentrated (having lost water, but not salt and other **solutes**), its solutes attract water out of the salivary glands. The mouth becomes dry as a result, and you drink to wet your mouth. The brain center known as the hypothalamus (described in Chapter 1) also monitors the solute concentration of the blood, and when it finds it too high, initiates impulses that stimulate drinking behavior. The blood volume also plays a role: thirsty animals drink until nerves in their hearts, known

ions (EYE-ons): electrically charged particles, such as sodium (positively charged) or chloride (negatively charged).

electrolytes: compounds that partly dissociate in water to form ions.

as stretch receptors, are stimulated enough to turn off the drinking.[1] Thirst adjusts to provide a water intake that exactly meets the need.

Thirst lags behind water lack, though. A water deficiency that develops slowly can switch on drinking behavior in time to prevent serious dehydration, but one that develops fast may not. Also, thirst itself does not remedy a water deficiency; drinking does. You have to notice that you are thirsty, pay attention, and take the time to get a drink. The athlete, the long-distance casual runner, the gardener in hot weather, and the elderly person whose attention wanders can experience serious dehydration; they need to learn to notice consciously their need for water and drink promptly in response to it. (Chapter 9 offers more on the fluid needs of active people.)

Water excretion is governed by the brain and the kidneys. The hypothalamus senses when the body's salt concentration is too high and calls forth a hormone from the pituitary gland that directs the kidneys to shift water back into the bloodstream from the pool destined for excretion. The kidneys themselves also respond to the salt concentration in the blood passing through them and secrete regulatory substances of their own. The net result is that the more water the body needs, the less it excretes. Still, there is a minimum amount of water that the body must excrete in order to carry off waste materials in the urine and feces, to generate sweat, and to evaporate in the lungs, and a minimum must be drunk each day to replace that water. Table 7–1 shows how intake and excretion naturally balance out.

It is never a bad idea to drink extra water. Water never accumulates in the body of a healthy person; the urine simply becomes more dilute. The only conceivable hazard is that in excreting the water, the body can lose too much salt, but normally, food intake ensures adequate salt intake.

About 40 percent of the body's water weight is found inside the cells, and about 15 percent bathes the outsides of the cells. The remainder is in the blood vessels. Special conditions are needed so that the cells do not collapse from water leaving them or swell up under the stress of too much water entering them. The cells cannot manage this by pumping water across their membranes, because water slips in and out freely. However, they can pump minerals across their membranes, and these minerals attract the water to come along with them. The cells use minerals for this purpose in a special form: as **ions** or **electrolytes**—single, electrically charged particles.

Table 7–1

Water Balance

Source	Water Received by the Body (ml)	Water Excreted by the Body (ml)	Excretion Route
Liquids	500 to 1500	500 to 1400	Urine
Foods	700 to 1000	350	Lungs
Water generated by the metabolism		150	Feces
of energy nutrients	200 to 300	450 to 900	Sweat
	1450 to 2800 (about 1 to 2 qt)	1450 to 2800 (about 1 to 2 qt)	

Figure 7–2 shows how the body uses electrolytes to move its fluids around. The result of the system's working properly is **fluid and electrolyte balance**—the proper amount and kind of fluid in every compartment of the body.

If something happens to overwhelm this balance, severe illness can result quickly, for fluid can shift rapidly from one compartment to another. For example, in vomiting or diarrhea, the loss of water from the intestinal tract pulls fluid from between the cells in every part of the body. Fluid then leaves the inside of the cells to restore balance. Meanwhile, the kidneys detect the water loss and attempt to retrieve water from the pool destined for excretion. To do this, they raise the sodium concentration outside the cells, and this pulls still more water out of them. When this happens, the very serious condition of **fluid and electrolyte imbalance** occurs. Water and minerals lost in vomiting or diarrhea ultimately drain every body cell.

The minerals help manage still another balancing act—the **acid-base balance,** already mentioned in Chapter 5. Among the major minerals, some give rise to acids, some to bases, when dissolved in water. A small percentage of water molecules (H_2O) also exist as positive and negative ions—H (positive) and OH (negative). Excess H ions in a solution make it an acid; excess OH ions make it a base.

The body's proteins and some of its minerals, as part of salts, prevent changes in the acid-base balance of its fluids by serving as **buffers**—molecules that gather up or release H ions as needed. The kidneys help control the balance by excreting more or less acid, and the lungs help control it by excreting more or less carbon dioxide (in solution in the blood, carbon dioxide forms an acid, carbonic acid). The maintenance of the acid-base balance by means of these tight controls permits all other life processes to take place.

fluid and electrolyte balance: maintenance of the proper amount and kind of fluid in each compartment of the body.

fluid and electrolyte imbalance: failure to maintain the proper amount and kind of fluid in every body compartment; a medical emergency.

acid-base balance: maintenance of the proper degree of acidity in each of the body's fluids.

buffers: compounds that can help keep the acidity of a solution from changing by neutralizing acids and bases.

Water makes up about 60% of the body's weight. Obligatory water losses amounting to over a quart a day necessitate daily consumption of the same amount. Electrolytes in the body fluid provide and help buffer the environment in which all life processes take place.

The Major Minerals

While all the major minerals help maintain water balance and acid-base balance, each also plays some special roles of its own. These roles are described in the following sections. The order does not imply that the first are the most important.

Calcium

Many people have the idea that calcium and phosphorus, once deposited in bone, stay there forever—that once a bone is built, it is inert, like a rock. Not so. Bones are in a state of constant flux, with formation and dissolution taking place every minute of the day and night.

Calcium is essential to the formation of bone (see Figure 7–3). As bones begin to form, calcium salts, along with some other minerals, particularly fluor-

Figure 7–2 Fluids and Electrolytes. Water goes where the dissolved particles are, because it is attracted to them. The body therefore regulates its water distribution by distributing its particles into the spaces where it "wants" water.

All matter is in constant motion; that is, the atoms and molecules of matter are in constant motion. This motion is not visible to the eye but is no less real. Because of it, the molecules of two adjacent liquids or solids mingle with each other. The direction of the **diffusion** of a substance is toward the place of lower concentration of the substance. For example, a person far from the kitchen can detect the frying of breakfast bacon. The molecules of the odor diffuse from the kitchen to the bedroom. Eventually, the bacon smell will be the same in both rooms, and although back-and-forth diffusion will continue, the odor will not again become concentrated in either room.

This movement of an odor in air is an example of a gas diffusing in a gas. You have seen a liquid diffuse in a liquid when you poured cream into a cup of coffee. Even without stirring, you could watch the cream molecules diffuse into the coffee. Two substances separated by a membrane can even diffuse through the membrane until their concentrations on both sides are equal.

Sometimes a membrane will allow water to pass through it, but will hold back certain particles. Then a force is created. The force is **osmotic pressure.** For example, if concentrated salt particles cannot flow out of a cell (because they cannot penetrate its membrane), then water will flow into the cell to dilute them. Water will move from a dilute solution to a strong solution until the *concentration* of particles is the same in both. There will then be more water where there are more particles and less water where there are fewer particles. The simplest way to state how osmotic pressure moves water from one side of a membrane to the other is to say that "water follows salt."

You have seen this force at work if you have ever salted a lettuce salad and let it stand a half hour before eating it. When you returned to it, the lettuce was wilted, and the salad bowl had water in it. The water had shifted out of the cells toward the higher concentration of salt. The lettuce cells had collapsed when they lost their fluid contents.

Water can flow freely across the membranes of most cells inside the body, but minerals cannot. Therefore, the cells use minerals to keep the water in the needed amounts in different places. The sodium ion is the main positive ion used for this purpose outside of cells, and the potassium ion is the main one used inside of cells. The negative chloride ion is used in association with both. Proteins in the cell membranes act as pumps to keep each ion in its proper compartment. As long as the body stays healthy, the cells' fluid contents will be maintained this way.

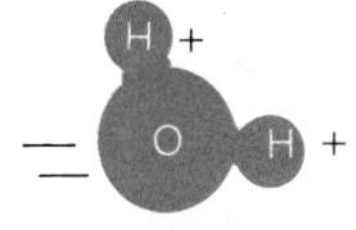

A. Water is electrically neutral but lopsided, so it has a positively charged side and a negatively charged side.

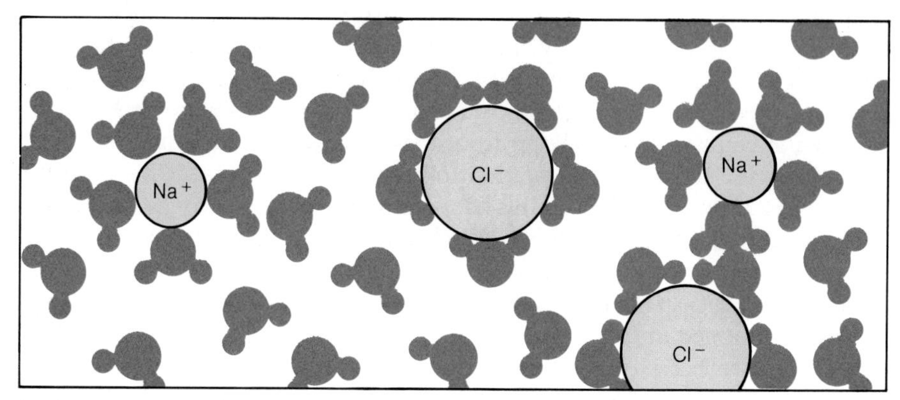

B. In an electrolyte solution, therefore, water molecules are attracted to both the positively and negatively charged ions. Notice that the negative oxygen atoms of the water molecules are drawn to the sodium ion (Na^+) here, while the positive sides of the water molecules are drawn to the chloride ions (Cl^-).

C. This is a simplified version of how water moves across boundaries to get next to dissolved particles.

1. With equal numbers of solute particles on both sides, there are equal amounts of water:

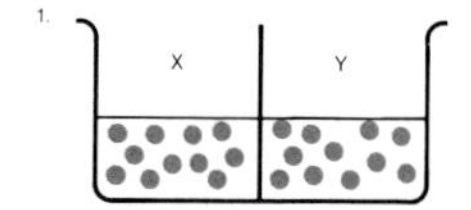

2. Now additional solute is added to side Y. Solute cannot flow across the divider:

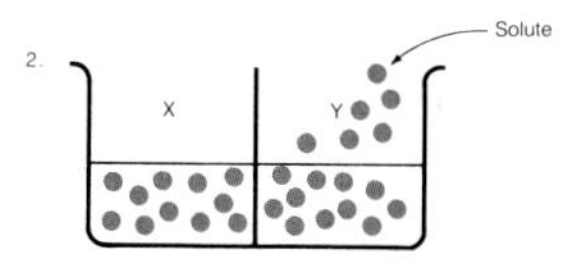

3. Water does flow across the divider, and it tends to remain on side Y, where there is more solute. The *volume* of water becomes greater on side Y, and the *concentrations* on sides X and Y become equal:

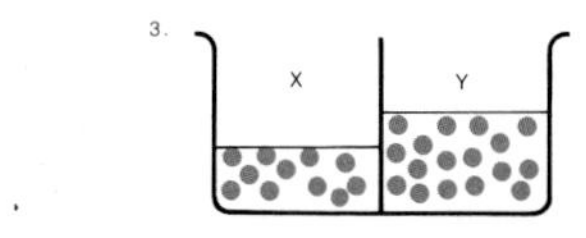

4. Now suppose that pressure (such as a pump) compresses the fluid on side Y. The amount of pressure just sufficient to restore the original volume would equal the *osmotic pressure* exerted by the added particles:

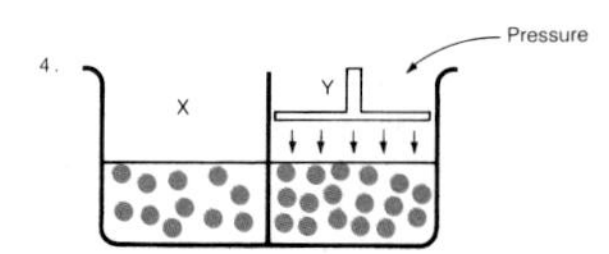

ide, lay down crystals on a foundation material composed of the protein collagen. These crystals, called **hydroxyapatite,** invade the collagen and gradually lend more and more rigidity to the maturing bones, until they are able to support the weight they will have to carry. Thus the long leg bones of children can support their weight by the time they have learned to walk. (Chapter 6 showed that the increase in length of the long bones involves a dismantling step for which vitamin A is essential, that vitamin C is needed for collagen to form, and that vitamin D helps make calcium available for the assembly process.)

The formation of teeth follows a pattern similar to that of bones (see Figure 7–4). Hydroxyapatite crystals form on a collagen matrix to create the enamel that gives strength to the teeth. Calcification of the "baby" teeth occurs in the gums during the latter half of the infant's time in the womb. The calcification of the permanent teeth takes place during early childhood, up to about the age of three; that of the "wisdom" teeth begins at about the age of ten. There is not such a rapid turnover of calcium in teeth as there is in bone, but some withdrawal and redepositing does take place throughout life. Fluoride hardens and stabilizes the crystals of both bones and teeth, opposing the withdrawal of minerals from them for excretion or use in other parts of the body.

About 99 percent of the calcium in the body is in the bones and teeth; less than 1 percent is in the fluid that bathes the cells; and an even smaller amount is inside the cells. These minute amounts play major roles, however. In addition to its structural roles, calcium:

- Regulates the transport of ions across cell membranes and is particularly important in nerve transmission.
- Helps maintain normal blood pressure (see Controversy 7).
- Is essential for muscle contraction and therefore for the maintenance of the heartbeat.
- Plays an essential role in the clotting of blood.
- Maintains the "glue" that holds cells together.

With such major roles to play, calcium must be furnished to the cells on demand. The body accomplishes this by maintaining a constant calcium con-

diffusion: the process by which a substance tends to distribute itself evenly throughout the available space.

osmotic (os-MOT-ic) **pressure, osmosis** (os-MOH-sis): the force that moves water into a space where a solute, such as sodium chloride, is more concentrated (*osmos* means "pushing").

hydroxyapatite: the chief crystal of bone, formed from calcium and phosphorus. (See also *fluorapatite*, p. 252.)

Blood travels in capillaries throughout the bone. It brings nutrients to the cells that maintain the bone's structure, and carries away waste materials from those cells. It picks up and deposits minerals as instructed by hormones.

This bone derives its structural strength from the lacy network of crystals that lie along the bone's lines of stress. If minerals are withdrawn to cover deficits elsewhere in the body, the bone will grow weak, and ultimately will crumble.

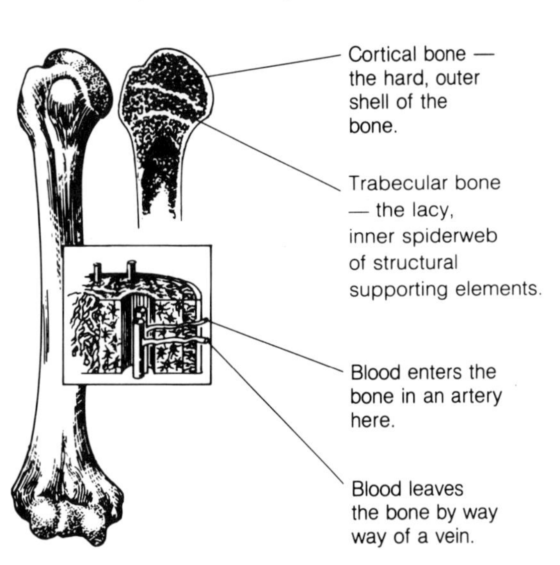

Figure 7–3 A Bone.

osteoporosis (OSS-tee-oh-pore-OH-sis), also known as **adult bone loss:** a disease of older persons in which the bone becomes porous and brittle (*osteo* means "bones"; *poros* means "porous").

centration in the blood. To this end, the skeleton serves as a bank: calcium can be borrowed and returned as needed. Withdrawals and deposits of calcium are not at the mercy of the amount taken in food but are regulated by hormones sensitive to blood levels of calcium.* This means you can go without dietary calcium for years and never suffer a noticeable symptom. Only late in life will you suddenly discover that your savings account has dwindled to the point where the integrity of your skeleton can no longer be maintained—that throughout your adult years you have been incurring **osteoporosis,** or **adult bone loss.** (The vitamin D deficiency diseases rickets in children and osteomalacia in adults involve softening and bending of the bones as described in Chapter 6; osteoporosis involves the bones' becoming brittle and shattering.)

Adult bone loss occurs in both sexes, but it is four times more prevalent in women than in men after age 50. It occurs in at least one out of every three people over the age of 65. Often it first becomes apparent when someone's hip suddenly gives way. People say, "She fell and broke her hip," but the fact of the matter may be that the hip was so fragile that it broke *before* she fell. Even the slight jarring from stepping down off a curb may be enough to shatter a bone made porous by loss of minerals. The break is not clean; it is an explosion into fragments so numerous and scattered that they cannot be reassembled. It is a struggle to remove them, and it takes major surgery to replace them with an artificial joint. Such a fracture condemns many older people to wheelchairs for the rest of their lives; they will never walk again. About a third die of complications within a year.

The spine is also susceptible to bone loss. Figure 7–5 shows the effect of the loss of spinal bone on a woman's height and posture. It is not inevitable that people "grow shorter" as they age, but it is more likely to happen if they don't take the measures necessary to prevent bone loss.

The consequences of bone loss dramatize the importance of an adequate calcium intake throughout life, but calcium is only one factor needed to prevent osteoporosis. Other nutrient deficiencies, and indeed many other factors, contribute to osteoporosis. Heredity, hormones, alcohol abuse, lack of exercise, prolonged use of prescription drugs, and other drugs all affect the bones. Other nutrients, especially fluoride and vitamin D, also play a role, but calcium deficiency is clearly one of the most important factors.

During periods of growth, intestinal absorption of calcium increases. Infants and children absorb up to 60 percent of ingested calcium; pregnant women, about 50 percent; and other adults, about 30 percent. Deprived of calcium for months or years, an adult may again become able to absorb as much as 60 percent of that available; when supplied for years with abundant calcium, the same person may absorb only 10 percent. It takes time to adjust to changing intakes. Thus it is impossible to rectify a calcium deficiency that has occurred over many years by taking massive supplements for only a few days or weeks.

Because human beings can adjust their calcium absorption to varying levels of intake, setting recommended allowances was difficult. The U.S. and Canadian recommendations for calcium intake are high compared with those of other countries, but are rightly so because most adults in the United States and Canada

Figure 7–4 A Tooth.
The inner layer of dentin is bonelike material that forms on a keratin matrix. The outer layer of enamel, which is harder than bone, forms on a collagen matrix. Both dentin and enamel contain hydroxyapatite crystals (made of calcium and phosphorus); those of enamel may harden with fluoride to become fluorapatite.

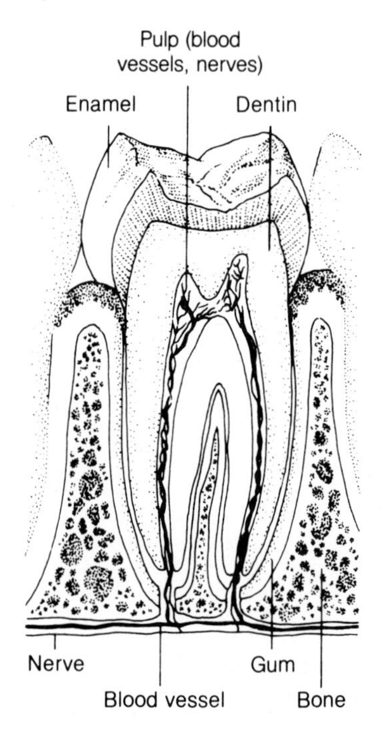

*Calcitonin, made in the thyroid gland, is secreted whenever the calcium concentration in the blood rises too high. It acts to stop withdrawal from bone and to slow absorption from the intestine. Parathormone, from the parathyroid glands, has the opposite effect.

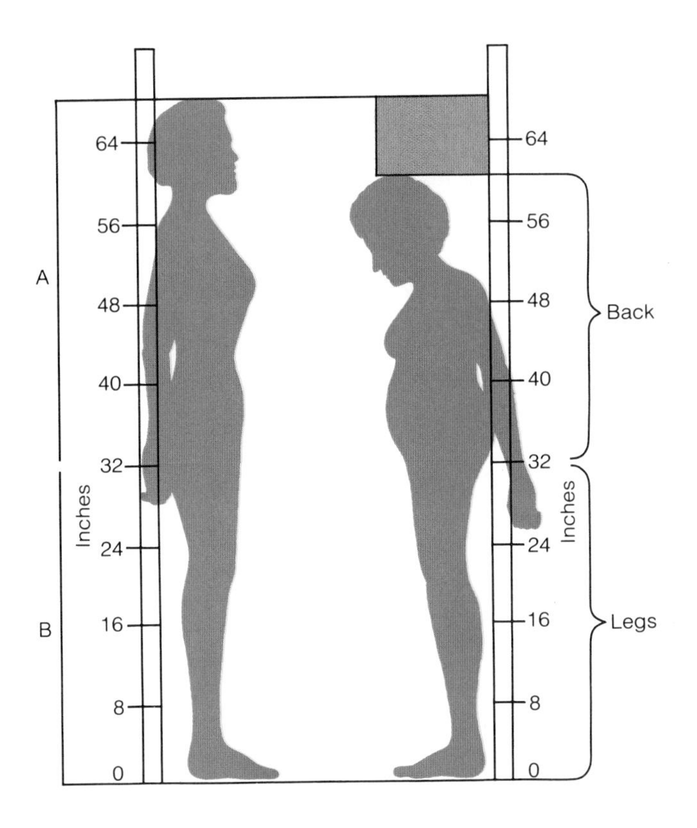

Figure 7–5 Loss of Height in a Woman Caused by Adult Bone Loss.
The woman on the left is about 50 years old. On the right, she is 80 years old. Her legs (B) have not grown shorter; only her back (A) has lost length, due to collapse of her spinal bones (vertebrae). Collapsed vertebrae cannot protect the spinal nerves from pressure that causes excruciating pain.

consume large quantities of meat and other protein-rich foods, which promote the excretion of calcium.

The RDA for calcium has been set at 800 milligrams daily for adults, but women's intakes should perhaps be even higher. More is recommended for a pregnant or lactating woman, because she is supplying calcium to another growing person. Around the time of menopause, women are advised to increase their calcium intakes to the level required during pregnancy, to prevent bone loss.

The simplest and most efficient way to obtain the calcium you need is to drink milk. Everyone knows that children need to drink milk because they are growing. Adults, however, switch to beverages they think are more appropriate to their age: coffee, iced tea, soft drinks, or alcoholic beverages. As they see it, their bones have stopped growing, and they no longer need the calcium milk provides. Nothing could be further from the truth. In fact, it is because high calcium intakes early in life are the best defense against osteoporosis, that this book deals with the disease in this chapter, rather than in the chapter on nutrition in later life. Tables 7–2 and 7–3 show that a reasonable amount of milk or milk products daily can most easily meet one's calcium needs.

People who dislike milk can find substitutes for it. Care is needed, though—*wise* substitutions must be made. Most of milk's many sisters are recommended choices: yogurt, kefir, buttermilk, cheese (especially the low-fat or nonfat varieties) and, for people who can afford the calories, ice milk. Even lactose-intolerant individuals can absorb significant quantities of calcium from milk or fermented milk products if they take them in small, divided doses throughout the day. Some highly reputed milk products are less-than-ideal sources, though. Cottage cheese is only fair, 2 cups being equivalent in calcium to 1 cup of milk.

Table 7–2

Recommended Fluid Milk Intakes

Age	Recommended Intake
Children under 9	2 to 3 c
Children 9 to 12	3+ c
Teenagers	4+ c
Adults	2 c
Pregnant women	3+ c
Lactating women	4+ c
Older women	3 to 5 c

Table 7–3

Food Sources of Calcium Selected to Show a Range of Values

If you eat this size serving of:	You will receive this % of your need[a] of CALCIUM:	If you want 100% of your need[a] of CALCIUM from this food:	You will have to eat this size serving:
Sardines, canned w/bones (3 oz, 175 cal)	37%	Bok choy cabbage, cooked	6 c (120 cal)
Kefir (1 c, 160 cal)	35	Turnip greens, cooked	5 c (145 cal)
Goat milk (1 c, 168 cal)	33	Spinach, canned	3.7 c (185 cal)
Shrimp, boiled (3.5 oz, 109 cal)	32	Dandelion greens, cooked	6.7 c (235 cal)
Romano cheese (1 oz, 110 cal)	30	Broccoli, cooked	5.5 c (253 cal)
Nonfat milk (1 c, 86 cal)	30	Nonfat milk	3.3 c (284 cal)
Swiss cheese (1 oz, 107 cal)	27	Shrimp, boiled	11 oz (338 cal)
Spinach, canned (1 c, 50 cal)	27	Romano cheese	3.3 oz (363 cal)
Cheddar cheese (1 oz, 114 cal)	20	Swiss cheese	3.7 oz (396 cal)
Oysters, raw (1 c, 160 cal)	20	Kefir	2.9 c (464 cal)
Turnip greens, cooked (1 c, 29 cal)	20	Sardines, canned w/bones	8 oz (473 cal)
Broccoli, cooked (1 c, 46 cal)	18	Goat milk	3 c (504 cal)
Salmon, canned w/bones (3 oz, 120 cal)	17	Cheddar cheese	5 oz (570 cal)
Bok choy cabbage, cooked (1 c, 20 cal)	16	Salmon, canned w/bones	17 oz (684 cal)
Dandelion greens, cooked (1 c, 35 cal)	15	Oysters, raw	5 c (800 cal)
Sirloin steak, lean (8 oz, 480 cal)	3	Whole wheat bread	50 sl (3500 cal)
Whole wheat bread (1 sl, 70 cal)	2	Apple, fresh medium	100 apples (8000 cal)
Sole/flounder, baked (3 oz, 120 cal)	1	Sole/flounder, baked	19 lb (12,000 cal)
Apple, fresh medium (1, 80 cal)	1	Sirloin steak, lean	17 lb (16,320 cal)

[a]For "your need" of calcium, the U.S. RDA of 1000 mg is used.

Butter, cream, and cream cheese contain negligible calcium, being almost pure fat.

If no calcium-rich milk product is acceptable as is, consider tinkering with it to make it work. Add chocolate to milk;[2] fruit to yogurt or kefir; or nonfat milk powder to *any* dish—meatloaf, cookies, hamburgers, gravies, soups, casseroles, sauces, milkshakes, even beverages such as coffee or tea, hot or iced. Only five heaping tablespoons are the equivalent of a cup of fresh milk. Make pudding, cream soups, macaroni and cheese.

Equal to milk and milk products in calcium richness are small fish such as sardines or herring prepared with the bones left in the meat; salmon (with the bones); or oysters. Another rich source of calcium is extracts made from bones. (Witches are said to make magic with such brews, but actually, wise food preparers of all cultures favor them, too. Chapter 2 explained that the Vietnamese people's tradition of making such stock helped account for their adequate calcium intakes without the use of milk.) Save the bones from chicken, turkey, pork, or fish dishes, soak them in vinegar, and boil them. The bones release their calcium into the acid medium, and the vinegar boils off, leaving no acid taste behind. Then use the stock in place of water to cook soup, vegetables, rice, or stew. One *tablespoon* of such stock may contain over 100 milligrams of calcium.

Other foods that appear equal to milk in calcium richness are dark green leafy vegetables, and some grains and legumes. Actually, however, many of these provide none or very little, because they contain calcium binders that hold onto the calcium and prevent its absorption. Exceptions are broccoli, beet greens, and kale, which are good sources of available calcium,[3] and probably some seaweeds, such as the **nori** popular in Japanese cookery. The presence of calcium binders does not make greens and grains inferior foods; dark greens are a superb source of riboflavin, virtually indispensable for the vegan or anyone else who drinks no milk. Greens also are rich in iron and dozens of other essential nutrients; and grains are excellent sources of complex carbohydrate and fiber; but with the exceptions noted, they cannot be relied on to provide calcium.

nori: a type of seaweed popular in Asian, particularly Japanese, cookery.

Next in order of preference among nonmilk sources of calcium are foods that contain large amounts of calcium salts by an accident of processing or by intentional fortification. In the processed category are bean curd (tofu—a calcium salt is used in the preparation); canned tomatoes (they offer 63 milligrams per cup); stone-ground or self-rising flour; stone-ground whole or self-rising cornmeal; and blackstrap molasses. Among food products specially fortified to add calcium to people's diets, the richest in calcium is high-calcium milk itself (a new product available from major dairies), which provides more calcium per cup than any natural milk—500 mg per 8 oz. Then there is calcium-fortified orange juice, with 300 mg per 8 oz—a good choice, because the bioavailability of its calcium compares favorably with that of milk. Calcium-fortified soy milk can also be prepared so that it contains more calcium than whole cow's milk.[4] Infant formula, based on soy, is fortified with calcium, and no law says adults can't use it in cooking for themselves. The vegan, especially, is urged to use such products regularly in ample quantities. Other products that may be fortified if demand warrants are soft drinks, breads, cereals, and others. These are not the equal of "real" foods as calcium sources, but they rank somewhere above supplements in most people's estimates, and they are certainly better than nothing.

Finally, there are supplements—not foods, but packages of nutrient preparations intended to meet the one need for calcium without regard to needs for energy or other nutrients. The box, "Calcium Supplements," provides pointers on choosing among them, should no other alternatives appear feasible.

We cannot close this section without a brief word about other osteoporosis risk factors. All persons should cut out bone toxins such as cigarettes and large amounts of alcohol. Women should consider estrogen therapy at menopause, and possibly starting even before, so as to catch the early, accelerated loss of calcium from bone that begins at menopause. No matter how high your calcium intake, it cannot override the influence of the estrogen lack that accelerates bone loss. Importantly, too, everyone should exercise regularly. No matter how many glasses of milk you drink in a day, the calcium will not be maximally deposited in bone unless you *work* your bones. Bones are like muscles; it takes regular exercise to make them strong and to keep them that way. Chapters 8 and 9 take up this theme again.

Calcium makes up bone and tooth structure and plays roles in nerve transmission, muscle contraction, and blood clotting. Calcium absorption increases when there is a deficiency or an increased need. The calcium deficiency disease is osteoporosis (adult bone loss). Milk and milk products are most people's chief calcium sources; the body may or may not absorb calcium from supplements, depending on the form of calcium in the supplement.

Powdered nonfat milk adds needed nutrients to any dish.

amino acid chelates: compounds of minerals (such as calcium) combined with amino acids in a form that favors their absorption. (A *chelating agent* is a molecule that surrounds another molecule, and therefore is useful for either promoting or preventing its movement from place to place.)

bone meal, powdered bone: crushed or ground bone preparations intended to supply calcium to the diet. Calcium from bone is not well absorbed, and is often contaminated with toxic materials.

oyster shell: a product made from the powdered shells of oysters, sold as a calcium supplement, but not well absorbed by the digestive system.

dolomite: a compound of minerals (calcium magnesium carbonate) found in limestone and marble. Dolomite is powdered and sold as a calcium-magnesium supplement, but may be contaminated with toxic minerals, is not well absorbed, and interacts adversely with absorption of other essential minerals.

Calcium Supplements

Calcium supplements have become popular among people who wish to prevent adult bone loss and who cannot or will not drink milk. There is no evidence that these supplements will prevent bone loss; at this point, the only evidence available is that low calcium intakes from food, early in life, correlate with osteoporosis late in life. Still, supplements may be worth considering. They are woefully inferior to milk for many reasons, but for the person who insists on using them, here are some facts about them.

First of all, regular vitamin-mineral pills contain no significant calcium at all, as you can tell from the label. Don't be fooled; the label may list some number of milligrams of calcium that sounds like a lot, but the U.S. RDA for calcium is a gram—a thousand milligrams. So let's start with a list of the possible candidates that will offer 1000 or so milligrams a day. (The 1984 Consensus Conference on Osteoporosis recommended that women consume 1000 to 1500 milligrams a day, and intakes of up to 2500 milligrams a day are known to be safe for healthy people.[5])

Calcium supplements are available in three forms. Simplest are the purified calcium compounds—such as calcium carbonate, citrate, gluconate, lactate, malate, phosphate or the like, and compounds of calcium with amino acids (called **amino acid chelates**). Then there are mixtures of calcium with other compounds—such as mixtures of calcium carbonate with magnesium carbonate, with aluminum salts (as in some antacids), or with vitamin D. Then there are powdered forms of calcium-rich materials—such as **bone meal, powdered bone, oyster shell,** or **dolomite** (limestone).

If you wanted a calcium supplement, which of these should you choose? In comparing them, you should address several questions.

Before comparing on any other basis, you should eliminate some right away as unsafe. Some preparations of bone meal and dolomite, for example, have been found to be contaminated with amounts of arsenic, cadmium, mercury, and lead high enough to cause a hazard to the health of the person who takes them routinely.[6] Antacids that contain aluminum and magnesium hydroxides can accelerate calcium loss (Rolaids are an example, Tums are not).[7] Supplements that contain vitamin D present a toxicity risk; the user must be careful to take an amount that will provide enough, but not too much, vitamin D, and to eliminate any other concentrated vitamin D sources. The risk of stone formation in kidneys may also be a problem: when rats were fed calcium phosphate dibasic as their sole calcium source, they deposited abnormal amounts of calcium in their kidneys.[8] Some people are genetically susceptible to stone formation; they need to know who they are and avoid calcium supplements.

The next question to ask is how well the body absorbs and uses the calcium from various supplements. Based on limited research to date, it seems that most healthy people absorb calcium equally well—and as well as from milk—from any of these supplements: amino acids chelated with calcium, calcium acetate, calcium carbonate, calcium citrate, calcium gluconate, calcium lactate, calcium phosphate dibasic, and oyster shell. People absorb calcium less well from a mixture of calcium carbonate and magnesium carbonate, from oyster-shell calcium fortified with inorganic magnesium, from a chelated calcium-magnesium combination, or from calcium carbonate fortified with vitamins and iron.[9] This raises the spectre of interactions, and with it, another question: do calcium supplements, themselves, interfere with the absorption of other nutrients?

The answer, unfortunately, is yes. Calcium phosphate dibasic inhibits magnesium absorption. The same amount of calcium in milk does not; score 1, here, for milk. If the calcium phosphate dibasic is fortified with magnesium, then it interferes with iron absorption. Calcium carbonate also interferes with iron absorption; so does calcium hydroxyapatite.[10] A way to get around this may be to take calcium supplements between, not with, meals—but for anyone with reduced stomach acid secretion, this is not a satisfactory solution, for only a meal stimulates the secretion of enough stomach acid to permit the absorption of the calcium. Score another point, here, for milk.

Another point for milk: *some* people absorb calcium better from it than from even the most absorbable supplements named above.[11] Still another comes from the finding that after absorption, the source affects the body's internal use of a nutrient. Only one study has been reported on calcium in this regard, but that study shows that the body makes better use of calcium from milk than from calcium carbonate.[12] (But we were supposed to be talking about supplements.)

Supposing that you can absorb the supplement taken between meals, and that your body will use it well, then the next question to ask is Which contains the most calcium per pill? The more calcium is in a single pill, the fewer pills you have to take. Read the label to find out. Calcium carbonate is 40 percent calcium; calcium gluconate, only 9 percent; so they vary a lot.

Finally, consider the cost and choose a supplement. Establish a routine so that you will not forget to take it. If you are young and digest food easily, take it between meals; if older, or if your stomach acid secretion is weak, take it with meals. Take it several times a day in divided doses rather than all at once; divided doses can increase absorption by up to 20 percent.[13] And do take it, it may do you some good.

But think one more time before you commit yourself to this course of action. You need 1000 or more milligrams of calcium every day for the rest of your life. Are you absolutely sure you cannot get it from milk, milk products, or other foods? Everyone seems to prefer that you use foods. The Consensus Conference on Osteoporosis recommended milk. The American Society for Bone and Mineral Research recommends foods as a source of calcium in preference to supplements.[14] Nutrition authorities Mayer and Goldberg, whose syndicated column on nutrition reaches newspaper readers nationwide, state, "We stand firmly in favor of dietary measures to meet the RDA . . . of calcium."[15] The writers of this book are so impressed by the importance of using abundant milk and milk products daily, that they have worked out a way to do so at every meal. Seldom is such a consensus seen among nutritionists.

(continued on following page)

Supplements contain only calcium; they don't offer the other nutrients that accompany it as fringe benefits in a food such as milk—thiamin, riboflavin, niacin, potassium, phosphorus, vitamin A, and all the rest. Therefore the person who omits milk and attempts to make up for it by taking supplements still is left with the task of obtaining all the other nutrients, and for some of these, milk is an excellent source. Milk's other essential nutrients are present in appropriate amounts; imbalances are not likely and overdoses are impossible. Milk's long-term safety is assured. The habit of drinking milk is easy to sustain, once established, because it fits with meals, provides calories, and can be served in delicious forms. It is low in cost, and fits well into a food budget. Milk drinking squares with the philosophy that using whole foods is preferable to taking supplements; pill-taking opposes that philosophy.

Whatever you do, though, do work out a way of getting your calcium daily in adequate amounts. When you walk tall and straight in your later years, you will thank your present self for it.

Sodium

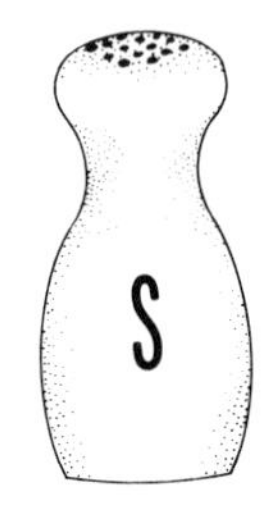

Sodium chloride.

Salt has been known throughout recorded history. The Bible's saying "You are the salt of the earth" means that a person is valuable. If, on the other hand, "you are not worth your salt," you are worthless. Even the word *salary* comes from the word *salt.** Sodium is the positive ion in the compound sodium chloride (table salt) and other salts, and contributes 40 percent of its weight. Thus, if a person consumes a gram of salt, that person has consumed 400 milligrams of sodium. As already mentioned, sodium is the chief ion used to maintain the volume of fluid outside cells.

The connection of salt with high blood pressure is well known, and most people have learned that they should not consume too much sodium. Some question has arisen recently, however, whether the culprit in relation to high blood pressure is sodium alone, the particular combination of sodium and chloride, or even the chloride ion alone. Controversy 7 describes the relationships of these and other factors to blood pressure.

A deficiency of sodium would be harmful, but there is seldom a sodium shortage in the diet. Foods usually include more salt than is needed, and the body absorbs it freely. The kidneys filter the surplus out of the blood into the urine. They can also sensitively conserve salt, and in the rare event of a deficiency they can return to the bloodstream the exact amount needed.** Normally, the amount excreted equals the amount ingested that day. About 30 to 40 percent

*To the chemist, a salt results from neutralization of an acid and a base. Sodium chloride—table salt—results from the reaction between hydrochloric acid and the base sodium hydroxide. The positive sodium ion unites with the negative chloride ion to form the salt, and the positive hydrogen ion unites with the negative hydroxide ion to form water.

Acid + base = salt + water.
Hydrochloric acid + sodium hydroxide = sodium chloride + water.

**The amount of sodium to be returned by the kidneys to the blood is under the control of an adrenal gland hormone, aldosterone.

of the body's sodium is thought to be stored on the surface of the bone crystals, where the body can easily draw upon it to replenish the blood concentration, is necessary.

For a brief summary of the kidney's action, see Chapter 1.

If the blood concentration of sodium rises, as it will after a person eats salted foods, thirst ensures that the person will drink water until the sodium-to-water ratio is constant. Then the kidneys can excrete the extra fluid along with the extra sodium.

Dieters sometimes think that eating too much salt or drinking too much water will make them gain weight, but they do not gain fat, of course. They gain water, but excess water is excreted immediately. Excess salt is excreted as soon as enough water is drunk to carry the salt out of the body. From this perspective, then, the way to keep body salt (and "water weight") under control is to drink more, not less, water.

If the blood concentration of sodium drops, both water and sodium must be replenished to avert emergency. Overly strict use of low-sodium diets in the treatment of kidney or heart disease can deplete the body of needed sodium; so can vomiting, diarrhea, or heavy sweating. Under normal conditions of sweating due to exercise, salt losses may easily be replaced later in the day with ordinary foods. Salt tablets are not recommended, because too much salt, especially if taken with too little water, incurs the risks of dehydration. If sweating has been extreme, and more than a gallon (about 4 liters) has been lost from the body, then salt may be needed. Guidelines for its replacement are in Chapter 9.

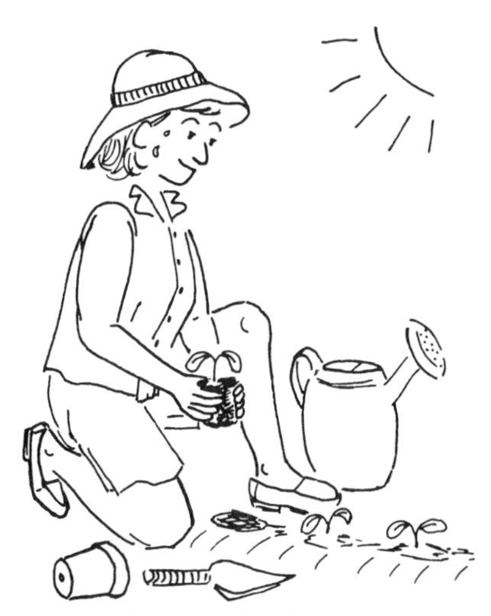

A person who sweats heavily needs to replenish sodium, and can do so by eating regular food.

Pregnant women used to be told to restrict their salt intakes to prevent pregnancy-induced hypertension (see Chapter 11). Now it is clear that they need not make special efforts to do so, but should eat a well-rounded diet of ordinary foods and avoid consuming salt in excess.

Chapter 9 recommends safe ways to replace fluid, sodium, and other minerals lost in sweat.

Intakes of sodium vary widely, especially because of cultural differences in diets. Asian people, whose staple sauces and flavorings are based on soy sauce and monosodium glutamate (MSG, or Accent), consume about 30 to 40 grams of salt per day; most people in the United States average about 6 to 18 grams of salt per day. It has been estimated, but not proven, that the upper limit of the safe and adequate range for daily sodium intake is 7 grams of salt, the equivalent of about 3 grams of sodium. The American Heart Association suggests keying salt intake to total food energy intake, and offers the guideline of 1 gram of sodium per 1000 calories, to a maximum of 3 grams per day.

One of the most important favors you can do yourself, especially if you have heart disease in your family, is to learn to control your salt intake. To stop salting foods in cooking and at the table is one step to take, but you can learn many other tactics besides. This chapter's Food Feature is devoted to controlling salt intake.

Sodium is the main positively charged ion outside the body's cells. Too much sodium may aggravate hypertension.

Potassium

Potassium is the principal positively charged ion inside body cells. It plays a major role in maintaining fluid and electrolyte balance and cell integrity. It is also critical to maintaining the heartbeat. The sudden deaths that occur during

diuretics (dye-you-RET-ics): medications causing increased water excretion (*dia* means "through"; *ouron* means "urine").

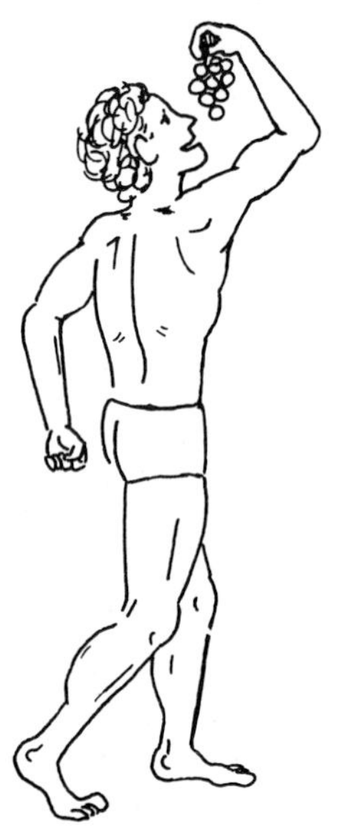

Body builders take note: fruit is a rich potassium source, so it may do as much for muscles as meat.

fasting or severe diarrhea and in kwashiorkor children are thought to be due to heart failure caused by potassium loss.

Dehydration leads to potassium loss from inside cells. It is especially dangerous because potassium loss from brain cells makes the victim unaware of the need for water. Because of this, adults are warned not to take **diuretics** (water pills) that cause potassium loss, except under the direction of a physician. When a person uses diuretics and consults another physician for a different health problem, that physician should be alerted to the diuretic use. Any physician prescribing diuretics will tell the client to eat potassium-rich foods to compensate for the losses and, depending on the diuretic, may advise a lowered sodium intake, too.

Gradual potassium depletion can occur when a person sweats profusely day after day and fails to replenish potassium stores. A person who sweats heavily and often should eat about five to eight servings of potassium-rich food each day—not hard to do as long as whole foods are used, for unbroken cells that have not been exposed to too much processing are rich in potassium. Table 7–4 shows the potassium contents of some foods selected to show a range of values. As you can see, while foods of all kinds offer abundant potassium; on a per-calorie basis, vegetables and fresh fruits are outstanding.

Potassium chloride is available freely over the counter and is sold in health food stores without a warning label, but should not be used except on a physician's advice. People's lives are not normally threatened by potassium overdoses as long as they are taken by mouth, because the presence of excess potassium in the stomach triggers a vomiting reflex that expels the unwanted substance. A person with a weak heart should not be put through this trauma, however, and a baby may not be able to withstand it.

Potassium is the major positive ion inside cells, important in many metabolic and structural functions. Diuretics can deplete potassium and so can be dangerous; potassium excess can also be dangerous.

Other Major Minerals

Magnesium barely qualifies as a major mineral: Only about $1\frac{3}{4}$ ounces are present in the body of a 130-pound person. Most of this is in the bones. Bone magnesium seems to be a storage reservoir to ensure that some will be on hand for vital cellular reactions regardless of recent dietary intake. The kidney acts to conserve magnesium; unabsorbed magnesium is excreted in the feces. Deficiency of magnesium may occur as a result of inadequate intake, vomiting, diarrhea, alcoholism, or protein malnutrition; in hospital clients who have been fed incomplete fluids into a vein for too long; or in persons using diuretics. It is not known to what extent magnesium deficiencies exist in the general population, but survey results show that the RDA is seldom met. Table 7–6 at the end of the chapter points out foods rich in magnesium, and Appendix A includes the magnesium contents of over 1000 foods. Severe magnesium deficiency, caused partly by low intake and partly by alcohol-induced magnesium excretion, is thought to cause the hallucinations experienced by alcohol addicts during withdrawal.

People whose drinking water has a high magnesium content experience a lower incidence of sudden death from heart failure than other people do. It

Table 7–4

Food Sources of Potassium Selected to Show a Range of Values

If you eat this size serving of:	You will receive this % of your need[a] of POTASSIUM:	If you wanted 100% of your need[a] of POTASSIUM from this food:	You will have to eat this size serving:
Peach halves, dried (10, 311 cal)	65%	Bok choy cabbage, cooked	3.1 c (62 cal)
Lima beans, cooked (1 c, 260 cal)	58	Spinach, cooked	2.4 c (98 cal)
Winter squash, baked (1 c, 96 cal)	54	Mushrooms, raw sliced	7.7 c (139 cal)
Pear halves, dried (10, 459 cal)	47	Cauliflower, cooked	5 c (150 cal)
Sirloin steak, lean (8 oz, 480 cal)	46	Winter squash, baked	1.9 c (182 cal)
Potato, microwaved w/skin (1, 212 cal)	45	Cantaloupe melon	1.2 melon (226 cal)
Pinto beans, cooked (1 c, 265 cal)	44	Dandelion greens, cooked	8.3 c (291 cal)
Spinach, cooked (1 c, 41 cal)	42	Broccoli, cooked	7.7 c (354 cal)
Cantaloupe melon (½, 94 cal)	41	Nonfat milk	5 c (430 cal)
Kidney beans, canned (1 c, 230 cal)	34	Lima beans, cooked	1.7 c (442 cal)
Bok choy cabbage, cooked (1 c, 20 cal)	32	Potato, microwaved w/skin	2.2 potato (466 cal)
Prunes, dried (10, 201 cal)	31	Peach halves, dried	15 halves (467 cal)
Nonfat milk (1 c, 86 cal)	20	Pinto beans, cooked	2.2 c (583 cal)
Cauliflower, cooked (1 c, 30 cal)	20	Prunes, dried	32 prunes (643 cal)
Oysters, raw (1c, 160 cal)	15	Kidney beans, canned	3 c (690 cal)
Sole/flounder, baked (3 oz, 120 cal)	14	Sole/flounder, baked	21 oz (840 cal)
Mushrooms, raw sliced (1 c, 18 cal)	13	Pear halves, dried	21 halves (964 cal)
Broccoli, cooked (1 c, 46 cal)	13	Sirloin steak, lean	17 oz (1008 cal)
Dandelion greens, cooked (1 c, 35 cal)	12	Apple, fresh medium	13 apples (1040 cal)
Apple, fresh medium (1, 80 cal)	8	Oysters, raw	6.7 c (1072 cal)
Whole wheat bread (1 sl, 70 cal)	3	Whole wheat bread	33 sl (2310 cal)
Cheddar cheese (1 oz, 114 cal)	1	Cheddar cheese	100 oz (11,400 cal)

[a]"Your need" of potassium is assumed to be about 2000 mg, near the midpoint of the safe and adequate daily dietary intake defined by the RDA committee.

seems likely that magnesium deficiency makes the heart unable to stop itself from going into spasms once it starts.[16]

The chloride ion is the major negative ion of the fluids outside the cells, where it is found mostly in association with sodium. As mentioned, it may have something to do with hypertension, either together with sodium or independently of it (see Controversy 7). The chloride ion can move freely across membranes and so is also found inside the cells, primarily in association with potassium. The chloride ion is also part of the hydrochloric acid that maintains the strong acidity of the stomach. In large doses, chlorine is deadly, and so is used as a disinfectant.

Sulfur plays no roles of its own, but forms part of proteins and other compounds; deficiencies are unknown. The summary table at the end of this chapter presents the main facts on the major minerals.

Magnesium is essential for cellular reactions; deficiencies can result from low intake, vomiting, diarrhea, alcoholism, or protein malnutrition. Chloride is the body's major negative ion inside and outside of cells. It is part of the stomach's hydrochloric acid, and is essential to the acid-base balance. Sulfur is also considered a major mineral, although it occurs only as part of other compounds such as protein.

goiter (GOY-ter): enlargement of the thyroid gland due to iodine deficiency.

cretinism (CREE-tin-ism): severe mental and physical retardation of an infant caused by iodine deficiency during pregnancy.

The Trace Minerals

Laboratory techniques developed in the last two decades have enabled scientists to detect minerals in smaller and smaller quantities in living cells. Knowledge of the "new" trace elements is coming out of this research. An obstacle to determining their precise roles lies in the difficult task of providing an experimental diet lacking in the one element under study. Thus research in this area is limited to study of laboratory animals, which can be fed highly refined, purified diets in environments that are free of all contamination. Whole books have been published on the trace minerals alone, and research is still rapidly expanding knowledge about them.

Iodine

Iodine occurs in the body in an infinitesimally small quantity, but its principal role in human nutrition is well known, and the amount needed is well established. Iodine is a part of thyroxine, the hormone responsible for regulating the basal metabolic rate.

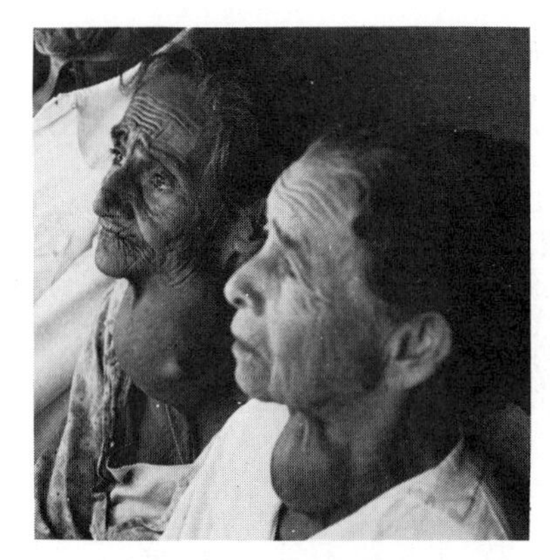

These people have goiter, enlargement of the thyroid gland due to iodine deficiency.

Iodine must be available for thyroxine to be synthesized. The amount in the diet is variable and generally reflects the soil in which plants are grown or on which animals graze. Iodine is plentiful in the ocean, so seafood is a completely dependable source. In the United States, in areas that were never under the ocean, the soil is iodine poor (most notably the Great Plains states and Oregon's Willamette valley). In those areas, the use of iodized salt and the consumption of foods shipped in from other, iodine-rich areas have been necessary to wipe out the iodine deficiency that once was widespread.

When the iodine level of the blood is low, the cells of the thyroid gland enlarge due to synthesis of a thyroxine precursor intended to trap as many particles of iodine as possible. If the gland enlarges until it is visible, it is called a **goiter.** In addition to causing sluggishness and weight gain, a thyroid deficiency may have serious effects on the development of an infant in the uterus. Severe iodine deficiency during pregnancy causes the extreme and irreversible mental and physical retardation known as **cretinism.** Much of the retardation can be averted by correction of the deficiency during pregnancy, but if it goes uncorrected, the child's IQ may be as low as 20 (100 is average).

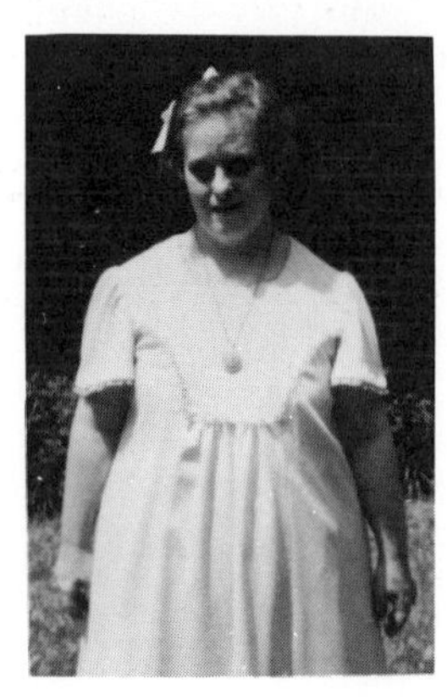

An adult cretin.

In most regions, the need for iodine is easily met by consuming seafood and vegetables grown in iodine-rich soil. In developed countries, food is shipped from place to place to such an extent that some iodine-rich food is likely to be available everywhere. In iodine-poor regions, the iodization of salt has all but eliminated the widespread misery caused there earlier by goiter and cretinism. However, goiter is still prevalent in primitive societies where people cannot read. Even among highly literate people, each new generation has to be taught to use iodized salt; otherwise the problem creeps back into their lives. In the United States you have to read the label to find out whether salt is iodized; in Canada all table salt is iodized.

People sometimes wonder whether sea salt, made by drying ocean water, is preferable to purified sodium chloride for use in the salt shaker. Sea salt does contain trace minerals, but its iodine becomes a gas and evaporates during the drying process. Thus in a region where iodine deficiency is a risk, iodized sodium chloride is the salt to choose.

Like chlorine and fluorine, iodine is a deadly poison in large amounts, even though traces of it are indispensable to life. Excessive intakes of iodine can cause an enlargement of the thyroid gland, resembling goiter, which in infants can be so severe as to block the airways and cause suffocation. A dramatic increase in iodine intakes in the United States concerns some observers. Average consumption rose from 150 micrograms per day in 1960 to over 450 in 1970, and reached an all-time high of over 800 micrograms per day in 1974; since then it has declined somewhat but still is several times the RDA. The toxic level at which detectable harm results is thought to be over 2000 micrograms per day for an adult, only a few times higher than current average consumption levels.[17]

Most of the excess iodine seems to be coming from iodates—dough conditioners used in the baking industry—and from milk produced in dairies that use iodine-containing medications for the cows and iodine-containing disinfectants on the milking equipment. Now that the problem has been identified, both industries have reduced their use of these compounds, but the sudden emergence of this problem points to a need for continued surveillance of the food supply.

Iodine is part of the hormone thyroxine, which controls energy metabolism. The deficiency diseases are goiter and cretinism. Iodine occurs in seafood and in foods grown on land that was once covered by oceans. Large amounts are poisonous.

hemoglobin (HEEM-oh-globe-in): the oxygen-carrying protein of the blood; found in the red blood cells (*hemo* means "blood"; *globin* means "spherical protein").

myoglobin (MYE-o-globe-in): the oxygen-holding protein of the muscles (*myo* means "muscle").

iron-deficiency anemia: reduction of the size of red blood cells and loss of their color because of iron deficiency. Accompanying symptoms are weakness, apathy, headaches, pallor, and in children inability to pay attention. (For *sports anemia,* see Chapter 9.)

Iron

Iron is probably the most widely known of all the essential minerals. Television viewers, particularly, hear that the woman who "takes good care of herself" takes iron supplements every day and that "you should, too."

Most of the iron in the body is a component of the proteins **hemoglobin** and **myoglobin.** Both these compounds carry oxygen in association with the iron they contain. Hemoglobin is the oxygen carrier in the red blood cells, and myoglobin is the oxygen reservoir in the muscle cells.

All the body cells use oxygen to combine with the carbon and hydrogen atoms released during breakdown of the energy-yielding nutrients. The carbon dioxide and water are then excreted; thus there is a constant need of fresh oxygen and nutrients to keep the energy-yielding pathways open so that cells can continue to function. Iron is also a part of many of the enzymes in energy pathways. As cells use up and excrete their oxygen (as carbon dioxide and water), the red blood cells shuttle between metabolizing tissues and lungs to bring in fresh oxygen supplies.

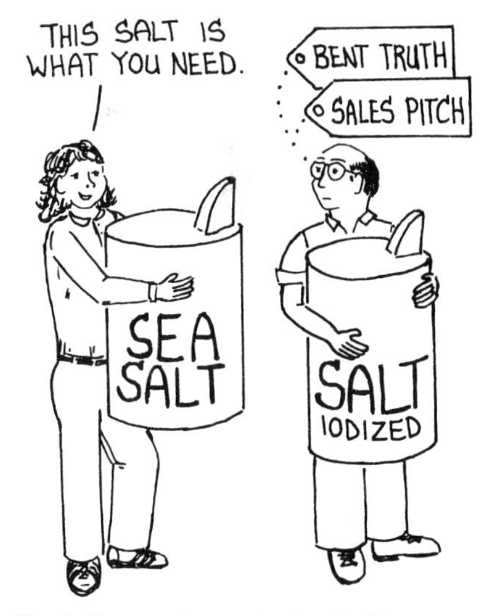

Ironically, sea salt contains less iodine.

In **iron-deficiency anemia** (which is only one of several types of anemias), the red blood cells contain too little hemoglobin and become unable to carry enough oxygen to meet the cells' energy needs. Some of the symptoms of iron deficiency are those of energy deficiency—tiredness and apathy. Others derive from failure to perform brain functions that iron supports—such as concentration. A sample of iron-deficient blood examined under the microscope shows smaller cells that are a lighter red than normal cells. To diagnose iron deficiency,

pica (PIE-ka): a craving for nonfood substances. Also known as **geophagia** (gee-oh-FAY-gee-uh) when referring to clay eating and **pagophagia** (pag-oh-FAY-gee-uh) when referring to ice craving (*picus* means "woodpecker" or "magpie"; *geo* means "earth"; *phagein* means "to eat"; *pago* means "frost").

the physician usually measures the blood hemoglobin concentration. Iron supplements will correct anemia—provided, of course, that iron deficiency has caused it (see the box entitled "Iron-Fortified Foods and Iron Supplements" later in the text).

Anemia can be caused by other nutrition problems. For example, a vitamin B_6 deficiency can indirectly cause anemia, because vitamin B_6 is required to make the iron-containing portion of the hemoglobin molecule. A vitamin E deficiency can cause anemia by making the red blood cell membranes so fragile that the cells lose their hemoglobin. A folacin deficiency also can cause it, because this vitamin is used in making new red blood cells to replace the old ones as they die. A vitamin B_{12} deficiency can cause it, because folacin can't work without B_{12}. Vitamin A, too, is involved in the making of red blood cells, and some people's low hemoglobin levels can be corrected only by administering vitamin A. Vitamin C deficiency makes the absorption of iron less than optimal and can cause anemia. The mineral copper is needed for the enzymes to make hemoglobin, and is low enough in some diets to cause cases of anemia. Still, iron deficiency is the most common cause of anemia.

A curious symptom seen in some iron-deficient subjects is an appetite for ice, clay, paste, and other nonnutritious substances. Such people have been known to eat as many as eight trays of ice in a day, for example. This behavior has been observed for years, especially in women and children of low-income groups who are deficient in either iron or zinc, and has been given the name **pica.** When caused by iron deficiency, pica clears up dramatically within days after iron is given, even if anemia is present and the red blood cells have not yet responded.

Millions of people the world over suffer from iron deficiency without the benefit of a diagnosis. Even in the United States and Canada, about 20 percent of all women and 3 percent of men have no iron in their body stores; some 8 percent of women and 1 percent of men are overtly anemic, experiencing fatigue, weakness, apathy, and headaches. Long before the mass of the red blood cells is affected, however, physical work capacity and productivity are impaired. Children deprived of iron become irritable, restless, and unable to concentrate. These symptoms are among the first to appear when the body's iron level begins to fall and among the first to disappear when iron intake is increased again.[18]

The impact of full-blown anemia can be stated (it is massive), but the impact of iron deficiency milder than anemia may be even greater, because it affects so many more people. Iron deficiency occurs in as many as *half* of all persons in some settings, even in developed countries—most predictably in inner-city and rural poor. With reduced energy available to work, plan, think, or learn, people simply do these things less. They don't appear to have an obvious deficiency disease; they just appear unmotivated and apathetic. Because they work and play less, they are less physically fit. The incidence of iron-deficiency anemia in developed countries ranges from 10 to 20 percent; it is even higher in the developing countries; and the incidence of undetected iron deficiency must be higher still.[19] If this one worldwide malnutrition problem could be alleviated, millions of people's lives would improve in quality.

The cause of iron deficiency is usually nutrition—that is, inadequate intake, either from sheer lack of food altogether or from high consumption of the wrong foods. In the western world, the cause is often displacement of iron-rich foods by foods high in sugar and fat. New vegetarians who design their own meal plans without traditional patterns often short themselves on iron, and are prone to anemia. Among nonnutritional causes of anemia, blood loss is the primary one, caused in many countries by parasitic infections of the digestive tract. In some countries, people go through their entire lives losing blood daily and do not know what it is like not to feel tired and unenergetic.

Periods of growth—infancy, childhood, adolescence, and pregnancy—involve enlargement of the blood volume to feed the new tissue. During such periods, the body increases iron absorption by making extra carrier proteins that pick up iron from the digestive tract. Often, however, the larger demands for iron are not met. At these times people must be sure to eat more iron-rich foods.

About 80 percent of the iron in the body is in the blood, so iron losses are greatest whenever blood is lost. Menstruation causes losses that make a woman's need for iron nearly twice as great as a man's.

Women are often told that they need more iron, yet they often have their blood cell count or blood hemoglobin pronounced normal. The key difference between them and men is a difference in their body *stores* of iron, which don't show up in these tests. Most men eat more food than women do, because they are bigger; and so their iron intakes are higher. Besides, women menstruate, and so their iron losses are greater. These two factors—lower intakes and higher losses—put women much closer to the borderline of deficiency. Even though they may not be overtly iron deficient, they are often deficiency prone. Should a woman lose blood for any reason (even by giving a blood donation) or become pregnant (so that her blood volume would need to increase), she would need to make a special effort to replenish her iron stores. The information about iron in foods that appears later is especially important to women.

Iron deficiency may also be caused by poor absorption of the iron that is in food. A normal, healthy person absorbs only about 10 percent of the iron from a mixed diet—about 2 to 10 percent from vegetables and about 10 to 30 percent from red meats. Increased absorption occurs when stores have been depleted, and also when vitamin C or meat, fish, or poultry is taken with other iron-rich food.

About 40 percent of the iron in meat, fish, and poultry is bound into molecules of **heme,** the iron-containing part of hemoglobin and myoglobin. Heme iron is much more absorbable (23 percent) than nonheme iron (2 to 10 percent). Meat, fish, and poultry also contain a factor (**MFP factor**) other than heme that promotes the absorption of nonheme iron, even that from other foods eaten with it. A system has been devised, based on all these factors, to calculate the amount of iron absorbed from a meal (see the Self-Study at the end of this chapter). Stomach acid also acts on iron to make it more absorbable. In fact, people with ulcers who have to take antacids readily develop iron-deficiency anemia. Other factors that reduce iron availability are tea, coffee, soy protein, wheat bran, and fiber.

Knowing how important adequate iron is to good health, you may think that a "wise" body would absorb *all* the iron in foods. But iron is toxic in large amounts, and once inside, it is difficult to excrete. The body's defense against iron poisoning is a control system: the intestinal cells trap some of the iron and hold it within their boundaries. When they are shed, these cells carry out of the intestinal tract the excess iron that they collected during their brief lives. When the intestinal lining is damaged (by alcohol abuse, for example), the body is vulnerable to poisoning by excess iron. Controversy 6 on vitamin-mineral supplements warns against taking those that contain high doses of iron unnecessarily.

heme (HEEM): the iron-containing portion of the hemoglobin and myoglobin molecules.

MFP factor: a factor (identity unknown) present in **M**eat, **F**ish, and **P**oultry that enhances the absorption of nonheme iron present in the same foods or in other foods eaten at the same time.

Factors that increase iron absorption:

- Vitamin C.
- MFP factor.
- Normal stomach acidity.

Factors that decrease iron absorption:

- Antacids.
- Tea.
- Coffee
- Soy protein.
- Wheat bran.
- Fiber.

iron overload: the state of having more iron in the body than it needs or can handle. Iron can become toxic in this situation.

Once inside the body, iron is hoarded as if it were gold. Red blood cells are manufactured using the iron that is kept in the bone marrow; then they are sent into the blood, where they live about three to four months. When they die and are broken down, the liver saves their iron and sends it to be deposited in the bone marrow for reuse. Only tiny losses occur in the clipping of nails, the cutting of hair, and the shedding of skin cells.

The iron RDA is 10 milligrams a day for adult males and older women. For women of childbearing age, the RDA is 18 milligrams. This amount is necessary to replace menstrual losses and to provide the extra iron needed during pregnancy. There is a general misunderstanding that only females need be concerned about their iron intakes. As a matter of fact, teenage males need the same 18 milligrams as females. This need stems from the enormous growth spurt that males achieve during their teen years. On the other hand, grown men experience iron-deficiency anemia rarely but may occasionally exhibit the toxicity condition, **iron overload.** When a man has low blood hemoglobin, this alerts his health care provider to examine him for a blood-loss site.

Iron from fortified foods and from supplements is poorly absorbed, even though they may contain as many as 50 milligrams per dose (see the box "Iron-Fortified Foods and Iron Supplements"). To be assured of meeting your iron needs, it is best to rely on foods. The usual Western mixed diet provides only about 5 to 6 milligrams of iron in each 1000 calories. Thus an adult man, whose RDA is 10 milligrams and who eats upwards of 2500 calories a day, has no trouble meeting his RDA. A woman whose RDA is 18 milligrams and who may eat fewer than 2000 calories a day understandably does have trouble. She must increase the iron-to-calorie ratio of her diet so that she will receive about double the average amount of iron, at least 10 milligrams per 1000 calories. It can be done by following guidelines long familiar to nutrition-minded consumers. From each food group, select those foods that are notable for their high iron density relative to calories.

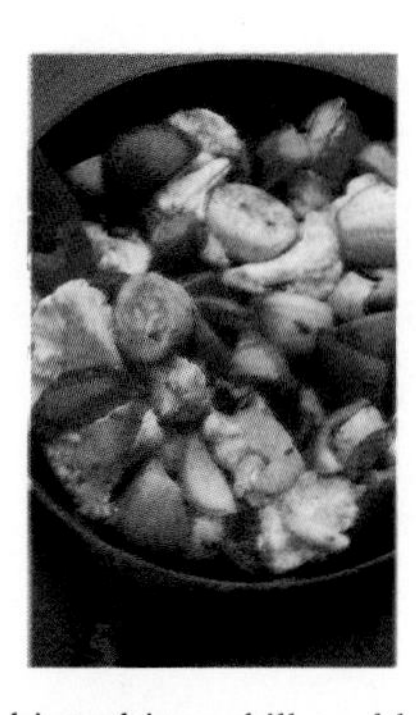

The old-fashioned iron skillet adds a much-needed nutrient to foods.

Table 7–5 shows how iron is distributed in foods. As you might expect, meats fall near the top of the left-hand column (iron per serving), and vegetables near the top of the right-hand column (iron per calorie). Clearly, iron is an expensive nutrient in terms of both total food and calories—you have to budget a sizable portion of your food allowance to meet the U.S. RDA.

Cooking utensils can enhance the amount of iron delivered by the diet. The iron content of 100 grams of spaghetti sauce simmered in a glass dish is 3 milligrams, but it is 87 milligrams when the sauce is cooked in an unenameled iron skillet. Even in the short time it takes to scramble eggs, their iron content can be tripled by cooking them in an iron pan. Similarly, the reasons why raisins contain more iron than grapes is because they are dried in iron pans. This iron is in the form of inorganic salts, and is not as well absorbed as that from meat, but some does get in. Foods containing 25 milligrams or more of vitamin C can more than double the amount of iron absorbed from nonheme iron sources eaten at the same meal. Therefore, two suggestions are:

- Cook with iron skillets whenever possible.
- Eat foods that contain small amounts of meat, fish, or poultry and vitamin C at every meal.

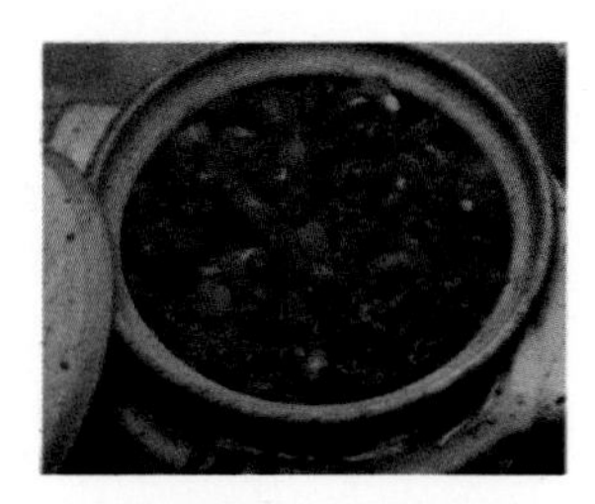

The meat and tomatoes in this chili help the eater absorb iron from the beans.

A few bits of pork or hotdogs added to a meal of baked beans, for example, will enhance iron absorption from the beans. A slice of tomato and a leaf of

Iron-Fortified Foods and Iron Supplements

Some people need iron in supplement form. The Committee on RDA acknowledges that pregnant women may need it; the Canadian RNI also includes this statement. However, the iron from supplements, similar to the inorganic iron from iron cookware, is far less well absorbed than that from food, so although the RDA for a woman is 18 mg/day, the amount of a supplement she may need may be as high as 50 mg/day. Absorption of iron from supplements is improved when they are taken with meat or with vitamin C–rich foods or juices. Look for the ferrous form, too; it is better absorbed than the ferric form.

The use of enriched or fortified foods is another option. Iron added to foods is similar to contamination iron; it may boost apparent intakes, but its absorption is poor. It is so poorly absorbed, in fact, that even prolonged use of enriched foods often seems to do little or nothing to improve people's iron status. In the right food carrier, though, it perhaps can make a difference. At present, 25 percent of all the iron consumed in the United States derives from foods to which iron has been added, including the familiar enriched breads and cereals, and fortified breakfast cereals that boast that they contain 100 percent of the RDA for iron. These food sources are important, because people eat so much of them as to derive significant iron from the total.

A number of proposals have been made for further fortification—of milk, fish, rice, infant foods, coffee, junk foods, salt, sugar, and soy sauce. Fortification of soy sauce could improve the iron status of a third of the world's people. A proposal to increase the iron level in enriched bread above that now in force has been defeated; that level of fortification is used in Sweden and is believed to account for that country's better iron status than the United States'. Whatever the iron in the food supply, though, it is clearly the responsibility of consumers themselves to see that they get enough iron.

In any case, foods are a better source of iron than fortification or supplements. Two stories illustrate this point—one set in the United States, the other in West Java. The first was a study of 200 adults in Boston who had hemoglobin levels below normal. Two-thirds were given iron-fortified foods for 6 to 8 months; the others were given the same foods without added iron. At the end of the study, *all* had higher hemoglobin levels. Food made the difference, with or without added iron.[20]

The study in West Java involved rubber plantation workers with iron-deficiency anemia. The more anemic they were, the less work they could do, and the more often they got sick with infections. Half were given an iron supplement, the other half a placebo—but *both* improved in work output. It turned out that, at first, the placebo effect had increased work output in both groups. This had led to increased pay, which they spent on food—food that supplied 3 to 5 extra milligrams of iron a day together with vitamin C.[21]

Table 7–5

Food Sources of Iron Selected to Show a Range of Values

If you eat this size serving of:	You will receive this % of your need[a] of IRON:	If you want 100% of your need[a] of IRON from this food:	You will have to eat this size serving:
Oysters, raw (1 c, 160 cal)	93%	Parsley, chopped fresh	5 c (100 cal)
Sirloin steak, lean (8 oz, 480 cal)	42	Spinach, cooked	2.9 c (119 cal)
Spinach, cooked (1 c, 41 cal)	35	Oysters, raw	1.1 c (176 cal)
Lima beans, cooked (1 c, 260 cal)	32	Bok choy cabbage, cooked	10 c (200 cal)
Braunschweiger sausage (2 pcs, 205 cal)	30	Beet greens, cooked	6.7 c (268 cal)
Beef liver, fried (3 oz, 185 cal)	29	Dandelion greens, cooked	10 c (350 cal)
Peach halves, dried (10, 311 cal)	29	Mushrooms, raw sliced	20 c (360 cal)
Navy beans, cooked dry (1 c, 225 cal)	28	Clams, raw meat only	21 oz (455 cal)
Soy beans, cooked dry (1 c, 235 cal)	27	Broccoli, cooked	10 c (460 cal)
Hamburger patty + bun (4 oz, 445 cal)	27	Beef liver, fried	10.3 oz (629 cal)
Kidney beans, canned (1 c, 230 cal)	25	Braunschweiger sausage	6.7 pcs (697 cal)
Parsley, chopped fresh (1 c, 20 cal)	20	Lima beans, cooked	3 c (780 cal)
Split peas, cooked (1 c, 230 cal)	19	Navy beans, cooked dry	3.6 c (810 cal)
Beet greens, cooked (1 c, 40 cal)	15	Soy beans, cooked dry	3.7 c (870 cal)
Clams, raw meat only (3 oz, 65 cal)	14	Kidney beans, canned	4 c (920 cal)
Dandelion greens, cooked (1 c, 35 cal)	10	Peach halves, dried	34 halves (1057 cal)
Broccoli, cooked (1 c, 46 cal)	10	Sirloin steak, lean	19 oz (1152 cal)
Bok choy cabbage, cooked (1 c, 20 cal)	10	Split peas, cooked	5.3 c (1219 cal)
Whole wheat bread (1 sl, 70 cal)	5	Whole wheat bread	20 sl (1400 cal)
Mushrooms, raw sliced (1 c, 18 cal)	5	Hamburger patty + bun	15 oz (1691 cal)
Sole/flounder, baked (3 oz, 120 cal)	2	Apple, fresh medium	100 apples (8000 cal)
Apple, fresh medium (1, 80 cal)	1	Cheddar cheese	100 oz (11,400 cal)
Cheddar cheese (1 oz, 114 cal)	1	Nonfat milk	too much (too many cal)
Nonfat milk (1 c, 86 cal)	<1	Sole/flounder, baked	too much (too many cal)

[a]"Your need" is defined here as the U.S. RDA, 18 mg of iron.

lettuce in a sandwich will enhance iron absorption from the bread. The meat and tomato in spaghetti sauce help the eater absorb the iron from the spaghetti. Meat iron is well absorbed regardless of context, but iron from vegetables, legumes, and grains needs help.

Most iron in the body is contained in hemoglobin and myoglobin or occurs as a part of enzymes in the energy-yielding pathways. Iron-deficiency anemia is a problem worldwide. Iron is lost through menstruation and other bleeding; the shedding of intestinal cells protects against overload. Too much iron is toxic. For optimal iron intake, use meat, vitamin C, and other iron sources together.

Zinc

Zinc occurs in a very small quantity but works with proteins in every corner of the body as a helper for some 70 enzymes. The summary table at the end of the chapter enumerates some of its many vital activities.

No nationwide survey has yet undertaken to assess the extent of zinc deficiency in the United States or Canada, but indications are that it does occur, especially where certain predisposing factors are present. A deficiency of zinc in human beings was first reported in the 1960s from studies with growing children and adolescent boys in Egypt, Iran, and Turkey. The native diets were typically low in animal protein and high in whole grains and beans; consequently they were high in fiber and other zinc-binding factors known as **phytates.** Furthermore, the bread they ate was unleavened; the phytates had not been broken down by yeast. The zinc deficiency was marked by severe growth retardation and arrested sexual maturation—symptoms that were responsive to zinc supplementation.

In the United States, too, poor growth, poor appetite, and impaired taste sensitivity may indicate zinc deficiency. When pediatricians or other health workers evaluating children's health note poor growth accompanied by poor appetite, they should think zinc.

Since the first reports, zinc deficiency has been recognized elsewhere, and it is known to affect much more than just growth. It alters digestive function profoundly and causes diarrhea, which worsens the malnutrition already present, with respect to not only zinc, but all nutrients. It drastically impairs the immune response, making infections likely—including infections of the intestinal tract, which worsen malnutrition, including zinc malnutrition (a classic evil cycle). It directly interferes with folacin absorption and impairs vitamin A metabolism, so the symptoms of those vitamin deficiencies often appear. (Recall from Chapter 6 that normal night vision depends on active vitamin A, which forms the visual pigment in the retina of the eye. Zinc is necessary, too, in the enzyme that activates vitamin A in the retina; so a zinc deficiency can bring about night blindness, even when vitamin A is abundant.) Zinc deficiency disturbs thyroid function and metabolic rate. It alters taste, causes anorexia, slows wound healing—in fact, its symptoms are so all-pervasive that generalized malnutrition and sickness are more likely to be the diagnosis than simple zinc deficiency.

Zinc can be toxic if consumed in large enough quantities. Toxicity can occur from use of zinc supplements or of acidic foods or drinks that have been allowed to stand in **galvanized** containers may contain toxic levels.

Doses of zinc only a few milligrams above the RDA lower the body's copper content—an effect that, in animals, leads to degeneration of the heart muscle. Higher doses affect cholesterol metabolism and appear to accelerate the development of atherosclerosis. Excess zinc intake may also interfere with the intestinal absorption of copper and calcium, which compete with zinc to be absorbed. Accidental consumption of zinc may cause vomiting, diarrhea, fever, exhaustion, muscle incoordination, dizziness, drowsiness, lethargy, kidney failure, anemia, and other symptoms; larger doses still can even be fatal.

Zinc enters the digestive tract not only in food, but also in zinc-rich juices that are secreted from the pancreas. Some of it is not reabsorbed but is excreted in the feces. Thus zinc has an escape route and does not pile up in the body's internal organs, as iron does.

Animal products and legumes are good sources of zinc (see Figure 7–6, opposite). Among plant sources, whole grains are richest in zinc, but it is not so well absorbed from them as from meat. The RDA of 15 milligrams per day for adults is probably not met by most people; the average intake is probably closer to 10 milligrams. Vegetarians are advised to eat varied diets that include whole-grain breads well leavened with yeast, which improves the availability of their zinc.

Zinc assists enzymes in all cells. Deficiency causes growth retardation with sexual immaturity. Animal foods are the best sources. Zinc is toxic in large amounts.

phytates: compounds present in plant foods (particularly whole grains and beans) that bind zinc and prevent its absorption.

galvanized: treated with zinc-containing coating to prevent rust. Metal containers are sometimes galvanized.

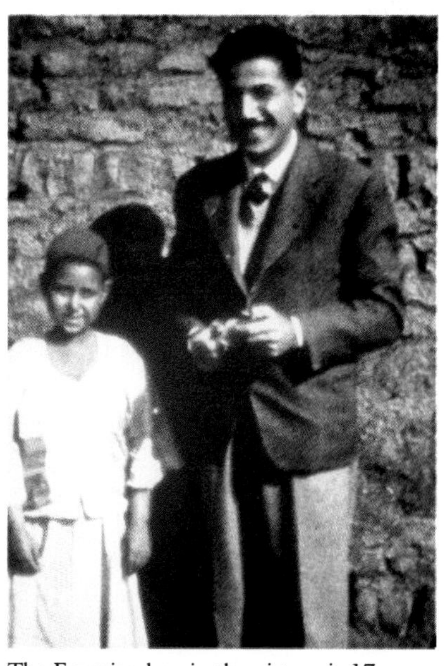

The Egyptian boy in the picture is 17 years old but is only 4 feet tall, like a 7-year-old in the United States. His genitalia are like those of a 6-year-old. The retardation is rightly ascribed to zinc deficiency, because it is partially reversible when zinc is restored to the diet.

Fluoride

fluorapatite (FLOOR-app-uh-tight): a crystal of bones and teeth, formed when fluoride displaces the hydroxy portion of hydroxyapatite (see p. 233). Fluorapatite resists being dissolved back into body fluid.

fluorosis (floor-OH-sis): discoloration of the teeth due to ingestion of too much fluoride during tooth development.

Fluoride has not been proven an essential nutrient.[22] Only a trace of fluoride occurs in the human body, but studies have demonstrated that with fluoride in the diet, the crystalline deposits in bones and teeth are larger and more perfectly formed. Fluoride replaces the hydroxy portion of hydroxyapatite (p. 233), forming **fluorapatite,** a crystal that is more resistant to decay.

Drinking water is the usual source of fluoride. In communities where the water contains too much—2 to 8 parts per million—discoloration of the teeth may occur; where fluoride is lacking, the incidence of dental decay is very high. Fluoridation of water, where needed to raise its fluoride concentration to 1 part per million, is recommended as an important public health measure. Not only does an intake of fluoride during childhood protect teeth from decay throughout life; it also helps make the bone crystals of older people resistant to the mineral loss of osteoporosis. Figure 7–7 shows the extent of fluoridation nationwide; states that have adopted fluoridation in more than half of their counties are shown in color.

Despite fluoride's value, violent disagreement often surrounds the introduction of fluoridation in a community. Proponents argue that fluoridation is an obvious, safe, and cost-effective measure to reduce the incidence of dental caries in the young and osteoporosis in older adults. Opponents argue that altering the community water supply is "unnatural" and deprives its consumers of their freedom of choice. Some say that "if God had wanted fluoride in the water supply, it would be there." They fear accidental overdoses, perhaps mistaking the relatively nontoxic salt sodium *fluoride* for the highly volatile gas *fluorine,* which is deadly in excess. They may claim that fluoridated communities have an increased cancer rate.

The first experiments in fluoridation, now famous, were performed in the 1940s in the paired communities of Kingston and Newburgh, New York, and in Grand Rapids and Muskegon, Michigan. In each instance, one of the two communities treated its water supply with fluoride, and the other did not. At the end of ten years, the dental records showed a reduction in the number of decayed, missing, and filled teeth of the Newburgh children (whose water was fluoridated) as compared with the children of Kingston. The youngest children (ages 6 to 9) showed the greatest improvement—about a 60 percent reduction—but even those aged 16 had benefited, with a 40 percent reduction. The medical team reported no significant differences in other aspects of the children's health and concluded that the fluoride had had no adverse side effects.[23] Similar results emerged from the Michigan studies and from others conducted thereafter. It seems from these experiments that fluoride helps prevent tooth decay.

Similar evidence has shown that osteoporosis is typically less extensive in communities with higher fluoride concentrations in their public water. Differing calcium intakes do not account for the differences; differing fluoride intakes seem to be responsible.

The Committee on RDA states that fluoride is present in all normal diets, is required for growth in animals, and is an essential nutrient for human beings. The committee points out that the amount consumed from fluoridated water is typically about 1 milligram a day, whereas chronic intakes, for years, of 20 to 80 milligrams a day are required to produce toxicity symptoms. The first identifiable indication of an excess is slight discoloration of the tooth enamel (**fluorosis**), and this, although unsightly, is not harmful to health.[24]

Figure 7–6 Zinc in Foods.
Most foods rich in zinc are from animal sources. Among plant foods, seeds are rich sources. The U.S. RDA for zinc is 15 milligrams. For more on the zinc contents of foods, see Appendix A.

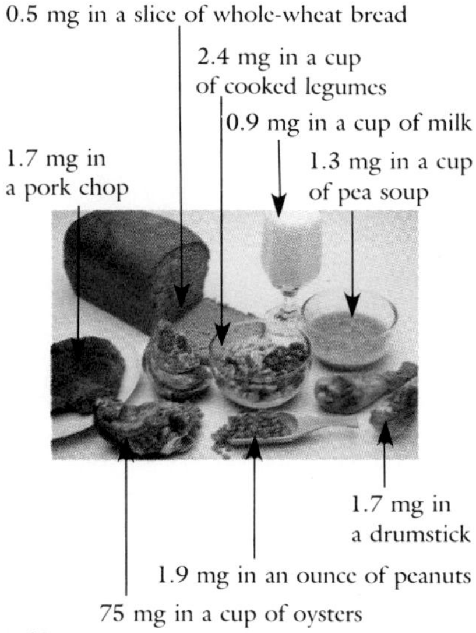

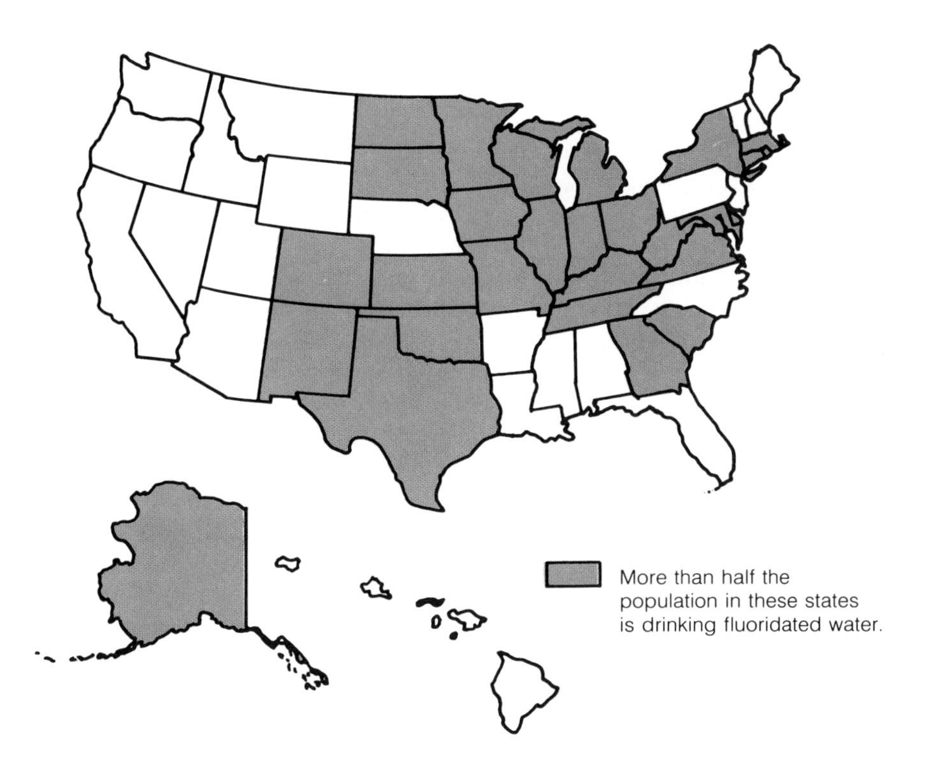

Figure 7–7 Fluoridation in the United States.
Source: U.S. Department of Health and Human Services, Public Health Service, Centers for Disease Control, Dental Disease Prevention Activity, Fluoridation Census, 1980, Figure 1.

On the basis of the accumulated evidence of its beneficial effects, fluoridation has been endorsed by the National Institute of Dental Health, the American Medical Association, the National Cancer Institute, and the National Nutrition Consortium. The allegation that it causes cancer has no identifiable basis in fact and has been refuted by the National Cancer Institute, the American Cancer Society, and the National Institute of Dental Research.

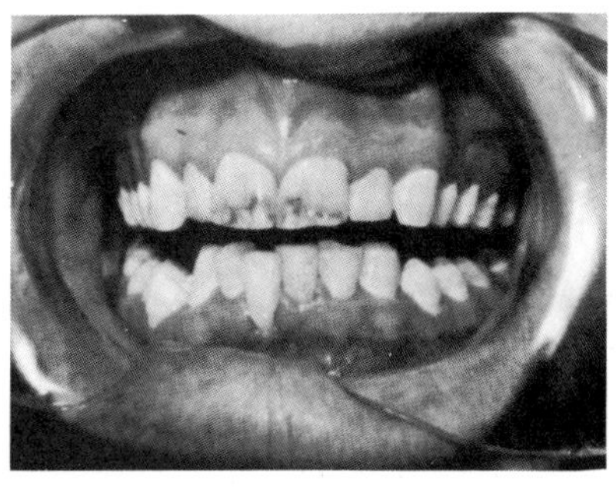

Fluorosis

Now that fluoride has been added to many water supplies, the amounts in foods processed in plants supplied by that water are increasing, so that the total fluoride consumed by certain populations may be greater than expected. No hazard exists at present levels of fluoride consumption, but continued monitoring is important.

In communities where fluoride in the water supply falls short of 1 part per million, individual consumers who want the protection provided by fluoride have several options. (One is, of course, to fight for fluoridation.) They can use fluoride toothpaste or tablets and can make sure their children do the same. During pregnancy, women can request a fluoride-containing supplement from their physicians and a similar one for their newborn infants. During their early years—up to 16—children should receive twice-yearly fluoride applications directly on their teeth as part of dental care.

Fluoride stabilizes bone and makes teeth resistant to decay. Excess fluoride discolors teeth; massive doses are toxic.

Other Trace Minerals

Experiments on animals have suggested that chromium works closely with the hormone insulin, facilitating the uptake of glucose into cells and the release of its energy. Chromium occurs in foods in association with several different com-

glucose tolerance factor (GTF): an organic compound containing chromium; found in foods.

plexes; the one that is best absorbed and most active is a small organic compound—the **glucose tolerance factor (GTF).** Depleted tissue concentrations of chromium in human beings have been linked to a diabetes-like condition in adults and growth failure in children with protein-energy malnutrition. There is some concern that chromium deficiency may be becoming a serious public health problem because of the increased refinement of foods and the resulting loss of their trace minerals.[25]

Copper helps form hemoglobin and collagen, and is needed in many enzymes. Selenium functions as part of an enzyme that acts as an antioxidant and can substitute for vitamin E in some of that vitamin's antioxidant activities; deficiency and toxicity of selenium have both been major public health problems in China. Nickel is now recognized as an essential nutrient, important for the health of many body tissues; deficiencies harm the liver and other organs.[26] Silicon is also essential, and is known to be involved in bone calcification, at least in animals.[27] Tin is necessary for growth in animals and probably in human beings. Vanadium, too, is necessary for growth and bone development and also for normal reproduction. Cobalt is recognized as the mineral in the large vitamin B_{12} molecule; the alternative name for vitamin B_{12}, cobalamin, reflects its presence. The future may reveal that many other trace minerals also play key roles: silver, mercury, lead, barium, cadmium. Even arsenic—known to be a poison and a carcinogen—may turn out to be essential in tiny quantities.

As research on the trace minerals continues, many interactions between them are also coming to light. An excess of one may cause a deficiency of another. (A slight manganese overload, for example, may aggravate an iron deficiency.) A deficiency of one may open the way for another to cause a toxic reaction. (Iron deficiency, for example, makes the body much more susceptible than normal to lead poisoning.) Good food sources of one are poor food sources of another, and factors that cooperate with some trace elements oppose others. (Vitamin C, for example, enhances the absorption of iron and depresses that of copper.) The continuous outpouring of new information about the trace minerals is a sign that we have much more to learn.

All of the trace minerals are toxic in excess. The hazards of overdoses are among the chief risks faced by people who take multiple nutrient supplements. The way to obtain the trace minerals is from food—not hard to do, as long as whole foods are eaten. To eat highly refined foods or empty-calorie fats and sugar is to risk trace mineral deficiency, however, because trace minerals are lost as these products are made. Some claim that organically grown foods contain more trace minerals than those grown on chemical fertilizers. Organic fertilizers do contain more trace minerals than do refined chemical fertilizers, and plants do take up some of the minerals they are given, so this claim may turn out to be valid.

Table 7–6 sums up what this chapter has said about the minerals and fills in some additional information.

Chromium may work with the hormone insulin to control blood glucose concentration. Copper helps make hemoglobin. Selenium is part of an antioxidant enzyme. Many other trace elements also play important roles in the body.

Table 7–6

The Minerals—A Summary

Mineral Name	Chief Functions in the Body	Deficiency Symptoms	Toxicity Symptoms	Significant Sources
Major Minerals				
Calcium, phosphorus	The principal minerals of bones and teeth. Calcium is also involved in normal muscle (including heart muscle) contraction and relaxation, proper nerve functioning, blood clotting, blood pressure, and immune defenses. Phosphorus is a part of every cell, important in the genetic material, as part of phospholipids, in energy transfer, and as buffering systems that maintain acid-base balance.	Calcium: stunted growth in children; bone loss (osteoporosis) in adults. Phosphorus deficiency unknown.	Excess calcium is excreted except in hormonal imbalance states (not caused by nutritional deficiency). Excess phosphorus may draw calcium out of the body in being excreted.	Calcium: milk and milk products, small fish (with bones), tofu (bean curd), greens, legumes. Phosphorus: all animal tissues.
Magnesium	Another factor involved in bone mineralization, the building of protein, enzyme action, normal muscular contraction, transmission of nerve impulses, and maintenance of teeth.	Weakness; confusion; depressed pancreatic hormone secretion; and, if extreme, convulsions, bizarre muscle movements (especially of the eye and facial muscles), hallucinations, and difficulty in swallowing. In children, growth failure.[a]	Not known; large doses have been taken in the form of the laxative Epsom salts, without ill effects except diarrhea.	Nuts, legumes, whole grains, dark green vegetables, seafoods, chocolate, cocoa.
Sodium	Sodium, chloride, and potassium are electrolytes that maintain normal fluid balance inside and outside cells and a proper balance of acids and bases in the body. Sodium is especially important in extracellular water balance and acid-base balance, and to nerve impulse transmission.	Muscle cramps, mental apathy, loss of appetite.	Hypertension.	Salt, soy sauce; moderate quantities in whole, unprocessed foods, large amounts in processed foods.
Chloride	Chloride is also part of the hydrochloric acid found in the stomach, necessary for proper digestion.	Growth failure in children; muscle cramps, mental apathy, loss of appetite; can cause death (uncommon).	Normally harmless (the gas chlorine is a poison but evaporates from water); can cause vomiting.	Salt, soy sauce; moderate quantities in whole, unprocessed foods, large amounts in processed foods.

[a]A still more severe deficiency causes tetany, an extreme, prolonged contraction of the muscles similar to that caused by low blood calcium.

(continued on following page)

Table 7–6

(continued)

Mineral Name	Chief Functions in the Body	Deficiency Symptoms	Toxicity Symptoms	Significant Sources
Potassium	Potassium also facilitates many reactions, including the making of protein; the maintenance of fluid and electrolyte balance, and support of cell integrity; the transmission of nerve impulses; and the contraction of muscles, including the heart.	Deficiency accompanies dehydration; causes muscular weakness, paralysis, and confusion; can cause death.	Causes muscular weakness; triggers vomiting; if given into a vein, can stop the heart.	All whole foods: meats, milk, fruits, vegetables, grains, legumes.
Sulfur	An element related to protein metabolism because it is a component of certain amino acids; part of the vitamins biotin and thiamin and the hormone insulin; involved in the body's detoxification processes, combines with toxic substances to form harmless compounds; also as part of proteins, stabilizes their shape by forming sulfur-sulfur bridges (see Figure 5–4 in Chapter 5).	None known; protein deficiency would occur first.	Would occur only if sulfur amino acids were eaten in excess; this (in animals) depresses growth.	All protein-containing foods.
Trace Minerals				
Iodine	A component of the thyroid hormone thyroxine, which helps to regulate growth, development, and metabolic rate.	Goiter, cretinism.	Very high intakes depress thyroid activity.	Iodized salt; seafood; plants grown in most parts of the country and animals fed those plants.
Iron	Part of the protein hemoglobin, which carries oxygen from place to place in the body; part of the protein myoglobin in muscles, which makes oxygen available for muscle contraction; necessary for the utilization of energy as part of the cells' metabolic machinery.	Anemia: weakness, pallor, headaches, reduced resistance to infection, inability to concentrate	Iron overload: infections, liver injury.	Red meats, fish, poultry, shellfish, eggs, legumes, dried fruits.
Zinc	A working part of many enzymes; present in the hormone insulin; involved in making genetic material and proteins, immune reactions, transport of vitamin A, taste perception, wound healing, the making of sperm, and the normal development of the fetus.	Growth failure in children, sexual retardation, loss of taste, poor wound healing.	Fever, nausea, vomiting, diarrhea.	Protein-containing foods: meats, fish, poultry, grains, vegetables.

Mineral Name	Chief Functions in the Body	Deficiency Symptoms	Toxicity Symptoms	Significant Sources
Copper	A factor necessary for the absorption and use of iron in the formation of hemoglobin; part of several enzymes; a factor that helps to form the protective covering of nerves.	Anemia, bone changes (rare in human beings).	Unknown except as part of a rare hereditary disease (Wilson's disease).	Meats, drinking water.
Fluoride	An element involved in the formation of bones and teeth. Helps to make teeth resistant to decay and bones resistant to loss of their minerals.	Susceptibility to tooth decay and bone loss.	Fluorosis: discoloration of teeth.	Drinking water (if naturally fluoride-containing or fluoridated), tea, seafood.
Selenium	Part of an enzyme that works with vitamin E to protect body compounds from oxidation.	Anemia (rare).	Digestive system disorders.	Seafood, meat, grains.
Chromium	Associated with insulin and required for the release of energy from glucose.	Diabetes-like condition marked by inability to use glucose normally.	Unknown as a nutrition disorder. Occupational exposures damage skin and kidneys.	Meats, unrefined foods, fats, vegetable oils.
Cobalt	Part of vitamin B_{12} and therefore involved in nerve cell function and in the process of blood formation.	Unknown in human beings except in vitamin B_{12} deficiency.	Unknown as a nutrition disorder. Occupational exposures damage skin and red blood cells.	Vitamin B_{12}-containing foods (meats, milk and milk products).
Molybdenum, manganese	Facilitators, with enzymes, of many cell processes.	Molybdenum: unknown. Manganese (in animals): poor growth, nervous system disorders, reproductive abnormalities.	Molybdenum: enzyme inhibition. Manganese: poisoning, nervous system disorders.	Molybdenum: legumes, cereals, organ meats. Manganese: widely distributed in foods.
Vanadium, tin, nickel, silicon, others	Necessary for many biological functions in animals.	Not reported in human beings.	Unknown as nutrition disorders. Industrial exposures cause poisoning via the lungs.	Widely distributed in foods.

Food Feature

Controlling Salt Intake

Figure 7–8 Sources of Sodium in the Diet.
To limit salt means, in general, to limit sodium. Use the foods in part A in liberal quantities. Restrict use of the foods in part B. Add salts and sauces (C) sparingly or not at all.

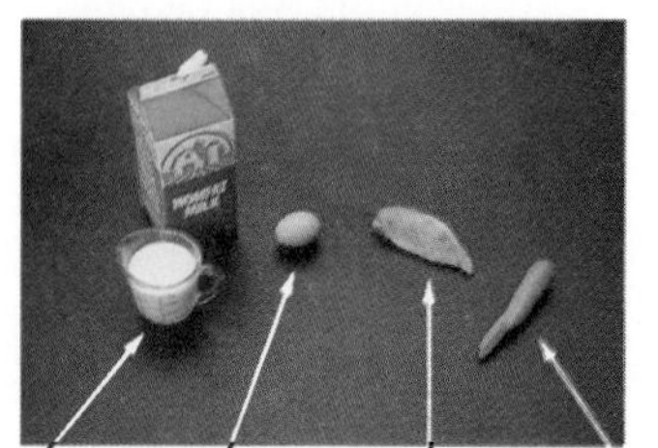

A. One-third is from natural sources.

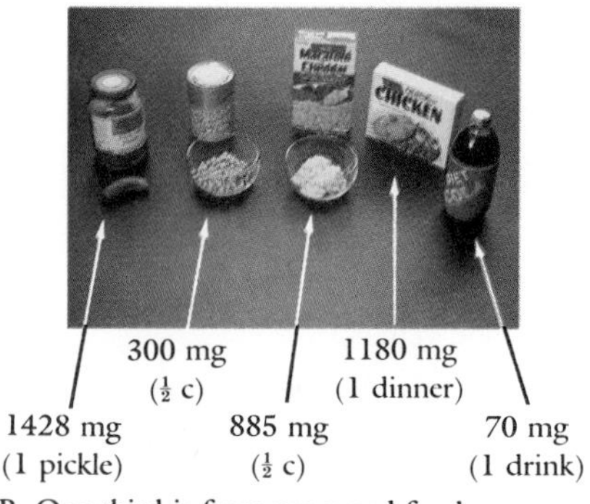

B. One-third is from processed foods.

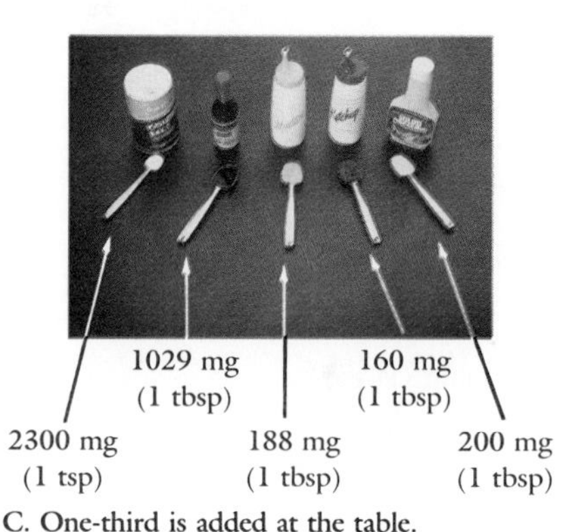

C. One-third is added at the table.

The role of diet in the prevention of hypertension remains a controversy. Most of the debate centers on whether a high-sodium diet causes hypertension and, conversely, whether a sodium-restricted diet can prevent it. The evidence is inconclusive. The value of a low-sodium diet in the treatment of *established* hypertension is unquestioned, however. Studies have shown that even mild restriction of sodium can produce a modest but definite fall in blood pressure in many people.

One of the problems that has plagued researchers investigating the links between salt and hypertension is that heretofore, they have not distinguished between *sodium* and *sodium chloride*, or salt. That distinction is just now being recognized, and its implications have not yet found their way into practical advice on food choices. Salt alone may be what people need to limit, but most advice is still phrased in terms of all sodium compounds. Such advice is useful, however, because most guidelines to reduce dietary sodium intake also reduce salt intake. For those who wish to limit their salt and sodium intakes, then, here are some recommendations.

First, as Figure 7–8 shows, be aware that what you pour from the salt shaker may be only a third of the total salt you consume. Another third comes from processed foods, to which salt was added before you brought them home. All the rest of the foods you consume—all the whole, unprocessed foods—contain only small amounts of sodium, naturally, and contribute only a third of your salt intake in a much larger volume of food. Use many more whole foods, then, such as those shown in part A of the figure, and you will have accomplished a tremendous reduction in your salt and sodium intake. Notice, too, from Table 7–7, that in each food group the least processed foods are not only lowest in sodium but also highest in potassium, an added benefit. No recommendation has been made for the potassium-to-sodium ratio of the diet, but the RDA tables indicate that a 2-to-1 ratio or higher is acceptable; lower might not be.

In reducing your intakes of processed foods, pay particular attention to those listed in Table 7–8. Also, note that processed foods don't always taste salty. Most people are surprised to learn that a serving of cornflakes contains more salt than a serving of cocktail peanuts—and that a serving of chocolate pudding contains still more. A perusal of the sodium (generally reflecting salt) contents of foods in Appendix A is well worth while for anyone wishing to prevent or reduce high blood pressure.

In cooking the foods you select, use only small amounts of added salt, and add little or no salt at the table. Learn to enjoy the unsalted flavors of foods, and to enhance them with salt-free spices such as cinnamon, curry, garlic, ginger, lemon, mustard powder, nutmeg, paprika, parsley, thyme, and vinegar. Table 7–9 offers hints on how to combine these and other spices to make tasty dishes without added salt.

It may take time to learn to enjoy salt-free cooking, so give it time. Sour flavors, such as lemon juice and vinegar, are especially useful in replacing salt, because they enhance whatever natural salty flavor a food may have. As salt

Table 7–7

How Processed Foods Gain Sodium and Lose Potassium

Food	Amount	Potassium (mg)	Sodium (mg)	Potassium-to-Sodium Ratio
Milk Foods				
Milk	1 c	370	122	3:1
Chocolate pudding (cooked from mix)	1 c	354	343	1:1
Chocolate pudding (instant)	1 c	335	820	1:2
Meats				
Beef roast (cooked)	3 oz	279	42	7:1
Corned beef (canned)	3 oz	51	803	1:16
Chipped beef	3 oz	170	3660	1:22
Vegetables				
Corn (cooked)	1 c	304	71	4.1
Creamed corn (canned)	1 c	248	671	1:3
Sugar-coated cornflakes	1 c	27	262	1:10
Fruits				
Peaches (fresh)	1 peach	202	1	202:1
Peaches (canned)	1	333	5	67:1
Peach pie	1 piece	201	201	1:1
Grains				
Whole-wheat flour	1 c	444	4	100:1
Whole-wheat bread	1 slice	68	132	1:2
Doughnut, snack cake	1	23	125	1:5

Table 7–8

Foods That Are High in Salt or Sodium

Foods prepared in brine, such as pickles, olives, and sauerkraut.

Salty or smoked meat, such as bologna, corned or chipped beef, frankfurters, ham, luncheon meats, salt pork, sausage, and smoked tongue.

Salty or smoked fish, such as anchovies, caviar, salted and dried cod, herring, sardines, and smoked salmon.

Snack items such as potato chips, pretzels, salted popcorn, and salted nuts and crackers.

Bouillon cubes; seasoned salts (including sea salt); soy, Worcestershire, and barbecue sauces.

Cheeses, especially processed types.

Canned and instant soups.

Prepared horseradish, catsup, and mustard.

Table 7–9

Spices to Enhance Salt-Free Dishes

For general seasoning purposes, use these mixed herbs (place in shaker):

Saltless surprise:	2 tsp garlic powder; 1 tsp each of basil, oregano, and powdered lemon rind (or dehydrated lemon juice). Blend, mix well, store in glass container with rice to prevent caking.
Pungent salt substitute:	3 tsp basil; 2 tsp each of savory, celery seed, ground cumin seed, marjoram, sage, lemon thyme. Mix well, then powder with a mortar and pestle.
Spicy salt substitute:	1 tsp each of cloves, pepper, and crushed coriander seed; 2 tsp paprika; 1 tbsp rosemary. Mix in a blender and store in an airtight container.

For specific seasoning purposes, use these herbs. Store together mixtures of those you especially like, and label them "soup blend," "beef blend," etc.

When you Serve:	Use:
Beef	Bay, chives, cloves, cumin, garlic, hot pepper, marjoram, rosemary, savory
Bread	Caraway, marjoram, oregano, poppy seed, rosemary, thyme
Cheese	Basil, chervil, chives, curry, dill, fennel, garlic chives, marjoram, oregano, parsley, sage, thyme
Fish	Chervil, dill, fennel, garlic, parsley, tarragon,[a] thyme
Fruit	Anise, cinnamon, cloves, coriander, ginger, lemon verbena, mint, rose geranium, sweet cicely
Lamb	Garlic, marjoram, oregano, rosemary, thyme (make little slits in lamb and insert herbs before roasting)
Pork	Coriander, cumin, garlic, ginger, hot peppers, pepper sage, savory, thyme
Poultry	Garlic, oregano, rosemary, sage, savory
Salads	Basil, borage, burnet, chives, garlic chives, parsley, rocket salad, sorrel[b]
Soups	Bay, chervil, marjoram, parsley, rosemary, savory, tarragon[a]
Vegetables	Basil, burnet, chervil, chives, dill, marjoram, mint, parsley, pepper, tarragon,[a] thyme

[a]French tarragon.

[b]Use these herbs fresh, if possible; if using dry, add to salad dressing. Use herb vinegars for extra flavor.

Source: Adapted from H. H. Shimizu, Do yourself a flavor, *FDA Consumer,* April 1984, pp. 16–19.

intake decreases, the taste buds adjust, and the taste of food with less salt becomes the preferred taste. Ease your way by reducing salt intake gradually to allow time to adjust to the flavor of unsalted foods. Many cookbooks with helpful tips are available.

Make substitutions, too. In particular, in place of bouillon or canned broths, use low-sodium bouillon and homemade stocks; to concentrate their flavors, reduce them by boiling until half the liquid evaporates.

Table 4–5 in Chapter 4 showed how easy it is to modify a recipe to reduce its sodium content. (While they were at it, the cooks reduced the fat content as well.) The lasagne shown can be made without the oil, with more vegetables, with less and leaner meat, with less salt, and with less cheese. It is still delicious, and substantially lower than the original in calories, fat, *and* salt.

When soft water is used in food products, it may contribute significantly to salt intake, so learn whether your water is hard or soft, and adjust your use accordingly. Be aware that medications, toothpastes, mouthwashes, and other nonfood products may also contain salt. Many low-sodium products are available, but in general, you can make a low-sodium diet attractive without using these products. Some people, however, like to use them to add variety.

In salt substitutes, the sodium is generally replaced by potassium. Some people don't like the taste of salt substitutes but may find them acceptable if used sparingly. (Don't heat them, though, because they turn bitter.) Often people find food more acceptable without any salt at all. The use of a potassium-containing salt substitute serves the dual purpose of increasing potassium intake while reducing sodium.* Some products contain a combination of half regular table salt and half salt substitute. Although these products may be more palatable, they also can contribute a significant amount of salt to the diet.

Besides all these considerations, many positive choices are possible. The person who wishes to use diet to prevent or reduce high blood pressure should emphasize these positive actions:

- Eat plenty of fresh fruits, vegetables, milk products, and meat, because these foods are especially rich in potassium.
- Be sure to eat a balanced diet, including good food sources of calcium and magnesium.
- Maintain appropriate weight.
- Use alcohol moderately, if at all.

These are explained further in the Controversy that follows this chapter.

*People with renal insufficiency should not use salt substitutes containing potassium.

shopping list:

two new herbs or spices each time you shop (until you have a variety that you like)
low-salt seasoning mixtures
garlic
lemons
vinegar
pepper
parsley

Notes

1. T. Vokes, Water homeostasis, *Annual Review of Nutrition* 7 (1987): 383–406.
2. L. K. DeBruyne and S. R. Rolfes, *Chocolate Milk: Sweet Treat or Good Food?,* a monograph available (1985) from The Nutrition Company, P.O. Box 11102, Tallahassee, FL 32303.
3. L. H. Allen, Calcium bioavailability and absorption: A review, *American Journal of Clinical Nutrition* 35 (1982): 798–808.
4. M. Hirotsuka and coauthors, Calcium fortification of soy milk with calcium-lecithin liposome system, *Journal of Food Science* 49 (1984): 1111–1112, 1127.
5. L. D. McBean, Food versus pills versus fortified foods, *Dairy Council Digest* 58, March–April 1987.
6. McBean, 1987.
7. B. G. Shah, Calcium supplementation with antacids, *Journal of the American Medical Association* 257 (1987): 541.
8. J. L. Greger, Food, supplements, and fortified foods: Scientific evaluations in regard to toxicology and nutrient bioavailability, *Journal of the American Dietetic Association* 87 (1987): 1369–1373.
9. Greger 1987; M. S. Sheikh and coauthors, Gastrointestinal absorption of calcium from milk and calcium salts, *New England Journal of Medicine* 317 (1987): 532–536.
10. McBean, 1987.
11. Greger, 1987.
12. McBean, 1987.
13. More on supplementation: Calcium redux, *Nutrition Action,* December 1984, pp. 12–13.
14. McBean, 1987.
15. J. Mayer and J. Goldberg, Sufficient calcium intake still a major problem, *Tallahassee Democrat,* 5 November 1987.
16. P. D. M. V. Turlapaty and B. M. Altura, Magnesium deficiency produces spasms of coronary arteries: Relationship to etiology of sudden death ischemic heart disease, *Science* 208 (1980): 198–200.
17. F. Taylor, Iodine: Going from hypo to hyper, *FDA Consumer,* April 1981, pp. 15–18.
18. L. Hallberg, Iron, Chapter 32 in *Present Knowledge in Nutrition,* 5th ed. (New York: Nutrition Foundation, 1984), pp. 459–478.

Self-Study

Evaluate Your Mineral Intakes

These exercises make use of the information you recorded on Form 3 in Appendix H.

1. Start with calcium. What percentage of your recommended intake did you consume? Was this enough? What foods contribute the greatest amount of calcium to your diet? If you consumed more than the recommendation, was this too much? Why or why not? In what ways would you change your diet to improve it in this respect?

2. With respect to sodium, the amounts you arrived at on Form 3 may not be meaningful, because different products contain vastly different amounts of salt, and different cooks and eaters add vastly different amounts of salt to foods. The amounts in the particular foods you ate may have differed from those in the tables. However, most of the sodium you consume comes from two sources: processed foods, and the salt shaker. Your food record contains an approximation of the contribution made by processed foods, and you can roughly estimate the amount of salt you add to foods if you are willing to observe yourself for (let's say) three days. Each time you salt your foods from the salt shaker, also sprinkle the same number of shakes onto a napkin, and collect the salt into a container. At the end of three days, measure the total amount of salt you have used. If you have access to a sensitive balance, use it; if not, you can use a measuring spoon. The procedure you are following is only approximate, anyway, and a spoon measure will not significantly reduce its accuracy. Each teaspoon represents about 5 grams of salt, or 2000 mg of sodium. Divide by 3 to obtain your daily average, and add this amount to the average on your food record (Form 3).

How does your intake of sodium compare with the safe and adequate intake, for an adult, of 1100 to 3300 mg of sodium?

3. Heighten your awareness of the sodium contents of processed foods. Look up the following foods in Appendix A and list their sodium contents: dill pickle, corn flakes, cottage cheese, hot dog, chicken pot pie, canned soup (your choice), a fast-food hamburger (your choice), margarine, potato chips, peanuts, chocolate pudding. What foods *you* like to eat are high in sodium? Is there another way you could enjoy these foods without so much salt?

4. Calculate your intakes of magnesium, phosphorus, and potassium, and compare them with the recommended intakes. If you need to improve your diet with respect to these minerals, how will you go about doing so?

5. Go on to iron. What percentage of your recommended intake did you consume? Was this enough? Which of the foods you eat supply the most iron? Rank your top five iron contributors. How many were meats? Legumes? Greens? Other? Are enriched or whole-grain products important to your iron intake?

6. Compute your iron absorption from a meal of your choosing, using the following method. First, inspect the foods you ate that contained iron and distinguish between the heme and nonheme iron. Remember that 40% of the iron in animal tissues is heme iron. Calculate the amount of iron from animal tissues (MFP), and take 40% of it to find the heme iron in the meal (use Form 6). Calculate the remaining iron, including 60% of the iron from animal tissues, to get nonheme iron. Also calculate the amount of vitamin C in the meal. Now determine if the nonheme iron is of high, medium, or low availability, based on either the vitamin C or the MFP factor in the meal, whichever gives the better score. Vitamin C provides high availability if there is more then 75 mg in the meal, medium if there is 25 to 75 mg, and low if there is less than 25 mg. MFP provides high availability if there is more than 3 oz of lean meat, fish, or poultry in the meal; medium if 1 to 3 oz; and low if less than 1 oz. Now calculate the amount of iron absorbed. For heme iron, use 23%. For nonheme iron, use 8% (high availability), 5% (medium availability), or 3% (low availability). Add the amounts of heme iron absorbed and nonheme iron absorbed to get total iron absorbed.[28]

The RDA assumes you will absorb 10% of the iron you ingest. Thus, if you are a man of any age or a woman over 50 (RDA 10 mg), you need to absorb 1 mg/day; if you are a woman 11 to 50 (RDA 18 mg), 1.8 mg/day. How could you eat differently to improve your iron absorption?

7. Now turn to zinc. What percentage of the recommendation did you consume? What were your best food sources of zinc? What guidelines do you need to follow to be sure of obtaining enough zinc from the foods you eat?

8. Iodine, fluoride, and other trace elements are not listed in Appendix A, but you can evaluate your intakes as follows. For iodine, answer these questions: Are you in an area of the country where the soil is iodine poor? If so, do you use iodized salt?

9. For fluoride: Is the water in your

Self-Study

county fluoridated? (Call the county health department.) If not, how do you and your family ensure that your intakes of fluoride are optimal?

10. For trace elements, try to get a sense of where your typical diet falls on the spectrum between all natural (whole) foods and processed foods. List, with their calorie amounts, the foods you ate in three days that were predominantly whole unprocessed foods like those on the exchange lists. List separately those that were highly processed foods, such as TV dinners, pastries, and instant gravies. What percentage of the calories you consume comes from whole, natural foods? What percentage from processed foods? In light of the fact that processed foods tend to lack trace elements, do you suppose you get enough trace elements in your diet?

19. N. S. Scrimshaw, Functional consequences of iron deficiency in human populations, *Journal of Nutrition Science and Vitaminology* 30 (1984): 47–63.
20. S. N. Gershoff and coauthors, Studies of the elderly in Boston: 1. The effects of iron fortification on moderately anemic people, *American Journal of Clinical Nutrition* 30 (1978): 134–141.
21. Scrimshaw, 1984.
22. F. H. Nielson, Ultratrace elements: Current status, in *Nutrition Update,* vol. 2, ed. J. Weininger and G. M. Briggs (New York: Wiley, 1985), pp. 107–126.
23. E. R. Schlesinger and coauthors, Newburgh-Kingston caries-fluorine study: 12. Pediatric findings after 10 years, *Journal of the American Dental Association* 52 (1956): 296–306.
24. Food and Nutrition Board, Committee on Recommended Allowances, *Recommended Dietary Allowances,* 9th ed. (Washington, D.C.: National Academy of Sciences, 1980), pp. 156–159.
25. W. Mertz, The essential trace elements, *Science* 213 (1981): 1332–1338.
26. Nielson, 1985.
27. Nielson, 1985.
28. E. R. Monsen and coauthors, Estimation of available dietary iron, *American Journal of Clinical Nutrition* 31 (1978): 134–141. Moderate iron stores assumed.

Nutrition and Hypertension

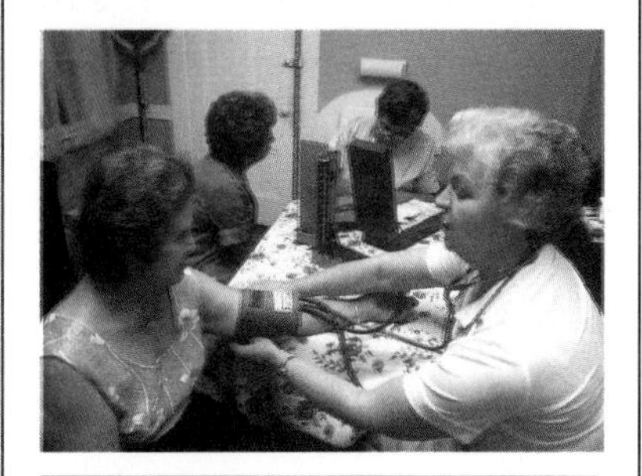

The most effective single measure you can take to protect yourself against high blood pressure is to know whether you have it or not.

You cannot tell if you have high blood pressure; it presents no symptoms you can feel. But if you do have it, it threatens to impair the quality of your life and even strike you down before your time. Chronic elevated blood pressure, or hypertension, is the most prevalent form of cardiovascular disease, believed to affect some 60 million people—more than a third of the entire adult population.[1] It contributes to half a million strokes and over a million heart attacks each year.[2] The higher the blood pressure above normal, the greater the risk of heart disease.

The most effective single step you can take toward protecting yourself from hypertension is to find out whether you have it or not. At checkup time, a health care professional can give you an accurate blood pressure reading. (Self-test machines in drugstores and other places can mislead you by reporting inaccurate readings.) If your blood pressure is above normal, the reading should be repeated before the diagnosis of hypertension is considered confirmed. Thereafter, it should be checked by means of additional readings at regular intervals.

When a blood pressure reading is taken, two numbers are important: the pressure in the arteries during contraction of the ventricles (the "dub" of the heartbeat), which is higher, and the pressure during relaxation of the ventricles (the "lub"), which is lower. The first number is the **systolic pressure,** and the second is the **diastolic pressure.**

Blood pressure should probably be around 120 over 70, ideally.* However, it is generally considered normal if it is less than 140 over 90. Above this level, the risks of heart attacks and strokes increase in direct proportion to increasing blood pressure, especially systolic pressure. Mild hypertension, which accounts for 75 percent of all blood pressure problems, involves a systolic pressure in the range of 140 to 160, and a diastolic pressure of 90 to 95. Severe hypertension is anything greater than 160/95.[3]

A word of caution about interpreting blood pressure readings: many factors can affect them. For example, your blood pressure rises when you speak, so it is important to remain silent as the reading is being taken. Body position, too, is important for accuracy: your blood pressure is lowest when you are lying down, higher when you are sitting up, and higher still when you are standing. The cuff should fit; people with excess body fat may sometimes get a falsely high blood pressure reading simply because the cuff is too small. A high reading should be confirmed on a separate occasion before it is believed.

*Blood pressure is read in millimeters of mercury. The silver column that rises on a blood pressure instrument is a column of mercury; the height to which it is pushed is marked off in millimeters.

How Hypertension Develops

A certain blood pressure is vital to life in the cells. The pressure of the blood against the walls of the arteries pushes fluids, carrying a cargo of nutrients and oxygen, out of the arteries into the tissues. By the time blood reaches the veins, much of its fluid has exited, and the concentration of cells and dissolved materials in the remaining blood is at a maximum. Fluids carrying wastes from the tissues are attracted by the concentrated blood and seep back into the veins. Thus the cells are nourished and cleansed.

The pressure the blood exerts on the inner walls of the arteries is the result of two forces acting together: the heart's pushing the blood into the arteries, and the smallest arteries and capillaries resisting its flow. The heart's push ensures that the blood circulates through the whole system; the **peripheral resistance** and resulting pressure ensure that some of the blood's components, including nutrients, are pushed through the capillary walls to feed the tissues. One other factor contributes to blood pressure: the volume of fluid in the vascular system—and that, in turn, is affected by the number of dissolved particles it contains. By the rule that "water follows salt," the more salt in the blood, the more water there will be. Figures 1–2 and 1–3 in Chapter 1 showed how the system works; Figure C7–1 shows the forces that contribute to blood pressure.

The kidneys depend on the blood pressure to help them filter waste materials out of the blood. (The pressure has to be high enough to force the blood's fluid out of the capillaries into the kidney's filtering network.) If the blood pressure is too low, the kidneys release substances to set things right: some of them constrict the peripheral blood vessels, and others lead to the retention of water in the body. These actions increase peripheral resistance and blood volume, and thus raise the blood pressure.

Figure C7–1 The Blood Pressure.
Two major contributors to the pressure inside an artery are the heart's pushing blood into it, and the small-diameter arteries and capillaries at its other end resisting the blood's flow (peripheral resistance). Another determining factor is the volume of fluid in the circulatory system, which depends in turn on the number of dissolved particles in that fluid; see Chapter 7.

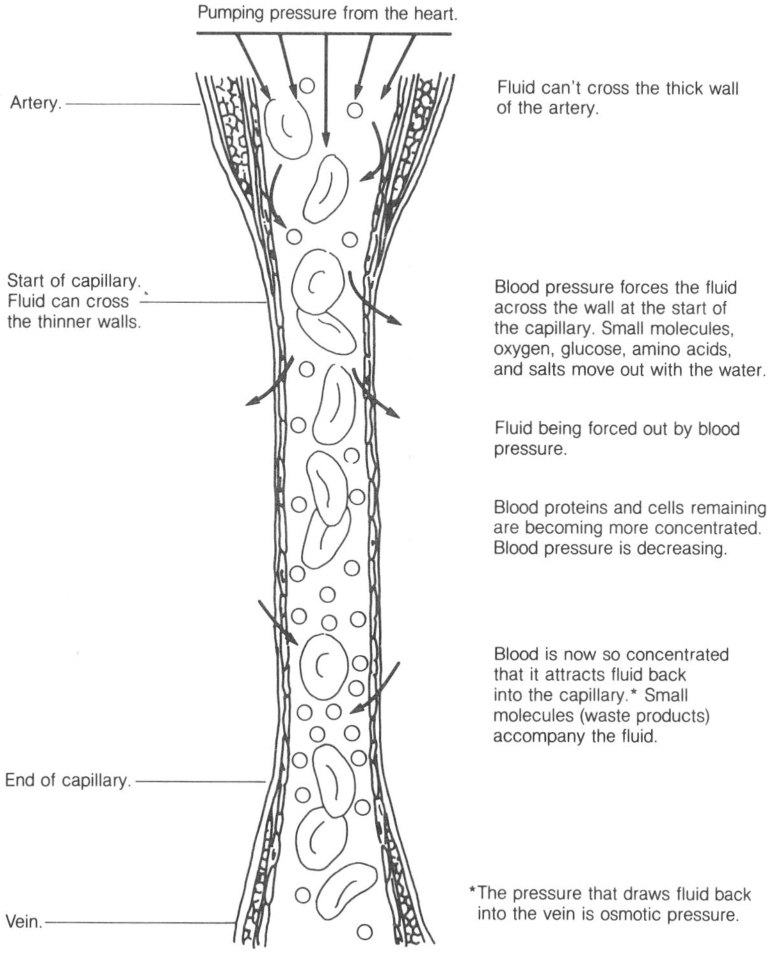

Normally, the blood pressure–raising action of the kidneys is beneficial. In dehydration, for example, a "water deficiency" exists. By constricting the blood vessels and conserving water and sodium, the kidneys ensure that blood pressure is maintained until the person can drink water. In hypertension, however, the kidneys are fooled: they react as if there were a "water deficiency," but there is none. Then their raising of the blood pressure has harmful effects.

It seems logical that something might be wrong in the kidneys of a person with hypertension, but fewer than 10 percent of all cases of hypertension are known to arise from kidney disorders. These cases are classified as **secondary hypertension** (meaning that kidney malfunction came first—that is, was primary). Treatment for people with secondary hypertension focuses on correcting the underlying disorder in the kidneys—infection, injury, or whatever. For the other 90 percent or more of all cases of hypertension, no cause is known; those are classified as cases of **essential** or **primary hypertension.**

The kidneys may be just as involved in essential hypertension as they are in secondary hypertension, but exactly how they are involved is not known. Essential hypertension may have more than one cause: suspected are genetic, environmental, nutrition, and life-style factors. One such factor is an imbalance among the eicosanoids that regulate blood pressure by dilating or constricting the narrow arteries[4] (see the box in Chapter 4). Added weight (obesity) raises blood pressure; extra adipose tissue means miles of extra capillaries through which the blood must be pumped. Another factor is atherosclerosis (hardening of the arteries), which reduces circulation to the tissues and deprives in kidneys of water just as dehydration does (thus fooling the kidneys into raising blood pressure as described earlier). Not only does atherosclerosis contribute to hypertension, but also the reverse. Hypertension promotes atherosclerosis by mechanically injuring the artery linings, making plaques likely to form.

The combination of hypertension, atherosclerosis, and obesity puts a severe strain on the heart and arteries, leading to many forms of cardiovascular disease and death. Some of the results were mentioned in the Miniglossary of Controversy 4. Strain on the heart's pump, the left ventricle, enlarges and weakens it, until finally it fails (heart failure). Pressure in the aorta causes it to balloon out and burst (aneurysm). Pressure in the small arteries of the brain makes them burst and bleed (stroke). The kidneys can be damaged when the heart is unable to adequately pump blood through them (kidney failure).

Epidemiologic studies have identified several risk factors to predict the development of hypertension, including:

- *Age.* Blood pressure levels increase with age; most people who develop essential hypertension do so in their 50s and 60s.
- *Family background.* A family history of hypertension and heart disease raises the risk of developing hypertension two to five times.
- *Obesity.* Obese people are more likely to develop hypertension.
- *Race.* Hypertension is twice as common among blacks as among whites; it tends to develop earlier and become more severe.

While researchers continue looking for the cause or causes, clearly it is urgent that we do what we can to detect and treat hypertension wherever it presents its deadly threat—or better still, that we prevent it. A major national effort has been made to identify and treat hypertension. Even mild hypertension can be dangerous; individuals who have it benefit from treatment, showing a reduced incidence of early death and illness.[5] Diet changes alone, even without the drugs used to reduce blood pressure, can bring about these benefits without the undesirable side effects of the drugs.

Authorities differ on the exact modes of treatment to select. Some say drugs should be used rather routinely; others advocate the aggressive use of diet therapy and other life-style changes (stress management, weight reduction, taking up regular exercise) in preference to the use of drugs.[6] This Controversy, of course, focuses on the diet, with a word or two about exercise along the way.[7]

What are the diet-related factors that affect blood pressure? Most people might respond "salt" (meaning sodium), without even thinking, but research into sodium's role has disappointed investigators who hoped they were on the track to a single answer. Other factors are obesity and exercise—or rather, lack of it. Other elements may be involved—notably, potassium, calcium, and chloride. Dietary fat, alcohol, and magnesium are also suspect.

Obesity Evidence supports a positive link between obesity and hypertension. (This is not to say that every obese person becomes hypertensive, or that all people with hypertension are overweight, but that those who are should sit up and take notice.)

Weight reduction in overweight people with hypertension significantly lowers blood pressure. This is so, even if the person does not go all the way to achieve ideal body weight. Those who are using drugs to control their blood pressure can often reduce or discontinue use of them.[8] Even a 10-pound weight loss more than doubles the chance that hypertensive people can normalize their blood pressure without drugs, even if they have been maintained on aggressive hypertensive drug therapy for five years.[9]

Researchers have wondered whether the weight loss itself brought the benefits mentioned, or whether, in restricting calories, people were actually eating a diet that was lower in salt or sodium, and *that* accounted for the results. Moderation in salt or sodium intake does help normalize blood pressure,[10] but people who lose weight can lower their blood pressure, even without altering their salt or sodium intakes. Thus weight loss alone may be one of the most effective nondrug treatments for hypertension.[11]

Exercise Exercise, of course, is part of the energy balance equation (see Chapters 8 and 9). The more you exercise, the more energy you spend, and the less fat you accumulate (or the more you take off). But moderate exercise of the right kind also helps directly to reduce hypertension. Although blood pressure rises temporarily at each bout of exercise, the effect in the long run is to lower the blood pressure significantly.[12]

The "right kind" of exercise is *not* the short-duration, heavy weightlifting type. It is the endurance type, such as jogging, undertaken faithfully as a daily or every-other-day routine, that strengthens the heart and blood vessels and permanently alters body composition in favor of lean over fat tissue. Such exercise training increases the volume of oxygen the heart can deliver to the tissues at each beat, reducing its work load. Such exercise also changes the hormonal climate in which the body does its work (it alters "sympathetic tone"—stress hormone secretion—in such a way as to lower blood pressure). It brings about a redistribution of body water, and it eases transit of the blood through the peripheral arteries.[13] The exercise to seek is that of great enough intensity to elevate the heart rate and speed up breathing, but of low enough intensity to be sustainable for 20 consecutive minutes. Chapter 9 gives details on this kind of exercise.

Exercise helps correct raised blood cholesterol levels, too, and if heart and artery disease has already set in, a monitored exercise program may actually help to reverse it.[14] When heart muscle tissue is threatened by a narrowed artery, the heart begins to compensate by finding alternate vessels through which to deliver the blood. These smaller **collateral blood vessels** in the heart act as a detour around the blockages, and many times they can avert much tissue death that otherwise would occur. Some evidence from studies using animals suggests that the heart forms new collateral vessels in response to exercise, especially in the young.[15] In human beings, the development of such vessels may be a factor in the excellent recovery seen in some heart attack victims who exercise.[16]

Sodium/Sodium Chloride Sodium clearly has something to do with blood pressure. In fact, for years, research on populations has seemed to indicate that high sodium intakes were "the" factor responsible for people's high blood pressure; but recently that notion has been falling into disfavor. Where does sodium fit in, now? And is it sodium in any form, or salt (sodium chloride) that is responsible for the effects seen? Positive and negative ions always travel together. They separate in water solution and may join up again in other combinations, but overwhelmingly, sodium's partner in foods and in the body fluids is the chloride ion. Thus, much of the early research that implicated sodium in hypertension's causation may have unwittingly uncovered the effects of sodium's silent partner, chloride. Apparently, sodium in combination with other negative ions causes water retention and certain hormonal responses, but sodium chloride, uniquely, seems to raise blood pressure.[17] Throughout the following discussions of research results formerly stated in terms of sodium, we have therefore had to add "and chloride" or "or salt."

The sodium (and chloride) concentration in the blood and other body tissues is maintained through an elaborate regulatory mechanism involving the kidneys, the adrenal glands, the pituitary gland, and other glands. Most people can therefore safely consume more salt than they need, and rely on these control mechanisms to regulate its excretion and retention as needed. "Sodium-sensitive" individuals, however, experience high blood pressure from excesses in sodium or salt intake. People with chronic renal disease, those whose parents (one or both) have hypertension, blacks, and persons over 50 years of age are most likely to be sodium (or salt) sensitive.[18]

How dietary sodium or salt contributes to hypertension in these people is unknown, but recent research suggests a chain of events that leads to contraction of the small arteries, increasing peripheral resistance. The chain may begin with an inherited or acquired defect in the kidneys.

When salt intake exceeds what the kidneys can excrete, sodium, chloride (and other negative ions), and water are retained in the blood (remember, "water follows salt"), and the blood volume expands. The extra fluid volume is thought to help bring about the secretion of a hormone **(natriuretic hormone)** not normally active, which enables the kidneys to excrete some of the excess. However, the same hormone moves sodium (and chloride and other negative ions) into the smooth muscle cells that line the arteries, and affects their membranes so that they bring in too much calcium, too. The more calcium, the more these muscle cells contract, the more peripheral resistance increases, and the higher the blood pressure rises.[19] In short, the hormone trades a wrong for a right; it reduces the blood volume, but it increases peripheral resistance so that blood pressure stays high.

This long chain of reasoning, worked out by medical researchers intent on getting to the bottom of the sodium-hypertension connection, promises to help in efforts to identify, treat, and perhaps prevent hypertension—but remember, it happens only in "sodium-sensitive" individuals. For them, it implies that eating a diet low in sodium, or at least salt, is a wise idea. But for others—the majority of people with hypertension—this may not be an effective diet strategy. Sodium restriction does not lower the blood pressure in half of the hypertensive people in whom it is tried.[20] It is important to look further to see what other dietary factors might be relevant.

Potassium When sodium is retained in the body, potassium is excreted. Some subjects with normal blood pressure, if fed very large quantities of sodium, ultimately show a rise in blood pressure—but at the same time, their potassium excretion is increasing. When fed potassium simultaneously with the sodium, they do not have a rise in blood pressure.[21] For this reason, many health care practitioners recommend that food sources of potassium be emphasized in the daily diet.

Population studies show sodium being traded for potassium in a different sense. People who eat many foods high in salt often happen to be eating fewer potassium-containing foods at the same time.[22] Table 7–7 showed that as the *same* food goes through several processing steps, it loses potassium as it gains sodium, so that its potassium-sodium ratio falls dramatically. Some authorities believe that it is important to obtain enough potassium for both prevention and treatment of hypertension.[23]

Potassium may be important in heart disease independently of its relationship to sodium. Even in people without high blood pressure, a high potassium intake protects against stoke.[24]

People using diuretics (see p. 242) to control hypertension should know that some cause potassium excretion and can induce a deficiency. Those using these drugs must be particularly careful to include rich sources of potassium in their daily diets.*

Calcium Calcium acts as a key element in maintaining normal tone and function of the circulatory system. Specifically, calcium affects blood pressure through its action on the muscle cells in the artery walls. An excess of calcium inside these muscle cells causes contraction, which narrows the arteries and elevates blood pressure. The contraction process involves other components as well: hormones, sodium, and potassium. A possible explanation for the calcium-hypertension connection is that when the dietary calcium is low, the artery muscle cells "hoard" the calcium and contract, raising blood pressure. If dietary calcium were at least adequate, the cells would limit their uptake of calcium, and the arteries would be relaxed, lowering blood pressure.[25] This may explain the finding, first reported years ago, that soft water (high in sodium) was linked to a higher heart disease death rate than hard water (high in calcium).

Calcium may play a role in pregnancy-related hypertension, too. Fewer than 1 in 200 pregnant women suffer from hypertension in areas where average calcium consumption exceeds 1000 milligrams per day. There is a five-fold to tenfold increase in the incidence of pregnancy-related hypertension where calcium intakes average less than 500 milligrams per day.[26]

Several surveys report that people with hypertension consume less calcium than those with normal blood pressure.[27] Surprisingly, they also consume ***less sodium*** than those without high blood pressure—but perhaps this is because they are trying to do so. (People on low-salt diets tend to avoid dairy products, since these contain significant amounts of sodium; consequently, they lower both their intakes of sodium and calcium.) In a major survey that undertook to determine the relationship of 17 nutrients and total calories to blood pressure levels in over 10,000 individuals 18 to 74 years old, calcium was the nutrient that distinguished those with hypertension from those without it. The survey evaluation revealed that hypertensive people reported consuming about 20 percent less calcium than those without hypertension; there appeared to be an inverse relationship between calcium and blood pressure. Based on these data, researchers estimated that people with the lowest calcium intakes (below 300 milligrams per day) had a twofold to threefold increase in risk of developing hypertension when compared with people with the highest calcium intakes (1200 milligrams per day).[28]

Calcium may be important in both the prevention and treatment of hypertension. For those at risk of developing it, increasing the amount of calcium in the diet may protect against hypertension. For people already diagnosed with hypertension, obtaining adequate calcium in the diet may lower blood pressure. One study shows that a calcium-rich diet reduced blood pressure in 44 percent of the people with hypertension studied. Of those with normal blood pressure, 19 percent also experienced reduction in their systolic pressure, the indicator most closely associated with risk of mortality.[29] It is recommended, therefore, that people with hypertension, or at risk of developing it, at least meet the current RDA for calcium—800 milligrams a day for adults. Dairy products are recommended, because they provide not only calcium, but also potassium and magnesium, which may also help keep blood pressure normal. Low-fat or nonfat dairy products have an added advantage (see next section).

Fat Fat is well known as a dietary factor contributing to atherosclerosis. Less well known is its independent role in relation to blood pressure. Diets high in saturated fat

*Another class of drugs used to treat hypertension is the adrenergic blockers. Adrenergic blockers interfere with a neurotransmitter to alter blood pressure.

are associated with hypertension. Populations that consume small quantities of animal products—vegetarians, for example—have a low incidence of hypertension. When people restrict their total dietary fat and increase the ratio of polyunsaturated to saturated fatty acids in the diet to 1.0 or above, their blood pressure falls, whether or not it was their intent to make it do so.[30]

This probably works at least partly by way of certain eicosanoids, which affect both hormonal control of sodium excretion and relaxation or constriction of the peripheral blood vessels. The essential fatty acid linoleic acid is a precursor of arachidonic acid, which in turn is a precursor of the prostaglandins. Research using animals shows that when dietary linoleic acid is restricted almost to the point of deficiency, synthesis of prostaglandins is suppressed, and blood pressure rises.[31] Linoleic acid may increase the synthesis of the prostaglandins that relax the blood vessels and therefore lower peripheral resistance or slow the long-term vascular changes associated with hypertension.[32] The effects are small, and not consistent from one study to the next.[33]

The implications of the findings suggesting a role for dietary fat in hypertension are not yet clear. Monounsaturated fat may work as well as polyunsaturated fat; oleic acid from olive oil seems to correlate inversely with blood pressure in the Mediterranean,[34] and research on omega-6 fatty acids from fish is under way. Many professionals are advising hypertensive clients to follow the same fat-controlled diet as is recommended to prevent atherosclerosis—reducing fat to 30 percent of calories, obtaining one third each from polyunsaturated, monounsaturated, and saturated sources, and limiting dietary cholesterol to 300 mg a day or less.[35] Hypertensive people are at greater-than-normal risk for developing heart disease anyway, and this diet may offer benefits for blood pressure control as well.

Alcohol Alcohol has several roles in relation to heart disease. In moderate doses, alcohol initially reduces pressure in the peripheral arteries and so reduces blood pressure, but high doses clearly raise blood pressure.[36] In fact, of people with alcoholism, 30 to 60 percent have hypertension.[37] The hypertension is apparently caused directly by the alcohol,[38] and it leads to cardiovascular disease as severe as hypertension caused by any other factor.[39] Immediately on withdrawal, in a heavy drinker, blood pressure soars, but stopping drinking restores normal blood pressure in most drinkers after a while.[40] Furthermore, alcohol causes strokes—even *without* hypertension.[41] Advice on alcohol use is quite straightforward, then: if you drink, do so in moderation (the words are those of the *Dietary Guidelines for Americans*, p. 39). *Moderation* means one to two drinks a day, not more.[42] (For more on alcohol and nutrition, read Controversy 12.)

Other Factors

Research is continuing to reveal relationships of other factors to hypertension. For example, magnesium seems to protect against it. Magnesium deficiency causes visible changes in the walls of arteries and capillaries and makes them tend to constrict, a possible mechanism for its hypertensive effect.[43] Also, a connection between hypertension and insulin resistance is coming to light; hypertension appears to be an insulin-resistant state. This is so, even in the

Miniglossary

collateral blood vessels: small blood vessels that form detours around blocked or narrowed larger arteries, permitting continued blood delivery and thus preventing much tissue death. Collateral vessels may also develop in response to exercise.

diastolic pressure: the second figure in a blood pressure reading (the "lub" of the heartbeat), which represents the arterial pressure when the heart is between beats.

essential (primary) hypertension: hypertension with no known cause; more than 90 percent of all cases of hypertension.

natriuretic hormone: a hormone (not yet fully characterized) that increases the rate of excretion of sodium in the urine (*natri* means "sodium"; *uresis* means "urinary excretion").

peripheral resistance: resistance to the flow of blood caused by a reduced diameter of the vessels at the periphery of the body—the smallest arteries and capillaries (see Chapter 1, Figure 1–3).

secondary hypertension: hypertension caused by kidney disease, accounting for about 10 percent of all cases of hypertension.

systolic pressure: the first figure in a blood pressure reading (the "dub" of the heartbeat), which represents arterial pressure caused by the contraction of the left ventricle of the heart.

absence of obesity and may reflect the operation of a factor common to both hypertension and diabetes. Perhaps insulin itself is, in some way, a causal agent of hypertension, sometimes.[44] A tantalizing bit of information that suggests the nature of the link is that insulin enhances the kidney's reabsorption of sodium.[45] Another is that it stimulates the activity of the hormones associated with the stress response.[46]

Diet in Prevention of Hypertension

The role of diet in *treatment* of hypertension is not questioned. The two most effective dietary measures the person with hypertension can take are to reduce weight if overweight, and to reduce sodium, or at least salt, intake (Chapter 7's Food Feature showed how). As for diet in *prevention* of hypertension, there is less agreement, but many professionals and agencies believe that enough evidence is available to warrant a recommendation to the general public to moderately restrict salt intake. They reason that, at worst, such a diet cannot be harmful.

It seems to us, however, that the person wishing to avoid hypertension can take many other dietary measures that may be more useful. Start with weight control. Expend energy, so as to earn the right to eat more nutrients—in other words, exercise. (If that benefit doesn't motivate you, then exercise to improve your circulation, reduce your weight, improve your morale, or make friends—but anyway, exercise.) Eat foods high in potassium (whole foods of all descriptions), high in calcium (dairy products and appropriate substitutes), low in fat, and high in fiber. Vary your diet. Not all the nutrients that affect blood pressure have been studied yet. (Others are cadmium, selenium, lead, caffeine, and protein—some perhaps needed in greater quantities and some in less, so exercise moderation.)[47] Use moderation with respect to alcohol, too. If the recommendations sound familiar, it may be because they have been made in relation to one health goal or another several times since the start of Chapter 1.

Notes

1. E. D. Frohlich, Physiological observations in essential hypertension, *Journal of the American Dietetic Association* 80 (1982): 18–20.
2. W. B. Kannel and T. J. Thom, Incidence, prevalence, and mortality of cardiovascular diseases, in *The Heart,* 6th ed., ed. J. W. Hurst (New York: McGraw-Hill, 1986), pp. 557–565.
3. D. A. McCarron and coauthors, Blood pressure and nutrient intake in the United States, *Science* 224 (1984): 1392–1398.
4. H. Sheldon, *Boyd's Introduction to the Study of Disease,* 9th ed. (Philadelphia: Lea and Febiger, 1984), pp. 120–121.
5. Hypertension Detection and Follow-up Program Cooperative Group, The effect of treatment on mortality in "mild" hypertension, *New England Journal of Medicine,* 307 (1982): 976–980.
6. N. M. Kaplan, Non-drug treatment of hypertension, *Annals of Internal Medicine* 402 (1985): 359–373.
7. This Controversy is adapted from M. A. Boyle and E. N. Whitney, *Nutrition and Hypertension* (a 1987 monograph in the *Nutrition Clinics* series available from Stickley Publishing Co., 210 Washington Square, Philadelphia, PA 19106).
8. E. Reisin and coauthors, Effect of weight loss without salt restriction on the reduction of blood pressure in overweight hypertensive patients, *New England Journal of Medicine* 298 (1978): 1–6.
9. H. G. Langford and coauthors, Dietary therapy slows the return of hypertension after stopping prolonged medication, *Journal of the American Medical Association* 253 (1985): 657–664.
10. Langford and coauthors, 1985.
11. S. Wassertheil and coauthors, Effective dietary intervention in hypertensives: Sodium restriction and weight reduction, *Journal of the American Dietetic Association* 85 (1985): 423–430.
12. C. M. Tipton, Exercise, training, and hypertension, *Exercise and Sports Sciences Reviews* 12 (1984): 245–306; R. S. Williams, R. A. McKinnis, and F. R. Cobb, Effects of physical conditioning on left ventricular ejection fraction in patients with coronary artery disease, *Circulation,* July 1984, pp. 69–75.
13. G. Nomura, Physical training in essential hypertension: Alone and in combination with dietary salt restriction, *Journal of Cardiac Rehabilitation* 4 (1984): 469–475.
14. Tipton, 1984.
15. T. B. Jacobs, R. D. Bell, and J. D. Clements, Exercise, age and the development of myocardial vasculature, *Growth* 48 (1984): 148–157.
16. K. Przyklenk and A. C. Groom, Effects of exercise frequency, intensity, and duration on revascularization in the transition zone of infarcted rat hearts, *Canadian Journal of Physiology and Pharmacology* 63 (1985): 273–278.
17. T. W. Kurtz, H. A. Al-Bander, and C. Morris, "Salt-sensitive" essential hypertension in men: Is the sodium ion alone important? *New England Journal of Medicine* 317 (1987): 1043–1048.
18. A. M. Altschul and J. K. Grommet, Sodium intake and sodium sensitivity, *Nutrition Reviews* 38 (1980): 393–402.
19. M. P. Blaustein and J. M. Hamlyn, Sodium transport inhibition, cell calcium, and hypertension: The natriuretic hormone/Na-Ca exchange/hypertension hypothesis, *American Journal of Medicine,* 77(4A) (1984): 45–59.
20. J. K. Huttunen and coauthors, Dietary factors and hypertension, *Acta Medica Scandinavica* (supplement) 701 (1985): 72–82.
21. G. Kolata, Value of low-sodium diets questioned (Research News), *Science* 216 (1982): 38–39.
22. H. G. Langford, Dietary potassium and hypertension: Epidemiologic data, *Annals of Internal Medicine* 98 (1983): 770–772.
23. Kolata, 1984.

24. K. T. Khaw and E. Barrett-Connor, Dietary potassium and stroke-associated mortality: A 12-year prospective population study, *New England Journal of Medicine* 316 (1987): 235–240.
25. Huttunen and coauthors, 1985.
26. J. M. Belizan and J. Villar, The relationship between calcium intake and edema-, proteinuria, and hypertension-gestosis: An hypothesis, *American Journal of Clinical Nutrition* (1980): 2202–2206.
27. H. Henry and coauthors, Increasing calcium intake lowers blood pressure: The literature reviewed, *Journal of the American Dietetic Association* 85 (1985): 182–185.
28. D. A. McCarron and coauthors, Blood pressure and nutrient intake in the United States, *Science* 224 (1984: 1392–1398.
29. D. A. McCarron and C. D. Morris, Blood pressure response to oral calcium in persons with mild to moderate hypertension: A randomized, double- blind, placebo-controlled, crossover trial, *Annals of Internal Medicine* 103 (1985): 825–831.
30. R. Weinsier, Recent developments in the etiology and treatment of hypertension: Dietary calcium, fat, and magnesium, *American Journal of Clinical Nutrition* 42 (1985): 1331–1338.
31. Weinsier, 1985.
32. Huttunen and coauthors, 1985.
33. P. Bursztyn, Does dietary linolenic acid influence blood pressure? (letter to the editor), *American Journal of Clinical Nutrition* 45 (1987): 1541–1542.
34. P. T. Williams and coauthors, Associations of dietary fat, regional adiposity, and blood pressure in men, *Journal of the American Medical Association* 257 (1987): 3251–3256.
35. Lowering blood cholesterol to prevent disease, NIH Consensus Conference, *Journal of The American Medical Association* 253 (1985): 2080–2086.
36. J. P. Knochel, Cardiovascular effects of alcohol, *Annals of Internal Medicine* 98 (1983): 849–854.
37. Knochel, 1983.
38. A. L. Klatsky, G. D. Friedman, and M. A. Armstrong, The relationships between alcoholic beverage use and other traits to blood pressure: A new Kaiser Permanente study, *Circulation* 73 (1986): 628–636.
39. G. D. Friedman, A. L. Klatsky, and A. B. Siegelaub, Alcohol intake and hypertension, *Annals of Internal Medicine* 98 (1983): 846–849.
40. Klatsky, Friedman, and Armstrong, 1986.
41. J. S. Gill and coauthors, Stroke and alcohol consumption, *New England Journal of Medicine* 315 (1986): 1041–1046.
42. A. L. Klatsky, M. A. Armstrong, and G. D. Friedman, Relationship of alcoholic beverage use to subsequent coronary artery disease hospitalization, *American Journal of Cardiology* 58 (1986): 710–714.
43. M. R. Joffres, D. M. Reed, and K. Yano, Relationship of magnesium intake and other dietary factors to blood pressure: The Honolulu heart study, *American Journal of Clinical Nutrition* 45 (1987): 469–475.
44. E. Ferrannini and coauthors, Insulin resistance in essential hypertension, *New England Journal of Medicine* 317 (1987): 350–357; L. Landsberg, Insulin and hypertension: Lessons from obesity (editorial), *New England Journal of Medicine* 317 (1987): 378–379.
45. Ferrannini and coauthors, 1987; Landsberg, 1987.
46. J. W. Rowe and coauthors, Effect of insulin and glucose infusions on sympathetic nervous system activity in normal man, *Diabetes* 30 (1981): 219–225, as cited by Landsberg, 1987.
47. J. Tuomilehto and coauthors, Nutrition-related determinants of blood pressure, *Preventive Medicine* 14 (1985): 413–427.

Chapter Eight

Contents

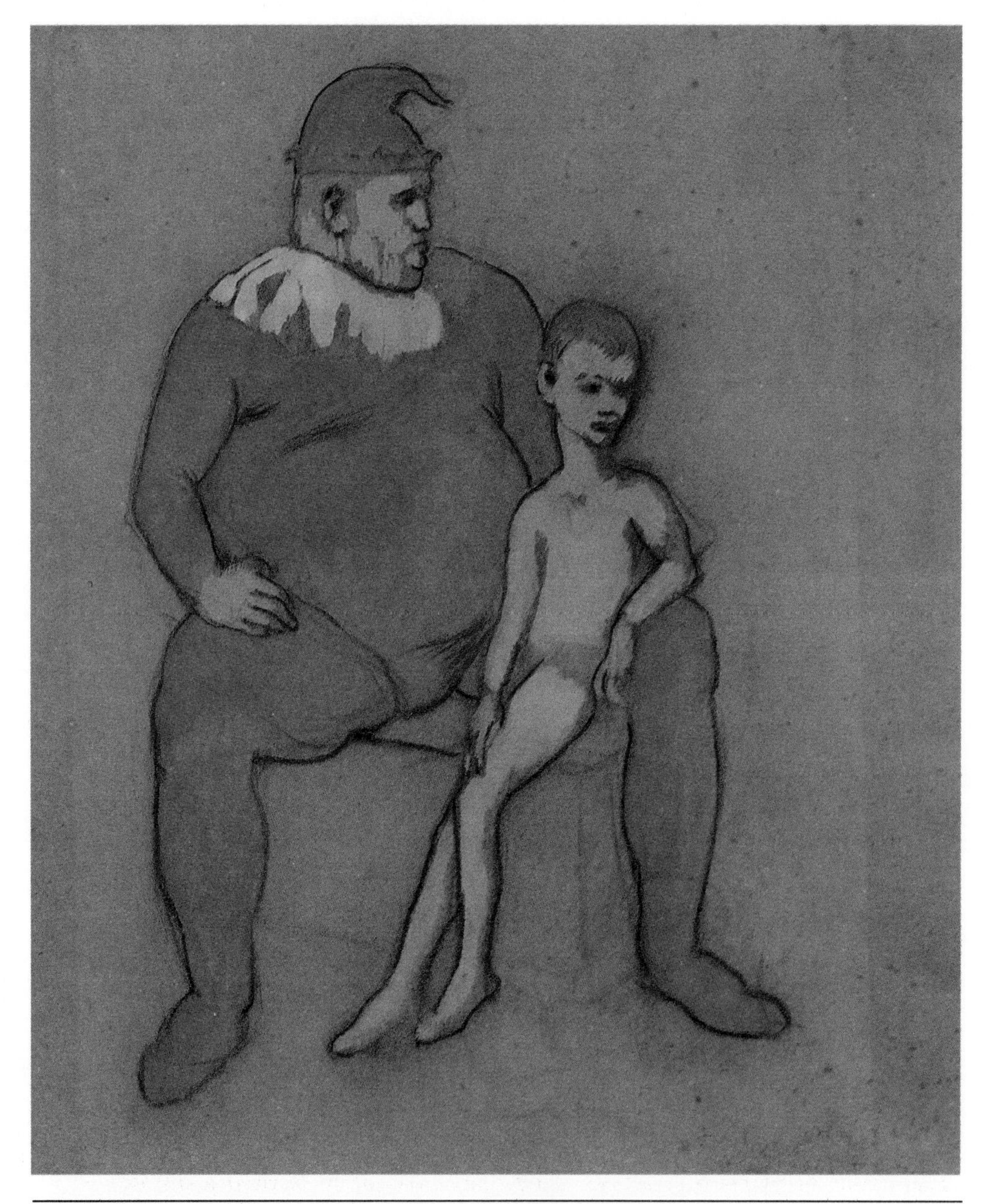

Seated Saltibanque with Boy by Pablo Picasso, 1905. The Baltimore Museum of Art: The Cone Collection, formed by Dr. Claribel Cone and Miss Etta Cone of Baltimore, Maryland. BMA 1950.270.

Energy Balance and Weight Control

Are you pleased with your body weight? If you answered yes, you are a rare individual. Nearly all people in our society think they should weigh more or less (mostly less) than they do. Usually, their primary reason is that they want to look acceptable by society's standards, but they often perceive, correctly, that physical health is also somehow related to weight.[1]

People also think of their weight as something they should control. They are right, but a pair of misconceptions makes their task difficult. The first is to focus on *weight;* the second is to focus on *controlling* weight. To put it simply, it isn't your weight you need to control; it's the fat in your body in proportion to the lean. And it isn't possible to control either one, directly; it is possible only to control your *behavior.* In other words, the title of this chapter is wrong; it should be renamed "Behavior to Promote Appropriate Body Composition." If it bore that name, though, hardly anyone would read it.

This chapter has two main missions. One is to present the problems associated with deficient and excessive body fat; the other is to present strategies for solving these problems.

Both deficient and excessive body fat present health risks. It has long been known that thin people will die first during a siege, in a famine, or in a concentration camp. A fact not always recognized, even by health care providers, is that overly thin people are also at a disadvantage in the hospital, where they may have to go for days without food so that they can undergo tests or surgery. Underweight also increases the risk for any person fighting a wasting disease. In fact, people with cancer often die from starvation, not from the cancer itself. Thus underweight people are urged to learn how to nourish themselves optimally—to gain body fat as an energy reserve, and to acquire protective amounts of all the nutrients that can be stored.

As for overfatness: for one thing, it can precipitate hypertension or make it worse. Often weight loss alone can normalize the blood pressure of an overfat person; some people with hypertension can tell you exactly at what weight their blood pressure begins to rise. Weight gain can also precipitate diabetes in genetically susceptible people. If hypertension or diabetes runs in your family, you urgently need to control your weight. Excess body fatness also increases the risk of heart disease by worsening atherosclerosis. Excess fat demands to be fed by miles of extra capillaries, increasing the heart's work load to the point of damaging it. Other conditions aggravated by overfatness include abdominal hernias, breast cancer, varicose veins, gout, gallbladder disease, arthritis, respiratory problems, complications in pregnancy, and even a high accident rate. The health risks of overfatness are so many that it has been declared a disease: **obesity.**[2] People who are obese are urged to reduce their weight. Their health risks are expected to normalize as they do.

obesity: overfatness with adverse health effects. Conventionally defined as weight 20% or more above the appropriate weight for height. Obesity also can be defined by body mass index; see p. 285.

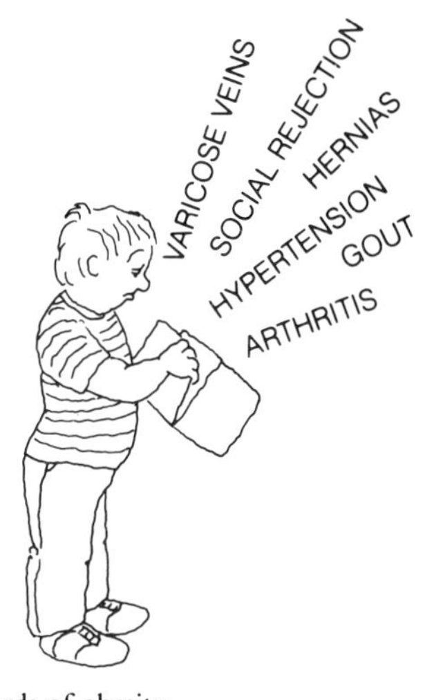

Hazards of obesity.

set-point theory: the theory that the body tends to maintain a certain weight by means of its own internal controls.

thermogenesis: the generation of heat by the body, a reflection of how much energy the body is spending.

basal thermogenesis: the heat generation associated with basal metabolism.

exercise-induced thermogenesis: heat generation by muscular activity.

A warning about weight reduction is in order, though: some fad diets are more hazardous to health than obesity itself. One survey of 29,000 weight-loss strategies found fewer than 6 percent of them effective—and 13 percent were dangerous![3] This chapter's Controversy is devoted to the fad diets; it filters out the valuable elements they have to offer and throws the rest away.

Some obese people can escape at least some of the health problems mentioned, but no one who is fat in our society quite escapes the social and economic handicaps. Fat people are less sought after for romance, less often hired, and less often admitted to college. They pay higher insurance premiums, and they pay more for clothing. Psychologically, too, a body size that embarrasses a person diminishes self-esteem. Why is it that some people develop too much body fat? Mysteries still surround that question, but some answers are beginning to come in.

Both deficient and excessive body fatness present health risks, and overfatness presents social and economic handicaps as well.

The Mystery of Obesity

Why do some people get fat? Why do some get thin? And most amazingly, how do some people—most people, in fact—stay at the same weight year after year? A single extra pat of butter each day might make them gain 5 pounds in a year, but if they overeat by that much one day, they work it off, somehow, or undereat by the same amount in the days that follow. In general, two schools of thought attempt to explain obesity. One attributes it to metabolic causes; the other, to behavioral factors.

Metabolic Causes

One currently popular metabolic theory is the so-called **set-point theory.** Researchers have noted that many people who lose weight on reducing diets subsequently return to their original weight. When fat tissue is surgically removed from animals, they compensate afterward by depositing more fat until they are back where they started from. The opposite is also seen: when subjects are made to overeat so that they gain weight, they spontaneously lose it again when the experiment ends. This suggests that somehow, the body chooses a weight that it wants to be, and defends that weight by regulating eating behaviors and hormonal actions. The theory implies that science should search inside obese people to find the causes of their problems—perhaps in their hunger-regulating mechanisms or in their systems of burning fuels.

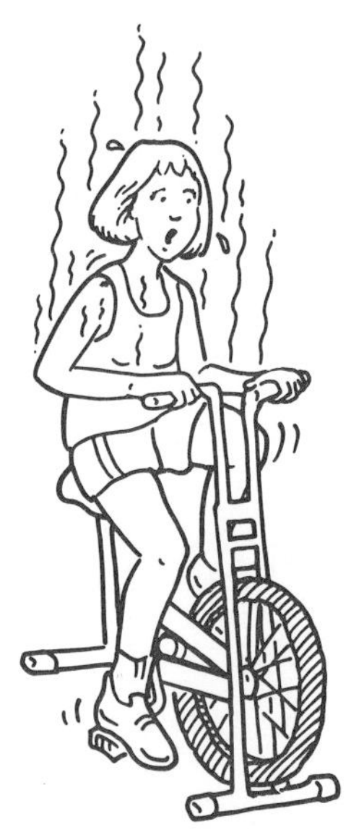
Some of the energy used by the muscles in exercise is released as heat.

A major way in which the body spends energy is in generating heat—**thermogenesis.** Some of this heat is produced as the body goes about the chemical business of supporting life—its metabolism, referred to later. This heat production maintains normal body temperature and is called **basal thermogenesis.** Some of the energy spent in exercise also appears as heat—**exercise-induced thermogenesis.** There are two minor categories of heat production by the body, which contribute little to the total energy output. They are usually ignored in rough estimates of energy needs. For completeness' sake, however, they are **diet-induced thermogenesis** and **adaptive thermogenesis.**

Diet-induced thermogenesis is associated with assimilating food. When food is taken into the body, many cells that have been dormant begin to be active. The muscles that move the food through the intestinal tract speed up their rhythmic contractions; the tissues that manufacture and secrete digestive juices begin their tasks. All these cells and others need extra energy as they come alive to participate in the digestion, absorption, and metabolism of food. Diet-induced thermogenesis is generally thought to amount to about 6 to 10 percent of the energy of the food taken in.

Related to diet-induced thermogenesis is the composition of the food eaten. The calories presented by the three energy-yielding nutrients seem to vary in their contributions to body fatness. Calories from fat or protein seem to contribute more to fat stores than calories from carbohydrate.[4] Perhaps the body doesn't "count" fat calories as well, and so more are eaten. Perhaps fat is metabolized more efficiently, and therefore provides more net calories. Perhaps carbohydrate triggers thermogenesis and so causes the body to expend more energy as heat. Individuals' metabolic systems vary, too—depending on heredity and customary energy intakes, people may use different energy fuels more or less efficiently.

Adaptive thermogenesis is of interest because of its possible relationship to body fat stores. When the body has to adapt to changed conditions, it has work to do, secreting the necessary hormones and enzymes, and making the physical adjustments to maintain body conditions in the face of a challenge. An example is seen in the person who attempts to gain weight by increasing food intake and sees no results at first. The body seems to waste some of the excess energy; in addition, much of the energy contributed by the added food is dedicated to supporting the adaptations needed to handle that food—such as the secretion of more digestive juices, the building of stomach muscles, and the enlargement of the digestive tract. While the work of adapting goes on, the person cannot store much energy as fat. (Persist; it will become easier after a while.)

Another example: if you were exposed to cold weather, producing body heat would become a top priority. In response, the body uses metabolic tricks that "waste" energy to produce only heat, instead of using energy to perform work or chemical reactions. A tissue that specializes in generating heat is **brown fat.** Regular white fat stores energy in its chemical bonds and has a slow metabolic rate; brown fat breaks those bonds and releases the energy they store as heat. Animals that hibernate for months in cold weather have a great deal of brown fat activity that generates heat while they sleep. Human babies are born with brown fat around their backs and shoulders, which protects their small bodies from brief exposures to cold; adults retain a little of this tissue. In lean animals, brown fat is more abundant and more active than in fat ones. Differences in brown fat's energy-use capacity, or in the amounts of brown fat in different people's bodies have been theorized to partly account for differences in their white-fat-storing tendencies.

Energy balance determines whether weight (body fat) is gained, maintained, or lost. The two major components of energy expenditure are basal metabolic energy and energy for activities; minor components are diet-induced and adaptive thermogenesis.

diet-induced thermogenesis: heat generation associated with assimilating food.

adaptive thermogenesis: heat generation associated with body adjustments to changed circumstances, such as to a cold environment, stress, or trauma.

brown fat: adipose tissue abundant in hibernating animals and human babies. The tissue is packed with pigmented, energy-burning enzymes that give it its characteristic brown color.

external cue theory: the theory that some people eat in response to such external factors as the presence of food or the time of day rather than in response to such internal factors as hunger.

hunger: as defined in Chapter 1, the physiological need to eat; an instinct and a negative sensation.

appetite: as defined in Chapter 1, the psychological desire to eat; a learned motivation and a positive sensation.

satiety (sah-TIE-uh-tee): as previously defined in Chapter 4, the feeling of fullness or satisfaction at the end of a meal, which prompts a person to stop eating.

endogenous (en-DODGE-en-us) **opiates:** compounds made in the brain in response to stimuli such as pain, stress, exercise, eating, and many others, that have a pain-killing or tranquilizing effect (*endo* means "within"; *gen* means "arising"; *opiate* means "painkiller").

Behavioral Causes

The other point of view is that obesity is determined by behavioral responses to environmental stimuli.[5] Proponents of this view hold that people overeat because they are susceptible to factors in their surroundings—foremost among them, the availability of a multitude of delectable foods. People who eat at mealtimes even though they aren't hungry, who clean their plates even though satisfied beforehand, and who partake of food "because it is there" are responding to environmental influences. The two views are not mutually exclusive. Both are usually operating, even in the same person, and of course, behavioral tendencies can have a genetic basis.

A few people easily resist external stimuli to eat, as though they had some sort of internal calorie counter. Others seem unable to do so. Of interest in this connection is the report of an experiment in which lean and fat people were confined in a setting where the availability of food could be completely controlled and were offered their meals in monotonous liquid form from a feeding station. The lean people ate enough to maintain their weight, but the fat people drastically reduced their food intake and lost weight. When calories were added to the formula, the lean people reduced their intake and continued maintaining weight. The obese people were unaware of the change, continued drinking the same amount of formula as before, and stopped losing weight. The obese people obtained no cues from the environment as to how many calories they were getting, and nothing inside them registered the change in the caloric density of the formula. In contrast, the normal-weight people seemed able to monitor their caloric intake somehow. This is the basis of the **external cue theory**—the theory that, at least in some people, outside-the-body influences override internal regulatory systems.

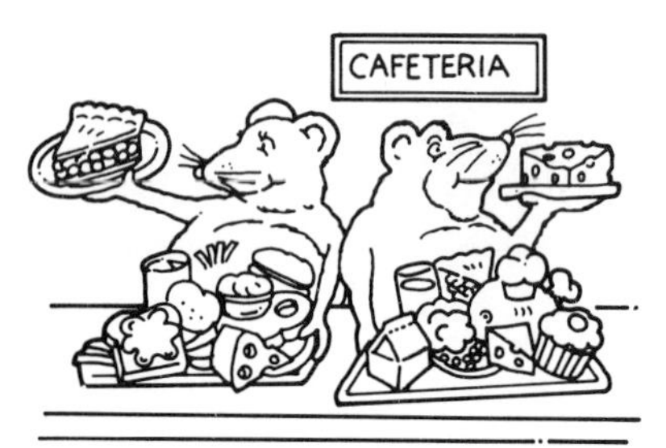

Cafeteria rats.

Experiments with "cafeteria rats" support the external cue theory. Ordinary rats, fed regular rat feed, maintain their weight, but if those very same rats are offered free access to a wide variety of tempting, rich, highly palatable foods, they greatly overeat and become obese. If you are an external cue responder (or a rat), you had better stay out of the cafeteria.

One way researchers have attempted to study what makes people overeat is to investigate **hunger, appetite,** and **satiety.** Hunger is a drive programmed into us by our heredity. Appetite, which is learned, can teach us to ignore hunger or over-respond to it. Hunger is physiological, while appetite is psychological, and the two do not always coincide. A person who has appetite without hunger says, "I'm not hungry, but I'd love to have some." The person who has hunger without appetite says, "I know I'm hungry, but I don't feel like eating." Hunger is a negative experience (you eat to avoid it); appetite is positive (you eat to enjoy it).

Satiety signals that it is time to stop eating. One view holds that eating behavior is turned on all the time, except when the satiety signal turns it off. But what is the satiety signal? Blood glucose is thought to signal satiety, and when your blood glucose level falls—or perhaps when liver glycogen is beginning to be exhausted—that signals hunger. Blood lipids, and possibly amino acids and other molecules, also play a role. When you eat carbohydrate, **endogenous opiates** are made in your brain; these have a tranquilizing effect, and it is thought that some people may eat in order to obtain this effect. (There's more about eating and mood in Controversy 13.) Satiety may also be signaled by one or more hormones; some 20 or 30 hormones are known to be secreted in response to eating.*

You might have heard that if you diet, your stomach shrinks, and then you don't want to eat as much. It may feel that way, because the stomach is involved in signaling satiety. The stomach's nerves perceive stretching, and you stop eating when your stomach feels stretched full.

Although we may have been born with the instinct to eat, we are not helpless when confronted with food. We also have the ability to override the instinct to eat. Psychologists who study behavior view the problem of overeating as a conditioned response to a variety of stimuli. Sometimes eating behavior tends to get turned on by the wrong triggers. A crying child with a skinned knee who is offered a lollipop to help soothe the hurt may learn to associate food with comfort and so seek food inappropriately when experiencing emotional pain later in life. To alter such inappropriate responses to life events, the psychologists use techniques called behavior modification. Later sections of this chapter show how behavior can be changed by changing the responses to cues to action and by arranging for consequences after the behavior.

Eating behavior may be a response not only to hunger, appetite, and other signals, but also to complex human sensations such as yearning, craving, addiction, or compulsion. For an emotionally insecure person, eating may be less threatening than calling a friend when lonely and risking rejection. Often, people eat to relieve boredom or to ward off depression.

Several studies illustrate how the emotions can affect eating. In one experiment, people were led to believe they were anxious by listening to recordings of rapid human heartbeats they had been told were their own. They were then given a faux breathing exercise to reduce the "anxiety." When the researchers slowed down the heartbeat recording in response to people's breathing efforts, the people ate a minimal amount of a snack that had been provided; when the speed of the tape remained unchanged, they ate more of the snack. Apparently, negative mental states such as anxiety, or even the *perception* of anxiety, can cause overeating, particularly when control measures appear to fail.[6] A second experiment showed that stress can cause an increase in appetite, possibly by way of internal chemical signals.[7] Another study has shown that positive emotions, too, can contribute to overeating, because people often celebrate with food.[8] All these experiments indicate that any kind of **arousal** can cause overeating, perhaps because the aroused emotional state is misinterpreted as hunger. The eating done in response to arousal is **stress eating.** Significantly, however, if people are able to give a name to their aroused condition, thereby gaining a feeling that they have some control over it, they are not as likely to overeat.[9] However, while some people overeat in response to stress, others cannot eat at all. It is not known why people react differently, but research continues.

Stress may also directly promote the accumulation of body fat. The stress hormones favor the breakdown of energy stores (glycogen and fat) to glucose fragments and fatty acid fragments that can be used to fuel the muscular activity of fight or flight (see Chapter 1). If a person fails to use the fuel in physical exertion, the body restores the fat fragments to fat, but cannot turn the glucose

arousal: heightened activity of certain brain centers associated with excitement and anxiety. The behavior known as **stress eating** is inappropriate eating in response to arousal.

*Among hormones secreted after eating are cholecystokinin (coal-ee-sis-to-KINE-in), produced in the brain as well as in the digestive tract in response to meals containing fat; and calcitonin, produced in both the thyroid gland and the brain when blood calcium rises.

frame size: the size of a person's bones and musculature. A person with a large frame can weight more than one the same height with a small frame before risk begins to increase.

fragments back into glycogen; it has no alternative but to convert them to fat, too. Each time glucose gets pulled out of storage and broken down in response to stress and then transformed into fat, the lowered glucose level or exhausted glycogen will signal hunger, and the person will eat again soon after.[10]

One other cause of obesity stands out—lack of exercise. The control of hunger/appetite appears to work well in most healthy, active people; few athletes are obese. But appetite control fails when activity falls below a certain minimum level. Some obese people eat less than lean people, but they are so extraordinarily inactive that they still manage to have an energy surplus. Some people move smoothly and efficiently; others are restless, and spend more energy fidgeting. Little bits of activity add up.

No two people are alike, either physically or psychologically, and the causes of obesity are varied, just as people are. Treatments must be multifaceted, too—but before discussing them, it is important to decide what weight to aim for.

Some of obesity's causes may be inappropriate responses to external cues. Among possible outside-the-body regulators of food intake are the sight, smell, and taste of foods, the fat content of meals, and stress. A major contributor to obesity is underactivity.

Definition of Appropriate Weight

Once upon a time, the definition of appropriate weight was simple. A person's weight could be compared with that in the "ideal weight" tables. If the actual weight were 20 percent or more above the "ideal weight," then the person was obese; if it was 10 percent under, the person was underweight. Now (to tell a long story in a few words), the term *ideal weight* is no longer in use, and the definition of obesity is no longer simple.

Among the problems were these. Weight depends on a person's **frame size**—but how do you measure frame size? Weight doesn't matter as much as body composition, and especially body fat content, but how do you measure body fat content? How much body fat there is doesn't matter as much as where it is located on the body, but how do you tie this to ideal weight and the definition of obesity? Anyway, the 1959 ideal weight tables listed the wrong weights; a reevaluation of the statistics on which they were based showed that the weights should have been higher, and higher weights were published in 1983. Then the basis on which the 1983 weights had been arrived at was challenged. No weight tables have ever met all three of these criteria:

- Controlling for cigarette smoking, which is strongly linked to lower body weight and, of course, makes lower weights appear to be associated with a high mortality risk.
- Controlling for hypertension and other physiological effects of obesity, which pull the other way, making obesity appear to be associated with a high mortality risk.
- Failure to distinguish low weight caused by disease from low weight in healthy people.[11]

Furthermore, fatness in women is tangled up with age and socioeconomic status: the daughters of wealthy families tend to be overweight, but to become thin as adults; the daughters of families in poverty tend to be thin and to become fat as adults.[12] These associations complicate the picture further.

After much discussion and review of the evidence at a Consensus Development Conference on Obesity in 1985, the experts have settled on some temporary working procedures and have agreed that more research is needed:

- They will continue defining obesity as 20 percent above the insurance company table weights, using either the 1959 tables or the 1983 tables.
- If a person is deemed obese by this rough indicator, the physician should apply a more sensitive indicator, the **body mass index (BMI).** A body mass index of greater than 27.2 in men or 26.9 in women indicates the need for weight reduction. No lower limit is set, for people who might need to gain weight.

$$\text{BMI} = \frac{\text{weight (kilograms)}}{\text{height}^2 \text{ (meters)}}.$$

- Diabetes (non-insulin-dependent type), hypertension, and high blood cholesterol also indicate the need for weight loss.
- The severity of the obesity also depends on factors associated with it, such as the distribution of the body fat; social, economic, and ethnic status; and age.[13]

body mass index (BMI): the weight in kilograms, divided by the square of the height (in meters), an indicator of obesity.

Figure 8–1 shows you how to use both the traditional tables and the body mass index, and guides you to a tentative answer to the question, "What is an appropriate weight for you?"

The problem of using weight as an indicator of health or risk status is greatest for weights near the average (presumably desirable) weights. The problem is that body weight says so little about body composition. A person who doesn't seem to weigh too much may be too fat; a person who does seem to weigh too much may not be. A dancer or an athlete, whose muscles are well developed and whose bones have become well mineralized by responding to constant stress, may weigh the same as a sedentary person with a similar figure, yet the dancer or athlete may be at the right weight, and the sedentary person may be too fat. There is no easy way to look inside a person and see the bones and muscles.

There are other problems with the ideal weight concept. Even supposing everyone had the same percentage of body fat, the use of the word *ideal* demands an answer to the question "ideal for what?" The weights in the tables were never shown to be ideal *for* anything; they were considered desirable on the basis of a correlation. They were, simply, the weight ranges that correlated with the greatest longevity in the population studied. The population studied was a population of insured people, and people who buy life insurance may be unlike others in terms of their health. Their weights had only been taken once, if ever; some had only reported their weights verbally and not been weighed. The weights were taken at the time they submitted their applications for life insurance, not years later when, by dying, they provided the statistics the life insurance companies used to generate the weight tables. All of this makes it clear that when a person's weight is compared with the table weight, it is not being

Figure 8–1

What Is an Appropriate Weight for You?

When physical health alone is considered, a wide range of weights is acceptable for a person of a given height. Within the safe range, the definition of appropriate weight is up to the individual, depending on factors such as family history, occupation, physical and recreational activities, and personal preferences.

1. Determine the safe range for a person your height and sex.

- Record your height: ________ ft, ________ inches.
- Determine your frame size, using Table 8–1. Record whether you have a small, medium, or large frame: ________ frame.
- Look up the appropriate weight for a person your height, sex, and frame size in the table on the inside back cover. (*Note*: The heights listed assume you were measured in shoes with 1-inch heels. If you wore no shoes to be measured, add an inch; if you wore shoes with heels higher or lower than an inch, adjust accordingly.) Record the entire range: ________ to ________ lb.
  Example: For a man 5 ft 7 inches tall (in shoes) with a small frame, the range of weights is 138 to 145 lb.
- Determine the bottom end of the safe range. A person who is more than 10% below the lowest indicated weight for height is considered underweight to a degree that might compromise health. Take 10% off the bottom end of your range: ________ lb.
  Example: 10% of 138 lb is 13.8 lb (rounded off to 14 lb). Bottom end of range is 138 minus 14, or 124 lb.
- Determine the top end of the safe range. A person who is more than 20% above the highest indicated weight for height is considered obese. Add 20% to the top end of your range: ________ lb.
  Example: 20% of 145 lb is 29 lb. The top end of the range is 145 plus 29, or 174 lb.
- Record your safe range here: ________ to ________ lb.
  Example: 124 to 174 lb.

2. If your weight is below the bottom end of this safe range, you need to gain weight for your health's sake. If your weight is above the top end of the range, determine your body mass index to obtain confirmation that you need to lose weight. (Refer to the nomogram opposite. Use your weight without clothing and your height without shoes.) A body mass index greater than 27.2 in men or 26.9 in women indicates the need for weight loss.

Example: A man 5 ft 6 inches tall (without shoes), according to this figure, would have a body mass index of 27.2 if he weighed 169 lb. This would be a more accurate upper limit of his safe weight range; he should not exceed this weight, unless advised by a health professional to do so. Revise the top end of your safe range if necessary.

3. Check your health history for further confirmation. A family or personal medical history of diabetes (non-insulin-dependent type), hypertension, or high blood cholesterol indicates the need for weight loss.
4. Choose a goal weight within the safe range. Answering the following questions should help you to determine where, within the safe range, your personal appropriate weight may be:

- Does your occupation demand that you have a certain body shape? Record the weight, within the safe range, that would most nearly approximate this body shape: ________ lb.
- Do you engage in a sport or other physical activity that requires a particular body weight for optimal performance? Consult your instructor or other expert in that sport or activity, and record the weight recommended on that basis: ________ lb.
- Do you hope to start a pregnancy soon? If so, consult your health care provider as the ideal weight with which to begin a pregnancy: ________ lb.
- Undress and stand before a mirror. Do you think you need to gain or lose weight? Add or subtract pounds to arrive at a personal goal weight (but be sure to stay within the safe range): ________ lb.

Based on all of these considerations, choose a final goal weight. No formula exists for this estimate, but don't choose a weight outside the safe range without a professional assessment.

Your goal weight: ________ lb.

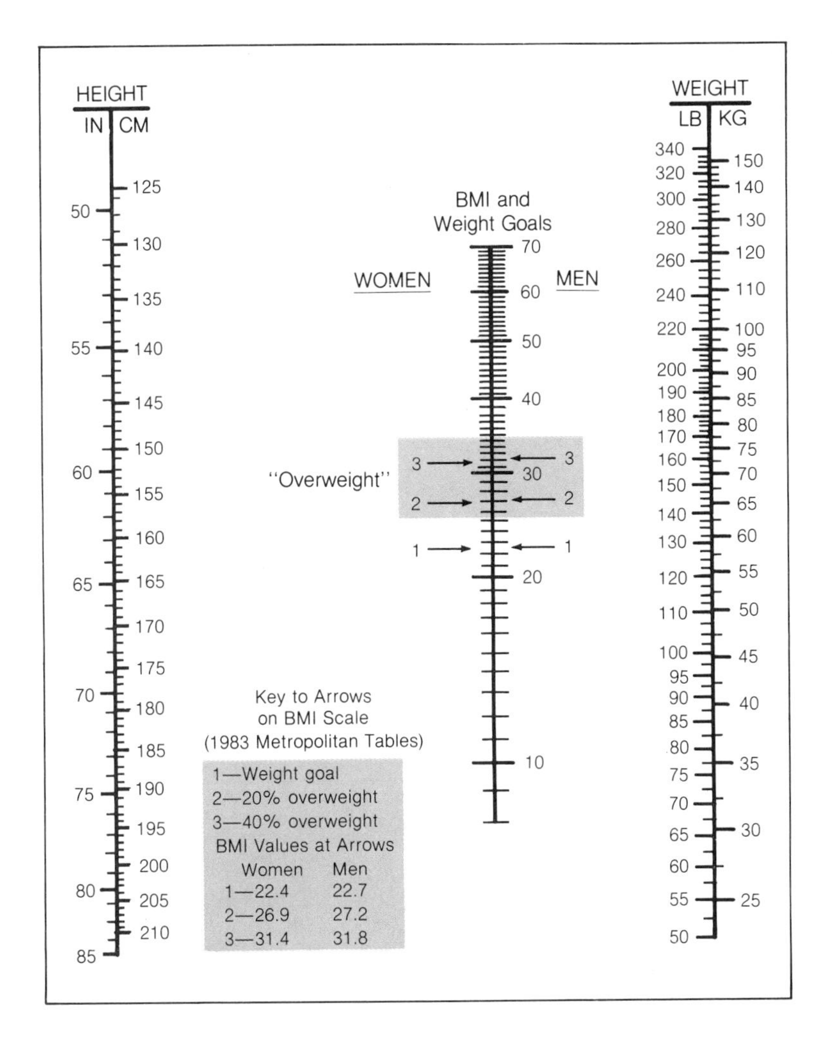

Figure 8–1 continued.
Nomogram for body mass index. Weights and heights are without clothing. With clothes, add 5 pounds for men or 3 pounds for women, and 1 inch in height for shoes. Draw a straight line or place a ruler from your height (left) to your weight (right). At the point where it crosses the BMI line, read your body mass index. A body mass index greater than 27.2 for men or 26.9 for women indicates obesity.

Source: From the 1983 Metropolitan Life Insurance Company tables, designed by B. T. Burton and W. R. Foster, Health implications of obesity, an NIH Consensus Development Conference, *Journal of the American Dietetic Association* 85 (1985): 1117–1121.

measured against a standard, but simply compared with the average weight found years ago in a population of people who lived quite long after that until they died.

The determination of frame size represents an attempt to deal with the problem of people's differing bone and muscle structures. Now: how to measure frame size? Researchers have attempted to answer several questions, in order to ensure that they are doing it right. First, does bone mass correlate with muscle mass (that is, do people with bigger bones also have greater muscle mass)? Reassuringly, the answer to that question seems to be yes.[14] That means it should be possible to measure a bone to obtain an estimate of the body's fat-free mass.

Next, what bone to measure? It has to be one that correlates with fat-free mass, but not with body fat. Six frame measures have been suggested, including the breadth of the elbow bone, the distance between the hip bones, the breadth of the wrist bone or that of the ankle bone, and measures at the shoulder and knee. The wrist and ankle breadths seem to be associated *least* with total body fat, but the insurance height-weight tables use the breadth of the elbow bone as an index of frame size (see Table 8–1). They chose this particular measurement

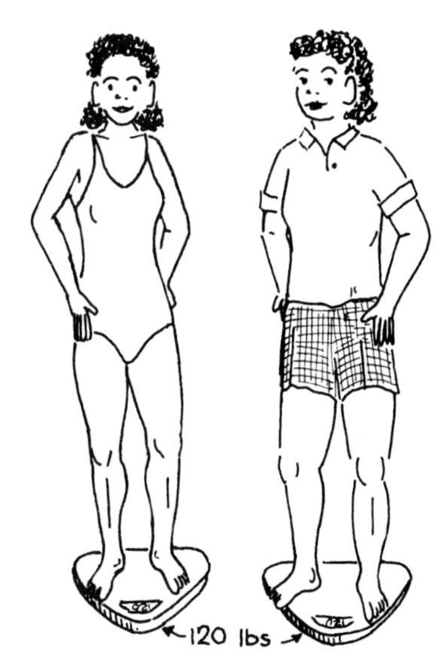

Both women weigh 120 pounds. One has more muscle and bone; the other, more fat.

because a recent survey had provided extensive reference values for elbow breadth in U.S. adults.[15] Unfortunately, though, elbow breadths tend to be greater in fatter people—or, to put it the other way around, people with larger elbow bones tend to be fatter. This may mean that a large frame, determined this way, is itself, a risk factor.[16]

The struggle continues. Research is directed toward making the height-weight tables useful in assessing obesity and its risks. Meanwhile, they have limited usefulness, but every bathroom and every doctor's office seems to have a scale, and the tables will doubtless continue to be used. If you choose to use them, be sure to add an inch to your barefoot height (you are assumed to be wearing shoes with one-inch heels), and adjust for clothing (the tables assume three to five pounds for clothes).

If the weight tables cause frustration in would-be users, perhaps that reaction brings with it a benefit—it leads them to ask deeper questions about the state of the body most compatible with good health and long life. Simple answers don't await the asker, but when answers do come, they will doubtless have to do with body composition.

The definition of appropriate weight based on frame size, weight, and standard tables is beset with problems. The currently preferred definition is based on body mass index.

Table 8–1

How to Determine Your Frame Size by Elbow Breadth

To make a simple approximation of your frame size:
Extend your arm, and bend the forearm upwards at a 90-degree angle. Keep the fingers straight, and turn the inside of your wrist away from your body. Place the thumb and index finger of your other hand on the two prominent bones on *either side* of your elbow. Measure the space between your fingers against a ruler or a tape measure.[a] Compare the measurements with the following standards.

These standards represent the elbow measurements for medium-framed men and women of various heights. Measurements smaller than those listed indicate you have a small frame, and larger measurements indicate a large frame.

Men

Height in 1-Inch Heels	*Elbow Breadth*
5 ft 2 inches to 5 ft 3 inches	2 1/2 to 2 7/8 inches
5 ft 4 inches to 5 ft 7 inches	2 5/8 to 2 7/8 inches
5 ft 8 inches to 5 ft 11 inches	2 3/4 to 3 inches
6 ft 0 inches to 6 ft 3 inches	2 3/4 to 3 1/8 inches
6 ft 4 inches and over	2 7/8 to 3 1/4 inches

Women

Height in 1-Inch Heels	*Elbow Breadth*
4 ft 10 inches to 4 ft 11 inches	2 1/4 to 2 1/2 inches
5 ft 0 inches to 5 ft 3 inches	2 1/4 to 2 1/2 inches
5 ft 4 inches to 5 ft 7 inches	2 3/8 to 2 5/8 inches
5 ft 8 inches to 5 ft 11 inches	2 3/8 to 2 5/8 inches
6 ft 0 inches and over	2 1/2 to 2 3/4 inches

[a]For the most accurate measurement, have your health care provider measure your elbow breadth with a caliper.

Source: Courtesy "Statistical Bulletin," Metropolitan Life Insurance Company.

Body Composition

fatfold test: a clinical test of body fatness in which the thickness of a fold of skin on the back of the arm (on the *triceps*), below the shoulder blade (*subscapular*), or in other places is measured with a caliper. The older, less preferred, term for this is *skinfold test.*

central obesity: excess fat around the trunk, as measured by subscapular fatfold.

Several laboratory techniques for estimating body fatness have been developed. One way is to determine the body's density (weight compared with volume). Lean tissue is denser than fat tissue, so the more dense a person's body is, the more lean tissue it must contain. Weight is measured with a scale; volume measurement involves submerging the whole body in a large tank of water and measuring the amount of water displaced. From the density, an estimate of the percentage of body fat can be derived. This technique is not available in the typical home or doctor's office, for obvious reasons, but is in wide use on university campuses that pursue exercise physiology research.

Another way to estimate body fat is to inject a water-soluble substance that is easy to detect and measure, and allow it to penetrate into the lean tissues (it will not mix into the fat tissues). A blood sample taken soon after will show the extent to which the substance has been diluted, providing an estimate of the amount of lean tissue. Still another way is based on the difference between the electrical impedance of fat and lean tissue; the ratio of the two in a person's body can be determined by an instrument that measures electrical conductivity.[17]

A simpler way to obtain an estimate of the amount of body fat is by taking a fatfold measure. The assessor lifts a fold of skin from the back of the arm, from the back, or from other body surfaces and measures its thickness with a caliper that applies a fixed amount of pressure. The fat under the skin in these regions represents about half of the body's total fat tissue, and on most people it is roughly proportional to total body fat. If the person gains body fat, the fatfold increases proportionately; if the person loses fat, it decreases. The **fatfold test** is a practical diagnostic procedure in the hands of trained people and is in increasingly wide use. Table 8–2 presents percentiles for fatfold measures for males and females. Generally speaking, people whose fatfold measurements exceed the 95th percentile are considered obese.

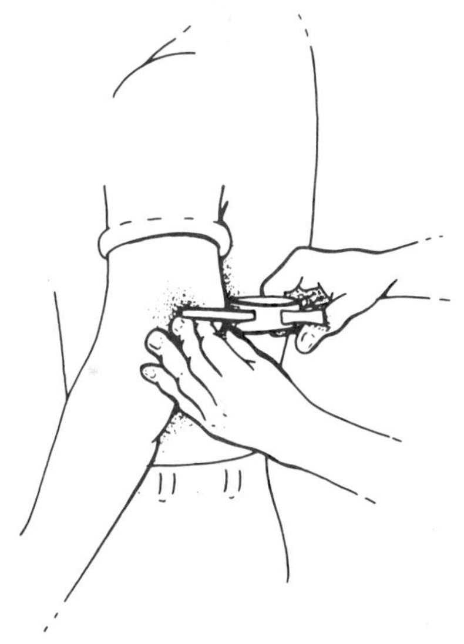

The fatfold test gives a fair approximation of total body fat.

The major limitation of the fatfold test is that fat may be thicker under the skin in one area than another. A pinch at the side of the waistline may not yield the same measurement as a pinch on the back of the arm. This limitation can be overcome by taking the average of a number of different fatfolds.

There is another complication, too: fat around the middle—**central obesity**—may represent a greater risk to health than fat elsewhere on the body. Abdominal fat is closest to the portal circulation; when it is mobilized, it goes directly to the liver, where it is made into cholesterol-carrying LDL; and it has been shown to correlate, more closely than fat located elsewhere on the body, with an increased incidence of diabetes and coronary heart disease.[18] Fatfold measurements do not take this fat distribution difference into account. A simple comparison of the waist to the hip measurement may become a standard part of the assessment of body fatness in years to come.[19]

Even after you have a body fatness estimate, problems arise. For example, how do you interpret it? What is the "ideal" amount of fat for a body to have? The question—ideal for what?—has to be answered first.

For competitive athletes, expecially endurance athletes, the ideal is relatively easy to define. The amount of fat in the body should be above the minimum needed for essential functions such as providing fuel, insulation, and normal fat-soluble hormone activity. Otherwise it should be as low as possible, so as not to contribute excess weight for the muscles to carry. A man of normal weight

Table 8–2

Triceps Fatfold Percentiles (millimeters) for Males and Females

	Male					Female				
Age	*5th*	*25th*	*50th*	*75th*	*95th*	*5th*	*25th*	*50th*	*75th*	*95th*
1– 1.9	6	8	10	12	16	6	8	10	12	16
2– 2.9	6	8	10	12	15	6	9	10	12	16
3– 3.9	6	8	10	11	15	7	9	11	12	15
4– 4.9	6	8	9	11	14	7	8	10	12	16
5– 5.9	6	8	9	11	15	6	8	10	12	18
6– 6.9	5	7	8	10	16	6	8	10	12	16
7– 7.9	5	7	9	12	17	6	9	11	13	18
8– 8.9	5	7	8	10	16	6	9	12	15	24
9– 9.9	6	7	10	13	18	8	10	13	16	22
10–10.9	6	8	10	14	21	7	10	12	17	27
11–11.9	6	8	11	16	24	7	10	13	18	28
12–12.9	6	8	11	14	28	8	11	14	18	27
13–13.9	5	7	10	14	26	8	12	15	21	30
14–14.9	4	7	9	14	24	9	13	16	21	28
15–15.9	4	6	8	11	24	8	12	17	21	32
16–16.9	4	6	8	12	22	10	15	18	22	31
17–17.9	5	6	8	12	19	10	13	19	24	37
18–18.9	4	6	9	13	24	10	15	18	22	30
19–24.9	4	7	10	15	22	10	14	18	24	34
25–34.9	5	8	12	16	24	10	16	21	27	37
35–44.9	5	8	12	16	23	12	18	23	29	38
45–54.9	6	8	12	15	25	12	20	25	30	40
55–64.9	5	8	11	14	22	12	20	25	31	38
65–74.9	4	8	11	15	22	12	18	24	29	36

Adapted from A. R. Frisancho, New norms of upper limb fat and muscle areas for assessment of nutritional status, *American Journal of Clinical Nutrition* 34 (1981):2540–2545. © American Society of Clinical Nutrition.

may have, on the average, 15 percent, and a woman, 20 percent of the body weight as fat. Endurance athletes consider it ideal to have lower fat percentages than these.

For an Alaskan fisherman, the ideal percentage of body fat is probably higher. Fat provides an insulating blanket, and in some settings, heat loss from the body handicaps performance. In those settings, such a blanket confers an advantage. For a woman starting a pregnancy, the ideal percentage of body fat may be different again; it is known that the outcome of pregnancy is compromised if the woman begins it with too little body fat. Below a certain threshold body fat content, some individuals become infertile, develop depression or abnormal hunger regulation, or become unable to keep warm. These thresholds are not the same for each function or in all individuals, and much remains to be learned about them.

Just as there is a minimum percentage of body fat that is ideal for a given individual, there is also a maximum, and this too may differ from person to person. One major factor that determines where to draw the line is the blood pressure. Some people can tell you exactly at what weight their blood pressure begins to rise; when they lose weight to below that threshold, their blood pressure becomes normal again. Other risk indicators also rise and fall with body fatness—blood glucose and blood cholesterol, for example. For those in whom these signs appear with added fat, weight reduction is most critical.

The uncertainties surrounding the definition of ideal body composition reflect the newness of the branch of nutrition science that studies body weight and its regulation. A better definition of obesity than the first approximation given on p. 273 would be body fatness significantly in excess of that consistent with optimal health, determined by a reliable measure, but the techniques to pinpoint it accurately are still to be worked out. With this understanding, you should be able to apply the appropriate number of grains of salt to rules of thumb such as these:

obesity: excessive body fatness, presently determined by comparing body weight with the life insurance tables. The person whose weight is 20% above the table weight is considered obese and should be evaluated further. Treatment is indicated if the body mass index exceeds 27.2 (men) or 26.9 (women) or if there is high blood pressure, high blood cholesterol, or diabetes.
Ten percent above the table weight is **overweight;** 10% below the table weight is **underweight.**

- Perform the "pinch test" (this is a fatfold measure without a skinfold caliper). Pick up the skin and fat at the back of either arm with the thumb and forefinger of the other hand. Keep your fingers still, so as not to lose the "measurement" when you pull them away from your arm. Measure the thickness on a ruler. A fatfold over an inch thick reflects obesity.
- Measure your waist compared with your chest (not bust). Every inch by which your waist measurement exceeds your chest measurement is said to take two years off your life.
- Lie down, relax, and place a ruler across your abdomen from one hipbone to the other. If it doesn't easily touch both bones while you're relaxing, you're too fat.

Besides having all the health implications that it does, body weight is also a social and personal matter. In some societies fatness is desired; it is equated with prosperity, comfort, and security. In others it is despised; it is considered undisciplined to be fat. The person seeking a single, authoritative answer to the question "How much should I weigh?" is therefore bound to be disappointed. No one can tell you *exactly* how much you should weigh—but with health as a value, at least you have a starting framework. Your weight should fall within a range. Below the bottom end or above the top end of the range, your athletic performance, fertility (in women), health, or longevity would be adversely affected. Within the range, the weight to pick is up to you. Your own standards are important.

Deciding to Gain Weight

The person who is underweight has a special problem—deciding whether, and how, to try to gain. The first question to ask is whether the underweight represents a healthy or unhealthy state. It is well known that to be slightly under the table weight, for most people, represents a desirable state. But if the underweight is due to anorexia nervosa (see Controversy 12) or a wasting disease such as tuberculosis or cancer, it may be a dangerous state, and weight gain, if possible, may be indicated. The answer, then, is: if you are healthy at your present weight, stay there; if you are at risk of illness, try to gain. Medical advice can help you make the distinction.

Some people may wish to gain weight for appearance's sake—provided that the gain is muscle and fat, not just fat. Athletes may wish, or be advised by their coaches, to gain weight to improve their performance. Such people need to be fully aware that such weight gain can only be achieved by physical conditioning combined with a high-calorie diet. A high-calorie diet alone will make a person gain fat only, and even if it makes the appearance look more acceptable in the person's own eyes, it is more likely to be detrimental than beneficial to health. Furthermore, some people are unalterably thin by reason of heredity or early environmental influences. Such people find it so difficult to gain weight, that it seems not worth the trouble. If such a person were to follow the guidelines for weight gain at the end of this chapter, and attempt to eat the many calorie-rich foods suggested there, the person might gain some fat and become uncomfortable, but would not achieve the desired change in body composition. In an athlete, such a weight gain might impair performance.

Weight gain is, like weight loss, a highly individual matter. In deciding whether to undertake it, be as aware as you can of what your body will permit and tolerate, and be willing to accept what you cannot change.

Appropriate weight would be best defined by determining a person's body composition (ratio of fat to lean tissue), but no simple way exists to do this. Available methods of estimating a safe range of appropriate weights are to use the weight tables with frame size measures, fatfold measures, or the body mass index; individual preferences can be applied within the safe range.

Energy Balance

Suppose you decide you are too fat or too thin. How did you get that way? By having an unbalanced energy budget—that is, by eating either more or less food energy than you spent.

Energy In versus Energy Out

A day's energy balance can be stated like this:

> Change in fat stores (energy) equals food energy taken in minus energy spent on metabolism and muscle activities.

More simply:

> Change in fat stores (energy) = energy in − energy out.

An apple provides you with 100 calories; an average candy bar, with 425 calories. You may already know that for each 3500 calories you eat in excess of expenditures, you store approximately 1 pound of body fat.*

1 lb body fat = 3500 cal.

For more on food energy, calories, and joules, see Chapter 2 and the inside back cover.

Food energy consumed in a day is the only contributor to the "energy in" side of the energy balance equation. Before asking the question, how much

*Pure fat is worth 9 calories per gram. A pound of it (450 grams), then, would store 4150 calories. A pound of body fat is not pure fat, though; it contains water, protein, and other materials (hence the lower calorie value).

energy you need in a day, you must first know about how energy is measured. To measure the energy in a food, a laboratory scientist can burn the food in a **bomb calorimeter.** Heat given off or oxygen consumed in the burning can be measured, and the amount is mathematically converted to represent the energy released. Burning a food in a calorimeter is not exactly the same as its use by the human body, because foods vary in digestibility. Values obtained in the laboratory are adjusted to correct for this and other factors. (The calorie values for several hundred foods in Appendix A of this book have been obtained in this way.)

If you do not happen to be a laboratory scientist with access to a bomb calorimeter, and if you have no time to look up in a table each food you eat, you can estimate food energy values from the values given for similar foods in the exchange system, which classes foods by their protein, fat, and carbohydrate contents. The exchange system provides a convenient estimate of the grams of energy-yielding nutrients in foods; you also have to add calories from alcohol if it is present. The Food Feature at the end of this chapter shows you how to use the exchange system to estimate calories quickly.

While it is easy to estimate the energy present in a meal or in a day's meals, it is not easy to determine the energy needs of an individual. The U.S. Committee on RDA and the Canadian Ministry of Health and Welfare have published recommended energy intakes for various age-sex groups in their populations. These are useful for population studies, but the range of energy needs for any one group is so broad that it is impossible even to guess an individual's needs from them without knowing something about the person's lifestyle. The U.S. recommendation for a woman, for example, which assumes that she is 20 years old, stands 5 feet 4 inches tall, weighs 124 pounds, is of average body fatness, and engages in light activity, still provides a wide margin of error: it states that she needs 2500 to 3300 calories of energy a day. Taller people, on average, need proportionately more, and shorter people proportionately less energy to balance their energy budgets. Older people generally need less, due to both slowed metabolism and reduced activity, with the number of calories diminishing by about 5 percent per decade beyond age 30. The day's activities, for both women and men, include sleeping or lying down for eight hours a day, sitting for seven hours, standing for five, walking for two, and spending two hours a day in light physical activity. Most adults fall within an 800-calorie span for energy needs, but some fall outside this range. In any group of 20 similar people with similar activity levels, one will expend twice as much energy per day as another.[20] Clearly, it is impossible to pinpoint any person's energy need within such a wide range without studying that person.

One way to obtain an estimate of your energy needs is to monitor your food intake and body weight over a period of time in which your activities are typical of your life-style. If you keep a strictly accurate record of all the food and beverages you consume for a week or two, and if your weight has not changed during the past few months, you can conclude that your energy budget is balanced. A week of record keeping is minimum, though, because intakes fluctuate from day to day. (On about half the days you eat less food energy than the average; on the other half, more.)

An alternative method of determining energy output is to compute the two components of energy expenditure separately and then add them together. The body spends energy in two major ways: (1) to fuel its **basal metabolism** and

bomb calorimeter: a device used to determine the calories in food by measuring the heat given off or the oxygen consumed when the food is burned.

basal metabolism: the sum total of all the cellular activities that are necessary to sustain life, including respiration, circulation, and new tissue synthesis, and excluding digestion and voluntary activities. Basal metabolism accounts for the largest component of the average person's daily energy expenditure. It is measured while lying down, awake, at least 12 hours after eating.

Remember these average values of the energy-yielding nutrients:

- 1 g carbohydrate = 4 cal.
- 1 g fat = 9 cal.
- 1 g protein = 4 cal.
- 1 g alcohol = 7 cal.

The energy RDA are presented in the inside front cover.

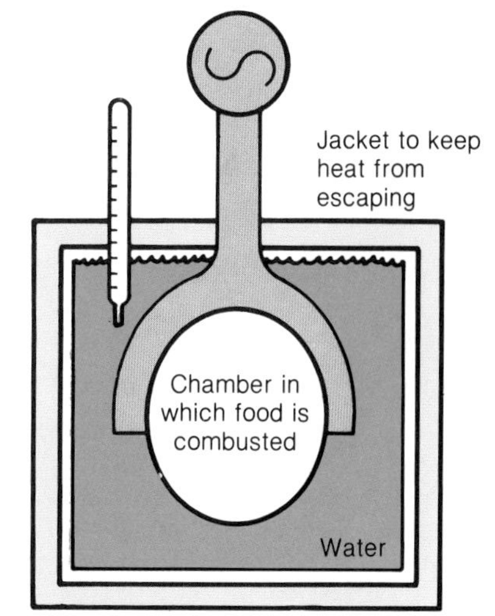

Bomb calorimeter.

basal metabolic rate (BMR): the rate at which the body uses energy to support its basal metabolism.

(2) to fuel its voluntary activities. You can change both of these to spend more or less energy in a day, as explained later.

The basal metabolism supports the work that goes on all the time, without conscious awareness. The beating of the heart, the inhaling and exhaling of air, the maintenance of body temperature (mentioned earlier as basal thermogenesis), and the sending of nerve and hormonal messages to direct these activities are the basal processes that maintain life. The **basal metabolic rate (BMR)** is surprisingly fast. A person whose total energy needs are 2000 calories a day spends as many as 1200 to 1400 of them to support basal metabolism. The thyroid hormone thyroxine directly controls basal metabolism—the less secreted, the lower the energy requirements for basal functions. Many other factors affect the BMR (see Table 8–3).

A typical breakdown of the total energy spent by a moderately active person (for example, a student who walks back and forth to classes) might look like this:

	BMR (cal)	Activity (cal)	Total energy spent (cal)
Male	1980	720	2700
Female	1170	430	1600

The first is the larger component, and you cannot change it much today. You can, however, change the second component—voluntary activities—and so spend more calories today. If you want to increase your basal metabolic output, make exercise a daily habit. Your body composition will change toward the lean, and your basal energy output will pick up the pace as well. The next section shows how to calculate an approximation of your daily energy output.

Table 8–3

Factors that Affect the BMR

Factor	Effect on BMR
Age	In youth, the BMR is higher; age brings less lean body mass and slows the BMR.
Height	Tall, thin people have higher BMRs.
Growth	Children and pregnant women have higher BMRs.
Body composition	The more lean tissue, the higher the BMR. The more fat tissue, the lower the BMR.
Fever	Fever raises the BMR.
Stress	Stress hormones raise the BMR.
Environmental temperature	Both heat and cold raise the BMR.
Fasting/starvation	Fasting/starvation hormones lower the BMR.
Malnutrition	Malnutrition lowers the BMR.
Thyroxine	The thyroid hormone thyroxine is a key BMR regulator; the more thyroxine produced, the higher the BMR is.

The exact amount of energy a voluntary activity will cost you depends on your personal style. For example, the larger the muscle mass you use to perform the activity, the heavier the weight of the body part being moved, and the longer the time you invest, the more calories you spend. During exercise, do you relax the muscles you are not working, or keep them tense? When you sit, are your muscles tense or relaxed? Are you well-trained or a novice? (The streamlined moves of an expert swimmer, for example, cost less than the movements of the untrained.) Do you have much lean tissue or only a little; a lot of fat or a little? All these factors and others bear on how much an activity will cost in terms of body fuel. Table 8–4 shows the approximate number of calories you might require to swim, bike, or run. Table 8–5 translates some activity values into food energy terms.

How much energy an activity costs also depends on how intense the exercise is and how often you do it. A football player may need close to 6000 calories a day during the season, and on some days he may need even more. A basketball player may need 5000 calories a day to play well and maintain her weight during the season. (After the season, it is equally important for an athlete to cut back to an energy intake that suits the off-season activity.)

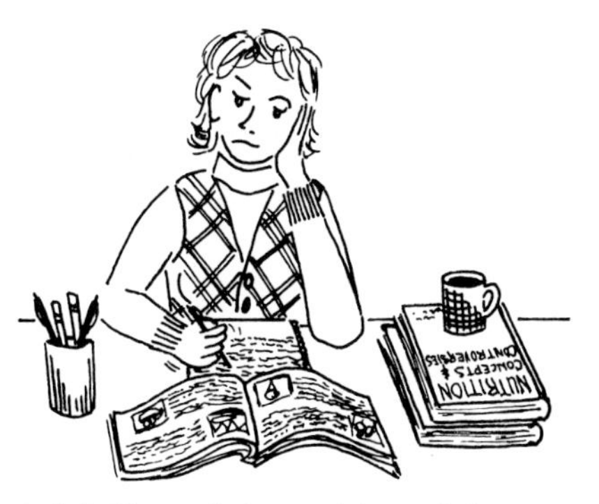

It feels like work, but studying only burns .011 calories per pound per minute.

The balance between food energy taken in and energy expended determines how much fat a person's body stores or uses up. Food energy (calories) can be measured using a bomb calorimeter or estimated from the exchange system or published tables. Energy expenditure can be estimated from tables of recommendations such as the RDA or by keeping records of food energy consumed and changes in body weight over time.

Table 8–4

Energy Demands of Activities

Activity	Intensity	Cal/Lb/Minute
Swimming (crawl)	20 yd/minute	0.032
	45 yd/minute	0.058
	50 yd/minute	0.070
Bicycling	13 mph	0.045
	15 mph	0.049
	17 mph	0.057
	19 mph	0.076
	21 mph	0.090
	23 mph	0.109
	25 mph	0.139
Running	11:30 minutes per mile—5.2 mph	0.061
	9:00 minutes per mile—6.7 mph	0.088
	8:00 minutes per mile—7.5 mph	0.094
	7:00 minutes per mile—9.0 mph	0.103
	6:00 minutes per mile—10.0 mph	0.114
	5:30 minutes per mile—11.0 mph	0.131
Studying		0.011

Note: Skiing, squash, and handball require about the same energy as biking at 13 mph.

Source: All data except that for studying from G. P. Town and K. B. Wheeler, Nutritional concerns for the endurance athlete, *Dietetic Currents*, 1986. Reprinted with the permission and available from Ross Laboratories, Columbus, OH 43216. Copyright 1986 Ross Labs.

Table 8–5

Activity Equivalents of Food Energy Values

Food	Calories	Activity Equivalent for a 150-Pound Person to Work Off the Calories (minutes)		
		Walk[a]	*Jog*[b]	*Wait*[c]
Apple, large	101	19	5	78
Regular beer, 1 glass	114	22	6	88
Cookie, chocolate chip	51	10	3	39
Ice cream, 1/6 qt	193	37	10	148
Steak, T-bone	235	45	12	181

[a]Energy cost of walking at 3.5 mph—5.2 calories per minute.
[b]Energy cost of running—19.4 calories per minute
[c]Energy cost of reclining—1.3 calories per minute.

Estimation of Energy Output

The first step in estimating energy output is to estimate the energy spent in basal metabolism. Use the factor 1.0 cal per kilogram of body weight per hour for men, or 0.9 for women (men usually have more muscles than women). Example (for a 150-lb man):

1. Change pounds to kilograms:

   150 pounds ÷ 2.2 pounds per kilogram = 68 kilograms.

2. Multiply weight in kilograms by the BMR factor:

   68 kilograms × 1 calorie per kilogram per hour = 68 calories per hour.

3. Multiply the calories used in one hour by the hours in a day:

   68 calories per hour × 24 hours per day = 1632 calories per day.

The second step is to estimate the energy spent on voluntary muscular activity. The following figures are crude approximations based on the amount of muscular work a person typically performs in a day. To select the one appropriate for you, remember to think in terms of the amount of *muscular* work performed; don't confuse being *busy* with being *active*.

- For sedentary (mostly sitting) activity (a typist), add 40 to 50% of the BMR.
- For light activity (a teacher), add 55 to 65%.
- For moderate activity (a nurse), add 65 to 70%.
- For heavy work (a roofer), add 75 to 100%.

If the man we used for an example were a clerk, we could estimate the energy he needed for activities by multiplying his BMR calories per day by 50%:

1632 calories per day × 50 percent = 816 calories per day.

Now, total the two components. The man in our example spends, in a day:

1632 calories per day + 816 calories per day = 2448 calories per day.

The exact figure is based on several estimates, so express the man's needs within a 100-cal range: 2400 to 2500 cal/day.

To estimate the energy spent on basal metabolism, use the factor (for men) 1.0 cal/kg/hr (or for women, 0.9 cal/kg/hr) for a 24-hour period. Then add an increment of 40 to 100%, depending on the extent of daily muscular activity.

Weight Gain and Loss

When you step on the scale and note that you weigh a pound or two more or less than you did the last time you weighed, this does not indicate that you have gained or lost body fat, for body fat cannot change that quickly. Changes in body weight reflect shifts in many different materials—not only fat, but large amounts of fluid, some bone minerals, and lean tissues such as muscles. It is important for people concerned with weight control to realize that quick changes in weight are not changes in fat.

An average man or woman about 5 feet 10 inches tall who weighs 150 pounds carries about 90 of those pounds as water and 30 as fat. The other 30 pounds are the so-called lean tissues—muscles; organs such as the heart, brain, and liver; and the bones of the skeleton.* Stripped of water and fat, then, the person weighs only 30 pounds! This lean tissue is vital to health. The person who seeks to lose weight wants, of course, to lose fat, not this precious lean tissue. And for someone who wants to gain weight, it is desirable to gain lean and fat in proportion, not just fat.

The type of tissue gained or lost depends on how the person goes about gaining or losing it. To lose fluid, for example, one can take a "water pill" (diuretic), causing the kidneys to siphon extra water from the blood into the urine. Or one can engage in heavy exercise while wearing thick clothing in the heat, losing abundant fluid in sweat. (Both practices are dangerous, incidentally, and are not being recommended here.) To gain water weight, a person can overconsume salt and water; for a few hours the body will then retain water until it manages to excrete the salt. (This, too, is not recommended.) Most quick-weight-loss diets promote large fluid losses that register temporary, dramatic changes on the scale but accomplish little loss of body fat. Worse, they also promote breakdown of lean tissue. A later section on strategy stresses exercise as a means of maintaining lean tissue during weight loss.

Weight Gain

When you eat more food than you need, where does it go in your body? Previous chapters provided the answer, which is reviewed here. The energy-yielding nutrients—carbohydrate, fat, and protein—contribute to body stores as follows:

- Carbohydrate (other than fiber) is broken down to sugars for absorption. In the body tissues, these may be built up to glycogen or converted to fat and stored.

*For a healthy woman or man 5 ft tall who weighs 100 lb, the comparable figures would be 60 lb of water, 20 lb of fat, 20 lb of lean.

- Fat is broken down to glycerol and fatty acids for absorption. In the body tissues, these may be recombined to make new fat for storage.
- Protein is broken down to amino acids for absorption. Inside the body, these may be used to replace lost body protein and, in a person who is exercising, to build new muscle and other lean tissue. Any extra amino acids have their nitrogen removed and are converted to fat.

Remember that, although three kinds of energy-yielding nutrients enter the body, they are stored there in only two forms: glycogen and fat. (Glycogen stores amount to about ¾ pound; fat stores can, of course, amount to many pounds.) Remember, too, that when excess protein is converted to fat, it cannot be recovered later as protein, because the nitrogen is stripped from the amino acids and excreted in the urine. No matter whether you are eating steak, brownies, or baked beans, then, if you eat enough of them, any excess protein will be turned to fat within hours.

It is important to repeat at this point that:

- Any food can make you fat. The net excess amount of energy is what makes the difference.
- Protein is not stored in the body except in response to exercise; it is present only as working tissue.* Some working protein tissue is lost each day and can be replaced only by protein eaten that day.

When energy balance is positive, the three energy-yielding nutrients are converted to glycogen or fat and stored. Protein cannot later be recovered as amino acids; only its energy value is recovered.

Weight Loss and Fasting

When the tables are turned and you eat less than you need, the body has to draw on its stored energy fuel to keep going. Nothing is wrong with this; in fact, it is a great advantage to us that we can eat periodically, store fuel, and then use up that fuel between meals. The between-meal interval is ideally about four to six hours—about the length of time it takes to use up most of the available liver glycogen—or 12 to 14 hours at night, when body systems are slowed down and the need is less. The major reason people who fast lose weight so dramatically within the first days is that they use up their glycogen. Since glycogen contains only half as many calories per pound as fat, it disappears twice as fast; and with the liver's ¾ pound of glycogen, 3 to 4 pounds of associated water are also lost.

If a person doesn't eat for, say, three whole days or a week, then the body makes one adjustment after another. After about a day, the liver's glycogen is essentially exhausted. Where, then, can the body obtain glucose to keep its nervous system going? Not from the muscles' glycogen, because that is reserved for the muscles' own use.

*Amino acids are present in all body fluids, performing such functions as maintaining the acid-base balance there. As an energy source, they are insignificant when compared with stored fat and glycogen.

An alternative source of energy might be the abundant fat stores most people carry, but at this stage, these are of no use to the nervous system. The muscles and other organs use fat as fuel, but the nervous system ordinarily cannot. Most importantly, the body's major fuel, fat, cannot be converted to glucose—the body possesses no enzymes to carry out this conversion. The liver, however, does possess enzymes that can convert protein to glucose. Therefore, to keep up its glucose supply, the underfed body must turn to the protein in its own lean tissues.

In early food deprivation:

- The nervous system cannot use fat as fuel, only glucose.
- Body fat cannot be converted to glucose.*
- Body protein can be converted to glucose.

One small qualification needs to be added to the statement that the body cannot convert fat to glucose. Glycerol, the small backbone of each triglyceride molecule, can be retrieved during fat breakdown, and two units of glycerol can be converted into one molecule of glucose. For each glycerol unit of three carbons that *can* be converted to glucose, however, there are three fatty acids from the triglyceride, containing perhaps 50 or 60 carbons, that *cannot* be converted to glucose. The fatty acids released from a triglyceride provide possibly 25 times the energy of the glycerol they were attached to. Glycerol from fat is therefore an insufficient source of glucose in the absence of other carbohydrate.

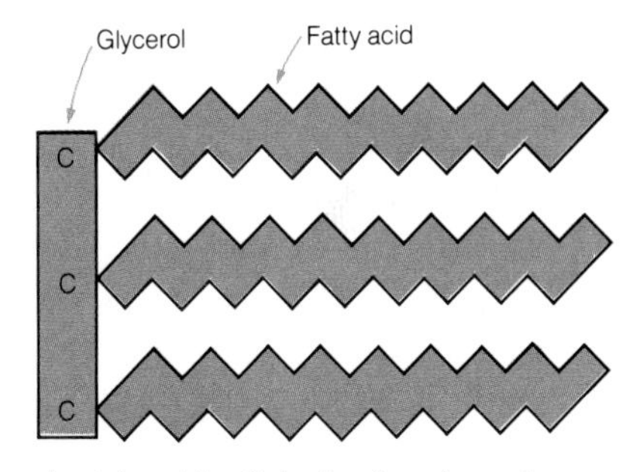

A triglyceride. Only the tiny glycerol backbone in each giant triglyceride molecule can be converted to glucose, and it takes two glycerols to make a single glucose unit. This is why the fats are such an inefficient source of glucose.

If the body were to continue to consume itself unchecked, death would ensue within about ten days. After all, not only skeletal muscle, but also the liver, the heart muscle, the lung tissue, the blood cells—all vital tissues—are being burned as fuel. (In fact, fasting or starving people remain alive only until their stores of fat are gone or until half their lean tissue is gone, whichever comes first.) To prevent this, the body plays its last ace: it begins converting fat into compounds that the nervous system can adapt to use and so forestall the end. This is ketosis, which was first mentioned in Chapter 3 as an adaptation to prolonged fasting or carbohydrate deprivation.

In ketosis, instead of breaking down fat molecules to carbon dioxide and water, as it normally does, the body takes partially broken down fat fragments, combines them to make ketone bodies** (compounds that are normally rare in the blood), and lets them circulate in the bloodstream. The advantage is that about half of the brain's cells can make the enzymes needed to use these compounds for energy. Within a few weeks, the brain can meet most of its energy needs using ketone bodies. Thus, indirectly, the nervous system begins to feed on the body's fat stores. This reduces the nervous system's need for glucose, it spares the muscle and other lean tissue from being devoured so quickly, and it prolongs the starving person's life. Thanks to ketosis, a healthy person starting with average body fat content can live totally deprived of food for as long as six to eight weeks. Figure 8–2 reviews how energy is used during both feasting and fasting, and in ketosis.

Fasting has been practiced as a periodic discipline by respected, wise people in many cultures. Clearly, the body tolerates short-term fasting, although there is no evidence that it benefits by being "cleansed," as some believe. And long-term ketosis may be harmful to the body. For the person who merely wants to lose weight, fasting is usually not the best way. The body's lean tissue continues to be degraded to supply glucose to those nervous system cells that cannot use ketone bodies as

*Glycerol, 5% of fat, can yield glucose, but is a negligible source.

Ketone bodies are energy-containing compounds, made by joining two or more fragments of fatty acids together. Some people call them ***ketones*, but not all of them fit the chemical definition of a ketone, so the preferred term is ***ketonelike compounds***, or ***ketone bodies***.

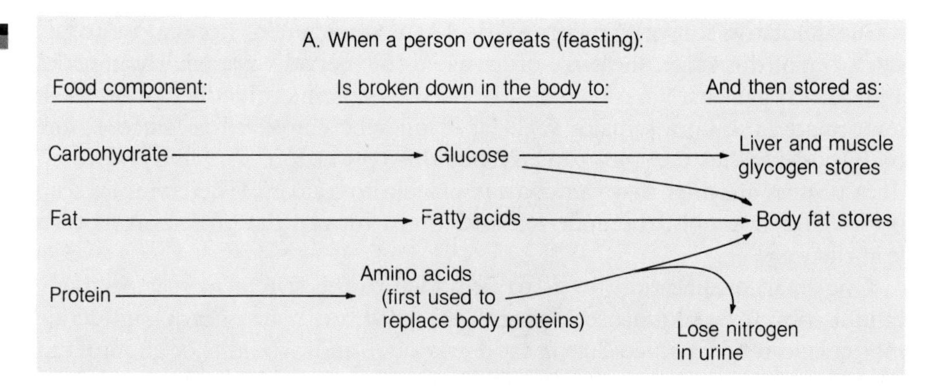

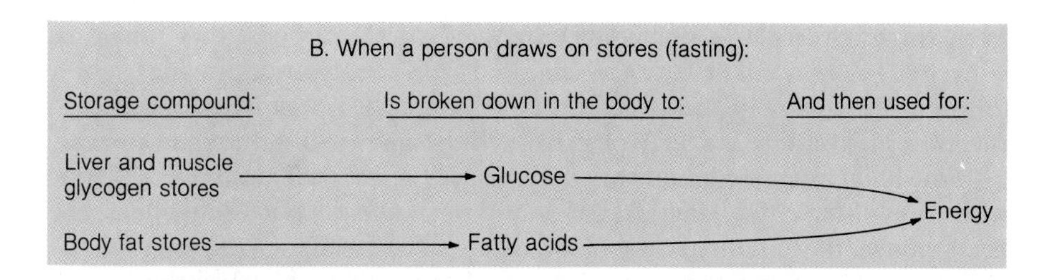

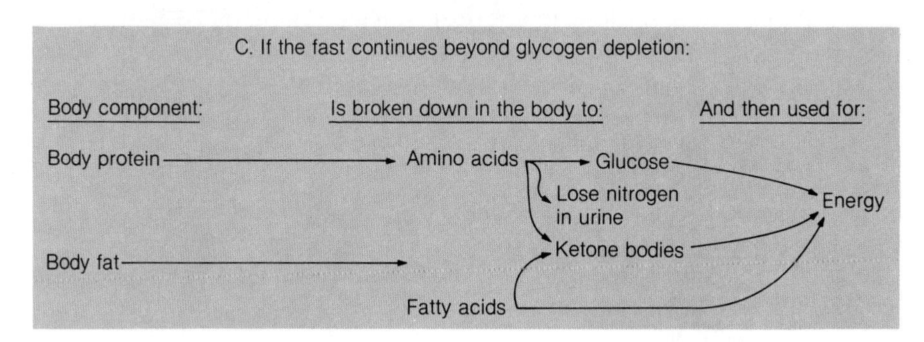

Figure 8–2 Feasting and Fasting.
In A, the person is storing energy. In B, the person is drawing on stored energy. In C, the person is in ketosis.

fuel. The body is deprived of nutrients it needs to assemble new enzymes, red and white blood cells, and other vital components. The body also slows its metabolism during a fast so as to conserve energy. (A low-calorie diet has actually been observed to promote the same rate of *weight* loss over the long run, and a faster rate of *fat* loss, than a total fast.[21]) Just how to design a low-calorie diet is the subject of a later section, but first the low-carbohydrate diets warrant a moment's attention. They are examples of how *not* to design a diet.

When energy balance is negative, glycogen returns glucose to the body; then body protein is called upon to do so. Fat also supplies fuel as fatty acids. In a fast, after carbohydrate runs out, fat supplies fuel as ketone bodies.

The Low-Carbohydrate Diet

Many low-carbohydrate diets have been promoted to the public in many different guises, and each has enjoyed a surge of popularity, thanks largely to the sizable initial weight loss they promote. They are designed to make a person go into ketosis. The sales pitch is that "you'll never feel hungry" and that "you'll lose weight fast—faster than you would on any ordinary diet." Both claims are true, but both are misleading. Loss of appetite accompanies any low-calorie diet. Fast weight loss means loss of water and lean tissue, both of which are rapidly regained upon refeeding. Perhaps most importantly, these diets, undertaken without medical supervision, are dangerous.

Since carbohydrate is in short supply, the body responds to a low-carbohydrate diet as it does to a fast. It is receiving protein and fat but it uses up its stored glycogen in a day. It then turns to protein to make the needed glucose. But why make the body convert protein into glucose? Why not just give it the protein it requires to meet its protein needs, and the carbohydrate it needs to meet its glucose needs? With enough of these two energy-yielding nutrients, the body will use its stored fat to supply energy at the maximal rate.

Low-carbohydrate diets have another disadvantage. When protein is converted to glucose, it loses its nitrogen, which has to be excreted. This and ketone bodies put a burden on the kidneys. The low-carbohydrate dieter who fails to drink abundant water is placing an unnecessary strain on the kidneys, by concentrating nitrogen wastes and ketone bodies.

Many other physiological hazards accompany low-carbohydrate diets: high blood cholesterol, hypoglycemia, mineral imbalances, and other metabolic abnormalities. Some low-carbohydrate diets, particularly the protein-sparing fast type, have caused heart failure. These diets are never recommended by legitimate practitioners—except under close medical supervision, as described next.

Unsupervised low-carbohydrate diets are popular because they promote rapid weight loss, but it is due largely to water and lean tissue loss. They are dangerous and, over the long term, ineffective.

Names of low-carbohydrate diets:

- Air Force Diet.
- Atkins Diet.
- Calories Don't Count Diet.
- Drinking Man's Diet.
- Herbalife Diet.
- Mayo Diet.
- Protein-sparing Fast.
- Scarsdale Diet.
- Simeons HCG Diet.
- Ski Team Diet.
- Stillman Diet.
- You Name It Diet.

Very-Low-Calorie Diets

If fasting is not safe, and low-carbohydrate diets are not safe, is there any quick-weight-loss method that *is* safe? Putting it another way, what is the maximum medically permissible rate of weight loss, and under what circumstances can it be advocated? Researchers and business people are trying hard to find out, for weight loss is big business in this country, and people always want to lose weight in a hurry. In the effort to find an answer, many very-low-calorie diets have been devised and tested on thousands of people. Since 1980, some success has been legitimately claimed—within limits that are important to acknowledge. A conference committee funded by the Cambridge Diet Plan in 1985 reviewed the evidence on very-low-calorie diets, and its findings are reported here.[22]

The goal of these diets is to maximize the rate of fat loss while preserving lean body tissue, normal blood chemistry, and overall good health. An understanding of how to achieve this goal will be realized when these issues are resolved:

- How much protein and carbohydrate to provide, from what sources, and in what forms.
- What other nutrients and ingredients (for example, fiber) to provide.

lipectomy: surgical removal of skin and fat.

suctioning: surgical removal of fat from beneath the skin.

- How to screen clients for entry into, or exclusion from, very-low-calorie diet programs.
- How long to allow dieters to stay on the diets.
- What medical tests to require and at what intervals.

As of 1985, the best approximations of medically acceptable, very-low-calorie diet plans seemed to be variations on a single theme. The diet would consist of a formula containing not less than the RDA of protein, typically from egg white, with carbohydrate added to approximate 400 to 500 calories a day; essential nutrients; fluid; and fiber. It would be taken in four to five equal portions a day. The plan's duration would be from 4 to 12 weeks. Medical tests of blood pressure and blood and urine chemistry would be required weekly or every other week, together with health care provider appointments. Only obese people that were otherwise healthy would be allowed to enter. Clients would be required either to go off the formula at intervals and eat meals of specified composition; or, during the diet, to eat one meal a day (say, one small portion each of fish, vegetables, salad, and fruit) while using the formula for the other meals. Typical weight loss rates would range from about 3 to 5 pounds a week for people having 50 to over 100 pounds to lose, to 1 to 3 pounds a week for people with fewer pounds to lose. Success in weight loss on some of these plans is considerable; success in maintenance of the lost weight averages about one-third (that is, one-third of those who lose the weight keep it off).

It is encouraging that progress is being made toward designing a plan that meets the demand for quick weight loss with a minimum of hazards, because people will demand it. Still, it is preferable to undertake the kind of plan that changes eating habits permanently, as described in the Food Feature.

Medically supervised very-low-calorie diets offer an alternative means of rapid weight loss that, for healthy people, sometimes proves successful.

Other Approaches (Not Recommended)

Other ways *not* to choose are water pills, diet pills, health spa regimens, muscle stimulators, hormones, and surgery. Brushes, sponges, and massages intended to break down "cellulite" do nothing of the kind, because there is no such thing as cellulite.[23] Water pills (diuretics) do nothing to solve a fat problem, although they may bring about the loss of a few pounds on the scale for half a day and cause dehydration. Diet pills have many strikes against them (see box, "Diet Pills and Other Aids"). Health spas may be a nice place to exercise, but you cannot "jiggle" or "melt" pounds away on their special machines. Muscle stimulators reduce body measurements by making muscles tighter, not by reducing their fat content—and only for an hour or so. Hormones are powerful body chemicals, and many affect fat metabolism, but all have proven ineffective and often hazardous as weight-loss aids.

"Cellulite" (SELL-you-leet) is supposedly a lumpy form of fat, but is actually a fraud. The skin sometimes appears lumpy in fatty areas of the body because strands of connective tissue attach the skin to underlying structures. These points of attachment may pull tight where the fat is thick, making lumps appear between them.

Cosmetic surgical approaches include **lipectomy** and **suctioning.** In lipectomy, a slice of loose skin with its underlying fat is removed and the remaining skin closed tightly over the area. This procedure is appropriate for people who have lost large amounts of weight and who are left with stretched skin that will not shrink to fit their smaller body size. It is not appropriate for the removal of large amounts of fat, and like all surgery, it entails the risks associated with anesthesia, infection, and disfigurement. Suctioning involves pushing a large-bore needle beneath the skin and vacuuming out the fat from a specific area. This procedure is appropriate for minor adjustments of trouble areas in people who want to remodel their figures, but is out of the question as a means to solve an obesity problem. Both procedures are expensive, and neither works without calorie control along with it. Some cosmetic surgeons run unethical practices; get at least two medical opinions before agreeing to have surgery.

Some obese people choose to have their jaws wired shut so that they will be forced to consume a liquid diet. This does bring about weight loss, but when the wires are removed, there is "relentless weight gain . . . until the prewiring weight has been reached."[30]

Surgery on the internal organs for obesity has dangerous side effects. Bypass surgery, which involves disconnecting or removing a portion of the small intestine to reduce absorption, is seldom performed any more, because results have been so disappointing and dangerous. Stapling the stomach to reduce its capacity is preferred, but not perfect: stomach tissue is damaged, scars are formed, and staples often pull loose. So little food can be eaten at one time that a person has to eat inconveniently often. Food leaves the stomach so quickly that it dumps into the intestine too suddenly, causing cramping, pain, and in some, a reactive hypoglycemia after each meal.

New approaches to limit the stomach's capacity are developed at intervals. One involves slipping a balloon-like device into the stomach and inflating it; the safety of this procedure is being reviewed by the FDA. It is not a trouble-free procedure, and it causes pain and ulcers in some.[31] Success, as measured by long-term weight maintenance, is seldom achieved by such methods.

Earlier, it was mentioned that a survey of weight-loss schemes found only a few to be effective, and many to be dangerous. People may respond to this fact with the question, Can't the government do something about that? The government is active in pursuing and cracking down on health swindles, but most agencies have insufficient staff and resources to handle the massive number of reported cases. They can eliminate only the most dangerous schemes at best. This results in a free market for other promoters who can rake in millions of dollars on products that are only slightly less dangerous than the worst ones. It is easy for a swindler to get a product on the market and time-consuming and costly for the government or other groups to get it off. That puts the burden of distinguishing frauds from reality on you, the consumer. To keep from getting taken in, remember: if it sounds too good to be true, it probably is.

A multitude of unsound weight-loss schemes are available. Many are expensive and some are dangerous.

the small society
by Brickman
BOOKS
NEW DIET BOOK $7.95
HOW MUCH DO YOU THINK I COULD LOSE WITH THAT?
SEVEN NINETY-FIVE –
11-5
BRICKMAN
Washington Star Syndicate, Inc.

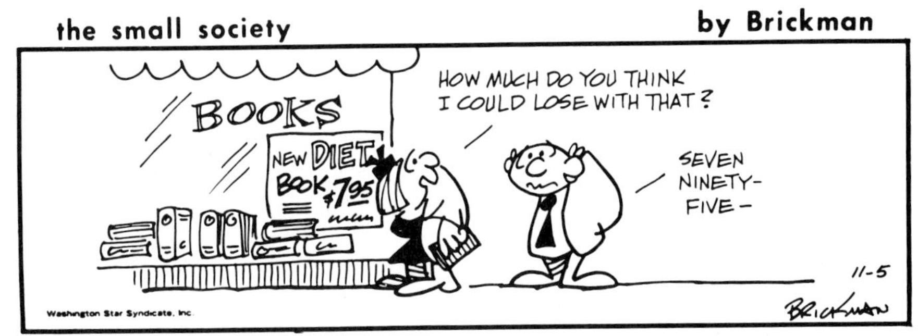

thyroxine: a hormone of the thyroid gland that regulates the body's metabolic rate; it promotes breakdown of glucose and protein, but not breakdown of fat. Thyroxine plays a role in remodeling of lean tissue during growth.

metabolic accelerator: a substance credited with speeding up the metabolic rate; in large amounts, oral doses of thyroxine have this effect.

human chorionic gonadotropin (HCG): a hormone from the placenta that supports early pregnancy, not useful in weight loss.

human growth hormone (HGH) releasers: amino acids that stimulate release of a pituitary hormone that promotes growth of human tissue. HGH promotes deposition of body protein and other lean tissue, and promotes breakdown of fat for energy. HGH is also called *somatotropin* (*soma* means "body"; *tropin* means "make more").

acromegaly (ack-ro-MEG-uh-lee): a disease caused by above-normal levels of HGH. A child with the condition is said to have *gigantism* (*acro* means "limb"; *mega* means "big").

cholecystokinin (CCK): a hormone secreted into the blood by the intestine in response to the arrival of fat, originally known to signal the gallbladder to release bile, now known also to reach the brain and create feelings of satiety.

Diet Pills and Other Aids

Wouldn't it be wonderful if people could lose weight just by taking a pill? Unfortunately, most such pills fall into three groups: some work but present health hazards; some are harmless but do not work; and some both do not work and are outright dangerous.

Hormones top the list of potentially harmful diet aids, and **thyroxine** tops the list of such hormones. Thyroxine has long been promoted as a **metabolic accelerator,** but it is dangerous in the amounts needed to overwhelm the human thyroid regulatory system. Its side effects include degradation of the body's lean tissue, including the heart muscle, and an irregular heart rate. At one point, a heart medicine and a diuretic were added to thyroxine to counter these effects, but they did not prevent the damage it caused, and some people even died from the combined effects of the drugs.[24]

Two other hormones follow thyroxine on the list: **human chorionic gonadotropin (HCG)** and **human growth hormone (HGH) releasers.** Schemes that require injections of HCG are not only expensive and useless, but also present a risk of illness and shock from infected serum or amateur administration. HGH releasers are really amino acids (arginine and ornithine) that supposedly correct a too-low level of HGH, and promote weight loss during sleep. It is true that some obese people secrete less HGH in response to an arginine dose than thin people do, but this fact only shows arginine is *not* effective, precisely in those who need it the most.[25] As for the hormone itself, a true overdose causes **acromegaly,** a disfiguring disease. In adults, acromegaly causes thickening of the bones of the hands, feet, cheeks, and jaw, thickening of the soft tissue of the eyelids, lips, tongue, and nose, and thickening and rumpling of the skin on the forehead and soles of the feet. Internally, the heart, liver, and other organs become distorted. In children, the bones grow abnormally long.

The hormone **cholecystokinin (CCK)** is worth a mention, because it is widely available in health-food stores. It is sold in pill form; the pills contain ground-up animal intestines (CCK is produced there), supposedly to provide CCK, supposedly to signal satiety. In reality, the amount of CCK in a pill's worth of animal intestine is almost too small to detect, let alone suppress appetite. Anyway, CCK is a protein and so it is destroyed by digestion in the stomach, and none is absorbed from an oral dose.[26]

Another class of useless and potentially harmful diet aids is the diuretics, or "water pills." These have a legitimate medical use in the treatment of hypertension caused by raised blood volume, but they are of no use in controlling body fatness. The wishful thought behind their use by dieters is that excess weight is due to water accumulation. If *water* retention is a problem, a diuretic and possibly a mild degree of salt restriction can help, but the obese—that is overfat—person has a *smaller* percentage of body water than the person of normal weight. If such a person takes a diuretic, the resulting weight loss will be water, not fat, it will be accompanied by dehydration and electrolyte loss, and it will last less than a day.

Similarly, laxatives may be safe and effective for their intended purpose, but not for weight loss, and herbs that are credited with satiety effects can be dangerous (see Controversy 10). Food products other than herbs are generally harmless, but not effective. Spirulina, a seaweed already described in Controversy 6, has no special talent for promoting weight loss, and as a nutritious food it is vastly overpriced. Another vegetable product, **glucomannan,** has been claimed by the Japanese to be an ancient weight-control aid, but in a controlled experiment reported in 1982, glucomannan was ineffective.[27] As for **bee pollen,** which is also highly regarded by some, it causes allergies, and it is very expensive—about $24 per pound. More to the point, it is almost pure sugar. So are the candies promoted as "appetite spoilers" (Aydes and others). These candies also contain a local anesthetic in an attempt to "deaden the taste buds," but efficacy for weight loss is probably due to the sugar content. As you will see in this chapter's Controversy, a little sugar can be useful in weight loss, but ordinary table sugar will do.

Only one drug, a nervous system stimulant that suppresses the appetite, has been deemed safe and effective by the FDA for use in over-the-counter diet pills. It is **phenylpropanolamine.** Seventy diet products with different names line the shelves of drug stores, but read the labels, and you'll find this one active ingredient. (Even "Amazing Grapefruit Pills" fail to amaze when you read their labels and find phenylpropanolamine.) You'll also find a warning that the drug might induce stroke in those with a history of hypertension, and may harm people who suffer from any of a number of diseases. Even healthy people risk brain hemorrhage from the drug, especially if they exceed the suggested dose or combine it with other common drugs such as oral contraceptives, cold and cough remedies, or even caffeine.[28]

A common over-the-counter drug used in cold and asthma medicines is **ephedrine.** This substance has been deemed safe for other uses, and shows promise of stimulating thermogenesis, thereby helping the body to spend energy, when administered with aspirin or caffeine.[29] In the future, ephedrine may offer another choice among the nonprescription diet aids.

Then there are **amphetamines**—powerful, addictive mind- and body-altering stimulants that reduce the appetite. When obesity is life-threatening, a physician may decide to prescribe them. Side effects include nervousness, sleeplessness, and irritability, among others. A tough question concerning amphetamines, and in fact, all legitimate diet aids, is How can a person get off such drugs without regaining weight? Short-term weight loss achieved by any means is not a permanent solution to a weight problem, and when achieved through drugs, can leave a person with two problems—the overweight and the drug.

glucomannan (gloo-co-MAN-an): a preparation derived from a vegetable (konjac tuber) used in Japanese cooking, and claimed to have weight-controlling properties; the claims have been tested and not confirmed.

bee pollen: a product sold with the claim that it aids in weight loss and boosts athletic performance, but that in reality has no such effect.

phenylpropanolamine (FEN-ill-prope-ah-NOLE-ah-meen): the active ingredient of over-the-counter diet pills, as well as an ingredient of many cold, cough, and allergy remedies.

ephedrine (eh-FED-rin): an ingredient in many cold, cough, and allergy medicines that produces energy wastage through increased thermogenesis, especially when the drug is combined with aspirin or caffeine. Not yet approved for use in diet pills.

amphetamines: a group of prescription drugs (popularly called "speed") that stimulate the nervous system and depress the appetite, used in cases of mental depression, hyperactivity in children, and obesity. Amphetamines are psychologically and physically addictive.

Food Feature

Planning a Weight Control Program

This Food Feature is for the person who is serious about weight change and is willing to adopt a lifelong plan. It concentrates on weight loss, because so many people want to achieve that, but weight gain is here, too. Many of the same strategies work well for both, and the secret is the same for both—a sensible approach (we didn't say *easy*) involving diet, exercise, and behavior modification. To accomplish either goal takes tremendous dedication, especially at first, for a person whose habits have all supported a particular body weight must adopt as habits a hundred or so new behaviors that will promote and maintain a different weight. When people succeed, they do so because they have employed many of the techniques described in this chapter.

To emphasize the personal nature of weight-control plans, the following sections are written in terms of advice to "you." This is intended to give you the illusion of listening in on a conversation in which a person is being competently counseled by someone familiar with the techniques known to be effective.

Strategies for diet planning:

1. Get involved personally.

2. Adopt a realistic plan.

Diet No particular food plan is magical, and no particular food must be either included or avoided. You are the one who will have to live with the plan, so you had better be involved in designing it. Don't think of yourself as going "on" a diet—because then you may be tempted to go "off." Think of yourself as adopting an eating plan for life. It must consist of foods that you like or can learn to like, that are available to you, and that are within your means.

Choose an energy level you can live with. For the person wanting to lose weight, a deficit of 500 calories a day for seven days (3500 calories a week) is enough to lose a pound a week of body fat. It is easiest to do this by both increasing activity (see next section, "Exercise") and reducing food intake, for it is urgent not to try to cut calories too far. Two risks spring from overly severe restriction of calories—one, that a person will spiral into anorexia nervosa, the other, that the person will experience an irresistable urge to binge, and repeatedly undo whatever progress is made. (Anorexia nervosa and bulimia are the subjects of Controversy 9). Also, severe calorie restriction slows the basal metabolic rate, making weight loss harder to achieve. A rule of thumb is that you need at least 10 calories per pound of current weight.

Anyway, there is no point in hurrying, because you will never go off the plan; you will only modify it slightly when you have reached your goal. Nutritional adequacy is hard to achieve on a low-calorie diet; even a small person should not try to get by on fewer than 1200 calories (1000 at the very least). A larger person should adjust the calories upwards; some people can lose weight steadily on diets of 1600 calories or more. For the lower ranges, it is appropriate to use a balance vitamin-mineral supplement; see Controversy 6 for how to choose one. Table 8–6 presents a sample balanced 1250 calorie weight-loss diet.

For the person who wants to gain weight, a combination of diet and exercise also is best, but different considerations apply. As you add exercise, you must eat additional calories to support that exercise—otherwise, you will lose weight (body fat). If you eat just enought to support the exercise, you will build muscle,

Table 8–6

A Sample Balanced Weight-Loss Diet

Exchange Item	Number of Exchanges	Carbohydrate (g)	Protein (g)	Fat (g)	Energy (cal)
Starch/bread	4	60	12	Trace	320
Meat (lean)	5	0	35	15	275
Vegetables	4	20	8	0	100
Fruit	4	60	0	0	240
Milk (nonfat)	2	24	16	Trace	180
Fat	3	0	0	15	135
Total		164 g	71 g	30 g	1250 cal

[a]This 1250-cal diet typifies the balance recommended for a weight-loss diet: approximately 50% carbohydrate, 25% protein, and 25% fat. (Carbohydrate supplies 656 cal; protein, 284 cal; and fat, 270 cal.) When the dieter returns to a maintenance plan by adding mostly carbohydrate foods, the ratio will resemble the 15% protein, 30% fat, and 55% carbohydrate recommended for a maintenance diet.

but at the expense of body fat; that is, fat will be burned to support the muscle building. If you eat more, you will gain both muscle and fat.

It takes an excess of about 2000 to 2500 calories, in theory, to support the gain of a pound of pure lean tissue.[32] The rate at which that tissue can be built depends on the person. Men and women with more male hormones build muscle more easily than others, but it is not known at what rate muscle can be built. Conventional advice on diet to the body builder is to eat about 700 to 1000 calories a day above normal energy needs. This is enough to support both the added exercise and the building of muscle. (Chapter 9 provides much more information on gaining fitness, as well as cautions on the use of steroid hormones.)

Counting the calories in foods is time consuming, and only the most motivated will persist at it for long. For the rest of us, some acquaintance with the exchange system (introduced in Chapter 2) provides a simpler method. The foods depicted in Figure 8–3 could be found one by one in Appendix A, but it is quicker to translate them into exchanges and add up the energy values to get a rough idea of the total. With some practice, you can look at any plate of food and "sense" the number of calories it represents. The energy amounts to remember are:

3. Keep track of calories.

- One nonfat milk exchange—90 calories (for lowfat milk, 120 calories; for whole milk, 150).
- One vegetable exchange—25 calories.
- One fruit exchange—60 calories.
- One starchy vegetable/bread exchange—80 calories.
- One lean meat exchange—55 calories (for medium-fat meat, 75 calories; for high-fat meat, 100 calories). Remember, one exchange of meat is one *ounce*.
- One fat exchange—45 calories.
- One teaspoon sugar—20 calories.

So how many calories are in the meal in Figure 8–3? The answer is at the end of this chapter.

Along with calories, put nutritional adequacy high on your list of priorities. This is a way of putting yourself first. "I like me, and I'm going to take good

Figure 8–3 Calorie Quiz.
In case you'd like to try guessing how many calories are in the meal depicted here, the answer is provided in Figure 8–6.

1 small baked potato
1 pat butter
Lemon
1 c low-fat milk (2%)
½ c green beans
4 oz fish fillet

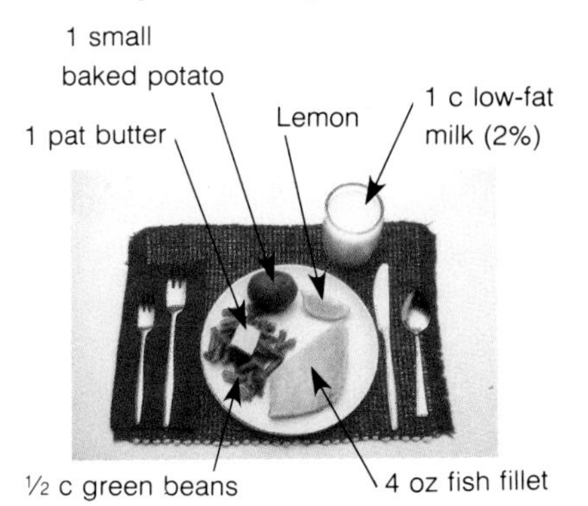

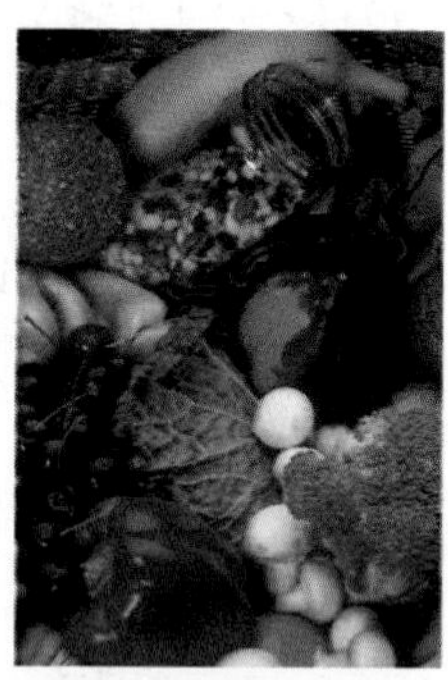

Crunchy, wholesome foods offer bulk and satiety for far fewer calories than smoothly refined foods.

4. Make the diet adequate.
5. Emphasize high nutrient density.
6. Individualize. Use foods you like.
7. Stress dos, not don'ts.

8. Eat regular meals with no skipping—at least three a day.

care of me" is the attitude to adopt. A plan that uses the minimum servings suggested in Four Food Group Plan (Chapter 2) without frills and allows a teaspoon of fat at each meal provides less than 1200 calories; most people could lose weight at a satisfactory rate following such a plan and meet most of their nutrient needs, too (women might well need an iron supplement, though). Within each category, search the exchange lists for a number of foods on each list that you like, and use them often. If you plan resolutely to include a certain number of servings of food from each food group each day, you may be so busy making sure you get what you need that you will have little time or appetite left for high-calorie or empty-calorie foods. Foods such as vegetables and whole grains take a lot of eating, too—crunchy, wholesome foods offer bulk and satiety for far fewer calories than smooth, refined foods. Limit your meats: an ounce of ham contains more calories than an ounce of bread, and many of them are from fat. Especially, don't lose track of the fat you add—as Chapter 4 stated, fat calories probably contribute more to body fat stores than do carbohydrate calories, and fat has so many calories per bite, it is easy to overload quickly. Just a few bites of fatty food can provide the whole allowance of calories for a meal before the diner has eaten enough food for satiety.

Three meals a day is standard for our society, but no law says you shouldn't have four or five meals—only be sure they are smaller, of course. What is important is to eat regularly and, if at all possible, to eat before you are very hungry. Make sure it is hunger, not appetite, urging you to eat. When you do decide to eat, eat the entire meal you have planned for yourself. Then don't eat again until the next meal. Save "free" or favorite foods or beverages for a planned snack at the end of the day, if you need insurance against late-evening hunger.

For person who wants to gain weight: you, too, must learn to eat different foods. No matter how many sticks of celery you consume, you won't gain weight very fast, because celery simply doesn't offer enough calories. The person who cannot eat much volume is encouraged to use calorie-dense foods in meals (the very ones the dieter is trying to stay away from). Yes, these foods are high in fat, but if they are contributing energy needed to spare protein, they won't contribute to heart disease. They will help you build a stronger body. Choose milk shakes instead of milk, peanut butter instead of lean meat, avocado instead of cucumber, whole-wheat muffins instead of whole wheat bread. When you do eat celery, put cream cheese on it; add cream and sugar to coffee; use creamy dressings on salads, whipped cream on fruit, sour cream on potatoes, and the like. (Because fat contains twice as many calories per teaspoon as sugar, it adds calories without adding much bulk.)

Eat more frequently. Make three sandwiches in the morning and eat them between classes in addition to the day's three regular meals. Spend more time eating each meal: if you fill up fast, eat the highest-calorie items first. Don't start with soup or salad; start with meaty appetizers or the main course. Drink between meals, not with them, to save space for higher-calorie foods. Ask your health-care provider for a liquid supplement to drink between meals. Always finish with dessert. Many an underweight person has simply been too busy (for months) to eat enough to gain or maintain weight. These strategies will help you change this behavior pattern.

Exercise The second component of a successful weight control program is exercise. Some people hate the very idea of exercise. Obese people often—

understandably—do not enjoy moving their bodies. They feel heavy, clumsy, even ridiculous. A word to reassure them: weight loss, at least to a point, is possible without exercise, but even if you choose not to alter your habits at first, let your mind be open to the possibility that you will want to take up some activity later on. As the pounds come off, moving your body will become a pleasure.

ratchet effect or **yoyo effect** (of dieting): the effect of repeated rounds of dieting; the person rebounds to a higher weight (and higher body fat content) at the end of each round.

For the person who wants to gain weight, exercise is indispensable to ensure that the gain will be at least partly lean tissue. Of the two options, endurance exercise and strength training, the former will build lean body mass slightly, but often is accompanied by a loss of fat, because the exercise uses up energy and depresses appetite. Strength training is recommended as a more efficient way of supporting weight gain; Chapter 9 provides details.[33]

Thinness is not the same as fitness. For a definition of fitness, see the next chapter.

Weight loss without exercise can have a negative effect on body composition, especially if the weight is regained. A person who diets without exercising loses both lean and fat tissue, as described earlier. If the person then gains weight without exercising, more fat than lean is gained. Fat tissue is less active metabolically than lean tissue, and so the person's daily energy expenditure is less. Each time a person loses weight and regains it without exercising, that person's metabolism requires fewer calories. If the person eats the same amount as before the last diet, the person will not maintain, but will gain weight. This is one explanation for the so-called **ratchet effect,** or **yoyo effect** of dieting (see Figure 8–4), and underlines the importance of exercise as part of a weight-loss plan.

Loss of metabolically active muscle tissue due to failure to exercise does not account completely for the ratchet effect.[34] Other effects must also be operating; perhaps obese people who have dieted repeatedly are metabolically different to begin with. In any case, it must be clear by now that exercise provides many benefits for as long as you keep your body conditioned. Among the benefits of exercise are:

Figure 8–4 The Ratchet Effect.
Each round of dieting, without exercise, is followed by a rebound of weight to a higher level than before. The body fat content increases and caloric needs fall after each round, making the next round of weight loss harder.

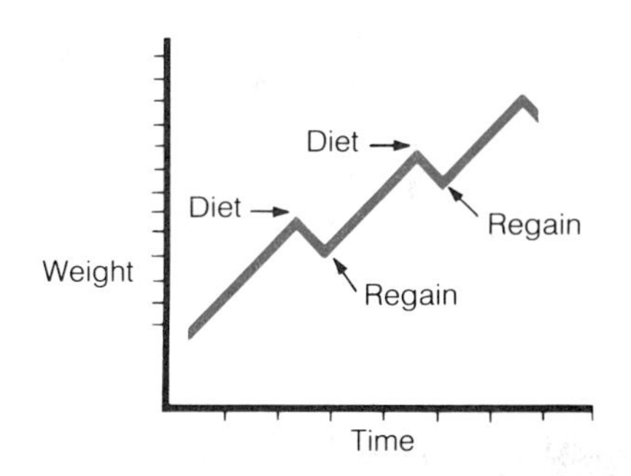

- Increased expenditure of energy.
- Long-term increase in resting metabolic rate.
- Appetite control.
- Control of stress and stress-induced over- or under-eating.
- Increased self-esteem.
- Psychological and physical well-being.

Chapter 9 provides more information on fat use, energy use, and exercise, but a few strategies are in order here. For one thing, you must keep in mind that if exercise is to help you with weight control, it must be active exercise—voluntary moving of muscles. Being moved passively, as by a machine at a health spa or by a massage, neither increases energy expenditure nor builds muscles. The more muscles you move, the more muscle tissue you build, and the more calories you spend.

Strategies for using exercise for weight control:
1. Choose active exercise; move large muscle groups.
2. Think in terms of quantity, not speed.

People sometimes think that workouts have to be fast-paced. This is not true. For example, whether you choose to walk or run a given distance, you will use up about the same amount of energy; walking will just take you longer.*

Another strategy is to incorporate more exercise into your daily schedule in many simple, small-scale ways. Park the car at the far end of the parking lot;

3. Exercise informally, in daily routines.

*Runners use about 10 percent more energy, because they push their weight up as well as forward with each step.

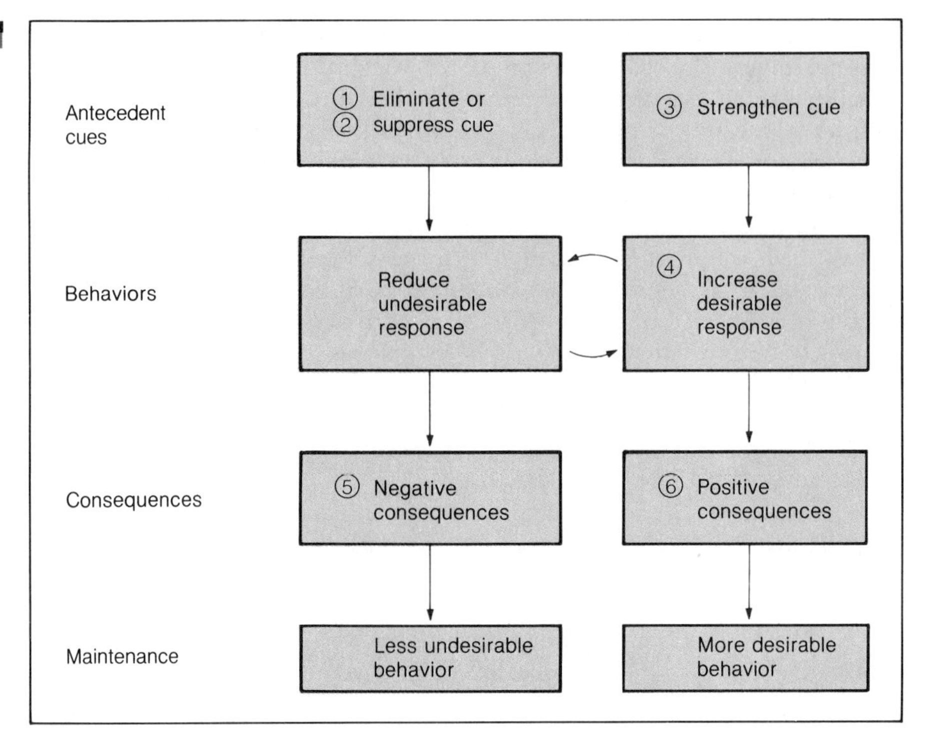

Figure 8–5 Behavior Modification Model. A behavior occurs in response to antecedents (cues or stimuli). The behavior leads to consequences, and the more intense these are, the more or less likely the behavior will occur again. The antecedents and consequences can be manipulated so as to favor the repeated occurrence of a desired behavior and to extinguish the occurrence of unwanted behavior.

Source: Adapted from R. B. Stuart and B. Davis, *Slim Chance in a Fat World: Behavioral Control of Obesity* (Champaign, Ill.: Research Press, 1972), Figure 2, p. 76.

use the stairs instead of the elevator; work your abdominal muscles while you stand in line; tighten your buttocks each time you get up from your chair. These activities add up to only a few calories each, but over a year's time they become significant.

Strategies to modify behavior:
1. Establish a baseline, and keep records.

Behavior modification The third component of a sound weight-control plan is behavior modification. Behavior modification works to cement into place the behaviors of eating and exercise that lead to and perpetuate apropriate body weight. Figure 8–5 shows six areas of changes to reduce the frequency of unwanted behaviors and increase the frequency of desired behaviors. The discussion that follows applies these six behavior modification principles mostly to weight loss and shows how some also apply to weight gain.

First, behavior modification experts say, you should establish a baseline, a record of your present eating behaviors against which to measure future progress. Keep a diary, so that you can learn what your particular eating stimuli, or cues, are. Continue recording as you embark on your plan. At first it may seem as if you have to spend all your waking hours thinking about and planning your meals. Such a massive effort is always required when a new skill is being learned. (You spent hours practicing writing the alphabet when you were in the first grade.) But after about three weeks, it will be much easier. Use positive imaging: see yourself as a person who "eats thin," or "eats hearty"—whichever you need to become. Your new eating pattern will become a habit.

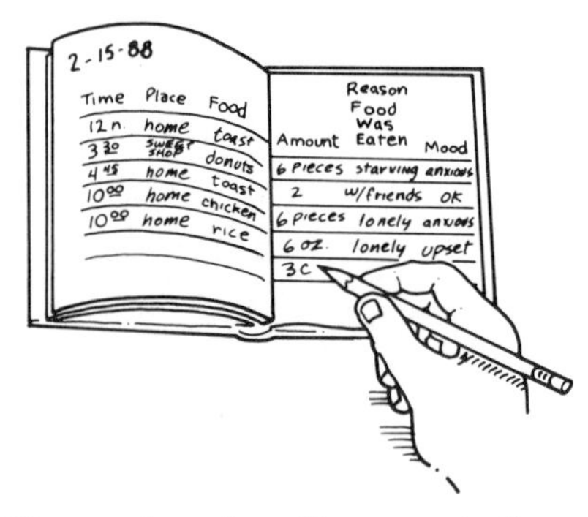

The record reveals problem areas, the first step toward solving problems.

Second, set about eliminating or suppressing the cues that prompt you to eat inappropriately. There may be many such cues in the overeater's life: watching television, talking on the telephone, passing a convenience store or a vending machine, being offered food, and many more. Resolve to respond no longer to the remaining cues by eating. Respond only to one set of cues designed by you: one particular place in one particular room. No other place should stimulate you to eat. To eliminate cues:

2. Eliminate or suppress cues to inappropriate eating.

- Eat only in one place, in one room.
- Don't buy problem foods (shop when you aren't hungry).
- Don't serve rich sauces and toppings.
- Let spouse and children buy, store, and serve their own sweets.
- Clear plates directly into the garbage.
- Create obstacles to the eating of problem foods (for example, make it necessary to unwrap, cook, and serve each one separately, allowing time for resistance to develop).

If some cues to inappropriate eating behavior can't be eliminated, suppress them:

- Minimize contact with excessive food (serve individual plates, don't put serving dishes on the table, leave the table when finished).
- Make small portions of food look large (spread food out, serve on small plates). Garnish empty spaces with lettuce.
- Control deprivation, so that you will not overeat to compensate (plan and eat regular meals, don't skip meals, avoid getting over-tired, avoid boredom by keeping cues to interesting activities in plain sight).
- Place the television in a cabinet behind doors.

Third, strengthen the cues to appropriate eating and exercise. The person who needs to gain weight might select many of those just identified (the ones the overeater is attempting to eliminate) and start using them as cues to eat. For example—*do* snack while watching television; make large portions of food look small, and so forth. Also:

3. Strengthen cues to appropriate behaviors.

- Encourage others to eat appropriate foods with you.
- Keep a variety of appropriate foods available.
- Learn appropriate portion sizes.
- Save permitted foods from meals for snacks (and these should be your only snacks).
- Prepare permitted foods attractively.
- Keep your ski poles (hiking boots, tennis racket) by the door.

Fourth, alter the response itself. Overeaters eat faster than others, so:

4. Slow down eating; move more.

- Slow down (pause for two to three minutes, put down utensils, swallow before reloading the fork, always use utensils).

Fat people tend to move their muscles minimally:

- Move more (shake a leg, pace, fidget, flex your muscles).

For weight-gain efforts, do the opposite: speed up eating, relax more.

5. Arrange negative consequences for negative behaviors.

Fifth, arrange as far as possible to have negative consequences follow inappropriate eating behavior and activity. Scolding is *not* a negative consequence (it is a form of attention-giving, which is positive), so don't ask to be scolded:

- Have others nearby when you eat.
- Ask that others respond neutrally to your deviations (make no comment). This is a negative consequence, because it withholds attention.
- If you slip, don't punish yourself.

Consider the last item. If you ate an extra 1000 calories yesterday, don't try to eat 1000 fewer calories today. Just go back to your plan. On the other hand, you can plan ahead and budget for special occasions. If you want to celebrate your birthday with cake and ice cream, cut the necessary calories from your bread and milk allowance for several days *beforehand*. Your weight loss will be as smooth as if you had stayed with the daily plan.

6. Reward yourself. Make rewards personal and immediate.

Sixth and finally, make sure that positive consequences, including material rewards, follow your exhibition of the desired behaviors. Rewards should be personal—they should give *you* pleasure; and they should be immediate. To acquire positive reinforcement, weigh yourself only every week or two. Gains or losses of a pound or more in a matter of days reverse themselves quickly; the smoothed-out average is what is real. Don't expect to lose continuously as fast as you did at first. A sizable water loss is common in the first week, but it will not happen again. If you have been working out lately, occasional weighings may show no loss or even a gain. This may reflect a welcome development: the gain of lean body mass—just what you want, if you want to be healthy.

- Update records of food intake, exercise, and weight change regularly.
- Arrange for material reinforcement—rewards (other than food) for each unit of behavior change or weight loss.
- Provide social reinforcement (ask to be encouraged).
- Take well-spaced weighings to avoid discouragement.

Many dieters experience a temporary plateau after about three weeks—not because they are slipping, but because they have gained water weight temporarily while they are still losing body fat. The fat they are hoping to lose must be used for energy. To use it, the body must combine it with oxygen (oxidize it) to make carbon dioxide and water. These compounds are heavier than the fat they are made from, because oxygen has been added to them.* The carbon dioxide will be exhaled quickly, but the water stays in the body for a longer time. The water takes a while to leave the cells, then makes its way into the spaces between them, and finally enters the bloodstream. Only after the water has arrived in the blood do the kidneys "see" it and send it to the bladder for excretion. Meanwhile, the dieter has a weight gain, but one day the plateau will break. The signal that this is happening is frequent urination.

You may have to get tough with yourself if you stop making progress. Ask yourself honestly, "What am I doing wrong?" (no one is listening in). Seldom does an unpredicted weight plateau of any duration have no explanation in the dieter's own choices.

Finally, if you stop making progress, be aware that this may be a good time to stop. Your weight may be at a point you are willing to accept, at least for

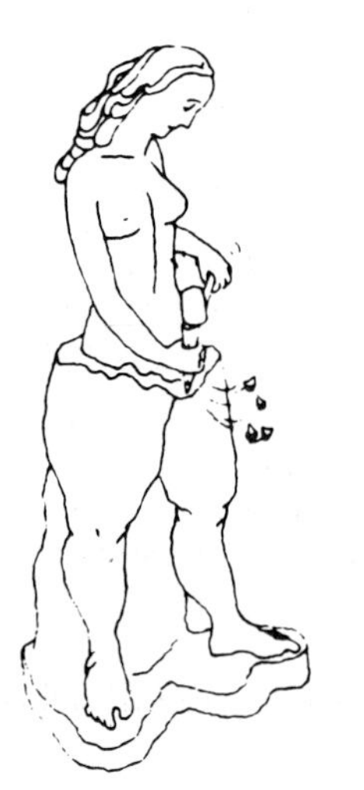

Inside every fat person is a fit person, struggling to be freed.

*Water weight accumulates during fat oxidation because one fatty acid weighing 284 units leaves behind water weighing 324 units, 14 percent more.

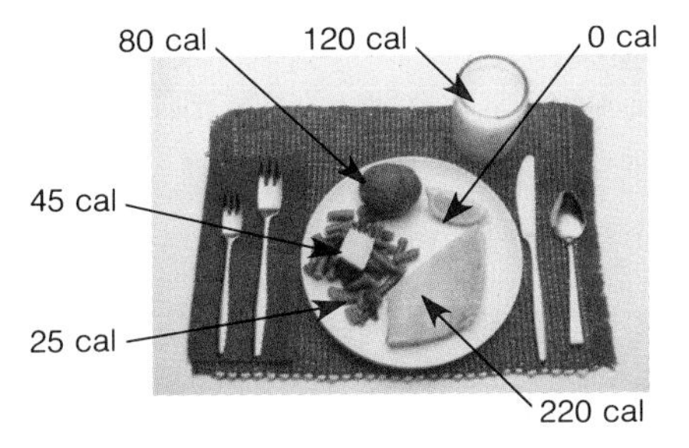

1 c low-fat milk	120 cal
½ c green beans	25
1 small potato (1 starchy vegetable)	80
1 pat butter (1 fat)	45
4 oz fish (4 oz lean meat, assuming no fat is added), at 55 cal/oz	220
Lemon wedge	0
	490 cal

Note: Appendix A values yield a total of about 432 cal, lower because these foods are low-calorie choices within the exchange groups. Any answer within about 50 to 100 cal of this is a good estimate.

Figure 8–6 Quiz Answers.
We figure about 490 calories for the meal.

the present. In fact, you may have come to realize that your original goal weight was unrealistic, or not worth the effort it would take to get there. Neither "thin" nor "muscular" is necessarily happy; and "fit and healthy" is a more desirable state, in any case. You may decide to join the ranks of people who have rejected the magazine-cover ideal, and opt for cheerful self-acceptance. Hold your head high and take the attitude, "This is the way I am choosing to be right now."

7. Maintain self-esteem.

Weight-losers may find it helpful to join a group such as TOPS (Take Off Pounds Sensibly), Weight Watchers, or Overeaters Anonymous. A modest expenditure for your own wellness is worthwhile (but avoid ripoffs, of course). Many dieters form their own self-help groups. If they are expecially sensitive to social situations where there is pressure to eat, it will also help to have some assertiveness training. Learning to say "No, thank you" might be one of your first objectives. Learning not to "clean your plate" might be another.

8. Learn and practice assertiveness.

9. Use small-step modification.

From all the available behavior changes, you choose the ones to begin with. Don't try to master them all at once. No one who attempts too many changes at one time is successful. Set your own priorities. Pick one behavior you can handle, start with that, and practice it until it is habitual and automatic. Then select another.

Enjoy your new, emerging self. Inside every overly fat or thin person is a healthier person, struggling to be freed. Get in touch with—reach out your hand to—that new self, and help that self to feel welcome in the light of day.

Finally, be aware that it can be harder to maintain a new weight than to achieve it. On arriving at the goal weight after months of self-discipline and new habit formation, the victor must at all costs avoid "celebrating" by resuming old eating habits. They are gone forever. Membership in an ongoing weight-control group and continued physical activity with others can provide needed support for the formerly fat or thin person who wants to remain fit.

Whether you need to gain, lose, or maintain weight, attention to eating and exercise can pay off. To enjoy life to the fullest, let a regular routine of balanced meals and exercise set the rhythm for your days. As you will see in the next chapter, the choice of kinds and amounts of exercise can be an art.

Did you guess how many calories were in the meal shown earlier in Figure 8–4? It is here, in Figure 8–6.

shopping list (for weight loss):

- milk group: low-fat favorite foods
- vegetables: several favorites
- fruits: several favorites
- grains/starches: fat-free favorites
- meat/meat alternate group: lean choices
- sweat band, socks, or other comforts for exercising
- rewards (other than food)
- brown bags or opaque boxes to store food out of sight

Self-Study

Practice Diet Planning

Diets can be planned using the exchange system to gain weight, lose weight, or stay the same. For practice in the use of this convenient system, try planning two diets, one for weight maintenance or gain, the other for weight loss.

Diet for Weight Maintenance or Gain

1. Determine your daily energy output, following the example on p. 290. If you choose to maintain weight, it should be equal to your daily energy output. If you wish to gain weight, it should be at least 500 calories above that.
2. Decide on the proportions in which protein, fat, and carbohydrate calories will be represented in the diet. A suggested ratio is about 10 to 15 percent of the energy from protein, not more than 30 percent from fat, and the rest from carbohydrate. Given the daily calorie level you chose, how many calories will you allot to each nutrient?
3. Translate these calorie amounts into grams. (Remember, 1 gram of protein or carbohydrate = 4 calories; 1 gram of fat = 9 calories.) Enter these gram amounts and your intended calorie total at the top of Form 6 (Appendix H).
4. Now decide how many exchanges of milk, vegetables, and fruit you'd like to have each day; enter these numbers in the form; and compute the number of grams of carbohydrate, protein, and fat they will deliver (don't compute calories yet). See p. 301 or Appendix E for the exchange system values. (Caution: use pencil. You'll want to change these numbers several times before you finalize your plan.)

Only one more set of foods—the starch/bread exchanges—contribute any carbohydrate to the diet. Select the number of starch/bread exchanges that will bring your total carbohydrate intake close to the amount you want. Adjust the numbers of these four exchanges until they seem reasonable to you.

Suggestions: Diets for adults should include two to three milk exchanges daily, two or more vegetable exchanges, and at least two, and preferably more, fruit exchanges. The number of starch/bread exchanges is variable, but the list includes many nutritious foods containing complex carbohydrates. It is not unusual for women's diets to include four to six starch/bread exchanges and for men's to include twice as many or even more. High-calorie diets can have many more of all of these carbohydrate-containing exchanges.

If you have a special fondness for sugar or sugar-containing foods, add a line to Form 6 under "Starch/bread," and allow yourself some "sugar exchanges" (see p. 301). At the end of this step, you should have a carbohydrate gram total within about 10 percent of the number you planned in step 3.
5. Subtotal the protein grams delivered by these four types of foods. Only one more list of foods—the meat exchanges—will contribute any protein to the diet. Select the number of meat exchanges you need to bring your total protein intake close to what you planned in step 3.

Note: The recommended intake of carbohydrate is high compared with what many people are used to. Planners often find that once they have completed step 4 of this procedure, they have almost used up their protein allowance and must therefore drastically limit their consumption of meat exchanges. If it works out this way for you, you have two choices. You can accept the dictates of this pattern and resolve to limit your intake of meats and meat alternates accordingly. Or you can increase the number of protein grams you will allow yourself (step 3) and reduce carabohydrate and/or fat to keep the calorie level within bounds.

At the end of this step, you should have a protein gram total that agrees (within 10 percent) with your plan of step 3.
6. Subtotal the fat grams delivered by these five categories of foods. Now use the fat exchanges to bring your total fat intake up to the level planned in step 3.
7. Fill in the calorie amounts contributed by the exchanges you have selected, and check to see that the total agrees (within 10 percent) with the calorie level you set in step 1. The completed form now indicates the total exchanges of each type that you will consume on each day of your diet.
8. Distribute the exchanges you have selected into a meal pattern like that on Form 7 in Appendix H. You may want to plan four to six meals a day or to have only one snack; if so, or if you have other preferences, make your own form.
9. Finally, to see how your diet plan might work out on an actual day, make a sample menu. Look over the exchange lists, and choose foods you would like to eat that fit the pattern you worked out in step 8. For example, your meal pattern for breakfast might specify:

- 1 fruit exchange.
- 2 starch/bread exchanges.
- 1 milk exchange.
- 1 sugar exchange.
- 1 fat exchange.

So you might choose:

- ½ cup orange juice.
- ¾ ounce dry cereal and 1 slice toast.

Self-Study

- ½ cup milk on the cereal and ½ cup milk in a glass.
- 1 teaspoon sugar on the cereal.
- 1 pat margarine on the toast.

Diet for Weight Loss

1. Pick a number of calories to consume each day, based on the rate of weight loss you would like to achieve. If you wish to lose a pound a week, set it 500 calories per day below your energy need. You could set it higher or lower than this, but on no account should you set it below 1000 calories per day, even if you are 5 feet tall.
2. Decide on the proportions in which protein, fat, and carbohydrate calories will be represented in the diet. A suggested ratio is that offered in Table 8–6: about 50 percent of the calories from carbohydrate, and 25 percent each from protein and fat.
3. Translate these calorie amounts into grams, as in the previous diet plan, and enter them and your energy level into Form 6.
4. Now, using pencil on Form 6, decide on the number of carbohydrate-containing exchanges you'll have, as in step 4 of the first plan. Try to include two milk, two vegetable, and at least two fruit exchanges, and make up the rest of your carbohydrate intake with starch/bread exchanges. Allow no sugar unless you really can't do without it. At the end of this step you should have a carbohydrate gram total within about 10 percent of the number you planned in step 3.
5. Now subtotal the protein grams you have so far, and bring your total protein intake up to the level of your plan by adding meat exchanges until you have arrived at the protein intake planned in step 3.
6. Now subtotal the fat grams you have so far, and add fat exchanges to bring your total fat intake up to the level planned in step 3.
7. Fill in the calorie amounts contributed by the exchanges you have selected, and check to see that the total agrees (within 10 percent) with the calorie level you set in step 1.
8. Distribute the exchanges into a meal pattern, using Form 7 or your own form based on your own preferences.
9. Make a day's sample menus, as in step 9 of the first plan.

Notes

1. Parts of this discussion are adapted from Chapter 6, Weight control, in *Life Choices: Health Concepts and Strategies,* by F. S. Sizer and E. N. Whitney (St. Paul, Minn.: West, 1988).
2. G. Kolata, Obesity declared a disease (Research News), *Science* 227 (1985): 1019–1020.
3. M. Simonton, An overview—Advances in research and treatment of obesity, *Food and Nutrition News,* March/April 1982.
4. G. A. Leveille and P. F. Cloutier, Isocaloric diets: effects of dietary changes, *American Journal of Clinical Nutrition* 45, supplement no. 1 (January 1987): 158–163.
5. This discussion of causes of obesity is adapted from Chapter 8, Energy balance and weight control, in *Understanding Nutrition,* 4th ed., by E. N. Whitney, E. M. N. Hamilton, and M. A. Boyle (St. Paul, Minn.: West, 1987).
6. J. Slochower and S. P. Kaplan, Anxiety, perceived control, and eating in obese and normal weight persons, *Appetite* 1 (1980): 75–83.
7. A. S. Levine and J. E. Morley, The shortening pathways to appetite control, *Nutrition Today* January/February 1983, pp. 6–14.
8. B. S. Rosenthal and R. D. Marx, Determinants of initial relapse episodes among dieters, *Obesity/Bariatric Medicine* 10 (1981): 94–97.
9. Slochower and Kaplan, 1980.
10. W. H. Griffith, Food as a regulator of metabolism, *American Journal of Clinical Nutrition* 17 (1965): 391–398.
11. Optimal body weight for greater longevity, Diet therapy/obesity update, a supplement to *Nutrition and the MD,* October 1987.
12. S. M. Garn, Family-line and socioeconomic factors in fatness and obesity, *Nutrition Reviews* 44 (1986): 381–386.
13. Consensus panel addresses obesity question, *Journal of the American Medical Association* 254 (1985): 1878; A. R. Frisancho and P. N. Flegel, Relative merits of old and new indices of body mass with reference to skinfold thickness, *American Journal of Clinical Nutrition* 36 (1982): 697–699.
14. T. B. Van Itallie, When the frame is part of the picture (editorial), *American Journal of Public Health* 75 (1985): 1054–1055.
15. First National Health and Nutrition Examination Survey (HANES I), as cited by Van Itallie, 1985.
16. J. H. Himes and C. Bouchard, Do the new Metropolitan Life Insurance weight-height tables correctly assess body frame and body fat relationships? *American Journal of Public Health* 75 (1985): 1076–1079.
17. M. D. Van Loan and coauthors, Use of total-body electrical conductivity for monitoring body composition changes during weight reduction, *American Journal of Clinical Nutrition* 46 (1987): 5–8; M. D. Van Loan and coauthors, TOBEC methodology for body composition assessment; A cross-validation study, *American Journal of Clinical Nutrition* 46 (1987): 9–12.

18. Consensus panel addresses obesity question, 1985; R. P. Donahue and coauthors, Central obesity and coronary heart disease in man, *Lancet,* 11 April 1987, pp. 821–824.
19. M. Ashwell, T. J. Cole, and A. K. Dixon, Obesity: New insight into the anthropometric classification of fat distribution shown by computed tomography, *British Medical Journal* 290 (1985): 1692–1694.
20. Refractory obesity and energy homeostasis, *Nutrition Reviews,* November 1983, pp. 349–351.
21. T. B. Van Itallie and M. U. Yang, Current concepts in nutrition and diet and weight loss, *New England Journal of Medicine* 297 (1977): 1158–1161; Evaluation of 3 weight-reducing diets, *Nutrition and the MD,* March 1978. An experiment in which fasting caused increased weight loss but decreased fat loss compared with a low-calorie mixed diet was reported in M. F. Ball, J. J. Canary, and L. H. Kyle, Comparative effects of caloric restriction and total starvation on body composition in obesity, *Annals of Internal Medicine* 67 (1967): 60–67.
22. G. L. Blackburn and G. A. Bray, Introduction, in *Management of Obesity by Severe Caloric Restriction,* eds. G. L. Blackburn and G. A. Bray (Littleton, Mass.: PSG Publishing, 1985).
23. D. C. Fletcher, What is cellulite? (letter to the editor), *Journal of the American Medical Asociation* 235 (1976): 2773. The FDA concurs, in its leaflet: L. Fenner, Cellulite: Hard to budge pudge, HHS publication no. FDA 80–1078 (Washington, D.C.: Government Printing Office), reprint from *FDA Consumer,* May 1980.
24. L. Lasagna, Drugs in the treatment of obesity, in *Obesity,* ed. A. J. Stunkard (Philadelphia: W. B. Saunders, 1980), p. 296.
25. J. Lowell, "Growth hormone releasers" don't cause weight loss, *Nutrition Forum,* December 1984, p. 24.
26. Cholecystokinin (CCK): weight-loss breakthrough or hoax?, *NCAHF Newsletter,* January/February 1985, p. 1.
27. L. Sanders, But do they work?, *Health,* September 1982, pp. 29, 52, 62.
28. Diet pills and stroke, *The American Journal of Nursing* 87 (1987): 1070.
29. A. G. Dulloo and D. S. Miller, Aspirin as a promoter of ephedrine-induced thermogenesis: Potential use in the treatment of obesity, *American Journal of Clinical Nutrition* 45 (1987): 564–569; A. G. Dulloo and D. S. Miller, The thermogenic properties of ephedrine/methylxanthine mixtures: Animal studies, *American Journal of Clinical Nutrition* 43 (1986): 388–394.
30. A. E. Kark, Jaw wiring, *American Journal of Clinical Nutrition* 33, supplement no. 2 (February 1980): 420–424.
31. E. Zamula, Stomach 'bubble': Diet device not without risks, *FDA Consumer,* April 1987, pp. 28–31.
32. W. D. McArdle, F. I. Katch, and V. L. Katch, *Exercise Physiology: Energy, Nutrition, and Human Performance,* 2nd ed. (Philadelphia: Lea & Febiger, 1986), Chapter 28, pp. 527–528.
33. McArdle, Katch, and Katch, 1986.
34. C. A. Geissler and coauthors, The daily metabolic rate of the post-obese and the lean, *American Journal of Clinical Nutrition* 45 (1987): 914–920.

Fad Diets—Fact *and* Fiction?

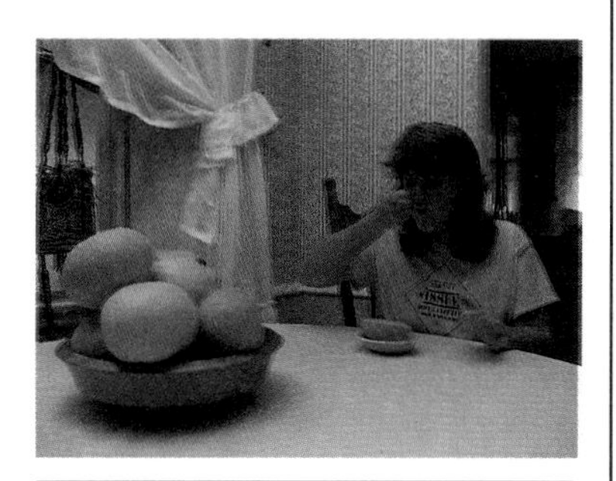

Grapefruits are a wonderful food—but so *many* grapefruits?

"I've only been on this diet a week, and I've lost 5 pounds!"

"That's terrific. What diet is it?"

"It's called the Twigfig Diet. You eat four meals a day of stems—celery, bamboo shoots, broccoli stalks—and then you can have one fig for dessert at each meal."

"That sounds terrible. You must be hungry all the time."

"Well, it's worth it to me to lose the weight."

"Surely you can find a safer way to lose weight. That diet sounds positively dangerous."

"Well, you don't see me dropping dead, do you? I have a friend who lost 30 pounds on this diet, and nothing bad happened to her."

Fad diets appeal to people, of course, because they promise quick and easy weight loss. They often do produce a brief weight loss early in the course of their use, but as the chapter explained, this loss is illusory—mostly lean tissue and water, not fat. It is quickly regained. People seldom stick to fad diets and often learn that they are not only ineffective, but dangerous. Yet fad diets never seem to fade away. As quickly as one loses popularity, another just like it pops up to take its place. Why do people keep turning to fad diets if they are known not to work, and to be hazardous?[1]

The dieter in the fictional dialogue above exemplifies the answer. Fad diets do not quite "not work." They often cause a large initial weight loss, some small fraction of which may actually be fat loss. They usually do not prove fatal, and the harm they do is usually not perceptible day by day to the dieter. Furthermore, some fad diets have things to offer dieters—such as foods or behaviors they have never tried before. They can then become experts (everyone enjoys being an expert) and turn around and instruct their friends. Before throwing out any newly popular diet merely because it is new and popular, a rational appraiser would examine it open-mindedly to see what its merits and demerits may be. A way to begin is to compare the diet to the guidelines presented in Table C8–1. If the diet fits any of these descriptions, it is probably more fiction than fact.

Demerits of Fad Diets

The first six of the seven questions that follow examine diets for their adequacy, balance, and variety. After all, inadequacy and lack of dietary balance and variety are negatives, notwithstanding our dieter's disregard of their adverse health effects. Each day on an inadequate or unbalanced diet is a day of dwindling nutrient stores; each week on a diet without variety increases the likelihood of nutrient deficiency or toxicity. The seventh question asks about the diet's long-term acceptability—for the ultimate criterion of success of a weight-loss diet is the extent to which it retrains eating habits to support maintenance of the lost weight.

Table C8–2 compares several popular diets according to these seven criteria. We started by giving each diet 100 points and subtracted wherever it fell short in these respects:

1. Does the diet provide a reasonable number of calories (not fewer than 1200 calories for an average-size person)? If not, give it a ***minus 10***.

2. Does it provide enough, but not too much, protein (at least the recommended intake or RDA, but not more than twice that much)? If no, ***minus 10***.

3. Does it provide enough fat for balance but not so much fat as to go against current recommendations (say, between 20 and 35 percent of the calories from fat)? If no, ***minus 10***.

4. Does it provide enough carbohydrate to spare protein and prevent ketosis (100 grams of carbohydrate for the average-size person)? Is it mostly complex carbohydrate (not more than 10 percent of the calories as concentrated sugar)? If no to either or both, ***minus 10***.

5. Does it offer a balanced assortment of vitamins and minerals—that is, foods from all food groups? If it omits a food group (for example, meats), does it provide a suitable substitute? Count five food groups in all: milk/milk products, meat/fish/poultry/eggs/legumes, fruits, vegetables, and starches/grains. For *each* food group omitted and not adequately substituted for, ***subtract 10 points***.

6. Does it offer variety, in the sense that different foods can be selected each day? If you'd class it as boring or monotonous, give it a ***minus 10***.

7. Does it consist of ordinary foods that are available locally (for example, in the main grocery stores) at the prices people normally pay? Or does the dieter have to buy special, expensive, or unusual foods to adhere to the diet? If you would class it as "bizarre" or "requiring unusual foods," *minus 10*.

Each of the diets shown in the table has enjoyed great popularity at one time or another.

Table C8–1

Guidelines for Evaluating Weight-Loss Promotions

1. Promise or imply dramatic, rapid weight loss (i.e., substantially more than one percent of total body weight per week).
2. Promote diets that are extremely low in calories (i.e., below 800 calories per day; 1200 calories per day diets are preferred) unless under the supervision of competent medical experts.
3. Attempt to make clients dependent upon special products rather than teaching how to make good choices from the conventional food supply (this does not condemn the marketing of low-calorie convenience foods which may be chosen by consumers).
4. Do not encourage permanent, realistic lifestyle changes including regular exercise and the behavioral aspects of eating wherein food may be used as a coping device (i.e., programs should focus upon changing the causes of overweight rather than simply the effects, which is the overweight itself).
5. Misrepresent salespeople as "counselors" supposedly qualified to give guidance in nutrition and/or general health. Even if adequately trained, such "counselors" would still be objectionable because of the obvious conflict of interest that exists when providers profit directly from products they recommend and sell.
6. Require large sums of money at the start or require that clients sign contracts for expensive, long-term programs. Such practices too often have been abused as salespeople focus attention upon signing up new people rather than delivering continuing, satisfactory service to consumers. Programs should be on a pay-as-you-go basis.
7. Fail to inform clients about the risks associated with weight loss in general, or the specific program being promoted.
8. Promote unproven or spurious weight-loss aids such as human chorionic gonadotrophin hormone (HCG), starch blockers, diuretics, sauna belts, body wraps, passive exercise, ear stapling, acupuncture, Electric Muscle Stimulating (EMS) devices, spirulina, amino acid supplements (e.g., arginine, ornithine), glucomannan, and so forth.
9. Claim that "cellulite" exists in the body.
10. Claim that use of an appetite suppressant or methylcellulose (a "bulking agent") enables a person to lose body fat without restricting accustomed caloric intake.
11. Claim that a weight-control product contains a unique ingredient or component unless it is unavailable in other weight-control products.

Source: Reprinted with permission from *National Council Against Health Fraud Newsletter,* March/April 1987.

As you can see, no diet scores a perfect 100 points, but most receive some points. They have some disadvantages, but they may also offer offsetting advantages.

What might the advantages be? The sections that follow present some scientific bases for giving credit (where credit is due) to a few kernels of truth amidst the chaff of the fad diets. Anyone wishing to construct a diet for personal use might wish to make use of the strategies they imply.

Merits of Fad Diets

The merits of fad diets discussed here are really applications of the rules of behavior modification introduced in Chapter 8 (see Figure 8–5, p. 304). They are summarized in Table C8–3, at the end of this Controversy. Each one implies a strategy that dieters can use, even if they do not use the diet. Occasionally, the strategies appear to contradict each other: for example, one is to employ monotony to reduce food consumption, while another suggests variety to prevent boredom. Both may be valid for different people at different times; people can choose among the techniques presented to find the ones best suited to their preferences and lifestyles. With that in mind, the first strategy might be "know yourself"—that is, get in touch with your own needs, because a weight-control plan that doesn't suit you will not work for you.

Diets centered on one basic food are among the most popular and long-lived of fads. The grapefruit diet is probably the most familiar among them; others use eggs, spinach, rice, and even ice cream. Many people associate grapefruit with weight loss, because grapefruit has been touted as a fat-burning agent that cancels the calories of other foods eaten with it. Promotors of grapefruit diet books claim that people can eat as they like without restriction, as long as this "magic" agent precedes every meal or snack throughout the day. Of course, these claims are false, but people do lose weight when they follow the instructions, because, as scientific studies show, monotony in the diet reduces food intake.

An experiment illustrates this principle: rats fed meals that included a variety of tasty foods ate more than if they were fed meals consisting of only one food, even when the food was a favorite.[2] Just being bored prompts some people to eat, and for them, the more interesting the foods, the more likely that they will eat beyond the amount that hunger alone would dictate. Conversely, when foods are boring, people eat less than hunger dictates. People who tend to overeat in the presence of a variety of foods can apply this principle to help with weight loss. In doing so, they are applying behavior modification rule 2 (p. 304), Eliminate or suppress cues to inappropriate eating. A word of caution, though—excessive monotony can impair nutrition status. Variety, after all, is a key to diet adequacy, so use monotony in moderation—if you'll pardon the expression.

Studies of rats have shown that the association of any unpleasant task with eating can help to produce an aversion to food.[3] Fads that apply this principle include the all-liquid diets and diets that substitute a liquid or solid meal replacement for one or more daily meals. These products may be available over the counter, from any of several diet organizations, or from door-to-door salespeople, but all the regimens are so monotonous that they may condition people who use them to dislike even the thought of eating except, minimally, to relieve hunger.

Many fad diets employ behavior modification rule 3 (p. 304)—Strengthen cues to appropriate behaviors—in the form of ritual. Rituals at mealtimes set the stage for the eating of planned meals and simultaneously help eliminate overeating.[4] They take many forms, but all of them serve as delaying tactics that give dieters the chance to think before they eat. Repetitive food preparation before a meal is a ritual. A grapefruit diet, for example, may require that at every meal the person take the time to pare a grapefruit, cut it up, dig out the seeds, throw away scraps, and then eat it before eating anything else. Other fad diets use rituals such as drinking water or eating bran before meals, eating only under certain social conditions, weighing food portions before eating, and keeping records, all of which delay the act of eating and help condition dieters to eat less.[5]

Fad diets also sometimes employ rule 4—Alter the eating behavior itself. An example is the use of fiber and water as fillers. Someone who fills up on high-fiber foods or low-calorie liquids will have less appetite for other foods. Some fad diets recommend fillers at the beginning of each meal, a technique known as preloading; others include liquid or solid fillers interspersed throughout the daily meal plan.

Most low-carbohydrate diets (see Chapter 8) call for a minimum of eight glasses of water a day and emphasize drinking some of it before meals. One good reason to drink a lot of water on these diets is that they cause ketosis; the water helps the body to excrete ketone bodies and waste products from protein breakdown. (This problem is seldom mentioned in the fad diet books, except when it is used to claim that these waste products carry off a lot of calories—and they do not. At most, ketone bodies excreted in a day add up to fewer than 100 calories.) Another reason for drinking fluid is that it gives a temporary feeling of fullness, helping to compensate for a diet plan that provides little food. Diets that recommend consuming soup before meals use this same principle; they have been found to reduce caloric intake and promote greater weight loss than diets that include no soup.[6] The other variation on preloading—filling up on low-calorie, bulky foods—works, too, because filling foods like grapefruit or rice at the beginning of the meal take up considerable room in the stomach; they also require more chewing than do refined foods, and so tire the jaw muscles. Diets that use this variation of preloading remain a popular choice, because dieters who use them can feel full for so few calories. Too much of low-calorie, high-bulk fillers, such as on the Twigfig diet, can cause diarrhea, nutrient losses, electrolyte imbalances, and irregularities of heart rhythms. Still, the filler strategies can be useful as part of sound weight-loss plans.

Another way of altering eating behavior, already mentioned in Chapter 8, is to slow the rate of eating. Some fad diets, whether intentionally or fortuitously, have this effect, for high-fiber fillers take time to eat. Soup, taken hot, slows eating, too. Eating slowly enables the first food eaten to reach the small intestine and signal satiety before an excess of calories is consumed. One study of rats showed that stimulation of a portion of the small intestine inhibits feeding behavior, particularly in rats that are obese.[7] When so stimulated, the intestine releases into the bloodstream chemicals called neuropeptides that

Table C8–2

Weight-Loss Diets Compared

Diet Description (for question, see text)	Question 1: Calories	Question 2: Protein
A low-carbohydrate/high-protein diet that allows unlimited protein and fat, but severely limits carbohydrate. In addition to the hazards of a low-carbohydrate diet, explained in Chapter 8, the diet is high in total fat, saturated fat, and cholesterol. The omission of breads and cereals and the large reduction of fruits, vegetables, and milk characterize the diet.	Yes	No, excessive protein MINUS 10
A diet of six bananas and three glasses of nonfat milk daily, plus vitamin and mineral supplements.	No, provides less than 1000 cal MINUS 10	No, low protein MINUS 10
A diet that allows, for the first ten days, no food other than specific fruits. Timing and combining of foods are claimed to cause weight loss, with no scientific basis for the claims. Sometimes causes diarrhea and excess gas in the digestive tract because of the laxative nature of fruit. Physicians warn that shock, low blood pressure, and perhaps death may result.	No, low calories MINUS 10	No, low protein MINUS 10
The plan is a two-weeks-on, two-weeks-off low-carbohydrate, ample-protein diet of about 1100 cal/day, touted as a no-hunger, no-pills way to lose 20 lb in two weeks. It includes plenty of meat, vegetables, fruits, and some starches, but no milk.	Yes	No, provides approximately 216% of the protein needs MINUS 10
A powdered formula sold directly to the public for use three times daily. One day's worth of the formula provides 33 g protein, 40 g carbohydrate, and 3 g fat, fortified with vitamins and minerals.	No MINUS 10	No, low protein MINUS 10
A fast in which only water is allowed.	No MINUS 10	No MINUS 10
A diet that requires the addition of 2 tsp of bran to be taken with water at each mealtime. The foods provided by the menus are low-fat, low-calorie items, with few milk products.	Yes	Yes
A strict diet built around the Four Food Group Plan, which alternates periods of 700 cal/day and 1500 cal/day.	The average intake is 1100 cal/day, but periods of severe restriction are included MINUS 5	Yes

Question 3: Fat	Question 4: Carbohydrate	Question 5: Food Groups	Question 6: Variety	Question 7: Ordinary Foods	Total Score
No, excessive fat MINUS 10	No, inadequate carbohydrate MINUS 10	No, three food groups omitted MINUS 30	No, monotonous MINUS 10	Yes	30 points
No, low fat MINUS 10	Yes	No, three food groups omitted MINUS 30	No, monotonous MINUS 10	Yes	30 points
No, low fat MINUS 10	No, no starch MINUS 10	No, four food groups omitted MINUS 40	No, monotonous; omits most food groups other than fruits MINUS 10	No, requires tropical fruits in large quantities and later suggests lobster and steak MINUS 10	0 points
No, meat has a high fat percentage MINUS 10	No, carbohydrate level is 30% of need MINUS 5	No, milk group omitted MINUS 10	Yes	Yes	65 points
No, low fat MINUS 10	No, low carbohydrate MINUS 10	No food allowed on a regular basis MINUS 50	No, monotonous MINUS 10	No ordinary food; expensive formula required MINUS 10	0 points
No MINUS 10	No MINUS 10	No MINUS 50	No MINUS 10	No MINUS 10	0 points
Yes	Yes	Half the milk allowance MINUS 5	Yes	Requires bran MINUS 5	90 points
Yes	Yes	Yes	Yes	Yes	95 points

(continued on following page)

Table C8–2

(continued)

Diet Description (for question, see text)	Question 1: Calories	Question 2: Protein
A diet that involves eating only rice and fruit. Vitamin and mineral supplements are recommended.	Yes	No, low protein MINUS 10
A very-low-carbohydrate, high-fat, high-meat, very-low-calorie diet with no milk. One-half grapefruit is required before each meal.	No MINUS 10	No, too high MINUS 10
A diet that severely restricts fat, limits protein to below the recommended levels, and limits dairy products severely. Several levels of calories are available from 700 to 1200 per day.	Choosing any plan except 1200 cal will not provide the recommended level MINUS 5	No, too low MINUS 10
A diet that uses the exchange system to ensure adequate nutrient intake, while emphasizing complex carbohydrate foods.	Yes	Yes
A diet that alternates 600, 900, and 1200 cal/day intakes (higher for men) in the first three weeks, then allows moderate intakes for a week, and starts over. It also includes unlimited quantities of selected fruits and vegetables.	Two weeks of severe calorie restriction is ill advised MINUS 5	Not likely to have sufficient protein, especially in view of carbohydrate restriction MINUS 5
A high-carbohydrate, low-protein diet that allows no meats or milk products.		No, too low MINUS 10
A diet of powdered herbs or other powders to replace food for one meal a day.	Likely to be inadequate MINUS 10	Depends on how much consumed from food in other meals

Question 3: Fat	Question 4: Carbohydrate	Question 5: Food Groups	Question 6: Variety	Question 7: Ordinary Foods	Total Score
No, low fat MINUS 10	Yes	No meat, milk, or vegetables allowed MINUS 30	No, monotonous MINUS 10	Yes	40 points
Yes, but so low in calories that total fat is low MINUS 10	No, too low MINUS 10	No milk or grains allowed MINUS 20	No, monotonous MINUS 10	Yes	30 points
No, too low MINUS 10	Yes	No, meat and milk groups restricted MINUS 5 MINUS 5	YES	No, dieters are urged to use special products MINUS 10	55 points
Yes	Yes	Yes	Yes	Yes	100 points
No, too little fat, half the time MINUS 5	No, too little carbohydrate, half the time MINUS 5	No, insufficient milk likely, half the time MINUS 5	Yes	Yes	75 points
No MINUS 10	Yes	No, meat and milk omitted MINUS 20	No, monotonous MINUS 10	Yes	50 points
Likely to be inadequate MINUS 10	Likely to be inadequate MINUS 10	One or more likely to be omitted MINUS 10	No, monotonous MINUS 10	No, dangerous; herbs can be toxic and cause adverse reactions MINUS 10	40 points or less; if meals are omitted and only the powder is taken, score the diet 0 points.

act as signals to the brain's hypothalamus that food has arrived. The hypothalamus responds by shutting down hunger. Another study found that people who were fed meals emphasizing bulky, unrefined foods reached satiety on about half the calories of a high-fat, high-sugar meal that included meat and dessert.[8]

High-carbohydrate and high-fiber diets can also automatically restrict people's fat intakes, a significant factor in weight control. As mentioned earlier, it is believed that carbohydrate and protein calories cause less of a weight gain than the same number of fat calories.[9] Conversely, a high-fat diet may also raise the set-point weight, at least in rats.[10] As a result, some researchers are predicting that the high-carbohydrate diet will replace the high-protein and high-fat fad diets that have been popular in the past.[11] People with diabetes or hypertension should approach these diets with caution; some research indicates that diets comprised of carbohydrates which elicit a strong glycemic response could alter blood lipoproteins adversely.[12]

Fad diets also offer many kinds of rewards (behavior modification rule 6—Provide positive consequences for desired behaviors). One is to allow sugar, in strictly defined forms and quantities, as part of meals. Some research vindicates the limited use of sugar in weight-loss diets. One study contradicts a common belief that foods high in sugar are overconsumed more readily than other foods. When rats' diets included foods that contained sucrose, dextrose, and fructose, they developed either modest or no obesity. In fact, the rats ate *less* of the high-sugar foods than the other foods they were offered, and researchers concluded that sugar's satiating effect outweighed the foods' increased palatability.[13]

That many fad diet products contain sugar may help explain their persistent popularity. Research suggests that sugar satisfies a craving for carbohydrate-rich foods that relates to the brain's neurotransmitters. One study showed that in fasting, neurotransmitters in the brain become unbalanced, and that when fasting people were fed a sugar meal, the imbalance in neurotransmitters righted itself.[14] Artificial sweeteners, on the other hand, probably would fail to correct the imbalance of neurotransmitters, because they are not carbohydrate sources. Over-the-counter liquid formula diets, both premixed and powdered, usually deliver most of their carbohydrate in the form of simple sugars; this may help explain why they have remained among the most popular of fads. Commercially available meal replacement such as "meal-in-a-bar" products and specially formulated cookies and wafers also contain a high percentage of sugar. So-called reducing candies, recommended by the maker to be eaten before meals, are little different from the regular confections they resemble. Not all such goodies are equally valuable (some are too palatable and too high in calories per bite), but including a little sugar in the diet for its satiety value can be a boon for some dieters. For people who choose sugary foods that are also high in fat, though, it is a bane.

The same principle applies to the use of fat. Rather than attempting to reduce fat in the diet to an absolute minimum, it may be wise to include small amounts of flavorful fats such as olive or sesame oil and avoid bland fats such as margarine or other vegetable oils. Studies show that people consume fewer calories from fat when they do so.[15] Again, this should only be used if it works.

Another way of obtaining a reward is to enlist the support of others. Some groups that promote "rotation"-type diets go so far as to sponsor local meetings for people who use the diets. Other promoters of fads require dieters to join a club, pay a membership fee that entitles them to purchase liquid formulas or special "diet" foods, and attend meetings. In both cases, success may come from the provision of some form of group support, a factor shown to promote greater weight loss for some people than individual effort alone.[16] Even programs that require no formal club meetings can create the illusion of a support network. They often use persuasive promotional techniques to gain media attention, so that it seems as if everyone is following the diet. This bandwagon effect gives people the feeling of being part of a group, even though they may never meet formally with others who are on the diet. Of course, many legitimate, reasonable weight-loss plans make use of this effect, too.

A different twist to the group support principle is used by the "socializing" diets. These plans capitalize on the claim that people who use their plans can drink alcoholic beverages, attend parties, and dine in restaurants, so long as they are together when they do so. Whatever success these diets have had may result partly from overeaters' feeling inhibited by the presence of other people. One study has shown that when dieters eat in the presence of observers, they conform to external norms for acceptable eating behavior rather than to their own internal demands to overeat.[17] These diets may also succeed because they permit people the pleasure and moral support of socializing with others. Learning to control food and alcohol consumption on special occasions is an important part of long-term weight control. Fad diets are not the only ones that can include social events and restaurant dinners; sound weight-loss plans can, too, and they serve the same purposes—to control, and to reward.

One feature some fad diets offer is not a behavior modification strategy, but a strategy that affects physiology. A key factor in weight loss is the individual's basal metabolic rate (BMR)—that is, the amount of energy required to maintain the basic life processes. One group of fad diets has gained popularity by claiming to raise the BMR. The so-called metabolic diets say they raise the BMR "naturally" while restricting calories, by providing small meals at frequent intervals throughout the day. Whatever success these plans have had can be explained in part by studies showing that eating frequent meals of small servings of food may raise the BMR more than eating three large meals does.[18]

Rotation diets claim to sustain a rapid metabolism by varying the calorie level from week to week, because reducing calories severely for extended periods reduces BMR—a disadvantage to the dieter. Some rotation-type diets alternate periods of very-low-calorie dieting with periods of "maintenance" or even unrestrained eating, claiming that the body will maintain a normal BMR because it has too little time to adapt to the energy deprivation as an ongoing state. The success of such diets can probably be attributed partly to the preloading principle—most plans include high-carbohydrate, low-fat foods that provide a lot of bulk for few calories. They may also relieve the boredom that would attend an unchanging diet, thus enhancing dieters' willingness to adhere to them for longer times.

The most healthful way to sustain a normal BMR is to eat a normal number of calories and to exercise regularly. Yet the fad dieter objects to eating too many calories, fearing that weight loss will be too slow. The solution is twofold: keep the calories coming to keep the BMR high and to deliver nutrients, and raise the BMR further through exercise.[19] Most fad diets mention exercise only as a token gesture to its importance and do not include physical activity formally in their plans, but the educated fitness-conscious person knows that both regular, aerobic exercise, and habitual "fidgeting" burn calories and support a raised BMR.[20] (See Controversy 10 for a note on the use of hot spices, too.)

In short, although not recommended without reservation, fad diets do have merits; they are not all bad. Table C8–3 summarizes the information presented here by providing a checklist of some long-lasting fad diets and the principles they use. Table C8–4 summarizes their merits, in hopes that the dieter will easily see that useful strategies can be extracted from their original packages and combined into a sound weight-control program that is likely to work over the long term. To put the fad diets in perspective, the last section criticizes weaknesses they all seem to share, and offers suggestions for improvement.

Fad Diets in Perspective

Almost all fad diets share one gimmick: they require strict adherence to a preset plan, claiming that deviance from the recommended combination of foods negates the diet's fat-burning properties. These diets may seem to succeed by sleight-of-hand, but the technique they use is straightforward: shortcutting. Instead of learning to select foods and plan meals wisely, a step necessary to long-term weight control, shortcutting techniques bypass it.

Many people who use fad diets would make unwise food choices if left to their own devices, whether from lack of knowledge or lack of motivation. Monotonous diets and diets that use commercial meal replacements or prepared meals can produce weight loss because they automatically limit food selections and hence the dieter's responsibility to choose wisely. In every case, these diets circumvent central issues in permanent weight loss: learning and behavior change. That most fad diets bypass this step through shortcuts only emphasizes its importance.

All fad diets owe some of their popularity to the various types of rewards they provide. Unfortunately, most offer only fleeting rewards; some even use food as reinforcement. High-protein diets and all diets that severely restrict calories produce a large initial weight loss and an immediate psychological boost. The loss is largely illusion, though, since more water is lost than fat. When the rate of weight loss slows, people become disillusioned and frequently abandon their diets.[21] Another immediate reward is the sensation of pleasure from consuming the sugar that so many fad diet products contain. In fact, sugar is such a powerful reward that it has been called a "supernormal reinforcer" of behavior.[22] "Controlled cheating" diets and rotation-type diets that alternate periods of restricted food intake with periods of unrestrained eating reward people with the very thing the diets are urging them to control. This condoned overindulgence also gives people the feeling of "getting away with something." When this feeling accompanies an act as pleasurable as eating, it

Table C8–3

Some Long-Lasting Fad Diets and Scientific Principles They Use

Fad Diet Types	Monotony	Aversive Conditioning	Ritual	Fillers	Slowed Eating Time	Fat Restriction
All-fruit crash diets	√	√	√	√	√	√
All-vegetable crash diets	√	√	√	√	√	√
Banana diets	√	√	√			√
Bran meal diets		√	√	√		
"Controlled cheating" diets						
Egg diets	√	√	√			
Fasts[c]	√	√		√		
Fiber supplement diets[d]		√	√	√		
Grapefruit diets	√	√	√	√	√	
High-carbohydrate diets				√	√	√
High-fiber diets				√	√	√
High-protein diets	√	√	√			
Ice cream diets	√	√	√			
Juice fasts	√	√	√	√		√
Liquid formula diets[e]	√	√	√			
Liquid protein diets	√	√	√	√		
"Macrobiotic" diets	√	√	√	√	√	√
"Metabolic" diets						
"Reducing candy" diets			√	√		
Rice diets	√	√	√	√	√	√
"Rotation"-type diets						
"Socializing" diets						
Solid meal replacement diets[f]	√	√	√			
Soup-including diets			√	√		
Spinach diets	√	√	√			
"State-of-mind" diets						
Water-drinking diets		√	√	√		

[a]This table denotes only those diets that include support as a formal element. However, as mentioned in the text, most fad diets create the illusion of group support through a "media blitz" of promotional techniques that sell a sense of group identity along with the diet.

[b]In most cases, the reward is the large initial weight loss that provides an immediate psychological boost to the dieter.

[c]This class of diets denotes fasts that permit only water.

Sugar	Meal Frequency	Alternation of Calorie Levels	Support[a]	Shortcuts	Reward[b]	Control of Attitude and Emotions
√				√	√	
				√	√	
√				√	√	
				√		
√		√		√	√	
				√	√	
				√	√	
				√		
√				√	√	
√				√		
				√		
	√			√	√	
√				√	√	
√				√	√	
√				√	√	
				√	√	
		√		√	√	
	√	√		√	√	
√				√	√	
				√	√	
		√	√	√	√	
			√	√	√	
√			√	√		
				√	√	
				√	√	
			√		√	√
				√	√	

[d]These diets require that an over-the-counter product such as fiber pills, wafers, or cookies be taken with water before meals.
[e]These include liquids and powders sold over-the-counter or by diet clubs, clinics, or distributors.
[f]These include bars or cookies sold over-the-counter or by grocery stores or distributors.
Note: The purpose of this table is to isolate some sound scientific principles within fad diets, not to encourage their use.
Source: D. K. Cowley and F. S. Sizer, *Fad Diets—Facts and Fictions* (a 1987 monograph available from Stickley Publishing Co., 210 W. Washington Sq., Philadelphia, PA 19106).

Table C8–4

Weight-Loss Strategies that Work

The following strategies promote weight loss, and they are based on sound principles that work. Some strategies on the list contradict each other (for example, compare the "Monotony" strategy with the last "Reward" strategy). Use these suggestions selectively—choose the strategies that best suit your personal preferences and life-style. Especially, select strategies that address any special concerns you might have.

Monotony:
- Limit the selection of foods to reduce temptation—choose several nutritious "key" foods, and use them often. (Do use foods from all food groups, though. Monotony becomes dangerous when it makes the diet unbalanced.)

Aversive Conditioning:
- Link an unpleasant task with eating—pay bills or do household chores before eating (this is particularly helpful if it is done before eating "problem" foods—for example, high-calorie foods or foods consistently overeaten).
- Eat least-liked foods in a meal first.

Ritual:
- Delay eating by performing some kind of ritual first (set the table with china, cloth napkins, and candles).
- Peel and chop fresh vegetables before each meal (prepare an appetizer of raw foods).
- Eat only in one place, and concentrate only on eating—exclude activities such as reading or watching television.
- Update food records meticulously before meals.

Fillers:
- Drink water or low-calorie liquids throughout the day, especially before meals.
- Consume a low-calorie soup, such as bouillon or vegetable soup, before meals.
- Eat a filling, low-calorie appetizer before meals—grapefruit, celery, or carrots with low-calorie sauce, a large salad with lemon dressing, or any similar combination (this is especially helpful before restaurant or dinner-party meals whose content cannot be controlled).

(When using any of the "filler" strategies, be sure to consume other foods, too—filling foods and liquids can somctimcs displace from the diet foods that offer other necessary nutrients.)

Slowed Eating Time:
- Choose bulky, high-fiber foods that require a lot of chewing: raw vegetables, certain fruits, whole-grain products, air-popped popcorn.
- Drink water between bites of food.
- Place eating utensils on the table after each bite; converse between bites.
- Serve food while still hot.

Fat Restriction:
- Plan meals around raw vegetables, fruits, whole-grain products, and any unrefined foods that are high in carbohydrates.
- Satisfy the taste buds by using small amounts of flavorful fats such as peanut, olive, or sesame oil rather than bland fats such as margarine or cooking oil. Studies show that people consume fewer calories from fat when they do so.
- Learn low-fat ways to prepare favorite foods.
- Substitute nonfat milk for whole milk; low-fat yogurt for sour cream; imitation butter flavoring or commercial butter replacement granules for butter; broth or cooking spray for frying fat.

Sugar:
- Include a moderate amount of sugar in the diet for its satiety value, but make sure it is not accompanied by a lot of fat.
- Eat fruits—they contain simple sugars as well as valuable nutrients.
- Emphasize carbohydrate-rich foods in meal plans; the starch in them may satisfy just as sugar does.

Metabolism:
- Exercise regularly. Aerobic exercise in particular helps raise the metabolic rate.
- Divide the daily food allowance into many small meals to be eaten at frequent intervals throughout the day.
- Emphasize unrefined foods that are low in fat and calories so more food can be eaten.
- Move around; move the arms and legs while sitting. Studies show that people who engage in spontaneous physical activity such as fidgeting burn more calories than those who do not.

Support:
- Join a weight-loss group, or start one.
- Enlist the help of friends, co-workers, or family members.
- Enjoy parties and other social events while limiting food and alcohol intake. (Choose appetizers and hors d'oeuvres such as raw vegetables and fruits; strictly limit alcohol consumption to one drink, choosing low-calorie mixes like club soda or tonic.)

Shortcuts:
- Learn legitimate shortcuts such as using an exchange system for balanced meal planning.
- Learn the calorie and nutrient values of foods.
- Learn to read and use the information on food labels.
- Learn to identify high-fat, high-sodium, and high-sugar foods; they frequently offer few nutrients for many calories.

Reward:
- Keep a weekly graph of weight loss.
- Plan for occasional sweet treats.
- List the positive changes that accompany weight loss: greater ease of breathing and ease of movement, better-fitting clothes, enhanced appearance, and the like.
- Plan frequent nonfood rewards such as material items or favorite activities.
- Vary menu plans from time to time to prevent boredom.

Control of Attitude and Emotions:
- Work toward developing a positive self-image—learn and use techniques such as positive imaging or positive self-talk.
- Learn and use a stress-reduction technique—exercise, progressive muscle relaxation (PMR), yoga, self-hypnosis, meditation, prayer—that promotes a sense of personal control over problems.
- Learn to distinguish between hunger and emotions and to respond appropriately to each.
- Learn constructive ways of ventilating emotions, particularly negative ones.
- Seek the help of a qualified counselor.

Source: D. K. Cowley and F. S. Sizer, *Fad Diets—Facts and Fictions* (a 1987 monograph available from Stickley Publishing Co., 210 W. Washington Sq., Philadelphia, PA 19106).

is indeed a powerful reinforcer.[23] Rewards are absolutely essential to sustain the motivation to lose weight, but unless they are chosen with care, they can undermine long-term weight control.

The factor most crucial to the success of any serious weight-loss effort, although less tangible and less easily manipulated than food choices, is attitude. The way dieters deal with their emotions helps determine not only whether they will lose weight, but whether they will maintain the loss. Hence one of the most important steps people can take is to learn to recognize and deal constructively with emotions and develop a positive attitude. A popular trend is the "state-of-mind" diets that recommend positive thinking, stress-reduction techniques, yoga, religion, philosophy, or other approaches that provide a sense of personal control.

When coupled with a sound weight-loss diet, this is ideal.

Fad diets of all kinds seem to hold special appeal for people who have tried diet after diet to no avail. The diets sell hope for weight loss, and hope is essential to the success of human efforts. Hopeful people feel less helpless and less anxious. Belief is equally essential to success, and fad promoters play upon people's desire to believe that their weight problem can be miraculously solved without effort. One basic principle of nearly all fad diets, and especially of those based on "new scientific findings," is the placebo effect—the ability of a person's belief in a method, even an outlandish one, to bolster motivation and promote weight loss where all else has failed. The placebo effect works by giving hope, reducing anxiety, and helping people feel in control.[24] Few people have the ability to evaluate scientific-sounding schemes—many simply choose to believe in them until they fail.

Fad diets fail for many reasons. First, they fail to reeducate: they respond to long-term problems with short-term solutions whose dazzle wears thin as the diet wears on. Their regimens are usually too inflexible to fit most people's lifestyles, and their gimmicks do little to prepare people for long-term weight maintenance. For the most part, they ignore internal factors such as emotional states that can provoke the desire to overeat, and they overlook most of the coping skills needed to deal with external life circumstances that can trigger overeating. Although the fad diets themselves fail, seeds of truth they contain can help the smart dieter to succeed.

Notes

1. This Controversy was adapted with permission from D. K. Cowley and F. S. Sizer, *Fad Diets—Facts and Fictions* (a monograph available, 1987, from Stickley Publishing Co., 210 Washington Sq., Philadelphia, PA 19106).
2. B. J. Rolls, Experimental analyses of the effects of variety in a meal on human feeding, *American Journal of Clinical Nutrition* 42 (1985): 932–939.
3. I. L. Bernstein, M. W. Vitiello, and R. A. Sigmundi, Effects of interference stimuli on the acquisiton of learned aversions to food in the rat, *Journal of Comparative and Physiological Psychology* 94 (1980): 921–931.
4. S. B. Penick and coauthors, Behavior modification in the treatment of obesity, *Psychosomatic Medicine* 33 (1971): 49–55.
5. J. Dwyer, Sixteen popular diets: Brief nutritional analyses, in *Obesity,* ed. A. J. Stunkard (Philadelphia: Saunders, 1980), p. 287.
6. H. A. Jordan and coauthors, Role of food characteristics in behavioral change and weight loss, *Journal of the American Dietetic Association* 79 (1981): 24–29.
7. H. S. Koopmans and coauthors, The effects of ileal transposition on food intake and body weight loss in VMH-obese rats, *American Journal of Clinical Nutrition* 35 (1982): 284–293.
8. K. H. Duncan and coauthors, The effects of high and low density diets on satiety, energy intake, and eating time of obese and nonobese subjects, *American Journal of Clinical Nutrition* 37 (1983): 763–767.
9. L. B. Oscai, M. M. Brown, and W. C. Miller, Effect of dietary fat on food intake, growth, and body composition in rats, *Growth* 48 (1984): 415–424.
10. S. W. Corbett, J. S. Stern, and R. E. Keesey, Energy expenditure in rats with diet-induced obesity, *The American Journal of Clinical Nutrition* 44 (1986): 173–180.
11. Corbett, Stern, and Keesey, 1986.
12. C. I. Waslien, The dangers of a high-carbohydrate diet, *Cereal Foods World* 32 (1987): 505.
13. A Sclafani, Dietary obesity, in *Obesity,* ed. A. J. Stunkard (Philadelphia: Saunders, 1980), pp. 166–181.
14. D. V. M. Ashley and coauthors, Evidence for diminished brain 5-hydroxytryptamine biosynthesis in obese diabetic and nondiabetic humans, *The American Journal of Clinical Nutrition* 42 (1985): 1240–1245.
15. S. S. Schiffman, Recent findings about taste: Important implications for dieters, *Cereal Foods World* 31 (1986): 300–302.
16. S. O. Adams and coauthors, Weight loss: A comparison of group and individual interventions, *Journal of the American Dietetic Association* 86 (1986): 485–490.
17. C. P. Herman and J. Polivy, Restrained eating, in *Obesity,* ed. A. J. Stunkard (Philadelphia: Saunders, 1980), p. 220.
18. P. Fabry, Metabolic consequences of the pattern of food intake, in *Handbook of Physiology: Alimentary Canal I,* ed. C. F. Code (Washington, D.C.: American Physiological Society, 1967), pp. 31–49.
19. P. D. Wood, The science of successful weight loss, in *Medical and Health Annual* (Chicago: Encyclopedia Britannica, 1984), pp. 126–141.
20. F. S. Sizer and E. N. Whitney, Chapter 6, Weight control, and Chapter 7, Fitness, in *Life Choices: Health Concepts and Strategies* (St. Paul, Minn.: West, 1988); E. Ravussin and coauthors, Determinants of 24-hour energy expenditure in man: Methods and results using a respiratory chamber, *Journal of Clinical Investigation* 78 (1986): 1568–1578.
21. R. B. Stuart, J. A. Jensen, and K. Guire, Weight loss over time, *Journal of the American Dietetic Association* 75 (1979): 258–261.
22. E. N. Whitney, E. M. N. Hamilton, and M. A. Boyle, Sugar—Why so powerful? in *Understanding Nutrition,* 4th ed. (St. Paul, Minn.: West, 1987) pp. 83–87.
23. J. D. Nash and L. O. Long, *Taking Charge of Your Weight and Well-being* (Palo Alto, Calif.: Bull Publishing, 1978), p. 46.
24. O. Fennema, The placebo effect of foods, *Food Technology,* December 1984, pp. 37–67.

Chapter Nine

Contents

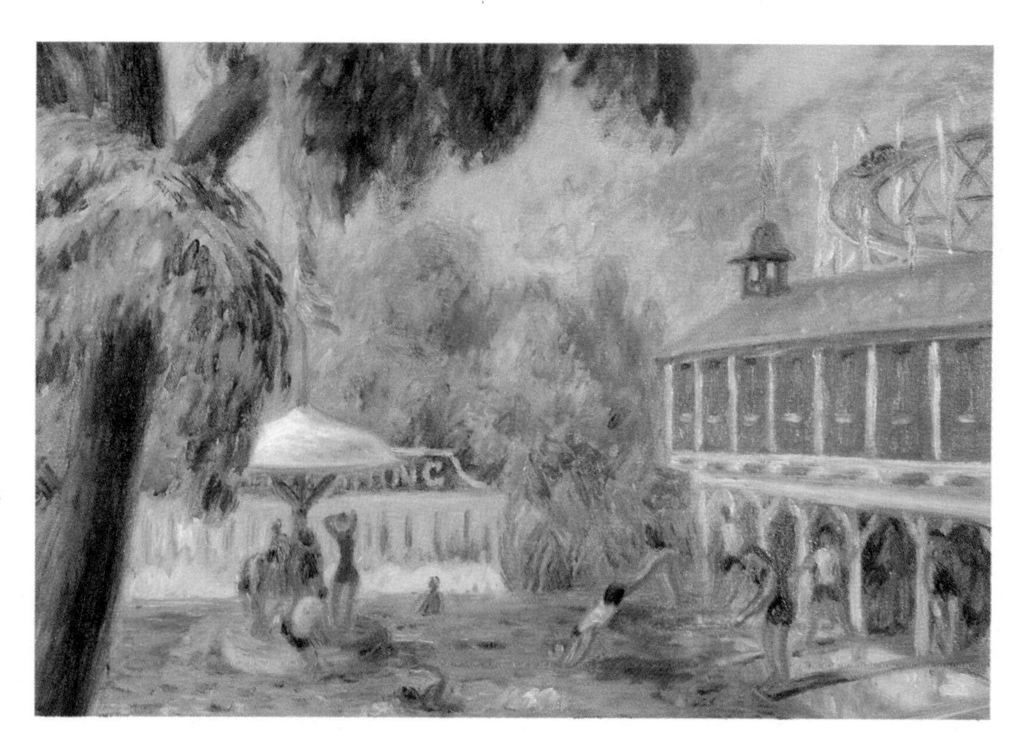

Palisades Amusement Park, 1934, by William Glackens. Virginia Museum of Art, Charlottesville, Virginia.

Fitness, Nutrition, and Exercise

Health seekers know that **fitness** is as important as nutrition or sleep.[1] Fitness also enhances appearance, but this is not to say that to be fit you have to develop a Ms. Olympia or Mr. Universe body. Rather, you need to achieve a reasonable weight and enough of the four components of physical fitness—**flexibility, strength, muscle endurance,** and **cardiovascular endurance**—to support optimal health. Athletes need not only these components, but also skill, balance, speed, and coordination—the fruits of practice and talent. Nutrition alone cannot endow you with fitness or athletic ability, but it can augment the effort you put forth to obtain them. Conversely, unwise food selections can stand in your way.

fitness: the body's ability to meet physical demands, composed of four components: flexibility, strength, muscle endurance, and cardiovascular endurance.

flexibility: the ability to bend without injury; it depends on the elasticity of muscles, tendons, and ligaments and on the condition of the joints.

strength: the ability of muscles to work against resistance.

endurance: the ability to sustain an effort for a long time.

muscle endurance: the ability of a muscle to contract repeatedly within a given time without becoming exhausted.

cardiovascular endurance: the ability of the cardiovascular system to sustain delivery of oxygen to the working muscles over a period of time.

exercise: physical effort of the body, which tends to maintain or improve fitness.

Why Exercise?

Heredity gave the Stone-Age people bodies that needed **exercise.** Yours does, too. The human body is designed to fight enemies; push, pull, and carry heavy objects; and run long distances. Modern people still need to develop the same bodily equipment, but modern life offers so many labor-saving conveniences that it usually doesn't involve as much physical exertion as we need to remain healthy. We therefore have to use our brains—the same ones that designed modern conveniences for us—to plan exercise into our days.

The benefits of regular exercise make up an impressive list, which is growing longer as new discoveries are made. People who exercise regularly can receive such benefits as:

- More enjoyable, perhaps even longer, life.[2]
- Improved mental outlook.[3]
- Improved mental capacity.
- Feeling of vigor.
- Feeling of belonging—the fun and companionship of sports.
- Improved self-image and self-confidence.
- Reduced incidence and severity of personality disorders.[4]
- Reduced fatness and increased lean body tissue.[5]
- Greater bone density (better protection against disabling bone loss).[6]
- Improved circulation, heart capacity, and lung function.[7]
- Sound, beneficial sleep.
- A youthful appearance; healthy skin; improved muscle tone.
- Reduced risk of cardiovascular disease.[8]

Components of fitness:
Flexibility.
Strength.
Muscle endurance.
Cardiovascular endurance.

use-disuse principle: the principle that fitness develops in response to demand and diminishes in response to a lack of demand.

overload: an extra physical demand placed on the body. A principle of training is that for a body system to improve, its workload must be increased by increments over time.

hypertrophy (high-PURR-tro-fee): to increase in size in response to use.

frequency: the number of occurrences per unit of time; in exercise, the number of repetitions of the work.

duration: length of time; time spent in an exercise session.

intensity: degree; the degree of exertion while exercising.

Blood lipids, including HDL, LDL, and other risk factors for heart disease, are discussed in Chapter 4 and Controversy 4.

- Slowed cardiovascular aging.[9]
- Reduced LDL cholesterol; raised HDL.
- Normalized blood pressure and slower resting pulse rates, indicators of a healthy cardiovascular system.[10]
- Reduced risk of stroke (even in oral contraceptive users, who experience an increased risk).
- Improvement of symptoms in some people with diabetes.[11]
- A lower incidence of constipation and colon disorders, including cancer.[12]
- Faster wound healing.
- Improvement or elimination of menstrual cramps.
- Improved resistance to colds and infections.[13]

Science cannot promise that you will receive all of these benefits if you exercise, but almost everyone who exercises reaps at least some of them. If even half of these rewards were yours for the asking, wouldn't you step up to claim them? Despite evidence of the benefits, not all of the population of the United States exercises regularly, although the number may be increasing.*

There is no RDA for exercise, but there probably should be one. The notion that a certain minimum daily average amount of exercise is indispensable to health is just now reaching public consciousness. Stretching the point, it is even possible to speak of "exercise deficiency," just as we speak of nutrient deficiencies. A consequence of such deficiency is accelerated development of the diseases associated with sedentary life—cardiovascular disease, intestinal disorders, and others (the opposite of the list of benefits of fitness). Researchers are searching for an optimum fitness level, and have yet to discover how little exercise is too little and how much might be too much. The standard advice has been that the minimum needed for cardiovascular endurance is 20 minutes of exercise that raises the heart rate, at least three times each week. Another recommendation states that if you expend 3500 calories a week in any kind of exercise, the heart will benefit. Table 9–1 shows which types of exercise generally enhance which type of fitness.

Occasionally, you may hear someone state that 30 minutes *a week* or just a few minutes a day is plenty of exercise. Indeed, there are a few individuals who seem to have the genetic disposition to be healthy no matter what they do, and for these few, the statement may be true. For most people, though, it is not true. A well-conditioned body costs time and effort. What is true for most people is that once a person builds up cardiovascular endurance, the benefits decline as gradually as they were gained, and at least some of the benefits persist for as long as six weeks during periods of inactivity.[14]

It seems obvious that people's bodies are shaped by what they do, but the principle governing this fact is often overlooked. The **use-disuse principle** is this: muscles respond to the **overload** of exercise by gaining strength, size, and ability to endure, a response called **hypertrophy.** Overload can consist of increased **frequency, duration,** or **intensity** of work. The converse is also true:

*In 1983, the proportion of adults aged 18 to 65 regularly exercising was estimated at just over 35 percent, with children participating in daily physical education programs at 33 percent, and 36 percent of adults over 65 taking regular walks. Public Health Service implementation plans for attaining the objectives for the nation, *Public Health Reports Supplement,* September-October 1983, p. 155. In 1987, a privately funded Gallup telephone poll indicated that 69 percent of adults reported taking some form of exercise regularly. Taking charge, *American Health,* March 1987, pp. 52–57.

Table 9–1

Activities to Develop the Components of Fitness

Fitness Component	Activity
Flexibility	Stretches will enhance flexibility. They should be long, luxurious, and pleasurable. Hold each for 10 to 15 seconds. Never use bouncy, choppy, or painful stretches that twist or put pressure on joints.
Strength	Calisthenic exercises such as pushups and situps and few repetitions with heavy weights increase muscle bulk—the key to strength. Use extreme caution when working with heavy weights or machines; without proper guidance, injury is likely.
Muscle endurance	Repetitive exercises such as push-ups, pull-ups, sit-ups (calisthenics), or many repetitions with light weights will build endurance of the muscle groups worked.
Cardiovascular endurance	Activities include swimming, rowing, fast walking, jogging, fast bicycling, soccer, hockey, basketball, water polo, lacrosse, rugby, and many more. These can provide the needed *sustained, submaximal* activity level, because they raise the heart rate for more than 20 minutes, and they use most of the large muscle groups of the body (legs, buttocks, abdomen).

atrophy (AT-tro-fee): a decrease in size because of disuse.

muscles, if not called on to perform, **atrophy**. Thus runners often have tough, muscled legs, but may have weak arm or chest muscles; a tennis player may have one arm that is superbly strong, while the other is just average. A swimmer usually develops in a balanced way—all limbs, chest, back, and so forth are called on to perform and so develop uniformly. This doesn't mean that everyone should give up tennis and running for swimming, but only that a variety of kinds of exercise will produce the most uniform overall fitness. This is why people are told to use different muscle groups in their exercise from day to day. It makes sense, because muscles are slightly damaged during bouts of exercise and exhaust their fuel stores. It takes a day or two to repair and refuel them.

Exercise benefits people's physical, psychological, and social well-being and improves their resistance to disease. A certain minimum amount of exercise is indispensable to health. To build fitness—whose components are flexibility, strength, and muscle and cardiovascular endurance—a person must apply overload in increments that increase with respect to frequency, duration, or intensity.

Exercise and Heart Health

Controversy 4 made clear that heart and artery disease kills more people in the United States than anything else. Of the actions you can take to protect yourself, exercise is among the most powerful. In this regard, not all exercises are equal.

Cardiovascular conditioning is characterized by:

- Increased blood volume and oxygen delivery.
- Increased heart strength and **stroke volume.**
- Slowed resting pulse.
- Increased breathing efficiency.
- Improved circulation.
- Reduced blood pressure.

Workouts to gain flexibility, strength and muscle bulk, or muscle endurance, if they do not exercise the heart, do not promote heart health effectively (but they do strengthen the joints and so reduce the likelihood of injury). One kind of exercise (aerobic) promotes cardiovascular endurance most efficiently.

Exercise that places demands on the heart, **aerobic** exercise, not only improves its condition, but also improves the condition of the lungs and all muscles of the body, whether or not they are directly involved in the exercise. For example, the muscles along the arteries and in the walls of the digestive tract become more fit, and able to work more effectively. This is conditioning—the microscopic nuts and bolts of fitness, entailing a multitude of adaptations cells make to facilitate the work that **training** demands of them. In **cardiovascular conditioning,** the total blood volume increases, so that the blood can carry more oxygen. The heart muscle becomes stronger and larger, and each beat empties the heart's chambers more completely, so that the heart pumps more blood per beat. This makes fewer beats necessary, so the pulse rate falls. The muscles that inflate and deflate the lungs gain strength and endurance, and breathing becomes more efficient. Blood moves easily through the body's arteries and veins, because the muscles of the arteries contract powerfully, and other muscles move the blood through the veins. The blood pressure falls, because vessel resistance is reduced. Figure 9–1 shows major relationships among the heart, circulatory system, and lungs.

An informal pulse check can give you some indication of how conditioned your heart is. As a rule of thumb, the average resting pulse rate for adults is around 70 beats per minute, but the rate can be higher or lower. Active people can have resting pulse rates of 50 or even lower. Instructions for taking your pulse are given in Figure 9–2.

Figure 9–1
Delivery of Oxygen by the Heart and Lungs to the Muscles.
The more fit a muscle is, the more oxygen it draws from the blood. That oxygen is drawn from the lungs, so the person with more fit muscles extracts from the inhaled air more oxygen than a person with less fit muscles. The cardiovascular system responds to the demand for oxygen by building up its capacity to deliver oxygen. Researchers can measure cardiovascular fitness by measuring the amount of oxygen a person consumes per minute while working out, a measure called the **VO_2 max.**

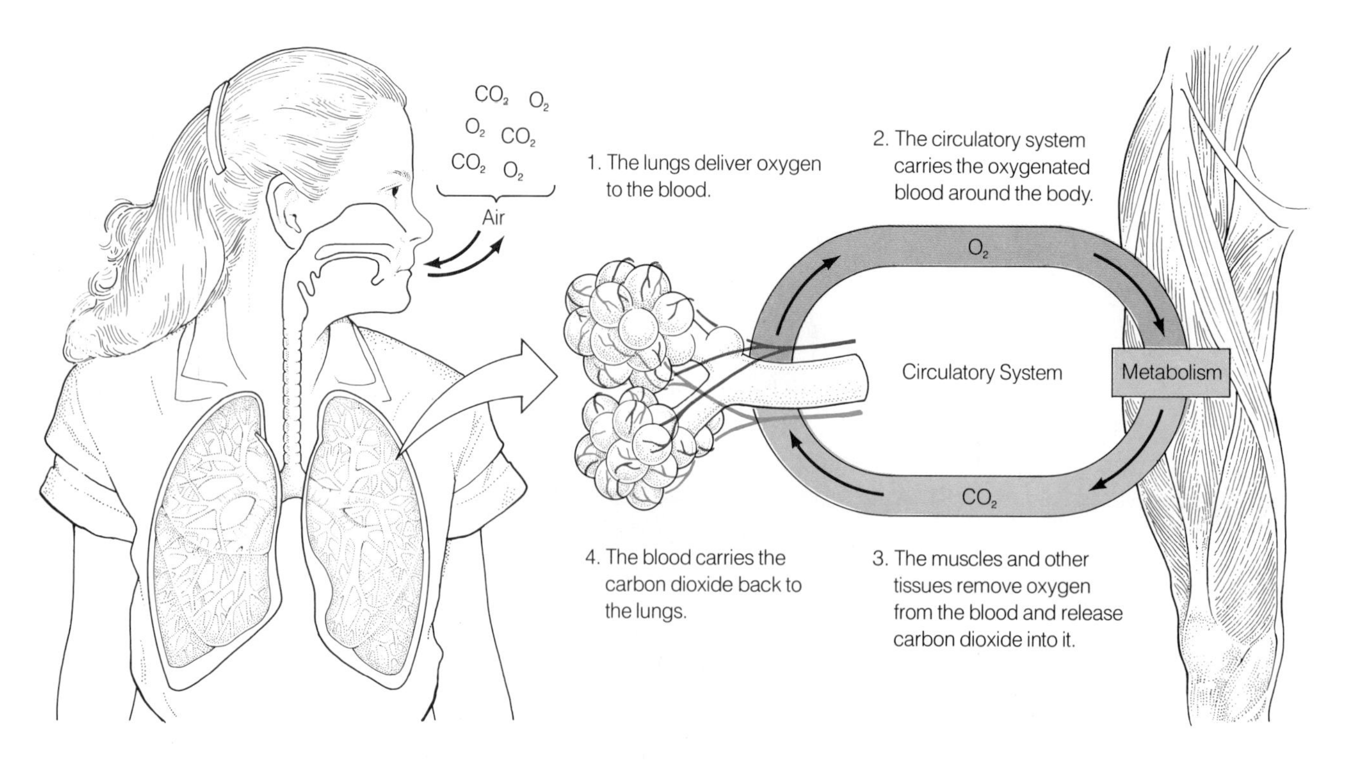

The other kind of exercise, **anaerobic** exercise, generally does not bring about cardiovascular conditioning, but develops strength and bulk of muscles. It involves sudden, all-out exertions of muscles that exceed the cardiovascular system's capacity to deliver oxygen. The distinctions between these two types of exercise, the fuels they require, and their relationships to oxygen are discussed later.

As important as cardiovascular conditioning is, it is only one facet of fitness. All fitness components are important to health and appearance. For balanced fitness, you might want to try light activity and stretching, to warm the muscles and connective tissues and prepare them for the activity ahead; then you might try a sport or jogging for cardiovascular endurance on some days, with weight work or calisthenics to build strength on other days. Table 9–2 rates fitness programs according to their completeness and safety.

Although running usually has a positive effect on heart health, occasional reports describe people suddenly struck down with heart attacks while running, most of whom had histories of heart problems. When heart attacks occur suddenly, without prior warning symptoms during a run, it is probably because the run elicits production of the body's natural painkilling drugs **endorphins** (endogenous opiates) that can mask the pain of the heart in trouble. These opium-like compounds, produced in the brain during exercise, suppress pain many times more effectively than the narcotic morphine. They may also produce the dreamy, pleasant state that has been dubbed "runner's high," and are thought to be related to "silent" or painless heart disease.

aerobic (air-ROE-bic): requiring oxygen.

training: following a goal-oriented activity program that develops desired physiological changes and that benefits performance.

cardiovascular conditioning: the effect of regular exercise on the cardiovascular system—including improvements in heart, lung, and muscle function and increased blood volume.

stroke volume: the amount of oxygenated blood ejected by the heart in a single beat.

VO_2 max: the maximum volume of oxygen consumed per minute of work (see Figure 9–1).

anaerobic (AN-air-ROE-bic): not requiring oxygen.

endorphins: painkilling compounds produced in the brain in response to exercise; one of several kinds of endogenous opiates (see p. 276).

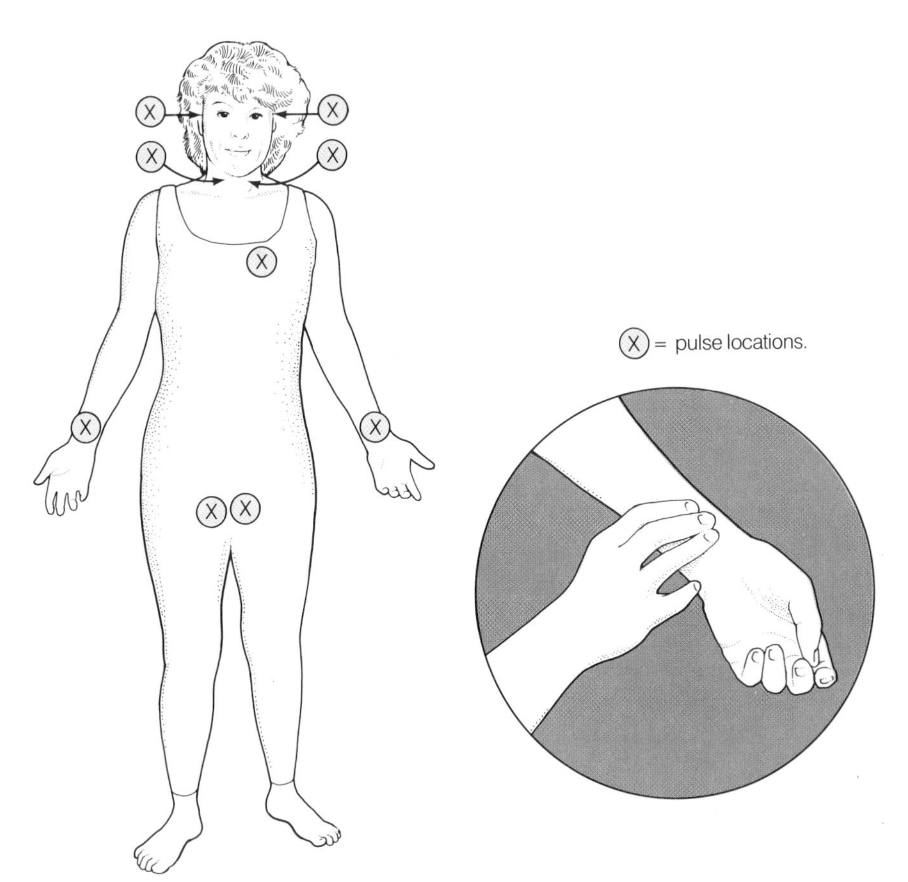

Figure 9–2
How to Take Your Pulse.
Get a watch or clock with a second hand. Rest a few minutes for a resting pulse; for an exercising pulse, take the reading immediately after stopping the work. Place your hand over your heart or your finger firmly over an artery in any pulse location that gives a clear rhythm. Start counting your pulse at a convenient second, and continue counting for 10 seconds. If a heartbeat occurs exactly on the tenth second, count it as one-half beat. Multiply by 6 to obtain the beats per minute.
To ensure a true count:

- Use only fingers, not your thumb, on the pulse point (the thumb has a pulse of its own).
- Press just firmly enough to feel the pulse. Too much pressure can interfere with the pulse rhythm.

Table 9–2

Fitness Programs Compared

You can evaluate fitness programs objectively by using your knowledge of what fitness is and how it is gained and maintained. The following are some questions that can help in your evaluation. Start with 100 points and subtract the points indicated for shortcomings.

1. Does the program include sufficient aerobic exercise for cardiovascular fitness (about 20 minutes, three days per week)? If not, ***minus 10.***
2. Does the program include exercises that promote muscle strength, such as sit-ups, push-ups, or weight training? If not, ***minus 5.*** Are strengthening exercises given for all large muscle groups? If some parts are left out, ***minus 5.***
3. Does the program include exercises for flexibility, such as gentle stretches? If not, ***minus 10.***
4. Does the program allow for varying initial fitness levels; that is, can you start out slowly and work your way up? If not, ***minus 10.***
5. Does the program give adequate exercises within a reasonable time each day—say at least 20 minutes, but less than an hour—at least three days per week? If not, ***minus 10.***

Fitness Program Name and Description	Question 1: Aerobic Exercise	Question 2: Muscle Strength	Question 3: Flexibility	Question 4: Initial Levels
The Aerobics Way (Dr. Kenneth Cooper). An aerobic system that favors cardiovascular over other fitness. It provides safety tips missing in previous versions. It is goal-oriented, and may lack fun for some, and it under-values some enjoyable activities such as soccer.	Yes	No, insufficient strength exercises MINUS 10	No, insuffi-cient flexibil-ity exercises MINUS 10	Yes
Jogging (Bill Bowerman and Dr. W. E. Harris). A book that provides three jogging plans for various fitness lev-els. It presents no other types of exercise.	Yes	No, no strength exercises MINUS 10	No, insuffi-cient flexibil-ity exercises MINUS 10	Yes
Total Fitness (Dr. Lawrence Morehouse). A program that promises an excellent fitness level in just 12 hr, with many pounds of weight loss.	No, insufficient aerobic exer-cises by current standards MINUS 10	No, insufficient strength exer-cises by current standards MINUS 10	No, insuffi-cient flexibil-ity exercises by current standards MINUS 10	Yes
The Official YMCA Physical Fitness Handbook (Dr. Clay-ton R. Myers). A balanced program of aerobics, muscle strength, and flexibility exercises. YMCA membership may be required, but the cost is low. The emphasis is on health, not beauty.	Yes	Yes	Yes	Yes
The Fit Kit (Recreation Canada). The official fitness program of the National Health and Welfare Depart-ment of Canada.	Yes	Yes	Yes	Yes
The Royal Canadian Air Force Programs. Programs de-signed to develop fitness in 11 minutes of vigorous ex-ercise each day. The programs are needlessly divided into sex groups and do not individualize advancement to higher levels.	No, only the advanced levels give sufficient aerobic work MINUS 10	Yes	Yes	Yes
Adult Physical Fitness (President's Council on Physical Fitness and Sports). A program intended to help men and women gain fitness at home. It needlessly separates men's and women's programs.	Yes, for ad-vanced men's level (for others, MINUS 10)	Yes	Yes	Yes
Vigor Regained (Dr. Herbert de Vries). A home exer-cise program for the out-of-shape older individual; em-phasizes good health by way of a fit body.	Yes	Yes	Yes	Yes

6. Does the program include a warm-up period? If no, *minus 10.*
7. Can the program be performed with only basic equipment, such as shoes, small weights, or a jump rope? Must you join an expensive club to participate? If specific or unusual products, perhaps sold by the promoters, must be used, or if a large membership fee is required, *minus 10.*
8. Is the program safe? If it suggests bouncy stretches or straight-leg sit-ups, give it a *minus 10.* If it advocates clearly hazardous practices, such as running in heavy or rubber clothing, don't even consider using it; its *total score is zero.*
9. Does the promoter make only claims backed up by legitimate research? If unorthodox claims are made, such as "no-work fitness," "redistribute your fat" (or cellulite), or "cures your heart disease" (or other diseases), *minus 10.*
10. Does the program promote a lifetime fitness plan based on a variety of enjoyable activities? If the program is monotonous, it will soon become boring and hard to stay with, so give it a *minus 10.*

Question 5: Reasonable Time	Question 6: Warm-up/ Cool-down	Question 7: Equipment/ Membership	Question 8: Safety	Question 9: Accuracy of Claims	Question 10: Ability to Hold Interest	Total Score
Yes	Yes	Yes	No, the uniform advancement rate may not be safe for all MINUS 10	No, may overstate helpfulness for heart disease MINUS 10	Yes, notes that different sports can lead to fitness, but deemphasizes them	60
Yes	Yes	Yes	Yes	Yes	No, monotonous MINUS 10	70
No, time required is insufficient MINUS 10	No, warm-up period is insufficient MINUS 10	Yes	Yes	No, makes unproved claims for fitness from minimal effort MINUS 10	No, doesn't include sports MINUS 10	30
Yes	Yes	Yes	No, includes some exercises of questionable safety MINUS 10	Yes	No, doesn't include sports MINUS 10	80
Yes	Yes	Yes	Yes	Yes	Yes	100
No, the 11 minutes per day is insufficient for aerobic work MINUS 10	No MINUS 10	Yes	Yes	Yes	No, a set routine is to be performed MINUS 10	60
No, too much of the 15 minutes per day is warm-up time MINUS 10	Yes	Yes	No, includes some exercises of questionable safety MINUS 10	Yes	Yes. Doesn't include sports, but does urge broadening of program	80 (70)
Yes	Yes	Yes	Yes	Yes	No, program repeats exercise routine MINUS 10	90

exercise stress test: a test that monitors heart function during exercise to detect abnormalities that may not show up under ordinary conditions; exercise physiologists and trained physicians or other health care professionals can administer the test.

In ancient days, the production of endorphins during exercise was probably life-saving, for a person injured by a carnivorous beast could not afford the luxury of limping to safety. Those who produced painkillers could reach safety despite minor injury. Today, the opiates are still produced in the brain during exercise, but their effect may sometimes threaten rather than preserve life by masking the pain that would otherwise warn of an impending heart attack. It is prudent to seek an **exercise stress test** before proceeding with a new plan for exercise, particularly for those over 35 years of age and those who have been sedentary for several previous years. That way, you won't have to rely on symptoms (that could be masked by endorphins) to warn you of danger. If during exercise, you notice *any* change in comfort or experience pain, stop exercising and consult a health care provider before continuing. Fitness should be built slowly. There is no rush to gain it, because like an adequate diet, it should become a part of the day as inevitable as the sunrise.

Sound fitness programs develop all aspects of fitness: flexibility, strength, and both muscle and cardiovascular endurance. To develop cardiovascular endurance is especially important. Before beginning a fitness program, a person should consult a health care provider.

Oxygen, Fuels, and Muscular Work

When you begin to exercise, the hormones epinephrine and norepinephrine, among others, begin to circulate in the bloodstream, signaling the liver and fat cells to liberate stored energy nutrients. These hormones are also released in response to stress, and the effect on the body is the same, with one important difference. Fuels called forth by stress are not fully used up by muscles, but continue cycling around the bloodstream until the stress ceases, hormones diminish, and the fuels are stored once more, perhaps in their original form, or perhaps after conversion to something else—glucose to fat, for example, or fat to cholesterol. In exercise, those same hormones set the table for the muscles' energy feast—the muscles pick up and use for energy the glucose and fatty acids liberated from storage. This is one reason why people under stress often find exercise to be a release—the body is primed for physical action, and action makes use of the fuels in the blood. It may also be a link to understanding how stress is related to heart disease—perhaps those circulating fuels, if not used for exercise, influence the advancement of plaques that ultimately clog the arteries.

The stress response is discussed in Chapter 1.

Most of what we know about fuel use during exercise comes from research on athletes, but anyone can make use of it. To burn fat and build lean tissue, anyone needs to know which types of exercises burn which fuels. Exercise metabolism requires that the muscles be supplied with three main things: oxygen, and the two muscle fuels, glucose and fatty acids. As Figure 9–1 showed, the oxygen comes from the lungs, which pass it to the blood, which carries it to the muscles. The glucose is derived chiefly from glycogen stored within the muscle itself; some comes from the liver, via the blood. The fatty acids come partly from fat inside the muscles, but mostly from fat that is released from the body's fat tissues and delivered by the blood.

Oxygen

During rest, your body uses both fat and glucose for energy. During exercise, though, oxygen availability in the muscles determines which of the two fuels will provide most of the energy to fuel the work. With ample oxygen, muscles can extract all available energy from glucose and fat by means of aerobic metabolism (see Figure 9–3, below). During moderate exercise, your lungs and circulatory system have no trouble keeping up with your muscles' need for oxygen. You breathe deeply and easily, and your heart beats steadily—the exercise is aerobic.

The heart and lungs can provide only so much oxygen, only so fast. When the muscles' exertion is great enough that their energy demand outstrips their oxygen supply, aerobic metabolism can no longer provide all the energy they need. Fat requires oxygen for breakdown (aerobic metabolism), so the muscles cannot meet their increased energy needs with fat. They must use a fuel that can be metabolized, at least partially, without oxygen—glucose. Figure 9–4 (next page) shows that fatty acids cannot enter the aerobic pathways for energy release without ample oxygen in the muscles, but that glucose can be partially broken down under these circumstances. At this point, your body is building up an **oxygen debt.** You may even have to slow down or even stop to catch your breath and replenish your oxygen supply. When you do, your body can rely on energy produced aerobically once more.

As you develop an oxygen debt, partly broken-down portions of glucose molecules accumulate; more oxygen is needed to completely break them down. The heart and lungs speed up, but a point comes at which they can't keep up.

You may have heard the name of one of the byproducts generated during oxygen debt: **lactic acid.** Its buildup causes burning pain in the muscles and

oxygen debt: a deficit of oxygen built up by a body performing exercise so demanding that the cardiovascular system cannot deliver oxygen fast enough to the muscles to support aerobic metabolism; the debt must be repaid by rapid breathing after the activity slows down or stops.

lactic acid: a fragment produced from glucose during anaerobic metabolism. When oxygen becomes available, lactic acid can be completely broken down to carbon dioxide and water.

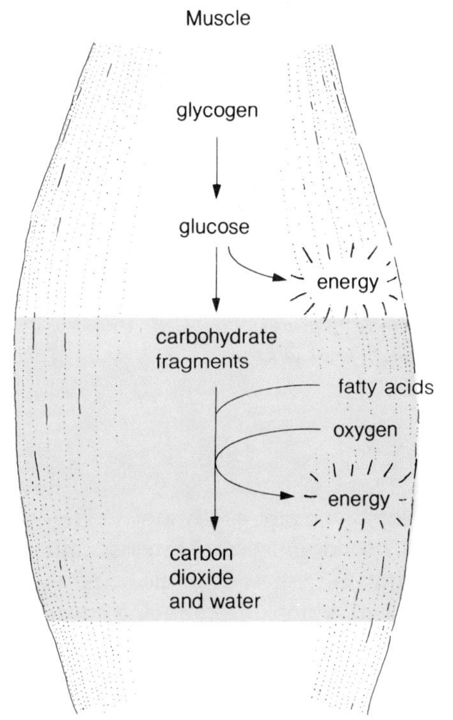

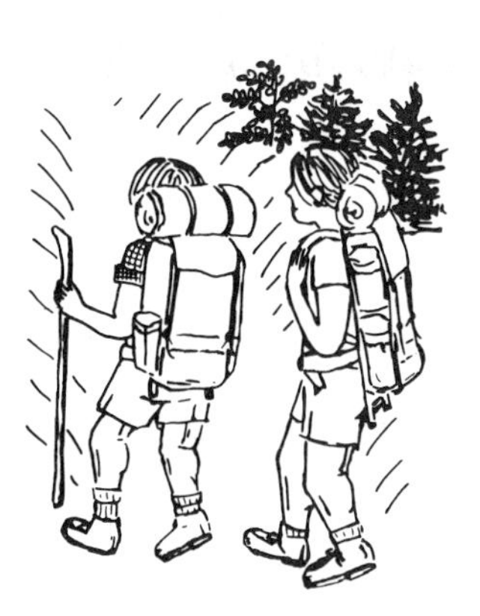

Slow, steady exercise produces lots of energy from body fuels aerobically.

Figure 9–3
The Aerobic Part of Energy Release. When oxygen is available, we get much energy from glucose molecules and from fatty acids.

Figure 9–4
Energy Release Partially Blocked by Lack of Oxygen.
During intense exercise, oxygen is used up quickly. When no more oxygen is available, glucose can only be broken down this far. When carbohydrate fragments start to build up, they are converted into lactic acid. Fatty acids cannot enter this breakdown pathway and are diverted.

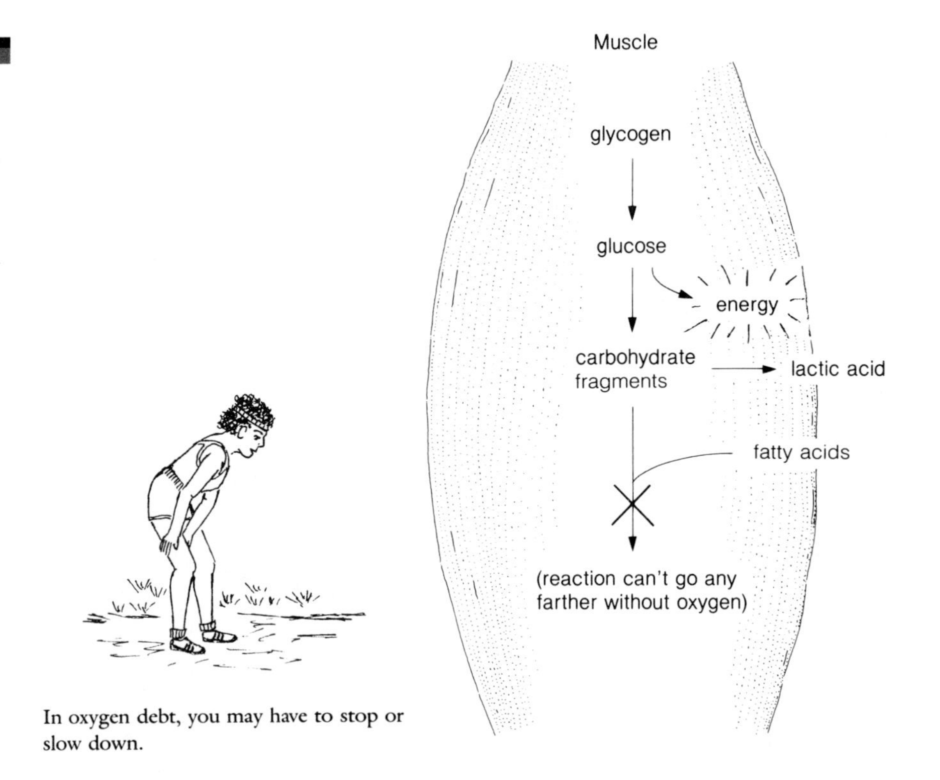

In oxygen debt, you may have to stop or slow down.

can lead to muscle exhaustion within seconds if it is not drained away. A strategy for dealing with lactic acid buildup is to relax the muscles at every opportunity, so that the circulating blood can carry it away and bring oxygen to support aerobic metabolism and reduce the oxygen debt. This is what mountaineers are doing when they relax their leg muscles at each step (the "mountain rest step").

The liver is the body's waste management specialist. Figure 9–5, opposite, shows that when oxygen is restored, lactic acid is routed to the liver, where it is converted to glucose. Meanwhile, the muscles can once again produce energy aerobically.

The energy demands of aerobic exercise are within the circulatory system's ability to supply oxygen. Anaerobic exercise demands energy beyond this point, and produces oxygen debt.

Exercise and Glucose Use

Glycogen was defined in Chapter 3.

The body stores just a small amount of carbohydrate as glycogen. The liver contains some glycogen, which it breaks apart into glucose and releases into the bloodstream when the body needs it. During exercise, the muscles pick up and use the glucose donated by the liver, along with glucose from their own private glycogen stores. Compared to fat, the carbohydrate sources of the body are limited. A person with 30 pounds of body fat to spare may have only a pound

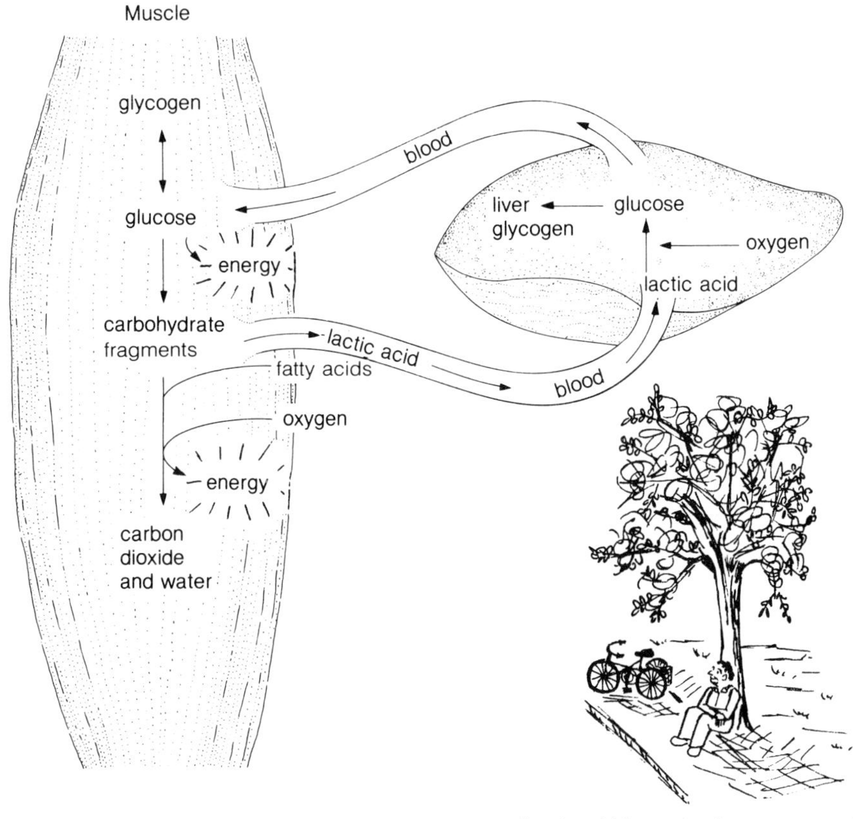

Lactic acid becomes glucose once again when oxygen is restored.

Figure 9–5
Energy Release Completed when Oxygen is Again Available.
The muscles are no longer forced to produce their energy anaerobically. Lactic acid that has traveled to the liver is converted back to glucose.

or so of glycogen to draw on. Furthermore, the body glycogen is constantly being used and replenished, and, unlike body fat, is closely related to the carbohydrate content of the diet. How much carbohydrate you eat determines how much glycogen you store, and it influences the rate at which you will use it in any given exercise.[15] The more glycogen you store, the longer the stores will last during exercise. The rate at which you use glucose also depends partly on the duration of the exercise and partly on its intensity. Some activities, such as sprinting, use the body's stores of glycogen very quickly. Others, such as jogging, are more conservative of glycogen, but joggers still use it, and eventually they can run out of it. Figure 9–6 shows how the proportions of fuels used during exercise change over time, according to the intensity of the exercise.

Within the first 20 minutes or so of moderate exercise the body uses up about a fifth of its stored glycogen.[16] If you tested the exercising person's blood glucose during this period, you would see it rise for a while, signaling that the liver is pouring out its stored carbohydrate for the muscles' use. The muscles, ravenous for glucose, increase their uptake 20-fold or more.[17] Blood glucose is thus kept from rising too high, and indeed, it will soon begin to decline.

As exercise continues, glycogen use slows down. The body begins to rely more on fat for fuel, to conserve the remaining glycogen supply. At some point beyond this, if exercise continues long enough and at a high enough intensity,

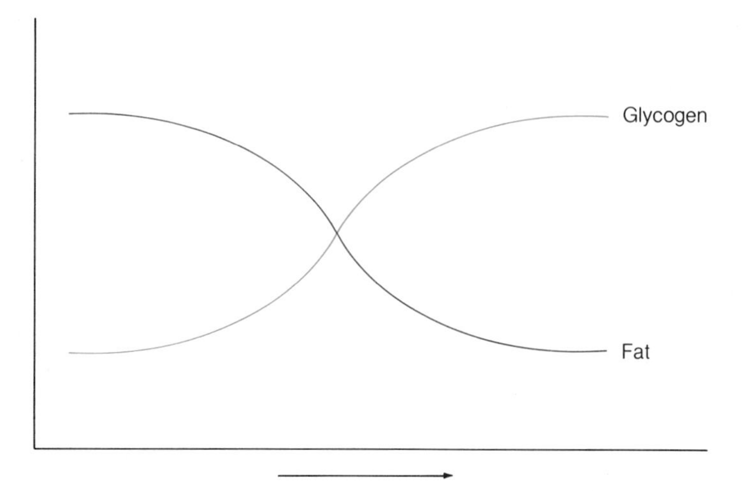

Figure 9–6
Fuels Used by the Muscles during Exercise.
Exercise of high intensity requires more glycogen per minute than does exercise of lower intensity.

glycogen will run out almost completely. Exercise can continue for a short time thereafter, only because the liver scrambles to produce the minimum amount of glucose needed to briefly forestall hypoglycemia. When hypoglycemia hits, it brings nervous system function almost to a halt, making exercise difficult, if not impossible. You may wonder, then, why weight lifters become fatigued after only a few heavy lifts—long before glycogen stores run out. Such fatigue is the result of lactic acid buildup (oxygen debt) and the depletion of metabolic energy-carrying compounds within each muscle cell.* Trained muscles can tolerate more lactic acid than untrained muscles, and so can exercise at high intensities somewhat longer, but eventually, even the best-trained heavyweight lifter succumbs to muscle fatigue.

Besides intensity and duration of exercise, another factor helps determine how much glycogen a person uses during exercise—how well-trained the person is to do the exercise at hand. When you first attempt an activity, you use much more glucose than an athlete who is trained to perform it. This is because glucose most quickly and easily yields the needed energy; processing fat takes longer and requires that the muscle cells be equipped with abundant fat-burning metabolic enzymes. Untrained muscles rely heavily on glucose, but with training they adapt, packing their cells with more fat-burning enzymes. As a result, trained muscles use more fat and conserve their glycogen. Training has another effect: hormone levels during exercise are lower in the trained person, slowing the glucose release from the liver and conserving its supply of glycogen. The person who wishes to burn fat by exercising can make use of this knowledge: patient, persistent, consistent low-intensity training, such as fast walking, is the road to maximum fat use and use of less carbohydrate.

People used to think that they should not consume sugar during exercise, for fear of stimulating the release of too much insulin (whose function is to

*The metabolic energy-carrying compounds referred to here are adenosine triphosphate (ATP) and creatine phosphate (CP), created during the breakdown of energy-yielding nutrients and immediately broken down themselves, providing energy for muscle contraction.

move glucose and other energy-yielding nutrients into cells). This was a logical thought, because insulin (see Chapter 3) normally causes all of the body's tissues to take up glucose from the blood and stow it away. This could bring on hypoglycemia, they reasoned, and limit endurance.

During exercise, though, other hormones moderate insulin's effects. These hormones keep the insulin level fairly constant, even if sugar is eaten. They also increase muscle sensitivity to insulin so that muscle tissue gobbles up any energy-yielding nutrients that happen by. Meanwhile, since the insulin level is normal, other body tissues, such as fat tissue, are not triggered to collect glucose from the blood. In fact, they respond to exercise by releasing fuels for the muscles' use. This increased sensitivity of muscles to insulin lasts beyond the exercise period, and is part of the training effect on the body. For this reason, exercise is helpful in the defense against the disease diabetes. People with diabetes who begin to exercise regularly can often reduce their daily requirements of insulin or insulin-eliciting drugs because their muscles adapt to the exercise and thereby respond to insulin more sensitively.

Exercise moderates insulin's effects by:

- Suppressing release of insulin, even if sugar is eaten.
- Sensitizing the muscles to insulin, and thereby greatly increasing their uptake of glucose and other energy-yielding nutrients.

Because of the moderating effect of exercise on the insulin response, sugar during exercise is no longer feared to impair performance. In fact, at critical moments late in endurance competition, some sugar may improve performance. Small amounts of glucose from slightly sweetened drinks taken during exercise slowly make their way from the digestive tract to the muscles, and augment the body's supply of glucose enough to postpone exhaustion.[18] The key phrase is *taken during exercise,* for any carbohydrate-containing nourishment taken within three hours *before* exercise will indeed bring about the feared result—elevated insulin levels, increased glucose uptake and storage by all the body tissues, hypoglycemia, and lessened release of fat stores.[19] Translation: poor athletic performance. In fact, research on runners shows that a sugar drink taken directly before exercise can reduce athletic performance by 25 percent.[20]

So, should exercisers rely on sugar for performance? Probably not. First, as just said, no one should take sugar within about three hours before beginning to exercise if they want to perform their best. Second, sugar during exercise helps only people who are exercising so strenuously and so long that they chance running out of glycogen, such as bikers finishing the Tour de France, triathletes in the Ironman competition, or racers in the Boston marathon. For most others, no additional sugar is needed to perform well; the glycogen stored from nourishing meals with abundant carbohydrate eaten earlier will sustain them. For people who exercise to control weight, sugar from any source is particularly detrimental, a source of unneeded nutrient-poor calories.

Some candy makers advertise their wares as energy-boosters. Sugar *is* the quick energy source for muscles, but you do not have to eat it for performance. Glycogen is the muscles' preferred sugar source, and regular food can supply it best. A later section gives details on how to eat to store glycogen, and the effects of sports drinks that provide sugar are discussed in a later box.

How quickly a person uses up glycogen during exercise depends on how much glycogen was stored to begin with, the intensity and duration of the exercise, and how well-trained the person is at the task. The hormones of exercise prevent wide swings in blood glucose, even when sugar is eaten; for most, ingesting carbohydrate during exercise is unnecessary.

Exercise and Fatty Acid Use

Compared with its stores of glycogen, the body's fat is almost unlimited. When you exercise, the fat your muscles burn comes from the fatty depots all over the body, especially from those with the greatest amounts of fat to spare, wherever it is stored. That's why fit people look trim all over—they reduce their fat stores all over the body, not just those overlying the working muscles.

People who wish to burn off body fat through exercise cherish this fact—slow and steady low-intensity exercise lasting longer than 20 minutes or so works best. During the early glycogen-dependent period, the fatty acid levels in the blood begin to drop—the muscles are using up the fatty acids already present there. If exercise continues, the fat cells get the message that fat is needed for energy, and they break apart their stored triglycerides rapidly, liberating fatty acids into the blood. Soon, the blood fatty acid concentration rises again and surpasses the normal resting concentration. It is during this phase of sustained, submaximal exercise that the fat cells begin to shrink in size as they empty out their lipid stores.

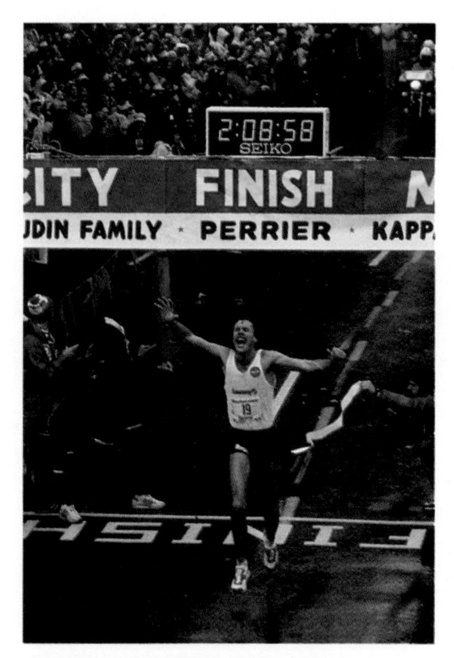

Running a marathon requires vast amounts of fuel, much of it fat.

People sometimes ask about "spot reducing." Can you lose fat in particular locations? Unfortunately, muscles do not "own" the fat that surrounds them. Fat cells release fat not into the underlying muscles, but into the blood, and the fat is shared by all the muscles. Spot-reducing exercises therefore do not work. Proof of this is found in a tennis player's arms—the fatfolds measure the same, even though the muscles of one arm are much better developed than those of the other. A balanced exercise program will, however, tighten muscles underneath the fat in trouble spots to improve their appearance.

To use fat during exercise, work at about half or less of your maximum capacity. At this intensity, you will draw heavily on fat stores. A rule of thumb for gauging intensity of workouts to exercise the heart and to burn fat is: if you can't talk normally, you are incurring oxygen debt and are burning more glucose than fat (so slow down); if you can sing, you aren't burning energy very quickly or working your heart (so speed up).

After exercise has ceased, fat use may continue at an accelerated rate for about a day. Metabolism is stimulated by about 25 percent for as long as three hours after intensive exercise and may still be running 10 percent faster two days later. It takes energy to link glucose molecules back into glycogen and to build new muscle tissue; fat supplies some of this energy. The hormones generated during exercise favor the continued liberation of stored fat, too.[21] When exercise becomes part of a person's life, the body changes to accommodate it. One of the changes is that muscles build up their supply of fat-burning enzymes, and so burn more fat all day long, not just during exercise.

Other molecules contribute only small amounts of energy to support exercise. Blood amino acids are one of these energy sources. These amino acids always travel free in the blood, so you need not worry that exercise breaks down your muscle and other lean tissue for fuel (as does starvation, described in Chapter 8).[22] The muscle breakdown observed after exercise most likely makes way for muscle remodeling to produce stronger trained muscles, and is not related to fuel use.

A word of caution is in order—anything, including exercise and weight control, can be carried to the extreme. Especially among women, it is common for athletes to engage in extreme dieting behavior[23] (as described in this Chapter's

Controversy). Ironically, athletes caught up in these destructive patterns seek from them improved athletic performance (not a particular body appearance). Of course, extremes in dieting have the exact opposite of the effect they seek—starvation weakens people. As you will see in the next section, any behavior that limits the vitamin and mineral contents of the diet also limits performance.

In exercise, the body draws on its vast stores of fat from all over the body. Sustained, moderate exercise uses up fat most efficiently, and accelerates metabolism. Persistent training increases the muscles' use of fat over glycogen.

Vitamins and Minerals—Keys to Energy Use

The interplay of glucose, fatty acids, and oxygen during exercise takes place in the muscles and depends on how well-stocked they are with the vitamins and minerals. Without adequate amounts of these critical nutrients, the body's work capacity is compromised.

Vitamins

A molecule of glucose or fat is of no value to an exercising muscle unless the molecule's bonds can be broken so that the muscle fibers can obtain and use the energy. Scientists are still working to clarify the roles of the vitamins; Table 9–3 (next page) shows some of the known roles of vitamins and minerals in exercise. As discoveries are made, a general trend has become apparent—with rare exceptions, suspicions that the exercising body needs more of the vitamins than a healthy diet can supply are being disproved, one by one. For example, thirty years ago, scientists used logic to reason that, since thiamin plays a role in energy production, and exercise uses up energy, people who exercise need more thiamin. (This logic is still used today by companies that sell vitamin pills.) When tested scientifically, however, it turned out that even people who train intensively need only the thiamin contained in a normal, adequate diet. More thiamin than that, taken in supplements, confers no performance benefits on people.[24]

This does not mean that thiamin or any of the other vitamins is not important. The words ***adequate diet*** are weighty in this regard, and they apply to all the nutrients discussed in this chapter. At least most of the athlete's extra energy needs must be met with nutrient-dense foods, not fats and sweets. Even sedentary people who consume a "junk" diet—that is, a diet of foods relatively empty of nutrients—can become thiamin deficient. This effect is magnified for the exerciser who spends many more calories of energy each day than do others.

Another B vitamin used in the release of energy is riboflavin. Studies of riboflavin needs in athletes have seemed to indicate that overweight women who begin an exercise regime need twice the RDA of riboflavin.[25] These studies show that a measurement of riboflavin activity remains normal during the early stages of training when riboflavin is supplemented, and that riboflavin's activity is not maintained when only the RDA amount of riboflavin was given. Contrary to what you might expect, the studies also show that the women taking supplemental riboflavin had no advantage over the nonsupplemented group in performance or condition. That is, when tested, women who did not take riboflavin supplements gained fitness and performed just as well as those who did take them. No one yet knows why performance is not affected by the drop in blood riboflavin activity. Perhaps the body sacrifices blood riboflavin in order to pack it into the riboflavin-containing muscle enzymes that do the work of exercise.

The human body is designed to work, and is healthiest when it is exercised. Adjustment after adjustment is made to accommodate increased activity. An example is in the handling of vitamin B_6, a vitamin critical to building the blood and muscle tissues needed in exercise. The body responds to exercise by conserving vitamin B_6. The livers of those who exercise store more vitamin B_6 than the livers of others.[26] Hence, exercisers need not take in more than the RDA of the vitamin—rather, their bodies excrete less. This sort of body wisdom has proven to be the case for other nutrients, too. The body conserves what it needs.

Niacin, another B vitamin, may affect exercise performance more directly than do the other vitamins, especially when it is taken in the form of supplements. Niacin taken before exercise suppresses the release of fatty acids, forcing muscles to use extra glycogen. Whether or not this impairs performance is unknown, but it probably shortens the time to glycogen depletion and makes the work seem more difficult to the exerciser.[27] Exercisers need no more niacin than that supplied by a nutrient-dense diet, and people who take niacin supplements before exercise are probably affecting their workouts for the worse.

Table 9–3

Exercise-Related Functions of Vitamins and Minerals

Vitamin or Mineral	Function
Thiamin, riboflavin, niacin, magnesium	Energy-releasing reactions
Vitamin B_6, zinc	Building of muscle protein
Folacin, vitamin B_{12}	Building of red blood cells to carry oxygen
Vitamin C	Collagen formation for joint and other tissue integrity; hormone synthesis
Iron	Transport of oxygen in blood and in muscle tissue; energy transformation reactions
Calcium, vitamin D, vitamin A, phosphorus	Building of bone structure; muscle contractions; nerve transmissions
Sodium, potassium, chloride	Maintenance of fluid balance; transmission of nerve impulses for muscle contraction
Chromium	Assistance in insulin's energy-storage function
Magnesium	Cardiac and other muscle contraction

Note: This is just a sampling. Other vitamins and minerals play equally indispensable roles in exercise.

Some theorists have thought of exercise as a form of stress, and because other stresses increase the destruction of vitamin C in the body, they have reasoned that exercisers might need extra vitamin C. Evidence that supports that notion comes from reports in the 1970s and early 1980s that noted increased excretion and reduced blood levels of vitamin C after exercise. This preliminary research suggests that vitamin C in amounts two or three times the RDA might turn out to best serve the needs of the athlete, but so far, further experimentation has not borne this out. The great bulk of work shows that vitamin C beyond that in an adequate diet has no beneficial effect on work performance.

Some vitamin C enthusiasts, however, encourage athletes to ingest huge quantities of vitamin C, measured in *grams*. The evidence so far does not conclusively prove that the RDA is sufficient, nor does it disprove it, but there is not a shred of evidence that even remotely suggests that large doses of the vitamin will improve athletic performance. When you consider the quantity of food an athlete must eat to meet energy requirements, that almost twice the RDA for vitamin C is provided by one serving of orange juice, and that substantial vitamin C is present in potatoes and other foods, it is clear that an athlete would have to try hard *not* to consume several times the RDA for vitamin C in a day, just eating normal, whole food.

Of the fat-soluble vitamins, supplemental A and D have been shown not to benefit athletic performance, and they are toxic in excess. Vitamin E in amounts beyond the RDA, although not as toxic as the other fat-soluble vitamins, has been shown to be useless in promoting athletic performance. Some early studies (1950s and 1960s) suggested an effect, but these studies were flawed in design or analysis. They are still used by the sellers of supplements, though, to market potions for athletes that contain vitamin E. Anyone wanting adequate intakes of vitamin E can easily obtain them—by including vegetable oil products, nuts, fruits and vegetables, and whole-wheat products in meals.

For the most part, then, studies indicate that athletes need no special supplements to maximize performance.[28] What the studies do not address, however, is that not all, or even most, athletes are well nourished, for people who consistently choose nutrient-poor foods cannot wring from them the nutrients they need. But, for the most part, active people who choose foods with care can be sure of meeting their vitamin needs without supplements. After all, vitamins and energy occur together in food. People who are active need to eat a greater quantity of food to maintain their weight. If the foods chosen are nutritious ones, the needed vitamins will be supplied adequately.

Vitamins are essential for releasing the energy trapped in energy-yielding nutrients, and for other functions that support exercise. Most active people can meet their vitamin needs with an ordinary diet of nutrient-dense foods sufficient to meet their energy needs.

Iron and Sports Anemia

Iron in hemoglobin is essential for carrying oxygen to the working muscles, and it is therefore critical to performance. Most active people do not need more than the RDA of iron, but many people do not obtain this amount, and athletes are among them. The accompanying box discusses supplements for athletes.

ergogenic: a term intended to imply that a food or supplement gives energy; usually a hoax (*ergo* means "work"; *genic* means "gives rise to").

Supplements Athletes Take

Different people tell you different things about nutrient supplements for performance. Some say to take protein supplements, carbohydrate drinks, and muscle-building powders, while others recommend electrolyte pills, vitamin pills, and "ergogenic" foods. The term **ergogenic,** often associated with supplements claimed to benefit athletes, implies that the products are energy-giving. Actually, no nutrient is ergogenic. When you hear such claims for supplements, remember to ask yourself who is speaking and what they may have to gain from a sale. Most nutrition experts agree that supplements do not help performance in a well-nourished person, and that if nutrients are lacking, they should be restored by way of diet. Clinical deficiency states, as identified by health professionals, should be treated medically—that is, with the appropriate nutrient supplements—and the diet should be corrected.

Many athletes make easy targets for quacks, because they have invested much time and effort in training, and they are open to wishful thinking. If a salesperson or advertisement can convince them that a product might provide their competitors a winning edge in their field, they may fear that by not using it, they will deny themselves equal advantage. Of course, simply purchasing and swallowing a product cannot provide competitors a winning edge, but the *fear* that it could is strong. Even casual exercisers are susceptible to unfounded product claims; they, too, are lured by promises of better performance through pills.

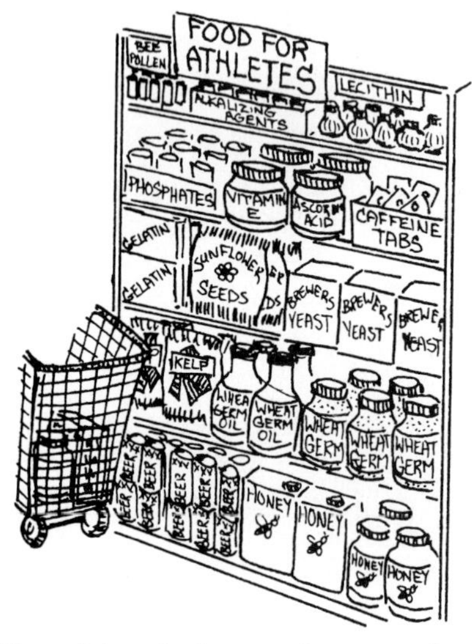

None of these foods or supplements confers any special athletic benefit, no matter what the ads tell you.

Among the pills and powders hawked to athletes and exercisers are amino acid supplements that are of no value, and that may be dangerous (see the box in Chapter 5, and see Controversy 13 for a discussion on how single amino acids interact with the brain). Then there are drinks that manufacturers claim provide "complete" nutrition. They are mixtures of carbohydrate, protein (usually amino acids), and certain vitamins and minerals. They are usually tasty, sweet with sugar, and rich in food energy, although they are not really "complete" nutrition; and they are of no use in boosting performance or building muscle when they are taken in addition to a balanced diet.

Special supplements are also sold in the form of pills, usually vitamins and minerals, under the pretext of being useful in the last hours before competition. The text explained that niacin before exercise could have negative results by suppressing fatty acid release. The taking of any vitamin and mineral supplements before competition as pregame "insurance" runs contrary to science: such products provide no energy, and their nutrients will not find their way to the enzymes they assist (presuming they were lacking there) in time to be useful. The body's enzymes can ensure successful performance only if they are fully supplied on a daily basis with all the vitamins and minerals they require, including the ones not present in supplements but only in whole foods.

A type of commercial drink could conceivably be of value. In the case of the nervous athlete who cannot tolerate solid food the day of an event, a liquid meal (that nutritionally "complete" supplement, mentioned earlier) three or four hours before the event can supply the needed fluid and carbohydrate to replace the pregame meal. Just as effective, a milk shake of nonfat milk and ice milk blended with sugar and flavorings could do the same thing, and less expensively.

There is one instance when an ordinary multivitamin and mineral supplement might be prudent: when an athlete's need for energy outstrips the ability to eat the quantity of food required to supply it. In this case, many athletes must turn to concentrated energy sources, such as candies and fats. While such foods supply abundant energy, they are practically devoid of vitamins and minerals. Thus, during the heaviest training, a supplement may be appropriate. Choose one on the basis of the information in Controversy 6—don't be led astray by the words "athlete" or "fitness" on a label.

One other instance justifies iron supplementation. Long-distance runners (especially females) may lose iron through red cell destruction, reduced absorption, and increased excretion so that their reserves become dangerously low and their performance in sports impaired. In these cases, treatment with iron reverses the condition, but the dosage should be individualized, and prescribed by a physician.

The overwhelming majority of potions sold for athletes are frauds. Wishful thinking will not substitute for hard training, adequate diet, and mental preparedness in competition. The placebo effect is strong at work in athletes, so even if a reliable source reports a performance boost from a newly tried product, give it time. Chances are excellent that the effect was simply the power of the mind over the body. Incidentally, don't discount that power, for it is formidable, and sports psychology is a field of study dedicated to harnessing it. You can use it by imagining yourself as a winner and visualizing yourself as capable in your sport. You don't have to turn to concoctions for an extra edge, because you already have one—your mind.

Source: D. W. Barnett and R. K. Conlee, The effects of a commercial dietary supplement on human performance, *American Journal of Clinical Nutrition* 40 (1984): 586–590; National Dairy Council, Diet, exercise, and health, *Dairy Council Digest,* May/June 1985; M. H. Williams, *Nutritional Aspects of Human Physical and Athletic Performance* (Springfield, Ill.: Charles C. Thomas, 1985), pp. 11–17.

sports anemia: a temporary condition of low hemoglobin in the blood, associated with the early stages of sports training or with other strenuous activity.

As you know from Chapter 7, iron-deficiency anemia is widespread. Iron-deficiency anemia hinders exercise performance by limiting the amount of oxygen available to muscles. A person with anemia slips into oxygen debt at even low-intensity work, feels exhausted, and cannot work nearly as long as people with full iron stores can. The more severe the anemia, the greater the hindrance of performance.[30]

People who begin exercising vigorously sometimes develop a particular kind of anemia—**sports anemia.** It is especially likely to develop in two groups with low iron intakes and high iron needs—teens and women involved in running and other strenuous sports. One other group, adult male runners, is also affected, even though iron intakes of this group are usually adequate. Sports anemia is

runners' anemia: a true iron-deficiency anemia that develops in many high-mileage runners.

stress fracture: bone damage or break caused by stress on bone surfaces during exercise.

not the same as iron-deficiency anemia, in that it does not hinder gains in fitness or the ability to perform work.[31]

Sports anemia can strike just about anyone who takes up vigorous exercise. It is not limited to elite athletes. It probably does not reflect a true iron-deficient state, but may be due to the body's adjustment of its blood volume in response to training. In order to increase the blood volume, it first must increase the plasma.[32] Clear, cell-free fluid flows into the vessels. Additional red blood cells, though, take time to produce, and for a while, the number of cells per volume of blood is less than ideal. In two or three weeks, the blood cell count catches up to the plasma volume, but if someone were to take a blood cell count during the lag time, it would indicate anemia. The transient nature of sports anemia supports this theory. Iron-related anemias do not clear up without treatment, but sports anemia always does. Iron supplements are needed when athletes or exercisers have *iron-deficiency* anemia. Sports anemia, while an interesting phenomenon, does not require treatment.

Elite runners and others who exercise heavily sometimes develop a true iron-deficiency anemia, called **runners' anemia.** Iron status might be affected by exercise in any of several ways. For example, it is known that at least a little iron is lost when people sweat, and exercisers sweat more than other people do, although their iron losses diminish with training.[33] Another way that athletes lose iron is by way of red blood cell destruction. When body parts (such as the soles of the feet) make contact with an unyielding surface (such as the ground), some of the blood cells trapped in that part of the body are squashed. The hemoglobin from those destroyed cells is degraded, some of the iron is excreted in the urine, and some is recycled for use by the body. On testing, though, such destruction of red blood cells does not appear to be significant enough to cause true iron-deficiency anemia. What may be more significant is reduced absorption of iron by some athletes and its increased use by muscles in training to make the iron-containing molecules of the muscle tissue needed for energy release.* Perhaps losses by all these routes work together to produce anemia. As you might expect, runners' anemia requires treatment with iron to reverse it.

Two types of anemia are associated with exercise: sports anemia and runners' anemia. The first type, sports anemia, reflects the body's adjustment to increased exercise and does not require treatment. The second type, runners' anemia, occurs in high-mileage runners and must be treated with iron supplements.

Calcium and the Bones

Bones absorb great stresses during exercise, and like the muscles, they respond by growing thicker and stronger along the lines of stress. Sometimes, though, a bone is not strong enough to withstand the strain placed on it by athletic exertion, and it can develop tiny, hairline cracks in what has become known as a **stress fracture.** When a person suffers such a fracture, there are three probable causes. One is unbalanced muscle development, which allows strong muscles to pull against bone opposed only by weaker, undeveloped muscles. Second,

*The molecules are myoglobin, an iron-containing protein, and mitochondrial cytochromes—iron-containing porphyrins.

bone weakness caused by inadequate calcium intake during bone remodeling, especially in young runners, makes bones give way under the pressure of exercise. Third might be a reduced estrogen concentration, which leads to bone mineral loss in women who have stopped menstruating.

Balanced muscle development can help protect the bones from undue stresses. Each set of muscles pulling on bones to bend a joint should be opposed by an equally strong set of muscles pulling to straighten the joint. No one in training should work a set of muscles without working the opposing muscles as well. Another strategy to spare the bones is to have patience in training—to give the bones and muscles plenty of time to build up to one level of performance before subjecting them to additional stress.

athletic amenorrhea (AY-men-o-REE-uh): cessation of menstruation associated with strenuous athletic training.

Some women who exercise strenuously cease to menstruate, a condition called **athletic amenorrhea.** Such women have lower than normal amounts of estrogen, a hormone essential for maintaining the integrity of the bones. With low estrogen levels, the mineral structures of the bones are rapidly dismantled, weakening the skeleton. Women who have athletic amenorrhea are more open to stress fractures now and to osteoporosis in later life.[34] To reverse the condition, they should not stop exercising altogether, for reasonable amounts of exercise may be a key defense against bone depletion. They should, however, seek evaluation from a health care provider who specializes in sports medicine to find the cause of their amenorrhea and to receive treatment.

Eating disorders are sometimes related to athletic amenorrhea, and a logical part of diagnosis is to inspect the diet carefully for adequacy.[35] It could be that a diet too low in calories, coupled with low body fat stores and strenuous exercise, sets the stage for athletic amenorrhea to develop. In such cases, calcium intakes between 1000 and 1500 milligrams per day may help protect the bones somewhat.[36]

Besides those mentioned here, other vitamins and minerals are important to fitness, but these sections have demonstrated the central point—that nutrition is vital to performance. Knowing this, we could easily bet which of two equally trained athletic teams would win a competition—the team whose members habitually consumed half or less of the needed nutrients, or the one whose members arrived with a long history of full nutrient stores and well-met metabolic needs.

During strenuous exercise, weak bones can develop stress fractures. Contributers to this are unbalanced muscle development, inadequate calcium intake, and reduced estrogen in women who have stopped menstruating. Moderate exercise with proper muscle development and high calcium intakes help maintain bone integrity.

Fluids and Electrolytes

The human body relies on watery fluids as the medium for all of its life-supporting chemistry, as Chapter 7 explained in detail. If the body loses too much water, as in dehydration, its chemistry is compromised. The first symptom of dehydration is fatigue. A rapid water loss equal to 5 percent of the body weight can reduce muscular work capacity by 20 to 30 percent.[37]

heat stroke: an acute and dangerous reaction to heat buildup in the body, characterized by high body temperature, loss of consciousness, low blood pressure, and possibly death. *Heat exhaustion* precedes it, with warning signs of fatigue, nausea, dizziness, and stomach cramps.

You know that water is lost from the body via sweat; second to that, breathing costs water, exhaled as vapor. In exercise, both routes can be significant, but sweat is the greater. Remember from Chapter 8 that working muscles produce heat—exercise-induced thermogenesis. Sweating serves to rid the body of its excess heat by evaporation.

In humid, hot weather, sweat doesn't evaporate well because the surrounding air is already laden with water. As body heat builds up, it triggers maximum sweating—the body's only defense against excess heat. Still, without much evaporation, little cooling takes place. In such conditions, active people must take precautions to prevent **heat stroke,** the dangerous accumulation of body heat with accompanying loss of body fluid. The only defense against it is to drink enough fluid before and during the activity, to rest in the shade when tired, and to wear lightweight clothing that encourages evaporation. Hence the danger of rubber or heavy suits sold supposedly to promote weight loss during exercise—they promote profuse sweating, prevent sweat evaporation, and invite heat stroke.

The recommended "enough fluid" to prevent heat stroke can be quite a bit. Even though they conserve water better than do others, athletes can lose 2 to 4 quarts of fluid *every hour* of heavy exercise. The digestive system can absorb a mere quart in an hour. Hence, the athlete must rehydrate before, during, and after exercise to prevent excessive loss. Even then, in heavy exercise in hot weather, the digestive tract may not be able to absorb enough water fast enough to keep up with an athlete's sweating losses, and some degree of dehydration becomes inevitable. Athletes who are preparing for competition are often advised to drink extra fluids in the few days before the event, especially if they are in training. Of course, extra water is not stored in the body, but drinking extra water ensures maximum levels of hydration at the start of the event. The athlete who arrives slightly dehydrated from chronic insufficient fluid intake arrives with a disadvantage. There is no harm in drinking a few extra glasses of water a day, and it may be protective.

Even casual exercisers must tend carefully to their fluid needs. Exercise blunts the thirst mechanism. During heavy exercise, thirst is unreliable as an indicator of how much to drink—it signals too late, after fluid stores are depleted, so during exercise, don't wait to feel thirsty before drinking. Plan in advance to drink enough. Table 9–4 presents one schedule of hydration for exercise. To find out how much water is needed to replenish losses after a workout, weigh yourself before and after—the difference is all water. One pound equals roughly 2 cups fluid (a quart equals 2 pounds).

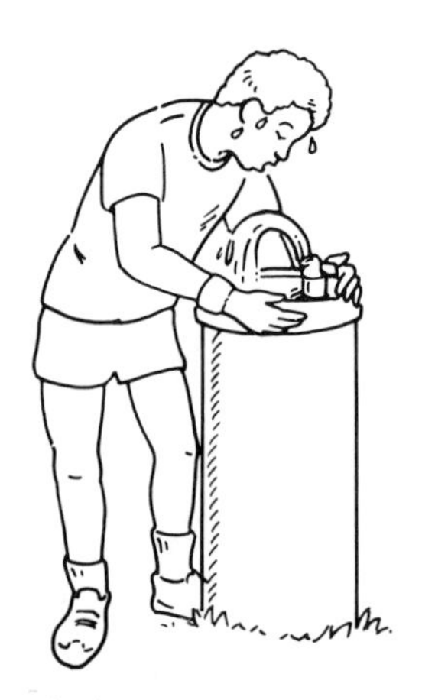

Cold water is the optimal beverage for replacing fluids.

Table 9–4

Schedule of Hydration Before and During Exercise

When to Drink	Amount of Fluid
2 hours before exercise	About 3 c
10 to 15 minutes before exercise	About 2 c
Every 10 to 20 minutes during exercise	About ½ c or more
After exercise	Replace each pound of body weight lost with 2 c fluid

Source: Adapted from J. B. Marcus, ed., *Sports Nutrition* (Chicago: American Dietetic Association, 1986), p. 57.

Sports Drinks

Many good-tasting drinks are marketed for active people. Manufacturers claim that if a drink tastes good, people will drink more, thereby ensuring adequate hydration. In addition, they say, the drinks duplicate the fluid lost in sweat, and so can facilitate performance. Furthermore, the drinks supply energy from carbohydrate—another proposed edge over plain water. Exercise physiologists counter most of these claims.

For one thing, immediate replacement of the minerals lost in sweat isn't necessary; hours after competition is soon enough. Further, a major ingredient in the drinks is salt, and most people eat diets that are already so high in salt that they can aggravate hypertension—a major health problem in this country. Salt-containing drinks could counteract the blood-pressure-normalizing effects of exercise. In rare cases of the most strenuous competition at the world-class level, heavy sweating for many days in a row has been reported to dilute the blood concentration of sodium, and in these few cases, sodium repletion was needed. For the average exerciser, though, salt in drinks is in excess and places an extra burden on the kidneys to excrete it.

On one aspect of the needs of the athlete, researchers agree with the companies: a beverage that supplies glucose in some form might be desirable during an endurance event that lasts more than just a couple of hours. In such cases, use a weak sugar solution (2 tablespoons table sugar or 1 cup of fruit juice in a quart of water), but not a commercially prepared sports drink, because it contains too much sugar that slows down its absorption. Some manufacturers of commercial sports beverages have changed their formulas to include starch-like **glucose polymers,** but whether these are more quickly absorbed than the glucose-containing ones is debatable. While carbohydrate is known to enhance the performance of an endurance athlete in grueling competitive events, such as marathon runs, it is of no value to the average exerciser, and is counterproductive if weight loss is a goal. Glucose is sugar, and like candy, provides the exerciser with only empty calories—no nutrients. Sports drinks contain about half the sugar of ordinary soft drinks, about five teaspoons in each twelve ounces.

The commercial drinks do provide a psychological edge for some people who equate the drinks with athletes and sports. The need to belong is valid, but it may be preferable to satisfy it with athletic equipment, clothing, or teammates, rather than with sports drinks. The fluid you choose should have a lower concentration of dissolved solids, such as sugars and salts, than does body fluid, because such a fluid enters the tissues most quickly. If the solution has too much dissolved solid, as do sports drinks, it will demand dilution in the digestive tract, pulling still more fluid from the tissues instead of replenishing it. Fructose is sometimes used in fluids to raise blood sugar before exercise. It does not elicit as high an insulin response as does glucose and so does not drive energy-yielding nutrients into cells. Fructose causes other problems, though. It often causes gas, and some people experience bloating, pain, and diarrhea after consuming it—a definite disadvantage to exercise performance.[38]

glucose polymers: compounds that supply glucose, not as single molecules, but linked in chains somewhat like starch. The object is to exert less attraction to water (osmotic attraction depends on the number, not the size of particles), and so not "pull" water from the body into the digestive tract.

What is the best fluid for your exercising body? Surprisingly, cold water, especially in warm weather. It is the optimal beverage for replacing fluids, because it leaves the digestive tract and so enters tissues faster than room temperature water, and it cools the body.[39] If the weather is cold and you are exercising outdoors, choose room temperature or warm beverages; the absorption advantages conferred by cold temperature are overshadowed by the threat of loss of too much body heat, a condition equally as dangerous as heat stroke.

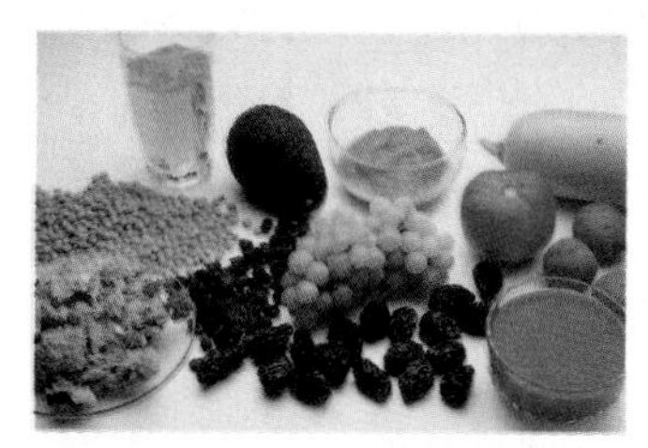

These foods are rich in potassium per calorie. Note that they are whole foods in several categories—not just fruits.

Electrolytes, the charged minerals sodium, potassium, magnesium, and chloride, are lost from the body in sweat. People who are just beginning an exercise regimen lose electrolytes to a much greater extent than do trained people; as the body trains, it becomes better at conserving them. An exception is magnesium; its losses in sweat are about the same for trained and untrained individuals. One study found magnesium levels in the cell-free blood to be lower in exercising people than in others; the effect remained even three months after exercise began.[40] This could mean that a magnesium deficiency was coming on, or it could mean that the magnesium had moved out of the blood and into the tissues in response to training.

As the box on sports drinks says, most times exercisers need make no special effort to replenish lost electrolytes; a regular diet that meets their energy and nutrient needs also supplies all the electrolytes they need. There is also no need to replace them during exercise, unless you work up a drenching sweat exceeding 3 percent of body weight (5 to 10 lost pounds) a day for several consecutive days. Under such conditions, a "sweat replacer" beverage, diluted with an equal volume of water, may be drunk for fluid replacement; a homemade mixture of 1 cup of fruit juice added to each quart of water will also serve the purpose. Avoid electrolyte tablets or salt tablets; they can irritate the stomach, can cause vomiting, encourage further potassium depletion, and always cause water to flow into the digestive tract from the tissues, thereby worsening dehydration and impairing performance.[41]

As for potassium, it usually remains safely inside the cells, where it does its work. However, in dehydration, it does migrate outside of cells, and if profuse sweating goes on day after day, potassium is lost. Even so, it is easily replaced with just a few servings of whole foods. The more processed a food, the lower its potassium content; whole, unprocessed foods of all kinds provide it abundantly, as Table 7–7 in Chapter 7 clearly shows. As already stated, potassium supplements are to be avoided unless prescribed by a physician, because, while they better some conditions, they worsen others.

Athletes, like others, sometimes drink beverages that contain alcohol or caffeine. Both are diuretics, and both promote the excretion of water, vitamins, and minerals—exactly the wrong effect for fluid balance and nutrition. Both also have other effects on performance. The accompanying box discusses the use of these and other practices that are best avoided, for health's sake.

Fluid is crucial to exercise performance, and must be provided before, during, and after activity. Heat stroke is a dangerous condition caused by fluid loss that inhibits the body's cooling system. Electrolytes are lost during exercise, but do not require replacement during activity.

Drugs, Blood Doping, and Hormones

Practices athletes follow may include not only the use of nutrients, but also the use of alcohol, caffeine, a technique known as blood doping, and self-administration of steroid drugs and growth hormone. Some of these practices are harmful; some, beneficial in some ways. None, however, is neutral.

The text mentioned that both alcohol and caffeine are diuretics and that they therefore adversely affect fluid balance. Aside from that, they have other effects. It may seem unimaginable that someone would drink a few beers before a run, but imagine a ski lodge party where hot toddies are available. In such a festive atmosphere, the person could easily be enticed to drink alcohol before skiing without even being conscious of doing so. Alcohol taken before sports slows reactions at a time when fast action is often needed, sometimes with disastrous results. Many sports-related fatalities involve alcohol or other drugs. (Read about the effects of alcohol on the brain in Controversy 12.)

As well as being a diuretic, caffeine is a stimulant, and athletes sometimes use it to enhance performance. In college, national, and international competitions, it is a forbidden drug in amounts greater than the equivalent of 2 cups of coffee. Taken in moderation before an event, caffeine offers one clear advantage: it mobilizes fat from stores, a process that normally does not become maximal until intense activity is under way. The competitor who drinks a cup or two of coffee 30 minutes to an hour before the start of an event will be using the most efficient fuel mixture right from the start and will conserve glycogen stores.[42] The casual exerciser might try working out an hour or so after drinking coffee in the morning to ease the start of the exercise session.

The technique known as **blood doping** sounds like drug use, but it actually has nothing to do with drugs. Blood doping is the practice of collecting one's own red blood cells and storing them for later use. A blood bank might do this for someone anticipating surgery, so that the person's own blood cells would be available if a transfusion were needed. An athlete practicing blood doping would save up red blood cells beforehand, and then, before a competitive event, receive a transfusion. Because the athlete has lost no blood, the added cells dramatically raise the blood count. Doped blood could, therefore, theoretically carry more oxygen to the muscles, enhancing performance. The evidence indicates that blood doping confers some degree of increased performance. Whether the practice is safe is unknown, but it has been deemed unethical. It also exposes the person's blood to the environment, thus incurring a health risk. It may be outlawed in competition, but methods for detecting red blood cells cannot indicate with certainty that cells have been added—that the blood was doped.

Long ago, people realized that men develop bulkier muscles in response to exercise than do women, because men produce larger amounts of certain **steroid hormones** in their bodies. Some people, both men and women, dose themselves with added steroid hormones in the attempt to grow bulkier muscles. Whether those muscles boost athletic performance is still

(continued on following page)

blood doping: an untested procedure that involves collecting and storing an athlete's own blood prior to competition, then adding it back to the person's blood supply in the attempt to overcome the limits on performance set by the oxygen-carrying capacity of the blood.

steroid hormones: hormones with a chemical structure similar to that of cholesterol; such hormones have wide-ranging effects on body functioning.

unproven, but the risks associated with steroid use are certain.[43] For one thing, all steroid users experience a sharp change in their blood lipid content to the type associated with high risk of heart disease.[44] In addition, some steroid users suffer impairment of liver function, cancerous liver tumors, liver rupture and hemorrhage, permanent changes in the reproductive system, and altered facial appearance.

Hormones other than steroids carry risks, too. Athletes who take human growth hormone to increase their muscle size develop symptoms of the disease acromegaly—huge body size and other deformities as described in the box of Chapter 8 (p. 298), and an increased likelihood of death before age 50.[45] This practice may be even more damaging to health than steroid use.

Steroid drug use has been ruled illegal by professional, collegiate, and Olympic athletic governing boards. Steroids are hard to detect, though, since their effects on the body remain long after the drugs themselves have disappeared from the body. Testing for these drugs at the time of the event is rarely effective.

Scientists do not yet know what symptoms may result from 20 years of steroid abuse, but they predict serious liver and bone disease, heart disease, and other severe health problems. For now, serious athletes must make a hard choice—to use no steroids and face what may be a field full of artificially endowed opponents, or to use the drugs and risk both their side effects and the punitive actions of athletic governing boards. Judging from estimates that from 50 to as many as 90 percent of professional athletes are using steroids, many must view the risks of steroid use to be less severe than the risks of even a theoretical disadvantage in competition.

Food for Performance

How should a person who wishes to eat for performance go about it? The most basic of all needs, nutrient adequacy, should undoubtedly be the first goal, for a lack of nutrients will undermine even the most carefully thought-out training plan. To review the foods in which nutrients reside, turn back to Chapter 2, and look again at the comparison of the high-fat and high-nutrient-density meals (pp. 56–57). For athletes, for fitness seekers, for everyone, the secret to adequate nourishment lies in selecting those foods that are not prefabricated, partitioned, and synthetic, but are whole—vegetables, meats, legumes, whole grains, starchy vegetables, fruits, and milk.

Athletes do not always choose so wisely, though. In a study of men athletes, only half knew basic nutrition facts.[46] In a study of women athletes, all who were questioned knew the importance of calcium, but only 12 percent chose diets that provided the RDA of calcium.[47] Reported intakes of some nutrients were not quite as dismal as for calcium—fewer than half of the women received the RDA for vitamin A, but most (69 percent) received enough vitamin C. Along with a host of other vitamins and minerals, chromium, magnesium, and iron are needed by athletes for critical steps in oxygen delivery and energy use, but few people get enough from the diets they choose. Most people, and especially active ones with high energy needs, can meet their nutrient needs by carefully choosing whole foods.[48]

glycogen loading: a technique of exercising, followed by eating a high-carbohydrate diet, that enables muscles to store glycogen beyond their normal capacity.

Planning the Diet

The diet recommended for most people in Chapter 3, a diet high in complex carbohydrates, is the best choice to ensure the full glycogen stores that endurance athletes require. Thus, the diet that provides the best balance of nutrients for just about anyone also supports physical activity best, as Figure 9–7 demonstrates.

Some endurance athletes use a technique called **glycogen loading** to trick their muscles into storing extra glycogen. When the technique was first introduced, athletes were taught a two-step procedure. First, they restricted their carbohydrate intake for several days by eating meals high in protein and fat; simultaneously, they exercised heavily to empty their muscles of glycogen. Then they reduced the intensity of the exercise and switched abruptly to a diet high in carbohydrate. Muscle glycogen stores rebounded to about two to four times the normal level.

Glycogen loading practiced this way may have side effects, including abnormal heartbeat; swollen, painful muscles (glycogen attracts and holds water); and weight gain immediately before competition. Most exercise physiologists now recommend a modified plan that confers similar benefits but that is not so extreme. The athlete exercises intensely without restricting carbohydrates, then

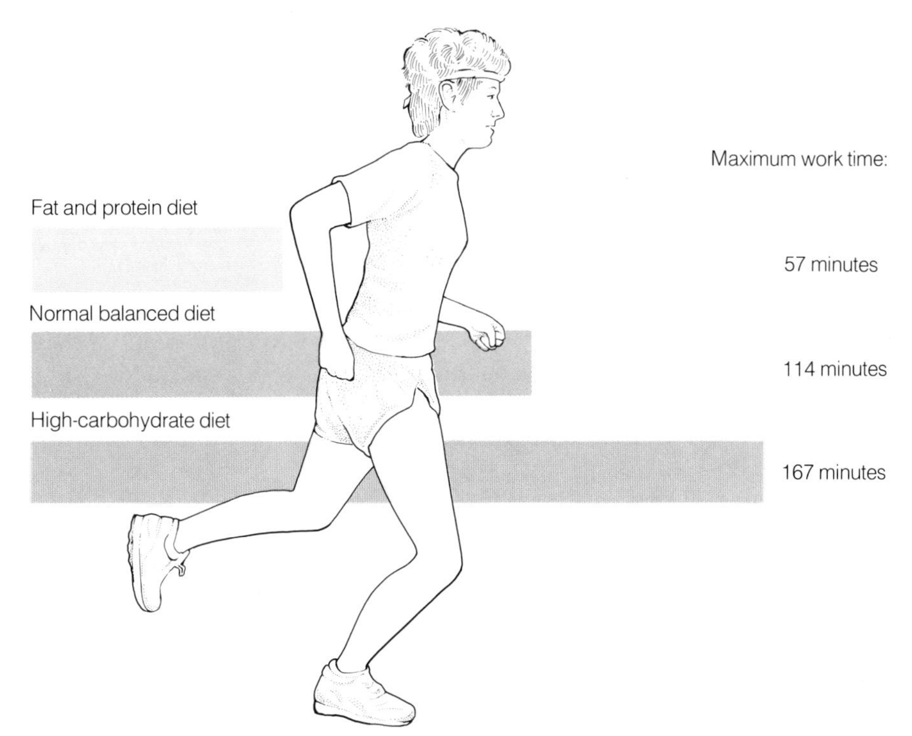

Figure 9–7
The Effect of Diet on Physical Endurance. A high-carbohydrate diet can triple an athlete's endurance.

Source: Data from P. Astrand, Something old and something new . . . very new, *Nutrition Today,* June 1968, pp. 9–11.

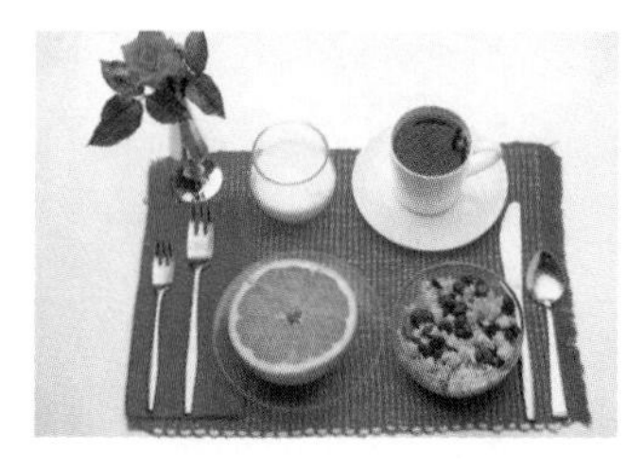

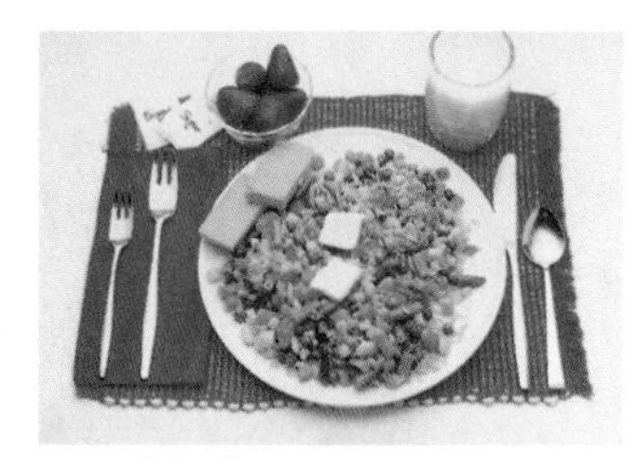

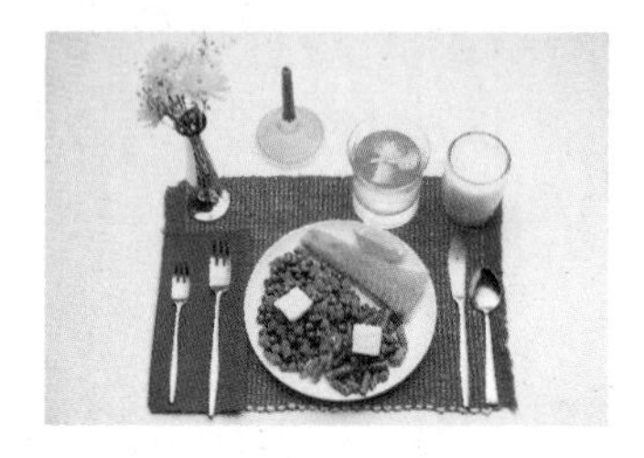

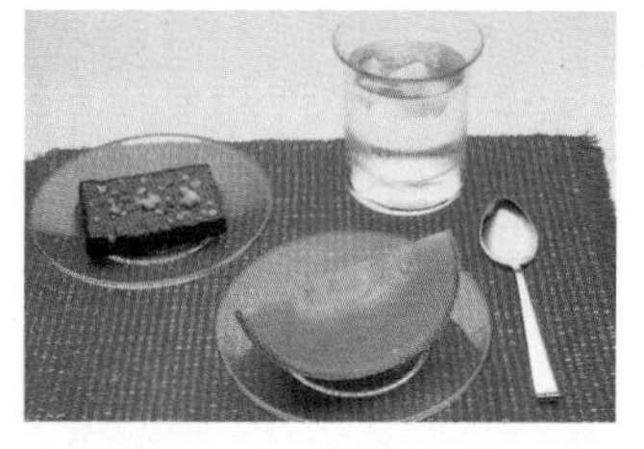

If you are looking for a diet to support performance, look no further than carbohydrate-rich, whole, nutrient-dense foods.

during the week before competition gradually cuts back on exercise, rests completely the day before, and eats a very-high-carbohydrate diet.[49] In the modified plan, carbohydrates are never restricted; only exercise levels are manipulated, and extra carbohydrate is packed in at the end. Endurance athletes who follow this plan can keep going longer than their competitors without ill effects. In a hot climate, extra glycogen confers an additional advantage; as glycogen breaks down, it releases water, which helps to meet the athlete's fluid needs.[50] For the regular, everyday exerciser, such extremes in glycogen storage are unnecessary. (Remember, glycogen isn't likely to run out in a short exercise session.) All that is necessary to provide consistently full glycogen stores for workouts is to eat a high-carbohydrate diet based on whole foods, and to allow muscle groups to recover fully before working them again. Full recovery of glycogen stores takes from 24 to 48 hours. This doesn't mean you can only work out every other day; it means you should vary your exercise routine from day to day as suggested earlier, work different groups of muscles on different days, and rest on one or two days each week.

Notice that the high-nutrient-density meals of Chapter 2, repeated here, provide 57 percent of their calories from carbohydrate. For most people, this is close to ideal. Athletes who wish to pack their muscles with extra glycogen are told to try for a diet that is even higher in carbohydrate, up to 80 percent. The exchange lists (Chapter 2) tell us that the food groups that donate the most carbohydrate are grains/starchy vegetables, fruits, and milk. Table 9–5 shows some sample diet plans for people who wish to increase their carbohydrate intakes along with their calories by using whole foods. These plans are not for glycogen loading before an event, but are for daily use by active people. In using them, choose whole foods to provide nutrients as well as calories—extra milk for calcium and riboflavin, many vegetables for vitamins A and C, B vitamins, and minerals, meat or meat alternates for iron and other vitamins and minerals,

Table 9–5

Diet Plans for High-Calorie, High-Carbohydrate Intakes

Use the number of exchanges indicated, to arrive at the specified energy levels.

	Energy Level				
Exchange	*3000 cal*	*3300 cal*	*3800 cal*	*4400 cal*	*5400 cal*
Nonfat milk	3	4	5	6	8
Vegetable	9	10	11	13	13
Fruit	8	8	10	12	16
Starchy vegetable/ grain	16	17	20	22	26
Lean meat	7	8	8	11	15
Fat	8	10	10	10	12

Note: These plans supply 55 to 60% of calories as carbohydrate and less than 30% as fat. To increase the carbohydrate content to over 60%, substitute ⅓-c servings of legumes for the meats. People who cannot eat these quantities of whole foods may have to replace some of them with refined sugars and fats in order to meet their energy needs.

and whole grains for magnesium and chromium. In addition, these foods provide plenty of sodium, potassium, and chloride.

Adding more carbohydrate-rich foods is a sound and reasonable option for increasing calories, up to a point. The point at which it becomes unreasonable is when the calories needed outnumber those the person can eat from such foods. At that point, the person must find ways of adding concentrated sources of energy to the diet, mostly through the addition of refined sugars and even some fat.

It is well and good to eat carbohydrate, you might think, but what about protein? Can a diet so rich in carbohydrate meet protein needs? Fit people have more muscle mass; exercise involves muscles; muscles are made largely of protein. It would seem, then, that to exercise, one might need to eat more protein than normal. Muscular, active people do use more protein in their activities than others.[51] But most people's diets—even the diets of vegetarians, and certainly those presented in Table 9–5—contain about twice as much protein as they can possibly use, no matter how active or muscular they are. They are actually using about half the protein they eat not to build lean tissue, but rather for energy. As shown in the Food Feature of Chapter 5, anyone who meets a day's energy needs with whole foods probably consumes double the RDA for protein—more than enough, even for elite athletes. The photo in the margin should drive this point home.

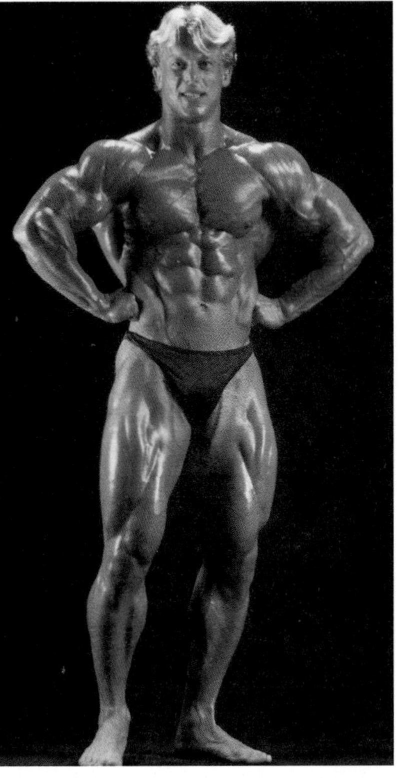

This is a body that vegetables built: Andreas Cahling, a vegetarian.

Wouldn't it be nice if we could force extra protein into our muscles just by eating more of it? Actually, cells don't respond to what's given to them by helplessly accepting it. They respond to the hormones that regulate them and to the demands put upon them, and they select the nutrients they need from what is offered. The way to make muscles grow is to put a demand on them—that is, to make them work. Active people, by eating the extra calories they need to sustain their activity, avoid having to use food protein for energy and can use it instead to replace lost muscle protein.

When the sport season is over, or when activity drops off for any reason, it is equally important to cut back food intake to avoid gaining body fat. A classic case is that of the ex-college athlete who complains that, in later years, all his muscle has "turned to fat." In response to sedentary life, muscle no longer needed for sports is broken down, and if the energy is not expended in activity, it can indeed be used to build fat. A bigger contributer to overfatness, though, is the failure of the athlete to cut back on food intake to match lower activity levels.

In summary, the diet that supports performance is similar in composition to the diet that best supports health. This diet also happens to be the one most protective against disease. Think back to the diet recommendations in Controversies 3, 4, 5, and 7—the ones to minimize risks of the diseases diabetes, atherosclerosis, cancer, and hypertension. Recommended in each case was a diet of whole, minimally processed foods, low in fat, sugar, and salt, and high in complex carbohydrates, vitamins, and minerals. The exerciser who needs more energy should meet the need with regular whole foods—milk, fruit, breads, and legumes—to provide carbohydrate along with protein, vitamins, and minerals. Only on certain occasions should people deviate from these recommendations. One case is during intensive training, when energy needs outstrip the capacity to eat enough whole foods; in that case, sugar and fat are also needed. Another special occasion is the pregame meal.

The Pregame Meal

Before a competitive event, is there any special way that a person should eat? Many coaches and athletes believe intensely in special food rituals—breakfasting on T-bones, avoiding milk because it causes mucus or "cotton mouth," or taking only liquids before the event. Do rituals work?

Scientifically, no particular food confers a special benefit before an athletic contest, but particular kinds of food make a difference. A meal of steak may boost morale, but it is high in fat and may take so long to digest that it hinders performance. The idea that milk causes cotton mouth is pure superstition; if low in fat, milk is perfectly permissible in the pregame meal. Fluids are essential before competition; a lack of fluid *can* cause "cotton mouth." Some foods are permissible, and perhaps even beneficial, up to three or four hours before the event although some successful athletes take a ritual fast in these "magic" hours.

On the other hand, most food rituals have little physical effect, and some can impair performance. If a harmless but scientifically unproven practice gives a competitor extra confidence, it can make the difference between winning and losing and so should be respected, but no foods actually have unusual power to promote performance.

Does it matter at all what the meal before an event consists of? Olympic training tables are laden with foods such as breads, pasta, rice, potatoes, and fruit juice. These are wise choices, for three reasons. They are high in carbohydrate—the fuel the athlete needs to store before the event. They are low in fat and have little protein, which would stay in the digestive tract too long. And they are low in fiber. Fiber is normally highly desirable, but not right before physical exertion, because it remains in the digestive tract and attracts water out of the blood. Any meal should be finished at least three or four hours before the event, for two reasons. First, digestion requires routing the blood supply to the digestive tract to pick up nutrients, and second, insulin levels should be back to normal so that they will not oppose fuel release.

The athlete may not want to have a meal before the event, but may choose a snack instead. The following Food Feature discusses snacks for the athlete, and for people in general.

A diet high in carbohydrate; adequate in protein, vitamins, and minerals; and low in fat best supports athletic performance. Such a diet is best constructed from whole, minimally processed foods. The pregame meal is an exception; it should emphasize digestibility and so can include refined foods and sugars, and it should be finished at least 3 to 4 hours before the start of the event.

Food Feature

Snacks, Snackers, and Snacking

Table 9–6 lists some small meals that meet the needs of the athlete before a game. Note that they all deliver fluid with carbohydrate, so that they will be absorbed quickly. Note, too, that they are all vitamin and mineral poor. They are not recommended for regular, daily consumption—just for the one meal

Table 9–6

Sample Pregame Snacks

These foods, to be eaten three to four hours before competition, do *not* have many vitamins or minerals for the most part, and should not be overemphasized in the daily diet. The hours before competition are too late for vitamins and minerals, but the special needs for energy and fluid can be met by eating the following snacks.

Food	Serving Size	Energy (cal)	Energy Donated by Carbohydrate (% of calories)
Sample Snack #1			
White bread	2 slices	140	74
Jam or jelly	2 tbsp	130	100
Gelatin dessert	1 c	70	97
Grape juice	1 c	165	100
Total		505	94
Sample Snack #2			
Spaghetti and tomato sauce (canned, plain)	1 c	190	80
Roll (white flour)	1	85	71
Popsicle (3 oz)	2	140	100
Limeade	1 c	100	100
Total		515	90
Sample Snack #3			
Banana	1	100	100
Sweetened dry cereal	¾ c	115	90
Nonfat milk	½ c	45	53
Cranberry juice cocktail	⅔ c	109	100
Gumdrops	1 oz	100	100
Total		469	95

Note: Substitutions can be made for cereal (1 c), spaghetti (1 c), or bread (2 slices):

- 1 c white or flavored rice.
- 1 3-inch-diameter muffin (plain).
- 1 piece angel food cake.
- 3 small pancakes and syrup.

To substitute liquids (gelatin, juices, limeade), use 1 c for each: 1 c any sugar-sweetened beverage.

before competition. For athletes at other times, and for people in general, a different mode of snacking is in order.

Another reason athletes snack is to pack in extra food. An athlete who cannot fit the needed food comfortably into three meals may need to consume it in six or eight meals each day, rather than three or four meals. Large between-meal snacks of milk shakes with egg, ice cream, and peanut butter added; dried fruits; peanut butter sandwiches; or cheese and crackers can add substantial food energy and nutrients to the day's intakes. The Food Feature of Chapter 8 provided hints to those who want to gain weight. Those hints are applicable to the athlete who needs to snack for energy, too.

A thread of moralizing seems to run through many people's pronouncements on snacking. You should eat three meals a day, shouldn't skip breakfast, shouldn't eat between meals, and so on. Some good reasons lie behind these commandments, but the rules may not apply in all cases. "Eat three meals a day" is an admonition based on the finding that people who skip breakfast and/or lunch often overeat or snack on nonnutritious foods when they do eat. That is, meal skippers are more likely to be obese, inadequately nourished, or both. The directive to eat breakfast comes from the observation that schoolchildren remain alert, maintain higher morale, perform better, and earn higher grades if they have eaten breakfast before their morning classes.[52]

grazing: eating small amounts of food at intervals all day, rather than, or in addition to, eating regular meals.

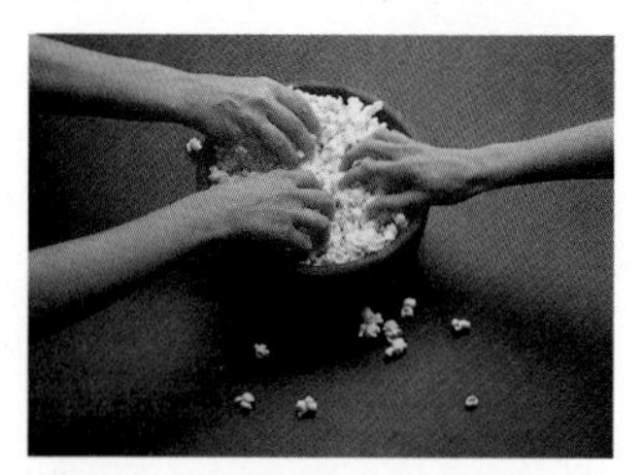

A complex-carbohydrate, high-fiber snack.

However, individuals differ. A meal skipper who makes a habit of **grazing** on many nutritious, moderate snacks that add up, within a day, to a balanced diet may well be neither too fat nor poorly nourished. The "don't snack" dictum is based on the assumption that snacks represent food eaten beyond need and therefore that they promote obesity, or that most snacks are composed of nonnutritious foods and so displace needed nutrients. Neither is necessarily the case, especially for a person who wants to *gain* weight. For such a person, many small meals throughout the day may best pack in extra calories and nutrients. Table 9–7 shows the calories in some common snack foods.

Table 9–7

Food Energy in Snacks

Snack	Food Energy (cal)
1 c air popped popcorn	30
1 c caramel corn	135
6 crackers	75
6 tsp dip	70
½ c nuts	400
8 oz commercial fruit yogurt	230
8 oz plain nonfat yogurt and ½ c fruit	150
1 egg roll	250

A study of snackers who live in the United States revealed that people's ideas of what constitutes a snack vary by sex, age, and income level, as well as by where people live and whether or not they are on weight-reduction diets.[53] People in the western states prefer fruit and vegetables, while people in the northeastern states prefer pizza and sandwiches. Women tend to eat more nutritious snack foods than do men, while older people and people on weight-reduction diets are most likely to choose brownies, pastries, cheesecake, and ice cream with toppings. Dieters rarely choose vegetables. Of people in all the income brackets, those with middle incomes do the most grazing.

shopping list:
fresh fruit
rice cakes, plain crackers, bagel chips
popcorn
plain yogurt (add your own fruit for sweetness)
crunchy vegetables
low-calorie dip, such as Mexican tomato sauce (salsa)

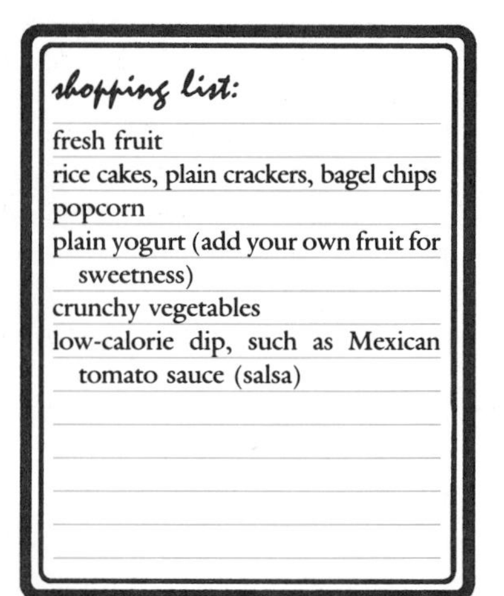

Whatever kind of snacker you are, the questions to ask are:

- What nutrients do the snacks contribute?
- Are the nutrients needed?
- How can meals and snacks be adjusted to provide the best total nutrition picture for the day?

If you like to snack, allow room in your diet for nutritious choices, purchase the foods you like, and eat them when you feel like it. Try to avoid impulsive snacks that are high in fat, sugar, or salt; eat the ones you've planned for.

Self-Study

Estimate Your Fitness Level

This exercise presents a simple method of estimating your fitness level. A human performance laboratory would perform actual tests and more extensive calculations.

Occupation and Daily Activities

1. I usually walk to and from work or shopping (at least 1/2 mile each way). 1 point

2. I usually take the stairs rather than use elevators or escalators. 1 point

3. The type of physical activity involved in my job or daily household routine is best described by the following statement (select one):

a. Most of my workday is spent in office work, light physical activity, or household chores. 0 points

b. Most of my workday is spent in farm activities, moderate physical activity, brisk walking, or comparable activities. 4 points

c. My typical workday includes several hours of heavy physical activity (shoveling, lifting, etc.) 9 points

Leisure Activities

4. I do several hours of gardening or lawn work each week. 1 point

5. I fish or hunt once a week or more, on the average. (Fishing must involve active work, such as rowing a boat. Dock sitting does not count.) 1 point

6. At least once a week, I participate for an hour or more in vigorous dancing like square or folk dancing. 1 point

7. In season, I play golf at least once a week, and I do not use a power cart. 2 points

8. I often walk for exercise or recreation. 1 point

9. When I feel bothered by pressures at work or home, I use exercise as a way to relax. 1 point

10. Two or more times a week, I perform calisthenic exercises (sit-ups, push-ups) for at least 10 minutes per session. 3 points

11. I regularly participate in yoga or perform stretching exercises. 2 points

12. I participate in active recreational sports such as tennis or handball:

a. About once a week. 2 points

b. About twice a week. 4 points

c. Three times a week or more. 7 points

13. I participate in vigorous fitness activities such as jogging or swimming (at least 20 continuous minutes per session):

a. About once a week. 3 points

b. About twice a week. 5 points

c. Three times a week or more. 10 points

Total points: ______

Scoring:

- 0 to 5 points: sedentary — This amount of exercise is inadequate and leads to a steady deterioration in fitness. Improvement is needed.
- 6 to 11 points: light activity — This level of activity slows the rate of fitness loss but will not maintain adequate fitness levels in most persons.
- 12 to 20 points: moderate activity — This amount of activity will maintain an acceptable level of physical fitness.
- 21 points and over: heavy activity — This level of activity will maintain a high state of physical fitness.

Source: Adapted with permission of Russell Pate Ph.D. (University of South Carolina, Columbia Human Performance Laboratory).

Notes

1. Much of the discussion about fitness is derived from Chapter 7, Fitness, in *Life Choices: Health Concepts and Strategies,* by F. S. Sizer and E. N. Whitney (St. Paul, Minn.: West, 1988).
2. R. S. Paffenbarger and coauthors, Physical activity, all-cause mortality, and longevity of college alumni, *New England Journal of Medicine* 314 (1986): 605–613.
3. V. Gurley, A. Neuringer, and J. Massee, Dance and sports compared: Effects on psychological well-being, *Journal of Sports Medicine* 24 (1984): 58–68.
4. K. T. Francis and R. Carter, Psychological characteristics of joggers, *Journal of Sports Medicine* 22 (1982): 386–391; R. M. Hayden and G. J. Allen, Relationship between aerobic exercise, anxiety, and depression: Convergent validation by knowledgeable informants, *Journal of Sports Medicine* 24 (1984): 69–74.
5. Quantity and quality of exercise for developing and maintaining fitness in healthy adults, a position paper of The American College of Sports Medicine, *Physician and Sportsmedicine* 6 (1978): 39–41.
6. N. E. Lane, D. A. Block, and H. H. Jones, Long distance running, bone density, and osteoarthritis, *Journal of the American Medical Association* 255 (1986): 1147–1151.
7. Quantity and quality of exercise, 1978.
8. S. Rainville and P. Vaccaro, Lipoprotein cholesterol levels, coronary artery disease and regular exercise: A review, *American Corrective Therapy Journal* 37 (1983): 161–165; B. Stamford, Improving coronary circulation, *Physician and Sportsmedicine* 11 (1983): 163.
9. N. B. Belloc and L. Breslow, Relationship of physical health status and health practices, *Preventive Medicine* 1 (1972): 409–421.
10. C. M. Tipton, Exercise, training, and hypertension, *Exercise and Sports Sciences Reviews* 12 (1984): 245–306.
11. K. Jung, Physical exercise therapy in juvenile diabetes mellitus, *Journal of Sports Medicine* 22 (1982): 23–31.
12. D. H. Garabrant and coauthors, Job activity and colon cancer risk, *American Journal of Epidemiology* 119 (1984): 1005–1014.
13. A. Viti and coauthors, Effect of exercise on plasma interferon levels, *Journal of Applied Physiology,* August 1985, pp. 426–428; H. B. Simon, The immunology of exercise, *Journal of the American Medical Association* 252 (1984): 2735–2738; J. G. Cannon and M. J. Kluger, Exercise enhances survival rate in mice infected with *Salmonella typhimurium, Proceedings of the Society for Experimental Biology and Medicine* 175 (1984): 518–521.
14. C. E. Thompson and coauthors, Response of HDL cholesterol, apoprotein A–1, and LCAT to exercise withdrawal, *Atherosclerosis* 54 (1985): 65–73.
15. J. P. Flatt, Dietary fat, carbohydrate balance, weight maintenance: Effects of exercise, *American Journal of Clinical Nutrition* 45 (1987): 296–306.
16. E. Jequier, Carbohydrates: Energetics and performance, *Nutrition Reviews* 44 (1986): 55–59.
17. R. C. Hickson, Carbohydrate metabolism in exercise, *Report of the Ross Symposium on Nutrient Utilization during Exercise* (Columbus, Ohio: Ross Laboratories, 1983), pp. 1–8.
18. J. L. Ivy and coauthors, Enhanced performance with carbohydrate supplements during endurance exercise, *Report of the Ross Symposium on Nutrient Utilization during Exercise* (Columbus, Ohio: Ross Laboratories, 1983), pp. 54–60.
19. Jequier, 1986.
20. K. Keller and R. Schwarzkopf, Preexercise snacks may decrease exercise performance, *Physician and Sportsmedicine* 12 (1984): 89–91.
21. R. Bielinski, Y. Schutz, and E. Jequier, Energy metabolism during the postexercise recovery in man, *American Journal of Clinical Nutrition* 42 (1985): 69–82.
22. G. L. Dohm, Protein metabolism in exercise, *Report of the Ross Symposium on Nutrient Utilization during Exercise* (Columbus, Ohio: Ross Laboratories, 1983), pp. 8–13.
23. L. W. Rosen and coauthors, Pathogenic weight-control behavior in female athletes, *Physician and Sportsmedicine* 14 (1986): 79–86.
24. M. H. Williams, *Nutritional Aspects of Human Physical and Athletic Performance* (Springfield, Illinois: Charles C. Thomas, 1985), pp. 152–155.
25. A. Z. Belko and coauthors, Effects of exercise on riboflavin requirements: Biological validation in weight reducing women, *American Journal of Clinical Nutrition* 41 (1985): 270–277.
26. D. M. Dreon and G. E. Butterfield, Vitamin B_6 utilization in active and inactive young men, *American Journal of Clinical Nutrition* 43 (1986): 816–824.
27. Williams, 1985, pp. 156–158.
28. M. H. Williams, Vitamin supplementation and physical performance, *Report of the Ross Symposium on Nutrient Utilization during Exercise* (Columbus, Ohio: Ross Laboratories, 1983), pp. 26–30.
29. F. T. O'Neil, M. T. Hynak-Hankinson, and J. Gorman, Research and application of current topics in sports nutrition, *Journal of the American Dietetic Association* 86 (1986): 1007–1015.
30. B. J. Koziol and coauthors, Changes in work tolerance associated with metabolic and physiological adjustment to moderate and severe iron deficiency anemia, *American Journal of Clinical Nutrition* 36 (1982): 830–839.
31. S. M. Blum, A. R. Sherman, and R. A. Boileau, The effects of fitness-type exercise on iron status in adult women, *American Journal of Clinical Nutrition* 43 (1986): 456–463.
32. R. H. Dressendorfer, C. E. Wade, and E. A. Amsterdam, Development of pseudoanemia in marathon runners during a 20-day road race, *Journal of the American Medical Association* 246 (1981): 1215–1218.
33. M. Brune and coauthors, Iron losses in sweat, *American Journal of Clinical Nutrition* 43 (1986): 438–443.
34. M. E. Nelson and coauthors, Diet and bone status in amenorrheic runners, *American Journal of Clinical Nutrition* 43 (1986): 910–916.
35. Nelson and coauthors, 1986.
36. Osteoporosis Consensus Conference, *Journal of the American Medical Association* 252 (1984): 799–802.
37. J. Bergstrom and E. Hultman, Nutrition for maximal sports performance, *Journal of the American Medical Association* 221 (1972): 999.
38. W. Hasler, Fructose and sorbitol, *American Family Physician,* October 1986, pp. 264, 266.
39. O'Neil, Hynak-Hankinson, and Gorman, 1986.
40. G. Stendig-Lindberg, Changes in serum magnesium concentration after strenuous exercise, *Journal of the American College of Nutrition* 6 (1987): 35–40.
41. O'Neil, Hynak-Hankinson, and Gorman, 1986.
42. W. M. Sherman and D. L. Costill, The marathon: Dietary manipulation to optimize performance, *American Journal of Sports Medicine* 12 (1984): 44–51.

43. H. Haupt and G. D. Rovere, Anabolic steroids: A review of the literature, *American Journal of Sports Medicine* 12 (1984): 469–484; D. R. Lamb, Anabolic steroids in athletics: How well do they work and how dangerous are they? *American Journal of Sports Medicine* 12 (1984): 31–38.
44. O. L. Webb, P. M. Laskarzewski, and C. J. Glueck, Severe depression of high-density lipoprotein cholesterol levels in weight lifters and body builders by self-administered exogenous testosterone and anabolic-androgenic steroids, *Metabolism* 33 (1984): 971–975; M. Alen and P. Rakhila, Reduced high-density lipoprotein-cholesterol in power athletes: Use of male sex hormone derivatives, an atherogenic factor, *International Journal of Sports Medicine* 5 (1984): 341–342.
45. Haupt and Rovere, 1984.
46. L. R. Shoaf, P. D. McClellan, and K. A. Birskovich, Nutrition knowledge, interests, and information sources of male athletes, *Journal of Nutrition Education* 18 (1986): 243–245.
47. M. Perron and J. Endres, Knowledge, attitudes, and dietary practices of female athletes, *Journal of the American Dietetic Association* 85 (1985): 573–576.
48. F. Hickson, J. Schrader, and L. C. Trischler, Dietary intakes of female basketball and gymnastics athletes, *Journal of the American Dietetic Association* 86 (1986): 251–253; Have you had your chromium today? Probably not (Brief Communications), *Journal of the American Dietetic Association* 86 (1986): 667; H. C. Lukaski, Maximal oxygen consumption as related to magnesium, copper, and zinc nutriture, *American Journal of Clinical Nutrition* 37 (1983): 407–415.
49. J. D. Cantwell, Carbohydrate loading (Questions and Answers), *Journal of the American Medical Association* 256 (1986): 3024.
50. G. R. Hagerman, Nutrition in part-time athletes, *Nutrition and the MD,* August 1981.
51. Protein needs higher for those who exercise (News Front), *Modern Medicine,* August 1986, p. 16; Position of the American Dietetic Association: Nutrition for physical fitness and athletic performance for adults, *Journal of the American Dietetic Association* 87 (1987): 933–939.
52. E. Pollitt, R. Leibel, and D. Greenfield, Brief fasting, stress and cognition in children, *American Journal of Clinical Nutrition* 34 (1981): 1526–1533.
53. *Snacking Trends,* MRCA Information Services, as cited in What you eat between meals depends upon where you live, survey says, *Journal of the American Dietetic Association* 85 (1985): 604.

Controversy 9

Eating Disorders and Society

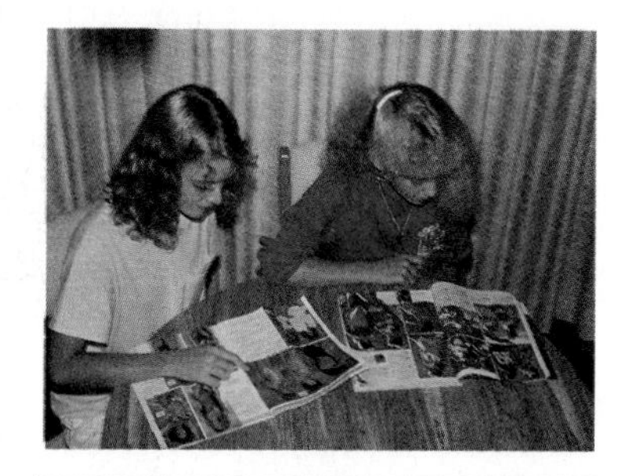

At a tender age, young women are already concerned about becoming thin.

Julie is 18 years old. She has always been a superachiever in school; she prides herself on her fine figure and watches her diet with great care. She exercises daily, maintaining a heroic schedule of self-discipline. She is thin, but she is not satisfied with her weight and is determined to lose more. She is 5 feet 6 inches tall and weighs 85 pounds. She has **anorexia nervosa.**

Julie is unaware that she is undernourished, and she sees no need to obtain treatment, but her friends and family have become concerned about her. She stopped menstruating (developed amenorrhea) several months ago and has become very moody. She insists that she is too fat, although her eyes lie in deep hollows in her face. She denies that she is ever tired, although she is obviously close to physical exhaustion. Her family is reluctant to push her, but has insisted that she see a psychiatrist. The psychiatrist has evaluated her case and has decided to hospitalize her. This step may save her life.

Anorexia Nervosa

The incidence of anorexia nervosa in our country and in other industrially advanced countries is steadily increasing. The disease now occurs in 1 or more of every 100 women.[1] Those who have studied it are convinced that the predisposition to it is inherited, and that our particular culture favors its development.[2] It is four to five times more common in identical than in nonidentical twins. People with anorexia nervosa often have a history of complications surrounding the time of their birth; they also have a higher birthweight and greater incidence of obesity before they become anorexic than do people who never develop the disease. Nineteen out of 20 people with anorexia are young women.

It is believed that a person's adult behavior, including eating behavior, is shaped at least partly by childhood experiences. A characteristic cluster of family and social circumstances often surrounds the person with anorexia. Such a family is described as being dominated by the mother and values achievement and outward appearances more than an inner sense of self-worth and self-actualization. The young person may value her parents' opinion highly and try to please them by working unrealistically hard—perfectionism.

Eating disorders, especially in children, can often be traced to parents' disharmony or personal conflicts.[3] Often such conflicts are projected onto a child; for example, a parent who is overweight may focus negative attention on a child's bodily appearance. A parent who perceives a child as too thin or too fat may attempt to severely control the child's normal food intake, thereby setting the stage for sneaky eating to satisfy hunger, or resistance to forced eating. Alternatively, a parent may deny a child's overweight or underweight when it exists, and provide too few limits. A child who experiences distorted parental perceptions about eating, or who experiences overcontrol or undercontrol of eating and other behavior, may develop a full-blown eating disorder that mirrors the disorder of family relations between parent and child.

An absentee or distant father is often associated with anorexia nervosa in young women. Young women look to their male parents for feedback on their self-worth, and when they don't receive it, tend to be oversensitive to negative cultural influences such as the drive for thinness and the view of emaciation as beautiful.[4] Julie's father has alcoholism, and her mother left him a year ago. Julie loves both parents and wants very much to please them. She identifies so strongly with their ideals and goals for her that she sometimes feels she has no identity of her own. She can't get in touch with her own feelings, and she sometimes feels like a robot. She earnestly desires to control her own destiny, but she feels controlled by others.

Anorexia resembles an addiction. The characteristic behavior is obsessive and compulsive, and often there are other addictions in the family, as exemplified by Julie's father's alcoholism. When Julie eats, she does so for external reasons. As a child, when she cried with hunger, her parents didn't respond by feeding her. Rather, they fed her on a rigid schedule. They forced food on her at times when she didn't want it, insisting that she eat it; and they withheld it when she was hungry, thus overriding her internal hunger signals. Julie lost the ability to detect her own hunger signals, and as she grew up, she became a person who felt she had to control her eating from outside, as her parents had done.

As almost always happens, Julie began to develop anorexia within half a year after her menstrual periods started. She was distressed by the signs that she was turning into a woman and afraid of the changes that were taking place in her body. If she remained thin, she felt, she might escape being enveloped in a woman's body with hips, belly, and breasts—which frightened and revolted her. Julie's anorexia has tightened the bonds between herself and her mother, stabilizing her in a juvenile state and making it unnecessary for either of them to deal with the other problems that they face in their lives.

You may wonder how a person as thin as Julie could possibly continue to diet. Julie controls her food intake with tremendous discipline. She avoids carbohydrates and fats as if they were poison and eats strictly limited amounts of lean meat and low-calorie vegetables. She knows the number of calories per serving of dozens of different foods, and thinks and talks about food constantly. She cooks elaborate meals for her mother and her mother's friends, but she never partakes of them herself. If she feels that she has gained an ounce of weight, she runs or jumps rope until she is sure she has exercised it off. Her favorite sports are solitary; she doesn't participate in team sports. Once in a while she slips and eats more than she intends to, and when she has done that, she takes laxatives to hasten the exit of the food from her system. She is unaware that this has no effect on body fat, because her other ways of staying thin are so effective. Her preoccupation with food reveals that she is starving and is desperately hungry; the reason she doesn't eat is because of her fierce determination to achieve self-control, not because she isn't hungry.

When Julie looks at herself in the mirror, she sees herself as fat. The psychiatrist who tested her gave her a visual self-image test, and she drew a picture of herself that was grossly distorted. The psychiatrist took this as an index of the severity of her illness, knowing that the more she overestimated her body size, the more resistant she would be to the treatment, and the more unwilling to examine her faulty values and misconceptions. When asked to draw her best friend, Julie rendered an accurate image.

Physical abnormalities in anorexia nervosa include many hormonal aberrations. Amenorrhea (cessation of menstruation) always accompanies the disorder in women, and in 25 percent of cases, that symptom precedes the weight loss. Young people of both sexes with the disorder lose their sex drive and become unable to function sexually. To resume normal cycling, a woman must gain body fat to at least 17 percent of her body weight. Sometimes it requires 22 percent fat content before periods may resume, and some never restart, even after they have gained the weight. It isn't clear whether the hormonal change is first to occur or whether stress precedes it. Up to three out of every four women in concentration camps and all women on death row have amenorrhea.[5] The early teen years are a stressful time, and many teen girls may be uncertain about their own ability to fill the all-encompassing female role in modern society—as homemaker, wife, mother, lover, professional, natural beauty, etc. Roles are changing much more rapidly for women than men today, and traditional guidelines no longer exist. The likely sequence in the development of anorexia nervosa is stress; then hormonal abnormalities; then food restriction, amenorrhea, and weight loss.[6]

Once the victim has undertaken her rigorous dieting routine, physical effects of starvation begin to set in. Thyroid hormone secretion becomes abnormal. Adrenal secretions, growth hormone, and blood pressure–regulating hormones also are abnormal. Heart function changes drastically. The heart pumps less efficiently, the muscle becomes weak and thin, the chambers diminish in size, and the blood pressure falls. Heart rhythms may change, with a characteristic abnormality appearing on the heart monitor. Sudden stopping of the heart, perhaps due to lean tissue loss and mineral deficiencies, accounts for many cases of sudden death among severely emaciated subjects.

The person with anorexia nervosa also has many abnormalities of immune function, but does not have more numerous infections than contemporaries. There may be anemia. As the person becomes thinner and thinner, abnormalities of the gastrointestinal system also occur. Peristalsis becomes sluggish, and if the person eats too fast, the stomach becomes overfull, because it empties abnormally slowly. The lining of the digestive tract atrophies, and on eating a normal amount of food again the person may have diarrhea, because the system can't absorb nutrients well. The pancreas becomes unable to secrete many enzymes, as does the lining of the intestinal tract.

Other starvation effects include altered serum lipid levels, high concentrations of vitamin A and carotene in the blood, reduced blood proteins, an increased amount of fine body hair, skin dryness, and decreased skin and core temperatures. The electrical activity of the brain becomes abnormal, sleep is disturbed, and bad dreams are common. The person with anorexia nervosa may complain of never feeling rested.

Anorexia nervosa is hard to diagnose, because nearly everyone in our society is engaged in the pursuit of thinness. Some women *without* weight loss meet all the criteria for the diagnosis of anorexia nervosa based on their eating attitudes and behaviors, as if they had a subclinical disorder or were starting to develop the disease. Anorexia-like thought patterns are common among fashion models, long-distance runners, and dancers. Because our society favors thinness, this behavior may even help a person to attain personal or vocational goals. Many young women, on learning of the disorder, state that they wish they had a touch of it, in order to get thin.

It takes a skilled clinician to make a diagnosis. Denial runs high among people with anorexia, and they deceive their families effectively. Usually, the clinician has to employ diagnostic tests to make a differential diagnosis using a scheme of comparisons between this disease and others involving thinness or less of appetite. Table C9–1 shows the diagnostic criteria for anorexia nervosa.

Therapies for anorexia nervosa include insight-oriented therapy, cognitive behavior therapy, behavior modification, and family therapy. When they are compared, it is found that the therapy itself is not the key factor, but the spirit in which it is given: "The effectiveness of the [therapist]-patient interaction determines the outcome."[7]

Treatment is aimed at avoiding medical complications, altering the psychological and environmental patterns that have supported or permitted the emergence of anorexia, and restoring adequate nutrition. Treatment programs of recent date have been more successful than in the past, and residential treatment centers specializing in eating disorders are often especially successful. Medical, psychiatric-psychological, and nutrition personnel are all needed and should work together as a team.[8] The person who works most closely with the client should aim at four goals:

- To support her own feeling of autonomy—her feeling that she can control her own life, feel her own feelings, and choose her own behaviors.
- To earn her trust by being honest, acknowledging that the treatment for anorexia may be uncomfortable at first, and that for a while things may seem worse before they begin to get better.
- To involve the other family members, so that they will not continue to reinforce maladaptive behavior, but will help the client gain weight by providing positive reinforcement.
- To make connections with other health care agencies, depending on individual needs.

Table C9–1

Diagnosis of Anorexia Nervosa

Refusal to maintain body weight over a minimal normal weight for age and height, e.g., weight loss leading to maintenance of body weight 15% below that expected; or failure to make expected weight gain during period of growth, leading to body weight 15% below that expected.
Intense fear of gaining weight or becoming fat, even though underweight.
Disturbance in the way in which one's body weight, size, or shape is experienced; e.g., the person claims to "feel fat" even when emaciated, or believes that one area of the body is "too fat" even when obviously underweight.
In females, absence of at least three consecutive menstrual cycles when otherwise expected to occur (primary or secondary amenorrhea). (A woman is considered to have amenorrhea if her periods occur only following hormone, e.g., estrogen, administration.)

Source: American Psychiatric Association, *Diagnostic and Statistical Manual of Mental Disorders,* 4th ed. (Washington, D.C.: American Psychiatric Association, 1987), p. 67, with permission.

Some people have to go to the hospital. The malnutrition of anorexia nervosa can be so severe as to throw a person into severe electrolyte imbalance, create tremendous metabolic stress by way of infection, cause depression to the point of suicide, and even stop the heart. Programs that force-feed by tube have not been successful and, in fact, may traumatize and cause further harm. Even if they bring about weight gain, it is only temporary. Psychiatric hospitalization may be considered, but will benefit the person only if it is part of a more general treatment program.

Appropriate nutritional treatment is crucial. It need not be as aggressive as the remediation of malnutrition caused by other medical conditions, but it must be tailored to the client's needs. People with anorexia nervosa are usually younger than people with other medical conditions and are usually not ill with other diseases, so they are under less physical stress. Seldom are they willing to feed themselves, but if they are, chances are they can recover without other interventions. It is suggested that subjects be classed as being at low, intermediate, or high risk, depending on how they score on several indicators of protein-energy malnutrition.* Low-risk people need nutrition counseling by a dietitian and psychological counseling simultaneously. Intermediate-risk people may need nutritional supplements such as high-calorie, high-protein formulas besides ordinary meals but may not have to be hospitalized. The initial goal is to provide 250 to 500 calories above the daily energy requirement—about the maximum that most people are willing and able to accept. Drugs may be used to improve gastric motility and help people become able to tolerate larger meals. If the risk is high, then hospitalization is indicated, daily calorie supplementation may be greater, and tube feeding may have to be instituted. The hope is that the person will gain about 1 to 2 kilograms (2 to 4 pounds) a month. For a person who refuses to eat, forcible methods may be necessary to forestall death. These are in the domain of physicians and will not be described here. Drug therapies may be used as accompaniment.

Treatment outcomes are better than they used to be. Three-quarters of those in treatment may regain at least some weight. Half to three-quarters may resume normal menstrual cycles. About two-thirds fail to eat normally on follow-up, but they may eat better than they did before. About 6 percent die, 1 percent by suicide.*

Social and family relationships may remain impaired. A person afflicted with an eating disorder may be adversely affected for life psychologically, and in social and family relationships. Table C9–2 shows the factors that predict the degree of recovery from anorexia nervosa.

Bulimia

Sophie is a charming, intelligent woman of normal weight who thinks constantly about food. She alternately starves herself and binges, and when she has eaten too much she vomits. Few people would fail to recognize these characteristics as the description of **bulimia**, for although the disease was recognized and named only in 1980, it has received much media attention. Until 1979 it was thought to be a variant of anorexia nervosa. Now it is generally recognized as a separate entity. Diagnosis is not difficult, because no other diseases present similar symptoms (see Table C9–3).

Sophie is typical of people with bulimia—single, Caucasian, and in her early 20s. She is well educated and close to her ideal body weight. She binges periodically, and when she does so, it is in secret, usually at night, and lasts an hour or more. Sophie seldom lets binging interfere with her work or social activities, although a third of all bingers do; she is like most people with bulimia (60 percent) in that she starts the binge after having gone through a period of rigid dieting, so that her eating is accelerated by her hunger. Each time, she eats anywhere from one thousand to many thousands of calories of food containing little fiber or water, smooth in texture, and high in sugar and fat, so that it is easy to consume vast amounts rapidly, with little chewing. Typically, she chooses rich cookies, cake, ice cream, or bread, although sometimes she binges on atypical foods—for example, vegetables—when she is dieting. After the binge, she pays the price of having swollen hands and feet, bloating, fatigue, headache, nausea, and pain.

The binge itself is not like normal eating. It is not primarily a response to hunger, apparently, and the food is not consumed for its nutritional value. It is a compulsion and usually occurs in several stages: "anticipation and planning, anxiety, urgency to begin, rapid and uncontrollable consumption of food, relief and relaxation, disappointment, and finally shame or disgust."[9]

As Sophie repeats and repeats this behavior, she faces more and more serious consequences, including medical ones. Fluid and electrolyte imbalance caused by vomiting can lead to abnormal heart rhythms and injury to the kidneys, which have to cope with the altered balance. Infections of the bladder and kidneys can lead to kidney failure. Vomiting causes irritation and infection of the pharynx, esophagus, and salivary glands; erosion of the teeth; and dental caries. The esophagus may

*Indicators of protein-energy malnutrition: the percentage of body fat, serum albumin and serum transferrin levels, and immune reactions.

*This is from a review of 19 studies on about 1000 clients over a five-year period. Other deaths are from infection; heart disease; lung disease; and iatrogenic causes including aspiration, electrolyte imbalance from intravenous therapy, and vitamin D poisoning. M. A. Balaa and D. A. Drossman, Anorexia nervosa and bulimia: The eating disorders, *Disease-a-Month* (Chicago: Year Book Medical Publishers, June 1985), p. 34.

rupture or tear, as may the stomach. Sometimes the eyes become red from pressure on vomiting. The hands may be bruised and lacerated from scraping on the teeth while inducing vomiting.

Some people use **cathartics**—violent laxatives that can injure the lower intestinal tract. Others use **emetics** to induce vomiting; it was these that caused the death of popular singer Karen Carpenter in 1983. The first-aid treatment for poisonings, syrup of ipecac, is toxic to the liver, kidneys, and heart when taken repeatedly.

Bulimia is more common than anorexia nervosa in women, and much more common in men. Still, women are the predominant sufferers. Men are less likely to seek treatment for the condition.[10] The possibility exists that only the reporting of bulimia, especially by women, is increasing, but the incidence seems to be rising. In any case, a survey of 300 middle- to upper-class suburban women shoppers in Boston taken in 1984 showed that over 10 percent reported a history of bulimia, and almost 5 percent were currently experiencing it.[11] Among college women, the incidence may range anywhere from 5 to 20 percent.

Bulimia occurs in women of all ages but is most common in those under 30 years old. Fewer than one-third discuss their eating difficulties with their health care providers, and only 2.5 percent receive medical treatment. Only 5 percent of people with bulimia meet the criteria for anorexia nervosa, and fewer than 1 percent are actively anorexic.

What makes a person become bulimic? Again Sophie is typical. From early in her childhood, she has been a high achiever, with a strong feeling of dependence on her parents. Her

Table C9–2

Long-Term Prognostic Factors in Anorexia Nervosa

Good prognosis
- High educational achievement
- Early age at onset
- Good educational adjustment
- Improvement in body image after weight gain

Poor prognosis
- Late age at onset
- Continued overestimation of body size
- Premorbid obesity
- Self-induced vomiting or bulimia
- Laxative abuse
- Low social class
- Long duration of illness
- Disturbed parental relationship
- Male sex
- Marriage
- Marked depression, obsessional behavior, or somatic complaints

No effect on prognosis
- Premorbid personality type or psychological disturbance
- Hyperactivity
- Degree of weight loss
- Pharmacotherapy

Source: D. A. Drossman, D. A. Ontjes, and W. D. Heizer, Anorexia nervosa, *Gastroenterology* 77 (1979): 1115. Copyright 1979 by the American Gastroenterological Association.

Table C9–3

Diagnosis of Bulimia

Recurrent episodes of binge eating (rapid consumption of a large amount of food in a discrete period of time).

A feeling of lack of control over eating behavior during the eating binges.

Regular practice of either self-induced vomiting, use of laxatives or diuretics, strict dieting or fasting, or vigorous exercise in order to prevent weight gain.

A minimum average of two binge eating episodes a week for at least three months.

Persistent overconcern with body shape and weight.

Source: American Psychiatric Association, *Diagnostic and Statistical Manual of Mental Disorders,* 4th ed. (Washington, D.C.: American Psychiatric Association, 1987), pp. 68–69, with permission.

mother is a bright, well-educated woman who abandoned a promising career in order to stay home and raise the family; she has taught her children a high degree of respect for their father, who is a powerful but distant figure. Sophie experiences considerable social anxiety and has difficulty in establishing personal relationships. She is sometimes depressed and often exhibits impulsive behavior. Some people with bulimia exhibit antisocial behavior, including drug abuse, kleptomania, and sexual promiscuity.

Unlike Julie, Sophie feels that her behavior is abnormal, is aware of the risks, and is deeply ashamed. She feels inadequate, unable even to control her eating, and so she tends to be passive and to look to men for confirmation of her sense of worth. When she is rejected, either in reality or in her imagination, her bulimia becomes worse; in fact, many women point to real or imagined male rejection as the event that triggered the first big diet and subsequently the first binge. If Sophie gets carried away by bulimia, she may not only experience a deepening of her depression, but may move on to drug abuse (including alcohol abuse) or suicide.

A food-centered society that favors thinness in women puts a woman in a bind. Bulimia has been described as socially sanctioned and almost required among upper-class women who must attend many dinners and cocktail parties. Typically, they have been raised in families that encouraged hearty eating, and there is much socializing around the dinner table. Food is always involved in celebrations and also is used to console the family during periods of mourning. When a child raised in such a setting is also made socially conscious and is told she must become thin, she may perceive that she has little alternative but to celebrate or mourn with the family; indulge in vast quantities of food; and then vomit, crash diet, or fast to "undo the damage."

If Lenny and my parents wouldn't give me any attention, I would turn to someone who could love me back. Food loved me back.
Richard Simmons

Although the psychosocial influences in bulimia are irrefutable, there is emerging a biological basis for the binge behavior, once started. Certain foods are known to trigger the brain's endogenous opiates, those chemicals that perform druglike functions such as painkilling. These foods also trigger the pleasure experience and stimulate the appetite. It could be that a person who suffers from bulimia is addicted to the endogenous opiates produced during the binge. In fact, when the blood levels of endorphins were measured, people with bulimia had lower levels than other people. The researchers speculate that the low levels of endorphins "underlie excessive thoughts of food and prompt binge eating as a means of elevating these levels, analogous to the drug addict's *hunger* for opiates during withdrawal."[12]

Bulimia is in many respects easier to treat than anorexia nervosa, because it seems to be more of a chosen behavior. People with bulimia know that their behavior is abnormal, and many are willing to try to cooperate. A number of approaches have been described, but little study has shown, yet, which might be most effective. It is suggested that the most important goal is to help the person gain control over binge eating—a task more easily assigned than carried out, since the trigger that starts the binge has not been identified. Warning signs are times of family stress, and especially times of real or perceived rejection. One strategy is obvious: since most binges begin after a round of strict dieting, the person needs to learn to eat a quantity of nutritious food sufficient to nourish her body and leave her satisfied without bringing on the anathema of weight gain. Such an approach has been used successfully in the treatment of many people with severe bulimia; it requires that they eat no less than 1500 calories a day.[13]

Drug therapy may accompany psychotherapy for bulimia. Almost 90 percent of people with bulimia are clinically depressed, and about half have a biochemical abnormality not otherwise seen except in severe undernutrition, although their body weights are near normal.* Antidepressant medication doesn't help them all, but is indicated and useful for some.

Long-term follow-up studies remain to be undertaken. It isn't clear what becomes of people with bulimia in later life. Possibly, there are roughly three categories: college students who engage in the disorder briefly and then recover, binge/vomiters who also begin during college and who require more intensive therapy and hospitalization, and older people who have chronic and stable bulimia and whose binge-eating and vomiting patterns are regular and established. These people might be said to be socially adjusted, in a way, because their behavior does not make it impossible for them to function socially. Somehow, they fit it in with their other activities.

Eating Disorders and Society

Both anorexia nervosa and bulimia are relatively new diseases. Anorexia

*The abnormality referred to is an abnormal dexamethasone suppression test result. Balaa and Drossman, 1985.

nervosa was first described 100 years ago; bulimia was first defined as a medical disorder only in 1980. Both are known only in developed nations and become more prevalent as wealth increases. Some people point to the vomitoriums of ancient peoples and claim that bulimia is nothing new, but the two are actually quite distinct. The ancient people were eating for pleasure, without guilt, and in the company of others; they vomited so that they could rejoin the feast. Bulimia is a disease of isolation and is always accompanied by self-hate and low self-esteem. The causes of both bulimia and anorexia nervosa are unknown, but one school of thought labels them social problems. The common negative experiences that lead privileged young women to self-destructive eating patterns include the internalization of a message of their own low worth, and the idealizing of some unachievable, "perfect" image.

If asked today, Julie might describe herself as proud of her achievements in dieting, eager to achieve more, and resentful of her confinement in the hospital. She has, after all, made significant progress toward achieving society's goal for her—to be thin. Sophie, on the other hand, would describe herself as unhappy, because she has failed to control her eating. She is longing for the time when she'll be happy—that is, when she's thin. It's not uncommon in our society for some women to develop a kind of Cinderella complex—to hide behind obstacles, real or imaginary, waiting and hoping for some event or some person to bring them happiness. The reasoning goes like this: "I'll be happy when someone marries me (or when I have more money, a house, a child). I can't find someone to marry me until I meet him/her. I can't meet new people because I'm shy. People reject me because I'm too fat (not beautiful, too thin, too poor, too short, too tall). Someday my problems will go away, someone will marry me, and *then* I'll be happy." Caught in a trap of her own making, waiting for a preconceived stamp of approval from outside herself, such a person cannot grow, and through stagnation and a negative attitude, she may repel the very people with whom she could otherwise share life's enjoyments.

Deep inside there had always been a small child begging for my attention. . . . All I gave her was food. Now I give her love.
Eda LeShan

At so tender an age as 12 years, beautifully growing, normal-weight female youngsters are already worried that they are too fat. Most teenage girls are "on diets," and they are terrified of being fat.[14] Magazines, newspapers, and television all present two-dimensional, contrived, camera-ready women, flaws concealed, unreasonably thin, worthy only so long as they are lovely to look at; these are perceived as ideal. The message is clear—only with *this* kind of body are you acceptable. The way you are isn't good enough. You should become like the cover girl who doesn't sweat; doesn't grow hair on her slender legs; has firm, small breasts, a flat stomach, a perfect face, and small feet; and is always perfectly happy. If *you*, young woman, are not perfectly happy, it is because your body is not beautiful enough. Anorexia nervosa and bulimia are not a form of rebellion against such unreasonable expectations, but rather the exaggerated acceptance of them. That is why, as the title of a popular book expresses it, fat is a feminist issue.* As women become more assertive, perhaps the issue will lose power.

Slowly, society is changing. Recognition of the success and desirability of a growing number of outstanding women in such traditionally male-dominated fields as athletics, science, law, and politics has raised women's collective self-esteem. Perhaps anorexia nervosa and bulimia are diseases of society in transition, and they may once again become unknown to medical literature as feminine roles and ideals

*S. Orbach, *Fat Is a Feminist Issue: The Anti-Diet Way to Permanent Weight Loss* (New York: Paddington Press, 1978).

Miniglossary

anorexia nervosa: a disorder seen (usually) in teenage girls, involving self-starvation to the extreme (*an* means "without"; *orex* means "mouth"; *nervos* means "of nervous origin").

bulimia (alternative spelling **bulemia**) (byoo-LEEM-ee-uh): recurring binge eating. Some people call this **bulimarexia** (byoo-lee-ma-REX-ee-uh); others reserve the latter term for bulimia with emaciation probably caused by purging (vomiting) after binging (*buli* means "ox"; *orex* means "mouth").

cathartics: strong laxatives. Also called **purgatives.**

emetics (em-ETT-ics): agents that cause vomiting.

change. Prevention may be most effective if begun very early in children's lives. Warnings to children that the advertisers' classic, emaciated female figure is simply an advertising gimmick designed to sell products, and not an ideal with which to compare one's own living body, may be of some help. The simple concept—to respect and value your own uniqueness—may be lifesaving for a future generation.

Notes

1. M. A. Balaa and D. A. Drossman, Anorexia nervosa and bulimia: The eating disorders, *Disease-a-Month* (Chicago: Year Book Medical Publishers, June 1985), pp. 1–52.
2. Balaa and Drossman, 1985, p. 12.
3. E. M. Satter, Childhood eating disorders, *Journal of the American Dietetic Association* 3 (1986): 357–361.
4. K. McCleary, Eating disorders: Daddy Dearest, *American Health,* January/February 1986, p. 86.
5. Balaa and Drossman, 1985, p.10.
6. Balaa and Drossman, 1985, p. 20.
7. Balaa and Drossman, 1985, p. 33.
8. Position of the American Dietetic Association: Nutrition intervention in the treatment of anorexia nervosa and bulimia nervosa, *Journal of the American Dietetic Association* 88 (1988): 68.
9. Balaa and Drossman, 1985, p. 38.
10. J. E. Mitchell and G. Goff, Bulimia in male patients, *Psychosomatics* 25 (1984): 909–913, as cited in *Modern Medicine,* July 1985, pp. 101–102.
11. H. G. Pope, Jr., J. I. Hudson, and D. Yurgelun-Todd, Anorexia nervosa and bulimia among 300 suburban women shoppers, *American Journal of Psychiatry* 141 (1984): 2, as cited by Balaa and Drossman, 1985.
12. D. A. Waller and coauthors, Eating behavior and plasma beta-endorphin in bulimia, *American Journal of Clinical Nutrition* 44 (1986): 20–23
13. S. Dalvit-McPhillips, A dietary approach to bulimia treatment, *Physiology and Behavior* 33 (1984): 769–775.
14. N. S. Moses, M. Banilivy, and F. Lifshitz, Fear of obesity among adolescent females (abstract), *American Journal of Clinical Nutrition* 43 (1986): 664.

Chapter Ten

Contents

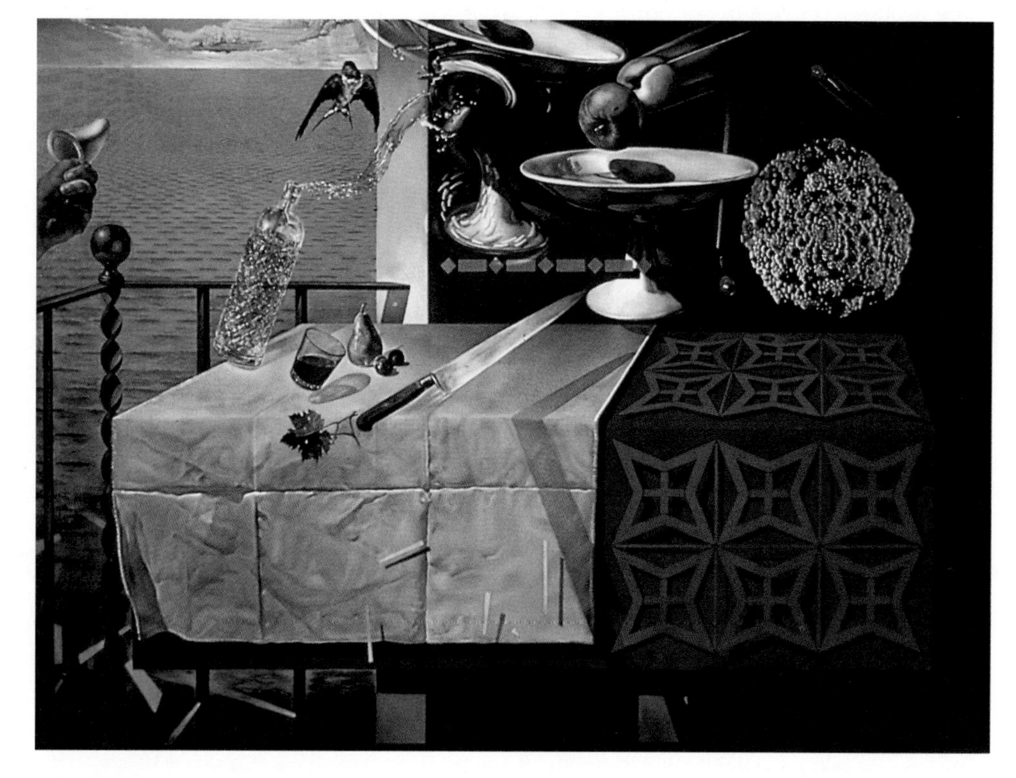

Nature Morte Vivante by Salvador Dalí, 1956, oil on canvas. The Salvador Dalí Museum, St. Petersburg, Florida, U.S.A.

Food Technology and Food Safety

The burden of solving today's problems in the nation's food supply rests largely with food technologists, scientists who work for large food companies. Corporate laboratories, operated for profit, work to improve products' taste, appearance, and keeping quality, and they compete with others to develop new products and so capture sales. Are today's new food products nutritious? Are the additives used to produce them safe? What about the contamination of fresh foods sold today? And who is looking out for the consumer?

In a free market, where food companies compete for sales, consumers receive benefits—the safest, most pleasing, and abundant food supply in the world. With these benefits comes the consumers' responsibility of looking out for their own best interests. This chapter provides the information you need to make your food purchasing decisions with confidence, starting with a class by class description of the food additives and their safety. It explains how different processing techniques affect nutrients; it gives perspective on the use of pesticides on foods, and it issues warnings about the dangers of contamination with environmental toxins or microorganisms. Finally, the Food Feature shows where to find pertinent information on food labels, and how to interpret what you find there. The Controversy that follows describes some chemicals other than nutrients that occur naturally in foods, that have effects, for better or worse, on the human body.

additives: substances not normally consumed as foods by themselves but added to food either intentionally or by accident. Some additives are defined in the accompanying Miniglossary, and many more are in Appendix G.

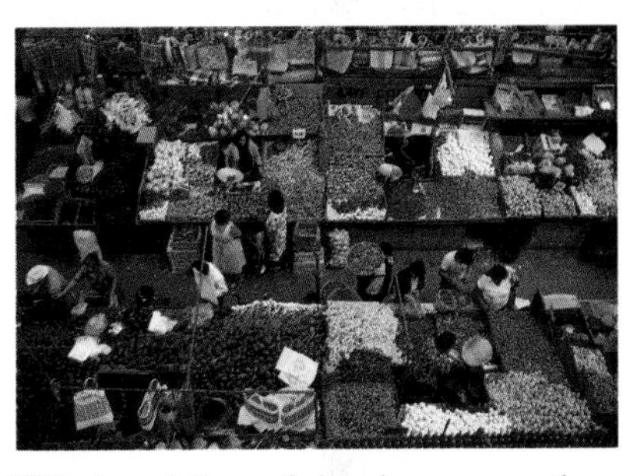

With the privilege of abundance comes the responsibility to choose wisely.

Food Additives

Most people want to know about **additives.** What are they, why are they there, and are they dangerous in any way? Are the foods labeled "no additives" better for health than others? Those questions are valid, but they ignore some other, more pressing concerns that may not receive the publicity that additives do. The Food and Drug Administration (FDA) lists hazards in order of impact on human health—that is, What about our food supply is actually causing, or has the potential to cause, the greatest harm to people? The safety of food additives is not first, or even third, on the FDA's list of priority concerns; it is sixth and last. This doesn't mean that additives are of no concern—they are, to many people. It does mean, though, that the other five hazards present greater causes for concern. The FDA prioritizes its list of food hazards as follows:

- Food poisoning, which is greatly increasing each year because increasing populations require large-scale food operations and multiple transfers involving handling.

intentional food additives: additives intentionally added to food, such as nutrients or colors.

incidental food additives: substances that can get into food not through intentional introduction but as a result of contact with the food during growing, processing, packaging, storing, or some other stage before the food is consumed. *Accidental* or *indirect additives* mean the same thing.

safety: the practical certainty that injury will not result from the use of a substance.

- Nutrition, which requires close attention as more and more artificially constituted foods appear on the market.
- Environmental contaminants, which are increasing yearly in number and concentration and whose consequences are difficult to foresee and forestall.
- Naturally occurring toxicants in foods, which occur randomly and constitute a hazard whenever people turn to consuming single foods either by choice (fad diets) or by necessity (poverty).
- Pesticide residues.
- Intentional food additives, listed last because so much is known about them, and because they are well regulated.

This chapter deals with all these concerns in reverse order, except for the naturally occurring toxicants, which are discussed in the Controversy that follows.

Some definitions will assist understanding of these crucial concerns. Substances put into foods on purpose are **intentional food additives,** while **incidental food additives** are those that may get in by accident during processing. This discussion begins with the intentional additives, and after taking them up class by class, goes on to the incidental additives.

Intentional food additives are substances put into foods to give them some desirable characteristic: color, flavor, texture, stability, or resistance to spoilage. Some are nutrients added to foods to increase their nutritional value, such as vitamin C added to fruit drinks or potassium iodide added to salt. The large categories of additives are listed in the Miniglossary, and each is treated in the following sections. In addition, numerous other additives, used in small quantities for miscellaneous other purposes, are listed in Appendix G along with other terms that appear on food and supplement labels.

Regulations Governing Additives

The agency charged with the responsibility of deciding what additives shall be in foods is the FDA. The FDA's authority over additives hinges primarily on their **safety.** A manufacturer has to go through a special procedure that can take many years to get permission to use a new additive in food products. The manufacturer must test it to satisfy the FDA that:

- It is effective (it does what it is supposed to do).
- It can be detected and measured in the final food product.

Then the manufacturer has to feed the additive in large doses to animals under strictly controlled conditions and prove that:

- It is safe (it causes no cancer, birth defects, or other injury).

Finally, the manufacturer must submit all test results to the FDA.

The FDA then calls a public hearing and announces the topic, date, and location in its official publication, *FDA Consumer.* Consumers are invited to participate at these hearings, where experts present testimony for and against granting permission to use the additive. Thus the consumer's rights and responsibilities are written into the provisions for deeming additives safe.

If the FDA approves the additive's use, that does not mean the manufacturer can add it in any amount to any food. On the contrary: the FDA writes a

Miniglossary of Intentional Food Additives

antimicrobial agents: preservatives that prevent microorganisms from growing.
antioxidants: chemicals that prevent rancidity in fats (see also definition in Chapter 4).
artificial colors: certified food colors, added to enhance appearance. (*Certified* means approved by the FDA.)
artificial flavors, flavor enhancers: chemicals that mimic natural flavors and those that enhance flavor.
nutrient additives: vitamins and minerals added to improve nutritive value.
Note: Examples of these are in Appendix G.

GRAS (generally recognized as safe) list: a list of food additives, established by the FDA, that had long been in use and were believed safe. The list is subject to revision as new facts become known.

Delaney Clause: a clause in the Food Additive Amendment to the Food, Drug, and Cosmetic Act that states that no substance that is known to cause cancer in animals or humans at any dose level shall be added to foods.

toxicity: the ability of a substance to harm living organisms. All substances are toxic if high enough concentrations are used.

hazard: state of danger; used to refer to any circumstances in which toxicity is possible under normal conditions of use.

margin of safety: as used when speaking of food additives, a zone between the concentration normally used and that at which a hazard exists. For common table salt, for example, the margin of safety is 1/5 (five times the concentration normally used would be hazardous).

regulation stating in what amounts, and in what foods, the additive may be used. No additives are permanently approved; all are periodically reviewed.

Many substances were exempted from complying with this procedure at the time it was first instituted, because they had been used a long time and there were no known hazards in their use. Some 700 substances in all were put on the **GRAS (generally recognized as safe) list.** However, any time substantial scientific evidence or public outcry has questioned the safety of any of the substances on the GRAS list, it has been reevaluated. All substances about which any legitimate question was raised have been removed or reclassified. A set of 2100 flavoring agents has similarly been reviewed, as well as some 200 coloring agents. Meanwhile, the entire GRAS list is subject to an ongoing review.

One of the criteria an additive must have met to be placed on the GRAS list is that it must not have been found to be a carcinogen in any test on animals or in human beings. The **Delaney Clause** (the part of a law on additives that states this criterion) is uncompromising in addressing carcinogens in food and drugs and has been under fire in recent years for being too strict.

A carcinogen is a cancer-causing agent. See the box in Controversy 5 for a discussion of the Delaney debate.

An additive's safety is determined based on a distinction between **toxicity** as a property of substances, and **hazard** associated with substances. "Toxicity—the capacity of a chemical substance to harm living organisms—is a general property of matter; hazard is the capacity of a chemical to produce injury under conditions of use. All substances are potentially toxic, but are hazardous only if consumed in sufficiently large quantities."[1] An additive is not considered to be a hazard if some immense amount that people never consume is toxic. The additive is a hazard only if it is toxic under the conditions of its actual use. Food additives are supposed to have wide margins of safety.

Most additives that involve risk are allowed in foods only at levels 100 times below those at which the risk is still known to be zero; their **margin of safety** is 1/100. Experiments to determine the extent of risk involve feeding test animals the substance at different concentrations throughout their lifetimes. The additive is then permitted in foods at 1/100 the level that can be fed under these conditions without causing any harmful effect whatever. In many foods, naturally occurring substances appear at levels that bring their margin of safety closer to 1/10. Even nutrients, as you have seen, involve risks at high dosage levels. The margin of safety for vitamins A and D is 1/25 to 1/40; it may be less than 1/10 in infants. For some trace elements, it is about 1/5. People consume common table salt daily in amounts only three to five times less than those that cause serious toxicity.

The margin-of-safety concept also applies to nutrients when they are used as additives. Iodine has been added to salt to prevent iodine deficiency, but it has had to be added with care, because it is a deadly poison in excess. Similarly, iron has been added to refined bread and other grains (enrichment) and has doubtless helped prevent many cases of iron-deficiency anemia in women and children who are prone to that disease. But the addition of too much iron could put men (who usually have enough) at risk for iron overload. The upper limit has to be remembered.

All the additives just named are in foods for a reason. They offer benefits that outweigh the risks they present, or make them worth taking. When the benefit to be gained from using an additive is small, as in the case of color additives that only enhance the appearance of foods but do not improve their health value or safety, then the risks may be deemed not worth taking. Only 33 of an original 200 color additives are still approved by the FDA for use in foods.

It is also the manufacturers' responsibility not to use more of an additive than is necessary to get the needed effect. Additives should also *not* be used:

- To disguise faulty or inferior products.
- To deceive the consumer.
- Where they significantly destroy nutrients.
- Where their effects can be achieved by economical, sound manufacturing processes.

The regulations governing the use of intentional additives are well-conceived, and have been effective, on the whole. Cutbacks in funding in the mid-1980s limit the watchdog capabilities of the FDA, however, and some mistakes and abuses are bound to slip by.

The following sections focus on a few individual food additives—notably, those that have received the most negative publicity, because people ask questions about them most often.

The use of intentional additives is regulated by the FDA; additives must be safe, effective, and measurable in the final product. Additives on the GRAS list are assumed to be safe because they have been long used. No additive may be used that has been found to cause cancer in animals or people, and those used must have wide margins of safety.

Antimicrobial Agents

Foods can go bad in two ways: one dangerous, one not. The dangerous way is by becoming hazardous to health; the other way is by losing their flavor and attractiveness. An example of the former: molds, bacteria, fungi, and yeasts growing in foods can cause food poisoning either by producing infections or by producing deadly toxins. Preservatives known as antimicrobial agents protect foods from these microbes.

The best known, most widely used antimicrobial agents are the two common substances salt and sugar. Salt has been added since before recorded history to preserve meat and fish; sugar serves the same purpose in canned and frozen fruits as well as jams and jellies. (Any jam or jelly that toots its "no preservatives" horn is exaggerating. There is no need to add extra preservatives, so most makers do not.) Both salt and sugar work by withdrawing water from the food; microbes cannot grow without water. Today, other additives such as potassium sorbate and sodium propionate are also used to extend the shelf life of baked goods, cheese, beverages, mayonnaise, margarine, and many other products.

Another group of antimicrobial agents is the **nitrites,** added to foods for three main purposes: to preserve their color (especially the pink color of hotdogs and other cured meats), to enhance their flavor by inhibiting rancidity (especially in cured meats), and to protect against bacterial growth. In amounts smaller than needed to confer color, nitrites prevent the growth of the bacteria that produce the deadly **botulinum** toxin, the most potent biological poison known. An amount of this toxin as tiny as a single crystal of salt can kill several people within an hour, and survivors still suffer the effects months or even years later.

Nitrites clearly perform important jobs, but they have been the object of controversy, because they can be converted in the human body to nitrosamines, and nitrosamines cause cancer in animals (see Controversy 5).

nitrites: salts added to food to prevent botulism. Compounds called **nitrosamines** (nigh-TROHS-uh-meens) are derivatives of nitrites that may be formed in the stomach when nitrites combine with amines, and nitrosamines are carcinogenic.

botulinum (bot-you-LINE-um) **toxin:** a toxin produced by bacteria that grow in meat, which causes *botulism* (BOTT-you-lism), a form of food poisoning.

sulfites: salts containing sulfur, added to fresh and frozen fruits and vegetables to prevent spoilage.

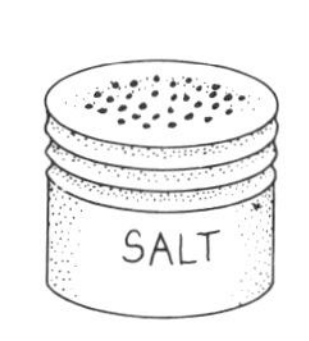

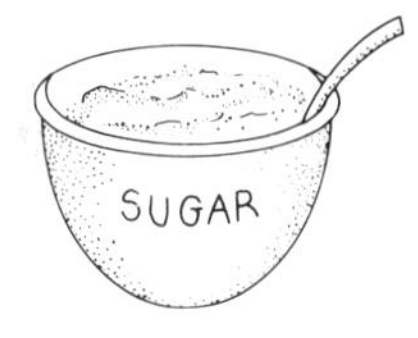

Two long-used preservatives.

Antioxidants

The other way in which food can go bad is by undergoing changes in color and flavor caused by exposure to air (oxidation). Oftentimes, these changes involve no hazard to health, but they damage the food's appearance, taste, and nutritional quality. Familiar examples of these changes are the ways sliced apples or potatoes turn brown, or oil goes rancid. Preservatives known as antioxidants protect food from this kind of spoilage.

A total of 27 antioxidants are approved for use in foods. Vitamin C (ascorbic acid) and vitamin E (tocopherol) are among them. Vitamin E is added to bacon to prevent nitrosamine formation while assisting nitrite's antioxidant activity. When the vitamin E additive is present in bacon along with the regular amount of nitrite preservative, nitrosamine formation is inhibited by more than half.*

Another group of preservatives is the **sulfites.** They are cheaper than the vitamins and are used to prevent oxidation in many processed foods, in alcoholic beverages (especially wine), and in drugs. They used to be popular with restaurant owners for use on salad bars, because they keep raw fruits and vegetables looking fresh, but this use has been banned. The ban came after some people experienced allergic reactions to the sulfites—reactions that were sometimes dangerous, and for a few, deadly.[2] The FDA has taken a number of steps to protect people who are allergic to sulfites. It prohibits sulfite use on food intended to be consumed raw (except grapes); it requires that foods declare sulfites in their ingredient lists, and that drug labels warn that sulfites are present. For most people, the sulfites do not pose a hazard in the amounts used in products,[3] but there is one more consideration: sulfiting agents destroy an appreciable

*The additive is Cure-trol, created by the Diamond Salt Company of St. Claire, Michigan.

amount of the vitamin thiamin in foods. A person choosing a food that contains sulfites should not count on that food to provide a share of the daily need for thiamin.

Two other antioxidants in wide use are the well-known BHA and BHT, which prevent rancidity in baked goods and snack foods. BHT provides a refreshing change from the tales of woe and cancer scares associated with many of the other additives. Among the many tests that were performed on BHT were several showing that animals fed large amounts of this substance developed *less* cancer when exposed to carcinogens and lived *longer* than controls. BHT apparently protects against cancer through its antioxidant effect, similar to that of vitamin E. To obtain this effect from BHT, though, a large amount of the substance must be present in the diet—larger by far than the amount in the U.S. diet. (A caution: at levels of intake even higher than this, the substance has experimentally *produced* cancer.) Vitamin E and vitamin C remain the most important dietary antioxidants to strengthen defenses against cancer.[4]

Upon learning of the studies that show BHA and BHT to inhibit cancer in rats, some people came to a wrong conclusion—that what works for rats must work for people, too. Manufacturers have begun marketing capsules of the preservatives as anticancer pills, and recommend taking amounts far beyond the FDA's limit of safety. In fact, the daily dose recommended by the makers of these pills is almost a lethal dose. Ironically, health food stores sell the capsules of BHT and BHA right alongside the packages of "no additives" foods.

This discussion provides the opportunity to mention an important point about additives. No two additives are alike, and therefore generalizations about them are meaningless. Whenever questions about the safety of "additives" are being discussed, you might as well leave the room, because no valid statement can be made that applies to the 3000-odd different substances commonly added to foods. Questions about which additives are safe, under what conditions of use, have to be asked and answered on an item-by-item basis.

Preservatives are added to food to prevent microbial spoilage; the most widely used of these are sugar and salt. Antioxidants, including vitamin E, prevent rancidity of fats; some have been found to prevent cancer in certain laboratory tests.

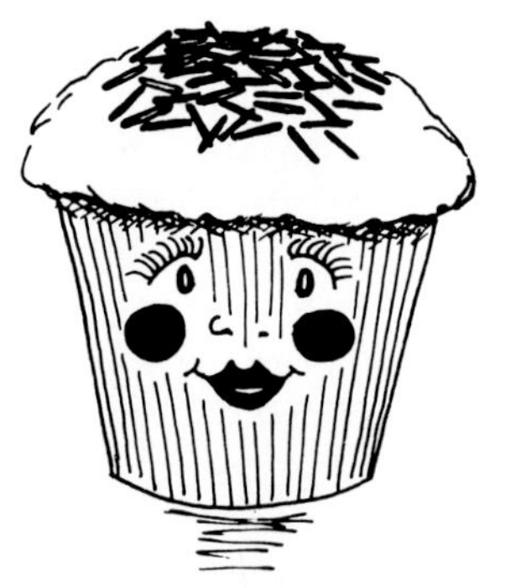

Some people think food colors are dispensable because they only make foods look pretty. Others say that because they make food more attractive, they are necessary.

Artificial Colors

As just mentioned, only 33 coloring agents are still on the GRAS list, a highly select group that has survived considerable screening. They are among the most intensively investigated of all additives. In fact, they are much better known than the *natural* pigments of plants, and we can state the limits on the safety of their use with greater certainty.[5]

Still, the food colors have been more heavily criticized than almost any other group of additives. This is because they are dispensable. Simply stated, they only make foods pretty, whereas other additives, such as preservatives, make foods safe. Hence with food colors we can afford to require that their use entail no risk, whereas with other additives we may have to compromise between the risks of using them and the risks of *not* using them.

An infamous food-coloring agent of an earlier time was red dye number 2, which came under suspicion as a carcinogen in 1970 on the basis of two studies conducted in Russia. It was never shown to cause cancer, but it proved impossible to demonstrate that it did *not* cause cancer, either, and so it was banned in the United States in 1976. On the same evidence, Canada concluded that it was not likely to cause cancer, and continued to permit its use. (Red candies in this country do not contain red dye number 2.)

More recently, the food color tartrazine (yellow number 5) has received a lot of publicity because it causes an allergic reaction in susceptible people. Symptoms include hives, itching, and nasal congestion, sometimes severe enough to require medical treatment. People who are allergic to aspirin are especially likely to be affected, but the tartrazine sensitivity also occurs in people without aspirin allergy. It is not a common problem; only one or two in 10,000 individuals may have the reaction, but still, that is over 20,000 individuals in the nation as a whole, and these people rightly demand to know where the dye is in foods so that they can avoid it. It is not enough to avoid yellow-colored foods, because tartrazine is used to confer turquoise, green, and maroon colors in foods and drugs as well.[6]

Tartrazine was for a while blamed for causing many (some people said most) cases of hyperactivity in children, and a special diet (the Feingold Diet), composed entirely of additive-free foods, was recommended for these children. By 1980 it was clear that the majority of cases of hyperactivity are not caused by tartrazine or other additives, but legislation is now in force requiring that tartrazine must be mentioned on all labels of foods that contain it so that consumers can avoid it if they wish.

Foods containing tartrazine:

- Orange drinks (Tang, Daybreak, Awake).
- Gatorade (lime flavored).
- Gelatin desserts (Jello, Royal).
- Golden Blend Italian dressing (Kraft).
- Some cake mixes and icings (Duncan Hines, Pillsbury, Cake Mate).
- Imitation banana or pineapple extract (McCormick).
- Seasoned salt (French's).
- Macaroni and cheese dinner (Kraft).
- "Cheez" curls and balls (Planter's).
- Fruit chews (Skittles).
- Butterscotch squares and candy corn (Brach's).

Chapter 12 addresses the idea that hyperactivity might be "cured" by diet.

Artificial Flavors and Flavor Enhancers

While only 33 colors are currently permitted in foods, there are close to 2000 flavoring agents, making them the largest single group of food additives. One of the best known members of this group is monosodium glutamate, or MSG (tradename, Accent)—the monosodium salt of the amino acid glutamic acid. MSG is used widely in restaurants, especially Asian restaurants. It is a flavor enhancer; it has no flavor of its own but increases the perception of flavor from the other substances present in food with it. MSG has received publicity because it may produce an adverse reaction in some individuals—the so-called Chinese restaurant syndrome—involving burning sensations, chest and facial flushing or pain, and throbbing headaches (see p. 198). MSG has been investigated extensively enough to be deemed safe for adults to use (except people who react adversely to it, of course), but it is kept out of foods for infants, because very large doses have been shown to destroy brain cells in developing mice. Infants' brains have not yet developed the capacity to fully exclude such substances as adult brains do, and so are more sensitive to them.

No one really knows how common Chinese restaurant syndrome is, or why it might occur. It may have some relationship to vitamin B_6 deficiency (see p. 198), but that does not account for all cases. Researchers are looking for a link between the development of the syndrome and elevated blood levels of the MSG fraction glutamate. So far, the results are mixed.

The placebo effect is discussed in Chapter 6.

Some of the research indicates that MSG is not the only cause of the syndrome and that if people do not know they are eating MSG, they may not have the symptoms.[7] This seems to indicate a strong placebo effect at work. In addition, it has been difficult to correlate blood glutamate levels with symptoms. Recently it was discovered that when MSG is administered along with some carbohydrate, as in a juice or other sweetened drink, the expected rise in blood glutamate does not occur.[8] When MSG is given with just water or broth, the blood glutamate zooms up.[9] This effect might explain some of the confusing results of early studies—when researchers delivered the MSG in water or broth, they reported elevated blood glutamate levels, but still had mixed results as to symptoms; those researchers who used sweet beverages reported no effects and little rise in blood glutamate levels.

There is still much to learn about Chinese restaurant syndrome, because it is still not known for certain whether only a few sensitive people are affected, whether the syndrome occurs universally with a high enough dose, or even whether elevated blood glutamate is the cause. However, it can do no harm to apply what is known to restaurant eating. For example, even if a restaurant chef has not added extra MSG, many industrial soup mixes and flavorings already contain it. Thus soups may contain substantial MSG even when the restaurant claims "no MSG added." Broth is one of the experimental fluids that allowed the blood glutamate levels to rise, so it would be prudent for a person who wishes to avoid Chinese restaurant syndrome to skip the soup, or to order the kind with noodles (carbohydrate). As for the rest of the meal, eat plenty of rice with each bite, as the Chinese themselves do, to provide carbohydrate.

Among colorings and flavorings added to foods, the yellow color Tartrazine and the flavoring MSG are suspected of causing reactions in people with sensitivities to them.

Nutrient Additives

COMPLETE FOOD BAR:
100% of EVERYTHING
BREAKFAST BAR
INGREDIENTS: SUGAR, VEGETABLE FAT, CHOCOLATE,

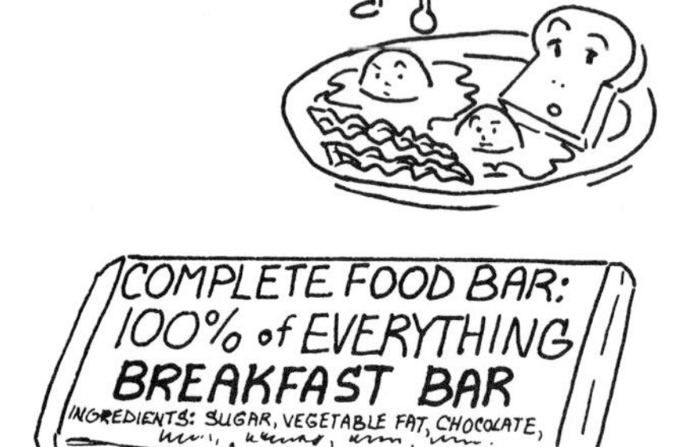

When nutrients are added, a nutrient-poor food can appear nutrient dense, but only in those nutrients chosen for addition.

Nutrients are sometimes added to improve or maintain the nutritional value of foods. Included among these are the four nutrients added to refined grains to enrich them; the iodine added to salt; vitamins A and D added to dairy products; and the nutrients added to fortified breakfast cereals. When nutrients are added to a nutrient-poor food, it may appear to the consumer to be nutrient-rich. It is, but only in those nutrients chosen for addition, and the absorption of these nutrients may be poor. Nutrients are sometimes also added for other purposes. Vitamins C and E are examples, already mentioned.

Nutrients are added to foods to enrich or fortify them, but still do not necessarily make them nutrient rich, except for the added vitamins and minerals.

Radiation

Ionizing radiation kills living cells.* Used in food processing, it kills microorganisms and insect pests, inhibits the growth of sprouts on potatoes and onions

*Ionizing rays include X rays, gamma rays, and beta rays (electrons). Radiation sources include x-ray machines and electron accelerators, or the source may be a radioactive isotope such as cobalt 60 or cesium 137.

by stopping cell division, and delays ripening in some fruits by interrupting enzymatic processes.[10]

People have learned to think of radiation as causing cancer, birth defects, and mutations; they think they should avoid all forms of radiation for their health's sake. When they hear talk of **irradiated food,** they naturally have doubts, if not strong emotions, about it. For example, some may fear that their food will be radioactive (hence the battle cry, "Don't nuke my food!"). Irradiating does not make foods radioactive, though; it takes stronger doses of radiation to do that. It is easy on foods—sterilizing them while leaving them attractive with their texture undisturbed and their flavor altered very little, if at all. Others may worry about the safety of irradiated food. Many different kinds of testing have revealed that there is no hazard to the consumer in foods that have been irradiated. The process is economically sound, too, because it cuts down on food wastage and replaces some costly pesticides that otherwise have to be used.

Radiation works by breaking up the cells' machinery (DNA and RNA) that is involved in reproduction and growth. As a result, tiny amounts of DNA and RNA derivatives remain in the food after the treatment is over, and this is why irradiation is considered an additive. The higher the dose of radiation, the more of these substances are formed. They are not unlike the substances that are present in food anyway, but a few are unique, and these have been carefully studied. Realistically, they too probably present no hazard.[11] These **unique radiolytic products (URPs)** are the same for all foods, because DNA and RNA are similar chemically no matter what living tissues they come from.

The FDA has approved irradiation in low doses to delay ripening of fruits and control sprouting of vegetables as mentioned earlier, to replace postharvest pesticide fumigation of certain foods, and to kill *Trichinella,* the dangerous parasitic worms that are sometimes found in pork. It has also approved high-dose treatment of dried spices, other seasonings, and teas to sterilize them. Milk products change flavor when irradiated, and so are not candidates for the treatment. (Incidentally, those boxes of milk kept at room temperature on the shelves of the grocery store are not irradiated, but treated with a process called **ultrahigh temperature;** the milk is exposed to temperatures above those of the normal milk treatment, **pasteurization,** for a short time—just long enough to sterilize it.)

The technology for food irradiation must be carefully scrutinized. Reports of accidental exposure of workers to radiation and liberation of radioactive waste from irradiation plants into public sewage and water systems are causes for concern.[12] There is no possibility of a meltdown or other nuclear disaster, because food irradiation plants are not nuclear reactors, but strict controls on irradiation facilities and the wastes they generate are needed to prevent hazards to workers and to the environment.

In the United States, the FDA has published regulations governing the use of irradiation.[13] Among requirements, each food treated with radiation must bear a label indicating that the food was "treated with radiation" or "treated by irradiation."[14] This informs consumers, but also could mislead them. Consumers could misinterpret the *absence* of the irradiation label to mean that the food was produced without treatment of any kind. This, of course, is not true; it is just that statements about the other treatments that perform similar functions, such as postharvest fumigation with pesticides, are not required on labels. Some people believe that if all treatment methods were declared, consumers could make fully informed choices.[15]

irradiated food: food that has been treated with radiation.

unique radiolytic (RAY-dee-oh-LIT-ic) **products (URPs):** products formed during the irradiation of food.

ultrahigh temperature: short-time exposure of a food to temperatures above those normally used, in order to sterilize it.

pasteurization: the treatment of milk with heat sufficient to kill certain pathogens (disease-causing microbes) commonly transmitted through milk, not a sterilization process. Pasteurized milk retains bacteria that causes milk spoilage. Raw milk, even if labeled "certified," transmits many foodborne diseases to people each year and should be avoided.

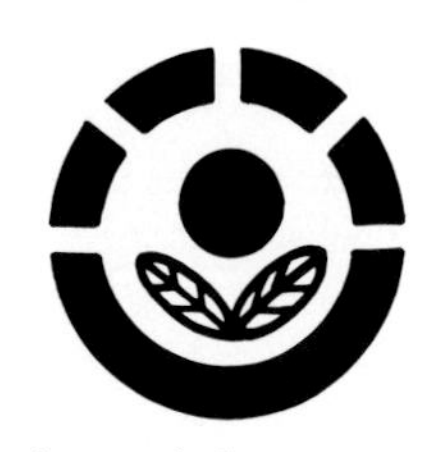

The irradiation symbol.

Related to irradiation by virtue of its creative use of radiation on food is the microwave oven. Like irradiation, microwaves sterilize foods. Unlike irradiation, though, microwaves cook the food as they pass through it.

All that has been said so far has indicated that, on the whole, the use of food additives seems to be justified by the benefits these additives offer, and that the risks associated with their use are small. All intentional additives are closely regulated and monitored. Still, some people wish to avoid them, and one way to do this is to eat a diet of mostly whole foods, as defined in Controversy 1—fresh fruits, vegetables, whole grains, fresh meats, and dairy products. That way, all you have to worry about are substances that get into food by accident, one of the more pressing concerns of the FDA.

Radiation is used to sterilize food after harvest, to kill Trichinella *worms in pork, to slow ripening, and to prevent sprouting. URPs are chemicals produced by the splitting of large molecules in foods by radiation; they have been tested and found safe in the quantities in which they occur in food.*

Incidental Food Additives

Incidental, accidental, or indirect additives are all substances that find their way into food as the result of some phase of production, harvesting, processing, storage, or packaging. For example, among incidental additives are tiny bits of plastic, glass, paper, tin, and other substances from packages, as well as chemicals from processing, such as the solvent used to decaffeinate some types of coffee.

Incidental additives are well regulated, just as intentional additives are. All food packagers are required to perform specific tests to discover whether materials such as these are migrating into foods; if they are, their safety must be confirmed by strict procedures similar to those governing intentional additives. Incidental additives sometimes find their way into foods, but adverse effects are rare.

A notable exception is lead, used to seal cans of food. This lead can dissolve into the food itself, especially if the food has a high acid content. The problems associated with lead exposure are discussed in a later section.

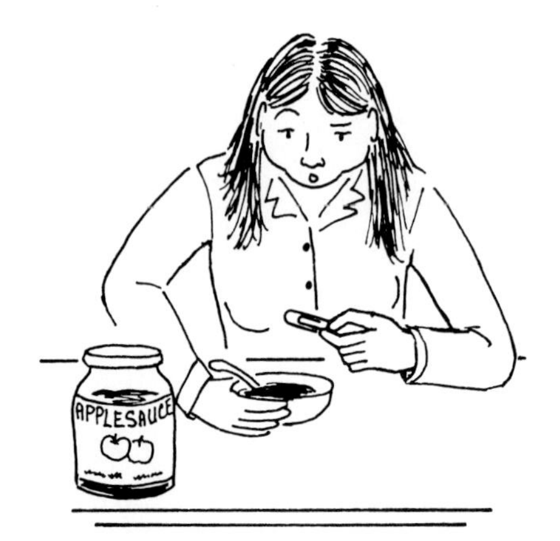

Incidental additives are substances that find their way into food as a result of production, processing, storage, or packaging.

Incidental additives are substances that get into food during processing. They are well regulated and most present no hazard.

Pesticides

Fifth on the FDA's list of concerns are the pesticides, unique among manmade chemicals used in relation to food because they are intended specifically to poison living things. Pesticides do occur in nature—the nicotine in tobacco is an example—but naturally occurring pesticides are far less lethal to other living things than the manmade chemicals. The ideal pesticide among manmade ones is one that destroys the pest and then quickly degenerates to other, nontoxic products. Table 10–1 lists a sampling of pesticides and their biological effects.

When pesticides were first used, it was considered desirable to use persistent ones—chemicals that would keep on killing for as long as they remained in the soil. Unfortunately, this was based on a simplistic idea—that they *would* remain in the soil. They did not. They washed into waterways, poisoned wild animals, contaminated the food supply, and would not go away. DDT, now no longer in use in the United States, was one such persistent pesticide, and after years of use, it began to show up in high concentrations in the body fat of animals. It threatened the survival of the American eagle by weakening eggshells to the point that they would collapse, killing the developing chicks. It showed up in big fish, carnivorous animals, and human beings, including human breast milk. Finally, after years of widespread agricultural use, DDT was banned. Substitutes have had to be found, but they have not always been as effective.

A lesson was learned in relation to substances like DDT: the extent to which it lingers in the body partly determines the potential harmfulness of a contaminant. If a contaminant enters the system and then is rapidly metabolized to some harmless compound, then its ingestion may not give cause for concern. If the contaminant is rapidly and preferentially excreted, then too the body may be able to survive a brief exposure time. But if it enters the body, interacts with the body's systems, is not metabolized or excreted, and fools the cells' proteins into accepting it as part of their structure, then it is dangerous. Additional doses will be piled on top of the first ones, and the contaminant will accumulate. All of these things are true of DDT, and that is why it is so deadly.

Table 10–1

A Sampling of Pesticides and Their Biological Effects

Type of Use	Common Names (examples)	Biological Effects
Insecticides	Parathion, Malathion	Toxic to nerves; acute poisoning causes respiratory failure.
	Aldicarb, Zectran	Toxic to nerves.
	DDT, Dieldrin, Heptachlor, Chlordane, Mirex	Accumulate in fatty tissues, inhibit electrolyte transport, impair reproduction in birds.
	Ethylene dibromide (EDB)	A carcinogen.
Herbicides	2,4,5-T	Toxic generally and to nerves.
	Paraquat	Toxic generally; causes edema in the lungs.
	Prophan	Allergenic.
	Simazine	Carcinogenic.
Fungicides	Captan	Causes birth defects.
	Pentachlorophenol (PCP)	Toxic generally.
Rodenticides	Warfarin	An anticoagulant.
	Red squill	Causes heart failure.
	Compounds 1080, 1081	Inhibit cellular respiration.
	ANTU	Causes edema in the lungs.

Source: Adapted from M. G. Mustafa, Agricultural chemicals, in *Adverse Effects of Foods,* eds. E. F. P. Jelliffe and D. B. Jelliffe (New York: Plenum Press, 1982), Table 1, pp. 112–113.

When a substance resists breakdown, either inside the body (by the body's enzymes) or outside (by microorganisms), and furthermore is stored in animals' bodies, it builds up in the food chain. Figure 10–1 shows the result.

The search for the perfect pesticide is continuing. Meanwhile, national and international agencies such as the Food and Agricultural Organization (FAO), the World Health Organization (WHO), the Environmental Protection Agency (EPA), and the FDA have adopted standards and attempt to regulate pesticide use. Pesticide use (including DDT use) worldwide is increasing and is not well monitored; the hazards of many of the chemicals in use today may be considerable and are unknown. The EPA monitors pesticide levels in fish, birds, and mammals; water, air, and food; and human beings.[16] The monitoring is not adequate, though, because new pesticides keep appearing before the EPA can act to monitor them, and because the maximum amounts allowed in a food assume that a person will only consume moderate quantities of that food; people sometimes overeat certain specific foods. Also, other countries use pesticides that are illegal for use here—some are even exported from here to those countries—and imported foods may not be tested for the presence of those pesticides.

Diagnosing toxic effects of pesticides is difficult. Many cause delayed reactions, especially those that poison the nerves. Toxins may collect in fatty tissues, sequestered away from the rest of the body—harmless until that fat becomes mobilized, as may occur in animals when food is scarce, or in people losing

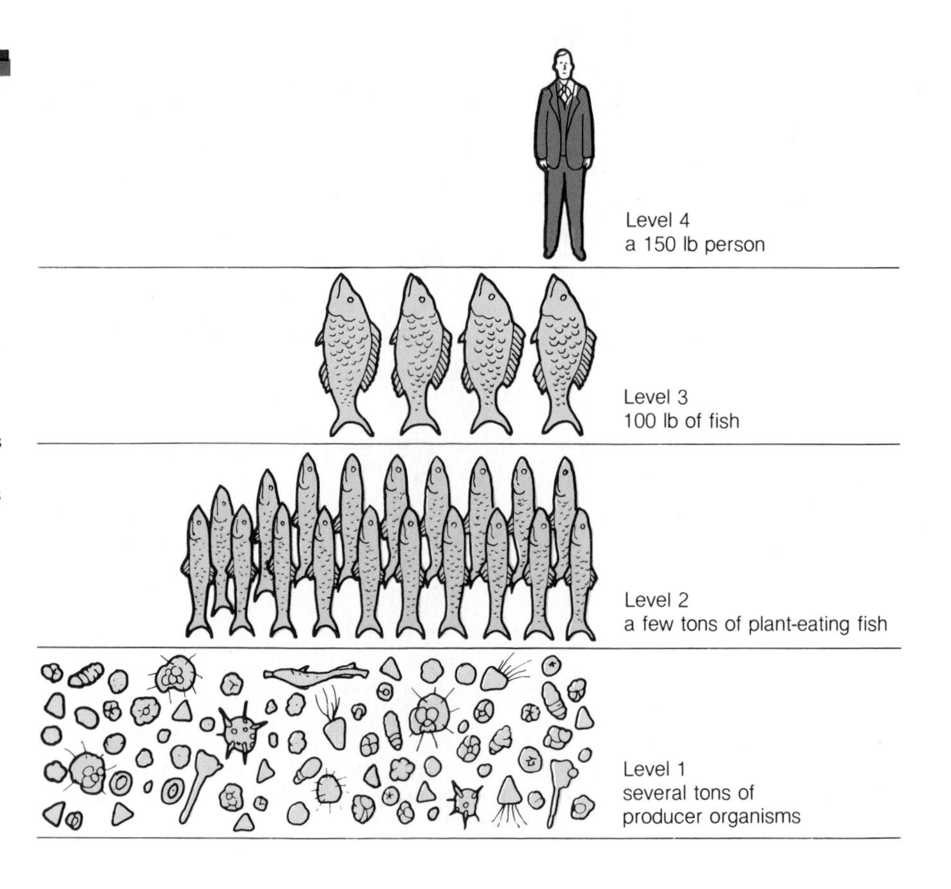

Figure 10–1
How a Food Chain Works.
A person whose principal animal protein source is fish may consume about 100 pounds of fish in a year. These fish will, in turn, have consumed a few tons of plant-eating fish in the course of their lifetimes. The plant eaters, in their lifetimes, will have consumed several tons of photosynthetic producer organisms. If the producer organisms have become contaminated with toxic chemicals, these chemicals become more concentrated in the bodies of the fish that consume them. If none of the chemicals are lost along the way, *one person* ultimately eats the same amount of contaminant as was present in the original *several tons* of producer organisms.

weight. Development of new pesticides and monitoring of their use is an ongoing activity that will require continued vigilance on the part of government agencies and consumers. Consumers should read reliable literature, discuss it with others, advise their government representatives on how pesticides should be handled, and apply pressure wherever it will help change procedures.

Meanwhile, how are consumers to avoid using foods containing unacceptably high levels of pesticides? Must they pay high prices for foods sold in special health-food stores and labeled *organic*—meaning "pesticide-free"? If all grocery-store foods were permeated with poisons and all organic foods were free of them, then that might be the obvious choice, but such is not the case. Two important considerations bear on the presence of pesticide residues in foods.

The first is the quantity of the poison present. Anything, even water, can be toxic if you consume enough of it. Whether a food has been exposed to pesticides at some time in the past is not the right question to ask about that food's effect on your health. The question to ask is how much residue remains in the food at the time you eat it, in relation to the threshold at which harm might occur. If a food has been sprayed and the poison has since evaporated, or changed into a nontoxic compound, or been diluted below the point at which it can do any harm, then the food may not be inferior to an unsprayed food; it may even be nutritionally superior, because it has not been weakened by attacks of pests.

Second, even though so-called organic foods sold in special stores claim not to have been sprayed, testing shows they sometimes contain pesticide residues in the same amounts as grocery store foods. Where these residues come from is not clear; perhaps in some cases farmers secretly spray them, perhaps in other cases pesticides drift onto farms that are not directly using them themselves, and perhaps in still other cases organic farms may be situated on pesticide-contaminated soil. The question is not what is on the label, then; the question is what is really in the food. Foods labeled "natural," "organic," or "health food" may not be superior to ordinary grocery store foods in terms of pesticide residues. People rightly fear ingesting poisons, and appropriately take the precaution of washing them in running water, scrubbing them with a vegetable brush, or soaking the uncut vegetables in a weak vinegar and water solution to remove pesticides. Irradiated fruits and vegetables are a reasonable choice in this regard, because they are spared post-harvest pesticide sprayings.

Next after pesticides, in order of the FDA's list of concerns, are naturally occurring toxins in foods. This topic receives treatment in Controversy 10 (see "Warnings") and will not be covered here. Instead, this chapter moves on to some chemicals that pose extreme hazards when they accidentally find their way into the food supply. They are third on the FDA's list of concerns—contaminants in foods.

Pesticides are used to control insects and other pests that would otherwise destroy food crops and food after harvest. Those in use have been tested for safety, although some, such as DDT, have had adverse effects when liberated into the environment. Those safest for human beings are those that break down quickly after use, but they are not always the most effective.

heavy metal: any of a number of mineral ions such as mercury and lead, so called because they are of relatively high atomic weight. Many heavy metals are poisonous.

organic halogen: an organic compound containing one or more atoms of a *halogen*—fluorine, chlorine, iodine, or bromine.

Contaminants in Foods

What are contaminants, and why are they considered so dangerous? They are the waste products of industry and other chemicals that are not normally present in amounts sufficient to cause harm, but that can and do occasionally break through safeguards intended to control them. A few examples will illustrate the problems they can cause.

In 1953, a number of people in Minamata, Japan, became ill with a disease no one had seen before. By 1960, 121 cases had been reported, including 23 in infants. Mortality was high; 46 died, and in the survivors the symptoms were ugly: "progressive blindness, deafness, incoordination, and intellectual deterioration."[17] The cause was ultimately revealed to be contamination of fish from the bay these people lived on. The infants who contracted the disease had not eaten any fish, but their mothers had, and even though the mothers exhibited no symptoms during their pregnancies, the poison had been affecting their unborn babies. Manufacturing plants in the region were discharging mercury into the waters of the bay, the mercury was turning to methylmercury on leaving the factories, and the fish in the bay were accumulating this poison in their bodies. Some of the families who were affected had been eating fish from the bay every day.[18]

In 1910, Dr. Alice Hamilton of the United States began documenting her observations of the toxicity to humans of another environmentally derived **heavy metal,** lead. Factory workers intoxicated with lead poisoning exhibited a wide variety of symptoms, she said, including anemia, constipation, loss of appetite, abnormal kidney function, jaundice due to liver damage, "wrist drop" (loss of muscular control of the hand), irritability, drowsiness, stupor, and coma. Mothers exposed to lead more often had abortions and stillbirths, and their children were more often sick.[19]

In 1973, in Michigan, half a ton of polybrominated biphenyl (PBB), a toxic chemical, was accidentally mixed into some livestock feed that was distributed throughout the state. The chemical found its way into millions of animals and then into people who ate their meat. The seriousness of the accident began to come to light when dairy farmers reported their cows going dry, aborting their calves, and developing abnormal growths on their hooves. Although more than 30,000 cattle, sheep, and swine and more than a million chickens were destroyed, effects on people were not prevented. By 1982 it was estimated that 97 percent of Michigan's residents had become contaminated with PBB. Nervous system aberrations and alterations in the liver and immune systems were among the effects in exposed residents.[20]

Mercury and lead are both heavy metals, and PBB is an **organic halogen.** These two classes of chemicals are among the most toxic and widespread in our environment. The number of contaminants and the amount of information available about them, is far beyond this book's scope. Instead of dealing superficially with many of them, it can illustrate principles that apply to all contaminants by giving details about just a few. A list of some of the chemical contaminants of greatest concern in foods is presented in Table 10–2. Table 10–3 gives more details on four of them.

Table 10–2

Chemical Contaminants of Concern in Foods, U.S., 1870–1980

Heavy Metals
Lead
Mercury
Cadmium
Selenium
Arsenic
Halogenated Compounds
Chlorine
Iodine
Vinyl chloride
Ethylene dichloride
Trichloroethylene
Polychlorinated biphenyls (PCBs)
Polybrominated biphenyls (PBBs)
Others
Asbestos
Dioxins
Acrilonitrile
Lysinoalanine
Diethylstilbestrol
Heat-induced mutagens
Antibiotics (in animal feed)

Source: E. M. Foster, How safe are our foods? *Nutrition Reviews* (supplement), January 1982, pp. 28–34.

Table 10–3

Examples of Contaminants in Foods

Name and Description	Sources	Toxic Effects	Typical Route to Food Chain
Cadmium (heavy metal)	Used in industrial processes including electroplating, plastics, batteries, alloys, pigments, smelters, and burning fuels. Present in cigarette smoke.	No immediately detectable symptoms; slowly and irreversibly damages kidneys and liver.	Enters air in smokestack emissions, settles on ground, absorbed into food plants, consumed by farm animals, and eaten in meat and vegetables by people. Sewage sludge and fertilizers leave large amounts in the soils; runoff contaminates shellfish.
Lead (heavy metal)	Added to gasoline, added to paints, used to seal cans of food (see text).	Displaces calcium, iron, zinc, and other minerals from their sites of action in the nervous system, bone marrow, kidneys, and liver, causing failure to function. Severe effects in fetuses, infants, and children who easily absorb and retain lead. Causes breakage of red blood cells (anemia) and interferes with the immune response.	Food can seals, air pollution, gasoline, water pipes, and others (see text).
Mercury (heavy metal)	Widely dispersed in gases from earth's crust; local high concentrations from industry, electrical equipment, paints, and agriculture.	Methylmercury poisons the nervous system, especially in fetuses (see text).	Inorganic mercury released into waterways by industry and acid rain is converted to methylmercury by bacteria and ingested by food species of fish (tuna, swordfish, and others).
Polychlorinated biphenyls (PCBs) (organic compounds)	No natural source; produced for used in electrical equipment (transformers, capacitors).	Long-lasting skin eruptions, eye irritations, growth retardation in children of exposed mothers, anorexia, fatigue, many others.	Discarded electrical equipment; accidental industrial leakage, or reuse of PCB containers for food.

On first studying this subject, a reader is likely to want the question answered, How serious is all this—how dangerous is it for *me*? Yet no one who has pursued the subject realistically expects to have that question answered in any simple way. It may be no problem in your area today, but it may become a severe problem tomorrow if there is a major accident. A general answer, then, is that the hazard is probably small, because most of the time, the chemicals are under control, but that in the event of an accident, the risk of toxicity can suddenly become very great. (Recall the meaning of *hazard* as opposed to *toxicity*, p. 373.)

Table 10–3 shows how pervasively a contaminant can affect the body. Look at the case of lead for a particularly telling example of how specific nutrients interact with heavy metals in specific ways. For further examples, total food intake; fat intake; and calcium, iron, and zinc intakes are known to alter animals' (and probably humans') susceptibility to lead toxicity:

- A diet low in calcium permits greater amounts of lead to accumulate in the body, probably by permitting more lead to be absorbed.
- Iron deficiency, even mild iron deficiency, permits greater lead intoxication. Iron deficiency in a nursing female makes her milk's lead content higher.
- Zinc status affects both tissue accumulation of lead and sensitivity to its effects.[21]
- The absorption of lead is greatest when the stomach is empty.[22]

The interaction of nutrients with contaminants like lead raises an important point. When an agency is charged with setting the "maximum permissible level" of an environmental contaminant, it sets about testing animals to see what levels bring about detectable ill effects. Usually these animals are being fed the standard laboratory chow—a very nutritious diet—and the only thing varied is their exposure to the contaminant. Healthy, well-nourished animals are likely to have considerably greater resistance to toxicity than they would if they were sick or malnourished, or if they were exposed to other toxins simultaneously. Yet the people to whom the results are applied may be neither healthy nor well nourished, and all probably encounter numerous toxins every day. These facts should be remembered when the limits are set.

In 1981, 535,000 U.S. children aged six months to five years were screened, and 22,000 were found to have symptoms caused by lead toxicity, reflecting a prevalent national health problem. In the same screening, an almost equal number of children—23,000—were found to need treatment for iron deficiency, a long-familiar, widespread public health problem. Thus lead toxicity ranks with iron deficiency in prevalence and severity and is more than just a theoretical hazard; 1 out of every 50 children in rural areas and more than 1 out of every 10 inner-city children are affected with lead poisoning.[23]

All foods contain some lead. Whether some of it is naturally present is not known, but much of it is known to come from industrial pollution. People use lead in gasoline, paint, batteries, and pesticides, and in industrial processes that release it into the air and water. Some domestic pipes are made of lead, and it dissolves into water—especially soft, acidic water. As mentioned, tin cans sealed with lead solder provide a major source of lead in canned food. Once opened, canned food should be immediately removed from the can, and always stored in a food storage container to minimize lead migration into the food. Lead in foods comes primarily from cans and from air pollution from gasoline, which works its way through rainfall and soil into plants and animals used as food.[24]

A standard has been recommended for weekly acceptable intakes of lead,* but no monitoring system keeps track of the amounts to which people are

*The World Health Organization suggests not more than 3 milligrams per individual per week for adults. Evaluation of mercury, lead, cadmium and the food additives amaranth, diethylpyrocarbonate and octyl gallate, *WHO Food Additives Series no. 4* (Geneva: WHO, 1972), as cited by D. G. Lindsay and J. C. Sherlock, Environmental contaminants, in *Adverse Effects of Foods,* eds. E. F. P. Jelliffe and D. B. Jelliffe (New York: Plenum Press, 1982), pp. 85–110.

actually exposed. Exposures are known to be higher in urban and industrial areas; near highways; and in slums, where children may accidentally ingest leaded paint by teething on old furniture, toys, and the railings of old buildings. The reduction of the use of leaded gasoline for automobiles and the application of new technology and material to the canning process are helping to limit the amounts of lead in the environment.

A popular new "therapy" to prevent or relieve "poisoning" by heavy metals is "chelation therapy," in which a person ingests a **chelating agent** and expects it to capture poisons and remove them from the body. You may remember from Chapter 9 that vitamin C helps iron to be absorbed into the body by chelating it; the principle of chelation therapy is to use an agent that is ***not*** absorbable but will carry heavy metals such as lead and mercury out of the body with the feces.

chelating agent: a chemical that sequesters another chemical; in nutrition, an agent that binds minerals and makes them unavailable for absorption.

The agent most often used is EDTA, ethylene diamine tetraacetic acid, a nonspecific chelating agent that grabs up positively charged molecules based only on their electrical charges. The trouble is that many nutrients have such charges, and EDTA does not distinguish ions you might want to absorb such as calcium, iron, magnesium, and copper from those you do not want, such as lead or mercury. Long-term use has been known to remove so much calcium from the bones that they no longer can support the body's weight. EDTA has legitimate uses; it can save the life of a child afflicted with metal poisoning, but it is also sometimes advertised by quacks who claim to be able to leach plaques out of your arteries, or do other such imaginary things.

It was said at the start that the hazard from contamination of food is probably small, and that the risk to individuals is from accidental gross contamination. However, this statement needs qualification. As mentioned, lead toxicity is a serious problem in many U.S. children today. As for other contaminants, much of what we know about them necessarily derives from episodes of acute contamination of limited populations. No one knows to what extent the total burden of contaminants accumulating in the environment may be reaching chronic levels that together pose a hazard to human beings. No one knows whether some individuals may be susceptible today to contamination levels in some areas. Another unknown factor is the question of interaction among contaminants. A substance that poses no threat by itself is chlorine in drinking water; however, when chlorine combines with organic wastes in the water, the chemicals join to form potent carcinogens. Another unknown is the time factor. Many substances of concern have been around for only a short time. What are the effects of prolonged exposure to them? Contaminants can be hard to identify; sometimes it is not even known that they are present, and so they are hard to regulate.

There is no systematic procedure for monitoring or controlling the presence of contaminants in food except in individual cases. Contaminants are unique in this respect. Additives and pesticides are intentionally used in or on foods, but contaminants are, of course, not. Additives and pesticides are subject to systematic testing, regulation, and monitoring; contaminants are not nearly so well watched. Examples have been given of attempts to quantify the risks associated with contamination of foods, but no across-the-board procedures are accepted and carried out. It will take effort and determination to detect these substances and control them appropriately.

An in-depth understanding of nutrition is essential to understanding the risks from contamination. Not 100 percent of the time, but more often than not, an adequate diet and optimal health help to protect against the toxicity of food

canning: preservation by killing all microorganisms present in food, and sealing out air. The food, its container, and its lid are heated until sterile; as the food cools, the lid makes an airtight seal, preventing contamination.

freezing: preservation by lowering food temperature to the point at which life processes cease. Microorganisms are not destroyed, but are held dormant as long as the food is frozen.

drying: preservation by removing sufficient water from food to inhibit microbial growth.

extrusion: a process by which the form of food is changed, such as changing corn to corn chips (see text); not a preservation measure.

high-temperature-short-time (HTST) principle: every 10° C (18° F) rise in processing temperature gives approximately a tenfold increase in microbial destruction, while it only doubles nutrient losses.

contaminants and other environmental pollutants. If you want to be well protected against possible exposure to toxic environmental contaminants in the future, you should look to your own nutritional health today. If you want your children to be protected, you should make sure that they receive an adequate and varied diet.

These thoughts bring us back to food selection. To be well-nourished, you must be able to choose intelligently among the foods presented to you in the grocery store.

Contaminants are potentially dangerous compounds that can accidentally find their way into food; lead is an example. Lead poisoning has widespread deleterious effects on many children who live in cities. Although maximum tolerance limits have been set, no monitoring system to detect levels that exceed these limits has been implemented. Regulating agencies do not yet have in place adequate monitoring systems to protect people from food contamination. The probabilities of toxic effects from day-to-day contact with small amounts of these substances are largely unknown. One defense against harm from small doses of toxins is adequate nutrition.

Food Processing and Nutrient Density

Uppermost in the minds of nutrition-conscious people is how processing affects the nutritional quality of the food they eat. The FDA ranks this concern number 2 in importance because of its far-reaching impact on health. A great percentage of the total food consumed, whether eaten in restaurants or at home, has been prepared in some way by industry. People often ask what processing does to foods, and which kinds of foods are most and least nutritious.

In general, food processing involves a trade-off: it makes food safer and gives it a longer usable lifetime than fresh food, but at the cost of some vitamin and mineral losses. In some instances, however, processed food has the edge over its unprocessed counterpart, even in terms of a nutrient or two. This section explains each of the processing techniques—**canning, freezing, drying,** and **extrusion**—and the effects they have on nutrients.

Which nutrients are affected by canning, and how are they affected? Canning is one of the more effective methods for preserving food against the microbes (bacteria, fungi, and yeasts) that might otherwise spoil it, but canned foods, unfortunately, do have fewer nutrients. Like other heat treatments, the canning process is based on time and temperature. Each small increase in temperature has a major killing effect on microbes with only a minor effect on nutrients. By contrast, long treatment times are costly in terms of nutrient losses. Therefore industry chooses treatments that employ the **high-temperature-short-time (HTST) principle** for canning.

To determine how much of a food's nutritional value is lost in canning, food scientists have performed many experiments. They have paid particular attention to three vulnerable water-soluble vitamins—thiamin, riboflavin, and vitamin C.

Acid stabilizes thiamin, but heat rapidly destroys it; therefore the foods that lose the most thiamin during canning are the low-acid foods like lima beans, corn, and meat. Up to half, or even more, of the thiamin in these foods can be lost during canning. Unlike thiamin, riboflavin is stable to heat, but sensitive to light; so glass-packed, not canned, foods are most likely to lose riboflavin. Vitamin C's special enemy is an enzyme (ascorbic acid oxidase) present in fruits and vegetables, as well as in microorganisms. By destroying this enzyme, HTST canning actually aid in preserving vitamin C, while the short time of treatment means less of the vitamin is destroyed. As for the fat-soluble vitamins, they are relatively stable and are not affected much by canning.

Minerals are unaffected by heat processing, because they cannot be destroyed, as vitamins can be. However, both minerals and vitamins can be lost when they leak into water that the consumer may throw away. Losses are closely related to the extent to which food tissues have been broken, cut, or chopped, and to the length of time the food is in the water.

Some minerals are added when foods are canned. Important in this regard is sodium chloride. In general, the more highly a food is processed, the more sodium chloride and the less potassium it is likely to contain. As Chapter 7 demonstrated, the person wishing to control salt intake is wise to use unprocessed food to the greatest extent possible.

In selecting brands of canned foods, keep in mind that high prices on nationally advertised brands reflect the cost of the advertising, not the nutritional quality of the products. As long as the ingredients are the same, the less expensive products with **generic names** provide comparable nutrients. Although taste differences may dictate a consumer's preference for one brand over another, the assumption that the less expensive brands are nutritionally inferior is incorrect.

An alternative to canning, as a means of preserving food, is freezing. People often ask how frozen foods compare with canned. In general, frozen foods' nutrient content is similar to that of fresh foods; losses are minimal. The freezing process itself does not destroy any nutrients, but some losses may occur during the steps taken in preparation for freezing, such as blanching, washing, trimming, or grinding. Vitamin C losses are especially likely, because they occur whenever tissues are broken and exposed to air (oxygen destroys vitamin C). Uncut fruits, especially if they are acidic, do not lose their vitamin C; strawberries, for example, may be kept frozen for over a year without losing any vitamin C.

Fresh foods are often shipped long distances, and to make the trip without bruising or spoiling, they are often harvested unripe. Frozen foods are shipped frozen, so produce is allowed to ripen in the field and develop nutrients to their fullest potential. If foods are frozen and stored under proper conditions, they will often contain more nutrients when served at the table than fresh fruits and vegetables that have stayed in the produce department of the grocery store even for a day.

Frozen foods have to be kept frozen to retain their nutrients. To be solidly frozen, a food has to be colder than 32 degrees Fahrenheit or 0 degrees Centigrade. Conversion of vitamin C to its inactive forms occurs rapidly at warmer temperatures. Food may seem frozen at 2 degrees Centigrade, but much of it is actually unfrozen, and enzyme-mediated changes occur more rapidly than if it were solidly frozen. Under these conditions, the vitamin C in a frozen food can be completely lost in as short a time as two months.

In general, for frozen foods, the lower the temperature, the longer the storage life and the greater the nutrient retention. If you want to maximize the nutritive

generic (jen-AIR-ic) **names:** the common names by which everyone recognizes products, as distinct from brand names. (Example: *seltzer water* is a generic name; Perrier is a brand name.)

To see the effect of canning on thiamin in foods, look at Appendix A, items 563 and 564 (3 oz of raw clams versus 3 oz of canned clams). Or check the thiamin in items 890 and 891 (½ c frozen green peas versus ½ c canned green peas). While you are looking, what other effects of canning on thiamin do you see?

value of the foods you store at home, invest in a freezer thermometer, monitor the temperature of your frozen-food storage place, and keep it below freezing.

Consumers wonder how dried or dehydrated foods compare with canned and frozen foods. Dried or dehydrated foods have their own special characteristics. Drying offers several advantages. It eliminates microbial spoilage (because microbes need water to grow), and it greatly reduces the weight and volume of foods (because foods are mostly water). Furthermore, drying does not cause major nutrient losses. Vacuum puff drying and freeze drying, which take place in cold temperatures, conserve nutrients especially well.

Sulfites, described earlier, are added during the drying of fruits such as peaches, grapes (raisins), and plums (prunes), to prevent browning. Sulfur dioxide happens to help preserve vitamin C as well, but it is highly destructive of thiamin. The overall effect of its addition is probably beneficial, because most dehydrated products with added sulfur dioxide are not major sources of thiamin anyway.

Some food products, particularly snack foods, have undergone the process known as extrusion. In this process, the food is heated, ground, and pushed through various kinds of screens to yield different shapes, usually bite-size or smaller, like pieces of breakfast cereal or the "bits" you sprinkle on salad—so-called food novelties. Considerable nutrient losses occur during extrusion processes, and nutrients are usually added to compensate. But foods this far removed from the original fresh state are still lacking significant nutrients (notably vitamin E) and consumers should not rely on them as staple foods. Enjoy them, but only as occasional snacks and as additions to enhance the appearance, taste, and variety of meals.

Should everyone avoid all processed food? The answer is not simple: it depends on the food and on the process. Consider the case of orange juice and vitamin C. Orange juice is available in several forms, each processed a different way. Fresh juice is simply squeezed from the orange—a process that extracts the fluid juice from the fibrous structures that contain it. The fresh-squeezed juice, per 100 calories, contains 111 milligrams of vitamin C. If this juice were condensed by heat, frozen, and then reconstituted, as is the juice in the freezer case of the grocery store, 100 calories of the reconstituted juice would contain just 88 milligrams of vitamin C—vitamin C is destroyed in the condensing process. Canning is even harder on the vitamin C content of orange juice—100 calories of canned juice has 82 milligrams of vitamin C.

These figures may seem to indicate that fresh juice is the superior food, and so it is—but consider this: the U.S. RDA for vitamin C is 60 milligrams, an amount covered single-handedly by one serving of any of the above choices. In this case, at least for vitamin C, the losses due to processing can be called negligible, and there is an enormous convenience and distribution advantage to the processing. Fresh orange juice spoils. Shipping it to distant points makes it much more expensive than frozen or canned juice. The fresh product cannot be stored indefinitely without compromising nutrient quality. Without canned or frozen juice, people who have no access to the fresh juice would be deprived of this excellent food.

Some processing stories are not so rosy. In Chapter 7, for instance, you saw how processed foods are often loaded with sodium as their potassium is leached away. A related mischief of processing is the addition of sugar and fat—palatable, high-calorie additives that reduce nutrient density. An example is nuts and raisins covered with natural "yogurt." This may sound like one healthy food being added to another, but a look at the ingredient panel warns that generous amounts of fat and sugar accompany the yogurt. About 75 percent of the weight of the product is fat and sugar, about 8 percent is yogurt. To pick just one nutrient for an example, here is what happens to the iron density of the raisins: 100 calories of raisins = 0.71 milligrams iron; 100 calories of "yogurt" raisins = 0.26 milligrams of iron. These foods taste so good that wishful thinking can easily take hold, but the reality is that fat- and sugar-coated food is candy. The word *yogurt* on the label means only that one of the ingredients of the candy coating is some small amount of yogurt. Names, even whole-food names, on labels do not prove that the foods so named confer any nutritional benefit on the consumer unless the foods themselves are nutritious.

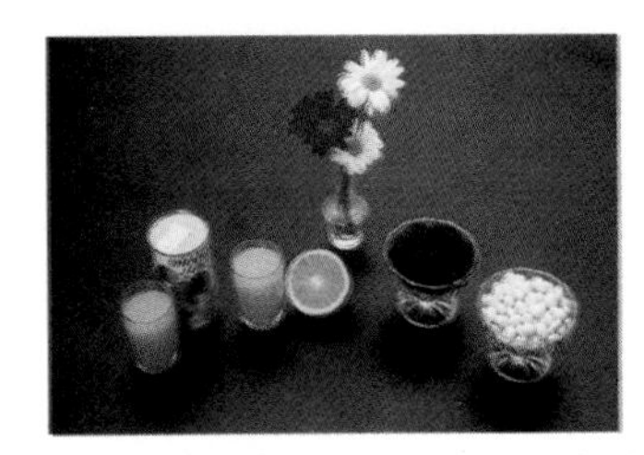

Canned juice may be as nutritious as fresh, but yogurt-coated raisins are *not* as nutritious as plain raisins.

(Incidentally, do not conclude from this example that raisins are a good source of iron. Compared with other food sources of iron on a per-calorie basis, raisins fall short. If you relied on raisins to supply 100 percent of the U.S. RDA for iron, you would have to eat 2600 calories of them. In contrast, 114 calories of spinach meets the U.S. RDA for iron. Table 7–5 in Chapter 7 shows how to select iron-rich foods.)

A generalization made many times before is worth repeating here—the more processed a food, the lower its nutrient value. But keep your mind open. Some processed foods are at least more nutritious than others. Consumers face the choice at the grocery store of selecting foods that are whole, those that have been minimally processed, and those are just parts of plant and animal tissues, the partitioned foods described in the first Controversy of this book. Two-thirds of the calories consumed in the U.S. diet come from the last type, the partitioned foods—fats, sugar, alcohol, and refined flour—foods completely, or almost completely empty of nutrients (unless you count energy as a nutrient). Only one-third of the calories in the U.S. diet come from relatively whole foods—whole in the sense of being unaltered from their original farm-grown state. These are the foods that contribute virtually all of our nutrients.

The implications for food choices are clear: for an optimally nutritious diet, choose whole foods to the greatest extent possible. Being realistic, few people have the time to bake all of their own bread from scratch, to shop every few days for fresh meats, or to wash, peel, chop, and cook fresh fruits and vegetables at each meal. And this is where food processing comes in—commercially prepared whole-grain breads, frozen cuts of meats, bags of frozen vegetables, and fruit juices do little disservice to nutrition and enable the consumer to eat a wide variety of lightly processed foods. The nutrient contents of processed foods exist on a continuum:

- Whole-grain bread > refined white bread > sugared doughnuts.
- Milk > fruit-flavored yogurt > canned chocolate pudding.
- Corn on the cob > canned creamed corn > caramel popcorn.
- Orange > orange juice > orange-flavored drink.
- Baked ham > deviled ham > fried pork rind.

Another continuum parallels it: that of the nutrition status of the consumer—the closer to the farm the foods you eat, the better nourished you are.

These pointers have answered the specific questions people most often ask about selecting processed foods. What about selecting fresh foods, then? A generalization you may find useful can be added to the previous pointers. As

food poisoning: illness transmitted to human beings through food, caused by a poisonous substance (*food intoxication*) or an infectious agent (*food-borne infection*).

food quality (appearance, taste, and texture) deteriorates, there is often a corresponding deterioration in nutrient content. For example, when a food smells bad, the odor reveals that oxidative or enzymatic changes have occurred—the same kinds of reactions as those that have adverse effects on nutrients. Thus, some unprocessed foods sold as "natural" foods may be a poor choice in spite of the claims made for them. If they have lost their freshness, they may well have lost their vitamins, too, because "no processing" means no measures have been taken to prevent oxidative and enzymatic changes. Thus your common sense, which tells you that a food "doesn't look quite right," can often be trusted to give you valid information.

In modern commercial processing, losses of vitamins seldom excceed 25 percent. In contrast, losses in food preparation at home can be 100 percent, and it is not unusual to see losses in the 60 to 75 percent range. These facts put the matter of food processing into perspective and reveal that while the kinds of foods you buy certainly make a difference, what you do with them in your kitchen makes a difference too. (See "Making Meals Rich in Vitamins," Chapter 6.)

Canning, freezing, and drying are three major means of preserving foods. Dried, frozen, and fresh foods have comparable nutrient contents. Canning causes some vitamin losses; however, canning companies add certain minerals, particularly sodium and chloride. Extrusion destroys many nutrients, and yields unique food forms.

Preventing Food Poisoning

The top item on the FDA's list of food hazards is **food poisoning,** which is estimated to cause 80 million cases of illness and many deaths every year. The overwhelming majority of mild cases are never reported because the victims pass them off as "flu." (Some viruses do cause intestinal distress, and those that do are usually transmitted via food; true influenza viruses cause symptoms primarily in the upper respiratory tract.) If you experience diarrhea, nausea, abdominal pain, or vomiting as the major or only symptoms of your next bout of "flu," chances are excellent that what you really have is food poisoning. If you take the proper precautions, you may never have it again.

The term *food poisoning* refers to ingestion of food that contains natural toxins or, more likely, is contaminated by microbes capable of causing illness. The microbes may produce toxins, or they may be infectious agents. Varieties of *Salmonella* are probably the most frequent causes of food-borne infections; those that are resistant to standard antibiotic therapy result from the overuse of antibiotics in animal feed and can be deadly. *Streptococcus* varieties produce toxins, and are also common. Much less common, and more deadly, is *Clostridium botulinum,* the organism that can grow in canned foods and that produces the deadly botulinum toxin mentioned earlier.

Foods can pick up microbes during processing, packaging, transport, storage, or preparation. Raw foods, especially meats and poultry, from the grocery store contain microbes, as all things do. Poultry is particularly likely to be contaminated with *Salmonella* bacteria. Whether or not those microbes multiply and cause illness is largely a matter of what you do or fail to do in your own kitchen.

Commercially prepared food is usually, but not always, safe. Batch numbering makes it possible to recall contaminated foods through public announcements via newspapers, television, and radio. The chance that someone may tamper with grocery store food is remote; to protect against this unlikely event, carefully inspect the seals and wrappers of packages. Jars should be firmly sealed (many have safety "buttons," areas of the lid designed to pop up once opened). Notice how the majority of the packages on the shelf appear. If the one you have chosen looks different, or if it has holes or tears, do not buy the product—turn it in to the store manager. A broken seal or mangled package is not doing its job of protecting the product from insects and spoilage, even if it hasn't been tampered with.

Food Safety in the Kitchen

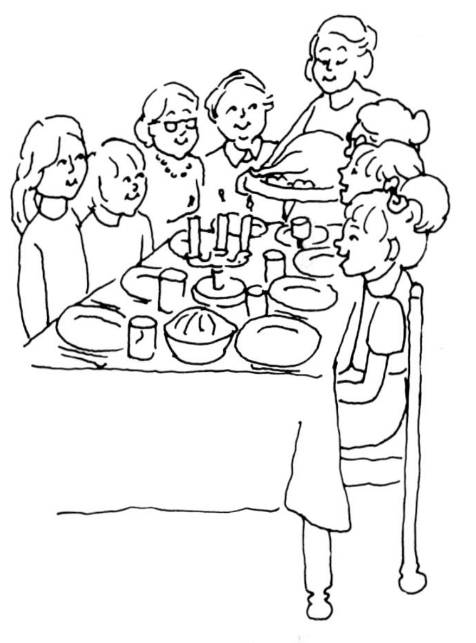

Food safety underlies eating pleasure.

Most cases of food poisoning that arise from kitchen mistakes can be averted by doing three simple things: keep hot food hot, keep cold food cold, and keep hands, utensils, and the kitchen clean. Keeping hot food hot includes allowing sufficient cooking time for food to reach safe internal temperatures during cooking (these temperatures are listed on meat thermometers), and holding it at a high enough temperature to prevent bacterial growth until served. Temperatures between 140 and 165 degrees Fahrenheit are usually safe for up to 2 hours. After that, the food should be chilled.

Keeping cold food cold starts when you leave the grocery store; if you are running errands, shop last, so the groceries do not stay in the car too long. Pack foods into the refrigerator or freezer immediately upon arrival at home.

A clean kitchen prevents contamination of otherwise wholesome foods. Wash the countertops, your hands, and utensils in warm, soapy water before each step of food preparation. Microbes love to nestle down in the fibers of wood cutting boards, kitchen cloths, and sponges. A microwave oven is handy for sterilizing wet sponges and clothes—after using, cook them on "high" until they are steamy and hot. Laundering with bleach will do the same thing; sponging bleach solution over the cutting board is a way to sterilize two kitchen items at once—the sponge and the board.

Meat requires special handling. It may contain all sorts of bacteria, and it provides a moist, nutritious environment—just right for microbial growth. If meat is marinated in a dish, wash that dish in hot, soapy water before reusing it to hold the cooked meat; otherwise, the bacteria inevitably left on the plate from the raw meat can contaminate and grow in the cooked product.

Especially susceptible to bacterial contamination is ground meat. It is handled more than other kinds of meat, and has much more surface exposed to the air for bacteria to land on. It is best to cook hamburgers to at least medium well done. For a meatloaf, use a thermometer to test the internal temperature.

An earlier section pointed out that fresh food smells fresh. It bears repeating that any food that has an off odor should not be used, but returned to the grocery store or thrown out. That odor is probably the result of bacterial wastes, and indicates that the number of bacteria in the food is dangerous. Not all types of food poisoning are detectable by odor, but if an abnormal odor exists, chances are excellent that the food is spoiled. Study Table 10–4; if you learn and follow the rules given there, you may save yourself the pain and inconvenience (and sometimes danger) of food-borne illness.

Picnics are fun and can be safe, too. Choose foods that last without refrigeration, such as fresh fruits and vegetables, breads and crackers, and canned spreads and cheeses that can be opened and used on the spot. Aged cheese, such as cheddar and Swiss, do well for an hour or two, but should be carried in an ice chest for longer periods. The advice not to add mayonnaise to picnic foods such as meat or pasta salads has been reversed by some who cite a study that found that mayonnaise was resistant to spoilage because of its acid content. Still, whether or not they contain mayonnaise, mixed salads of chopped ingredients spoil easily because they have extensive surface area for bacteria to invade, and they have been in contact with cutting boards, hands, and kitchen utensils that easily transmit bacteria to food. Chill them well before, during, and after the picnic. Mayonnaise itself must be kept cold.

Another danger concerns honey. Honey has been found to contain dormant bacterial spores, which can awaken in the human body to produce botulism, mentioned earlier. In adults, this is not a hazard, but infants less than a year old should never be fed honey.[25] (It can also be contaminated with environmental pollutants picked up by the bees.) Honey has been implicated in several cases of sudden infant death.[26]

For adults and children alike, eating raw or lightly steamed seafood is a risky proposition. As population density increases along the shores of seafood-harvesting waters, pollution of those waters inevitably invades the seafood living there. Watchdog agencies try to monitor the waters and keep harvesters out of the worst areas, but these efforts are often insufficient to ensure the wholesomeness of the food.[27] The food-borne infections that lurk in normal-appearing seafood can be much worse than those of spoilage—hepatitis, worms and parasites, severe viral intestinal disorders, and other diseases. (AIDS is not transmitted through seafood.)* Hepatitis is a prolonged illness, of months' or years' duration, and greatly increases the risk of liver cancer later. People who love raw seafood and have eaten it for years may try to brush off these threats because they have never experienced serious illness. Now, though, experts are suggesting that the risks are increasing to the point of being unacceptably high and it may be time to warn people to cook all seafood thoroughly before eating it.

Disease and illness can be transmitted to people through foods that harbor microbes or their toxins. Almost all cases of food poisoning can be averted by following the rules of safe food preparation, storage, and cleanliness. Organisms in seafood may cause serious illness, unless the seafood is thoroughly cooked.

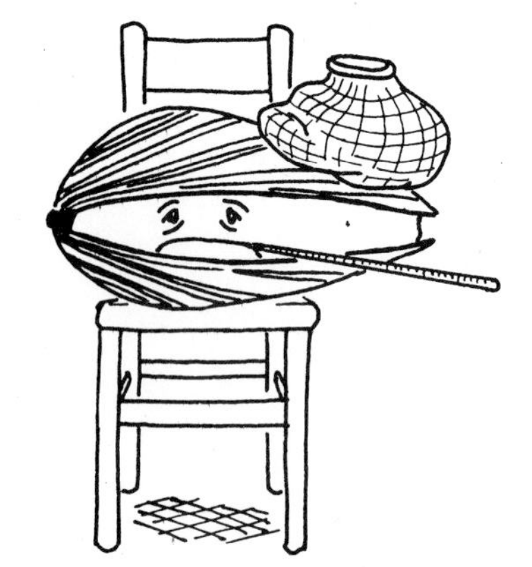

Shellfish can transmit diseases to people.

*AIDS is acquired immune deficiency syndrome, a viral infection that is transmitted by sexual contact and by needles shared among drug users. It is spreading rapidly worldwide among all people who have multiple sex partners, and among those who inject drugs. It is invariably fatal and thought to be preventable by the use of condoms during sexual intercourse and by the use of sterile needles in drug use.

Table 10–4

How to Prevent Food Poisoning

To prevent illness from *Salmonella* and *Streptococcus* varieties:

- Avoid transferring contamination: use hot, soapy water to wash hands, utensils, cutting boards, or countertops that have been in contact with raw meats, poultry, or eggs.
- Thaw meats or poultry in the refrigerator, not at room temperature. If you must hasten the thawing, use cool running water or a microwave oven.
- Stuff poultry just prior to cooking, or cook the stuffing separately. Use a meat thermometer to avoid undercooking. Insert the thermometer between the thigh and the body of a turkey, or in the thickest part of other meats, making sure the tip is not in contact with bone. Cook to the temperature shown for that meat on the thermometer.
- Refrigerate leftovers promptly, and heat them thoroughly before serving.
- Use clean eggs with intact shells, and cook eggs before eating.
- Keep susceptible foods at temperatures colder or hotter than room temperature. Keep hot foods at 140° F or more. Keep cold foods at 40° F or less.
- Mix foods with utensils, not hands; keep hands and utensils away from mouth, nose, and hair.
- A person with a skin infection or infectious disease should not prepare food. Anyone, though, may be a carrier of bacteria and should avoid coughing or sneezing over food.

To prevent poisoning from *Clostridium botulinum:*

- Before canning anything, seek professional advice. The U.S. Department of Agriculture Extension Service provides such information free of charge.
- Throw out food with off odors. (An off odor, however, is not necessarily detectable in a food containing toxins.)
- Do not even taste food that is suspect. If you are in doubt about the home-canning procedure used, and if you absolutely must eat the food, boil meats, poultry, corn, or spinach for 20 minutes and other vegetables for at least 10 minutes.
- Discard food from cans that leak or bulge. Dispose of the food in a manner that will protect other people and pets from its accidental use.

Some final reminders:

- Buy only those foods stored below the frost line in store freezers.
- Do not buy or use items that appear to have been opened or tampered with.
- When running errands, make the grocery store your last stop. Take the groceries out of the car when you get home, and refrigerate perishables immediately.
- Follow label instructions for storing and preparing packaged and frozen foods.
- When serving, keep hot foods at 140° F or higher and cold foods at 40° F.
- Cooked foods that are not to be served right away should be refrigerated immediately. Use shallow, not deep, containers—the foods will cool faster.
- Maintain a clean, dry kitchen that is free of flies and insects. Wash or replace dirty sponges and towels; clean up food spills and crumb-filled crevices. Use hot, soapy water for countertops, as well as for dirty dishes. Hot water and soap will immobilize bacteria and wash them away; cold water will not.

Food Safety While Traveling

If you are planning to travel far from home, you can take steps to protect your health by avoiding some pitfalls that can ruin a trip. One is digestive infections caused by organisms not found at home.

A person traveling to a less-developed country may find that the public health services we take for granted are not a reality there. The result can be a sometimes serious, always annoying bacterial infection of the digestive tract: traveler's diarrhea. It can most often be prevented if the traveler learns some simple rules about food and water, and follows them closely:

- Wash your hands often with soap and water, especially before handling food or eating.
- Eat only cooked food and canned items. Eat raw fruit or vegetables only if you have washed and peeled them yourself. Skip salads.
- Drink only boiled, canned, or bottled beverages and drink them without ice, even if they are not chilled to your liking. Avoid using the local water supply, even if you are just brushing your teeth, unless you boil it first. Take along a tiny hot plate or an element that boils water in a cup to use for oral hygiene.
- Check with your physician before you leave on the trip for recommendations on which medicines to take with you, in case your efforts to avoid illness fail.

Do not take medicines in hopes of warding off food-borne illness unless your physician directs you to do so. Chances are excellent, if you follow the rules above, that you will remain well.

Food Feature

Reading Food Labels

Up to this point, the Food Feature sections have been directed to the selection and handling of foods and the planning of diets that are adequate in nutrients. This Food Feature provides the background to fully understand in advance the contents of a box or package of prepared or processed food, before you include it in your diet.

The person who wants to read food labels intelligently needs to know some facts about the labeling laws. First of all, according to law, every food label must state:

- The common name of the product.
- The name and address of the manufacturer, packer, or distributor.
- The net contents in terms of weight, measure, or count.

Then, unless the food has a standard of identity (explained later), the label must list:

- The ingredients, in descending order of predominance by weight.

This information has to be prominently displayed, and must be expressed in ordinary words. That is all there is to the required label—but if you know how to read the front and side of a package, you are already a step ahead of the naive buyer. This is particularly true in regard to the ingredient list. Whatever is listed first is the ingredient that predominates, by weight. Consider the following ingredient lists:

- An orange powder that contains "sugar, citric acid, orange flavor . . ." versus a canned juice that contains "water, tomato concentrate, concentrated juices of carrots, celery. . . ."
- A cereal that contains "puffed milled corn, sugar, corn syrup, molasses, salt . . ." versus one that contains "100 percent rolled oats."
- A canned fruit that contains nothing but "apples, water."

If you read the label, you know what you are getting, and what the main ingredient is. (Look up ingredients you do not recognize in Appendix G.) Figure 10–2 demonstrates the reading of a label.

Labels often tell you more than the minimum, however. If a nutrient is added to a food (for example, vitamin C to a breakfast drink), or if an advertising claim is made (for example, that a food is a good source of vitamin A), then the package must provide an information panel that complies *fully* with the nutrition labeling requirements. Without a complete information panel, nutrition claims could deceive the consumer.

Several types of claims may not be made on labels:

1. That a food is effective as a treatment for disease.
2. That a balanced diet of ordinary foods cannot supply adequate amounts of nutrients (excepting the iron requirements of infants, children, and pregnant or lactating women).

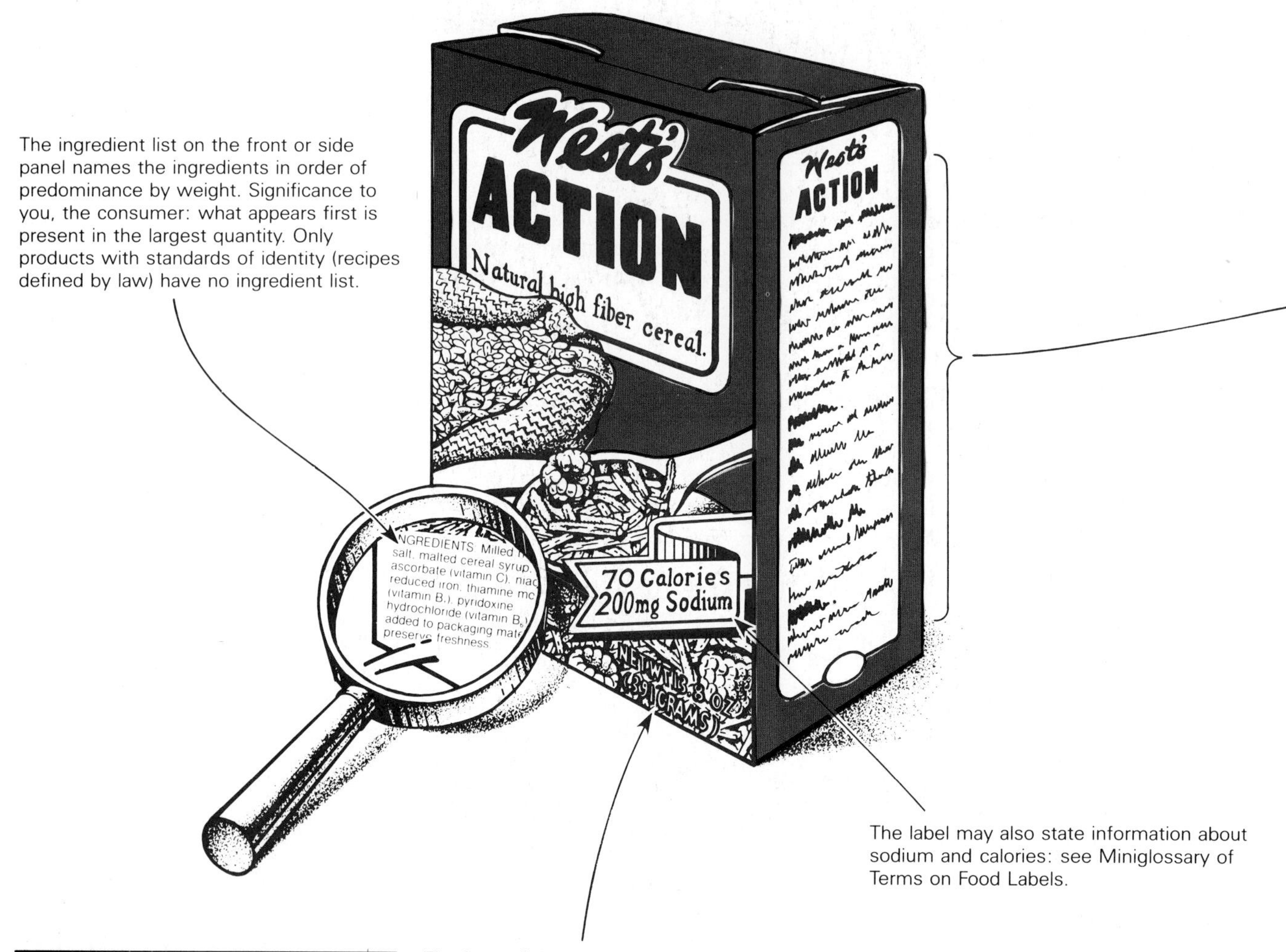

Figure 10–2
How to Read a Food Label
The ingredient list on the front or side panel names the ingredients in order of predominance. Significance to you, the consumer: what appears first is present in the largest quantity. Only products with standards of identity (recipes defined by law) have no ingredient list.

3. That the soil on which food is grown may be responsible for deficiencies in quality.
4. That storage, transportation, processing, or cooking of a food may be responsible for deficiencies in its quality.
5. That a food has particular dietary qualities when such qualities have not been shown to be significant in human nutrition.
6. That a natural vitamin is superior to a synthetic vitamin.

The nutrition labeling section of the law then states that, if any nutrition information or claim is made on the label of a food package, it must conform to the following format under the heading "Nutrition Information":

- Serving or portion size.
- Servings or portions per container.
- Food energy (in calories) per serving.

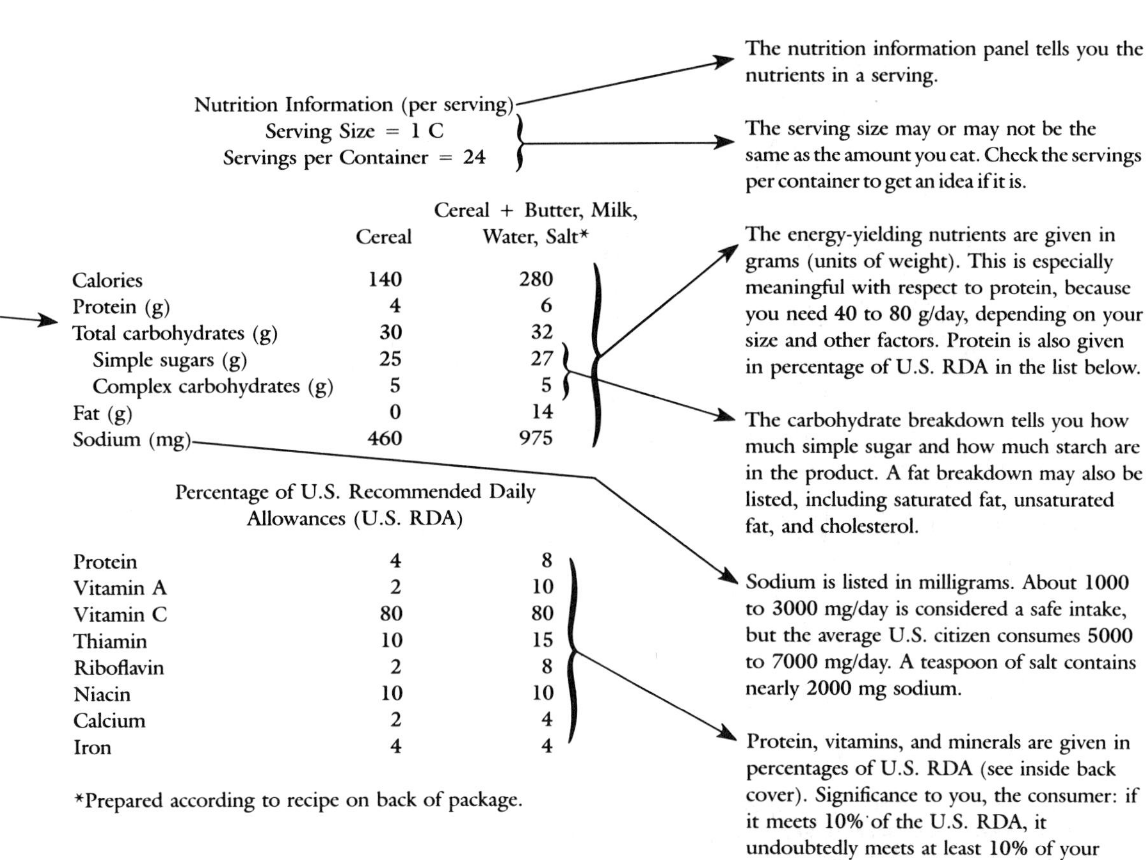

- Protein (grams) per serving.
- Carbohydrate (grams) per serving.
- Fat (grams) per serving.
- Protein, vitamins, and minerals as percentages of the U.S. RDA. (No claim may be made that a food is a significant source of a nutrient unless it provides at least 10 percent of the U.S. RDA of that nutrient in a serving.)

The side panel of the box of cooked cereal shown in Figure 10–2 provides all this information.

With an understanding of the U.S. RDA (see Chapter 2, p. 37), you can extract a lot of information from a nutrition label. The percentage of the U.S. RDA tells you generally what amounts of nutrients are in the package, and if you want to know exactly how many units of a nutrient are in a serving, you can do a simple calculation. Suppose a serving provides 25 percent of the U.S. RDA for vitamin A, for example. Turn to the U.S. RDA table to find out that the U.S. RDA is 1000 RE, and figure that 25 percent of that is 250 RE. For the nutrients included in the RDA tables, then, all the information is there that most consumers might want.

Labeling laws also specify just what labels may say about a food's energy and sodium contents (see Figure 10–2). Furthermore, wherever additives are listed on labels, their functions must be stated.

Miniglossary of Terms on Food Labels

Sodium terms:

sodium free: less than 5 mg per serving.

very low sodium: 35 mg or less per serving.

low sodium: 140 mg or less per serving.

reduced sodium: processed to reduce the usual level of sodium by 75%.

unsalted: processed without the normally used salt.

low salt: made with less salt than the regular variety of the same food.

Energy terms:

diet, dietetic: terms used to indicate that a food is either *low in calories* or a *reduced calorie* food.

low in calories: no more than 40 cal per serving or 0.9 cal/g.

reduced calorie: containing at least a third fewer calories than the food it most closely resembles.

Fat terms:

low fat: made with less fat than the regular variety of the same food.

lean: 90% fat-free.[a]

extra lean: 95% fat-free.

Weight terms:

gram: a unit of weight. A teaspoon of any dry powder (such as salt) weighs about 5 g. A half-cup of food (such as vegetables) or liquid (such as milk or juice) weighs about 100 g. Many food servings are 100-g servings; for photos of some, see p. 41.

milligram: 1/1000 of a gram.

[a]The word *lean* as part of the brand name (as in "Lean Supreme") indicates that the product is 25 percent lower in fat than the regular variety.

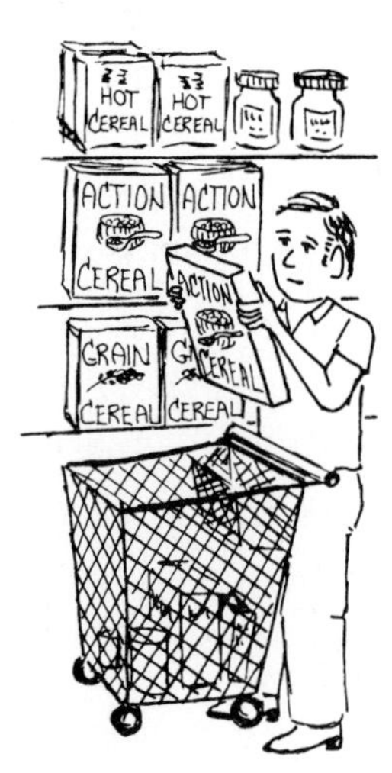

To know whether a food is really nutritious, you have to know more than just what's on the label.

The information just presented helps you with packaged foods that present information panels, such as breakfast cereals. But what about packaged foods that simply say "TV dinner" or "macaroni and cheese"? The FDA has devised nutritional quality guidelines for the nutrient contents of many kinds of convenience foods: frozen dinners, breakfast cereals, vitamin C–fortified beverages, and main dishes such as pizza or macaroni and cheese. If a product complies with the nutritional quality guidelines, it may carry on its label the statement that it "provides nutrients in amounts appropriate for this class of food as determined by the U.S. government."*

*For example, frozen dinners must contain one or more sources of protein from meat, poultry, fish, cheese, or eggs, and these must make up at least 70 percent of the total protein; they must include one or more vegetables or vegetable mixtures other than potatoes, rice, or cereal-based products; and they must have a certain minimum nutrient level for each 100 calories.

What if the label says nothing more than a name, such as *mayonnaise*? For some items the law provides **standards of identity,** mentioned earlier, and excuses manufacturers from the requirement of listing ingredients. Standards of identity exist for such foods as bread and mayonnaise—common foods that at one time were often prepared at home, so that the basic recipe was understood by almost everyone. Now, though, few people make these foods at home, and commercial recipes may include additives as well as the original recipe ingredients. Certain ingredients must be present in a specific percentage before the food may use the standard name.*

Another class of foods that concerns consumers is made up of foods developed in imitation of, and as substitutes for, familiar foods. With the new food technology, many **imitation foods** on the market may be superior to traditional foods; so it is misleading to the consumer to imply that they are inferior. (Egg replacers for those who wish to reduce their cholesterol intakes, for example, may be superior to eggs.) For this reason, the law requires that the word *imitation* be used on the label only if the product is "a substitute for and resembles another food but is *nutritionally inferior* to the food imitated. . . . Nutritional inferiority is defined as a reduction in the content of an essential vitamin or mineral or of protein that amounts to 10 percent or more of the U.S. RDA."

Another term you often see on labels is **fortified.** A fortified food is like an enriched food (Chapter 3, p. 76) in that nutrients have been added to it, but is different in that the nutrients added may or may not have been there in the original product. Examples are:

- Milk, to which vitamims A and D may be added.
- Soy milk, to which calcium and vitamin B_{12} are added.
- Salt, to which iodine is added.
- A sweetened drink, to which vitamin C is added.

As mentioned earlier, fortified foods may appear to be nutritious because of all the nutrients listed on their labels, but they may not contain the several dozen other nutrients that natural, whole foods have. To know whether a food is really nutritious, you have to know more than just what is on the label.

Among the most highly fortified of all foods on the market today are breakfast cereals, some of which have every vitamin and mineral of the U.S. RDA tables added to them. When a food has nutrients added in amounts greater than 50 percent above the U.S. RDA, it has to be labeled as a **supplement,** the same term as is used to describe a vitamin-mineral pill or powder. Thus some breakfast cereals (those made from refined flour and described as supplements on their labels) are more like pills disguised as cereal than like whole grains. They are nutritious—with respect to the nutrients added—but they may not contain the full spectrum of nutrients that an unrefined whole food (or better, a mixture of such foods) might have.

standards of identity: standards for the recipes manufacturers must use if they are to be permitted to use certain common names (example, *mayonnaise*) on labels.

imitation foods: processed foods that resemble ordinary foods, but that are significantly lower in an essential nutrient or in protein.

fortified: a term referring to the addition of nutrients to a food, often not originally present, and often added in amounts greater than might be found there naturally. The term *enriched* sometimes also has this meaning, but also means that four specific nutrients have been added, as explained on p. 76.

supplement: already defined in Controversy 6 as pills, liquids, or powders that contain nutrients, this term also has a meaning when used on food labels: it means that nutrients have been added in amounts greater than 50% above the U.S. RDA.

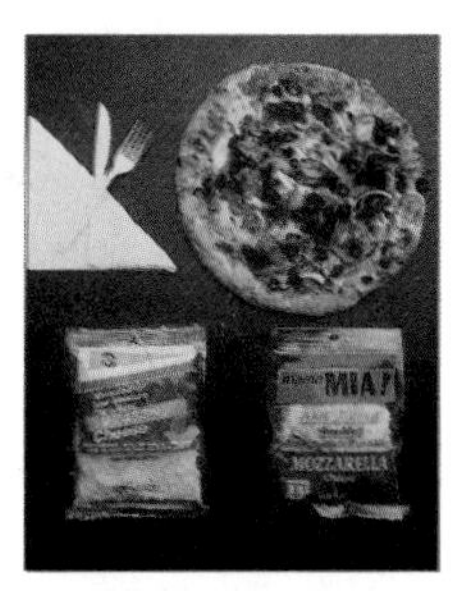

An imitation food is nutritionally inferior to the real thing.

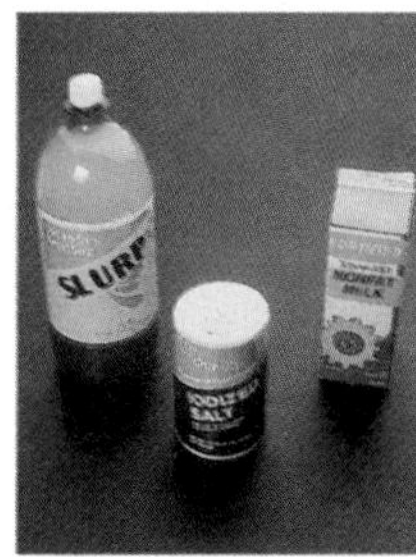

Fortified products.

*Any product like mayonnaise, for example, may use that name on the label only if it contains 65 percent by weight of vegetable oil, either vinegar or lemon juice, and egg yolk. The FDA does not have the authority to require that ingredients be listed for these foods, but it urges manufacturers to give the consumer more detailed information, and many manufacturers do so voluntarily. The FDA supplies copies of a fact sheet stating the required ingredients for any food with a standard of identity. Appendix F lists the FDA's address.

natural food: a food that has been altered as little as possible from the original farm-grown state (see also p. 23). As used on labels, this term may misleadingly imply unusual power to promote health. It has not been legally defined.

health food: a misleading term used on labels, usually of organic or natural foods, to imply unusual power to promote health. This term has no legal definition.

organic food: the chemist's definition of *organic* is given on page 31. The popular definition is a food or nutrient produced without the use of chemical fertilizers, pesticides, or additives. As used on labels, this term may misleadingly imply unusual power to promote health. It has not been legally defined.

lite, light: terms with no legal meaning, used on labels to imply that foods are low in calories, light in color, or low in alcohol content.

shopping list:

nothing to buy today

Some terms on labels only have meaning because they are popularly understood, not because they are legally defined. One such term is **natural food,** already discussed in Controversy 1. Others are **health food** and **organic food.** *Health food* is a term often used misleadingly on labels to imply unusual power to promote health; it has no legal definition. Used accurately, though, it could be informative. The term *organic* as used by a chemist denotes the presence of molecules with carbon atoms in them, but it also has a popular definition: a food or nutrient produced without the use of chemical fertilizers, pesticides, or additives. As used on labels, this term may misleadingly imply unusual power to promote health. It has not been legally defined, either. Foods labeled *organic* are often more expensive than their ordinary grocery-store counterparts, and they are sometimes (as in the case of herbal preparations) even dangerous to use. They may not even be pesticide-free, as already explained.

Although there is no legal definition of the word *natural* as used on food labels, the National Advertising Division of the Council of Better Business Bureaus has voluntarily adopted some guidelines. They are logical, but they permit use of the word under conditions that might surprise consumers. Foods that can, under these guidelines, be labeled "natural" include ice cream, carbonated beverages, chewing gum, syrup, flavored drink mixes, pan spray coating, and purified fructose—even though they contain added refined sugar, added salt, added fat, or no nutrients at all.[28]

Another ambiguous term is **lite** or **light.** People hope these words mean that their favorite treats have been formulated with less of the ingredients that may harm their health or add unnecessary calories: less fat, less cholesterol, less salt, fewer calories, or less sugar. Some of the products may indeed be just what the doctor ordered, like thinly sliced whole-grain breads and fruits packed in their own juice without added sugar. Others, such as light potato chips may contain a few less calories per serving than the originals, but still provide plenty of fat and salt with only traces of nutrients. Their overconsumption would encourage overweight, undernutrition, or both.

FDA has recently ruled to permit scientifically-based health statements on labels, provided that they are approved individually by the FDA and that they emphasize the importance of the total diet. It is permissible to state on the label of a high-fiber cereal, for example, that "A high-fiber diet may reduce your risk of some kinds of cancer." The statement is true, and it is phrased in terms of total diet, not in terms of the particular cereal in the box.[29] There is potential for abuse of this rule. Scientific truths might be stretched to attract consumer's grocery store dollars. Ideally, though, future refinements on the ruling will allow for delivery of responsible nutrition education to the public, while screening out false or premature claims.

Self-Study

Evaluate Your Food Choices

1. The preceding Self-Studies have revealed the strengths and weaknesses of your nutrient intakes and energy balance. By now, you may be looking at foods in a new light. Knowing what nutrients your diet tends to lack, you may be interested in finding foods that are especially rich in those nutrients. If you need to limit calories, you may need to find foods that supply those nutrients for the lowest possible calorie cost. You will recognize this description as the definition of a *nutrient-dense food* (Chapter 2).

Review your food records, looking for the three nutrients that your diet supplies in the smallest quantities relative to your need. (For many young women, these nutrients might be vitamin A, calcium, and iron.) Enter the names of these nutrients in the spaces provided at the tops of columns A, B, and C in Form 8 (Appendix H). Now make a list of ten foods you like and would be willing to eat frequently, that might supply these nutrients in significant quantities. List these foods in the first column of Form 8. List the size of the serving of each food that you would eat, and look up the amounts of nutrients #1, #2, and #3 and of calories that the serving would supply. Express the amount of nutrient #1 as a percentage of your RDA, round it off to the nearest whole number, and enter it in column A of the form. (For example, suppose you selected vitamin A as a nutrient of importance to you, and your RDA was 800 RE. Suppose you chose 1 peach as a food you might like to eat. Appendix A reveals that 1 peach offers 47 RE of vitamin A. That's 5.875 percent of your RDA—the calculation is 47 divided by 800, times 100. Round off to 6, and enter that number in column A of the form.) Perform a similar calculation for nutrients #2 and #3, and enter the results in columns B and C of the form.

Now express the amount of calories the food would supply as a percentage of your recommended intake of energy, and enter the result in column D of the form. (Example: Suppose your recommended intake of energy is 2000 calories. A peach supplies 37 calories. That's about 2 percent of your energy need for the day.)

Divide A by D, and enter the result in column E. This number represents the amount of nutrient #1 the food supplies relative to your need, compared with the amount of energy the food supplies relative to your need. (Example: A peach offers 6 percent of your need for Vitamin A and only 2 percent of the calories you can eat, so it gets a 3 for this nutrient.) Divide B by D and enter in column F; and divide C by D and enter in column G, to obtain similar scores for the next two nutrients. Now add columns E, F, and G to obtain a nutrient score for the food. This score, which is arbitrary (created by us), serves as a basis for comparing this food with other foods as a source of the nutrients you most need. The higher this score is, the more of that food you can eat without running through your calorie allowance before you have met your nutrient needs.

Don't stop at ten foods, if this exercise interests you. Don't stop at three nutrients, either. (We did, only because we ran out of horizontal space on the page.) You have much to learn about the virtues of food for meeting your particular nutrient needs by making comparisons of this kind.

2. Finally, you can go back to answer the question suggested at the very beginning of the first Self-Study: Do you need a supplement? Review your records once again. In light of the food choices you now are making, is there any nutrient in which your diet consistently falls short of the RDA? If so, describe the supplement you would need, and set about obtaining it.

Notes

1. F. M. Strong, Toxicants occurring naturally in foods, in *Nutrition Reviews' Present Knowledge in Nutrition,* 4th ed. (Washington, D.C.: Nutrition Foundation, 1976), pp. 516–527.
2. C. W. Lecos, Sulfites: FDA limits uses, broadens labeling, *FDA Consumer,* October 1986, pp. 10–13.
3. S. L. Taylor and R. K. Bush, Sulfites as food ingredients, *Contemporary Nutrition,* a publication (1986) available from the Nutrition Department, General Mills, Inc., P.O. Box 1172, Minneapolis, MN 55440.
4. W. F. Wilkens and J. I. Gray, Reduce N-nitrosamine formation in bacon, *Food Engineering* 58 (1986): 68–69; E. N. Frankel, Lipid oxidation: Mechanisms, products and biological significance, *Journal of the American Oil Chemists' Society* 61 (1984): 1908–1917.
5. T. M. Parkinson and J. P. Brown, Metabolic fate of food colorants, *Annual Reviews of Nutrition* 1 (1981): 175–205.
6. Tartrazine, *Nutrition and the MD,* January 1983.
7. M. Gore, The Chinese restaurant syndrome, in *Adverse Effects of Foods,* eds. E. F. P. Jelliffe and D. B. Jelliffe (New York: Plenum Press, 1982), pp. 211–223.
8. L. D. Stegink and coauthors, Effect of sucrose ingestion on plasma glutamate concentrations in humans administered monosodium L-glutamate, *American Journal of Clinical Nutrition* 43 (1986): 510–515.
9. L. D. Stegink, L. J. Filer, and G. L. Baker, Plasma glutamate concentrations in adult subjects ingesting monosodium L-glutamate in consommé, *American Journal of Clinical Nutrition* 42 (1985): 220–225.
10. Irradiated foods, a report (July 1985) by the American Council on Science and Health, available from the ACSH at 1995 Broadway, New York, NY 10023.
11. Select Committee on Health Aspects of Irradiated Beef, *Evaluation of the Health Aspects of Certain Compounds Found in Irradiated Beef* (Bethesda, Md.: Life Sciences Research Office, Federation of American Societies for Experimental Biology, 1977, 1979), as cited by ACSH, 1985.
12. E. Blume and M. F. Jacobson, Food irradiation: Is the time ripe? *Nutrition Action,* November 1986, pp. 1–7.
13. *Federal Register,* 27 March 1981, as cited in Food irradiation: Ready for a comeback, *Food Engineering,* April 1982, pp. 71–80.
14. C. W. Lecos, The growing use of irradiation to preserve food, *FDA Consumer,* July-August 1986, pp. 12–15.
15. Food irradiation under attack, *Nutrition Forum,* October 1986, p. 79.
16. M. G. Mustafa, Agricultural chemicals, in *Adverse Effects of Foods,* eds. E. F. P. Jelliffe and D. B. Jelliffe (New York: Plenum Press, 1982), pp. 111–128.
17. W. A. Krehl, Mercury, the slippery metal, *Nutrition Today,* November/December 1972, pp. 4–15.
18. Krehl, 1972.
19. M. A. Wessel and A. Dominski, Our children's daily lead, *American Scientist* 65 (1977): 294–298.
20. 97% of Michigan population contaminated by 1973 spills, *Tallahassee Democrat,* 16 April 1982.
21. K. R. Mahaffey, Nutritional factors in lead poisoning, *Nutrition Reviews* 39 (1981): 353–362.
22. M. B. Rabinowitz, J. D. Kopple, and G. W. Wetherill, Effect of food intake and fasting on gastrointestinal lead absorption in humans, *American Journal of Clinical Nutrition* 33 (1980): 1784–1788.
23. Update: Childhood lead poisoning, *Journal of the American Dietetic Association* 80 (1982): 592, 594.
24. D. G. Lindsay and J. C. Sherlock, Environmental contaminants, in *Adverse Effects of Foods,* eds. E. F. P. Jelliffe and D. B. Jelliffe (New York: Plenum Press, 1982), pp. 85–110.
25. Corn syrup can also be contaminated with *C. botulinum* spores. D. A. Kautter and coauthors, *Clostridium botulinum* spores in infant foods—a survey, *Journal of Food Protection* 45 (1982): 1028–1029.
26. I. B. Vyhmeister, What about honey? *Life and Health,* August 1980, pp. 5–7; R. W. Miller, Honey: Making sure it's pure, *FDA Consumer,* September 1979, pp. 12–13.
27. D. L. Morse and coauthors, Widespread outbreaks of clam- and oyster-associated gastroenteritis: role of Norwalk virus, *New England Journal of Medicine* 314 (1986): 678–681; H. L. Dupont, Consumption of raw shellfish—is the risk now unacceptable? (editorial), *New England Journal of Medicine* 314 (1986): 707–708; Sushi lovers: beware of parasites, *Science News,* 2 March 1985, p. 141.
28. Food cases involving "natural" claims, *NAD Case Report* (a newsletter from the Council of Better Business Bureaus, 845 Third Ave., New York, NY 10022), October 1984.
29. U.S. wants to lift health label ban, *New York Times,* 5 August 1987.

Nonnutrients in Foods

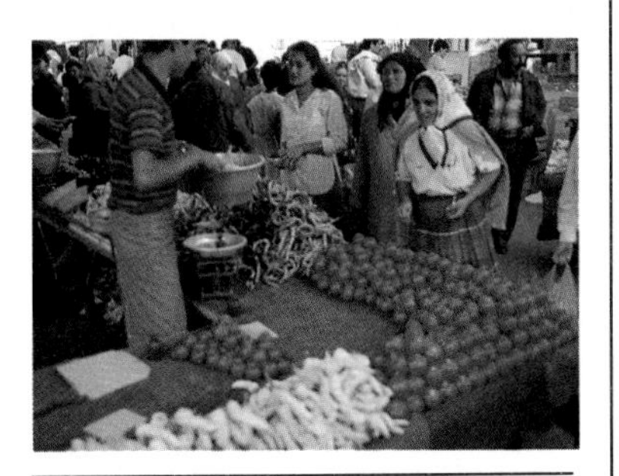

When you buy foods, buy variety.

> [20,000 years ago] The camp was quiet, settling down for the night. By the dim glow of hot coals, Iza checked the contents of several small pouches spread out in orderly rows on her cloak. . . . Earlier, she had inspected the vegetation growing around the cave, wanting to know the availability of plants to replenish and enlarge her pharmacopoeia. She always carried certain things with her in the otter-skin bag, but to her, the small pouches of dried leaves, flowers, roots, seeds, and barks in her medicine bag were only first aid. In the new cave she would have room for greater quantity and variety.
>
> —J. M. Auel,
> *The Clan of the Cave Bear*
> Crown Publishers, N.Y.

From earliest times, human beings have valued plants and animals not only for the nourishment they convey, but for other properties. Substances from both flora and fauna have offered ways to stop bleeding, to relieve pain, to quell coughing, to calm inflammation, to fight infection, to soften dry skin, and to ease the way to sleep, as well as many other remedies. And in the last hundred years, many of the active ingredients from plant and animal tissues have been isolated and identified and are now sold by pharmacists in purified form, in standard formulations, and in measured doses. Many of today's drugs are produced synthetically, but they still mimic drugs that occur naturally in **herbs** and other plants, and in animal tissues.[1]

Nutrients are thus not the only chemicals in foods, although they are by far the best-known ones. Foods, after all, come from the tissues of living things. Living tissues contain thousands of different chemicals, only some 40-odd of which happen to serve as nutrients for the human body. Among the familiar nonnutrients are fibers (in plants), a constituent vital to human nutrition, although not nourishing in the sense of directly promoting growth or repair of body tissues (see Chapter 3). The fibers of legumes and oats lower blood cholesterol, as reported in Controversy 4. Foods also contain pigments, such as chlorophyll, hemoglobin, myoglobin, and others, which give them their green, red, and other hues. They also contain poisons, including the toxins of poisonous mushrooms and many others. Then there are the subjects of the present discussion.

The subjects of this discussion are those nonnutrient components of foods other than fiber that are reputed to have beneficial health effects. Among these are some microbes; stimulants, including the familiar and universally popular stimulant caffeine; and other molecules that have a variety of physiological effects. Technically, because "a molecule with a physiological effect" is the definition of a drug, these latter compounds should all be called drugs—although in many cases their identity is not yet known, and they make their presence apparent only as "something in the food."

Nonnutrient food constituents that have beneficial health effects have led people to believe, wrongly, that certain *foods* have special power to promote health. They do not, but because they contain physiologically active substances, they may be "better for you," as many knowledgeable nutritionists like to proclaim, than nutrient supplements are. By eating a variety of foods, a person receives a variety of both nutrients and nonnutrients.

Seriously ill people in hospitals drink all-synthetic liquid diets described as "nutritionally complete"—meaning that they contain all of the essential nutrients in the amounts needed to support life. On such diets, people maintain physical well-being for up to six months.[2] Yet real food apparently supports health better. Foods convey more value than just that carried by the nutrients in them, although it is not clear just how they do so.[3] Certainly, one possibility is that a variety of nonnutrients confer extra benefits.

Warnings

Let us begin with a few warnings. Warning #1: when people consume plant or animal tissues in order to obtain a specific physiological effect, they don't always get the substance they think they are getting. Neither can they always know its concentration in a food when it is present. Foods vary from batch to batch, from strain to strain, from one part of a plant or animal to another, from season to season, from one geographical region to another, and from one preparation method to the next. When foods are transformed into powders and potions, their ingredients change, and so do their effects. Unlike the chemical composition of standardized drugs, that of foods taken from plants and animals is unreliable and unpredictable. The potential dangers are amplified when a food is mislabeled or misidentified. A root sold as the rare and expensive ginseng root may actually be that of a different plant, indistinguishable to an untrained eye.

As an example of the mistaking of one herb for another, a man confused **foxglove** (from which the potent heart medication digoxin is extracted) with **comfrey** (a plant popular for making tea). He brewed a tea from the foxglove and drank a little more than a quart of it over several days. As a result, he suffered digoxin poisoning.[4] Comfrey itself becomes toxic when used regularly (see later), but foxglove is even more so. Such stories involving the use of herbal preparations are common.

Warning #2: people differ in their reactions to biologically active compounds. Children are particularly susceptible to the effects of biologically active compounds, and special care must be taken when feeding children foods that contain them. Adults, too, can suffer from the careless use of natural sources of drugs, especially if they have current disease or inherited disease susceptibility.

Warning #3: when people consume plant or animal tissues in order to obtain a specific physiological effect, they may not get anything—that is, the effect may be neutral. Some foods for which special health-promoting claims are made do *not* contain chemical components that benefit the human body—or at least not in quantities or potencies worth anyone's special attention.

Warning #4: when people consume plant or animal tissues in order to obtain a specific physiological effect, they may get an unexpected, even harmful, effect. Whenever a food is prized for one compound it contains, the likelihood exists that it contains others for which it might be condemned. Many commonly used plants and plant products contain naturally occurring toxic substances. Mushrooms are a familiar example; but a number of other common foods have been observed to cause toxic effects. Consider this list:

- Cabbage, mustard, and other plants contain goitrogens; if these plants are consumed as a steady diet, they can enlarge the thyroid gland.
- Spinach and rhubarb contain oxalates, tolerable as usually consumed; but one normal serving of rhubarb contains one-fifth the toxic dose for humans.
- Potatoes contain solanine, a powerful inhibitor of nerve impulses; ordinary consumption of potatoes delivers one-tenth the dose of solanine that would be toxic.[5] When potatoes are exposed to light, they develop more solanine; it is in the green layer that develops just beneath the skin. Throw such potatoes away; don't eat them.
- Honey can be a host to the botulinum organism and can accumulate enough toxin to kill an infant.[6]

Some 700 other plants have caused serious illnesses or deaths in the Western hemisphere.[7] Some fish are also naturally toxic, presenting hazards from mild illness to instant death. A well-known environmental scientist has said, "One can predict that if the standards used to test manmade chemicals were applied to 'natural' foods, fully half of the human food supply would have to be banned."[8]

These warnings translate into a pair of questions any health-minded person would be wise to ask in relation to any food for which health effects are claimed. Examine the available scientific evidence, and ask:

1. Does it really do what is claimed? (Is there scientifically valid evidence that conclusively demonstrates that the claimed benefits are real?)
2. Does it do any harm? (Be sure that harmful effects have been looked for.)

When the answer to the first question is affirmative, other questions arise. At what concentration does the substance provide the beneficial effect? Is the concentration of the substance in the food, when the food is consumed in ordinary amounts, great enough to produce the desired effect? Even if it is, the chemical interactions that accompany digestion of the food and the body's handling of the components might interfere with the physiological action, thus altering the effect. This leads us to Warning #5: before nonnutrients can be assumed safe to take for their drug effects, their absorption and metabolism must be understood.

Keep in mind, too, that in many instances, the reported benefits of a food came from serendipitous observations and personal accounts, or even wishful thinking. Findings from studies conducted by individuals using questionable methods and published in journals without peer review cannot be accepted as valid. Unfortunately, the periodic publication of bits of new information about the true, beneficial effects of food components on health sets people up to believe larger claims made by misguided or unscrupulous individuals. The object, here, is to sort valid, useful information from the unfounded claims. Within this perspective, then, this Controversy looks at some foods that contain nutrients with supposedly beneficial effects and asks what significance, if any, the available information has for consumers.

Alfalfa

The **alfalfa** plant is a good example of a food for which claims have been overly enthusiastic. Like any plant, alfalfa contains hundreds of chemicals, including proteins, fats, organic acids, vitamins, minerals, fibers, pigments, and others. Alfalfa is a forage plant, and it supports the healthy growth of cattle both when they graze on it in summer and when they eat the dried hay in winter. Promoters of alfalfa claim that if it is good for cattle, it must be good for people, too—but that people should eat its nutrients directly, not "via the steer." Such a viewpoint may appeal to people consuming a vegetarian diet, but to equate the nutritional benefits of an alfalfa salad with those of beef from a cow that grazed on alfalfa is to overlook many biochemical transformations. (Alfalfa promoters do argue a valid point, however—that the earth benefits when people eat plants instead of animal-derived products. Plants require less land to produce a given amount of protein and food energy than animals do.)

Claims that alfalfa cures arthritis, reduces blood cholesterol, treats diabetes, stimulates the appetite, and acts as a general tonic are overstated. For example, in a test tube, alfalfa saponins bind with cholesterol; in a rat, the effect is evident, but insignificant.[9] To claim beneficial effects in human beings at this time is to exaggerate the research findings.

Like the positive physiological effects of alfalfa, the negative effects are minimal, if any, and so alfalfa is safe to consume. Indeed, consumers should feel free to eat alfalfa sprouts (and mung bean sprouts, and wheat berry sprouts, and radish seed sprouts, and a variety of other sprouts—in moderation, of course). Sprouted seeds are reasonably nutritious. Like most seeds and sprouts, alfalfa sprouts contain a variety of vitamins and minerals and provide relatively few calories. They are also, like all plant-derived foods, rich in fibers. However, even with these nutrition benefits, alfalfa has no health-promoting powers greater than other plants.

Although the alfalfa *plant* is neither particularly effective in promoting health nor particularly hazardous when consumed in moderation, alfalfa *tablets,* which are made from the crushed, dehydrated plant, are a different story. They deliver much more alfalfa, enough to be hazardous, particularly for people with systemic lupus erythematosus (SLE), a rare disease involving inflammation of the joints. A study of two people whose SLE had been in remission showed that the disease was reactivated after they had been taking doses of 8 to 15 tablets daily for a long time. Researchers found that the alfalfa tablets contained a substance that was shown to reactivate SLE in susceptible animals.[10] For most healthy people, though, taking the tablets a few at a time does little harm except to the pocketbook.

The unexpected harmful effect of alfalfa tablets illustrates the warnings issued at the start. First (recall Warning #1), the effects of a plant may differ from the effects of that same plant after it has been processed. The chemical compositions and concentrations of oils, extracts, and powders are not necessarily the same as those of their sources. Also (Warning #2), what is good, bad, or neutral for one person may not be for another. Each individual has a unique genetic endowment and health status that influence the body's reactions to various compounds. Still another lesson is a variation of "if it's not broken, don't fix it." For people to consume products on a whim or on the advice of a friend, store clerk, or advertisement is to play Russian roulette. The chances of receiving beneficial, neutral, or harmful reactions from a product are, for the most part, unknown (Warnings #3 and #4).

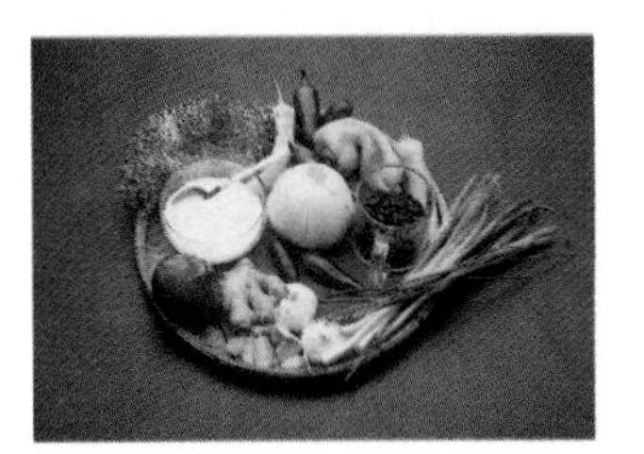

Some foods offer more than just nutrients.

Ginseng

The root of the wild, slow-growing **ginseng** plant (actually several species of plants) is so valued for its supposed antifatigue and aphrodisiac properties that it has been gathered almost to extinction. In the United States, ginseng has been declared an endangered species. Ginseng has been intensively studied, and over a thousand books and papers have been written about it, but much of the writing has been in the tradition of folklore and Oriental mysticism. Scientific work is incomplete.

The answers to two important questions about ginseng are apparent, though. To the question of whether it offers any beneficial health effects, the answer is yes; and to the question of whether it does any harm, the answer is also yes.

Like alfalfa, ginseng plants contain saponins—a family of chemicals that affect specific body functions—that is, they act as drugs. This makes ginseng, just like the multitude of other plants from which drugs are derived, both potentially valuable and potentially dangerous, for drugs can be misused or abused. Chinese folklore credits ginseng for providing health, strength, and happiness to people who are exhausted by stress, injury, or fatigue.

Like those in alfalfa, ginseng's saponins are largely responsible for its pharmacological activities. Saponin extracts of ginseng have been reported to be effective in relieving inflammation in rats (depending on the particular batch from which they are made). In the test tube, their inhibitory effect on the reaction of human white blood cells to a stressor proves more potent than that of hydrocortisone (a common anti-inflammatory drug).[11] Chewing the ginseng root is reported to be effective in raising HDL cholesterol levels and reducing cardiovascular disease risk ratings (as estimated from HDL) from high to zero.[12]

These reported effects of ginseng must be considered with caution. They are unpredictable—probably because ginseng potencies and chemical composition vary according to the strain, the part of the plant used, the season, and the mode of preparation. Thus ginseng has also been observed to raise blood pressure and to cause insomnia, nervousness, confusion, and depression—a cluster of symptoms observed often enough to be worth naming the **ginseng abuse syndrome.**[13] Many of these harmful effects appear to be due to a physiological action like that of the stress hormones or the female hormone estrogen. Excessive use of ginseng is associated with physiological changes in the vaginal mucosa in women, and one case is reported in which a daily ginseng tablet was associated with vaginal bleeding in an elderly woman.[14]

Ginseng is not commonly eaten as a food. Its druglike components can be extracted by chewing the root or by chemical processing. Ginseng teas and sodas are also available. When consumed for specific physiological actions, ginseng is a drug—a drug that does not work as desired, because its side effects can occur at about the same dose levels as its desired effects. The cost of purifying the chemicals from ginseng is high, and they are not in wide use pharmaceutically.

The cases of alfalfa and ginseng illustrate two different sets of answers to the questions asked at the start (Does the food do what is claimed? Does it do any harm?). In the case of alfalfa, the answers to both questions are no; in the case of ginseng, the answers to both are a qualified yes, although much of the evidence has been obtained from studies on animals, not human beings.

Caffeine-containing Foods

The drug **caffeine** occurs in several plants, including the familiar coffee bean and tea leaf—and the cocoa bean, from which chocolate is made. A true stimulant drug, caffeine increases the respiration rate, heart rate, blood pressure, and secretion of stress and other hormones. It stimulates the digestive tract, promoting efficient elimination, and its "wake-up" effect is well known. Nearly every human society uses one or another plant that delivers caffeine.

Caffeine seems to be relatively harmless when used in moderate doses (the equivalent of fewer than, say, two to four average-sized cups of coffee a day). In amounts greater than this, it can cause the symptoms associated with anxiety—sweating, tenseness, and inability to concentrate—and is suspected of increasing the risk for cardiovascular disease and heart attack, as well as the possibly painful but benign fibrocystic breast disease. (Chapter 13 provides more details about caffeine's safety record and about where it is found in foods.)

Caffeine is useful to illustrate two principles. First, caffeine-containing plants might be said to "work," in the sense that ginseng does not work—in that the druglike effects are obtained from the plant as normally used, usually without side effects. People seek coffee and tea specifically for the caffeine effects. The second point: it is mainly the caffeine within the coffee or tea that is valued; the taste is secondary, and the beverage is only a vehicle for its delivery. (People who use decaffeinated coffee are seeking to continue using a familiar beverage while consciously choosing to avoid caffeine.) This discussion has not yet named a single *food* that is unique in its beneficial properties—nor will it do so. The biological activity comes from chemicals within the foods.

Wine

One of the most potent and dangerous drugs used by human beings arises in plants when their carbohydrates are fermented by microorganisms—namely, alcohol. Its effects are too numerous, and its impacts too great, for the scope of this discussion. Controversy 12 provides greater insights into the effects of alcohol on the brain and on nutrition status. Setting alcohol aside, though, and granting that its moderate use may not be harmful, we might ask whether fermented beverages have special health effects. Wine, in particular, is certainly credited with many such effects—naturally, many of them claimed by wine makers and merchants, but some that have been scientifically validated. Test tube experiments suggest that grape juice has an antiviral effect that carries over (to a lesser extent) when the grape juice is made into wine.[15] The substance responsible for inactivating viruses is found in the skin of grapes, which explains why red wines are more antiviral than white. (White wines are fermented from the juice only, while red wines are made from the entire grape.) Strawberries and several other fruits also provide an antiviral effect.

Alcoholic beverages also affect the appetite. Usually, they take the edge off people's hunger by providing a few calories and a measure of relaxation. Sometimes, because they can be high in calories, they contribute to obesity. In people who are tense and unable to eat, though, small doses of wine taken 20 minutes before meals help because they stimulate the appetite. Acid compounds in the wine that are known as **congeners** are credited with this effect. For undernourished people and for people with severely depressed appetites, wine may facilitate eating even when psychotherapy fails to do so. At the same time, because it relaxes people, wine may help obese people lose weight. Its success in that connection is thought to stem from its ability to relieve emotional stress, which is a common reason for overeating. Certain of the congeners in wine may contribute to the tranquilizing effect, and some are said to be nearly 100 times more effective than alcohol.[16] French wine also contains a compound known to lower liver lipids and cholesterol in rats.[17]

It goes without saying that people need not drink wine to obtain many of these effects. The chemicals responsible for them are present in the original juice from which the wine was fermented, and they are still present when the alcohol is again removed from the wine. If people who drink wine give it up, they can still enjoy its benefits by learning to drink moderate amounts of fruit juices or dealcoholized wine in its place—or, of course, by eating grapes. The point of discussing wine rather than grape juice or grapes is to give another example of how science can help to sift reality out of folklore. The folklore surrounds the wine, but science finds the truth in the grapes.

How, then, would wine be evaluated in response to the two questions asked at the start? Does it really do what is claimed? Yes—although grape juice, grapes, or other fruits do many of the same things as well or better. Does it do any harm? Since the harmful effects of overconsumption of alcohol are well known, this question might have to be answered by saying yes, possibly so; and grape juice, grapes, or other fruits would not. In short, use wine in moderation, if at all, but do eat a variety of fruits—boring advice, perhaps, but safe and beneficial to health.

Garlic

People who are seeking an edge over heart disease have been looking to garlic for its nonnutrient effects on heart health. Garlic has been considered a "magic" food for centuries—the first Olympic athletes believed it conferred stamina, and they chewed it before competitive events. For those ancients who perceived themselves to be pestered by vampires, garlic was a well-known repellent. These claims remain untested, but the effect of garlic on blood lipids is supported by some research. The essential oil of garlic (equivalent to about 1 ounce, or one bulb, of raw garlic a day) appears not only to lower the blood lipids associated with heart disease, but also to oppose clot formation.[18] The effect is seen in both healthy people and in people with coronary heart disease, and is maintained for two months after garlic treatments are discontinued.

When people learned of the effects of garlic on blood lipids, many wanted to employ it for its heart health benefits. However, large quantities of garlic may bring more than the desired results (Warning #3). The effects may include gastric distress and excessive intestinal gas. Garlicky body odor is noticeable in people who regularly consume large quantities, and the immediate breath odor is unmistakable and considered unpleasant. (To improve garlic breath, brush the teeth and tongue after eating, and chew some fresh parsley. The chlorophyll in the parsley *may* help eliminate the garlic odor compounds, although this effect is more hearsay than science.[19]) Capsules of odorless garlic extract available at health-food stores are untested, and they are likely to lack the very chemicals that are candidates for imparting health benefits.

Garlic is commonly used to enhance the flavor of foods. When used in small quantities on an occasional basis, garlic confers minimal, if any, health benefits. However, when used in larger quantities on a regular basis, its components reach concentrations that do have both beneficial drug effects and unpleasant side effects. Thus, like ginseng, it does not work well as a drug. To minimize its potential for harm, moderate use is recommended—use at a level such that its benefits, other than its pleasing taste, may be insignificant as well.

Hot Peppers

Some groups of people have low incidences of the fatal blood clotting associated with heart and artery disease. A food associated with this effect is hot peppers, as indicated by reports from Thailand, Mexico, and Hungary, where these peppers are dietary staples. For example, Thai people eat hot peppers many times a day. Each time they eat them, a temporary anticlotting action takes place in their blood.[20] This effect is attributed to the pungent principle **capsaicin** in the hot peppers. Conceivably, this anticlotting action, repeated several times daily, is sufficient to reduce the risk of fatal blood clotting.

Hot peppers have another interesting effect: immediately after a person eats a meal spiced with them, the person's basal metabolic rate (BMR) rises by up to 65 percent, whereas the meal alone raises BMR by only 40 percent. The increased rate continues for three hours or more.[21] This makes a difference of only a few calories in the day's energy total (we calculate that a 25 percent rise in BMR might amount to a pound of fat every three months), but for the person concerned with weight control, the difference is in the right direction.

Hot peppers irritate the digestive tract, and treatment for ulcers includes avoiding them. There is speculation that such irritation could damage the digestive tract. Again, caution is necessary when using the components in foods to achieve an effect. Advantages and disadvantages must be weighed carefully. Asking Question 1 of hot peppers, then, we might respond that there appear to be small but real benefits. To Question 2: moderation is recommended.

Hot peppers and garlic are only two of the foods related to reducing the risk of heart disease. Unprocessed or lightly processed fruits, vegetables, legumes, and grains all play a role, thanks to the actions of their fibers—and possibly other constituents. These and other foods also play roles in defenses against cancer, as the following sections suggest.

Cabbages and Their Relatives

In the last 20 years, it has become apparent that many cancers originate from causes that are within people's power to control—food choices among them. Among dietary factors related to cancer are the diet's fat content; deficiencies of nutrients such as calcium, vitamin C, folacin, vitamin A, and its precursor carotene;[22] food additives (to a limited extent); food contaminants; and nonnutrients in foods. Controversy 5 mentioned each of these, but it is useful to look in depth at several candidates among the nonnutrients that may help prevent cancer: among them, the **indoles**[23] and **dithiolthiones**[24] among the cruciferous vegetables, and enzyme inhibitors in seeds and grains.

A table of the cruciferous vegetables appears in Controversy 5. They include broccoli, cauliflower, brussels sprouts, and other vegetables with cross-shaped flowers. The observation of their relationship to cancer originates with epidemiological research indicating that people who consume large amounts of these vegetables have lower cancer rates than those who do not.[25] This finding has led to studies of the vegetables themselves, and to the further finding that the indoles and dithiolthiones they contain induce the activity of certain enzymes in the liver. These enzymes, among other things, inactivate certain carcinogens (cancer-causing chemicals).[26] Often such effects are seen only in compounds purified and concentrated from plants, but the dithiolthiones in cabbage have this effect in mice even when the cabbage is fed in amounts comparable to servings people could normally eat.[27] It seems, therefore, that consuming these vegetables could tend to tip the balance toward a slightly lower likelihood of contracting cancer, but direct confirmation or rejection by way of experiments on human beings is not possible for ethical reasons.

Other vegetables contain other constituents that may activate the enzyme system that degrades carcinogens.[28] These constituents are so widespread among plants that the single most valuable application of the information obtained to date is *not* to eat cabbages in particular, but to eat a wide variety of vegetables in generous quantities. Balancing this advice, notice that the next section advocates the use of grains and seeds, and the next one, milk and milk products—so that, in the end, the tried-and-true recommendation to eat a balanced diet also seems to apply to the person wishing to avoid cancer.

Seeds and Grains

Another class of foods that may contain cancer-fighting substances is the **seed foods,** including grains, nuts, and legumes. Many of them contain **protease inhibitors**—substances that prevent digestive enzymes from doing their work.[29] These inhibitors prevent digestion of the seeds themselves, or at least enough of them to ensure passage intact through the digestive tract, so that they can return to the soil and sprout. However, the inhibitors also prevent digestion of other proteins. The inhibitor in raw soybeans is so powerful that it can prevent digestion of other foods eaten with the soybeans—the basis for the imperative that soybeans must be eaten cooked. Some investigators believe that these inhibitors may convey an anticancer advantage,[30] although whether they could convey this advantage as eaten is an unanswered question. Among the plants under study are soybeans, lima beans, other beans, and potatoes (in which the eyes are similar to seeds), all of which contain factors that may inhibit the process by which carcinogens are formed.[31] Answers to the interesting question of whether these foods play a role in cancer prevention are still to come, but some practical implications are apparent. Seed foods add variety to the diet and can be eaten in moderation. Overconsumption is probably possible, and would have adverse effects. Remember that both cabbages and potatoes were cited at the start as containing natural toxicants.

Yogurt

Years ago, when some long-lived people of another culture were asked their longevity secret, they gave the credit to their daily meals of yogurt—hence the start of yogurt mania in developed countries. Since then, researchers have studied both yogurt and yogurt-eating people to try to detect whether yogurt has health-promoting qualities.

Yogurt is made from milk that has been fermented by the **Lactobacillus** bacteria group, so it is nutritionally equivalent to the same quantity of milk, except that some of the lactose has been fermented to lactic acid. (This makes it useful for some people with lactose intolerance.) It is rich in calcium, protein, and the other nutrients normally found in milk. Its high calcium content may help protect against cancer, for diets high in calcium seem to protect against cancer generally, especially that of the colon (large intestine).[32] *Fermented* milk products (yogurt, buttermilk, kefir, and others) contain, in addition to nutrients, the bacteria from which they were made, and these bacteria, or products of their metabolism, seem to have additional special effects of their own. Specific strains of the yogurt-making bacteria produce enzymes that act against a number of transplanted and chemically induced cancers in animals, although exactly how they work is not yet known.[33]

Groups of people who include yogurt as a staple food suffer less colon cancer than people who do not. This is so even if their diets are high enough in fat to be expected to promote a high cancer rate. The bacteria of yogurt are known to survive the digestion process and take up residence in the large intestine, so it seems logical to look to bacterial action in the colon for an explanation of yogurt's anticancer effect. Researchers studying the colon contents of yogurt-eating people have found that they contain fewer enzyme-produced carcinogens than the colons of other people. It seems that *Lactobacillus* bacteria growing in the intestine inhibit those intestinal enzymes that convert at least some food chemicals into carcinogens in the colon.[34] In a study of mice, intestinal tumors stopped growing when the mice ate yogurt, presenting another possibility—that the by-products of bacterial growth inhibit tumor growth after it has begun.[35]

This is not to say that these researchers have proven that yogurt can prevent cancer. Their findings must be followed by more research, particularly research that uses the commercially available yogurt ordinarily consumed by people, to determine whether the products on the grocery store shelves have the anticancer effect. Assuming, though, that the *Lactobacillus* bacteria do inhibit carcinogen production in the colon, how can consumers apply this information?

The bacterial strain present in yogurt takes up only temporary residence in the digestive tract. It must be included in the diet regularly (reintroduced periodically) to achieve any possible benefits. Also, the yogurt must contain live cultures[36] (some manufacturers provide this information on the label).

Two other products also deliver *Lactobacillus:* **acidophilus milk** and acidophilus tablets. *Lactobacillus acidophilus* bacteria are grown in a medium, then harvested and added to milk. The bacteria are not grown in the milk, where they would ferment the lactose, for if they did, they would produce a sour by-product—lactic acid. The lactose content of acidophilus milk is therefore the same as that of milk, but it provides the beneficial bacteria, together with a medium suitable for their growth within the digestive tract. Acidophilus tablets taken without a milk product do not supply the needed medium in which the bacteria can multiply, and so do not establish a large *Lactobacillus* colony in the intestine.

Other research has led to other claims for yogurt. For example, yogurt cultures fed to rats produce and secrete an antibiotic effective against *other* bacteria that might cause harm—such as the ones that cause food poisoning.[37] Although supported by some research, these claims were derived from research in animals. Like all such claims, they need further investigation before they can be applied to human health.

Milk group foods may confer advantages against heart disease, too. Milk contains both saturated fat and cholesterol, which might be expected to raise blood cholesterol, and yet both milk and yogurt (even whole milk and yogurt in some experiments) have been shown to *lower* blood cholesterol.[38] (Nonfat milk would be preferable, of course, for the person seeking to escape the cancer-promoting effects of fat.) Among compounds present in milk that may account for the cholesterol-lowering effect are lactose[39] and two acids that, when purified and fed in higher doses, lower blood cholesterol.[40] Cheese also buffers salivary pH, inhibiting the caries-producing action of mouth bacteria. This makes it a good choice for a snack for people who can't brush their teeth right after eating—if they can afford the calories.[41]

It is a disservice to one's nutrition to overemphasize yogurt and milk at the expense of other, equally valuable foods from other food groups. But for calcium nutrition's sake, people are advised to include a minimum of two or more servings of yogurt or milk a day among the foods they choose. The possible nonnutrient benefits these foods convey make both of them excellent choices.

Other Foods

This discussion has left out some foods that have popular reputations the reader might wonder about. What about brewer's yeast, honey, wheat germ, chocolate, and other foods considered by some to be especially health promoting? Perhaps a word about each might not be amiss. In the old days, **brewer's yeast** was a byproduct of beer making; dead, bitter-tasting yeasts would settle to the bottom of the vats. Today, cultures of nonbitter yeasts are grown by a somewhat different method for use as food supplements and are still called brewer's yeast, or nutritional yeast. Since the yeast cells harvested from this process are dead, they do not make bread rise. Brewer's yeast is a source of B vitamins, iron, and protein (1 tablespoon has 3 grams of usable protein, or about 5 percent of the recommended amount for adults), and can be used to improve the quality of a vegetarian diet. Cereal grains combined with brewer's yeast are especially nutritious. Many vegetarian recipes for breads, cereals, soups, and rice dishes therefore recommend the addition of 1 to 2 tablespoons of yeast to their other ingredients. Brewer's yeast is highly nutritious, but for now, it seems to be true that it exerts health benefits only by donating the traditional nutrients. For example, people who lack the mineral chromium in their diets may suffer from high blood pressure or from a diabetes-like condition caused by resistance to the hormone insulin (insulin needs chromium in order to do its work). These conditions may be corrected by adding brewer's yeast or any other high-chromium food to the diet.

As for honey, it confers no proven benefits, although some people like to believe that eating locally harvested honey can reduce hay fever by introducing small amounts of the local pollens into the system, much as allergy shots do. It seems equally possible, though, that exposure to local pollens could aggravate hay fever and bee pollen is known to do so. Pollens also pick up high concentrations of environment contaminants. Spores of the organism that causes botulism, a deadly form of food poisoning, can get into honey, and parents are warned not to feed it to infants. Given the high sugar, low nutrient content of honey and the risk of botulism, honey remains in its proper place as an occasional treat, and only for older children and adults.

Wheat germ is high in B vitamins, magnesium, iron, and zinc and has a justified place in the diet of those who enjoy it, but it has no demonstrated nonnutrient benefits, either. Wheat germ oil is nutritionally inferior to wheat germ itself; it is much more expensive than other oils; and it has no apparent advantage over any other equally unsaturated oil.

And chocolate? Rumor has it that it relieves depression, but there is no proof that it does so physiologically. It does contain phenylethylamine, which is a biologically active amine, and could conceivably have an effect on mood. However, a search through the literature cited in support of the rumor reveals no connections established by actual research—doubtless a disappointment to chocoholics everywhere.[42] Perhaps chocolate's caffeine content, together with the sugar that is always added to it, accounts for its perceived effects on mood. (Controversy 13 discusses the effects of carbohydrate on mood.)

Many other foods contain substances that have nonnutrient effects. A fun example is the old Jewish remedy for a cold—chicken soup, which helps to speed the flow of mucus, ridding the body of infection.[43] Cinnamon, cloves, cranberries, and other plants contain benzoic acid and its esters, which act as preservatives, preventing microbial action in foods. The herb thyme contains one or more compounds that kill certain bacteria in food, as do cloves and clove oil. The herb ginger may prove to contain an effective motion-sickness drug.[44] However, as mentioned earlier, herbs can be misused and can cause harm. Like many other foods, and like drugs, herbs require the user to have adequate knowledge to use them properly. Unfortunately, because of the rampant quackery associated with herbs, that knowledge is not easy for users to sort out from the accompanying misinformation. This Controversy's reference, *The Honest Herbal,* is refreshingly different from most.*

Health-food stores sell a variety of herbal preparations to "remedy" a multitude of problems. One example is the use of comfrey capsules and tablets, prepared from the leaves or the roots of the comfrey plant, to aid digestion. A woman took two such tablets with each meal for four months. She became ill with liver disease due to the accumulation of a toxin in comfrey.**[45] Comfrey tea is carcinogenic in rats, and its use is discouraged because of its reported toxicity in human beings.[46]

The spices and herbs mentioned here are only a few among the many plants that people use in hopes of reaping health benefits. Table C2–1 presents some other plants that have been said to benefit health, and readers are referred to its source for further information.

Conclusions

That many foods contain compounds that have real physiological effects in people is interesting. A rational response to this reality is to keep an open mind, at first, about all such claims. That is, neither reject nor accept a newly reported food effect until it has been scientifically studied. Wait until the evidence is in. Although claims of special effects of foods are usually surrounded by a

*V. E. Tyler, *The New Honest Herbal: A Sensible Guide to Herbs and Related Remedies* (Philadelphia: Stickley, 1987). Varro E. Tyler, Ph.D. (pharmacognosy), formerly on the faculties of the Universities of Nebraska and Washington, is Dean of the Schools of Pharmacy, Nursing, and Health Services at Purdue University.

**The toxic substances found in comfrey are pyrrolizidine alkaloids. Tyler, 1987, p. 77.

Miniglossary

acidophilus milk: milk to which a culture of *Lactobacillus acidophilus* has been added (but not allowed to grow).

alfalfa: a perennial herb, used as cattle fodder and as food for people (as seeds or sprouts); claims of extraordinary health benefits from alfalfa are unfounded.

brewer's yeast: a preparation of yeast cells, often praised for its high nutrient content. It is especially rich in B vitamins, as are many other foods. Also called nutritional yeast, it is not useful for making bread rise.

capsaicin (cap-SAY-ih-sin): the chemical in peppers responsible for their "hot" taste.

caffeine: a natural stimulant found in many plants, including coffee, tea, and the cocoa bean (from which chocolate is made).

comfrey: an herb, used mostly for making tea.

congeners (CON-jen-erz): chemical substances other than alcohol that account for the physiological effects, such as taste and aftereffects, that are unique to different alcoholic beverages.

dithiolthiones: a class of chemical compounds, significant in this discussion because those occurring in the cruciferous vegetables are believed to exhibit some anticancer action.

foxglove: a plant (digitalis) containing a chemical (digoxin) of value as a drug for heart clients.

ginseng (JIN-seng): a plant containing chemicals that have physiological effects on human beings.

ginseng abuse syndrome: a cluster of symptoms associated with the overuse of ginseng, including high blood pressure, insomnia, nervousness, confusion, and depression.

herbs: nonwoody plants or plant parts valued for their flavor, aroma, or medicinal qualities.

indoles: a class of chemical compounds, significant in this discussion because those occurring in the cruciferous vegetables are believed to exhibit some anticancer action.

Lactobacillus: a genus of bacteria that includes several species that grow in milk and in the human intestine. *Lactobacillus acidophilus* is one of these species, sometimes added to milk to help ferment the sugar lactose in the intestine and so make the milk usable by people who cannot digest that sugar.

laetrile (LAY-uh-tril): the name given to a substance extracted from apricot pits, for which claims were made that it was a cancer cure. It is not, and it is poisonous.

protease inhibitors: chemicals that inhibit the action of enzymes that break down proteins. The inhibitors referred to here are those found in some seed foods; they make seed foods somewhat indigestible, a benefit to the seed but a hindrance to the eater's nutrition.

seed foods: foods made from seeds—grains, nuts, beans, peas, and the like.

Table C10–1

A Sampling of Plants for Which Claims of Nonnutrient Benefits are Made.

Selected are some of the more familiar plants of the more than 100 reviewed by Tyler (see source note). The judgments are Tyler's, and they are based on an honest scientific scrutiny of thousands of papers, books, and articles, many of which, however, are more in the realm of folklore than of science. The judgments are based on uses of the plants as described in Tyler's book (indiscriminate use of a plant called "safe," here, would not necessarily be safe). Much remains to be learned about these plants and the constituents responsible for their effects.

Common Name	Claim Made	Effective? (from available evidence)	Safe? (from available evidence)
Alfalfa (leaves and tops)	Cures arthritis	No	Yes
	Lowers blood cholesterol	No	Yes
Aloe (fresh juice)	Heals wounds and burns when applied to skin	Yes	Yes
Apricot pits (**laetrile**)	Cures cancer	No	No
Caffeine-containing plant parts	Acts as a stimulant	Yes	Yes/no
Chamomile (flowers)	Relieves intestinal gas	Yes	Yes[a]
	Soothes inflammation	Yes	Yes[a]
	Prevents or relieves spasms	Yes	Yes[a]
	Acts against infection	Yes	Yes[a]
Comfrey (roots, leaves)	Aids healing generally	Yes	No
Fennel (fruits, seeds)	Stimulates the stomach	Yes	Yes
	Relieves intestinal gas	Yes	Yes
Garlic and other onionlike bulbs	Reduces high blood pressure	Yes	Yes
Gentian (roots)	Stimulates the appetite	Yes	Yes
	Aids digestion	Yes	Yes
Hawthorn (fruits, leaves, flowers)	Dilates blood vessels, lowers blood pressure	Yes	Yes
Hibiscus (flowers)	Acts as a laxative, diuretic	Yes (?)	Yes
Honey	Cures arthritis	No	Yes
	Acts as a sedative	No	Yes
Hops (fruits)	Acts as a sedative, sleep aid	Yes (?)	Yes (?)
Horehound (leaves, tops)	Acts as an expectorant (causes productive coughing)	Yes	Yes
Papaya (dried leaves)	Aids digestion	No	Yes
	Expels intestinal worms	No	Yes
Peppermint (leaves)	Stimulates the stomach	Yes	Yes
	Relieves intestinal gas	Yes	Yes
Sassafras (root bark)	Acts as a stimulant	No	No
	Prevents or relieves spasms	No	No
	Produces sweating	No	No
	Relieves rheumatism	No	No
	Acts as a general tonic	No	No
Savory (above-ground plant)	Relieves intestinal gas	Yes	Yes
	Stimulates appetite	Yes	Yes
	Opposes diarrhea	Yes	Yes
	Acts as an aphrodisiac	No	Yes
	Reduces sex drive	No	Yes
Valerian (roots)	Tranquilizes, calms	Yes	Yes

[a]Except for allergic reactions.

Source: Adapted from V. E. Tyler, *The New Honest Herbal: A Sensible Guide to Herbs and Related Remedies* (Philadelphia: Stickley, 1987), with permission.

chaff of speculation, they may contain kernels of truth, and it is becoming increasingly interesting to watch the research sift them out. Maintain a healthy skepticism, and evaluate the sources from which claims come; scientists have much to learn about foods and their effects, but true scientists will be the first to tell you so.

Meanwhile, to apply the information now available: strive for variety in the foods you choose to eat. Even if scientific research supports the claims associated with the foods discussed here, it is unwise to eat the same foods day after day. To opt for the benefits of only a few to the exclusion of many others is to put all your health eggs in one basket, and perhaps to deny yourself many benefits not yet discovered. By eating a variety of foods, you can diversify your investment, obtain maximum benefits, and at the same time dilute the undesirable substances in all the foods consumed. Notice that the foods that seem to have won most endorsement in this discussion are members of every major food group except meat (we have nothing against meat; it just did not turn up among the foods for which health claims are most often made). They include vegetables, fruits, nuts, seeds, grains, and milk products, as well as herbs. So make selections from all of these categories, just as you would for nutrient adequacy.

Also, stay with whole foods, as close to the unrefined farm-grown products as possible, because they are the ones most likely to contain both needed trace nutrients and beneficial nonnutrients. This or that fraction extracted from a food may not be an improvement upon the food itself. Chances are, the beneficial effect of a food depends on a synergy among its nutrients, its structure, and its active nonnutrient components.

Notes

1. This discussion is adapted from E. N. Whitney, S. R. Rolfes, and F. S. Sizer, *Nonnutrients in Foods,* a monograph (1987) available from the Stickley Publishing Co., 210 Washington Sq., Philadelphia, PA 19106.
2. R. L. Koretz and J. H. Meyer, Elemental diets—facts and fantasies, *Gastroenterology* 78 (1980): 393–410
3. F. D. Moore, Current thoughts on malabsorption: Parenteral, enteral, and oral feeding (commentary), *Journal of the American Dietetic Association* 86 (1986): 1169–1170.
4. R. J. I. Bain, Accidental digitalis poisoning due to drinking herbal tea (letter to the editor), *British Medical Journal* 290 (1985): 1624.
5. E. N. Whitney, E. M. N. Hamilton, and M. A. Boyle, *Understanding Nutrition,* 4th ed. (St. Paul: West, 1987), p. 451.
6. R. W. Miller, Honey: Making sure it's pure, *FDA Consumer,* September 1979, pp. 12–13; I. B. Vyhmeister, What about honey? *Life and Health,* August 1980, pp. 5–7.
7. A. Brynjolfsson, Food irradiation and nutrition, *Professional Nutritionist,* Fall 1979, pp. 7–10.
8. R. Dubos, The intellectual basis of nutrition science and practice. Paper presented at the NIH Conference on the Biomedical and Behavioral Basis of Clinical Nutrition, 19 June 1978, in Bethesda, Md., and reprinted in *Nutrition Today,* July/August 1979, pp. 31–34.
9. J. A. Story and coauthors, Interactions of alfalfa plant and sprout saponins with cholesterol in vitro and in cholesterol-fed rats, *American Journal of Clinical Nutrition* 39 (1984): 917–929.
10. The substance the alfalfa tablets contained was an amino acid not normally found in proteins, L-canavanine. One person's SLE was reactivated after taking 15 tablets daily for nine months; the other person's, after taking eight tablets daily for two and a half years. J. L. Roberts and J. A. Hayashi, Exacerbation of SLE associated with alfalfa ingestion (letter to the editor), *New England Journal of Medicine* 308 (1983): 1361.
11. S. K. F. Chong and coauthors, Effect of ginseng saponins and hydrocortisone on phytohaemagglutinin transformation of lymphocytes, *Lancet,* 18 September 1982, pp. 662–663.
12. F. H. Schultz, Jr., R. Lowe, and R. A. Woodley, A possible effect of ginseng on serum HDL cholesterol (abstract no. 1522), *Federation Proceedings* 39, 1 March 1980.
13. M. A. Dubick, Historical perspectives on the use of herbal preparations to promote health, *Journal of Nutrition* 116 (1986): 1348–1354.
14. V. E. Tyler, *The New Honest Herbal: A Sensible Guide to the Use of Herbs and Related Remedies* (Philadelphia: Stickley, 1987), p. 113; E. M. Greenspan, Ginseng and vaginal bleeding (letter to the editor), *Journal of the American Medical Association* 249 (1983): 2018.
15. J. Konowalchuk and J. I. Speirs, Virus inactivation by grapes and wines, *Applied and Environmental Microbiology,* December 1976, pp. 757–763; A vintage medicine, *New York Times,* 12 June 1977, p. E7.
16. D. J. Forkner, Should wine be on your menu? *Professional Nutritionist,* Spring 1982, pp. 1–3.
17. P. N. Chaudhari and V. G. Hatwalne, Effect of epicatechin on liver lipids of rats fed with choline deficient diet, *Indian Journal of Nutrition and Dietetics* 14 (1977): 136–139.
18. A. Bordia, Effect of garlic on blood lipids in patients with coronary heart disease, *American Journal of Clinical Nutrition* 34 (1981): 2100–2103; A. Bordia, Effect of garlic on human platelet aggregation in vitro, *Atherosclerosis* 30 (1978): 355–360; A. A. Qureshi and coauthors, Suppression of avian hepatic lipid metabolism by solvent extracts of garlic: Impact on serum lipids, *Journal of Nutrition* 113 (1983): 1746–1755.
19. Garlic, *Journal of Nutrition Education* 15 (1983): 124.
20. S. Visudhiphan and coauthors, The relationship between high fibrinolytic activity and daily capsicum ingestion in Thais, *American Journal of Clinical Nutrition* 35 (1982): 1452–1458.
21. C. J. K. Henry and B. Emery, Effect of spiced food on metabolic rate, *Human*

Nutrition: Clinical Nutrition 40C (1986): 165–168.

22. G. A. Colditz and coauthors, Increased green and yellow vegetable intake and lowered cancer deaths in an elderly population, *American Journal of Clinical Nutrition* 41 (1985): 32–36.

23. L. W. Wattenberg, Inhibition of neoplasia by minor dietary constituents, *Cancer Research* 43 (1983): 24485–24535.

24. S. S. Ansher, P. Dolan, and E. Bueding, Biochemical effects of dithiolthiones, *Food and Chemical Toxicology* 24 (1986): 405–415.

25. B. S. Reddy and coauthors, Nutrition and its relationship to cancer, *Advances in Cancer Research* 32 (1980): 238–345.

26. The enzymes are the microsomal mixed-function oxidases, and in particular, aryl hydrocarbon hydroxylase. L. W. Wattenberg and coauthors, Dietary constitutents altering the responses to chemical carcinogens, *Federation Proceedings* 35 (1976): 1327–1331; L. W. Wattenburg and W. D. Loub, Inhibition of polycyclic aromatic hydrocarbon-induced neoplasia by naturally occurring indoles, *Cancer Research* 38 (1978): 1410–1413.

27. S. J. Stohs and coauthors, Effects of oltipraz, BHA, ADT and cabbage on glutathione metabolism, DNA damage and lipid peroxidation in old mice, *Mechanisms of Aging and Development* 37 (1986): 137–145.

28. Among the other inducers of the mixed-function oxidase system, found in plants, are flavones, aromatic isothiocyanates, coumarin, and selenium salts. Wattenberg and Loub, 1978.

29. W. Troll, K. Frenkel, and R. Wiesner, Protease inhibitors: Their role as modifiers of carcinogenic processes, in *Nutritional and Toxicological Significance of Enzyme Inhibitors in Foods,* ed. M. Friedman (New York: Plenum Press, 1986), pp. 153–165.

30. B. Merz, Adding seeds to the diet may keep cancer at bay, *Journal of the American Medical Association* 249 (1983): 2746.

31. J. Lauerman, A nutritional block against cancer? *Harvard Magazine,* May/June 1987, pp. 41–42.

32. M. Lipkin and H. Newmark, Effect of added dietary calcium on colonic epithelial-cell proliferation in subjects at high risk for familial colonic cancer, *New England Journal of Medicine* 313 (1985): 1381–1384.

33. B. A. Friend and K. M. Shahani, Antitumor properties of lactobacilli and dairy products fermented by lactobacilli, *Journal of Food Protection* 47 (1984): 717–723.

34. B. R. Goldin and S. L. Gorbach, The effect of milk and *Lactobacillus* feeding on human intestinal bacterial enzyme activity, *American Journal of Clinical Nutrition* 39 (1984): 756–761.

35. G. V. Reddy and coauthors, Antitumor activity of yogurt compounds, *Journal of Food Protection* 46 (1983): 8–11.

36. Goldin and Gorbach, 1984.

37. A. D. Hitchins and coauthors, Amelioration of the adverse effect of a gastrointestinal challenge with *Salmonella enteritidis* on weanling rats by a yogurt diet, *American Journal of Clinical Nutrition* 41 (1985): 92–100.

38. In an experiment using rats, both whole and nonfat milk lowered serum cholesterol significantly. D. Kritchevsky and coauthors, Influence of whole or skim milk on cholesterol metabolism in rats, *American Journal of Clinical Nutrition* 32 (1979): 597–600. In adolescent boys, nonfat milk, but not whole milk, lowered serum cholesterol. J. E. Rossouw and coauthors, The effect of skim milk, yoghurt, and full cream milk on human serum lipids, *American Journal of Clinical Nutrition* 34 (1981): 351–356.

39. B. D. Agarwal and coauthors, Effect of lactose on serum lipids in cases of coronary artery disease, *Journal of the Indian Medical Association* 75 (1980): 153–156.

40. These acids are hydroxymethylglutaric acid and orotic acid. L. Aftergood and R. B. Alfin-Slater, Adverse effects of some food lipids, in *Adverse Effect of Foods,* eds. E. F. P. Jelliffe and D. B. Jelliffe (New York: Plenum Press, 1982), p. 498.

41. N. Jenkins, Diet and dental caries, *Food and Nutrition News,* November/December 1984, p. 1.

42. R. Tomelleri and K. K. Grunewald, Menstrual cycle and food cravings in young college women, *Journal of the American Dietetic Association* 87 (1987): 311–315; W. J. Hurst, R. A. Martin, and B. L. Zoumas, Biogenic amines in chocolate—a review, *Nutrition Reports International* 26 (1982): 1081–1086; J. H. Burn and M. J. Rand, The action of sympathomimetic amines in animals treated with reserpine, *Journal of Physiology* 144 (1958): 314–336; B. Blackwell, Hypertensive crisis due to monoamine oxidase inhibitors, *Lancet* 2 (1963): 849–851; M. D. McDougal and G. B. West, The inhibition of the peristaltic reflex by sympathomimetic amines, *British Journal of Pharmacology* 9 (1954): 131–137.

43. Tidbits and morsels, *Nutrition and the MD,* January 1979.

44. Ginger aid, *Health,* August 1982, p. 14.

45. P. M. Ridker and coauthors, Hepatic venocclusive disease associated with the consumption of pyrrolizidine-containing dietary supplements, *Gastroenterology* 88 (1985): 1050–1054, as cited in R. J. Huxtable, J. Luthy, and U. Zweifel, Toxicity of comfrey-pepsin preparations, *New England Journal of Medicine* 315 (1986): 1095.

46. Questions and answers, *Nutrition and the MD,* December 1982.

Chapter Eleven

Contents

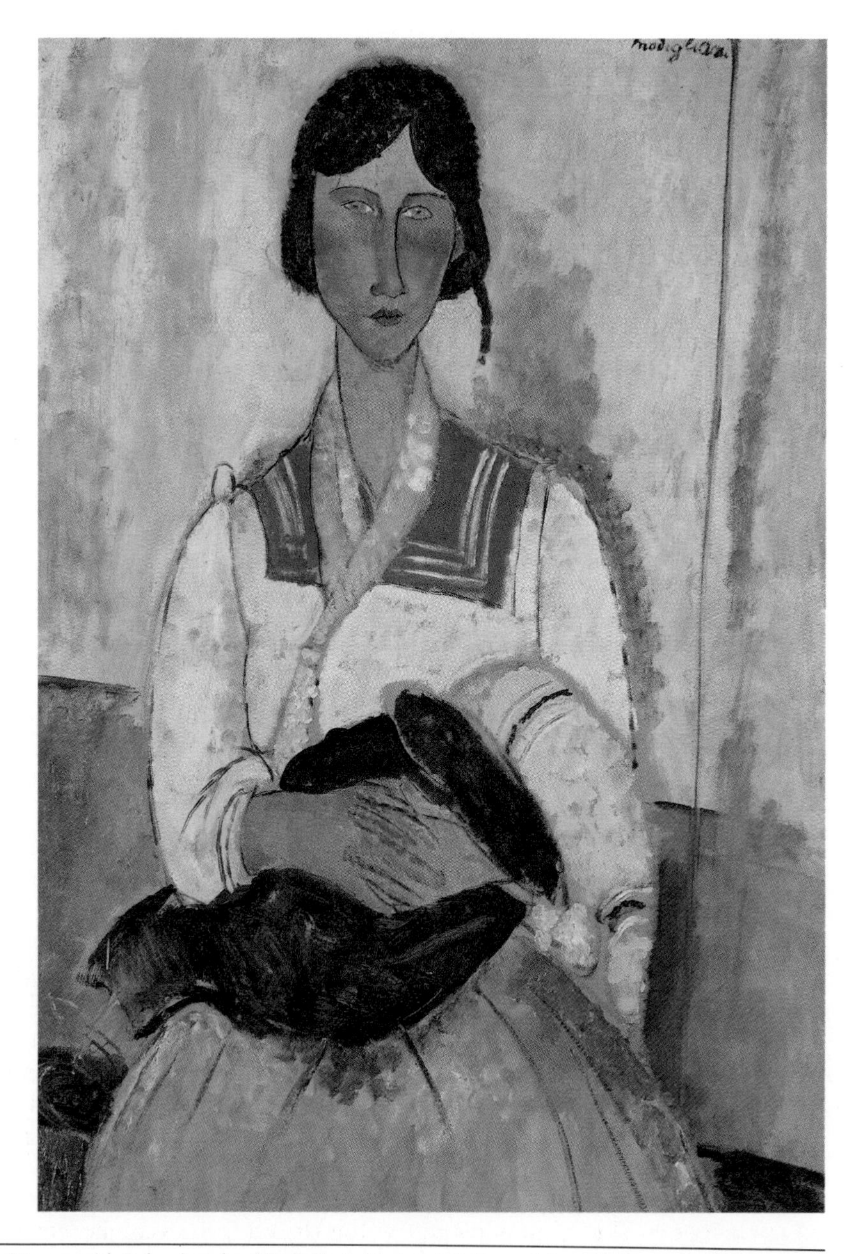

Gypsy Woman with Baby: Amedeo Modigliani; National Gallery of Art, Washington; Chester Dale Collection (Date: 1919; Canvas; 1.159 × 0.730 ($45\frac{5}{8} \times 28\frac{3}{4}$ in.))

Mother and Newborn Infant

The effects of nutrition extend over years. The woman who is expecting a baby and the health professional advising her will be strongly motivated to attend to the pregnant woman's nutrition needs if they understand how critical the nutrients are to the normal course of events in prenatal development, as well as to the health of the child for years to come.

The course and outcome of pregnancy are affected by many different events and circumstances. Some of these events are controllable; some are not. Nutrition throughout a woman's teenage and adult life, including pregnancy, is within her control. She can nourish herself optimally, given the knowledge, financial means, and motivation.

low birthweight (LBW): a birthweight of 5 ½ lb (2500 g) or less, used as a predictor of poor health in the newborn and as a probable indicator of poor nutrition status of the mother during and/or before pregnancy. Low-birthweight infants are of two different types. Some are **premature**; they are born early and are the right size for their gestational age. Others have suffered growth failure in the uterus; they may or may not be born early, but they are **small for gestational age (small for date)**.

Pregnancy: The Impact of Nutrition on the Future

To be sure of nourishing herself optimally for pregnancy, a woman must start beforehand. In the early weeks, significant developmental changes occur that depend on her nutrition status at a time when she may not even be aware that she is pregnant. A woman who eats nutrient-dense, whole foods prior to pregnancy establishes eating habits that will optimally nourish the growing fetus and herself. If nutrient supplementation is needed, the family-planning period is a good time to get it started.

Appropriate weight for height prior to pregnancy is also beneficial to pregnancy outcome. A strong correlation exists between prepregnancy weight and infant birthweight. In turn, infant birthweight is the most potent single indicator of the infant's future health status. A **low-birthweight (LBW)** baby, defined as one who weighs less than 5 ½ pounds (2500 grams), has a statistically greater chance than a normal-weight baby of contracting diseases and of dying early in life. Such a baby also is likely to be unable to do its job of obtaining nourishment by sucking and to win its mother's attention by energetic, vigorous cries and other healthy behavior. The low-birthweight baby can therefore become an apathetic, neglected baby, and this compounds the original malnutrition problem. Thus, for many reasons, babies of normal weight are usually more healthy. Nutritional deficiency, coupled with low birthweight, is the underlying or associated cause of more than half of all the deaths, worldwide, of children under five years old, and is responsible for the United States's relatively high infant mortality rate.[1] (The infant death rate in the United States is higher than in 13 other countries.)

placenta (pla-SEN-tuh): the organ inside the uterus in which the mother's and fetus's circulatory systems intertwine and in which exchange of materials between maternal and fetal blood takes place. The fetus receives nutrients and oxygen across the placenta; the mother's blood picks up carbon dioxide and other waste materials to be excreted via her lungs and kidneys.

uterus (YOO-ter-us): the womb, the muscular organ within which the infant develops before birth.

implantation: the stage of development in which the fertilized egg embeds itself in the wall of the uterus and begins to develop, during the first two weeks after conception.

ovum: the egg, produced by the mother, which unites with a sperm from the father to produce a new individual.

zygote (ZYE-goat): the term that describes the product of the union of ovum and sperm during the first two weeks after fertilization.

critical period: a finite period during development in which certain events may occur that will have irreversible, determining effects on later developmental stages. A critical period is usually a period of cell division in a body organ.

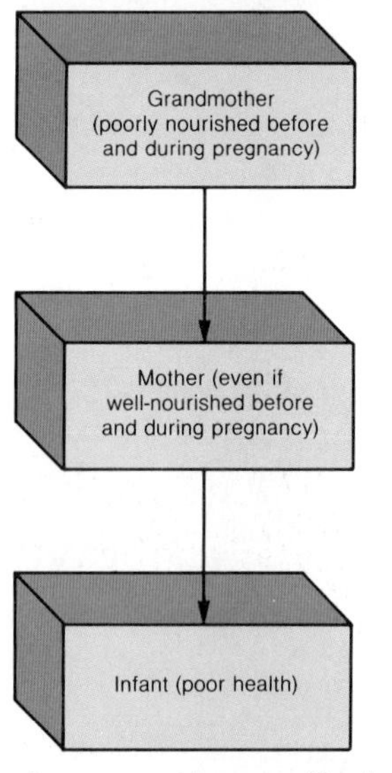

A woman's poor nutrition can affect her *grandchild* adversely.

Women who enter pregnancy 10 percent or more below or 20 percent or more above standard weight for height and age face a greater risk of impaired pregnancy outcome.[2] Underweight women are therefore advised to try to gain weight before becoming pregnant, and overweight women are wise to lose excess weight, to maximize the chances of having healthy babies as well as to maintain their own good health.

A major reason why the mother's prepregnancy nutrition is so crucial to a healthy pregnancy is that it determines whether she will be able to grow a healthy **placenta** or not. The only way nutrients can reach the developing infant in the **uterus** is through the placenta, a whole new organ that develops in the first month. The placenta is shown in Figure 11–1; it is a sort of cushion in which the mother's and baby's blood vessels intertwine and exchange materials—nutrients and oxygen going into the baby's system, wastes leaving it to be excreted by the mother.

Far from being passive in its transport of molecules, the placenta is a highly metabolic organ with some 60 enzymes. Much like muscles or other body tissues, it uses energy fuels to support its work. The placenta's work consists of actively gathering up maternally produced hormones, nutrients of all descriptions, large protein molecules such as antibodies, and other necessary items and forcing them into the fetal bloodstream. It also produces an array of hormones and factors, itself, that maintain pregnancy and prepare the mother's breasts for lactation. The placenta must develop normally if the developing fetus is to attain its genetic potential. If the placenta works perfectly, the fetus wants for nothing; if it doesn't, however, no alternative source of sustenance is available.

If the mother's nutrient stores are inadequate during the time when the placenta is developing, then the placenta will develop poorly. As a consequence, no matter how well she eats later, her unborn baby will not receive optimum nourishment. The infant is likely to be a low-birthweight baby, with a risk of attendant health consequences. After getting such a poor start on life, a girl child may be ill equipped, even as an adult, to store sufficient nutrients, and so may also be unable to grow an adequate placenta. In her turn, she may bear an infant who is unable to reach full developmental potential. Thus the poor nutrition of a woman during her early pregnancy can theoretically have an impact on the health of her *grandchild*, even after that child has become an *adult*.[3]

Not all cases of low birthweight reflect poor nutrition. Other factors that can damage the health of a low-birthweight baby are genetics, disease conditions, smoking, and drug (including alcohol) use during pregnancy. Even with optimal nutrition and health during pregnancy, some women give birth to small infants, for reasons unknown. Still, poor nutrition is the major factor, and ideally, an avoidable one.

Adequate nutrition before pregnancy establishes habits that best support fetal growth. Babies who weigh less than 5½ pounds at birth face greater health risks than normal weight babies.

Implantation and Embryonic Development

It is **implantation** of the newly fertilized **ovum**, or **zygote**, in the uterine wall that induces the uterus to grow a placenta, and this event, too, depends on conditions in the uterus at the time of conception. During the two weeks following fertilization, the zygote divides into many cells, and these cells sort themselves into three layers. Minimal growth in size takes place at this time, but it is a **critical period** developmentally. Adverse influences such as smoking, drug abuse, and severe malnutrition at this time lead to failure to implant or to other disturbances so severe as to cause loss of the zygote, possibly even before the woman knows she is pregnant. Many drugs affect the earliest intrauterine events and later cross the placenta freely. A prudent course of action for a potential mother is to avoid all drugs, including nicotine, alcohol, and even familiar over-the-counter drugs. Both mother and child will benefit most from an optimal supply of nutrients uncontaminated by other materials.

embryo (EM-bree-oh): the developing infant during its third to eighth week after conception.

fetus (FEET-us): the developing infant from eight weeks after conception until its birth.

hyperplasia (high-per-PLAY-zee-uh): an increase in cell number.

hypertrophy (high-PER-tro-fee): an increase in cell size.

The next six weeks, the period of embryonic development, register astonishing physical changes (see Figure 11–2). From the outermost layer of cells, the nervous system and skin begin to develop; from the middle layer, the muscles and internal organ systems; and from the innermost layer, the glands and linings of the digestive, respiratory, and excretory systems. At eight weeks, the 3-centimeter-long **embryo** has a complete central nervous system, a beating heart, a fully formed digestive system, and the beginnings of facial features. Already, an embryonic tail has formed and almost completely disappeared again, and the fingers and toes are well defined.

The growth of each organ and tissue type has its own characteristic pattern and timing. In the **fetus**, for example, the heart and brain develop early, the lungs much later. After birth, the brain doubles in weight within the first year, and by age five it has tripled. Thereafter, it slows considerably.[4] In contrast, the muscles start growing more slowly and develop for a longer time, becoming more than 30 times heavier at maturity than at birth.

Each organ is most dependent on an adequate supply of nutrients during its own intensive growth period. Thus a nutrient deficiency during one stage of development might affect the heart, and at another might affect the developing limbs. For example, the phase of brain growth most susceptible to malnutrition seems to be during the brain's growth spurt, defined as the period in which brain weight increases most rapidly.[5] In human beings, the brain's growth spurt begins in midpregnancy and continues into the second year of life.[6] The brain also goes through a phase of multiplication of cell contacts, which depends on both nutrition and social stimulation (learning). Undernutrition or lack of social stimulation at this time may have irreversible effects on some aspects of the brain's development.

The cells of a single developing organ also follow a schedule unique to them. The growth of all organs occurs by the processes of cell division, during which cells are increasing dramatically in *number* (**hyperplasia**), as well as cell growth, when cell *size* increases (**hypertrophy**). These two processes may occur simultaneously, or else separately, one preceding or following the other.

The period of increase in cell size appears to be the time when the most intensive growth appears to be going on. But actually, critical periods of cell division and differentiation may already be over. As mentioned, because events during a critical period can occur at only that time, and at no other, early malnutrition can have irreversible effects. Some of these effects may not become fully apparent until the person reaches maturity—for example, adults who suffered malnutrition in infancy may be shorter in stature than they would otherwise have been.

Figure 11–1
The Placenta.
The placenta is a sort of pillow of tissue in which maternal blood vessels lie side by side with fetal blood vessels entering it through the umbilical cord. This close association between the two circulatory systems permits the mother's bloodstream to deliver nutrients and oxygen to the fetus and carry fetal waste products away.

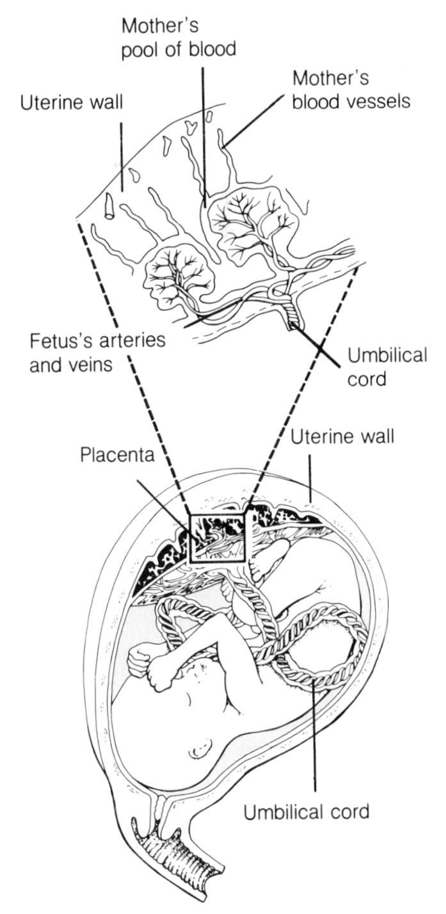

amniotic (am-nee-OTT-ic) **sac:** the "bag of waters" in the uterus, in which the fetus floats.

gestational diabetes: abnormal glucose tolerance appearing during pregnancy, with subsequent return to normal after the end of pregnancy.

The effect of malnutrition during critical periods is seen in the shorter height of people who were undernourished in their early years; in the delayed sexual development of those undernourished during early adolescence; in the poor dental health of children whose mothers were malnourished during pregnancy; and in the smaller brain cell number of children who have suffered from episodes of marasmus. The irreversibility of these effects is obvious when abundant, nourishing food fed after the critical time fails to remedy the growth deficit. Among the many Korean orphans adopted by U.S. families after the Korean War, for example, several years of catch-up growth occurred but did not completely make up for the growth retardation caused by early malnutrition.

Nutrition before and during pregnancy affects both present and future development of the infant. Placenta development, implantation, and early critical periods depend on nutrient supply, and in turn affect future growth and developmental events.

Figure 11–2
Stages of Fetal Development.
Only a little more than an inch long, the eight-week-old embryo has a complete central nervous system, a beating heart, a fully formed digestive system, and the beginnings of facial features. From eight weeks to term, it will grow 24 times longer and 50 times heavier.

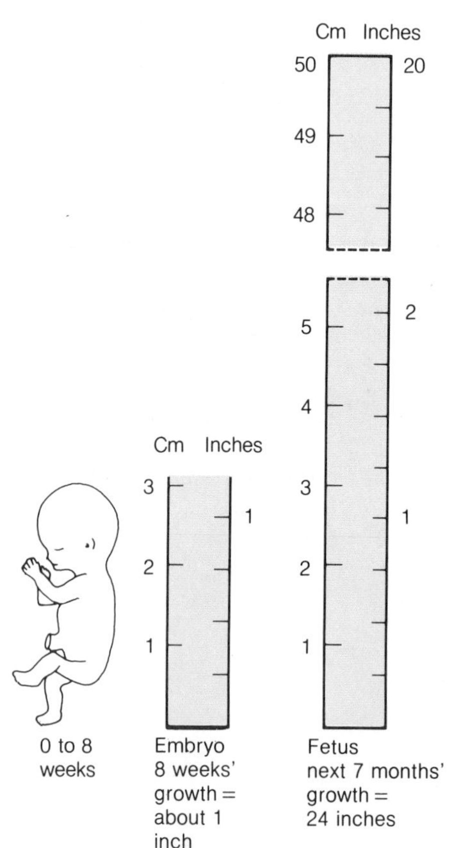

Maternal Physiological Adjustments

The last seven months of pregnancy, the fetal period, bring about a tremendous increase in the size of the fetus. Critical periods of cell division and development occur in organ after organ.

Meanwhile, the mother's body has been undergoing changes. As already mentioned, she has grown the placenta. The **amniotic sac** has filled with fluid to cushion the infant. The mother's uterus and its supporting muscles have increased greatly in size, her breasts have changed and grown in preparation for lactation, and her blood volume has increased by half to accommodate the added load of materials it must carry.

A mother's physiology changes so much during pregnancy that a naive observer might think that she was ill. She develops an apparent anemia, she may have edema, and her carbohydrate metabolism changes as if she were diabetic. These and other changes are, in most cases, normal for her altered state. Sometimes, however, the onset of diabetes occurs during pregnancy. This condition is known as **gestational diabetes**. If gestational diabetes is not properly managed, infant sickness and death is more likely than in normal pregnancies. Women who develop gestational diabetes are more likely than other women to develop permanent diabetes.

The "physiological anemia of pregnancy" results from an increase of about 50 percent in the mother's blood volume. The volume occupied by the red blood cells increases less—about 20 to 30 percent—so the number of red blood cells per milliliter is low compared with the nonpregnant state. Values for protein, iron, folacin, and other nutrients are correspondingly lowered, while other values rise (cholesterol and fat-soluble vitamins are examples). The clinician who assesses a pregnant woman's nutrition status therefore uses a set of standards specific for pregnancy.

The edema of pregnancy is also physiological (that is, expected and normal)—provided that it is not accompanied by high blood pressure or protein in the urine (see "Troubleshooting," later in this chapter). This normal edema results from the raised secretion of the hormone estrogen, which promotes water retention and helps, toward the end of pregnancy, to ready the uterus for delivery.

The altered carbohydrate metabolism of pregnancy resembles that of diabetes, but is normal for pregnancy. An untrained observer, however, could easily make an inappropriate diagnosis. These examples are intended to caution the reader who is unfamiliar with the special standards applicable to pregnancy not to jump to conclusions regarding out-of-line lab test values.

Nutrient Needs

Nutrient needs during periods of intensive growth are greater than at any other time and are greater for certain nutrients than for others, as shown in Figure 11–3. A study of the figure reveals some of the key needs.

One of the smallest increases apparent is in energy: a daily increase of 300 calories (during the second and third trimesters) above the allowance for nonpregnant women is recommended. For a woman of average size and moderate physical activity, this represents only about a 15 percent increase above nonpregnant energy needs. Compared with the needed increase in nutrients, this increase in energy need seems small, but in terms of pregnancy outcome, the importance of adequate maternal energy intake is great. The pregnant teenager or physically active woman may require more. In each case, enough calories are needed to spare protein for its all-important tissue-building work. A recommended average intake is 40 calories per kilogram of body weight, and energy intake should never fall below 36 calories per kilogram.[7] This is true for all women, even those who are overweight or obese. The increased recommendation for protein is more dramatic—from about 45 grams in a nonpregnant woman to about 75 grams per day for a pregnant woman, or about 30 additional grams of protein. The results of food consumption surveys, however, indicate that many women in the United States exceed the recommended protein intake each day.[8] Thus some women may not need the full 30 grams of additional daily protein recommended during pregnancy. Adequate protein consumption during pregnancy is important, but excessive protein may have adverse effects. Generous

Most severe risk factors for malnutrition in pregnancy:

- Age 15 or under.
- Unwanted pregnancy.
- Many pregnancies at intervals of less than a year (this depletes nutrient stores).
- History of poor outcome.
- Poverty and lack of family support.
- Food faddism.
- Heavy smoking.
- Drug addiction.
- Alcohol abuse.
- Chronic disease requiring special diet.
- More than 15% underweight.
- More than 15% overweight.

These factors at the start of pregnancy indicate that poor nutrition is likely to be present and to affect the pregnancy adversely.

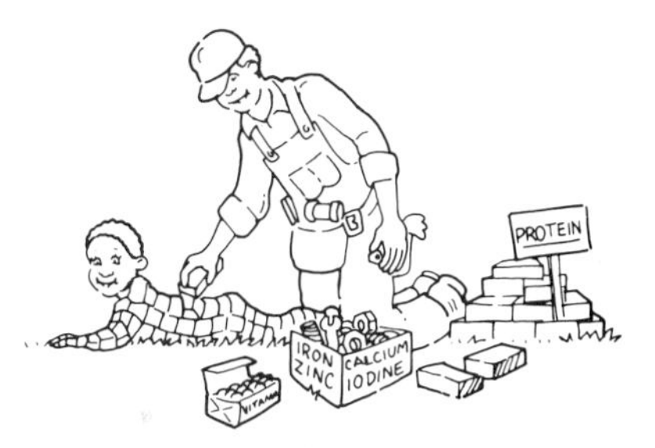

Baby building

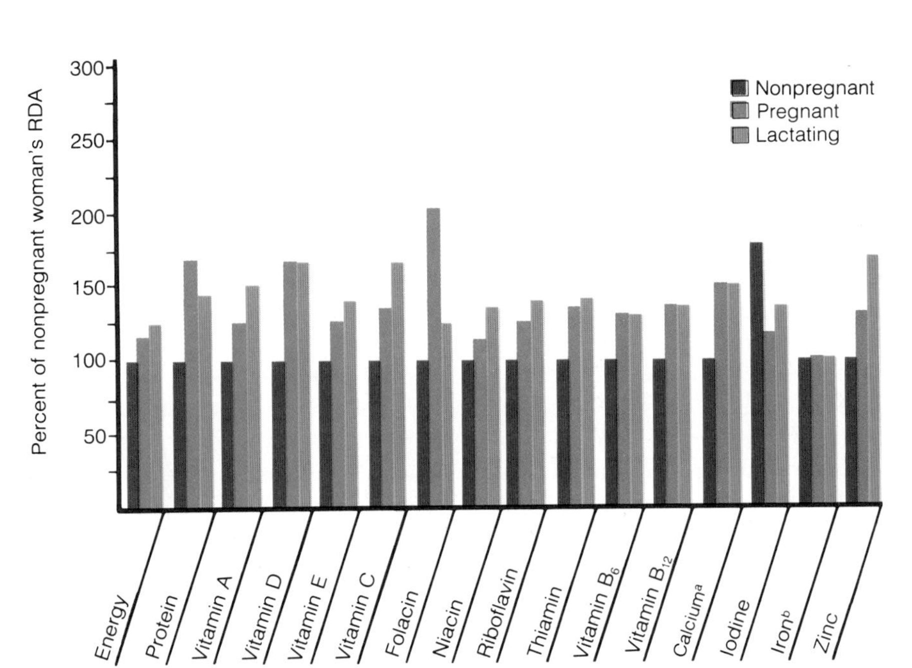

Figure 11–3
Nutrient Needs of Nonpregnant, Pregnant, and Lactating Women Compared.
The nonpregnant woman's nutrient recommendations are set at 100 percent (see RDA table, inside front cover).

[a]Recommended intakes of phosphorus and magnesium change similarly.
[b]The pregnant woman may need to take an iron supplement.

Recommended energy intake during pregnancy: 40 cal/kg (18 cal/lb).
Minimum energy intake: 36 cal/kg (17 cal/lb).
For a 120-lb woman, this represents at least 2000 cal/day, and preferably 2200 cal/day.
Recommended protein intake: 75 g/day.
Each of the following foods is equivalent to 15 g protein with accompanying calorie content as shown:

- 2 large eggs (160 cal).
- 1 c legumes (250 cal).
- 2 c nonfat milk (180 cal).
- 2 oz lean meat or fish (110 cal).
- 3 tbsp peanut butter (285 cal).
- ½ c cottage cheese (100 cal).

Two such selections over and above normal intake will therefore provide the additional 30 g protein recommended daily during pregnancy. The legumes are higher in calories then some of the other selections, but they are excellent sources of complex carbohydrate, vitamins, and minerals.

Recommended carbohydrate intake: about 50% of energy intake. In a 2000 cal/day intake, this represents 1000 cal of carbohydrate, or about 250 g. Four cups of milk a day will contribute about 50 g carbohydrate. An apple provides 10 g carbohydrate, and a slice of bread provides 15 g, so generous intakes of fruit and bread exchanges are clearly beneficial.

Foods containing vitamin B_6:

- Green leafy vegetables.
- Bananas.
- Salmon.
- Legumes.
- Beef.
- Chicken.

Foods containing folacin:

- Green, leafy vegetables.
- Legumes.
- Liver.
- Orange juice and cantaloupe.
- Other vegetables.
- Whole-wheat products.

Foods containing calcium:
Four cups of milk a day will supply 1.2 g calcium. For other food sources, see Chapter 7. The milk should be fortified with vitamin D; if it is not, a vitamin D supplement may be needed.

amounts of carbohydrate are needed to spare the protein. If added energy is needed, it is best obtained from carbohydrate.

Some vegetarian women choose to exclude all foods of animal origin from their diets. For these individuals, the selection of protein-rich foods is limited, and the need for abundant high-quality protein during pregnancy demands careful attention. The inclusion of adequate food energy each day and several servings of plant-protein foods such as legumes, whole grains, nuts, and seeds in generous quantities are imperative. In some instances, it may be advisable to supplement meals with a soy-based protein powder to ensure adequate protein intake.

The growing fetus and the altered hormonal activity of pregnancy increase the metabolic demand for vitamin B_6. Low intakes of vitamin B_6 have been reported in pregnant and lactating women. Foods rich in vitamin B_6 are shown in the margin.[9]

The pregnant woman's extraordinary need for folacin is due to the great increase in her blood volume and the rapid growth of the fetus. It is possible, but not easy, to obtain the recommended folacin amounts from foods; many diets are inadequate in this respect. Folacin deficiency is common during pregnancy, and folacin supplements are often prescribed for the pregnant woman. As you might expect, vitamin B_{12} is also needed in large amounts, because it assists folacin in the manufacture of red blood cells. Vitamin B_{12} is unique in that it is found almost exclusively in foods of animal origin. People who eat meat, eggs, and dairy products, or any combination thereof, are therefore protected from deficiency. If foods of animal origin are excluded from the diet, then vitamin B_{12}–fortified soy milk or supplements are recommended.

Among the minerals, those involved in building the skeleton—calcium, phosphorus, and magnesium—are in great demand during pregnancy, and increases of about 50 percent above nonpregnant intakes are recommended. Intestinal absorption of calcium doubles early in pregnancy, and the mineral is stored in the mother's bones. Later, as the fetal bones begin to calcify, there is a dramatic shift of calcium across the placenta, and the mother's bone stores are drawn upon. Because many women's diets are notoriously low in calcium and because pregnancy and breastfeeding draw on women's skeletal reserves, most mothers' intakes have to be increased well above the prepregnancy levels.

The body conserves iron even more than usual during pregnancy: menstruation ceases, and absorption of iron increases up to threefold due to a rise in the level of the blood's iron-absorbing and carrier protein, transferrin. However, iron stores dwindle during pregnancy and at the time of birth. The developing fetus draws on its mother's iron stores to create stores of its own to carry it through the first three to six months of life. This drain on the mother's supply may precipitate a deficiency; furthermore, the mother loses blood as she gives birth. Few women enter pregnancy with adequate stores to meet these demands, so the Committee on RDA recommends an iron supplement throughout pregnancy and for two to three months after delivery.[10] The exact amount of the iron supplement is determined by the physician administering prenatal care.

The most absorbable iron is that of red meat. Iron absorption from plant foods such as legumes and dark green vegetables is tripled in a meal containing meat, fish, or poultry (MFP; see Chapter 7). Vitamin C in fruits and vegetables can also triple absorption from nonmeat foods eaten at the same meal. Thus the pregnant woman is wise to include small bits of meat, fish, or poultry in every meal, or if her diet excludes all MFP, to eat abundant vitamin C–rich fruits and vegetables.

Zinc is another nutrient of vital importance in pregnancy. Zinc is most abundant in foods of high protein content, such as shellfish, meat, and nuts, but the presence of other trace elements and fiber in foods may adversely affect zinc absorption. One study of pregnant women found that their dietary zinc intake was, on the average, less than two-thirds of the RDA.[11] Zinc nutrition is the focus of intense study at the present time, and many questions remain to be answered regarding zinc metabolism and availability from foods. In the meantime, however, daily consumption of zinc-rich foods is no doubt beneficial to the pregnant woman and her fetus.

Calcification of the baby teeth begins in the third month after conception; 32 teeth are well along in development before birth. For these teeth and for the bones, fluoride may be needed. It is not clear from research whether supplemental fluoride crosses the placenta, but some evidence suggests that it does. Children whose mothers received 1 milligram of fluoride daily in addition to using fluoridated water have been observed to have more decay-free teeth at five to nine years of age compared with children whose mothers only used fluoridated water.[12] Foods that can be relied on to provide fluoride are few (their fluoride content depends on where they were produced), but small ocean fish and tea are known to be good sources. If the water is not fluoridated, then a prescribed supplement may be desirable.

Just as pregnancy is a time of increased nutrient needs, so is it a time when emotional and financial needs are increased. The pregnant women needs all the support and understanding that family and friends can provide. This is especially true for the woman facing the birth of her child without a partner.

Low-income pregnant women and their children may be eligible for financial assistance programs. At the community level, the Agricultural Extension Service provides educational services and materials, including nutrition, food budgeting, and shopping information. At the Federal level, the Women's, Infants', and Children's Supplemental Feeding (WIC) program provides nutrition counseling and low-cost nutritious foods to pregnant women and their children.

Ordinarily, a hemoglobin level below 13 g/100 ml is considered low for a woman. In pregnancy, values of 12 g are not unusual, and 11 g is where the line defining "too low" is often drawn. It is usually desirable to use more sensitive measures than hemoglobin if questions about the woman's iron status arise.

Food sources of iron:

- Liver and oysters.
- Red meat, fish, and other meat.
- Dried fruits.
- Legumes.
- Dark green vegetables.

Best food sources of zinc:

- Oysters, crabmeat, and other shellfish.
- Red meat.
- Legumes.

Pregnancy induces maternal physiologic adjustments, including altered blood composition, increased blood volume, and gain of supporting tissues. These developments demand increased intakes of energy, and more greatly increased intakes of nutrients.

Eating Pattern and Weight Gain

If the woman's dietary pattern is already adequate at the start of pregnancy, she can simply increase her servings of nutritious foods to meet the nutrient demands of pregnancy. The nutrients she needs the most are best provided by foods in the milk, meat/meat alternate, and vegetable categories.

Because energy needs increase less than nutrient needs, the pregnant woman must select foods of high nutrient density. For most women, appropriate choices include foods like nonfat milk, low-fat cottage cheese, lean meats, legumes, eggs, liver, dark green vegetables, and whole-grain breads and cereals. Vitamin C-rich foods in generous quantities should be present at every meal. A suggested food pattern is shown in Table 11–1.

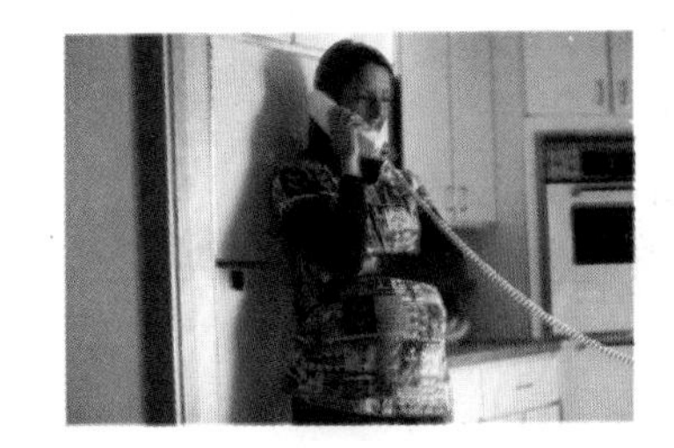

Pregnancy is a time to choose foods with special care.

Table 11–1

Daily Food Guides for Pregnant and Lactating Women

Food	Number of Servings		
	Nonpregnant Woman	*Pregnant Woman*[a]	*Lactating Woman*
Protein foods			
Animal (2-oz serving)	2	2 (2+)	2
Vegetable (at least one serving of legumes)	2	2	2
Milk and milk products	2	4 (4+)	5
Enriched or whole-grain breads and cereals	4	4 (5 to 6)	4
Vitamin C–rich fruits and vegetables	1	1 (1+)	1
Dark green vegetables	1	1	1
Other fruits and vegetables	1	1 (2+)	1

[a]Numbers in parentheses indicate number of servings recommended for the pregnant teenager.
Source: Adapted from California Department of Health, as cited in Nutrition and the pregnant obese woman, *Nutrition and the MD,* January 1978.

Individual food cravings during pregnancy do not seem to reflect real physiological needs. In other words, a woman who craves ice cream (the most common food craving) is not necessarily in need of calcium, but cravings in general may reflect a nutrient-poor diet. Food aversions and cravings may arise during pregnancy due to changes in taste and smell sensitivities.

A pregnant woman may crave and eat clay, ice, cornstarch, and other nonnutritious substances. This is pica (recall Chapter 7) and may reflect a need for iron or zinc. The behavior is not adaptive; the substances she craves do not deliver the nutrients she needs.

The pregnant woman must gain weight. Ideally, she will have begun her pregnancy at the appropriate weight for her height and will gain about 25 pounds, most of it in the second half of pregnancy. The ideal pattern is thought to be about 2 to 4 pounds during the first three months and a pound per week thereafter. Underweight women and teenagers need to gain more. Pregnancy weight gains between 16 and 24 pounds (depending on prepregnancy weight) are recommended for women who are 10 percent or more above the standard weight for height at the start of pregnancy.[13] A pregnancy weight gain of 22 to 28 pounds is recommended for most women (see Table 11–2).

Recently, some researchers have suggested that new weight-gain standards for pregnancy, based on larger, more diverse groups of women, are desirable.[14] They suggest that new pregnancy weight-gain charts be made for adolescents, obese and underweight women, and women who are carrying more than one fetus.

The weight the pregnant woman puts on is nearly all lean tissue: placenta, uterus, blood, and milk-producing glands, and of course, the baby itself. Thus little room is available in the diet for empty calories such as sugar, fat, and alcohol, which provide no nutrients to support the growth of these tissues and only contribute to fat accumulation beyond that needed to provide energy for labor and lactation. Some of the weight gained during pregnancy is lost at delivery; most of the remainder is generally lost within a few weeks or months, as blood volume returns to normal and accumulated fluids are lost.

Table 11–2

Weight Gain during Pregnancy

Development	Weight Gain (lb)
Infant at birth	7½
Placenta	1
Increase in mother's blood volume to supply placenta	4
Increase in size of mother's uterus and muscles to support it	2½
Increase in size of mother's breasts	3
Fluid to surround infant in amniotic sac	2
Mother's fat stores	2 to 8
Total	22 to 28

Note: The pattern of gain should be about a pound a month for the first three months, and a pound a week thereafter. Different patterns of weight gain are suggested for underweight, normal-weight, and overweight women, described by E. McCarthy, Report of a Montreal Diet Dispensary experience, *Journal of the Canadian Dietetic Association* 44 (1983): 71–75.

If a woman has gained more than the expected amount of weight early in pregnancy, dieting in the last weeks does not compensate, nor is it recommended. Women have been known to gain up to 60 pounds in pregnancy without ill effects. (A *sudden* large weight gain, however, is a danger signal that may indicate the onset of pregnancy-induced hypertension; see "Troubleshooting.")

Weight gain during pregnancy, like prepregnancy weight, is directly related to infant birthweight.[15] If the mother does not gain the full amount of weight recommended, she may give birth to an underweight baby. To the uninitiated, this may seem like no catastrophe, and in some instances it is not. A small mother may give birth to a small, normal, alert, and healthy baby. Nothing is wrong with that. On the other hand, a low-birthweight baby may be a malnourished baby, one who is more likely to get sick, as described earlier.

Another life-style component that is equally important in the promotion of health and well-being is exercise. Pregnancy does not necessitate inactivity. The active, physically fit woman experiencing a normal pregnancy can continue to enjoy the benefits of exercise throughout the pregnancy, adjusting the duration and intensity as needed. Common sense and consultation with the health care provider are recommended.

Some general rules for exercise during pregnancy:

- Stop exercising if you feel overheated.
- Drink plenty of fluids before you exercise.
- Avoid exercising in hot, humid weather.
- Protect the abdomen from injury, especially in games like baseball or basketball in which accidents are likely.
- Discontinue any exercise that causes discomfort.
- Do not exercise while lying on your back after about the fourth month.
- Do not allow your heart rate to exceed 140 beats per minute.

Practices to Avoid

A general guideline can be offered to the pregnant woman: eat a normal, healthy diet, and practice moderation. Some substances are truly harmful, though, and their potential impact is too great to risk.

One member of this group of substances to avoid is caffeine. One or two cups of coffee or tea a day or the equivalent are probably within safe limits, but caffeine is a drug, and excesses should be avoided. Many studies have shown intakes of up to four cups of coffee or tea a day to be associated with no increased risk, but one recent study links the use of 2 cups' worth of caffeine or more per day to an increased risk of spontaneous abortion in women.[16] A table of the caffeine amounts in beverages and medications is provided in Chapter 13.

A clearly harmful practice is smoking. Smoking restricts the blood supply to the growing fetus and so limits the delivery of oxygen and nutrients and the removal of wastes. It stunts growth, thus increasing the risk of retarded development and complications at birth. As this is written, alarming facts about the effects of smoking during pregnancy continue to be revealed. One study found that the incidence of cancer and leukemia in children of women who smoked while pregnant was twice as high as normal.[17]

Other drugs taken during pregnancy can cause serious birth defects. We live in a society in which the use of over-the-counter drugs is routine for many people, and abuse of drugs is a major problem. Without prior physician consultation, the use of any drugs or even vitamin supplements is inadvisable.

Dieting, even for short periods, is hazardous. Low-carbohydrate diets or fasts that cause ketosis deprive the growing brain of needed glucose and may impair its development.[18] Such diets are also likely to be deficient in other nutrients vital to fetal growth. Energy restriction during pregnancy is dangerous for all women, regardless of their prepregnancy weight. One study has shown that even in overweight women, those with the smallest pregnancy weight gains are twice as likely to experience impaired pregnancy outcomes.[19] The pregnant,

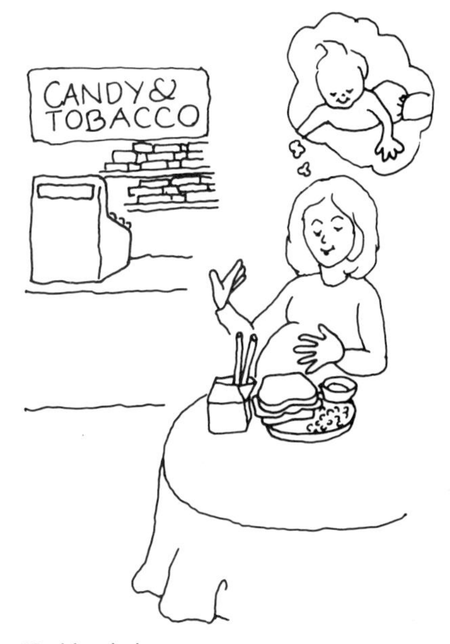

Healthy choices.

fetal alcohol syndrome: the cluster of symptoms seen in an infant or child whose mother consumed excess alcohol during her pregnancy; includes mental and physical retardation with facial and other body deformities.

pregnancy-induced hypertension (PIH): a cluster of symptoms seen in pregnancy, including edema, hypertension, and kidney complications. PIH was formerly known as *toxemia*. Other terms associated with PIH are *eclampsia* (symptoms include convulsions and coma, associated with high blood pressure, edema, and protein in the urine) and its predecessor, *preeclampsia*, characterized by edema, increasing hypertension, and protein in the urine.

overweight woman must therefore take special care in selecting those foods that will best promote optimal fetal growth and gradual weight gain—nutrient-dense foods.

The consequences of protein deprivation can be severe. This has been observed most frequently in the underdeveloped countries, but it has also been seen among food faddists who adopted an untested vegetarian diet. Their children's height and head circumference were markedly and irreversibly diminished. Iron deficiency during pregnancy in animals has been seen to give rise to offspring whose brain cells could never store the needed iron thereafter.[20] In human beings, fetal deaths, prematurity, and low birthweight occur more frequently when maternal iron status (by tests of hemoglobin or hematocrit) is poor.[21]

Most importantly, alcohol consumption can cause irreversible brain damage and mental and physical retardation in the fetus (**fetal alcohol syndrome**). The damage can occur with as few as two drinks a day, and its most severe impact is likely to be in the first month, before the woman even is sure she is pregnant. About 1 in every 750 children born in the United States is a victim of this preventable damage.[22] Fetal alcohol syndrome is the most common cause of mental illness from birth. This chapter's Controversy is devoted to the consequences of drinking during pregnancy.

The pregnant woman should gain 22 to 28 pounds during pregnancy, by eating a balanced diet of nutrient-dense foods. Recommended is avoidance of caffeine, smoking, other drugs, dieting, and especially alcohol consumption.

Troubleshooting

To avoid the most common problems encountered during pregnancy, some additional measures are helpful. Pregnancy precipitates the onset of diabetes in some women; it is recommended that all pregnant women be screened for diabetes at about the sixth month. Thereafter, at every checkup, routine testing of urine for ketone bodies is in order. Ketonuria may be a clue to diabetes or may warn of the starvation ketosis of ill-advised dieting.

The normal edema of pregnancy responds to gravity; blood pools in the ankles. The edema of PIH is a generalized edema. The distinction helps with diagnosis.

A certain degree of edema is to be expected in late pregnancy, as mentioned, but in a poorly nourished woman, it is often part of a larger problem known as **pregnancy-induced hypertension** (**PIH**) (formerly known as *toxemia*). Preexisting hypertension and PIH are the most common medical complications of pregnancy. They can cause maternal death, infant death, retarded growth, lung problems, and other birth defects. It is important to keep track of maternal blood pressure throughout pregnancy, and if PIH is indicated, to initiate treatment promptly.* Treatment is medical, and salt restriction is not a part of treatment until and unless the kidneys prove unable to handle a normal sodium load. A normal salt intake is necessary for health.[23]

*Blood pressure of 140/90 millimeters of mercury during the second half of pregnancy in a woman who has not previously exhibited hypertension indicates PIH. So does a rise in systolic blood pressure of 30 millimeters in diastolic blood pressure of 15 millimeters on at least two occasions more than six hours apart. R. J. Worley, Pathophysiology of pregnancy-induced hypertension, *Clinical Obstetrics and Gynecology* 27 (1984): 821–835.

The nausea of "morning" (actually, anytime) sickness seems unavoidable, because it arises from the hormonal changes taking place early in pregnancy, but it can often be alleviated. A strategy some expectant mothers have found effective in quelling nausea is to start the day with a few sips of water and a few nibbles of a soda cracker or other bland carbohydrate food, to get something in their stomachs before getting out of bed. Carbonated beverages also may help.

Later, as the hormones of pregnancy alter her muscle tone and the thriving infant crowds her intestinal organs, an expectant mother may complain of constipation. A high-fiber diet and a plentiful water intake will help to relieve this condition. Daily exercise, if the physician approves, may also be beneficial. The woman should use laxatives only if the physician prescribes them and determines the type to take.

Pregnancy for many women is a time of adjustment to major changes. The woman who is expecting to bear a baby is a growing person in more ways than one. Not only physically, but also emotionally, her needs are changing. If it is her first baby, she senses that her life-style will have to change as she takes on the new responsibility of caring for a child. Ideally, she will be encouraged to develop this sense of responsibility by caring for herself during pregnancy. The expectant mother needs support in thinking of herself as a worthwhile and important person with a new and challenging task that she can and will perform well. Oftentimes, as a young adult, she is still working out her relationship with her mate, and they both know that the coming of a first baby will affect that relationship profoundly. There is a need for sensitive communication and understanding on both parts in this time of transition.

This is only the briefest summary of the nutrient needs in pregnancy. But with all of this to think about, can a woman relax and enjoy expecting her baby? Of course she can. With the care and guidance of capable health professionals, and the love and support of family and friends, awaiting the birth of a child can be a special experience.

Common medical problems associated with pregnancy are gestational diabetes and pregnancy-induced hypertension (PIH). These should be caught and managed to minimize associated risks.

Preparing for Breastfeeding

Toward the end of her pregnancy, a woman who plans to breastfeed her baby should begin to prepare. No elaborate or expensive procedures are necessary, but breastfeeding in human beings involves many behaviors and attitudes that require learning, and it usually goes more smoothly for the mother who prepares than for the one who expects it to happen automatically. More is involved than can be discussed in detail here; it is recommended that the expectant mother read at least one of the many handbooks available on breastfeeding.* Talking

---

*An international organization of women who believe in breastfeeding and who help each other with related concerns is the LaLeche League. The main office is at 9616 Minneapolis Avenue, Franklin Park, IL 60131; there are branches in many cities. Among the League's publications are the *La Leche League News* (a newsletter), and *The Womanly Art of Breastfeeding* (a manual). The league also highly endorses the manual by P. B. Brewster, *You Can Breastfeed Your Baby . . . Even in Special Situations* (Emmaus, Pa.: Rodale Press, 1979).

with or observing women who breastfeed their babies successfully is also helpful, as is having a family and medical team support system.

As far as possible, the mother should discuss her plans in advance with the members of that support system, whoever they may be—her husband, her mother, her other grown children, the physician, the midwife, or a nurse. One of the most significant factors for successful lactation is the length of time between the baby's birth and the first nursing. The earlier breastfeeding is attempted after birth, the greater the likelihood that the baby will be solely breastfed at ten weeks of age.[24] In other words, breastfeeding success and duration are greatly facilitated when the baby is put to the breast as soon as possible after birth. Thus the cooperation of hospital or birthing facility staff is imperative. The mother's awareness before the birth that she may encounter problems related to breastfeeding will best enable her to deal with the problems, should they arise. Adherence to feeding schedules and early supplementation with breast milk substitutes adversely affect the duration of lactation. So does the exaggerated hope that rapid maternal weight loss will result from breastfeeding, for when this does not occur, women give up breastfeeding.

Before the birth time, the mother-to-be should buy two or more nursing bras—the kind that give good support and that have drop-flaps so that either breast can be freed for nursing. Also, if the nipples are tender, they can be toughened prior to or during lactation by the following means:

- Stop using soap on the breasts for the last three months of pregnancy so that the skin's own protective secretions can make the nipple area strong and resistant to irritation.
- Let the nipples rub against the outer clothing (wear the nursing bra open, or cut holes in an older bra for each nipple) so that they will be chafed.

A woman with flat or inverted nipples may want to manipulate her breasts by hand to help correct this condition or obtain a nipple shield that will help the nipple evert.

Preparation for breastfeeding begins before the end of pregnancy.

Breastfeeding: The Mother's Nutrition Needs

The mother who chooses to breastfeed her infant needs her nutrient supplies to support the infant's development, and her own health, even after birth. Adequate nutrition of the mother makes a highly significant contribution to successful lactation; without it, lactation is likely to falter or fail. An inadequate diet is incompatible with the stamina and patience that nursing a baby demands. By continuing to eat high-quality foods to the end of pregnancy and enjoying ample food and fluid at frequent intervals throughout lactation, the mother who chooses to breastfeed her baby will be nutritionally prepared to do so.

A nursing mother may produce approximately 30 ounces of milk a day (the amount varies). At 20 calories per ounce, this milk output amounts to 600 calories per day. In addition, energy is needed to produce this milk; so the energy allowance for a lactating woman is a generous 750 calories a day above her ordinary need. The RDA table suggests that 500 calories come from added food, and the rest from the stores of fat her body accumulated during pregnancy for that purpose. Recently it has been suggested that for some women, energy needed for milk production may be less than current recommendations.[25] Severe calorie restriction, however, will hinder milk production.

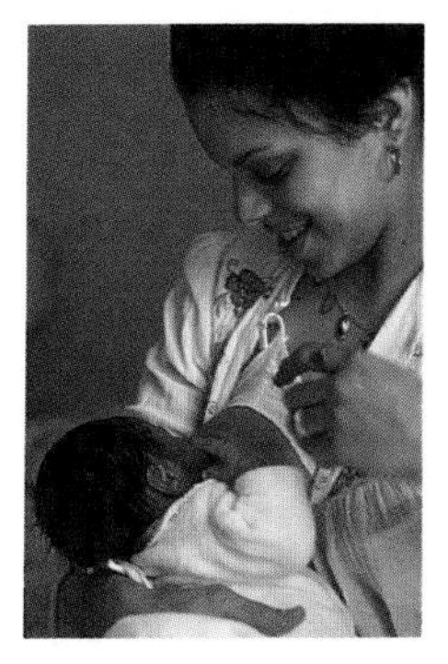

Nutrition supports lactation.

The calories consumed by the nursing mother should carry with them abundant nutrients—especially those needed to make milk, such as calcium, protein, magnesium, zinc, and plenty of fluid. Figure 11–3 shows the differences between a lactating woman's nutrient needs and those of a nonpregnant woman, and Table 11–1 shows a food pattern that would meet them.

Logically, the food best suited to support the mother's making of milk is milk, or something that resembles it in composition. The obvious choice is cow's milk. The nursing mother who can't drink milk needs to find nutritionally similar foods such as cheese, calcium-fortified soy milk, or the milk substitutes mentioned in Chapter 7. As during pregnancy, nutritious foods should make up the remainder of the needed calorie increase. Despite previous misconceptions, increasing maternal fluid intake does not increase breast milk volume.[26] The mother who is nursing a baby is nevertheless advised to drink at least 2 quarts of liquids each day to protect herself from dehydration. A convenient way to ensure adequate fluid consumption is to drink a glass of milk, juice, or water each time the baby nurses, as well as at mealtimes.

Alcohol easily enters breast milk. Large amounts consumed over a short time are thus readily available to the nursing infant. Large amounts of alcohol also decrease milk production, but an occasional glass of wine or beer is within safe limits. Excessive caffeine consumption during lactation may cause irritability and wakefulness in the breastfed baby. The use of illegal drugs is incompatible with breastfeeding, and prescription medications should be taken only after physician consultation.

The question is often raised whether a mother's milk may lack a nutrient if she is not getting enough in her diet. The answer differs from one nutrient to the next, but in general, the effect of nutritional deprivation of the mother is to reduce the quantity, not the quality, of her milk. For protein, carbohydrate, and most minerals, the milk of a healthy mother has a fairly constant composition. The levels of fat-soluble vitamins in human milk can be altered by excessive or deficient intakes of the mother. For example, large doses of vitamin A correspondingly raise the concentration of this vitamin in breast milk. The mother's diet may make her blood cholesterol higher or lower to some extent but seems not to affect her breast milk cholesterol. The fatty acid composition of breast milk, however, does respond to the mother's diet. The taking of a vitamin-mineral supplement that contains nutrient levels close to 100 percent of the RDA seems not to raise nutrient concentrations in the breast milk of an otherwise well-nourished mother. The breast milk concentrations of some of the water-soluble vitamins reach saturation levels in well-nourished women. Vitamin supplementation of *undernourished* women, however, does appear to raise the vitamin concentration of their milk, and may be beneficial.[27] It is best to avoid megadoses of vitamins or other nutrients, of course.

The period of lactation is the natural time for a woman to lose the extra body fat she accumulated during pregnancy. If her choice of foods is judicious, she can tolerate an energy deficit and a gradual loss of weight (1 pound per week) without any effect on her milk output. Fat can only be mobilized slowly, though, and too large an energy deficit, especially early on, will inhibit lactation. On the other hand, if a mother does not breastfeed, she may not as easily lose the fat she gained during pregnancy.

A woman who is nursing her baby is often the recipient of unsolicited, "friendly" advice as to what she should or should not eat, in order to avoid causing distress to her infant. Such advice may be well intended, but is frequently incorrect. It is true that some foods with strong flavors, such as garlic, may affect the baby's liking for the milk, but this depends on the individual baby. The same is true for other foods that have gained a reputation for irritating the infant's digestive tract or altering the taste of the milk.

Infants who are sensitive to particular foods such as cow's milk protein may become uncomfortable when they are included in the mother's diet. While this may be true of a few babies, it is not a reason for all nursing mothers to avoid cow's milk. The nutrients provided by dairy products make a significant contribution to the infant's and the mother's health. A mother who is nursing her baby is advised to eat whatever nutritious foods she chooses; then, if she suspects a particular food of causing the infant discomfort, she can try eliminating that food from her diet and see if the problem goes away.

The lactating woman needs extra fluid, and the energy and nutrients needed to make 30 ounces of milk a day. Avoidance of drugs, including alcohol, is recommended. Malnutrition can diminish the quantity and/or impair the quality of the milk produced.

Feeding the Infant

Once the baby is born, one of the many challenges parents face is providing the baby with the optimal nutrition that a brand-new life so well deserves. The nutritional health of the infant, as well as the nurturing of the child's whole self, is the responsibility of the parents for years to come; at times such responsibility can be overwhelming. Since sound nutrition is the basis of a healthy body and mind, all those involved need to know how to feed the infant.

Infant nutrient and feeding recommendations keep changing as new knowledge is gained. For example, breastfeeding has regained favor in recent years, after a trend toward the use of formula that began about 50 years ago. Recommendations as to the timing of the introduction of solid foods to the infant's diet have changed repeatedly over the years. At any given time, one or more aspects of infant feeding are always controversial and subject to disagreement, even among the experts. Parents can feel confused and frustrated when deciding how and what to feed their babies. The impact of ever-changing infant feeding recommendations, however, goes much further than confusion and frustration. That infant feeding practices are continuously being modified only serves to emphasize the experts' recognition of nutrition's crucial importance during the first year of life. Not only does early nutrition affect later development, but also, infancy sets the stage for eating habits that will affect nutrition status for a lifetime. Never fear: while the trends change and experts argue about the fine points, properly nourishing a baby is relatively simple, overall. Common sense in the selection of infant foods and a nurturing, relaxed environment go far to promote the infant's health and well-being.

A baby grows faster during the first year of life than ever again, as Figure 11–4 shows. The growth of infants and children directly reflects their nutritional well-being and is an important parameter in assessing their nutrition status. The birthweight doubles around four months of age, and has tripled by the age of one year. (If a ten-year-old child were to do this, the child's weight would increase from 70 to 210 pounds in a single year.) By the end of the first year, the growth rate slows considerably, so that between the first and second birthdays, the weight gained amounts to only about 5 pounds.

Nutrient Needs

The rapid growth and metabolism of the infant demands an ample supply of *all* the nutrients. However, the energy nutrients and those vitamins and minerals critical to the growth process, such as vitamin A, vitamin D, calcium, and iron, have special importance during infancy.

Babies, because they are small, need smaller total amounts of these nutrients than adults do; but as a percentage of body weight, babies need over twice as much of most nutrients. Figure 11–5.compares a three-month-old baby's needs with those of an adult man. As you can see, some of the differences are extraordinary. After six months, energy needs increase less rapidly as the growth rate begins to slow down, but some of the energy saved by slower growth is spent in increased activity.

Baby's metabolism:
Heart rate: 120 to 140 beats per minute.
Respiration rate: 20 per minute.

Adult's metabolism:
Heart rate: 70 to 80 beats per minute.
Respiration rate: 12 to 14 per minute.

At six months, the infant's energy needs are reduced by slower growth but increased by greater activity.

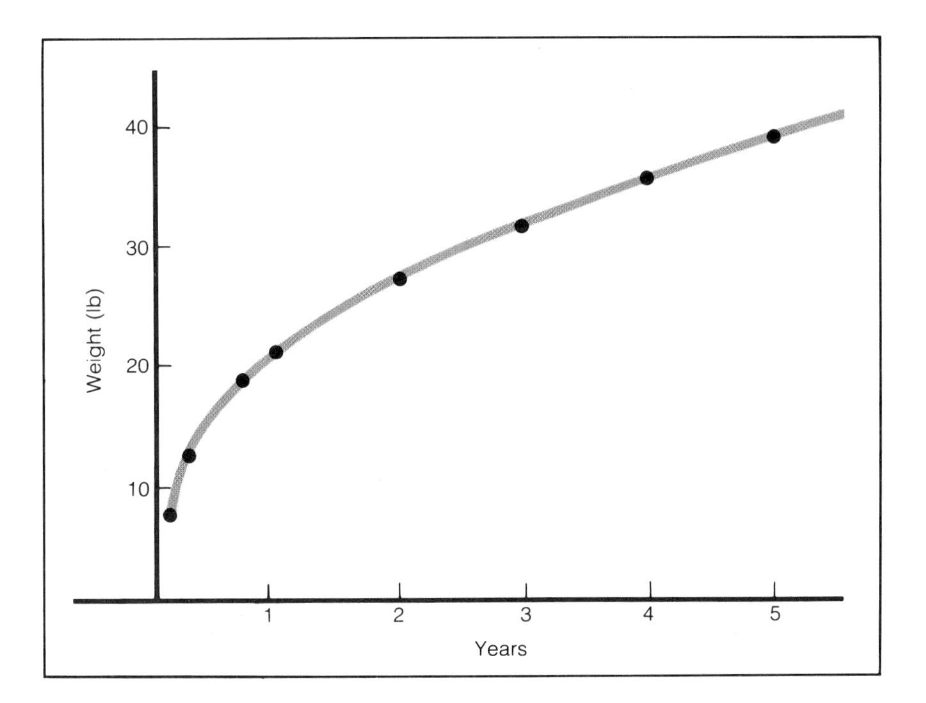

Figure 11–4
Weight Gain of Human Infants (Boys) in the First Five Years.
A baby grows faster during the first year than ever again.

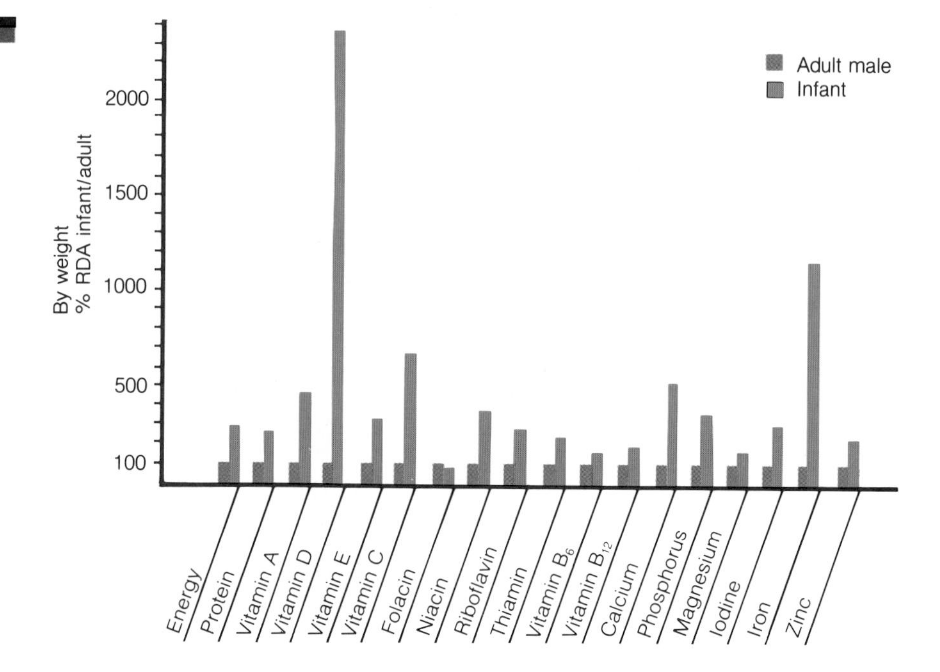

Figure 11–5
Nutrient Needs of a Three-Month-Old Infant Compared with Those of a Man, per Unit of Body Weight.
The man's needs are set at 100 percent (see RDA table, inside front cover).

At six months, the infant's energy needs are reduced by slower growth but increased by greater activity.

Wide variations in actual energy intakes of infants have been observed. Current recommendations reflect a decrease in energy intake at six months of age, but a study of breastfed infants in the United States and Canada indicates that the decline in infants' energy intakes may occur earlier.[28]

Nutrient allowances for infants are based on the average amounts of nutrients consumed by thriving infants who are breastfed by healthy, well-nourished mothers. The Recommended Dietary Allowances (RDA), the standard in the United States, and the Recommended Nutrient Intakes (RNI), the standard in Canada, are recommendations for nutrient intakes of population groups that take into account individual variability. Variations in growth rates, activity levels, sizes, metabolic rates, environments, and other factors in infants' lives make it impossible to establish one standard for all. Nevertheless, it is useful to have guidelines for estimating nutrient adequacy and planning when to introduce supplemental foods for infants.

The most important nutrient of all, for infants as for everyone, is the one easiest to forget: water. The younger a child, the greater the percentage of the body weight is water, and the more rapid the turnover. Proportionately more of the infant's body water than the adult's is between the cells and in the vascular space, so this water is easy to lose. Conditions that cause fluid loss, such as vomiting, diarrhea, sweating, or obligatory urinary loss without replacement can rapidly propel an infant into life-threatening dehydration. Fluid and electrolyte imbalances, caused by infection, kill more of the world's children than any other disease or disaster. Infants can cry, but cannot tell you what they are crying for; remember that they may need fluid, and let them drink it until their thirst is quenched.

In early infancy, breast milk or infant formula normally provides enough water for a healthy infant to replace water losses from the skin, lungs, feces, and urine.[29] If an infant is exposed to hot weather, has diarrhea, or vomits repeatedly, supplemental water is needed to prevent dehydration.

Supplemental water is required for all infants once solid foods are added to the diet. Foods with a high protein or electrolyte content, such as meat and eggs, in the absence of adequate water, can promote water loss to the point of dehydration. Water also provides fluid without additional food energy. Many adults today would no doubt be healthier had they learned early to quench their thirst with water.

For the most part, foods supply nutrients in combination. Thus a baby who consumes adequate amounts of a variety of the foods recommended during infancy receives all the nutrients needed and then some. Unfortunately, though, nutrient deficiencies do occur in infancy. In developed, well-nourished societies, such as the United States and Canada, the nutrition practices that influence infants' nutrition status the most center upon which type of milk is provided to the infant and the age at which solid foods are introduced. The remainder of this discussion is devoted to feeding the infant and identifying the nutrients most often deficient in infant diets.

Infants' rapid growth and development depend heavily on adequate nutrient supplies. Adequate water is also crucial.

rooting reflex: a reflex that makes a newborn turn toward whichever cheek is touched and search for the nipple.

let-down reflex: a reflex that forces milk to the front of the breast when the infant begins to nurse.

alpha-lactalbumin (lact-AL-byoo-min): the chief protein in human breast milk, as opposed to **casein** (CAY-seen), the chief protein in cow's milk.

Breastfeeding

Breast milk is considered the most desirable source of nutrients for the young infant. The Committee on Nutrition of the American Academy of Pediatrics (AAP) and the Nutrition Committee of the Canadian Pediatric Society have issued this joint statement: "Breastfeeding is strongly recommended for full-term infants, except in the few instances where specific contraindications exist."[30]

Breastfeeding the infant as soon as possible after birth facilitates successful lactation. Newborn infants adapt readily to breastfeeding; they are born with a **rooting reflex** that enables them to suckle right away. When the infant begins to nurse, the mother responds with a reflex of her own, the **let-down reflex,** which forces milk to the front of the breast. Let-down allows the infant to obtain milk easily. If it is slow, the infant may become irritable and tire before receiving enough milk. Let-down occurs less readily when the mother is tired or anxious than when she is rested and serene. A glass of water just before or during nursing may help relax her.

The infant's sucking and emptying of the breast stimulates lactation. Demand feedings, at least six a day, promote optimal milk production and infant growth. The infant is encouraged to nurse 8 to 12 minutes on each breast. Nursing sessions start on alternate breasts to ensure that each breast is emptied regularly.

Breast milk is tailor-made to meet the nutrient needs of the human infant. It offers its carbohydrate as lactose and its fat as a mixture with a generous proportion of the essential fatty acid, linoleic acid. The unique composition of the fat in breast milk, in combination with the fat-digesting enzymes present, contributes to highly efficient fat absorption by the breast-fed infant. The protein in breast milk is largely **alpha-lactalbumin,** a protein the human infant can easily digest.

The vitamin content of breast milk is ample. Even vitamin C, for which cow's milk is not a good source, is supplied generously by breast milk. The concentration of vitamin D in breast milk, however, is low. Reports of biologically

colostrum (co-LAHS-trum): a milklike secretion from the breast, rich in protective factors, present during the first day or so after delivery, before milk appears.

bifidus (BIFF-id-us, by-FEED-us) **factors:** factors in colostrum and breast milk that favor the growth, in the infant's intestinal tract, of the "friendly" bacteria *Lactobacillus* (lack-toh-ba-SILL-us) *bifidus*, so that other, less desirable intestinal inhabitants will not flourish.

lactoferrin (lak-toe-FERR-in): a factor in breast milk that binds iron, helps the intestine absorb it, and keeps it from supporting the growth of infectious intestinal bacteria.

active vitamin D sulfate in breast milk have not been confirmed. Vitamin D deficiency causes impaired bone mineralization in children. Cow's milk and infant formulas are fortified with vitamin D, but the concentration in breast milk falls short of adequacy. The vitamin is formed by the action of sunlight on the skin, but the amount formed depends on skin color, exposure time, atmospheric pollution, time of year (summer versus winter), and latitude (how far from the sun). Lack of daily sunlight exposure; prolonged, unsupplemented breastfeeding; and pigmented skin are risk factors for vitamin D deficiency in infants. For this reason, vitamin D supplements are routinely prescribed for breastfed infants in the United States and Canada.

As for minerals, the 2-to-1 calcium-to-phosphorus ratio of breast milk is ideal for the absorption of calcium. Both of these minerals and magnesium are present in amounts appropriate for the rate of growth expected in a human infant. Breast milk is also low in sodium. The iron in breast milk is highly absorbable, and its zinc, too, is absorbed better than from cow's milk, thanks to the presence of a zinc-binding protein.[31] Normally, given the nutrient composition of breast milk, nutrient supplements are not necessary, with the possible exceptions of vitamin D, fluoride, and iron (see the box, "Supplements for the Infant").

Besides nutrients, breast milk offers many other beneficial substances. During the first two or three days of lactation, the breasts produce **colostrum**, a premilk substance containing antibodies and white cells from the mother's blood. Colostrum is relatively sterile as it leaves the breast, and the baby cannot contract a bacterial infection from it even if the mother has one. Thus colostrum helps protect the newborn infant from those infections against which the mother has developed immunity. These diseases are the ones in her environment, and precisely those against which the infant needs protection. Entering the infant's body with the milk, these antibodies inactivate bacteria within the digestive tract, where they would otherwise cause harm. Some of the antibodies also "leak" into the bloodstream, because the infant's immature digestive tract cannot completely exclude whole proteins. These antibodies provide additional protection against polio and other diseases. Breast milk also contains antibodies, although not as many as colostrum.

Powerful agents against bacterial infection also occur in breast milk. Colostrum and breast milk contain factors (**bifidus factors**) that favor the growth of the "friendly" bacteria *Lactobacillus bifidus* in the infant's digestive tract, so that other, harmful bacteria cannot grow there. Another factor present in colostrum and breast milk stimulates the development of the infant's digestive tract.[32] Damaged cells in the infant's digestive tract are promptly replaced, and the protective factors within the tract remain intact.

Another component of breast milk, **lactoferrin**, indirectly benefits the baby's iron nutrition and, at the same time, acts as an antibacterial agent. Lactoferrin is an iron-grabbing compound that keeps bacteria from getting the iron they need to grow on, helps absorb iron into the infant's bloodstream, and also works directly to kill some intestinal bacteria.[33]

Other factors in breast milk include several enzymes, several hormones (including thyroid hormone and prostaglandins), and lipids that protect the infant against infection.[34] Much remains to be learned about the composition and characteristics of human milk, but clearly it is a very special substance.

Supplements for the Infant

A mother who is breastfeeding her healthy, full-term, newborn infant need not offer supplements of most nutrients. Breast milk and the infant's own internal stores will ensure that most nutrient needs are met for the first four to six months of life. At this time, the introduction of intelligently chosen juices and foods will keep up with changing nutrient requirements. The only exceptions to this statement have to do with vitamin D, fluoride, and possibly iron.

Most experts agree that breast milk does not provide enough vitamin D for the infant who has little exposure to sunlight. A light-skinned baby wearing just a diaper in strong summer sun and clear air might make enough vitamin D in a few minutes to meet daily needs. A dark-skinned baby wrapped up for cold weather in a smoggy city might not make enough even if outside for several hours. Because so many variables exist regarding vitamin D and sunlight exposure, the American Academy of Pediatrics (AAP) recommends vitamin D supplementation for breastfed babies beginning at birth.[35]

If the baby's only source of fluoride is breast milk, then the pediatrician is likely to prescribe fluoride supplements, too. Fluoride does not appear to be secreted into breast milk even if the mother's fluoride supply is ample.[36] As for iron, it may be desirable to begin iron supplements for the breastfed infant at about four months, especially if solid foods have not been introduced.[37] Once iron-fortified infant cereal is an established part of the baby's diet, iron supplementation is no longer necessary.

For the formula-fed infant, the makeup of the formula determines what further supplementation may be necessary. The AAP recommends the use of iron-fortified infant formula by four months of age. Most pediatricians recommend iron-fortified formula from birth, although some infants are fed non-iron-fortified formula for the first few months. For these infants, either iron-fortified formula, iron-fortified infant cereal, or a combination of the two are recommended by four months of age.

Fluoride supplement recommendations for the infant receiving formula are similar to those for the breastfed infant. Infants who consume formula that is mixed with fluoridated water do not need additional fluoride. For those who consume ready-to-use formula made without fluoridated water, fluoride supplementation may be desirable until they begin drinking water on a regular basis. For infants in areas of nonfluoridated water, fluoride supplementation is recommended.

Thus, with the possible exception of fluoride, formula-fed infants who consume adequate amounts of formula in appropriate combination with solid foods do not need nutrient supplementation during the first year of life. The pediatrician is the expert to consult on local needs.

bonding: the forming of an emotional tie between mother and infant.

Breastfeeding may provide still other benefits. Emotional **bonding** is facilitated by many events and behaviors of mother and infant during the early months and years; one of the first can be breastfeeding, beginning right after birth. A critical event in bonding, thought to be mediated by chemical messengers in breast milk, may occur in the first 45 minutes after birth, so this may be an especially important feeding time.[38] Prolonged breastfeeding (six months or more) has been shown to decrease the incidence of allergic disease in babies with a family history of allergies.[39] The act of suckling favors normal tooth and jaw alignment. Breastfeeding may have other advantages, too; some studies suggest that mothers who breastfeed are less likely to develop breast cancer and to form unwanted clots in the bloodstream after delivery. A woman who wants to breastfeed can derive justification and satisfaction from all these advantages.

When Breastfeeding Is Preferred Under most circumstances, a woman can freely choose to feed breast milk or formula, knowing that either mode of feeding is adequate to meet the infant's nutrient needs. However, if the infant is premature, if the family is poor, or if other factors act to the baby's disadvantage, then breastfeeding becomes the preferred choice.

For the premature infant, most authorities recommend the mother's own milk as soon as possible, even if the mother can't nurse. That is, if the baby is being kept sealed away in an incubator in the intensive care unit, the mother can express her milk with her hands or a breast pump and carry the milk to the intensive care unit to be fed to the baby. Her own milk is thought to be better for the baby than that of a full-term mother, because its composition is better suited to a premature infant's needs. Electronic breast pumps, available at most hospitals, facilitate efficient expression of breast milk.

Some communities maintain breast milk "banks"—storage and delivery facilities for breast milk. Mothers who have milk to spare donate it to the bank; others can obtain it when it is needed. Success and safety in milk banking require that the donor keep her milk sanitary while collecting it, and freeze it promptly. Breast milk can be stored safely in the freezer for up to six months, provided that it stays solidly frozen (below 0 degrees Fahrenheit).[40] Most home freezers are not kept that cold, and some sources urge that it not be stored for more than two to six weeks.

A premature baby receiving breast milk may be given a supplement of special formula for premature infants, depending on the philosophy of the clinic responsible for its care. Babies not receiving breast milk can be successfully nourished on this formula alone, and even on total parenteral nutrition (nutrients delivered directly into a central vein).

When Not to Breastfeed If a woman has a communicable disease such as tuberculosis or hepatitis that could threaten the infant's health, then mother and child have to be separated. Breastfeeding would be possible only by pumping the woman's breasts several times a day, something of a struggle. Similarly, if she must take medication that is secreted in breast milk and that is known to affect the infant, then breastfeeding is contraindicated. If drug therapy is temporary, it is possible to express milk during treatment to maintain the demand that will ensure a continued supply of breast milk after the drug therapy ends. Drug addicts, including alcohol abusers, are capable of taking such high doses that their infants can become addicts by way of breast milk; in these cases, breastfeeding is completely contraindicated. Prescription drugs should be taken on a physician's order only. Smoking is incompatible with the optimal health of both mother and child. If a woman has an ordinary cold, she can go on nursing without worry. If susceptible, the infant will catch it from her anyway, and thanks to immunologic protection, a breastfed baby may be less susceptible than a bottle-fed baby would be.

A woman sometimes hesitates to breastfeed because she has heard that environmental contaminants may enter her milk and harm her baby. The decision whether to breastfeed on this basis might best be made after consultation with a physician or dietitian familiar with the local circumstances.

An environmental contaminant that has caused concern is the PCBs, which are found in rivers and waterways polluted by industry. PCBs are stored in body fat and remain in the body; they are excreted only in the fat of breast milk. According to the Committee on Environmental Hazards of the American Academy of Pediatrics, women need not fear contamination of their breast milk with PCBs unless they have eaten large amounts of fish caught in PCB-contaminated rivers, such as the Saint Lawrence Seaway, or have been directly exposed because of their occupations.

For more about contaminants and nutrition, turn to Chapter 10.

Another contaminant of concern is dioxin, which has contaminated some mothers' milk in the south-central states to an extent incompatible with breastfeeding. A woman who has questions about PCBs, dioxin, or other contaminants in her breast milk is advised to consult the local state health department.

Breast milk is normally the ideal food for infants. It contains not only the needed nutrients in the right proportions but also protective factors. It is especially valuable for premature infants; it is inadvisable if contaminated with drugs or environmental pollutants.

Formula Feeding

The substitution of formula feeding for breastfeeding involves copying nature as closely as possible. Human and cow's milks differ; cow's milk is significantly higher in protein, calcium, and phosphorus, for example, to support the calf's faster growth rate. But a formula can be prepared from cow's milk that does not differ significantly from human milk in these respects; the formula makers first dilute the milk and then add carbohydrate and nutrients to make it nutritionally comparable to human milk.

The antibodies in cow's milk do not protect the human baby from disease (they protect the calf from cattle diseases), but the high level of preventive medical care (vaccinations) and public health measures achieved in the developed countries, especially in the United States and Canada, make this consideration less important than it was in the past. Safety and sanitation can be achieved with either mode of feeding by the informed mother whose water supply is reliable.

In developing countries, however, breastfeeding remains the preferred mode of infant feeding. It provides infants with a sterile, steady supply of nutrients and protective factors. It was, until recently, the traditional method of feeding infants for most or all of the first year or two, and as a result, infant nutrition problems were delayed until weaning, sometime during the second year of life. Now, as people have moved from rural settings into cities, formula feeding has become more common. In many instances, women prepare formulas incorrectly—they are wrongly diluted and unsanitary. As a result, malnutrition and infant disease are more prevalent, and occur at an earlier age, than in the past.

Like the breastfeeding mother, the mother who feeds formula deserves support in her choice. Bearing and nurturing a baby involve much more than merely pouring nutrients in, in whatever form. The mother who offers formula to her baby has valid reasons for making her choice, and her feelings should be honored. She and the baby can benefit in many ways from the supportive approval of those around them.

One of the major advantages of formula feeding is that gained by the mother whose attempts at breastfeeding have met with frustration. If she truly doesn't want to breastfeed, or worse, if she earnestly does want to and can't, continuing to try is an agonizing course, as hard on the baby as on the mother. When the mother finally accepts the necessity of formula feeding and weans the baby to the bottle, a period of anguish for both may be followed by the onset of peace and the first real opportunity to develop the all-important mother-child love. Other advantages:

- The mother can see that the baby is getting enough milk.
- She can offer the same closeness, warmth, and stimulation during feedings as the breastfeeding mother does.
- Other family members can get close to the baby and develop a warm relationship in feeding sessions.
- The mother will be free, sooner, to give time to her other children.
- The child can easily be cared for by others while the mother works.

The attendant who is asked to advise on breastfeeding versus formula feeding is obliged to remember the advantages of both. In fact, when addressing any audience, keep in mind that some members will be women who bottle-fed their babies. To praise breastfeeding out of proportion or without qualification can only make them feel guilty or angry.

Many mothers choose to breastfeed at first but wean within the first one to six months. This is a nice compromise. Even a few weeks of breastfeeding will significantly reduce the likelihood of the baby's developing an allergy to cow's milk when it is introduced, and this advantage alone is important if such an allergy is likely. Furthermore, the baby gets the immunological protection and all the special advantages of breastfeeding during the most critical first few weeks or months. Then the mother can choose to shift to the bottle and can know she has already given the baby those benefits. Prior to six months of age, it is imperative that the baby be weaned onto *formula*, not onto plain milk of any kind—whole, low fat, or skim. Only formula contains enough iron (to name but one of many, many factors) to support normal development in the baby's first months of life. Many physicians discourage the use of plain milk for babies before the end of the first year. Table 11–3 shows appropriate transitions in milk feeding.

National and international standards have been set for the nutrient contents of infant formulas. The Infant Formula Act of 1980 requires that formulas meet nutrient standards based on the American Academy of Pediatrics recommendations, and in 1982 the FDA adopted quality control procedures to be sure that they do. Formulas that meet the standards are nutritionally similar; small differences in nutrient content are sometimes confusing, but not usually important.

Table 11–3

Transitions in Milk Feeding

Before Six Months	After Six Months	After One Year
Breastfed infant should receive: Breast milk. Vitamin D. Fluoride and iron at pediatrician's discretion. Formula-fed infant should receive: Iron-fortified formula. Vitamins A, C, and D in formula or separately. Fluoride at pediatrician's discretion. If weaning from breast milk before six months, wean to formula as above. Wait to wean from formula until at least six months.	If weaning from breast milk after six months, wean to formula or whole cow's milk with supplementation. Whole cow's milk (may be fresh or evaporated) should be supplemented with: Vitamins A and D if not fortified. Iron and/or iron-fortified cereals. Vitamin C or C–rich foods or juices. Fluoride at pediatrician's discretion.	When all four food groups are eaten daily, whole or low-fat cow's milk is acceptable. Continue checking diet for vitamin C, iron, and all nutrients. Continue fluoride supplements if necessary.

Source: Adapted from recommendations made in *Pediatrics* 62 (1978): 733 and *Nutrition and the MD*, March 1980.

renal solute load: a measure of the concentration of all dissolved substances in the urine resulting from feeding a milk, formula, or diet. As the kidneys mature, they can handle higher solute loads; the low solute load of breast milk is ideal for the infant, especially the premature infant. A formula with too high a renal solute load can cause dehydration, a life-threatening condition in the infant, by incurring too great an obligatory water excretion.

Table 11–4 shows characteristics of human, cow's, and goat's milk, along with those of a formula prepared from modified cow's milk. The animal milks clearly differ significantly from human milk in many respects; you can see that the formula is similar to the animal milks in some ways, and to human milk in others. The formula resembles cow's milk in type and ratio of proteins, total fat, and calcium-to-phosphorus ratio but has been adjusted to resemble human milk in total protein, carbohydrate, linoleic acid, major minerals, and **renal solute load**. While obviously not identical to human milk, formula presents the same nutrients in roughly the same proportions for the most part.

Table 11–5 shows the AAP standard for the bulk ingredients of infant formulas and permits comparison with human milk and typical formulas. As you can see, the AAP standard recommends higher protein than is in human milk; this is because the cow's milk protein does not present as perfect a balance of amino acids for the human infant. You can also see that the formulas meet the AAP standard for the nutrients listed. The rest of the AAP recommendations for vitamins and minerals are shown in Table 11–6 to facilitate comparison with any formula chosen.

For infants with special problems, formulas can be adapted to make them closer in composition to human milk (adjusted protein ratio, lower linoleic acid, lower sodium and other minerals). For premature babies, special premature formulas are available. Special formulas based on soy protein are available for infants allergic to milk protein, and formulas with the lactose replaced can be used for infants with lactose intolerance. For infants with other special needs, many other variations are available.

Infant formulas are designed to resemble breast milk, and must meet an American Academy of Pediatrics standard for nutrient composition. Special formulas are available for premature babies, allergic babies, and others.

Weaning to Milk

As long as breast milk or formula is the baby's major food, ordinary milk is an inappropriate replacement—primarily because the milk provides insufficient vi-

Table 11–4

Human Milk, Other Milks, and Infant Formula Compared

Characteristic	Human Milk	Cow's Milk	Goat's Milk	Formula[a]
Carbohydrate (g/100 ml)	7.2	5.0	4.7	7.0–7.2
Energy (cal/100 ml)	74	67	76	68
Fat (g/100 ml)	2.7–4.6	3.5	4.1	3.6–3.7
Linoleic acid (% of total fatty acids)	10–15	4	—	13–23
Minerals				
Calcium (mg/1)	340	1200	1300	510–550
Calcium-to-phosphorus ratio	2.4	1.3	1.2	1.2–1.3
Iron (mg/1)	0.2–1.0	0.5	0.5	12 or 1.5[b]
Phosphorus (mg/1)	140	955	1060	390–460
Potassium (mEq/1)[e]	13	35	46	18–20
Sodium (mEq/1)[e]	7	25	18	11–12
Protein (g/100 ml)	1.1	3.5	3.3	1.5–1.6
Renal solute load (mOsm/1)[c]	74	220	—	105–108
Vitamins (per 100 ml)				
Folacin (μg)	2–5	0.3	0.2	5–11
Niacin (mg)	0.15–0.18	0.09	0.2	0.7–1.3
Pantothenic acid (mg)	0.18–0.23	0.4	0.3	0.30–0.32
Riboflavin (μg)	36–37	175	184	63–100
Thiamin (μg)	14–16	44	40	53–65
Vitamin A (IU)	190–250	103 or 190[d]	207	169–250
Vitamin B_6 (μg)	10–11	64	7	40
Vitamin B_{12} (μg)	0.03–0.05	0.4	0.06	0.15–0.21
Vitamin C (mg))	4.3–5.2	1.1	1.5	5.5
Vitamin D (IU)	2.2	1.3 or 38[d]	2.4	40–42

[a]These numbers represent two formulas, Similac and Enfamil.

[b]These formulas are available unfortified or with iron fortification.

[c]The ability of solutes to cause osmosis is measured in terms of *osmols;* the osmol is a measure of the total number of particles. A *milliosmol* equals 1/1000 of an osmol. Renal solute load is measured in milliosmols per liter of solution ((mOsm/l).

[d]The higher value represents fortified milk, which should contain 2000 IU vitamin A and 400 IU vitamin D per quart (1900 and 375 IU/l, respectively).

[e]Milliequivalents per liter of formula. A milliequivalent is the amount of a substance that contains the same number of charges as 1 mg of hydrogen—a useful measure, because the number of charges present is an index of the osmotic pressure the solution will exert.

Source: Adapted from K. Brostrom, Human milk and infant formulas: Nutritional and immunological characteristics, in *Textbook of Pediatric Nutrition,* ed. R. M. Suskind (New York: Raven Press, 1981); *Milk-based and Soy-based Formulations Used for Feeding Newborns in the Hospital,* an information sheet (January 1979) available from Ross Laboratories, Columbus, OH 43216. Data on goat's milk and on vitamins for all milks are adapted from S. J. Fomon, Milks and milk-based formulas, in *Infant Nutrition* (Philadelphia: Saunders, 1967), pp. 195–224.

Table 11–5

AAP Standard Compared with Human Milk and Infant Formula

Content	Mature Human Milk	AAP Standard	Infant Formula[a]
Energy (cal/100 ml)	67–75	60–80	67
Protein (% of cal)	5.2	7–18	9
Fat (% of cal)	35–58	30–55	47–50
Carbohydrate (% of cal)	35–44	35–50	41–43

[a]Five formulas were used to generate these data: Similac (Ross), Similac 60/40 (Ross), Enfamil (Mead Johnson), SMA (Wyeth), and Nan (Nestlé).

Source: Adapted from K. Brostrom, Human milk and infant formulas: Nutritional and immunological characteristics, in *Textbook of Pediatric Nutrition,* ed. R. M. Suskind (New York: Raven Press, 1981).

tamin C and iron. Once the baby is obtaining at least a third of the total daily food energy from a balanced mixture of cereal, vegetables, fruits, and other foods, then whole cow's milk in any form, fortified with vitamins A and D, is acceptable as an accompanying beverage.[41] The AAP recommends the introduction of cow's milk at six months, but many pediatricians advise continued use of breast milk or formula throughout the first year because of the iron it provides. (Don't offer plain cow's milk before six months, though, because the infant's digestive tract may be sensitive to its protein, and if so, may bleed.)

Cow's milk comes in many forms: pasteurized, homogenized, evaporated, powdered, and others. (The terms are defined in the Miniglossary of Milks.) Any pasteurized milk that has nutritional value equivalent or superior to whole cow's milk is acceptable, but the American Academy of Pediatrics recommends against the use of low-fat or nonfat milk with infants or children under two years old; they need the fat of whole milk.[42] Powdered milk is usually skimmed, but fat-containing varieties are available. Parents are advised to use vitamin A and D–fortified whole milk and avoid canned milk. Although lead solder has been eliminated from use in most cans used for food, canned milk products are still a major source of lead in the diets of infants and children.[43] Chapter 10 describes the devastating effects of lead on development and learning ability.

Formula preparation:

- Liquid concentrate (inexpensive, relatively easy)—mix with equal part water.
- Powdered formula (cheapest, lightest for travel)—read label directions.
- Ready-to-feed (easiest, most expensive)—pour directly into clean bottles.
- Whole milk—do not use before six months.

In a baby's first six months, the choice of formula is important, because whatever is chosen must supply the nutrients of human milk in similar forms and proportions. If supplements are necessary in addition, the type of formula determines what they should be (see the box, "Supplements for the Infant"). After the first year, the exact formulation of the milk selected is not so critical, but the choice is still important, because milk or its substitute occupies a place in the diet that no other type of food can fill.

Formula should be replaced with milk only after the baby is deriving significant amounts of energy and nutrients from a balanced assortment of foods. The earliest replacement time is 6 months; a year is preferred.

First Foods

Changes in body organs during the first year affect the baby's readiness to accept solid foods. At first, sucking is all that can be accomplished (and powerfully, at that), and only liquids that are well back in the throat can be swallowed. Later (at two months or so) the baby's tongue can move against the palate to swallow semisolid food. Still later, the first teeth erupt, but it is not until sometime during the second year that a baby can begin to handle chewy food. The stomach and intestines are immature at first; they can digest milk sugar (lactose), but can't manufacture significant quantities of the starch-digesting enzyme, amylase, until somewhat later. Thus they can't digest starch until about three months, with some variation depending on the individual baby.

The baby's kidneys are unable to concentrate waste efficiently, so a baby must excrete relatively more water than an adult to carry off a comparable amount

Table 11–6

AAP Recommendations for Nutrient Levels in Formulas

Nutrient	Amount Recommended (per 100 cal)
Protein (g)	1.8–4.5
Fat (g)	3.3–6.0
Essential fatty acid (linoleic acid)(mg)	300
Vitamins	
Vitamin A (μg or RE)	75–225
Vitamin D (μg)	1.0–2.5
Vitamin K (μg)	4
Vitamin E (mg tocopherol equivalent)	0.5
Vitamin C (mg)	8
Thiamin (μg)	40
Riboflavin (μg)	60
Vitamin B_6 (μg)	35 (with 15 μg/g protein in formula)
Vitamin B_{12} (μg)	0.15
Niacin (μg equivalent)	250
Folacin (μg)	4
Pantothenic acid (μg)	300
Biotin (μg)	1.5
Choline (mg)	7.0
Inositol (mg)	4.0
Minerals	
Calcium (mg)	60
Phosphorus (mg)	30
Calcium-to-phosphorus ratio	1.1–2.1
Magnesium (mg)	6
Iron (mg)	0.15
Iodine (μg)	5
Zinc (mg)	0.5
Copper (μg)	60
Manganese (μg)	5.0
Sodium (mg)	20 (6 mEq[c])
Potassium (mg)	80 (14 mEq[c])
Chloride (mg)	55 (11 mEq[c])

Source: Adapted from American Academy of Pediatrics, Committee on Nutrition, Commentary on breast feeding and infant formulas, including proposed standards for formulas, in *Pediatric Nutrition Handbook* (Elk Grove Village, Ill.: American Academy of Pediatrics, 1985), pp. 356–357.

Miniglossary of Milks

casein or sodium caseinate: the principal protein of cow's milk. Other milk proteins, found in a higher percentage in human milk, are *whey* and *lactalbumin*.

condensed milk: evaporated milk to which sugar (sucrose) is added before processing, as a preservative. The percentages of calories from protein, fat, and carbohydrate in condensed milk are 10, 24.5, and 65.5, respectively. Condensed milk contains 321 cal/100 ml and is more than twice as concentrated as evaporated milk (146 cal/100 ml). Accidental use of condensed milk in preparation of infant formula can cause dehydration.

evaporated milk: milk concentrated by evaporation. The milk is preheated (for example, at 120° C, or 248° F, for three minutes) and then run aseptically into cans. The ratio of fat to nonfat solids is the same as in the original milk. By adding water, you derive standard milk; the taste, however, is altered by this process. Whole or nonfat milk from any species (cow, goat, or other) can be evaporated.

evaporated milk formula: formula made at home from evaporated milk, sugar, and water—seldom used today.

fortified (with respect to milk): milk to which vitamins A and D have been added so that a quart contains 2000 IU vitamin A and 400 IU vitamin D.

homogenized milk: milk treated to mix the fat evenly with the watery part (fat ordinarily floats to the top as cream). Heated milk is forced under high pressure through small openings to break up the fat into small particles, which then remain dispersed throughout the milk. Whole or partially skimmed milk from any species (cow, goat, or other) can be homogenized.

lactalbumin: see *casein*.

pasteurized milk: milk that is heat treated to reduce its bacterial count to an acceptable level. Methods vary; a common one is to heat the milk to at least 72° C (161° F), hold it at or above this temperature for 15 seconds, and then cool it rapidly to 50° C (148° F) or lower. Whole or nonfat milk from any species (cow, goat, or other) can be pasteurized.

powdered milk: completely dehydrated milk solids produced by a variety of processes. Some powdered milks are processed to rehydrate easily (instant milk); others require extensive blending. Both whole and nonfat milks can be powdered.

whey: see *casein*.

whole milk: cow's milk from which the fat has not been removed. The standard of identity for whole milk in most states requires that milk labeled "*whole*" contain not less than 3.25% milk fat and not less than 8.25% nonfat milk solids.

of waste. This means that dehydration, which can be dangerous, can occur more easily in an infant than in an adult. As mentioned earlier, a crying infant may be crying for fluid.

Iron deficiency is a common nutrition problem, especially in young children, throughout the world. The deficiency affects infants' behavior, even if it is not severe enough to cause anemia. Given a test of mental development, infants with iron deficiency scored low; given iron supplements, they improved rapidly over a ten-day period. The investigators who performed this research compared preschool children with and without iron deficiency, and found that those that were deficient were "less likely to pay attention to relevant cues in problem-solving situations."[44] For early learning ability, then, it is important to prevent iron deficiency, or to remedy it wherever it occurs.

Iron deficiency is most prevalent in children between the ages of six months and three years due to their rapid growth rate and the significant place that milk has in their diets. Whole cow's milk is a poor source of iron. By the end of the first year, half or more of all infants are receiving less than the RDA for iron, and one-fourth are receiving less than two-thirds of the RDA. Iron is the nutrient most needing attention in infant nutrition.[45]

The timing for adding solid foods to a baby's diet depends on several factors. If the baby is formula fed, or breastfed by a healthy, well-nourished mother, additions to the diet are not needed until four to six months, but babies not fed solid foods before the end of the first year suffer delayed growth.[46] Foods should be started gradually, beginning between four and six months, depending on readiness. Any of the following is an indication of readiness:

- When the infant has doubled its birth weight.
- When the infant can consume 8 ounces of formula and is hungry again in less than four hours.
- When the infant is consuming 32 ounces of formula a day and wanting more.
- When the infant is six months old.

Solids should not be introduced too early, because infants are most likely to develop allergies to them in the early months. But all babies are different, and the program of additions depends on the individual baby's developmental readiness, not on any rigid schedule. Table 11–7 presents a suggested sequence.

The addition of foods to a baby's diet should be governed by three considerations: the baby's nutrient needs, the baby's physical readiness to handle different forms of foods, and the need to detect and control allergic reactions. With respect to nutrient needs, the nutrient needed earliest from food is iron, next is vitamin C. A baby's stored iron supply from before birth runs out after the birthweight doubles, so formula with iron; iron-fortified cereals; and later, meat or meat alternates such as legumes, are recommended.

It has been suggested that the early introduction of sweet fruits to babies' diets might favor their developing a preference for sweets and lessen their liking for vegetables introduced later. To prevent this, the order can be reversed, vegetables first, fruits later. This practice now has a wide following. As for sweets of any other kind (including baby food "desserts"), they have no place in a baby's life. The added food energy they contribute can promote obesity, and they convey no nutrients to support growth.

Physical readiness develops in many small steps. For example, the ability to swallow solid food develops at around four to six months, and experience with solid food at that time helps to develop swallowing ability by desensitizing the

Table 11–7

First Foods for the Infant

Age (months)	Addition
4–6	Iron-fortified rice cereal, followed by other cereals (for iron; baby can swallow and can digest starch now)[a]
5–7	Strained vegetables and/or fruits and their juices,[b] one by one (perhaps vegetables before fruits, so the baby will learn to like their less sweet flavors)
6–8	Protein foods (cheese, yogurt, tofu, cooked beans, meat, fish, chicken, egg yolk)
9	Finely chopped meat (baby can chew now), toast, teething crackers (for emerging teeth)
10–12	Whole egg (allergies less likely now), whole milk

[a]Later you can change cereals, but don't forget to keep on using the iron-fortified varieties. According to *Nutrition and the MD,* April 1981, the iron in cereal specially prepared for babies is so bioavailable that three level tablespoons a day is all they need.

[b]All baby juices are fortified with vitamin C. Orange juice causes allergies in some babies; apple juice is often recommended as the first juice to feed. Juices should be offered in a cup, not a bottle, to prevent nursing bottle syndrome.

Source: Adapted from the 1979 *Recommendations for Infant Feeding Practices of the California Department of Health Services,* as presented in Current infant feeding practices, *Nutrition and the MD,* January 1980.

gag reflex. Later still, a baby can sit up, can handle finger foods, and is teething; then hard crackers and other hard finger foods may be introduced under the watchful eye of an adult. They promote the development of manual dexterity and control of the jaw muscles, but the infant can also choke on them.

Some parents want to feed solids at an earlier age, on the theory that "stuffing the baby" at bedtime promotes sleeping through the night. There is no proof for this theory. On the average, babies start to sleep through the night at about the same age, regardless of when solid foods are introduced, and by three months, 75 percent are sleeping through the night whether or not they are receiving any solid foods.[47]

New foods should be introduced singly and slowly, so that allergies can be detected. For example, when cereals are introduced, try rice cereal first for several days; it causes allergy least often. Try wheat cereal last; it is the most common offender. If a cereal causes an allergic reaction (irritability due to skin rash, digestive upset, or respiratory discomfort), discontinue its use before going on to the next food. About nine times out of ten, the allergy won't be evident immediately, but will manifest itself in vague symptoms occurring up to five days after the offending food is eaten, so it isn't easy to detect. If there is a family history of allergies, even greater care should attend the introduction of new foods. If parents detect allergies in an infant's early life, they can spare the whole family much grief. (Chapter 12 offers more information on allergies.)

As for the choice of foods, baby foods commercially prepared in the United States and Canada are generally safe, nutritious, and of high quality. In response to consumer demand, baby food companies have removed much of the added salt and sugar their products contained in the past, and baby foods also contain few or no additives. They generally have high nutrient density, except for mixed dinners and heavily sweetened desserts. Parents using commercial baby food

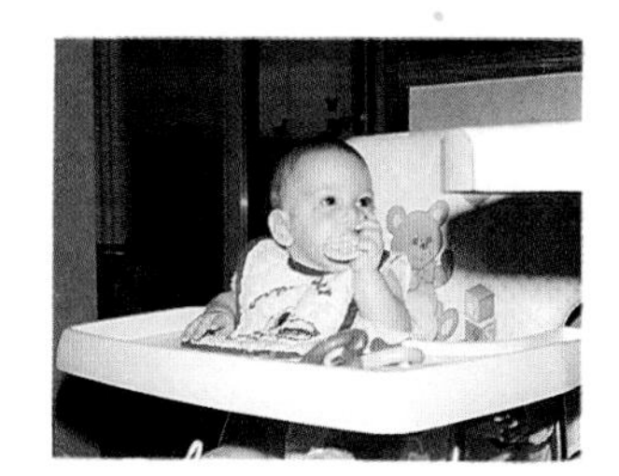

Ideally, the one-year-old eats many of the same foods everyone else eats.

milk anemia: iron-deficiency anemia caused by drinking so much milk that iron-rich foods are displaced from the diet.

should not feed directly from the jar, but should remove the portion to be fed to a dish for feeding, so as not to contaminate the unused food that will be stored in the jar.

An alternative to commercial baby food for the parent who wants the baby to have family foods is to "blenderize" a small portion of the table food at each meal. This necessitates cooking without salt, though. Foods adults prepare for themselves often contain much more salt than commercial baby foods. Besides, when foods are not salted, deep fried, or heavily seasoned, the taste of the food itself is allowed to come through. A baby will learn to like sweet potatoes because they taste like sweet potatoes rather than like brown sugar, butter, salt, or anything else. The adults can season their own food after taking out the baby's portion.

Canned vegetables are never appropriate for babies; not only is the sodium content too high, but also the risk of lead contamination is present. Awareness of food poisoning and precautions against it are imperative. Also avoid the use of vegetables in which nitrites are likely to form—notably, home-prepared carrots, beets, and spinach. Honey should never be fed to infants because of the risk of botulism. Babies and even young children have difficulty swallowing popcorn and nuts. An infant can easily choke on these foods; they are not worth the risk.

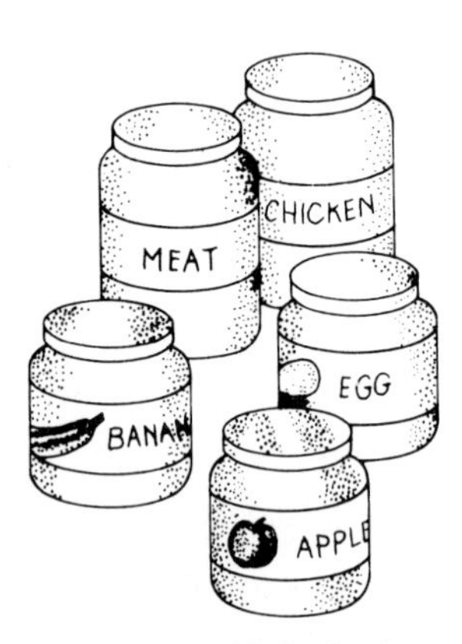

Commercially prepared baby foods are generally safe, nutritious, and of high quality.

At a year of age, the obvious food to supply most of the nutrients the baby needs is still milk; 2 to 3 ½ cups a day are now sufficient. More milk than this displaces foods necessary to provide iron and can cause the iron-deficiency anemia known as **milk anemia**. The other foods—meat, iron-fortified cereal, enriched or whole-grain bread, fruits, and vegetables—should be supplied in variety and in amounts sufficient to round out total energy needs. Ideally, the one-year-old is sitting at the table, eating many of the same foods everyone else eats, and drinking liquids from a cup—not a bottle. Soft drinks are never appropriate for infants and young children. This includes sugar-free types, caffeine-free types, all types. Infants and children thrive best on water, milk, or juice. A meal plan that meets the requirements for the one-year-old is shown in Table 11–8.

Solid food additions to a baby's diet should begin at about half a year and should be governed by the baby's nutrient needs and readiness to consume them. By one year, the baby should be receiving 2 to 3 ½ cups of milk a day and foods from all food groups.

Looking Ahead

The first year of a baby's life is the time to lay the foundation for future health. From the nutrition standpoint, the relevant problems most common in later years are obesity and dental disease. Prevention of obesity can also help prevent the development of the obesity-related diseases—atherosclerosis, diabetes, and cancer.

Infant obesity should be avoided. Probably the most important single measure to undertake during the first year is to encourage eating habits that will support continued normal weight as the child grows. Primarily, this means introducing a variety of nutritious foods in an inviting way, not forcing the baby to finish the bottle or the baby food jar, avoiding concentrated sweets and empty-calorie foods, and encouraging vigorous physical activity.

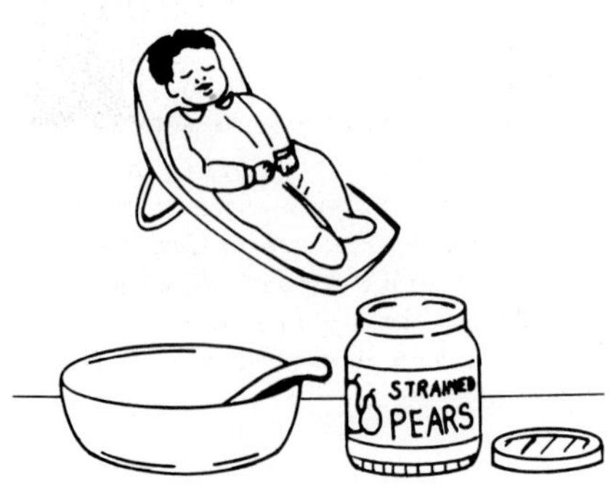

A baby stops eating when its stomach is full.

To discourage development of the behaviors and attitudes that plague the obese, parents should avoid teaching babies to seek food as a reward, to expect food as

Table 11–8

Meal Plan for a One-Year-Old

Breakfast	Snack
1 c milk 3 tbsp cereal 2–3 tbsp strained fruit Teething crackers	½ c milk Teething crackers
Lunch	**Supper**
1 c milk 2–3 tbsp vegetables Chopped meat or well-cooked, mashed legumes 2–3 tbsp pudding	1 c milk 1 egg 2 tbsp cereal or potato 2–3 tbsp cooked fruit Teething crackers

comfort for unhappiness, or to associate food deprivation with punishment. If they cry for thirst, give them water, not milk or juice. Babies seem to have no internal "calorie counter," and they stop eating when their stomachs are full, so nutrient-dense, low-calorie foods will satisfy as long as they provide bulk.

Babies develop sensitivity to their own satiety (see p. 276) at about ten months, another example of developmental readiness for solid foods.

Beyond these recommendations, some thought has been given to the idea of a "prudent diet" for infants, like that recommended for heart clients: restrict fat, increase the ratio of polyunsaturated to saturated fat, and reduce cholesterol intake. The AAP recommends against a fat-modified diet during infancy, stating that the evidence in its favor so far is insufficient and does not warrant dietary manipulation to lower blood cholesterol.[48] Dietary fat is necessary for proper development of the central nervous system. Further, growth failure has been observed in children on fat-restricted diets even when energy from other sources was constant.

For more about diet advice for children, turn to Controversy 4.

Babies need the food energy and fat of normal milk, and most experts agree that they should be fed whole or at least low-fat—not nonfat—milk until 2 years of age. The only exception might be the seriously obese baby, a case that would require physician consultation. Tampering with the amount of protein in a baby's diet could be especially risky. Protein is the single most important nutrient for growth.

Normal dental development is promoted by the same strategies outlined above: supplying nutritious foods, avoiding sweets, and discouraging the association of food with reward or comfort. In addition, the practice of giving a baby a bottle as a pacifier is strongly discouraged by dentists on the grounds that sucking for long periods of time pushes the normal jawline out of shape and causes the bucktoothed profile: protruding upper and receding lower teeth. Further, prolonged sucking on a bottle of milk or juice bathes the upper teeth in a carbohydrate-rich fluid that favors the growth of decay-producing bacteria. Babies permitted to do this are sometimes seen with their upper teeth decayed all the way to the gum line.

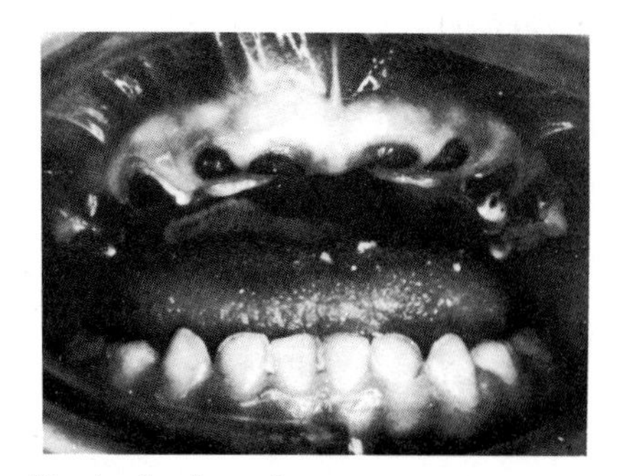

Nursing bottle syndrome, an extreme example. This child was frequently put to bed sucking on a baby bottle filled with apple juice, so that the teeth were bathed in carbohydrate for long periods of time—a perfect medium for bacterial growth. The upper teeth have decayed all the way to the gum line.

The early feeding of the infant lays the foundation for lifelong eating habits. It is desirable to foster preferences that will, throughout life, support normal weight and development and help avert common lifestyle diseases.

Food Feature

Mealtimes with Infants

The wise parent of a one-year-old offers nutrition and love together. Both promote growth. It is literally true that "feeding with love" produces better growth in both weight and height of children than feeding the same food in an emotionally negative climate.[49] It also promotes better brain development. The formation of nerve-to-nerve connections in the brain depends both on nutrients and on environmental stimulation.[50]

The person feeding a one-year-old has to be aware that this is a period in the child's life when exploring and experimenting are normal and desirable behaviors. The child is developing a sense of autonomy that, if allowed to flower, will provide the foundation for later assertiveness in choosing when and how much to eat and when to stop eating, as well as general confidence and effectiveness as an individual. The child's impulses, if consistently denied, can turn to shame and self-doubt. In light of the developmental and nutrient needs of one-year-olds, and in the face of their often contrary and willful behavior, a few feeding guidelines may be helpful. Following are several problem situations with suggestions for handling them:

- *He stands and plays at the table instead of eating.* Don't let him. This is unacceptable behavior and should be firmly discouraged. Put him down, and let him wait until later to eat again. Be consistent and firm, not punitive. If he is really hungry, he will soon learn to sit still while eating. A baby's appetite is less keen at a year than at eight months, and his energy needs are relatively lower. A one-year-old will get enough to eat if he lets his own hunger be his guide.
- *She wants to poke her fingers into her food.* Let her. She has much to learn from feeling the texture of her food. When she knows all about it, she'll naturally graduate to the use of a spoon.
- *He wants to manage the spoon himself, but can't handle it.* Let him try. As he masters it, withdraw gradually until he is feeding himself competently. This is the age at which a baby can learn to feed himself and is most strongly motivated to do so. He will spill, of course, but he'll grow out of it soon enough.
- *She refuses food that her mother knows is good for her.* This way of demonstrating autonomy, one of the few available to the one-year-old, is most satisfying. Don't force. It is in the one- to two-year-old stage that most of the feeding problems develop that can last throughout life. As long as she is getting enough milk and is offered a variety of nutritious foods to choose from, she will gradually acquire a taste for different foods—provided that she feels she is making the choice. This year is the most important year of a child's life in establishing future food preferences. If a baby refuses milk, an alternative source of the bone- and muscle-building nutrients it supplies must be provided. Milk-based puddings, custards, and cheese are often successful substitutes. For the baby who is allergic to milk, soy milk and other formulas are available.

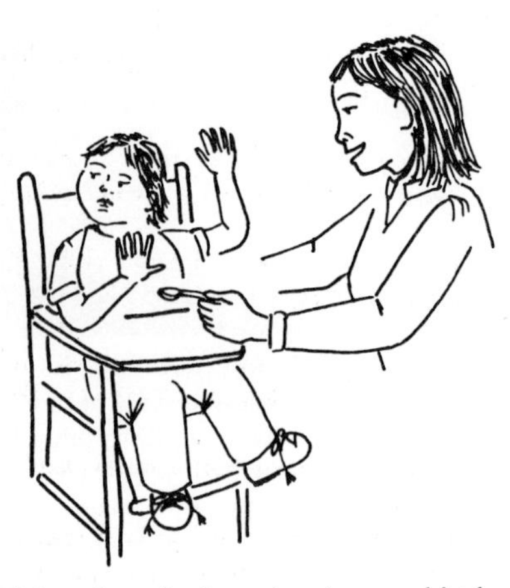

If she refuses food, put her down and let her wait until the next meal.

- *He prefers sweets—candy and sugary confections—to foods containing more nutrients.* Human beings of all races and cultures have a natural inborn preference for sweet-tasting foods. Limit them strictly. If they are kept in the house, keep them out of sight. There is no room in a baby's daily 1000 calories for the calories from sweets, except occasionally. The meal plan shown in Table 11–8 provides more than 500 calories from milk; one or two servings of each of the other types of food provide the other 500. If a candy bar were substituted for any of these foods, the baby would lose out on valuable nutrients; if it were added daily, the baby would gradually become obese.

These recommendations reflect a spirit of tolerance that serves the best interest of the child emotionally as well as physically. This tolerance also helps foster optimal physical development, for it is literally true that "feeding with love" produces better growth in both weight and height of children than feeding the same food in an emotionally negative climate.[51] The wise parent of a one-year-old offers nutrition and love together.

shopping list:
- iron-fortified infant cereal
- strained vegetables and fruits
- fruit juices
- mild cheeses
- yogurt
- tofu
- cooked beans
- meat, fish, poultry
- eggs
- bread (for toasting)
- teething crackers
- whole milk (after weaning)

Notes

1. A. Petros-Barvazian and M. Béhar, Low birth weight: What should be done to deal with this global problem? *WHO Chronicle* 32 (1978): 231–232; *New Trends and Approaches in the Delivery of Maternal and Child Care in Health Services* (sixth report of the WHO Expert Committee on Maternal and Child Health), as cited in *Journal of the American Dietetic Association* 71 (1977): 357; U.S. Department of Health and Human Services, *Facts about Premature Birth* (National Institute of Child Health and Human Development, publication no. 461-338—814/25324).
2. R. M. Pitkin, Assessment of nutritional status of mother, fetus, and newborn, *American Journal of Clinical Nutrition* 34 (1981): 658–668.
3. E. Hackman and coauthors, Maternal birth weight and subsequent pregnancy outcome, *Journal of the American Medical Association* 250 (1983): 2016–2019.
4. D. Sinclair, *Human Growth after Birth,* 4th ed. (New York: Oxford University Press, 1985), p. 85.
5. L. S. Hurley, *Developmental Nutrition* (Englewood Cliffs, N.J.: Prentice-Hall, 1980), p. 85.
6. J. Dobbing, Infant nutrition and later achievement, *Nutrition Reviews* 42 (1984): 1–7.
7. National Academy of Sciences, Committee on Dietary Allowances, *Recommended Dietary Allowances,* 9th ed. (Washington, D.C.: National Academy of Sciences, 1980), p. 26.
8. B. H. Dennis and coauthors, Nutrient intakes among selected North American populations in the Lipid Research Clinics prevalence study: Composition of energy intake, *American Journal of Clinical Nutrition* 41 (1985): 312–329.
9. R. D. Reynolds, M. Polansky, and P. B. Moser, Analyzed vitamin B_6 intakes of pregnant and postpartum lactating and nonlactating women, *Journal of the American Dietetic Association* 84 (1984): 1339–1344.
10. National Academy of Sciences, 1980, p. 138.
11. K. M. Hambidge and coauthors, Zinc nutritional status during pregnancy: A longitudinal study, *American Journal of Clinical Nutrition* 37 (1983): 429–442.
12. F. B. Glenn, W. D. Glenn, and R. C. Duncan, Fluoride tablet supplementation during pregnancy for caries immunity: A study of the offspring produced, *American Journal of Obstetrics and Gynecology* 143 (1982): 560–564.
13. R. L. Naeye, Weight gain and the outcome of pregnancy, *American Journal of Obstetrics and Gynecology* 135 (1979): 3–9; J. E. Brown and coauthors, Prenatal weight gains related to the birth of healthy-sized infants to low-income women, *Journal of the American Dietetic Association* 86 (1986): 1679–1683.
14. P. Rosso, A new chart to monitor weight gain during pregnancy, *American Journal of Clinical Nutrition* 41 (1985): 644–652.
15. B. Luke, M. A. Jonaitis, and R. H. Petrie, A consideration of height as a function of prepregnancy nutritional background and its potential influence on birth weight, *Journal of the American Dietetic Association* 84 (1984): 176–181.
16. W. Srisuphon and M. B. Bracken, Caffeine consumption during pregnancy and association with late spontaneous abortion, *American Journal of Obstetrics and Gynecology* 154 (1986) 14–20.
17. M. Stjernfeldt and coauthors, Maternal smoking during pregnancy and risk of childhood cancer, *Lancet* 1 (1986): 1350–1352.
18. National Dairy Council, Nutrition and pregnancy outcome, *Dairy Council Digest,* May/June 1983, pp. 13–18.
19. Naeye, 1979.
20. R. L. Leibel, Behavioral and biochemical correlations of iron deficiency: A review, *Journal of the American Dietetic Association* 71 (1977): 399–404.
21. S. M. Garn, M. T. Keating, and F. Falkner, Hematological status and pregnancy outcomes, *American Journal of Clinical Nutrition* 34 (1981): 115–117.
22. K. K. Sulik, M. C. Johnston, and M. A. Webb, Fetal alcohol syndrome: Embryogenesis in a mouse model, *Science* 214 (1981): 936–938.
23. F. P. Zuspan, Chronic hypertension in pregnancy, *Clinical Obstetrics and Gynecology* 27 (1984): 854–873.
24. A. Ferris and coauthors, Biological and sociocultural determinants of successful lactation among women in eastern Connecticut, *Journal of the American Dietetic Association* 87 (1987): 316–321.

25. N. Butte and coauthors, Effect of maternal diet and body composition on lactational performance, *American Journal of Clinical Nutrition* 39 (1984): 296–306.
26. Maternal nutrition during lactation, *Nutrition and the MD,* February 1987.
27. Maternal nutrition, 1987.
28. R. G. Whitehead and coauthors, A critical analysis of measured food energy intakes during infancy and early childhood in comparison with current international recommendations, *Journal of Human Nutrition* 35 (1981): 339–348.
29. American Academy of Pediatrics, Committee on Nutrition, *Pediatric Nutrition Handbook,* 2d ed. (Elk Grove Village, Ill.: American Academy of Pediatrics, 1985), p. 31.
30. American Academy of Pediatrics, Committee on Nutrition, and Nutrition Committee of the Canadian Pediatric Society, Breastfeeding: A commentary in celebration of the International Year of the Child, 1979, *Pediatrics* 62 (1978): 591–601.
31. C. Eckhert, Isolation of a protein from human milk that enhances zinc absorption in humans, *Biochemical and Biophysical Research Communications* 130 (1985): 264–269.
32. G. Carpenter, Epidermal growth factor is a major growth-promoting agent in human milk, *Science* 210 (1980): 198–199.
33. B. Lonnerdal, Biochemistry and physiological function of human milk proteins, *American Journal of Clinical Nutrition* 42 (1985): 1299–1317.
34. K. M. Shahani, A. J. Kwan, and B. A. Friend, Role and significance of enzymes in human milk, *American Journal of Clinical Nutrition* 33 (1980): 1861–1868; Thyroid hormones in human milk, *Nutrition Reviews* 37 (1979): 140–141; Prostaglandins in human milk, *Nutrition Reviews* 39 (1981): 302–303; J. J. Kabara, Lipids as host-resistance factors of human milk, *Nutrition Reviews* 38 (1980): 65–73.
35. American Academy of Pediatrics, 1985, p. 40.
36. J. Ekstrand, No evidence of transfer of fluoride from plasma to breast milk, *British Medical Journal* 283 (1981): 761–764.
37. Dr. James C. Penrod, pediatrician, Tallahassee, Florida (personal communication, June 1983).
38. B. J. Myers, Mother-infant bonding: Rejoinder to Kennell and Klaus, *Developmental Review* 4 (1984): 283–288.
39. C. Briggs, Recent developments in infant feeding and nutrition, in *Nutrition Update: 1,* eds. J. Weininger and G. M. Briggs (New York: Wiley, 1983), pp. 227–261.
40. Questions readers ask, *Nutrition and the MD,* December 1981.
41. American Academy of Pediatrics, Committee on Nutrition, The use of whole cow's milk in infancy, *Pediatrics* 72 (1983): 253–255.
42. S. Fomon, Do infant feeding practices lead to adult obesity? A speech presented at the American Dietetic Association National Conference, 19 October 1987.
43. Y. H. Neggers and K. R. Stitt, Effects of high lead intake in children, *Journal of the American Dietetic Association* 86 (1986): 938–940.
44. E. Pollitt and coauthors, Iron deficiency and behavioral development in infants and preschool children, *American Journal of Clinical Nutrition* 43 (1986): 555-565.
45. G. H. Johnson, G. A. Purvis, and R. D. Wallace, What nutrients do our infants really get? *Nutrition Today,* July/August 1981, pp. 4–10, 23–26.
46. M. Winick, Infant nutrition: Formula or breast feeding? *Professional Nutritionist,* Spring 1980, pp. 1–3.
47. L. L. Clark and V. A. Beal, Age at introduction of solid food to infants in Manitoba, *Journal of the Canadian Dietetic Association* 42 (1981): 72–78.
48. A "prudent diet" for infants? *Nutrition and the MD,* May 1983.
49. E. M. Widdowson, Mental contentment and physical growth, *Lancet* 1 (1951): 1316–1318.
50. J. Cravioto, Nutrition, stimulation, mental development and learning, *Nutrition Today,* September/October 1981, pp. 4–8, 10–15.
51. E. M. Widdowson, Mental contentment and physical growth, *Lancet* 1 (1951): 1316–1318.

Drinking during Pregnancy

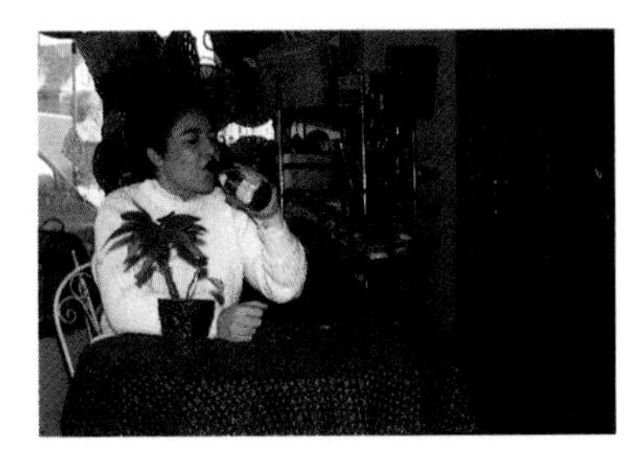

Both parents can raise the odds in favor of having a healthy infant by drinking nonalcoholic beverages before pregnancy.

Drinking excess alcohol during pregnancy endangers both the mother and her fetus. One consequence has already been mentioned in Chapter 11—the irreversible brain damage and mental and physical retardation known as fetal alcohol syndrome or FAS. The fetal brain is extremely vulnerable to a glucose or oxygen deficit, and alcohol causes both. In addition, alcohol itself crosses the placenta freely and is directly toxic to the fetal brain. Other consequences also follow upon overconsumption of alcohol during pregnancy. For women who want to drink during their pregnancies, then, the question is important, how much alcohol is too much.

Clearly, 3 ounces of alcohol (about 6 drinks) a day is too much early in pregnancy, even if the woman stops drinking immediately after she learns that she is pregnant.[1] Birth defects have been observed in the children of some women who drank 2 ounces (four drinks) of alcohol daily during pregnancy. Low birthweight (often associated with increased risk to the newborn) has been observed in infants born to some women who drank 1 ounce (two drinks) per day during pregnancy. At that level of alcohol intake, a sizable and significant increase occurs in the rate of spontaneous abortions, perhaps by poisoning of the fetus.[2] Also, in a study of 12,000 women, an intake of 2 drinks a day was found to be significantly associated with detachment of the placenta.[3] The damage of fetal alcohol syndrome is also known to occur with as few as 2 drinks a day.[4] Its most severe impact is likely to be in the first month, even before the woman is sure she is pregnant.[5] One study presents evidence of an association between two drinks a *week* and miscarriages.[6]

An individual exposed to alcohol before birth may respond differently to it in adulthood than if no exposure had occurred—and also to drugs for which alcohol causes cross-tolerance.[7] Research using animals shows that one-fifth of the level of alcohol needed to produce major, outwardly visible defects will surely produce learning impairment in the offspring. No sign of this impairment will be apparent on the outside, but the damage will be there on the inside.[8] Experiments using animals have even shown that alcohol in the female *before fertilization* may damage the ovum, and so lead to abnormalities. In males, the same is true—drinking before impregnation damages sperm and can also produce an abnormal pregnancy.[9]

At its most severe, fetal alcohol syndrome involves:

- Prenatal and postnatal growth retardation.
- Impairment of the brain and nerves, with consequent mental retardation, poor coordination, and hyperactivity.
- Abnormalities of the face and skull.
- Increased frequency of major birth defects (cleft palate and defects in major organ systems—heart, ears, genitals, urinary system).

About 1 in every 750 children born in the United States is a victim of this preventable damage.[10] Moreover, for every baby born with these symptoms, several others are born with **subclinical FAS**. The mothers of these children drank, but not enough to cause visible, obvious effects.

The many abnormalities associated with subclinical FAS are subtle, hidden under a normal-looking exterior. Without the clue from the classic facial abnormalities to alert them to the condition's presence, parents may not suspect the presence of defects, yet they may exist, and they can be devastating: learning disabilities, behavioral abnormalities, motor impairments, and more.

Thus, apparently, even moderate drinking can affect a woman's offspring negatively. This is true especially during the first month of pregnancy. Oxygen is indispensable, on a minute-to-minute basis, to the development of the fetus's central nervous system, and a sudden dose of alcohol can halt the delivery of oxygen through the umbilical cord.[11] During the first month of pregnancy, even a few minutes of such exposure can have a major effect on the fetal brain, which at that time is growing at the rate of 100,000 new brain cells a minute. The editors of the *Journal of the American Medical Association* have therefore taken the position that women should stop drinking as soon as they *plan* to become pregnant.[12] The editors of *Nutrition Today* magazine have stated that:

- The pregnant woman who drinks is more likely to give birth to a baby with FAS defects.
- The woman who is pregnant should not drink.
- The woman who is addicted to alcohol should be advised to avoid pregnancy at all costs.
- If, however, a woman addicted to alcohol becomes pregnant, she should be urged to have a preventive abortion.[13]

It is important to know, though, that if a woman has drunk heavily during the first two-thirds of her pregnancy, she can still prevent some damage by stopping heavy drinking during the third trimester.[14]

Not everyone agrees that women need to abstain totally from using alcohol during pregnancy. The American Council on Science and Health (ACSH) took the position, for a while, that women who drank only a little during pregnancy should not be harassed with overly conservative advice or made to feel guilty for a health habit that is insignificant in comparison with most others. Recently, however, the ACSH has modified this opinion. It now says, "Undoubtedly, there is a level of alcohol intake, as yet undetermined, that is not hazardous during pregnancy. Probably an occasional glass of beer or wine is tolerable in pregnancy, just as in the case of driving an automobile, provided that one drink does not lead to another. Total prohibition of drinking is an unacceptable rule for many people. Nevertheless, we believe that many pregnant women will prefer to give up drinking 'for the duration.' "[15]

We do too. It is a personal choice, but if we had it to make, we would opt for the healthy baby. We would

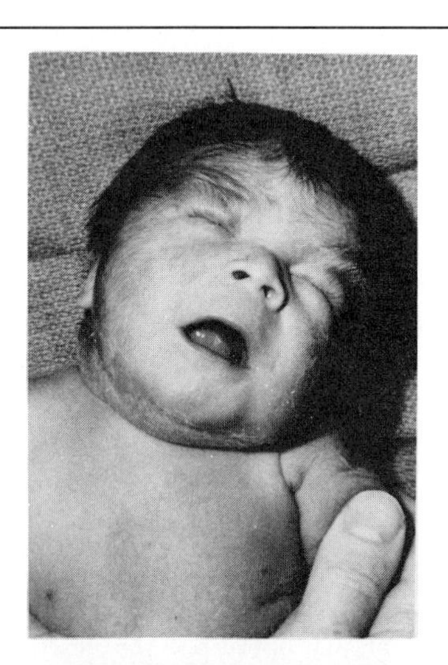
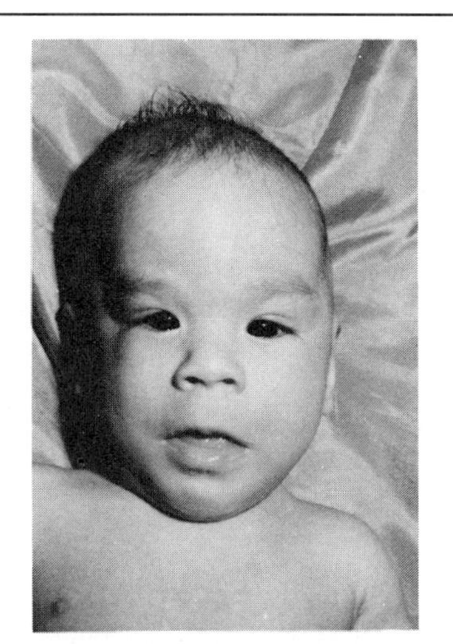
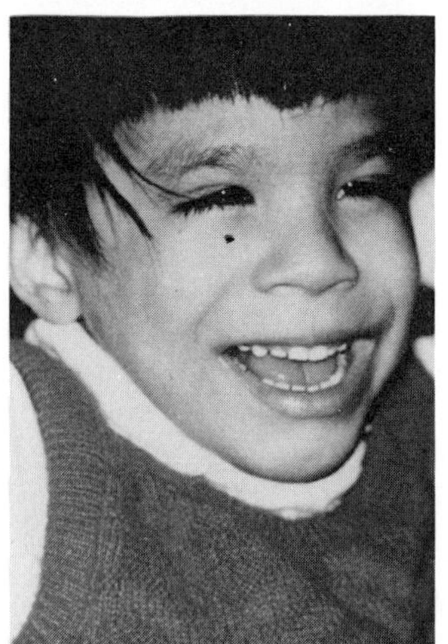
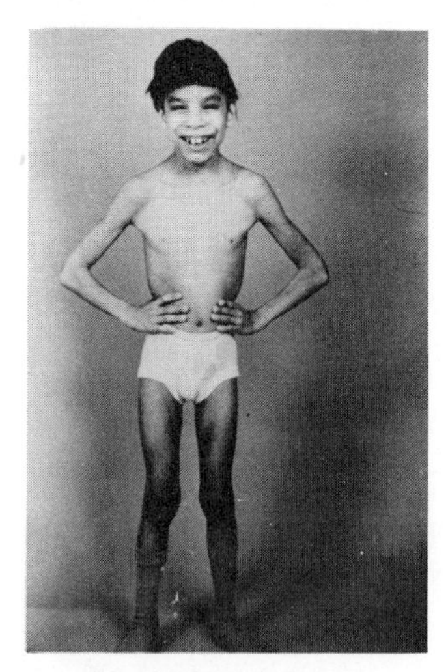

These facial traits reflect fetal alcohol syndrome, caused by drinking early in pregnancy. Irreversible abnormalities of the brain and internal organs accompany these surface features.

Miniglossary

fetal alcohol syndrome (FAS): the cluster of symptoms seen in an infant or child whose mother consumed excess alcohol during her pregnancy; includes mental and physical retardation with facial and other body deformities.

subclinical FAS: a subtle version of FAS, with hidden defects including learning disabilities, behavioral abnormalities, and motor impairments.

give up even the pleasure of wine with meals for the duration of pregnancy and drink a modest portion of alcohol only to celebrate after the baby's birth, if at all.

Notes

1. Alcohol and pregnancy, *Nutrition and the MD,* August 1984.
2. J. Kline and coauthors, Drinking during pregnancy and spontaneous abortion, *Lancet,* 26 July 1980, pp. 176–180.
3. M. C. Marbury and coauthors, The association of alcohol consumption with outcome of pregnancy, *American Journal of Public Health* 73 (1983) 1165.
4. Pregnancy and alcohol warning, *FDA Consumer,* October 1981, p. 2.
5. Fetal alcohol syndrome, *Nutrition and the MD,* July 1978.
6. Kline and coauthors, 1980.
7. E. L. Abel, R. Bush, and B. A. Dintcheff, Exposure of rats to alcohol in utero alters drug sensitivity in adulthood, *Science* 212 (1981): 1531–1533.
8. F. L. Iber, Fetal alcohol syndrome, *Nutrition Today,* September/October 1980, pp. 3–11.
9. M. H. Kaufman, Ethanol-induced chromosomal abnormalities at conception, *Nature* 302 (1983): 258–260.
10. K. K. Sulik, M. C. Johnston, and M. A. Webb, Fetal alcohol syndrome: Embryogenesis in a mouse model, *Science* 214 (1981): 936–938.
11. A. B. Mukherjee and G. D. Hodgen, Maternal ethanol exposure induces transient impairment of umbilical circulation and fetal hypoxia in monkeys, *Science* 218 (1982): 700–702.
12. Even moderate drinking may be hazardous to maturing fetus (Medical News), *Journal of the American Medical Association* 237 (1977): 2535.
13. *Nutrition Today* letter, 8 April 1981.
14. H. L. Rosett, L. Weiner, and K. C. Edelin, Treatment experience with pregnant problem drinkers, *Journal of the American Medical Association* 249 (1983): 2029–2033.
15. *Alcohol Use during Pregnancy,* December 1981 (a booklet available from the American Council on Science and Health, 47 Maple St., Summit, NJ 07901).

Chapter Twelve

Contents

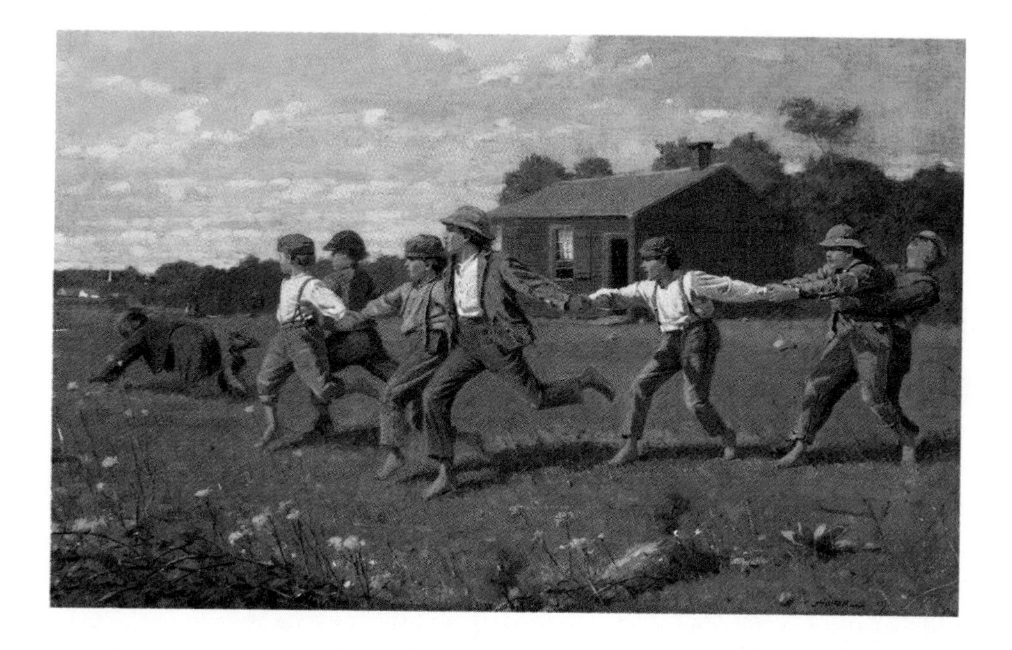

Snap the Whip by Winslow Homer, 1872. Oil on canvas, 12 × 20 inches. Reproduced with permission. The Metropolitan Museum of Art. Gift of Christian A. Zabriskie, 1950.

Child and Teen

The years of life described in this chapter—ages 1 to 18—are often called "the growing years," although, as we have seen, the year before birth and the first year after it are the most growing years of all. Still, there is more to come. From age 1 to 18 or thereabouts, height more than doubles, and weight increases up to sixfold or more. Optimal nutrition permits development to realize its full potential.

Growth Trends

Not everyone—indeed, not every population—enjoys the benefits of optimal nutrition. Observations of populations during times of change in their foodways have demonstrated that altered nutrition profoundly affects the timing and extent of young people's maturation.

Among the developmental characteristics that respond to environmental factors are rate of sexual maturation, rate of skeletal maturation, and ultimate height achieved. They respond to many factors, including improvements in medical care and sanitation, which help to prevent disease. Whatever improves socioeconomic status also permits children to mature faster and more fully than their parents; conversely, socioeconomic setbacks such as natural disasters or wars limit the growth and maturation rates of young people. Among these factors, though, nutrition is among the most significant.

Ultimately, when all environmental conditions are ideal, a population can realize its full genetic potential, but until then it is impossible to know what that potential may be. Take the rate of sexual maturation, for example. In 1880, people in the United States might have thought that women always started having menstrual periods at age 15.[1] In 1930, however, their granddaughters

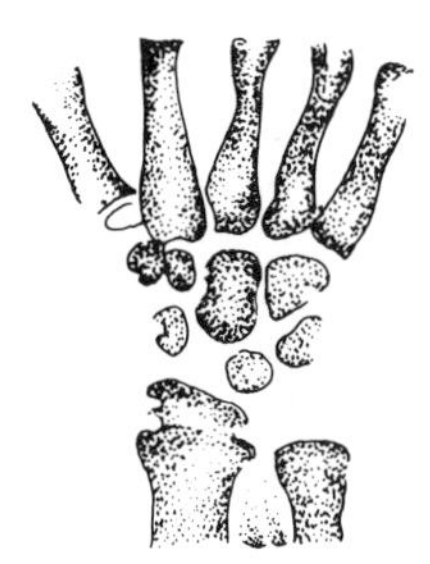

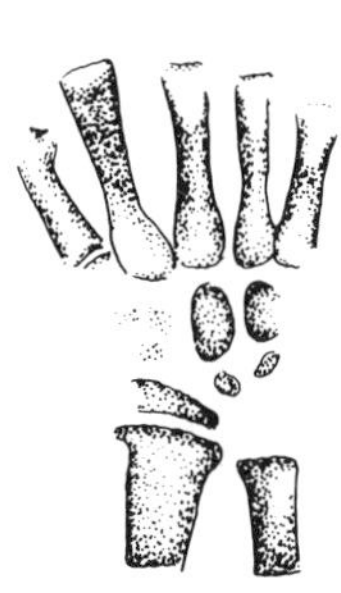

Skeletal maturity can be measured by x-raying the bones of the hand and and wrist to see how completely formed they are. Here, eight developing bony centers of two different children are shown. They are markedly more fully mineralized in one child's hand than in the other, although both children are six years old.

menarche (MEN-ark): the age at which the first menstrual period occurs (*mens* means "month"; *arche* means "beginning").

reached **menarche** between 13 and 14. This trend paralleled the accumulation of many economic advantages and ceased in the 1940s—presumably because the limits of genetic possibility had then been reached. A similar trend was seen in Europe, but the average ages were approximately one year higher than in the United States.

Height, too, responds to changes in socioeconomic conditions. Both the rate at which growth in height occurs and the ultimate height achieved have changed since 100 years ago. Children are completing more of their total growth at earlier ages, and are reaching greater adult heights than earlier in this century. Today, most young women arrive at their full height by the age of 16 or 17, and most young men by 17 or 18, whereas early in this century most men reached their full height at 25 years of age.[2]

All of this is not to say that all people "should" attain the same heights at the same ages or at maturity. Different races have different genetic potentials. Some are smaller, some taller, because they have inherited different genes for height. Several U.S. surveys have shown that blacks mature earlier and grow taller than whites, all else (including income) being equal. However, such differences in physical development can be attributed to differing genetic heritages only after environmental influences, including the adequacy and constancy of the food supply, have equalized. The case of the Japanese provides an example of a population that, until recently, had not reached its genetic potential for height.

In Japan, both the adverse effects of times of deprivation and the benefits of improved nutrition have been demonstrated in secular trends within this century. The heights of children at each age have steadily increased since 1900, probably mostly as a result of increased protein intakes—except during the Second World War, when food deprivation was severe. The effects are shown in Figure 12–1.

The rest of this chapter describes the growth and development of children in the context of advanced, industrialized societies like the United States and Canada, in which even the poor, compared with those of other countries, are not much poorer than the middle class. In other countries, poverty is so much more extreme that many parents' expectations for the physical and mental development of their children cannot realistically be as high as they are here.

Growth in children improves with socioeconomic status, and responds particularly to improved nutrition.

Figure 12–1
Effect of the War Years on Heights of Japanese Boys
The decline in growth is most dramatic at age 14—the age of maximum growth for adolescent males. The faster the boys were growing, the more severely they were affected. The figure also shows that boys at each age were taller in 1970 than boys of those ages were in 1900—believed to be an effect of improved protein nutrition. (The same effects were seen in girls.)

Source: Adapted from E. A. Martin and V. A. Beal, *Roberts' Nutrition Work with Children,* 4th ed. (Chicago: University of Chicago Press, 1978), p. 147, as adapted in turn from Helen S. Mitchell.

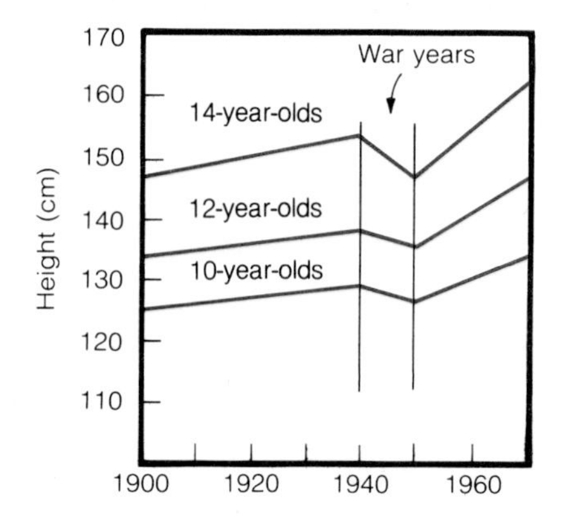

The Early Years

Nutrient needs change steadily throughout life and vary from individual to individual, depending on the rate of growth, the sex, the previous nutrition and health history, and many other factors. This section takes a general look at preschool and school-age children's needs, and later sections are devoted to the special concerns of teenagers.

Growth and Nutrient Needs

After the age of one, a child's growth rate slows, but the body continues to change dramatically. At one, babies have just learned to stand and toddle; by two, they can take long strides with confidence and are learning to run, jump, and climb. These new accomplishments are possible, thanks to the accumulation of a larger mass and greater density of bone and muscle tissue. Thereafter, the same trend—a lengthening of the long bones and an increase in musculature—continues, unevenly and more slowly, until adolescence. Growth comes in small spurts; a six-year-old child may wear the same pair of shoes for a year, then need new shoes twice in the next four months.

Appetite decreases markedly around the age of one year, in line with the great reduction in growth rate. An overzealous mother, unaware that her one-year-old is supposed to slow down, may begin a lifelong conflict over food by trying to force more on the child than the child feels like eating. Thereafter, the appetite fluctuates; at times children's appetites seem to be insatiable, and at other times the same children seem to live on air and water. Parents need not worry about this—a child will need and demand more food during periods of rapid growth than during slow periods. The perfection of appetite regulation in children of normal weight guarantees that their calorie intakes will be right for each stage of growth. As long as the calories they do consume are from nutritious foods, they are well provided for. (Two cautions: wandering school-age children may be spending pocket money at the nearby candy store; overweight children may eat in response to external cues, disregarding appetite regulation signals.)

A one-year-old child needs perhaps 1000 calories a day; a three-year-old needs only 300 to 500 calories more. At age ten a child needs an additional 1000 calories a day, for a total of about 2300 to 2500 calories, on the average. The total energy needs increase slightly with age, but energy needs decline gradually per pound of body weight. The wide variation in the physical activity

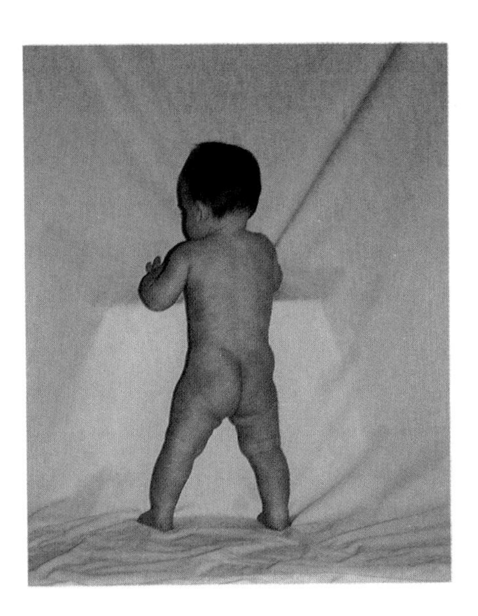

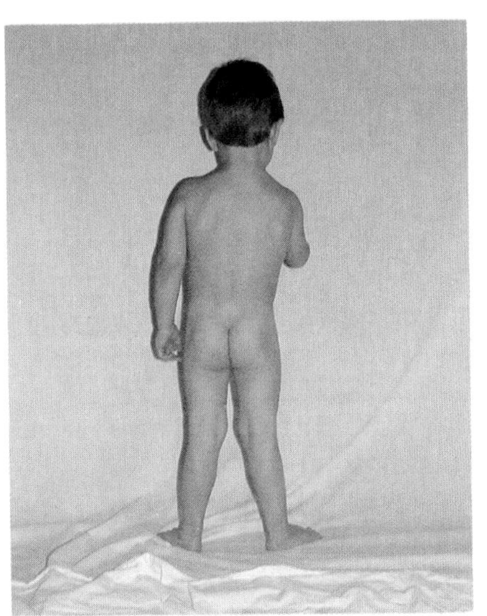

One-year-old and two-year-old shown for comparison of body shape. The two-year-old has lost much of the baby fat; the muscles (especially in the back, buttocks, and legs) have firmed and strengthened, and the leg bones have lengthened and increased in density.

of children requires judgment in determining an individual child's energy needs. An inactive child can become obese even when consuming a diet that is below average in calories.

Children gather their forces for the adolescent growth spurt by accumulating stores of nutrients that will be needed in the coming years. When they take off on that growth spurt, there will be a period during which their nutrient intakes cannot meet the demands of rapid growth. They will need to draw on these nutrient stores. This is especially true of calcium; the denser the bones are in childhood, the better prepared they will be to withstand bone loss in later life. The RDA table and the RNI for Canadians are averages of the nutrient needs for each span of three years.

One nutrient deserves special attention—iron. Iron-deficiency anemia is the most prevalent nutrient deficiency disease among children and adolescents in the United States.[3] As children grow older, they should receive 5.5 milligrams of iron or more from each 1000 calories of food. To achieve this goal, the diet must be balanced—with enough low-iron dairy products to ensure adequate calcium and riboflavin intakes, but no more. If nonfat or low-fat milk is used instead of whole milk, saved calories can be invested in such iron-rich foods as lean meats, fish, poultry, and legumes. Whole-grain or enriched products also contribute iron.

To provide all the needed nutrients, a variety of foods from each of the food groups is recommended. Table 12–1 offers a daily food pattern for children. The serving sizes increase with the child's age. To estimate serving sizes for meat, fruits, and vegetables, a serving is loosely defined as 1 tablespoon per year. Thus at four years of age, a serving of any of these foods would be 4 tablespoons (¼ cup). Because the serving sizes adjust as the child grows older, this rule of thumb is appropriate from age two to the teen years.

Careful food selection is essential to ensure adequate nutrition. To illustrate this point, consider the hypothetical case of a mother who makes an effort to deliver meat, milk, and whole–grain products to her child and still fails to achieve adequate nutrient intakes:

- *Breakfast:* ¼ cup of cereal with ½ cup of whole milk; fresh unpeeled apple slices.
- *Lunch:* Bologna sandwich with 1 slice bologna and 2 slices of whole-wheat bread; 1 bag of pretzels; 1 cup of whole milk.
- *Supper:* 2 fried chicken drumsticks; about 20 french fries; 1 dinner roll; a 12-ounce carbonated beverage; and ½ cup of gelatin with nondairy topping (from a fast-food restaurant).
- *Snack:* 4 chocolate sandwich cookies.

Table 12–2 compares the RDA for a 5-year-old with the nutrients provided by these meals. Assuming that the RDA are a reasonable standard, the table shows that the child failed to get enough of several nutrients.

A comparison between the recommended food pattern in Table 12–1 and this sample day's menus reveals that some foods are missing, and these account for the missing nutrients. In the milk and cheese group, only half of the recommended servings were consumed; as a result, calcium intake for the day was too low. The protein and cereal food groups were adequately represented on this day; as a consequence, the thiamin, riboflavin, iron, and zinc intakes were sufficient. Fruits and vegetables were scarce. An apple and a few french fries

Table 12–1

Children's Daily Food Pattern for Good Nutrition

Food Group	Servings per Day	Average Size of Serving: *1 to 3 Years*	*4 to 5 Years*	*6 to 12 Years*
Milk and cheese (1 oz cheese = 1 c milk)	4	½–¾ c	¾ c	¾–1 c
Protein foods	3 or more			
Eggs		1	1	1
Lean meat, fish, poultry, legumes (liver once a week)		2 tbsp	4 tbsp	2–4 oz
Peanut butter		0–1 tbsp	2 tbsp	2–3 tbsp
Fruits and vegetables	4; more recommended			
Vitamin C source (citrus fruits, berries, tomatoes, cabbage, cantaloupe)	1 or more	⅓–½ c	½ c	1 medium orange
Vitamin A source (green or orange fruits/vegetables)	1 or more	2–3 tbsp	4 tbsp	¼–⅓ c
Other vegetables (including potatoes)	2	2–3 tbsp	4 tbsp (¼ c)	⅓–½ c
Other fruits		¼–⅓ c	½ c	1 medium
Cereals (whole grain or enriched)	4; more recommended			
Bread, buns, pizza		½-1 slice	1½ slices	1 to 2 slices
Ready-to-eat cereals		½–¾ oz	1 oz	1 oz
Cooked grains (cereals, macaroni, grits, rice)		¼–⅓ c	½ c	½–¾ c
Fats and sugars	**Optional** These foods can be used to meet energy needs when the required servings of nutritious foods do not. Serving sizes listed here are maximum.			
Butter, margarine, mayonnaise, oils	1	1 tbsp	1 tbsp	2 tbsp
Desserts and sweets (100-calorie portions)[a]	1	1–1½ portions	1½ portions	3 portions

[a]⅓ c pudding or ice cream; 2 to 3 cookies; 1 oz cake; 1⅓ oz pie; or 2 tbsp jelly, jam, honey, sugar

Source: Adapted from B. B. Alford and M. L. Bogle, *Nutrition during the Life Cycle* (Englewood Cliffs, N.J.: Prentice-Hall, 1982), pp. 60–61. Originally from Behrman and Nelson *Textbook of Pediatrics,* 13/e 1987; Table 3–7.

offer minimal amounts of vitamins A, C, and folacin—nutrients that are provided almost exclusively by fruits and vegetables. Had this child eaten two more servings of fruits and vegetables (preferably a vitamin C source and a vitamin A source), as recommended in Table 12–1, the nutrient intakes provided by this day's meals would have been adequate.

Table 12–2

Typical Child's Nutrient Intakes[a]

RDA for 5-Year-Old		This Day's Meals Provided	
Protein	30 g	78 g	259% of RDA—higher than necessary
Vitamin A	500 RE	159 RE	32%—too low
Thiamin	0.9 mg	1.1 mg	129%—adequate
Riboflavin	1.0 mg	1.53 mg	150%—adequate
Folacin	200 μg	119 μg	60%—too low
Vitamin C	45 mg	23.5 mg	52%—too low
Calcium	800 mg	644 mg	81%—marginal
Iron	10 mg	9.3 mg	93%—marginal
Zinc	10 mg	8.6 mg	88%—marginal

[a]A key point to remember: the nutrients noted here are just a sampling. This child's diet probably lacks others, too.

Even so, the child did at least have three meals and a snack on this day. Imagine how much worse the picture is when a child skips breakfast, or when more sugary foods take the place of some of the nourishing ones. Chances are, the nutrients missed from a skipped breakfast won't be "made up" at lunch and dinner, but will be completely left out that day.

Experimentation with children's food patterns shows that candy, cola, and other concentrated sweets must be limited in a child's diet if the needed nutrients are to be supplied. (Table 12–1 notes that these optional high-calorie foods may be included only in addition to the required servings of nutritious foods, and then only in small portions.) A nonobese active child can enjoy the higher-calorie nutritious foods in each category: ice cream or pudding in the milk group, cake and cookies (whole grain or enriched only, however) in the bread group. These foods, made from milk and grain, carry valuable nutrients and encourage a child to learn, appropriately, that eating is fun. A child can't be trusted to choose nutritious foods on the basis of taste alone; the preference for sweets is innate. If such foods are permitted in large quantities, the only possible outcomes are nutrient deficiencies and/or obesity.

Growth occurs in spurts, and nutrition needs ebb and flow in response. The nutrient standards are averages of nutrient needs. Careful food choices ensure adequate nutrition.

The Effects of Nutrient Deficiencies on Behavior

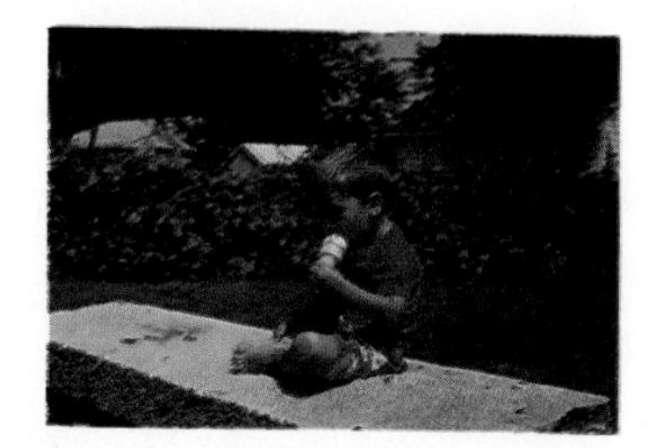

Calcium and riboflavin in a delicious form.

Nutrient deficiencies bring a host of physical symptoms, many of which are described in earlier chapters. Of particular interest to people concerned with caring for children is that nutrient deficiencies might also have behavioral symptoms.

Most people are familiar with the role of iron in carrying oxygen in the blood. A less known, but extremely important, function of iron is transporting that oxygen within cells, where it is used to help produce energy. A lack of iron not only causes an energy crisis, but also directly affects behavior, mood, attention span, and learning ability. Iron is involved in the functioning of many molecules in the brain and nervous system. Deficiencies of iron produced experimentally in animals have caused abnormal synthesis and degradation of neurotransmitters, and notably those that regulate the ability to pay attention, crucial to learning.[4]

Iron deficiency is usually diagnosed by use of iron indicators in the *blood* when it has progressed all the way to overt anemia. A child's *brain,* however, is sensitive to slightly lowered iron levels long before the blood effects appear. Iron's effects are hard to distinguish from the effects of other factors in children's lives, but it is likely that iron deficiency manifests itself in a lowering of the "motivation to persist in intellectually challenging tasks," a shortening of the attention span, and a reduction of overall intellectual performance. Anemic children perform less well on tests and have more conduct disturbances than their classmates.[5]

Iron is only one of several dozen nutrients that can be displaced from a diet high in empty-calorie foods. Any of the others may be lacking as well, and the deficiencies of those nutrients may also cause behavioral, as well as physical, symptoms.

A child with the behavioral symptoms of nutrient deficiencies might be irritable, aggressive, disagreeable, or sad and withdrawn. One might label such a child "hyperactive," "depressed," or "unlikable," when in fact the cause for these behaviors is simple, albeit marginal, malnutrition. In any such case, inspection of the child's diet by someone knowledgeable about children's nutrient needs is clearly in order. Should suspicion of nutrient deficiencies be raised, no matter what other causes may be implicated, the people responsible for feeding the child should take steps to correct those deficiencies promptly.

Irregularity of meals can also affect children's behavior. Children who eat no breakfast perform poorly in tasks of concentration, their attention spans are shorter, and they even show lower IQs on testing than their well-fed peers.[6] Common sense tells us that it is unreasonable to expect anyone to learn and perform work when no fuel has been provided. By the late morning, discomfort from hunger may become distracting even if a child has eaten breakfast.

The problem that arises for children who attempt morning schoolwork on an empty stomach appears to be at least partly due to hypoglycemia. The average child up to the age of ten or so needs to eat every four to six hours to maintain a blood glucose concentration high enough to support the activity of the brain and nervous system. A child's brain is as big as an adult's, and the brain is the body's chief glucose consumer. A child's liver is considerably smaller—and the liver is the organ responsible for storing glucose (as glycogen) and releasing it into the blood as needed. A child's liver can't store more than about four hours' worth of glycogen—hence the need to eat fairly often. Teachers aware of the late-morning slump in their classrooms wisely request that a midmorning snack be provided; it improves classroom performance all the way to lunchtime. But for the child who hasn't had breakfast, the morning is lost altogether.

Malnutrition is quite often a complex condition involving multiple nutrients and other factors. To give just one example of a possible complicating factor: lead poisoning can cause iron-deficiency anemia, and iron deficiency impairs the body's defenses against absorption of lead. The anemia brought on by lead poisoning may be mistaken for a simple iron deficiency. Lead toxicity symptoms are widespread among children—1 out of every 50 children in rural areas and more than 1 out of every 10 inner-city children are affected with lead poisoning.[7] Such problems are important to identify, but still, even while they are being investigated, the child should be fed properly.

Figure 12–2
The Malnourished versus the Well-Nourished Child.

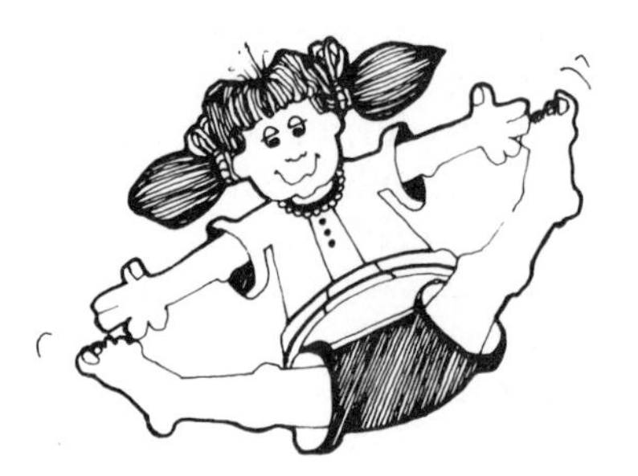

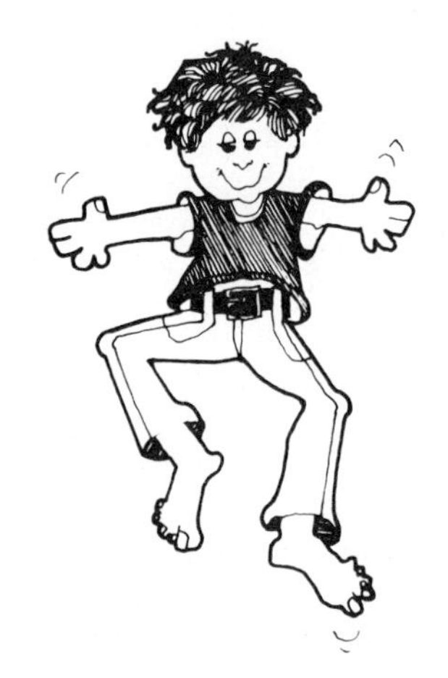

Normal hair: Shiny, firm in the scalp
Malnourished hair: Dull, brittle, dry, loose and falls out

Normal face: Good complexion
Malnourished face: Off color; scaly, flaky, cracked skin

Normal glands: No lumps
Malnourished glands: Swollen at front of neck, cheeks

Normal skin: Smooth, firm, good color
Malnourished skin: dry, rough, "sandpaper" feel, spotty, or sores; lack of fat under the skin

Normal nails: firm, pink
Malnourished nails: Spoon-shaped, brittle, ridged

Normal eyes: Bright, clear, pink membranes, adjust easily to darkness
Malnourished eyes: Pale membranes, spots, redness, adjust slowly to darkness

Normal lips: Smooth, good color
Malnourished lips: Red, swollen, cracks at corners of mouth

Normal tongue: Red, rough, bumpy
Malnourished tongue: Sore, smooth, purplish, swollen

Normal teeth and gums: No pain or cavities, gums firm, teeth bright
Malnourished teeth and gums: Missing, discolored, decayed teeth; gums bleed easily, swollen, spongy

Normal behavior: Alert, attentive, cheerful
Malnourished behavior: Irritable, apathetic, inattentive, hyperactive

Normal internal systems: Heart rate, rhythm, and blood pressure normal; normal digestive function; reflexes, psychological development normal
Malnourished internal systems: Heart rate, rhythm, or blood pressure abnormal; liver, spleen enlarged, abnormal digestion; mental irritability, confusion; burning, tingling of hands, feet; loss of balance, coordination.

Normal muscles and bones: Good muscle tone, posture; long bones straight
Malnourished muscles and bones: "Wasted" appearance of muscles, swollen bumps on skull or ends of bones, small bumps on ribs, bowed legs or knock-knees, pain

Source: From a wall poster available from The Nutrition Company, P.O. Box 11102, Tallahassee, FL 32302. Used with permission. Copies available for $3 plus $1.50 postage.

Parents and medical practitioners often overlook the possibility that malnutrition may account for abnormalities of appearance and behavior. Consider the behavior of a well-nourished child: alert, energetic, responsive to external stimuli; in other words, healthy. Any departure from normal, healthy appearance and behavior is a possible sign of poor nutrition. Figure 12–2 identifies physical signs of malnutrition in children.

All nutrients are important for normal growth; iron is most often in short supply. Regular meals support normal activity in children. Even mild malnutrition can manifest itself in behavior problems.

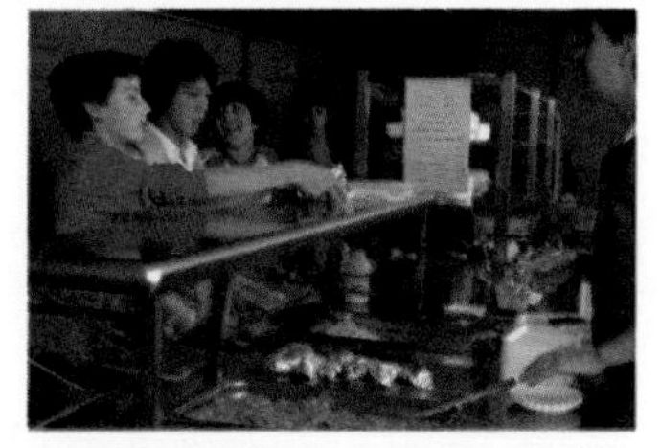

School lunch is available to 90 percent of all U.S. schoolchildren.

Nutrition at School

While parents are doing what they can to establish favorable eating behaviors during the transition from infancy to childhood, other factors are entering the picture. During preschool or grade school, the child encounters foods prepared and served by outsiders. The U.S. government funds several programs to provide nutritious, high-quality meals for children at school. (School lunches in Canada are administered locally and therefore vary from area to area.) School lunches are designed to meet certain requirements. They must include specified servings of milk, protein-rich foods (meat, poultry, fish, cheese, eggs, legumes, or peanut butter), vegetables, fruits, and breads or other grain foods. The design is intended to provide at least a third of the RDA for each of the nutrients. The U.S. school lunch pattern is split into several patterns so as to provide for the needs of different ages (see Table 12–3).

Parents rely on the school lunch program to meet a significant part of their children's nutrient needs on school days. Indeed, students participating in the school lunch program have higher intakes of energy and nutrients than students who do not. Children don't always like what they are served, and school lunch programs attempt to feed them both what they want and what will nourish them. In response to children's differing needs and tastes, the trend is:

- To increase the variety of offerings and allow children to choose what they are served.
- To vary portion sizes, so that little children may take little servings.
- To involve students (in secondary schools) in the planning of menus.
- To improve the scheduling of lunches so that children can eat when they are hungry and can have enough time to eat well.

Many schools are attempting to meet today's ideals of healthful food. They offer low-fat or nonfat milk instead of whole milk. To economize, they do not require

Table 12–3

School Lunch Patterns

	Preschool		**Grades**		
	Ages 1 to 2	*Ages 3 to 4*	*K to 3*	*4 to 12*	*7 to 12*
Meat or meat alternate					
One serving:					
Lean meat, poultry, or fish	1 oz	1½ oz	1½ oz	2 oz	3 oz
Cheese	1 oz	1½ oz	1½ oz	2 oz	3 oz
Large egg(s)	1	1½	1½	2	3
Cooked dried beans or peas	½ c	¾ c	¾ c	1 c	1½ c
Peanut butter	2 tbsp	3 tbsp	3 tbsp	4 tbsp	6 tbsp
Vegetable and/or fruit					
Two or more servings, both to total	½ c	½ c	½ c	¾ c	¾ c
Bread or bread alternate Servings[a]	5 per week	8 per week	8 per week	8 per week	10 per week
Milk					
A serving of fluid milk	¾ c	¾ c	1 c	1 c	1 c

[a]A serving is 1 slice of whole-grain or enriched bread; a whole-grain or enriched biscuit, roll, muffin, etc.; ½ c cooked pasta or other cereal grain such as bulgur or grits.

Source: Adapted from School lunch patterns: Ready, set, go! *School Food Service Journal,* August 1980, p. 31.

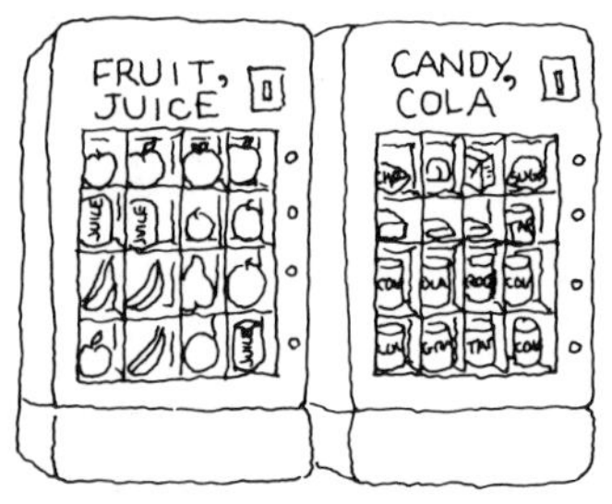

When fruits and juices are available in vending machines, candy and cola sales fall.

that children be served every item, but permit them to select what they will eat, so that little food will be wasted. Many schools offer salad bars, potato bars, and taco bars, providing students an opportunity to create their own meals from a selection of nutritious foods.

Whether to eat the school's lunch is not the only choice facing children in the school. Some children bring lunch from home; others rely on vending machines. Many health professionals and parents would like to eliminate the sale of confections as snacks in schools, but so far such efforts have met with little success. Most progress has been made by way of individual, voluntary initiatives. Experiments have shown that children choose more nutritious snacks if they are offered side by side with sugary foods. When apples are made available in vending machines, children choose chocolate bars less often. When milk is made available, soft drink use drops considerably.

Coincident with the school lunch program is a program of nutrition education and training (NET program) in all the public schools. Originally allocated 50 cents per year per child, this program was cut in 1980 to 9 cents per child, but program administrators are highly motivated and have been ingenious and creative in accomplishing the program's highest-priority objectives.[8]

Creative methods for teaching nutrition to children include stories, puppets, and games. For classes with computers, a number of nutrition education programs are available beginning at the preschool level. One way in which children can learn about nutrition, sometimes with only small expense to the school, is to take field trips to nearby food operations facilities. Among the possible places to visit are those listed in the margin. At the very least, children can go to the depots where the school food comes in and to the kitchens where it is prepared. Knowledgeable teachers can then use the questions that arise as opportunities to teach nutrition. Children need not only to be fed well, but to learn enough about nutrition to become able to make healthy food choices when the choices become theirs to make.

Children can learn from:

- Bakeries.
- Mills.
- Dairy farms.
- Milk-bottling plants.
- Farmers markets.
- Vegetable farms and fields.
- Food-processing plants.
- Fast-food places.
- Institutional kitchens.
- Supermarkets.
- Convenience stores.
- Neighborhood gardens.
- Natural-food stores.
- Food salvage banks.

School lunches are designed to meet the needs of growing children. Schools also have the responsibility of offering nutrition education.

Television's Influence on Nutrition

On the average, children in the United States spend as much time watching television as they do attending school. Little wonder that television viewing has become associated with a variety of child and teen behaviors. Television's influence is evident in childhood obesity and dental health.

Several effects of watching TV contribute to obesity. First, TV viewing requires no energy beyond the resting metabolic rate. Second, it replaces time spent in more vigorous activities. Physical inactivity may be the most important environmental factor contributing to obesity. Third, watching TV correlates with between-meal snacking on calorically dense foods most heavily advertised on children's programs. The more television children view, the greater the incidence of obesity among them. In fact, the incidence of obesity increases by 2 percent for each hour of television viewed.[9]

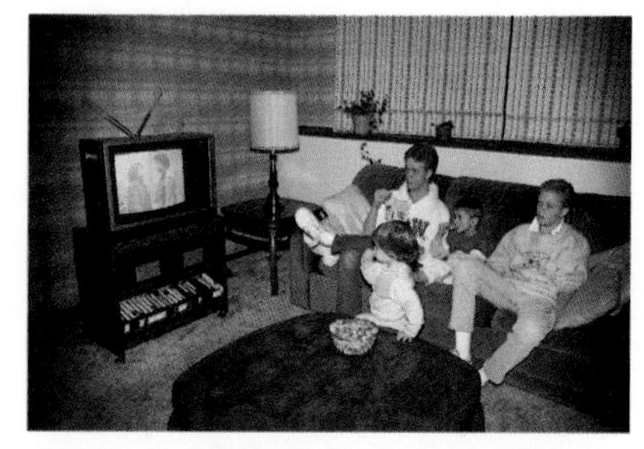

TV is a major influence in a child's life.

Television viewing also affects dental health. Frequent snacking on high-sugar foods is a major factor in **caries** development and TV-watchers snack on them often. Sugar that is eaten between meals poses a greater risk of dental caries than does sugar eaten with meals. Sticky, sugary foods left on the teeth provide an ideal environment for the growth of mouth bacteria and the formation of caries.

The average television-watching child sees more than 20,000 commercials a year. Approximately half are for foods and beverages, most of which contain sugar. Food companies spend several million dollars a year selling these foods to children. Their tantalizing messages about high-sugar (and therefore low-nutrient) foods take unfair advantage of an impressionable, nutritionally naive audience. Take a moment to consider this naive audience. They spend about 70 hours a year learning about foods by way of television commercials—information that is almost invariably misleading. Compare that with the number of hours parents, teachers, physicians, and dentists spend each year providing chldren with sound nutrition, health, and dental information. Television commercials do not offer nutrition education, nor do they warn of problems certain foods pose to health. Not only commercials, but also TV programs themselves mislead children. Children may miss the message that eating and drinking high-calorie, high-sugar foods will effect weight gain and rot teeth, when they see TV stars with sparkling white teeth indulging in such behavior and remaining thin. (See Controversy 3 for more on sugar and dental caries.)

No regulations to prevent the promotion of sticky, sugary foods are in force, however. Parents and health professionals need to compensate for the slanted information provided by advertisements. To promote dental health, they need to teach children to:

- Restrict sweets to mealtimes, if possible.
- Brush teeth or rinse the mouth with water after eating snacks.
- Limit the duration of time the teeth are exposed to sticky foods.
- Brush and floss daily.
- Rinse with water after eating when brushing and flossing are not possible.
- Eat foods rich in calcium and phosphorus.
- Eat a variety of firm, fibrous foods to brush over the teeth and stimulate the rinsing action of the salivary glands.

Dentists, especially, have the obligation to educate their clients individually as long as misleading claims continue to appear on national television. A selection of foods that favor dental health is shown in Table 12–4.

Television advertising of sugary foods promotes sugar consumption and tooth decay.

Food Allergies

Food allergies are frequently blamed for physical and behavioral abnormalities in children. A true food allergy occurs when a whole food protein molecule or other large molecule enters the system. (Recall that large molecules of food are normally dismantled in the digestive tract to smaller ones that can be absorbed.) The body's immune system reacts to a food protein or other large molecule as it does to an antigen—by producing antibodies (see Chapter 1), or other defensive agents such as **histamine.**

caries (KARE-eez): gradual decay and disintegration of a tooth (*carius* means "rottenness").

histamine: a substance produced by cells of the immune system as part of a local immune reaction to an antigen; participates in causing inflammation.

allergy: an immune reaction to a foreign substance (such as some component of food) in which antibodies are produced. (An immune reaction not involving antibody production is termed **sensitivity** by some researchers.) Allergies may be **symptomatic** or **asymptomatic.**

anaphylactic (an-AFF-ill-LAC-tic) **shock:** a whole-body allergic reaction to an offending substance. Symptoms: abdominal pain, nausea, vomiting, diarrhea, inflamed nasal membranes, chest pain, hives, swelling, low blood pressure.

Table 12–4

Dietary Recommendations for Controlling Dental Caries

Food Group	Frequent Use Recommended	Infrequent Use Suggested[a]
Dairy	Milk, cheese, plain yogurt	Chocolate milk, ice cream, ice milk, milk shakes, fruited yogurt
Meat/meat alternates	Lean meat, fish, poultry; eggs; legumes	Peanut butter with added sugar, lunch meats with added sugar, meats with sugared glazes
Fruits	Fresh or packed in water	Dried, packed in syrup or juice, jams, jellies, preserves, fruit juices or drinks
Vegetables	Salad greens, cauliflower, cucumbers, radishes, carrots, celery	Candied sweet potatoes, glazed carrots
Bread/cereal	Popcorn, soda crackers, toast, hard rolls, pretzels, potato chips, corn chips, pizza	Cookies, sweet rolls, pies, cakes, ready-to-eat sweetened cereals as between-meal snacks
Other	Sugarless gum, coffee or tea without sugar	Sugared soft drinks, candy, fudge, caramels, honey, sugars, syrups

[a]It is particularly important to practice good oral hygiene after eating those foods.
Source: S. R. Rolfes and E. N. Whitney, *Say Cheese and Smile: The Nutrition and Oral Health Picture,* a monograph (1988) available from Stickley Publishing Co., 210 Washington Sq., Philadelphia, PA 19106.

The term **allergy** has two components—antibodies and symptoms. A person may produce antibodies *without* having any symptoms (known as **asymptomatic allergy**) or may produce antibodies *and* have symptoms (known as **symptomatic allergy).** Symptoms without antibody production are *not* due to allergy.

Depending on its location in the body, the allergic reaction causes different symptoms. In the digestive tract, it causes nausea or vomiting; in the skin, it causes rashes; and in the nasal passages and lungs, it causes inflammation or asthma. A generalized, all-systems reaction is **anaphylactic shock.**

Allergic reactions to food occur with different timings, simply classified as immediate and delayed. In both, the interaction of the antigen with the immune system is immediate, but the appearance of symptoms may come within minutes or after several (up to 24) hours.[10] Diagnosis of an immediate allergic reaction is easy, because symptoms correlate closely with the eating of the offending food. Diagnosis of delayed reactions is more difficult, because the symptoms may not appear until a day after the offending food is eaten; by this time many other foods will have been eaten, too, complicating the picture.

The foods that most often cause immediate hypersensitivity reactions are listed in Table 12–5. According to one investigator, 91 percent of adverse reactions are caused by only four major foods—nuts (43 percent), eggs (21 percent), milk (18 percent), and soy (9 percent).[11] Sensitivity or allergic reactions to single foods are common. Reactions to multiple foods are the exception, not the rule.

A number of tests and food challenges are required to identify a true food allergy. A simple **elimination diet** that enables the person to avoid the offending food is the preferred test diet.[12] This requires the elimination of the suspected food for a week or two. If the symptoms do not disappear, the suspected food is not guilty. If symptoms resolve, the food is reintroduced into the diet in small quantities. If there is a reaction, the food is eliminated for a month or two and then reintroduced. Unless the reaction is severe, food challenges are performed at regular intervals until the food is either tolerated or it becomes clear that it will never be tolerated. A large majority of allergic reactions resolve themselves.[13] Allergies are not always diagnosed by these time-consuming, laborious methods, however. A number of unreliable tests, such as cytotoxic tests or skin tests, offer people quick, unfounded results.

The term *food allergy* is used loosely, even by many health providers, as a catchall term for any unexplained adverse reaction to foods. Thus a parent whose child has any kind of discomfort after eating—stomachache, headache, pain, rapid pulse rate, nausea, wheezing, hives, bronchial irritation, cough, or any other—may conclude that an allergy is responsible, when in fact it is something else entirely. Only careful, skilled testing can distinguish the many possibilities, and such testing is seldom done.

When parents conclude that their child has a food allergy, they stop serving the offending food. In so doing, they risk feeding the child an unbalanced diet, which could lead to nutrient deficiencies. Whenever a food is excluded from the diet, care must be taken to include other foods that offer the same nutrients as the omitted food contains.

Parents are advised to watch for signs of food dislikes and take them seriously: "Dislike of a food may be only a whim or fancy, but it should be regarded as significant until proven otherwise."[14] Although many cases of suspected allergies turn out to be something else, real allergies do exist. Don't prejudge, in any case. Test.

Food allergies cause illness and diagnosis can be difficult. Elimination diets can help pinpoint the cause.

Hyperactivity and Diet

In searching for explanations for a child's misbehavior, many people have looked to the kitchen. One such attempt is to blame food for the **hyperactivity syndrome.** Hyperactivity, one kind of **learning disability,** occurs in 5 to 10 percent of young school-age children—that is, in one or two in every classroom of 20 children. It can lead to academic failure and major behavior problems. Parents and teachers need to deal effectively with it wherever it appears, to avert the grief that can otherwise result.

elimination diet: a diet, used to diagnose food allergy, in which the suspected food is eliminated from and then reintroduced into the diet.

hyperactivity syndrome in children: a cluster of symptoms in which "the essential features are signs of developmentally inappropriate inattention, impulsivity, and hyperactivity." Other important features are onset before age seven, duration of six months or more, and proven absence of mental illness or mental retardation.[15] Other names associated with hyperactivity: attention deficit disorder, hyperkinesis, minimal brain damage, minimal brain dysfunction, minor cerebral dysfunction. Hyperactivity has nothing to do with autism. (A **syndrome** is a cluster of symptoms.)

learning disability: a defect in the ability to learn basic cognitive skills such as reading, writing, and mathematics; causes vary.

Table 12–5

Foods That Most Often Cause Immediate Hypersensitivity Reactions

Nuts	Peanuts
Eggs	Chicken
Milk	Fish
Soybeans	Shellfish
Wheat	Mollusks

Source: Information from F. M. Atkins, The basis of immediate hypersensitivity reactions to foods, *Nutrition Reviews* 41 (1983): 229–234.

In the average classroom of 20 children, aged five to eight or so, one or two will be hyperactive.

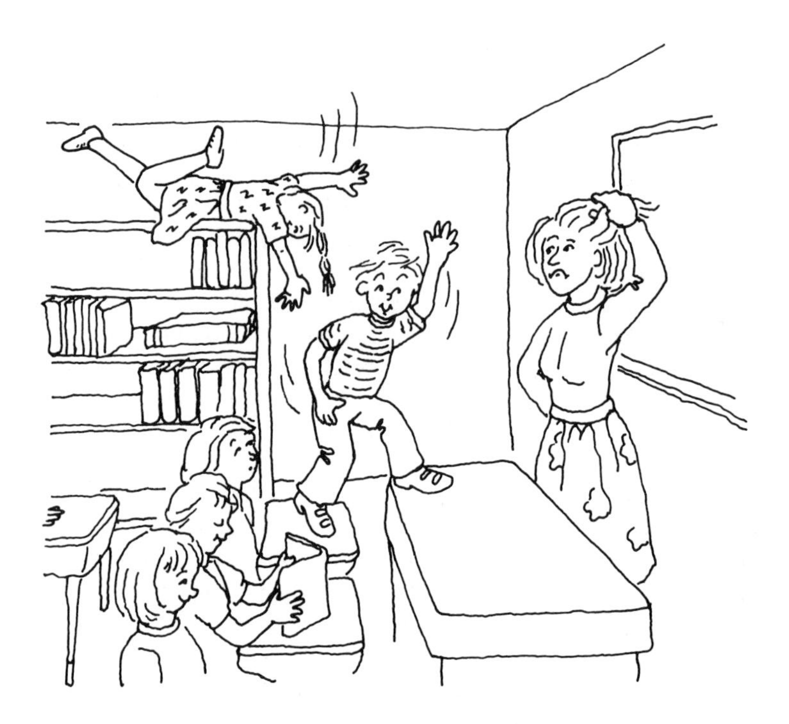

The idea that hyperactivity might be caused by diet became popular in 1973, when Dr. Benjamin Feingold proposed that hyperactive children suffer adverse reactions to the artificial flavors and colors in foods. He proposed that children be fed a diet free of all additives—which means, essentially, a diet prepared almost entirely from whole, unprocessed foods. However, when controlled, double-blind experiments with additive-containing and additive-free foods are conducted, the benefits of the Feingold diet do not materialize as they do in some individual family situations. In family situations in which the Feingold diet is introduced, diet is not the only thing that changes. Children receive special attention along with the special diet, and this may well have beneficial effects on their behavior. Both the children and their parents and teachers are likely to be influenced by the hope that the experiment will work—and by suggestibility, a factor that is difficult to rule out.[16]

The dietary approach to hyperactivity seems to work mostly by suggestion, if it works at all.[17] A child who has been deemed hyperactive "learns" that the food causes the hyperactive behavior. From now on the child and family are going to eat differently—no more junk foods, no more processed convenience foods, no more casual snacks. Foods will be prepared from scratch at home and eaten together. The whole family's lifestyle will change, and the child's behavior is expected to improve. It does improve—but in response to what? Not only are the family members eating differently, they are living differently, and the child is receiving more attention, more parental energy, and more structure than before. It is not the additive-free nature of the diet that works, but the changed lifestyle that the diet demands.[18]

One method physicians use to diagnose hyperactivity is to conduct a trial with stimulant drugs. If the child responds by calming down, then the drugs are used to help control the behavior problems. *In children who are responsive,* prescription medication is considered an integral part of treatment. Such treatment is accepted by the medical profession as a safe and effective means of treating hyperactivity in children. The most common side effects, insomnia and anorexia, usually disappear within a week or two.[19]

Understandably, many parents oppose the use of drugs to treat a behavior problem, especially when they believe a solution may be found by manipulating the diet. Diet is one aspect of a child's life over which parents feel they can have some control. If problems can be solved by adding carrots or deleting cookies, then parents are eager to give diet advice a try. The addition of whole foods and elimination of processed foods is sure to improve the diet. At least there is no harm in eliminating foods with artificial colors and flavors. Diet should be considered whenever a person's physical or mental health is less than optimal; caution is advised not to jump at appealing solutions that are unfounded and possibly harmful. If a wholesome diet elicits improved behavior, then obviously that is the treatment of choice.

Caffeine is often overlooked as a source of hyperactive behavior in children, but it is a matter of some concern to pediatricians. A 12-ounce cola beverage may contain as much as 50 milligrams of caffeine; two or more such beverages are equivalent in the body of a 60-pound child to the caffeine in 8 cups of coffee for a 175-pound man. Chocolate bars also contribute caffeine. Children who are troubled by sleeplessness, restlessness, and irregular heartbeats may need to control their caffeine consumption. (A table of caffeine contents of beverages and medications appears in the next chapter.) As long as such undeniably attractive temptations as cola beverages and candy bars surround children, barriers against their abuse have to be provided by adults until the children learn to control their own intakes.

Without any magical answers, parents still have to deal with excitable, rambunctious, and unruly children. Common sense says that all children misbehave at times. There are many normal, everyday causes of such behavior:

- Attempt to get attention.
- Lack of sleep.
- Overstimulation.
- Too much TV.
- Lack of exercise.

Together, these produce the **tension-fatigue syndrome,** which can be relieved by giving more consistent care to the child's welfare. It helps especially to insist on regular hours of sleep, regular mealtimes, and regular outdoor exercise.

tension-fatigue syndrome: apparent hyperactivity produced in a child by the combination of lack of sleep and overstimulation with anxiety.

Hyperactivity is not caused by poor nutrition, but may reflect genetics, poor management of the child, or other causes.

Looking Ahead

The childhood years are a parent's last chance to influence food choices. In addition to providing healthy foods, parents need to foster the development of healthy eating habits, by teaching children to like and select nutritious foods. Eatings habits help determine whether health develops positively or negatively.

To avoid obesity, train preschool children to "eat thin." Teach children to eat slowly, to pause and enjoy their table companions, and to stop eating when

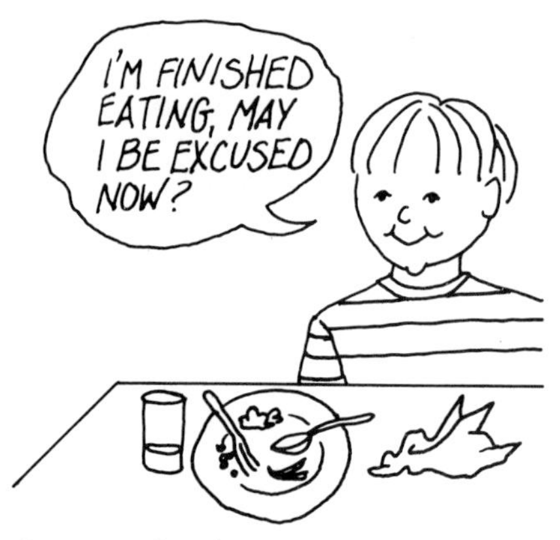

Stamp out the "clean your plate" dictum for all time.

they are full. Stamp out the "clean your plate" dictum for all time, and in its place learn to serve smaller portions that can be followed by additional servings, if needed. Allow children to determine their own limits—what, when, and how much to eat—within reason. Encourage physical activity on a daily basis to promote strong skeletal and muscular development and to establish habits that will undergird good health throughout life.

The child who is already obese needs careful handling. As in pregnancy, weight loss may easily have a harmful effect on growth in children. It is best that they be fed so as to maintain a constant weight while they grow. The object is to restrict the multiplication of fat cells while promoting normal lean body development. Thus children can "grow out" of their obesity.

Cardiovascular disease is another condition to prevent. Atherosclerosis begins in childhood, and many experts seem to agree that early childhood is the time to put practices into effect that until recently were recommended only for adults. Discourage snacking on high-fat, high-sugar, and high-salt foods, because it sets a pattern that favors the development of atherosclerosis and hypertension. Instead, follow recommendations like those of the *Dietary Guidelines for Americans,* emphasizing foods with high nutrient density.

As mentioned in Chapter 11, some nutrition experts suggest that children would be wise to follow a diet similar to that recommended for preventing heart disease in adults (Controversy 4)—a diet low in fat, saturated fat, and cholesterol, with polyunsaturated fat replacing some saturated fat. However, risks and benefits of such a diet for children have not been established, and the American Academy of Pediatrics advises *against* a fat-restricted diet in children under two. Regular screening of all children can determine what conditions each of them are likely to develop so that appropriate dietary and medical intervention can be implemented on an individual basis. (Figure 12–3 outlines the screening process.) Thus it would be advisable to feed the child of a parent with high blood pressure a diet relatively low in salt; the child of a parent with diabetes

Figure 12–3
Nutritional Screening of Children.

Source: From S. J. Fomon and coauthors, *Nutritional Disorders of Children: Prevention, Screening, and Followup,* DHHS publication no. (HSA) 76–5612 (Washington, D.C.: Government Printing Office), inside front cover.

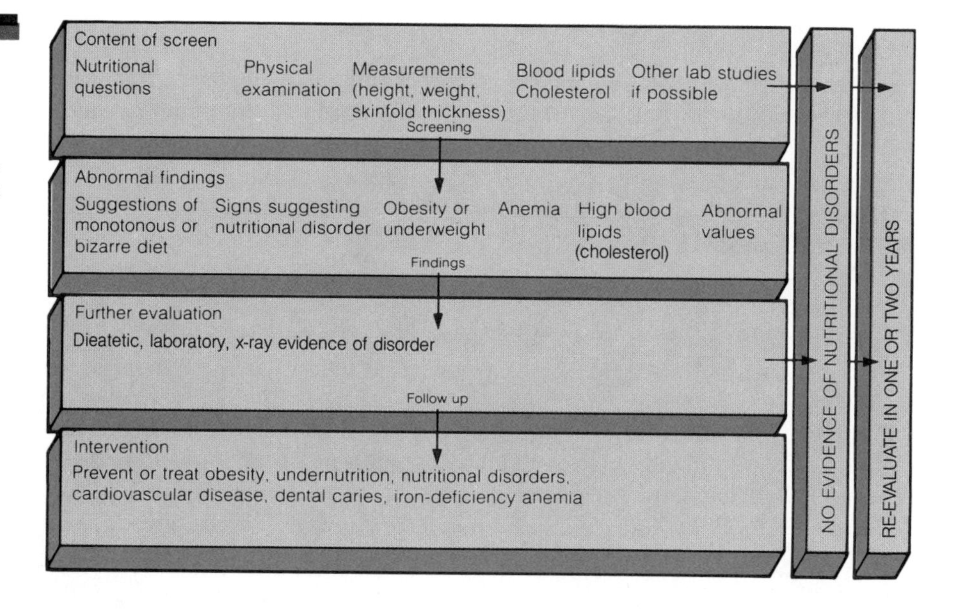

a diet high in complex carbohydrates; and the child of a parent with coronary artery disease a diet low in fat—especially saturated fat—and possibly low in cholesterol. In all these situations, the greatest success is likely to be achieved if the whole family, and not just the child, follows the recommended dietary guidelines.

Like atherosclerosis, osteoporosis is an adult disease that may reflect a person's childhood dietary habits. Milk consumption is encouraged during childhood primarily to provide the calcium needed for skeletal growth, but the benefits of young people's consuming calcium-rich foods reach far into the future. Frequent and adequate milk consumption throughout life encourages optimal bone density (within genetic limits, of course).[20] Bones grow not only in length, but also in density; bone density is the major determinant of osteoporotic fractures. High bone density maintains skeletal integrity and defends against bone loss in later life.

Poor dental health is another preventable condition. The measures recommended for its prevention center around two objectives. First, adequate nutrition is needed to help the mouth and teeth develop properly. This means providing an adequate diet, especially in terms of protein; calcium; vitamins A, C, and D; and fluoride. Where local water supplies are not fluoridated, direct application of fluoride to the teeth at intervals may be necessary. Second, it is important to restrict the supply of carbohydrate foods to the bacteria that cause tooth decay. This means brushing the teeth or rinsing the mouth with water after meals (especially meals high in carbohydrate), avoiding snacks that contain sticky carbohydrate, and dislodging persistent particles with dental floss.

It may be difficult to convince a young person to invest in tomorrow's health, but there is little question that prevention is the best treatment of obesity, cancer, atherosclerosis, osteoporosis, and dental caries. No doubt, developing healthful habits is easier than changing poor habits later.

Childhood nutrition lays the foundation for health in adulthood. Healthy eating habits learned in childhood can help forestall many lifestyle diseases of adulthood, including obesity, cardiovascular disease, cancer, osteoporosis, and dental caries.

The Teen Years

Few teenagers become interested in nutrition for its contribution to growth and health. Lessons (and misinformation) in nutrition attract teens if they relate to personal experiences (how diet can improve their lives now)—they crash diet in order to fit into a new bathing suit, avoid greasy foods in an effort to clear acne, or eat a large steak dinner in preparation for the big sporting event. The next few sections examine the nutrient needs and food intakes of adolescents.

Chapter 8 and Controversy 8 discuss fad diets. A box in this chapter describes the development and treatment of acne. Chapter 9 provides tips for the pregame meal.

Growth and Nutrient Needs

The fairly steady rate of growth throughout childhood increases rather abruptly and dramatically with the onset of **adolescence.**. Prior to adolescence, the dif-

adolescence: the period from the beginning of puberty until maturity.

acne: a chronic inflammation of the skin's follicles and oil-producing glands that involves the accumulation of sebum inside the ducts that surround hairs, usually associated with the maturation of young adults.

sebum: the skin's natural mixture of oils and waxes that helps keep skin and hair moist.

whitehead: a pimple caused by the plugging of an oil-gland duct with shed material from the duct lining.

cyst: an enlarged, deep pimple.

blackhead: an open lesion with an accumulation of the natural, dark pigment of the skin (not dirt) in its opening.

Acne

Most young people with **acne** are willing to go to considerable trouble and expense to find a remedy. But what is the remedy? To wash constantly? To sunbathe? To have the skin sanded? To take antibiotics? To spread vitamin A acid on the skin? To stop eating certain foods and drinking certain beverages? Or to try to find relief from stress? All of these approaches have been suggested, and each has helped some people in individual cases. But while advances are being made that give hope for the treatment of acne in the future, there is as yet no surefire way to get rid of it.

No one knows why some people get acne while others do not, but heredity plays a role—acne runs in families. The hormones of adolescence also play a role by increasing the activity of the glands in the skin. The skin's natural oil, **sebum,** is made in deep glands and is supposed to flow out through the tiny ducts around the hairs to the skin surface. In acne, the oily secretion is not brought to the surface of the skin.

Inside each of the ducts is a skinlike lining that regularly scales and flakes. The scales or flakes mix with the oil and then are pushed to the surface of the skin. At times, the scales stick together and form a plug, which may enlarge and weaken the duct, allowing oil and skin surface bacteria to leak into the surrounding skin. The oil and bacterial enzymes are irritating and cause redness, swelling, pus formation—and the beginning of a **whitehead,** or pimple. A **cyst** may be formed—a sort of enlarged, deep pimple. Or the skin may open above the plug, revealing an accumulation of dark skin pigments just below the surface—a **blackhead.**

Note that acne is not caused by the skin bacteria, although once the process has begun, they make it worse. Also note that the color of a blackhead is caused by skin pigments, not by dirt. Squeezing or picking at the lesions of acne in an attempt to remove their contents can cause more scars than the acne.

How, then, can acne be treated? Among the over-the-counter acne treatments, preparations that contain benzoyl peroxide are safe and effective. The remedies mentioned at the start are sometimes helpful, too. Careful washing helps remove skin-surface bacteria and oil and keeps the oil ducts open; surface treatment with antibiotics also helps control the bacteria. A cream or gel containing retinoic acid (a member of the vitamin A family) can help: retinoic acid loosens the plugs that form in the ducts, allowing the oil to flow again so that the ducts will not burst. But care is necessary, because the acid may burn the skin and even cause pimples to form, making the acne look worse rather than better at first.

Vitamin A supplements taken internally have no beneficial effect on acne, but they may cause the symptoms of vitamin A toxicity. The belief that vitamin A cures acne arises from the knowledge that it is needed for the health of the skin. Similar claims have been made for zinc because of its relation with vitamin A. (The interrelationship of zinc with vitamin A is described on p. 251.) As with all nutrients, however, vitamins and minerals promote health when enough are supplied; at pharmacological levels, some nutrients have therapeutic effects, but beyond that, they cause harm.

A topical acne medicine, Accutane, is made from vitamin A but is chemically different from over-the-counter vitamin A. Accutane is effective against the deep lesions of cystic acne. It is highly toxic, especially during growth, and causes serious birth defects in the infants of women who have taken it during their pregnancies. An effective form of contraception is advised beginning one month before and continuing until one month after Accutane's use. Another prescription treatment, a topical antibiotic lotion, works well, and may be safer than Accutane.

At the end of adolescence, when the acne has subsided, a surgical procedure known as **dermabrasion,** or skin planing, can remove the scars—in some cases. (Be sure to request a second opinion beforehand, and select a dermatologist or plastic surgeon with a reputation for skill in this procedure.)

Prevention of acne has long been sought. Among foods charged with aggravating acne are chocolate, cola beverages, fatty or greasy foods, milk, nuts, sugar, and foods or salt containing iodine. None of these foods has been shown to worsen acne, and two have been shown not to worsen it—chocolate and sugar.

Stress, with its accompanying hormonal secretions, clearly worsens acne. Vacations from school pressures help to bring acne relief. The sun, the beach, and swimming also help, perhaps because they are relaxing, and also because the sun's rays kill bacteria and water cleanses the skin.

One remedy always works: time. While waiting for acne to clear up, keep the symptoms under control by using preparations with benzoyl peroxide; even more important, prevent scarring by refraining from probing or picking at the skin. Also, keep a hopeful eye on the latest scientific developments.

dermabrasion: a technique used for removal of acne scars that involves planing the skin; it is a procedure that requires skill and one that works only on certain kinds of scars (*derm* means "skin"; *abrasion* means "sanding, planing").

puberty: the period of life in which a person becomes physically capable of reproduction.

ferences between female and male growth patterns are minimal; with the onset of **puberty,** differences become evident. For females, the adolescent growth spurt begins at 10 or 11 and reaches its peak at 12. In males, it begins at 12 or 13 and peaks at 14. Gender differences in the skeletal system, lean body mass, and fat stores become apparent during the adolescent growth spurt. In females, fat becomes a larger percentage of the total body weight, and in males, the lean body mass—muscle and bone—becomes much greater. This intensive growth period brings not only a dramatic increase in height and weight, but also hormonal changes that profoundly affect every organ of the body (including the brain) and that culminate in the emergence of physically mature adults within two or three years.

Tremendous individual variation occurs in teenagers' rates and patterns of growth. Growth charts used for children must be abandoned when the signs of puberty begin to appear. Chronological age is an inadequate indicator of development. The only way to be sure a teenager is growing normally is to compare his or her height and weight with previous measures taken at intervals and to note whether reasonably smooth progress is being made. Teenagers who want to know what they "should" weigh are best reassured that any of a wide range of weights is considered normal at this time in life.

premenstrual syndrome (PMS): a cluster of symptoms, including both physical and emotional pain, that some women experience prior to and during menstruation.

The rapid growth during adolescence is reflected in the high energy needs of this period. A rapidly growing, active boy of 15 may need 4000 calories or more a day just to maintain his weight. At the same age, girls have stopped growing, and a girl of 15 may need fewer than 2000 calories if she is not to become obese. Thus there is tremendous variation in the energy needs of adolescents.

Total nutrient needs are greater during adolescence than at any other time of life, with the exception of pregnancy and lactation. Again, iron deserves special mention. Iron needs are high during adolescence due to the onset of menstruation in females and to the great increase in lean body mass in males. These special needs augment the already high iron requirement created by a rapidly growing body. Other nutrients are also required in greater quantities during adolescence than in childhood. These nutrient requirements are either maintained or they diminish only slightly as the adolescent passes into adulthood.

Teenagers as a group do have nutritional problems. Nearly every nutrient can be found lacking in one or another group: iron in young women, calories in young men (especially blacks), vitamin A in young women (especially Hispanics), calcium, riboflavin, vitamin C, and even protein. The insidious problem of obesity becomes more apparent in adolescence and it often continues into adulthood, mostly in females, and especially in black females. Girls who become interested in nutrition may make choices that will benefit their health, or may become obsessed with weight control (see Controversy 9).

Growth and nutrient needs vary widely in the teen years. Nutrition problems of many kinds can occur.

Nutrition and the Menstrual Cycle

One of the many changes girls face as they become women is the onset of menstruation. The hormones that regulate the menstrual cycle are powerful, and they affect more than just the uterus and the ovaries. They alter the metabolic rate, glucose tolerance, appetite, food intake, mood, and behavior. Most women live easily with the cyclic rhythm of the menstrual cycle, but some are afflicted with physical and emotional pain prior to menstruation, a condition given the name **premenstrual syndrome,** or **PMS.**

All menstruating women can benefit from some recent findings on nutrition and the menstrual cycle. Many women just plain get hungry during the week or two before menstruation. Reliable research shows that two things happen during that time:

- Basal metabolic rate speeds up.[21]
- Appetite and calorie intake pick up.[22]

About 20 percent of the women in two studies indicated, when asked, that their appetites increased before menstruation,[23] but in fact most or all women may actually eat more during this time without being aware that they do. They report that they crave sweets, and when their food intakes are actually measured, they are seen to be eating an average of 500 calories a day more during the ten days prior to menstruation than during the ten days after—principally from carbohydrate.[24]

At least one application of these findings seems obvious at first glance. Many women attempt to restrict their calories, sometimes severely, in the effort to control their weight. During the two weeks following menstruation, they may find this relatively easy to do, but during the two weeks before the next menstruation, they may find it hard, because they are fighting a natural, hormone-governed increase in metabolic rate, appetite, and even craving for carbohydrate. Given the complex, sometimes guilt-ridden feelings about food that many women have (see Controversy 9), they are at a great disadvantage trying to fight these forces. Women need to know that the increased hunger and carbohydrate craving that precede menstruation are natural, probably universal biological phenomena, and not signs of their own incompetence, inadequacy, or neuroticism. Rather than attempt to restrict calorie intakes rigidly to some fixed amount throughout the month, any woman whose appetite is affected by the cyclic rhythm of her hormones would do better to relax and go with it: increase calories during the two weeks before menstruation, and reduce them during the two weeks after.

For the few women who suffer from physical pain before and during the menstrual period, it is important to know that it can have a wide variety of causes, some of which should clearly *not* be labeled PMS. Inflammation or infection of the lining of the uterus, a potentially dangerous condition, can cause symptoms like those ascribed to PMS—but a diagnosis and treatment are imperative. Muscular abnormalities of the uterus and its opening (the cervix) can cause cramping during menstruation; again, treatment depends on diagnosis. Once these causes are ruled out, cases remain that are, at least for the present, grouped together as PMS.

A woman suffering from PMS may complain of any or all of the following symptoms: cramps and aches in the abdomen; back pain; headaches; acne; swelling of face and limbs associated with water retention; food cravings, especially for sweets; abnormal thirst; pain and lumps in the breasts; diarrhea; and mood changes, including both nervousness and depression. Some researchers are attempting to define clusters of these symptoms, in hopes of assigning each cluster to a different cause.

Among the candidates for causes are abnormal secretion of prostaglandins (see Controversy 4); an altered secretion of the two major regulatory hormones associated with the menstrual cycle, estrogens and progesterone; an abnormality of the muscle tissue; emotional illness; or lack of exercise. Lack of exercise deserves attention because so many women lead sedentary lives. Many women find that taking up regular exercise greatly reduces menstrual discomfort, and for some, a brisk walk can relieve the symptom completely. Medical therapies can be useful in some cases of PMS.[25] For example, aspirin works by reducing prostaglandin action and is alone effective against the symptoms of PMS in many cases. An aspirin relative, ibuprofen, works even better.* Prescriptions of hormones seem to help in some cases (see box, "Oral Contraceptives"). Muscle relaxants relieve cramps. Physicians sometimes prescribe tranquilizers such as Valium (diazepam) to relax muscles. These seem to work, but they may do so by putting the woman out of touch with the problem rather than solving it; they also can cause a dangerous dependency.

Do emotional problems contribute to PMS? Researchers believe that at least some PMS may be psychological in origin, but it is hard to tell. After all, people are suggestible, and PMS is something of a fad. When women are expecting their periods, they may have learned to expect PMS. They may experience only

*Ibuprofen is sold under the names Advil, Motrin, Nuprin, and Rufen.

oral contraceptives: hormones taken in pill form to prevent conception.

Oral Contraceptives

About one in every five women in the United States uses **oral contraceptives.** Most use them, of course, to prevent unwanted pregnancy; some use them, as mentioned, to normalize their hormonal cycles and so relieve PMS. Do oral contraceptives affect women's nutrition? They have been in use only since the late 1950s, and so there have been only three decades in which to study them, but hundreds of studies have been conducted, and the answers are already clear enough to make some conclusions possible.

Oral contraceptives work by mimicking pregnancy—that is, by creating a hormonal climate similar to that of pregnancy. Because pregnancy imposes special nutritional needs on women, researchers wonder if nonpregnant women taking oral contraceptives might need to make special efforts to avoid deficiencies.

Oral contraceptives clearly do alter the blood concentrations of both vitamins and minerals in the body. For example, they depress blood concentrations of vitamin B_6, vitamin C, and zinc, while they raise blood concentrations of vitamin K, iron, and copper. At first glance this might seem to indicate that women using them are at risk for deficiency of the first six nutrients named, but have somehow increased their body stores of the last three. However, a closer look at the basis for these changes reveals that the changed blood concentrations may reflect a changed distribution of these nutrients within the body, and not a changed total body content.

Take vitamin A, for example. Its blood concentration rises, probably because the hormone progesterone impairs its storage in the liver. The body responds by destroying or excreting more of the vitamin than normal, and so the need for vitamin A may actually be raised by oral contraceptives. In contrast, iron's blood concentration also rises, but this is probably due to true conservation. Oral contraceptive use brings about both less blood loss in menstruation, and greater absorption of iron in the intestine.

Each nutrient responds differently to oral contraceptive use. There may be a real risk of deficiencies of riboflavin, vitamin B_6, folacin, vitamin B_{12}, and vitamin C. There seems to be no risk of vitamin E deficiency, and the need for vitamin K may actually be reduced. As for minerals, it seems that the body may conserve copper as it does iron; but may need more zinc.[26]

Users of oral contraceptives would be hard put to learn all these details, and should not be expected to do so. The general message that is clear from all of them is that, like all women, women using oral contraceptives should make the effort to eat adequate diets. If a woman becomes ill, she should seek diagnosis from a competent health care professional, and remind the professional that she takes oral contraceptives. If a deficiency is diagnosed, she should make every effort to improve her diet, and, if recommended, she should take a vitamin-mineral supplement that will provide RDA levels of a balanced assortment of nutrients.

One other item about oral contraceptives is noteworthy. They do increase the risk of clot formation in the blood vessels, and if a woman who uses them also smokes, her risk of heart attack and stroke rises dramatically.[27] No supplement will protect against these effects. To bring the risk back into line, the woman should first stop smoking, and then start exercising.

normal day-to-day fluctuations in sensation and mood, but they may think, wrongly, that they are worse at that time of the month than at other times.

In some cases, it seems apparent that psychological factors do contribute to PMS. Traditional housewives suffer more PMS, as well as other psychological disorders such as depression, than do women who work outside the home. Women of certain religious groups also have more problems with PMS. On the other hand, both exercise and orgasm sometimes relieve PMS. Perhaps in those cases the problem is simply one of muscle cramping. As for nutrition-related causes, this chapter devotes a box ("Nutrition and Premenstrual Syndrome") to them, because they often lead people to consider taking supplements.

One thing seems clear: the woman with PMS should look to her total lifestyle, diet being only one part of it. She may not have complete control over her condition, but many aspects of her lifestyle *are* under her control. If she has any nutrient deficiencies, then she isn't doing all she can to help herself be well. She should also be sure to get adequate sleep. Exercise helps, too; she should exercise regularly. She should be sensible about her intakes of sugar, caffeine, salt, alcohol, and any other abusable substances. If she has reason to think her nutrient intakes are inadequate and she cannot rectify them by eating foods, then she should fall back on a daily supplement for a while. But (see Controversy 6 and, for vitamin B_6, Chapter 6) she should avoid megadoses and stay with the moderate amounts available in an ordinary multivitamin-mineral supplement. She should watch out for snake-oil salespeople selling PMS "cures"—there are a lot of them out there.

The menstrual cycle affects women's metabolism and appetites in a cyclic fashion. Some women have the uncomfortable symptoms associated with the cycle—so-called premenstrual syndrome (PMS), which is probably a diverse set of conditions with no single cause. A sound diet without extremes is part of the recommended lifestyle to minimize PMS.

Teenage Pregnancy

Teenage pregnancy presents a special case of nutrient needs. Even when a teenage girl is not pregnant, she is hard put to meet her own nutrient needs at this time of maximal growth. Nourishing a growing fetus adds to her burden.

The high nutrient requirements of the rapidly growing young teenager compete with those of the rapidly growing fetus. Young teenagers (13 to 16 years old) are encouraged to gain approximately 35 pounds during pregnancy in order to deliver a baby of optimal birthweight. Young teenagers who gain the same amount of weight during pregnancy (24 pounds) as older teens and adults (17 to 25 years old) have smaller newborns. As discussed in the previous chapter, small newborns have a high risk of disease and death.

Unfortunately, little information is available on the specific nutrient needs of pregnant adolescents. Estimates of these needs are usually made by adding the increment for the pregnant adult woman to the RDA for the nonpregnant teenager 15 to 18 years of age. Figure 12–4 shows that a pregnant teenager's needs for many nutrients double, while her calorie allowance increases less. In the case of a girl who begins pregnancy with inadequate nutrient stores or who lacks the education, resources, and support she needs, these problems are compounded.

Nutrition and Premenstrual Syndrome

As the accompanying text made clear, PMS has many possible causes, nutrition being only one among them. Among nutrition possibilities, one is sodium and water retention caused by the hormones that dominate the premenstrual weeks. Some doctors prescribe diuretics to get rid of the excess sodium and water, and some researchers have reported that diuretics relieve all PMS symptoms except painful breasts; others, though, have tried to confirm this finding and failed. Possibly the placebo effect has confounded the work: it is extraordinarily powerful in PMS, so much so that even an agent that appears to relieve PMS symptoms for several months in a row may not in reality be a cure for the symptoms.[28] Diuretic therapy has been criticized on the basis that it may cause losses of needed minerals such as potassium or magnesium, possibly making PMS symptoms worse. Also, if women *do* retain sodium and water just before menstruation, it may be a normal and desirable state. In pregnancy, the accumulation of a certain amount of fluids is supposed to occur and should not be medically "corrected."[29]

Another nutrient that may have some connection with PMS is magnesium. When magnesium status was studied in "normal" and PMS subjects, the levels of this mineral in the red blood cells were found to be lower in the PMS group.[30] The naive reader might jump to the conclusion that people with PMS need more magnesium, but this may not be the case at all. The subjects' diets weren't studied, so it is impossible to tell whether they had a dietary deficiency, were absorbing less, or were excreting more magnesium. In fact, it is possible that the women's total body contents of magnesium hadn't changed but that there had been a shift of magnesium from the red blood cells into some other body compartment. Red blood cells, like all cells, "decide" what their contents should be; that is, they actively take in or reject available substances in response to signals from elsewhere—hormones, for example. The PMS group might have too much or too litle of some other substance, and this difference might cause their red blood cells to take up less magnesium. Clearly, on the basis of the one finding, it is impossible to say whether people with PMS need more magnesium or less, or more or less of something else.

In these studies, the researchers measured inside-the-body indicators of nutrition status in PMS sufferers versus those in other women. Other research has involved simply trying different agents and asking the women by questionnaire how they felt in response. One nutrient researched in this fashion has been vitamin B_6.

The logic of ascribing PMS to a vitamin B_6 deficiency is that women with PMS may have abnormal levels of hormones that regulate the menstrual cycle—hormones that require vitamin B_6 for their action. One of the symptoms of PMS is depression, a disorder of mood that many people, both male and female, experience under a wide variety of conditions and in many different physical and mental disorders. Vitamin B_6 deficiency has been implicated as one of many possible causes of depression, too.[31]

Trials of vitamin B_6 in PMS have had mixed results, at best. Typical is one study in which the researchers attempted to use vitamin B_6 to relieve premenstrual depression and found a dramatic positive response in only 1 of 13 women and a slight positive response in 4—balanced by a positive response in 5 women on placebo medication, no response in 2, and a strong *negative* response in 1![32]

We might conclude from this that vitamin B_6 is not effective in PMS, but it is also possible to conclude that it may occasionally be just what is needed—witness the one woman who did respond positively. Confirming this, another pair of researchers tested a particular woman who claimed to be responsive to vitamin B_6. They gave her the vitamin (50 mg/day) and a placebo in alternate months for six months without telling her and also without knowing, themselves, which was which until the end of the study (a double-blind experiment). She experienced relief from her symptoms, consistently with the vitamin and not with the placebo, showing clearly that in her case PMS was related to vitamin B_6.[33] It is possible that "the cause" of PMS is not the same in all women. For some women, a relative or absolute vitamin B_6 deficiency may aggravate or even cause PMS, whereas for others, it might have no relation to the syndrome.

Note that the effective dose mentioned above was 50 mg a day. No need exists for megadoses of vitamin B_6, and the hazards associated with such doses are well documented (p. 200). Vitamin E deficiency is another candidate for contributor to PMS, and one creditable attempt has demonstrated that vitamin E has some effectiveness in relieving one symptom often experienced in PMS—sore breasts. The research involved 75 women; it was a double-blind, placebo-controlled study; and its results suggested that vitamin E (300 IU) brought relief, while the placebo did not.[34] However, some women *without* PMS also have sore breasts that can sometimes be relieved by vitamin E.[35] Possibly the correct logic is that vitamin E deficiency can cause sore breasts and the menstrual cycle can make them worse, but not that vitamin E deficiency causes PMS.

Vitamin A deficiency, too, has been blamed for PMS. Vitamin A helped a woman once in 1947, and occasional other such reports have appeared since then. Surely, though, the past 40 years would have been enough time to confirm, if it were so, that vitamin A deficiency was the cause of PMS, or that vitamin A megadoses would cure it. Attempts to demonstrate these possibilities have failed, and no recommendations regarding vitamin A should be made on the basis of evidence collected to date.[36]

Before we can really know what to recommend to women who suffer with PMS, several kinds of studies will have to be done. One type of study will have to answer the question, How do the diets of women with PMS differ from those of women unaffected by PMS? One report suggests that women with PMS eat more refined sugar and salt, and less of several nutrients, than other women—in other words, that they tend to choose foods of lower nutrient density and have lower intakes of B vitamins, iron, and zinc as a consequence.[37] However, the study may be biased because its chief author is employed by a company that sells nutrient supplements. Without several more such studies, carefully performed by a variety of independent investigators, we cannot really know what the typical nutrition status of PMS women is. It seems far too early for any woman who thinks she suffers from PMS to leap to the conclusion that she needs a particular supplement. She had better see a competent health care provider and find out what the real possibilities are.

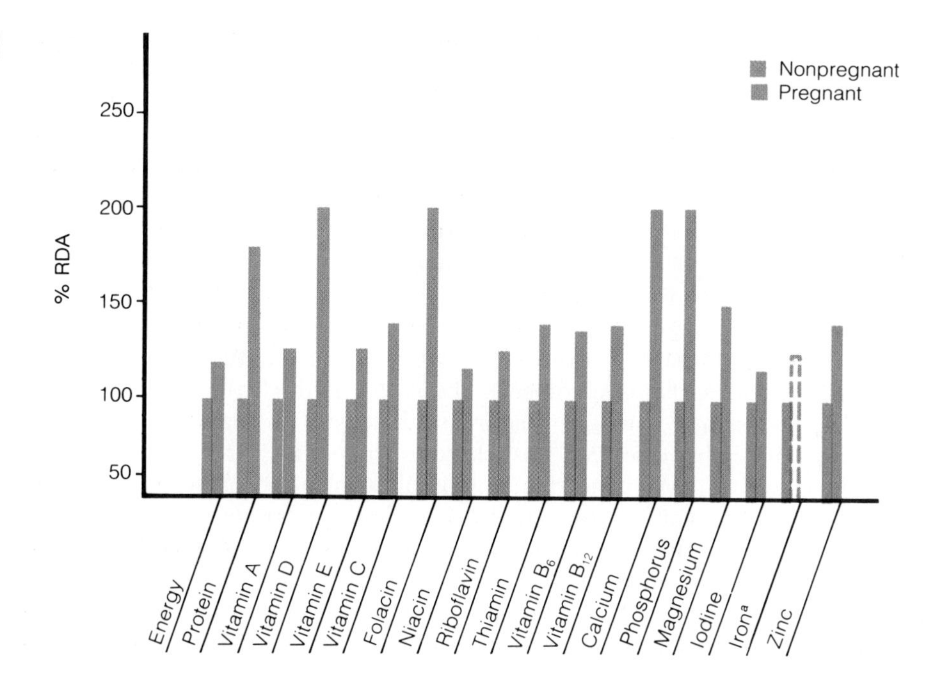

Figure 12–4
Comparison of the Nutrient Needs of a 15-Year Old Pregnant Girl with Those of a 23-Year-Old Nonpregnant Woman.

[a]The pregnant woman may need to take an iron supplement

The complications of pregnancy and the acute and long-lasting consequences of poor nutrition are discussed in Chapter 11. Complications are common in pregnant teenagers, with infant mortality 30 percent greater and maternal mortality 40 percent greater than for mothers who are in their next decade of life. Pregnancy-induced hypertension occurs in about one out of every five pregnant girls under the age of 15. If one pregnancy is followed by another, the stage is set for kidney damage that may be irreversible.

Teenage pregnancy is common. About one out of every five babies is born to a teenager, and more than a tenth of these mothers are 15 or younger. Emphasis on preparing adolescents for future pregnancy is needed in public schools and public health programs. Faced with her parents' and classmates' often insensitive reactions, a pregnant girl is likely to wind up alone, with little or no money to buy food and no motivation to seek prenatal care. She urgently needs programs addressed to all her problems, including medical attention, nutrition guidance, emotional support, and continued schooling. A model program for giving nutritional help to teenage mothers, among others, is the WIC (Women's, Infants' and Children's) program, a federally funded program that provides nutrition information and low-cost nutritious foods to low-income pregnant women and their children.

Pregnancy imposes tremendous nutrient needs on a growing teenaged girl. Support of all kinds, including nutrition support, is needed.

Eating Patterns and Food Choices

Teenagers are not fed; they eat. For the first time in their lives, they assume primary responsibility for their own food intakes. Teenagers come and go as they choose and eat what they want when they have time. With a multitude of after-school, social, and job activities, they almost inevitably fall into irregular eating habits. The adult becomes a gatekeeper, controlling the availability, but not the consumption, of food in the teenager's environment. The adult can't nag, scold, or pressure teenagers into eating, because teens typically turn a deaf ear to coercion, and often to persuasion. To "feed" effectively, the gatekeeper must make every effort to allow these young people independence while providing a physical environment that favors healthy development and an emotional climate that encourages adaptive choices.

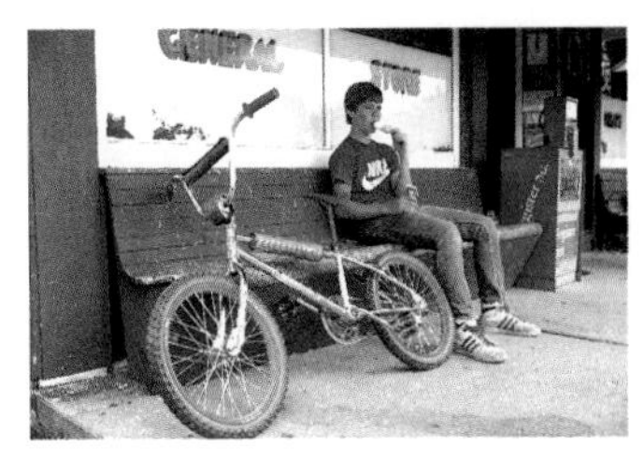

Teenagers often grab snacks on the run.

As with younger children, a wise maneuver is to provide access to nutritious and economical energy foods that are low in sugar and fat at home. The snacker—and a well-established characteristic of teenagers is that they are snackers—who finds only nutritious foods around the house is well provided for.

On the average, about a fourth of teenagers' total daily food energy intake comes from snacks. Their irregular schedules may worry adults who think teenagers are feeding themselves poorly, but usually the snacks they eat are fairly nutritious. They receive substantial amounts of protein, thiamin, riboflavin, vitamin B_6, magnesium, zinc, and even calcium (if they snack on dairy products). The nutrients they most often fail to obtain are vitamin A and folacin. Protein usually need not be stressed, but many teenagers need to be encouraged to consume more dairy products (for calcium) and more vegetables (for vitamin A and folacin).

For more on snacks and snackers, see Chapter 9's Food Feature.

Inevitably, teenagers will do a lot of eating away from home. There, as well as at home, their nutritional welfare can be favored or hindered by the choices they make. A lunch of a hamburger, a chocolate shake, and french fries supplies nutrients in the amounts shown in Table 12–6, at a calorie cost of 780. Teenagers consuming such fast food meals regularly risk overconsumption of fat, sodium, and calories.

This is not to say that fast foods have no place in the teen diet. For the most part, they contribute substantial percentages of recommended intakes at a calorie cost many teenagers can afford. Depending on how they adjust their breakfast and dinner choices, teenagers may meet their nutritional needs more than adequately with this sort of lunch. They need only select fruits and vegetables (for folacin and vitamins A and C), good fiber sources, and more good iron and zinc sources at their other meals.

The nutritive value of selected fast foods is presented in Appendix A.

The teenager's iron needs are a special problem, caused by several factors. In addition to the teenager's burgeoning iron needs, other factors are the lack of iron in traditional snack foods, the overemphasis on dairy products by some teenagers, the adoption of a vegetarian diet, and the low contribution made by fast foods to iron intakes. A National Academy of Sciences committee, writing on this special problem, finds it doubtful that long-term administration of iron tablets is practical and advises against the measure of fortifying snacks and other foods with iron. Instead, the committee recommends that physicians and clinics screen all teenagers for low levels of iron in the blood. Their report stresses that the best dietary source of absorbable iron is meats of all varieties, a point to stress in the nutrition education of teenagers.[38]

Another problem nutrient for teenagers is calcium. The requirement for calcium reaches its peak during these years. Unfortunately, many teens reject milk as a "child's drink" and opt instead for soft drinks with their lunches, dinners, and snacks. As might be expected, the more soft drinks teenagers drink, the less likely they are to meet their RDA for calcium.[39]

Table 12–6

Nutrients in a Hamburger, Chocolate Shake, and Fries

Nutrient	% of RDA[a]
Protein	45
Calcium	48
Iron	21
Zinc	25
Vitamin A	13
Thiamin	33
Riboflavin	38
Niacin	36
Folacin	15
Vitamin C	28

[a]RDA for an 18-year-old young man, except for iron, where the RDA for a young woman is used.

Teenagers are intensely involved in day-to-day life with their peers and in preparation for their future lives as adults. It is a time of experimenting with "adult" behaviors. Social pressures thrust choices at them: whether to drink alcohol, to drink coffee, to smoke marijuana or cigarettes, to experiment with cocaine, to practice birth control, to starve their bodies to meet extreme ideals of slimness. Each of these practices influences nutrition and is discussed elsewhere. Alcohol's effects on nutrition are described in Controversy 12; the effects of other drugs are discussed in Chapter 13; and eating disorders are the subject of Controversy 9.

Peer pressure and time pressures influence teens' nutrition. Teens determine their own food intakes, to a great extent, and the snacks they choose make a difference to their nutrition status. Among problem nutrients in the teen years are iron and calcium.

Food Feature

Mealtimes with Children

It is desirable for children to learn to like nutritious foods in all the food groups. With one exception, this liking usually develops naturally. The exception is vegetables, which young children frequently dislike and refuse. Even a tiny serving of spinach, cooked carrots, or squash may elicit an expression that registers the utmost in negative feelings (as well as great pride in the ability to make an ugly face). Since most youngsters need to eat more vegetables, the next few paragraphs are addressed to this problem.

Try to remember how you felt when first offered a cup of vegetable soup, a serving of runny spinach, or a pile of peas and carrots. If the soup burned your tongue, it may have been years before you were willing to try it again. As for the spinach, it was suspiciously murky looking. (Who could tell what might be lurking in that dark, stringy stuff?) The peas and carrots troubled your sense of order. Before you could eat them, you felt compelled to sort the peas onto one side of the plate and the carrots onto the other. Then you had to separate, into a reject pile, all those that got mashed in the process or contaminated with gravy from the mashed potatoes. Only then might you be willing to eat the intact, clean peas and carrots one by one—perhaps with your fingers, since the peas, especially, kept rolling off the fork.

Why children respond in this way to foods that look off or messy to them is a matter for conjecture. Parents need only be aware that this is how many children feel and then honor these feelings. Researchers attempting to explain children's food preferences are met with contradictions. Children describe liking colorful foods, yet vegetables are most often rejected, and brown peanut butter and white potatoes, apple wedges, and bread are among their favorites. Raw vegetables are better accepted than cooked ones, so it is wise to offer vegetables that are raw or slightly undercooked and crunchy, bright in color, served separately, and easy to eat. They should be warm, not hot, because a child's mouth is much more sensitive than an adult's. The flavor should be mild, and smooth foods such as mashed potatoes or pea soup should have no lumps in them (a child wonders, with some disgust, what the lumps might be). Irrational as the fear of strangeness may seem, the parent must realize that it is practically universal among children and often does have a biological basis. A child has more taste buds than an adult and they are more sensitive. Strong flavors are repulsive to them.

When feeding children, parents must always be alert to the dangers of choking. A choking child is a silent child—an adult should be present whenever a child is eating. Encouraging the child to sit when eating is also a good practice. The possibility of choking is more likely when a child is running or falling. Round foods such as grapes, nuts, hard candies, and hotdog pieces are difficult to control in a mouth with few teeth and can easily become lodged in the small opening of a child's trachea. Other potentially dangerous foods include tough meat, popcorn, and chips.

Wise parents allow children to help make the family's choices, including sometimes giving them the right to refuse food—at the same time, of course, sensibly preventing them from dominating the family. Allowing children to help

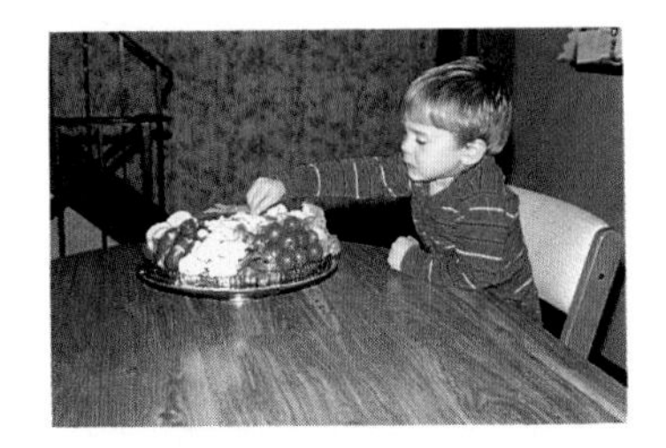

Children prefer vegetables that are crunchy, attractive in color and shape, and easy to eat.

plan and prepare the family's meals provides enjoyable learning experiences that encourage children to eat the foods they have prepared. Vegetables are pretty, especially when fresh, and provide opportunities to learn about color, about growing things and their seeds, about shapes and textures—all of which are fascinating to young children. Measuring, stirring, decorating, cutting, and arranging vegetables are skills even a young child can practice with enjoyment and pride.

Before sitting down to eat, small children should be helped to wash their hands and faces thoroughly. Ideally, outdoor playtime will have preceded the meal. If fun and games *follow* the meal, children are likely to hurry out to play, leaving food on their plates that they were hungry for and would otherwise have eaten.

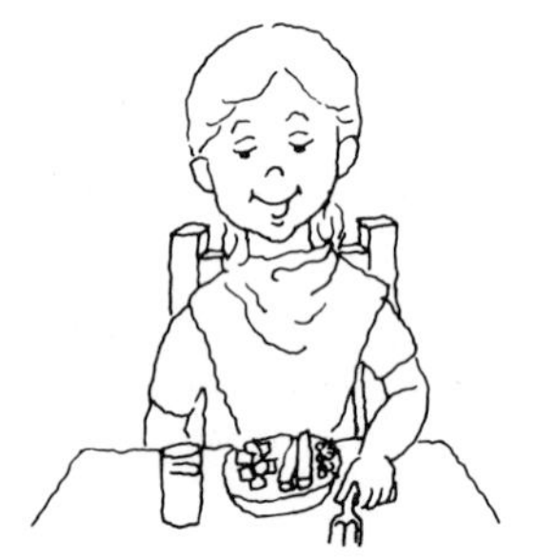

Little children like to eat small servings of food.

Little children like to eat at little tables and to be served little portions of food. Teaching children how to serve themselves the quantity they will eat minimizes waste. Parents need to remember that food is wasted whether it is dumped in the garbage or stored as excess fat on the child. Never force children to clean their plates. This practice can lead to behaviors that encourage obesity. Instead, allowing children to stop eating when they are full encourages them to listen to their bodies. The remaining food can be recycled as leftovers for another meal or as food for the family pet. One word of caution is in order: children who are too full to eat their dinner must also be too full to eat dessert.

Children like to eat with other children and have been observed to stay at the table longer and eat much more when in the company of their peers. Children are also more likely to eat nonpreferred foods when their peers are eating those foods. Eating is fun. It is healthy to look forward to and enjoy meals.

When introducing new foods at the table, parents are advised to offer them one at a time—and only a small amount at first. The more often a food is presented to a young child, the more likely the child will like that food. Whenever possible, the new food should be presented at the beginning of the meal, when the child is hungry. Offer the new food, and allow the child to make the decision. Never make an issue of food acceptance, not even to reward it. Rewards deliver the wrong messages. For example, if parents say, "When you finish eating your spinach, you will be allowed to watch television," then children learn that they must work to earn the reward. In this case, the work is spinach, and if it is work, it must not be desirable. Sometimes parents use foods as rewards to train their children to perform specific tasks: "When you finish putting your toys away, you will be allowed to eat ice cream." In this case, the child learns to give ice cream an enhanced preference.

Parents may find that their children often snack so much that they are not hungry at mealtimes. Some parents find they can live with the philosophy not of teaching children *not* to snack, but on teaching them *how* to snack. Provide snacks that are as nutritious as the foods served at mealtime. Snacks can even be mealtime foods that are served individually over time, instead of all at once on one plate. When providing snacks to children, a smart parent thinks of the four food groups and offers pieces of cheese, tangerine slices, carrot sticks, and peanut butter on whole-wheat crackers. Milk and water are appropriate beverages at snack time. Sweet drinks, including fruit juices, contribute to problems of dental caries and obesity. Snacks need to be easy to prepare and readily available to children. This is particularly important to children who return home after school without parental supervision.

A bright, unhurried atmosphere free of conflict is conducive to good appetite. Parents who serve meals in a relaxed and casual manner, without anxiety, provide the climate in which a child's negative emotions will be minimized. Conflicts can be promoted by unaware parents, even if they have the best of intentions. Parents who beg, cajole, and demand their child to eat deny the child an opportunity to develop self-control. Instead, the child enters a battle that takes on more importance than hunger. The power struggle almost invariably results in a confirmed pattern of resistance and a permanently closed mind on the child's part. Mealtimes can be nightmarish for the child who is struggling with personal and parental problems. If, as a child sits down to the table, a barrage of accusations are shouted—"Your hands are filthy . . . your report card . . . and clean your plate! Your mother cooked that food!"—mealtimes may be unbearable. The stomach may recoil, because the body as well as the mind reacts to stress of this kind.

In an effort to practice these many tips, parents may overlook perhaps the single most important influence on their child's food habits—themselves. Parents who don't eat carrots shouldn't be surprised when their child refuses to eat carrots. Likewise, parents who comment on the odor of brussels sprouts do not convince a child that those vegetables should be eaten. Much of the learning a child accomplishes is through imitation. By setting an example, parents can show children how to enjoy nutritious foods.

At each age, food can be served and enjoyed in the context of encouraging emotional as well as physical growth. If the beginnings are right, children will grow without the kind of conflict and confusion over food that can lead to nutrition problems. In the interest of promoting both a positive self-concept and a positive attitude toward food, it is important for parents to help their children remember that they are good kids. What they *do* may sometimes be unacceptable; but what they *are,* on the inside, are normal, healthy, growing, fine human beings.

shopping list:

small plates, cups, forks, spoons
bright-colored vegetables
booster seat or small table and chair

Notes

1. G. Wyshak and R. E. Frisch, Evidence for a secular trend in age of menarche, *New England Journal of Medicine* 306 (1982): 1033–1035, as cited by R. E. Frisch, Body fat, menarche, and reproductive ability, *Seminars in Reproductive Endocrinology* 3 (1985): 45–54.
2. D. Sinclair, *Human Growth after Birth,* 4th ed. (Oxford, England: Oxford University Press, 1985), pp. 28–31, 163.
3. *Iron Nutrition Revisited—Infancy, Childhood, Adolescence,* report of the 82d Ross Conference on Pediatric Research (Columbus, Ohio: Ross Laboratories, 1981), p. 1.
4. D. M. Tucker and H. H. Sandstead, Body iron stores and cortical arousal, in *Iron Deficiency: Brain Biochemistry and Behavior,* eds. E. Pollitt and R. L. Leibel (New York: Raven, 1982), pp. 161–182; Iron deficiency and brain proteins, *Nutrition Reviews* 45 (1987): 317–319.
5. R. L. Leibel, Behavioral and biochemical correlates of iron deficiency: A review, *Journal of the American Dietetic Association* 71 (1977): 399–404.
6. E. Pollitt, R. Leibel, and D. Greenfield, Brief fasting, stress and cognition in children, *American Journal of Clinical Nutrition* 34 (1981): 1526–1533.
7. These figures were obtained from the *Journal of the American Dietetic Association* 80 (1982): 591, 594. A complete discussion of lead and other contaminants in foods is found in E. N. Whitney, E. M. N. Hamilton, and M. A. Boyle, *Understanding Nutrition,* 4th ed. (St. Paul, Minn.: West, 1984), pp. 461–467.
8. H. R. Armstrong and D. B. Root, Managing a lean NET program, *Community Nutritionist* 2 (1983): 8–10.
9. W. H. Dietz, Jr., and S. L. Gortmaker, Do we fatten our children at the television set? Obesity and television viewing in children and adolescents, *Pediatrics* 75 (1985): 807–812.
10. S. L. Taylor, Food allergy: The enigma and some potential solutions, *Journal of Food Protection* 43 (1980): 300–306.
11. C. D. May, Food allergy: Perspective, principles, practical management, *Nutrition Today,* November/December 1980, pp. 28–31.
12. R. L. Lee, Environmental hypersensitivity: Would we really accept

the results of sound research? *Canadian Medical Association Journal* 134 (1986): 1333–1336.
13. S. A. Bock, The natural history of adverse reactions to foods in young children, an address presented at the American Dietetic Association 70th annual meeting, 19 October 1987, in Atlanta, Georgia.
14. V. J. Fontana and F. Moreno-Pagan, Allergy and diet, in *Modern Nutrition in Health and Disease,* eds. R. S. Goodhart and M. E. Shils, 6th ed. (Philadelphia: Lea and Febiger, 1980), 1071–1081.
15. American Psychiatric Association, *Diagnostic and Statistical Manual of Mental Disorders,* 3d ed. (Washington, D.C.: American Psychiatric Association, 1980), p. 41.
16. National Advisory Committee on Hyperkinesis and Food Additives, *Final Report to the Nutrition Foundation,* (New York: Nutrition Foundation, Inc., 1980).
17. National Advisory Committee, 1980; National Institutes of Health Consensus Development Panel, Consensus development conference statement: Defined diets and childhood hyperactivity, *American Journal of Clinical Nutrition* 37 (1983): 161–165.
18. In 1982, a review panel was assembled by the National Institutes of Health consisting of laypersons, biomedical researchers, pediatricians, nutritionists, immunologists, allergists, clinical pharmacologists, psychiatrists, behaviorists, geneticists, educators, epidemiologists, biostatisticians, environmental health specialists, and lawyers, "all relevant," they said, "to a study of childhood hyperactivity." Defined diets and childhood hyperactivity, *Journal of the American Medical Association* 248 (1982): 290–292.
19. L. Eisenberg, Clinical use of stimulant drugs in children, *Pediatrics* 49 (1972): 709–715.
20. R. B. Sandler and coauthors, Postmenopausal bone density and milk consumption in childhood and adolescence, *American Journal of Clinical Nutrition* 42 (1985): 270–274.
21. S. J. Solomon, M. S. Kurzer, and D. H. Calloway, Menstrual cycle and basal metabolic rate in women, *American Journal of Clinical Nutrition* 36 (1982): 611–616.
22. S. P. Dalvit, The effect of the menstrual cycle on patterns of food intake, *American Journal of Clinical Nutrition* 34 (1981): 1811–1815.
23. J. H. Morton and coauthors, A clinical study of premenstrual tension, *American Journal of Obstetrics and Gynecology* 65 (1953): 1182–1191; H. Sutherland and I. Stewart, A critical analysis of the premenstrual syndrome, *Lancet* 1 (1965): 1180–1183, as cited by D. Y. Jones and S. K. Kumanyika, Premenstrual syndrome: A review of possible dietary influences, *Journal of the Canadian Dietetic Association* 44 (1983): 194–203.
24. S. P. Dalvit-McPhillips, The effect of the human menstrual cycle on nutrient intake, *Physiology and Behavior* 31 (1983): 209–212.
25. Emotional problems, Chapter 4 in F. S. Sizer and E. N. Whitney, *Life Choices: Health Concepts and Strategies* (St. Paul, Minn.: West, 1988), pp. 88–89.
26. J. L. Webb, Nutritional effects of oral contraceptive use: A review, *Journal of Reproductive Medicine* 25 (October 1980): 150–156.
27. K. C. Dale, Facts: Some hazards of cigarette smoking, *ACSH News and Views,* May/June 1982, p. 10.
28. "There is a very striking placebo effect in this disorder. Symptoms often disappear during a woman's first month on sugar pills," but gradually return over the next four to five months. R. L. Reid, as quoted by E. R. Gonzalez, Premenstrual syndrome, an ancient woe deserving of modern scrutiny (Medical News), *Journal of the American Medical Association* 245 (1981): 1393–1396.
29. Jones and Kumanyika, 1983.
30. G. E. Abraham and M. M. Lubran, Serum and red cell magnesium levels in patients with premenstrual tension, *American Journal of Clinical Nutrition* 34 (1981): 2364–2366.
31. C. S. Russ and coauthors, Vitamin B_6 status of depressed and obsessive-compulsive patients, *Nutrition Reports International* 27 (1983): 867–873.
32. J. Stokes and J. Mendels, Pyridoxine and premenstrual tension (letter to the editor), *Lancet* 1 (1972): 1177–1178.
33. J. A. Mattes and D. Martin, Pyridoxine in premenstrual tension, *Human Nutrition: Applied Nutrition* 36A (1982): 131–133.
34. R. S. London and coauthors, The effect of alpha-tocopherol on premenstrual symptomatology, a double-blind study, *Journal of the American College of Nutrition* 2 (1983): 115–122.
35. E. R. Gonzalez, Vitamin E relieves most cystic breast disease; may alter lipids, hormones (Medical News), *Journal of the American Medical Association* 244 (1980): 1077–1078.
36. R. L. Reid and S. S. C. Yen, Premenstrual syndrome, *American Journal of Obstetrics and Gynecology* 139 (1981): 85–104.
37. G. S. Goei, J. L. Ralston, and G. E. Abraham, Dietary patterns of patients with premenstrual tension, *Journal of Applied Nutrition* 34 (1982): 4–11.
38. National Academy of Sciences, Food and Nutrition Board, Committee on Nutrition of the Mother and Preschool Child, *Iron Nutriture in Adolescence,* DHHS publication no. (HSA) 77–5100, 1977.
39. P. M. Guenther, Beverages in the diets of American teenagers, *Journal of the American Dietetic Association* 86 (1986): 493–499.

Alcohol and Nutrition

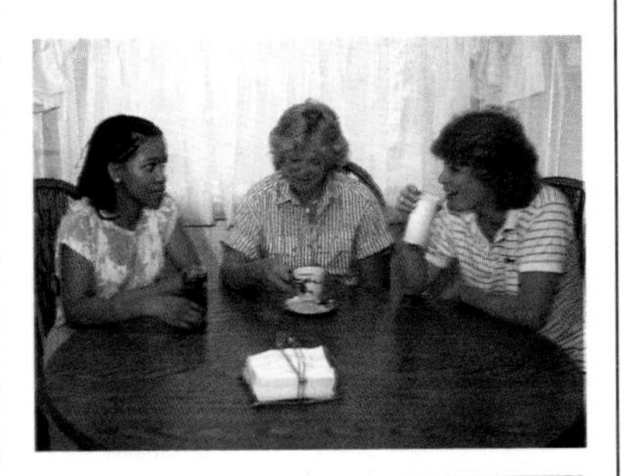

All beverages ease conversation, with or without alcohol.

Everything we do throughout our lives affects our bodies. Some of the effects are temporary: wounds heal, toxins are rendered inert and are excreted, infections are resisted and overcome. But these and other episodes usually leave traces that do not completely disappear.

As a person grows older, the effects of habits and experiences accumulate. While a single night's banquet may leave but a fraction of an ounce of extra fat on the body, a lifetime of overindulgence in rich food may render it grossly obese, with severe health handicaps. Nutrient deficiencies, ever so slight to begin with, may be magnified over the years to take a heavy toll. Your body in your later years will be the product of decades of daily choices that together add up to have a tremendous impact on your health and the quality of your life.

One of the choices that people first make in their teens or in early adulthood is the choice whether to make alcohol a regular part of their lives, to use it only occasionally, or not to use it at all. A person making an educated choice would want to know the immediate effects of alcohol when drinking, and also the long-term effects when a person has used alcohol over a lifetime. This discussion begins with the immediate effects, and starts at the point where alcohol enters the body.

Alcohol Enters the Body

From the moment alcohol enters the body in a beverage, it is treated as if it has special privileges. Foods sit around in the stomach for a while, but not alcohol. Alcohol molecules are tiny, and they need no digestion; they can diffuse as soon as they arrive, right through the walls of the stomach, and they reach the brain within a minute. You can become intoxicated right away when you drink, especially if your stomach is empty. When your stomach is full of food, the molecules of alcohol have less chance of touching the walls and diffusing through, so you don't feel the effects of alcohol so quickly. (By the time the stomach contents are emptied into the small intestine, it doesn't matter that plenty of food is mixed with the alcohol. The alcohol is absorbed rapidly anyway; it bumps all other nutrients out of the way and grabs first place.)

A practical pointer derives from this information. If you want to drink socially and not become intoxicated, you should eat the snacks provided by the host. Carbohydrate snacks are best suited for slowing alcohol absorption. High-fat snacks help, too, because they slow peristalsis.[1] This keeps the alcohol in the stomach longer.

If you drink slowly enough, the alcohol you absorb will be collected

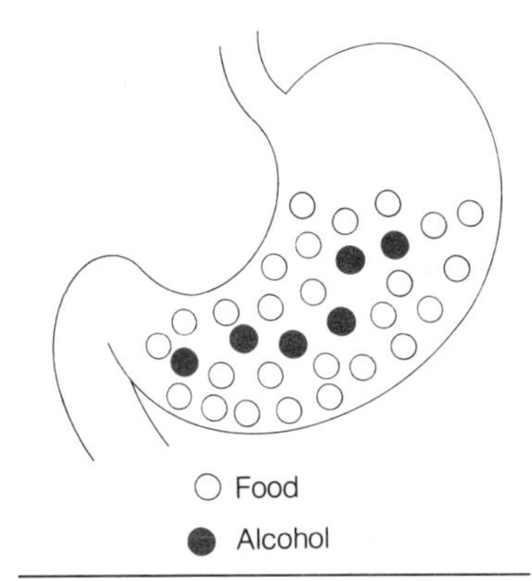

The alcohol in a stomach filled with food has a low probability of touching the walls and diffusing through.

in the liver and processed without much affecting other parts of the body. If you drink more rapidly, however, some of the alcohol bypasses the liver and flows for a while through the rest of the body and the brain.

Alcohol Arrives in the Brain

Alcohol depresses the nervous system's activity. It was used for centuries as an anesthetic because of its ability to deaden pain, but it wasn't a very good one, because it was unpredictable. One could never be sure how much a person would need and how much would be a lethal dose. As more predictable anesthetics were discovered, they quickly replaced alcohol. However, alcohol continues to be used today as a kind of social anesthetic, to help people relax or to relieve anxiety. People think that alcohol is a stimulant, because it seems to make them lively and uninhibited at first. Actually, though, the way it does this is by sedating *inhibitory*

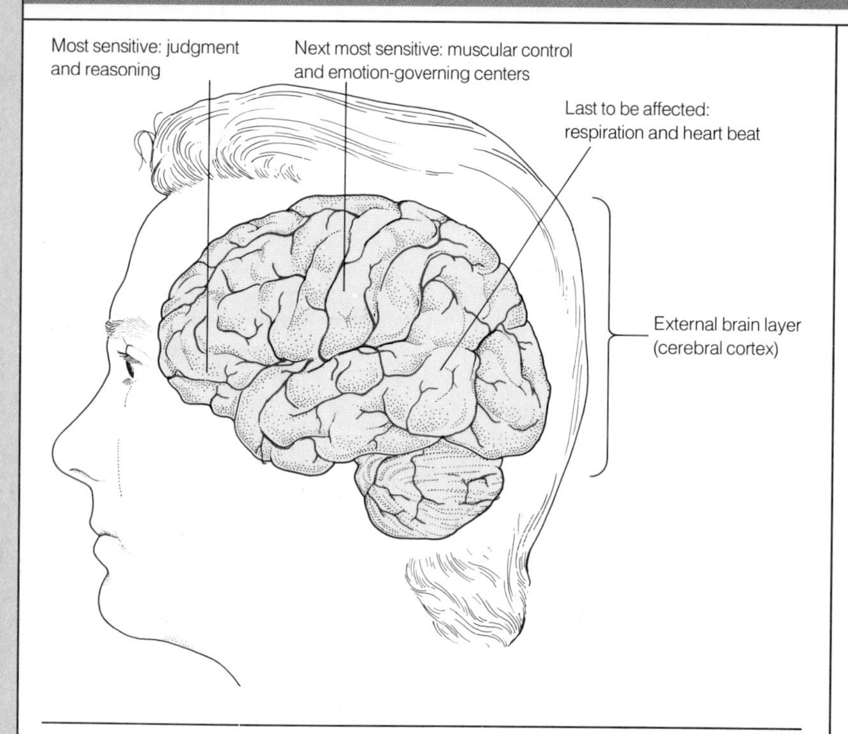

Alcohol's effects on the brain. Alcohol is rightly termed an anesthetic, because it puts brain centers to sleep in order: first the judgment-governing center; then the centers that govern emotions and muscular control; and finally, deep centers that control respiration and heartbeat.

nerves, which are more numerous than excitatory nerves. Ultimately, alcohol acts as a depressant and sedates all the nerve cells.

When alcohol flows to the brain, it sedates the frontal lobe first, the reasoning part. As the alcohol molecules diffuse into the cells of this lobe, they interfere with reasoning and judgment. If the drinker drinks faster than the rate at which the liver can oxidize the alcohol, then the speech and vision centers of the brain become narcotized, and the area that governs reasoning becomes more incapacitated. Later, the cells of the brain responsible for large-muscle control are affected; at this point, people under the influence stagger or weave when they try to walk. Finally, the conscious brain is completely subdued, and the person passes out. Now the person can drink no more; this is lucky, because a higher doses's anesthetic effect could reach the deepest brain centers that control breathing and heartbeat, and the person could die. Table C12–1 shows the blood alcohol levels that correspond with progressively greater intoxication.

We've called it lucky that the brain centers respond to alcohol in the order just described, because people pass out before they can drink a lethal dose. It is possible, though, for people to drink fast enough that the effects of alcohol continue to accelerate after they have gone to sleep. The occasional death that takes place during a drinking contest is attributed to this effect. The drinker drinks fast enough, before passing out, to receive a lethal dose.

Brain cells are sensitive to excessive exposure to alcohol, and when they have died, no others can multiply to replace them. That there is no regeneration of brain cells is one reason for the permanent brain damage observed in some heavy drinkers.

Alcohol depresses production of **antidiuretic hormone (ADH)** by the pituitary gland in the brain. All people who drink have observed the increase in urination that accompanies drinking, but they may not realize that they can easily get into a vicious cycle as a result. Loss of body water leads to thirst. Thirst leads to more drinking—but drinking of what? The only fluid that will relieve dehydration is water, but the thirsty person welcomes any cold fluid, even concentrated alcohol, because it relieves the dry mouth associated with thirst. If a person tries to use concentrated alcoholic beverages to quench thirst, however, it only becomes worse. The smart drinker, then, alternates alcoholic beverages with non-alcoholic choices, and when thirsty, chooses the latter.

The water loss caused by depression of antidiuretic hormone involves loss of more than just water and some alcohol. With water loss there is a loss of such important minerals as magnesium, potassium, calcium, and zinc (see Chapter 7). These minerals are vital to the maintenance of fluid balance and to nerve and muscle action and coordination.

Alcohol Arrives in the Liver

The capillaries that surround the digestive tract merge into the veins that carry the alcohol-laden blood to

Table C12–1

Alcohol Doses and Brain Responses

Number of Drinks[a]	Blood Alcohol Level (%)	Brain Response
2	0.05	Judgment impaired
4	0.10	Emotional control impaired
6	0.15	Muscle coordination and reflexes impaired
8	0.20	Vision impaired
12	0.30	Drunk, totally out of control
14	0.35	Stupor
More than 14	0.50 to 0.60	Total loss of consciousness, finally death

[a]Taken within an hour or so.

the liver. Here the veins branch and rebranch into capillaries that touch every liver cell. The liver cells make nearly all of the body's alcohol-processing machinery, and the routing of blood through the liver allows the cells to go right to work on the alcohol.

The liver makes and maintains two sets of equipment for metabolizing alcohol. One is a pair of enzymes that remove hydrogens from alcohols in the process of breaking them down; we can call them the **alcohol dehydrogenase (ADH)** enzymes 1 and 2.* They handle 80 percent of the alcohol delivered to them. The other alcohol-metabolizing equipment is a chain of enzymes (known as the MEOS) that handles 20 percent of the alcohol. The MEOS becomes important in the alcohol abuser's responses to drugs, as will be shown later, but let us look at the ADH system first.

*Enzyme 1, alcohol dehydrogenase, converts alcohol to acetaldehyde. Enzyme 2, acetaldehyde dehydrogenase, converts acetaldehyde to a common body compound, acetyl CoA, identical to that derived from carbohydrate and fat during their breakdown.

There is a limit to the amount of alcohol anyone can process in a given time. This limit is set by the number of molecules of the ADH enzymes that reside in the liver. If more molecules of alcohol arrive at the liver cells than the enzymes can handle, the extra alcohol must wait. It enters the general circulation and is carried to all parts of the body, circulating again and again through the liver until enzymes are available to degrade it.

The types of enzymes produced vary with individuals, depending on the genes they have inherited. Some racial groups—for example, Asians—have genetic information that causes them to produce atypical forms of the ADH enzymes, and this explains why some persons are made too uncomfortable by alcohol to become addicted.[2] High levels of intermediate products in the brain and other tissues are responsible for many of the punishing effects of alcohol abuse.

The amount of ADH enzymes present is also affected by whether you eat or not. Fasting for as little as a day causes degradation of body proteins, including the ADH enzymes in the liver, and this can reduce the rate of alcohol metabolism by half. Drinking on an empty stomach thus not only lets the drinker feel the effects more promptly, but also brings about higher blood alcohol levels for longer periods of time and increases the effect of alcohol in anesthetizing the brain.

Another lesson for the drinker emerges from these facts. Spacing of drinks is important. It takes about an hour and a half to metabolize one drink, depending on your body size, on previous drinking experience, on how recently you have eaten, and on how you are feeling at the time. Also, since the liver is the only organ that can dispose of significant quantities of alcohol, and since its maximum rate of action is fixed, you cannot sober up by walking around the block. Muscles can't metabolize alcohol. Time is the only thing that will do the job—time for the liver to do its work. Nor will it help to drink a cup of coffee. Caffeine is a stimulant, but it won't speed up the metabolism of alcohol. The police say ruefully that a cup of coffee will only make a sleepy drunk into a wide-awake drunk.

Alcohol is cleared in two other ways besides through metabolism by liver enzymes. About 10 percent is excreted through the breath and in the urine. This fact is the basis for the breathalyzer test that law enforcement officers administer when they suspect someone of driving under the influence of alcohol. But loss of alcohol by these routes is not sufficient to make a difference in the amount of time it takes to sober up after becoming drunk.

As the ADH enzymes break alcohol down, they produce hydrogen ions (acid), which must be picked up by a niacin-containing compound known as NAD. Normally, NAD shuttles this acid to a metabolic pathway where it is disposed of, but when alcohol is present in the system, this pathway shuts down. NAD remains loaded with hyrogens that it cannot get rid of, and so becomes unavailable for the multitude of reactions for which it is required.

As a result, dietary glucose and dietary fat cannot be metabolized as they normally are. They are diverted into the making of body fat, which accumulates in the liver cells, waiting to be carried away to permanent storage deposits.[3]

The synthesis of fatty acids also accelerates as a result of the liver's exposure to alcohol. Fat accumulation can be seen in the liver after a single night of heavy drinking. The first stage of liver deterioration seen in heavy drinkers is **fatty liver,** which interferes with the distribution of nutrients and oxygen to the liver cells. If the condition lasts long enough, the liver cells will die, and the area will be invaded by fibrous scar tissue—the second stage of liver deterioration, called **fibrosis.** Fibrosis is reversible with good nutrition and abstinence from alcohol, but the next (last) stage—**cirrhosis**—is not. All of this points to the importance of moderation in the use of alcohol.

The body's increased acid burden interferes with the process by which the liver generates glucose from protein. The unavailability of glucose from this source, together with the overabundance of fragments from glucose and fat flowing into the fat-making process, sets the stage for a shift into ketosis. The making of ketone bodies uses up some fragments, but some ketone bodies are acids, so they push the acid-base balance further toward acid. The surplus of loaded NAD also favors the making of lactic acid and other acids. This adds still further to the body's acid burden and interferes with the secretion of uric acid, causing symptoms like those of **gout.**

The presence of alcohol alters amino acid metabolism in the liver cells. Synthesis of some proteins important in the immune system slows down, weakening the body's defenses against infection. Synthesis of lipoproteins speeds up, increasing blood triglyceride levels.

Protein deficiency can develop in heavy drinkers, both from the depression of protein synthesis in the cells and from poor diet. Normally the cells would at least use the amino acids that happened to be eaten, but the drinker's liver takes the amino acids apart and uses many of the pieces to make fat or ketones. Eating well does not protect the drinker from protein depletion. One has to stop drinking alcohol for complete protection.

Benefits of Moderate Alcohol Use

The effects of wine, beer, and other fermented beverages have been known to human societies for over 5000 years. Taken in moderation, alcohol relaxes people, reduces their inhibitions, and encourages desirable social interactions.

The term *moderation* is important in the statement just made. Just what is moderation in the use of alcohol? We can't name an exact amount of alcohol per day that would be appropriate for everyone, because people differ in their tolerance levels, but authorities have attempted to set a limit that is appropriate for most healthy people: not more than three drinks a day for the average-sized, healthy man, or two drinks a day for the average-sized, healthy woman. (See the definition of a **drink** in the Miniglossary.) This amount is supposed to be enough to produce an elevation of mood without incurring any long-term harm to health. Doubtless some people could consume slightly more; others could definitely not handle nearly so much without significant risk.

Alcohol in any beverage has the same sought-after effects. In addition, wine in particular is credited with some special effects. Grape juice has a proven antiviral effect that carries over when the grape juice is made into wine.[4] The high potassium content of grape juice is beneficial to people with high blood pressure; when the grape juice is made into wine, the potassium remains in the wine, so this effect also carries over. In fact, since alcohol raises blood pressure (see Controvery 7), the grape juice is more beneficial than the wine.

Dealcoholized wine also increases the absorption of potassium, calcium, phosphorus, magnesium, and zinc; so does wine, but the alcohol in it promotes the *excretion* of these minerals, so the dealcoholized version is preferred.[5] If people who are accustomed to drinking wine give it up, they can still enjoy these benefits by learning to drink moderate amounts of fruit juices or dealcoholized wine in its place.

Alcoholic beverages also affect the appetite. Usually, they reduce it, making people unaware that they are hungry, but in people who are tense and unable to eat, small doses of wine taken 20 minutes before meals improve the appetite. Certain acid compounds in the wine, known as congeners, are credited with this effect. For undernourished people and for people with severely depressed appetites, wine may facilitate eating even when psychotherapy fails to do so. At the same time, because it relaxes people, wine may help obese people lose weight. Its success in that connection is thought to stem from its ability to relieve emotional stress, which is a common reason for overeating. Again, certain congeners in wine may contribute to the tranquilizing effect; some are said to be nearly 100 times more effective than alcohol.[6] French wine also contains a compound that is known to lower liver lipids and cholesterol.[7]

Several research studies have also shown that wine and beer contribute an important trace mineral—silicon—to people's diets. In wine-drinking countries, this is thought to be a factor that contributes to favorable cardiovascular mortality. This doesn't mean that people have to drink wine to obtain the silicon they need, of course, but where their diets lack silicon and their wine happens to supply it, the wine gets the credit.[8] Most wines are also low in sodium and high in potassium, and some are low enough in sugar to be useful in the diets of persons with diabetes. Wine adds calories, of course, but there is something to be said for its calories as opposed to those of, say, sour cream. (Sour cream is almost pure fat and is virtually empty of nutrients.) People who want to enhance their meals with a luxury item they enjoy could easily do worse than to add a glass of wine.*

An example of the beneficial use of alcohol is provided by the experience of the staff at a hospital for the aging,** where three-fourths of the male clients were incontinent (unable to control their bladders) and needed safety restraints to hold them in their wheelchairs. Needless to say, these clients became depressed. The staff decided to serve beer, cheese, and crackers six times a week in the late afternoon in hopes that this would improve morale and perhaps encourage the men to enjoy themselves and socialize more. Within two months, only one-fourth were incontinent, only 12 percent needed safety restraints, and most had become able to walk around unaided. Group activity more than tripled. The staff attributed the change to the "socializing" effect of the cocktail hour.[9]

This example shows that alcoholic beverages can be beneficial when used to improve people's morale. Another example: after President Eisenhower had his first heart attack, his physician recommended that he have a drink or two of cognac every evening. The purpose was to relax him and enable him to achieve a daily escape from the pressures of the presidency. Such uses of alcohol can prolong life and good health, although a person might be even better off learning how to relax without chemical help in the face of such pressures.

Alcohol's Long-Term Effects

By far the longest-term effects of alcohol are those felt by the child of a woman who drank during pregnancy. This is a topic so important it is given a space of its own (Controversy 11), and the recommendation is made that pregnant women should not drink at all. For nonpregnant adults, however, what are the effects of alcohol over the long term?

A couple of drinks set in motion many destructive processes in the body, but the next day's abstinence reverses them. As long as the doses taken are moderate, time between them is ample, and nutrition is adequate meanwhile, recovery is complete. Moderate drinking can be beneficial not only to a person's social life, but also to health.

If the doses of alcohol are heavy and the time between them is short, complete recovery cannot take place, and repeated onslaughts of alcohol gradually take a toll on the body. Cirrhosis takes 10 to 20 years to develop from the additive effects of frequent heavy drinking episodes.

The more alcohol a person drinks, the less likely that he or she will eat enough food to obtain adequate nutrients. Alcohol is empty calories, like pure sugar and pure fat; it displaces nutrients. In a sense, each time you drink 150 calories of alcohol, you are spending those calories on a luxury item and getting no nutritional value in return. The more calories you spend this way, the fewer you have left to spend on nutritious foods. Table C12–2 shows the calorie amounts of typical alcoholic beverages.

Alcohol abuse not only displaces nutrients from the diet, but also affects every tissue's metabolism of nutrients. Stomach cells oversecrete acid and the immune system's inflammation-producing agent, histamine, becoming vulnerable to ulcer formation. Intestinal cells fail to absorb thiamin, folacin, and vitamin B_{12} (see Figure C12–1). Liver cells lose efficiency in activating vitamin D, and they alter their production and excretion of bile. Rod cells in the retina, which normally process vitamin A alcohol (retinol) to the form needed in vision (retinal), find themselves processing drinking alcohol (Figure C12–2). The kidney excretes magnesium, calcium, potassium, and zinc.

*Wine has 200 other substances in it, some of which may be beneficial. It is low in sodium and in some cases may be high in calcium, iron, or other valuable nutrients. The virtues of wine are well described (possibly even without bias) by the Wine Institute in its publication *Wine and Medical Practice: A Summary* (San Francisco: Wine Institute, 1979) (for distribution only to the medical profession).

**The hospital described here is the Cushing Hospital, near Boston.

Table C12–2

Calories in Alcoholic Beverages and Mixers

Beverage	Amount (oz)	Energy (cal)
Beer	12	150
Gin, rum, vodka, whiskey (86 proof)	1½	105
Dessert wine	3½	140
Table wine	3½	85
Tonic, ginger ale, other sweetened carbonated waters	8	80
Cola, root beer	8	100
Fruit-flavored soda, Tom Collins mix	8	115
Club soda, plain seltzer, diet drinks	8	1

Figure C12–1
Alcohol's Effect on Vitamin Absorption (Example).
In the presence of alcohol, intestinal cells fail to absorb thiamin, except at very high concentrations.

Source: A. M. Hoyumpa, Mechanisms of thiamin deficiency in chronic alcoholism, *American Journal of Clinical Nutrition* 33 (1980): 2750–2761.

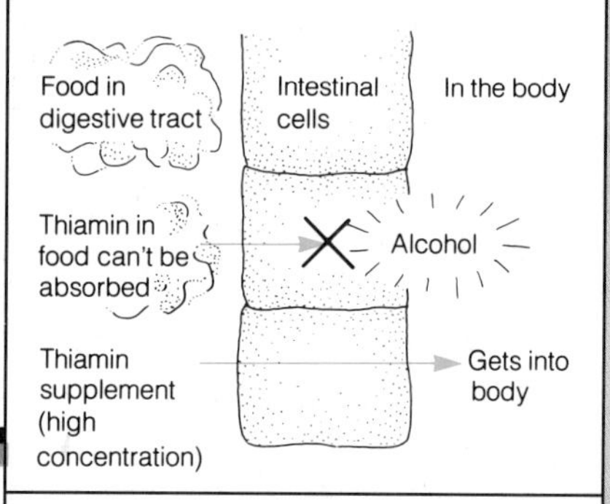

Miniglossary

alcohol dehydrogenase (ADH): an enzyme that breaks down alcohol. The two such enzymes in the liver are termed ADH enzymes 1 and 2 for purposes of this discussion.

antidiuretic hormone (ADH): a hormone produced by the pituitary gland in response to dehydration (or a high sodium concentration in the blood); it stimulates the kidneys to reabsorb more water and so excrete less. This ADH should not be confused with the enzyme alcohol dehydrogenase, which is sometimes also abbreviated *ADH*.

cirrhosis (seer-OH-sis): advanced liver disease, in which liver cells have died, hardened, and turned orange; often associated with alcoholism (*cirrhos* means "an orange").

drink: a dose of any alcoholic beverage that delivers ½ oz of pure ethanol:
- 3 to 4 oz of wine.
- 10 oz wine cooler
- 8 to 12 oz of beer.
- 1 oz distilled liquor (whiskey, scotch, rum, or vodka).

A term that describes the alcohol content of distilled liquor is **proof:** liquor that is 50% alcohol is 100 proof, 45% is 90 proof, and so forth.

fatty liver: an early stage of liver deterioration seen in several diseases, including kwashiorkor and alcoholic liver disease. Fatty liver is characterized by accumulation of fat in the liver cells.

fibrosis: an intermediate stage of liver deterioration seen in several diseases, including viral hepatitis and alcoholic liver disease. In fibrosis, the liver cells lose their function and assume the characteristics of connective tissue cells (fibers).

gout (GOWT): accumulation of uric acid crystals in the joints.

MEOS (microsomal ethand oxidizing system): a system of enzymes in the liver that oxidize not only alcohol, but also several classes of drugs. (The *microsomes* are tiny particles of membranes with associated enzymes that can be collected from broken-up cells; *micro* means "tiny"; *soma* means "body").

Alcohol's intermediate products interfere with metabolism, too. They dislodge vitamin B_6 from its protective binding protein so that it is destroyed, causing a vitamin B_6 deficiency and, thereby, lowered production of red blood cells.

Most dramatic is alcohol's effect on folacin. When alcohol is present, it is as though the body were actively trying to expel folacin from all its sites of action and storage. The liver, which normally contains enough folacin to meet all needs, leaks folacin into the blood. As the blood folacin level rises, the kidneys are deceived into excreting it, as though it were in excess. The intestine normally releases and retrieves folacin continuously, but it becomes damaged by folacin deficiency and alcohol toxicity, so it fails to retrieve its own folacin and misses out on any that may trickle in from food as well. Alcohol also interferes with the action of what little folacin is left, and this inhibits the production of new cells, espe-

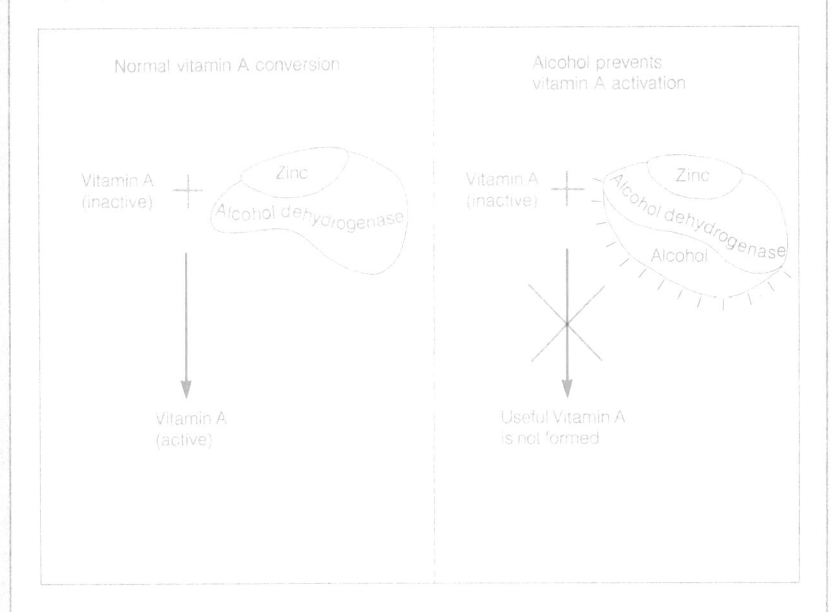

Figure C12–2
Alcohol, Zinc, and the Eye.
In the presence of alcohol, the eye can't produce active vitamin A for use in vision.

Source: R. M. Russell, Vitamin A and zinc metabolism in alcoholism, *American Journal of Clinical Nutrition* 33 (1980): 2741–2749.

cially the rapidly dividing cells of the intestine and the blood. Alcohol abuse causes a folacin deficiency that devastates digestive system function.

Nutrient deficiencies are thus a virtually inevitable consequence of alcohol abuse, not only because alcohol displaces food, but also because alcohol directly interferes with the body's use of nutrients, making them ineffective even if they are present. Over a lifetime, immoderate drinking, whether or not accompanied by attention to nutrition, brings about deficits of all of the nutrients mentioned and many more besides.

Alcohol and Drugs

The liver's reaction to alcohol is reflected in its handling of drugs, as well as nutrients. In addition to the ADH enzymes, the liver possesses an enzyme system that metabolizes *both* alcohol and drugs—any compounds that have certain chemical features in common. Called the **MEOS (microsomal ethanol oxidizing system)**, this system handles only about 20 percent of the total alcohol a person consumes, but the MEOS enlarges if repeatedly exposed to alcohol. This may not make the drinker able to handle much more alcohol at a time than before, because the total alcohol-metabolizing ability of the MEOS is small, but the effect on the ability to metabolize drugs is considerable.

When the MEOS enlarges, it makes the body able to metabolize drugs much faster than before. This can make it confusing and tricky to work out the correct dosages of medications. The doctor who prescribes sedatives every four hours, for example, assumes that the MEOS will dispose of the drug at a certain predicted rate. Well and good; but in a client who is a heavy drinker, the MEOS is adapted to metabolizing large quantities of alcohol. It therefore metabolizes the drug extra fast. The drug's effects wear off unexpectedly fast, leaving the client undersedated. Imagine the doctor's alarm if a client wakes up on the table during an operation! A skilled anesthesiologist always asks clients about their drinking patterns before putting them to sleep.

An enlarged MEOS will oxidize drugs faster than expected, but only as long as there is no alcohol in the system. If the person drinks and uses a drug at the same time, the drug will be metabolized more *slowly* and so will be much more potent. The MEOS is busy disposing of alcohol, so the drug can't be handled till later; and the dose may build up to where it greatly oversedates, or even kills, the user.

You may have heard the story of the country woman who kept saying "Amen!" as the preacher ranted about one sin after another; but when he got to her favorite sin, she whispered to her husband that the preacher had "quit preachin' and gone to meddlin'." We've tried to stick to scientific facts, so the only meddlin' that we'll do is to urge you to look again at the accompanying drawing of the brain and note that judgment is affected first when someone drinks. A person's judgment may tell him that he should limit himself to two drinks at a party, but the first drink may take his judgment away, so that he has many more. The failure to stop drinking as planned, on repeated occasions, is a danger sign that indicates that the person should not drink at all.

Notes

1. A. B. Eisenstein, Nutritional and metabolic effects of alcohol, *Journal of the American Dietetic Association* 81 (1982): 247–251.
2. D. P. Agarwal, S. Harada, and H. W. Goedde, Racial differences in biological sensitivity to ethanol: The role of alcohol dehydrogenase and acetaldehyde dehydrogenase enzymes, *Alcoholism: Clinical and Experimental Research* 5 (1981): 12–16.
3. C. S. Lieber, Liver adaptation and injury in alcoholism, *New England Journal of Medicine* 288 (1973): 356–361.
4. J. Konowalchuk and J. I. Speirs, Virus inactivation by grapes and wines, *Applied and Environmental Microbiology,* December 1976, pp. 757–763; A vintage medicine, *New York Times,* 12 June 1977, p. E7.
5. J. B. McDonald, Not by alcohol alone, *Nutrition Today,* January/February 1979, pp. 14–19.
6. D. J. Forkner, Should wine be on your menu? *Professional Nutritionist,* Spring 1982, pp. 1–3.
7. P. N. Chaudhari and V. G. Hatwalne, Effect of epicatechin on liver lipids of rats fed with choline deficient diet, *The Indian Journal of Nutrition and Dietetics* 14 (1977): 136–139.
8. R. M. Parr, Silicon, wine, and the heart, *Lancet,* 17 May 1980, p. 1087.
9. W. J. Darby, The benefits of drink, *Human Nature,* November 1978, pp. 31–37.

Chapter Thirteen

Contents

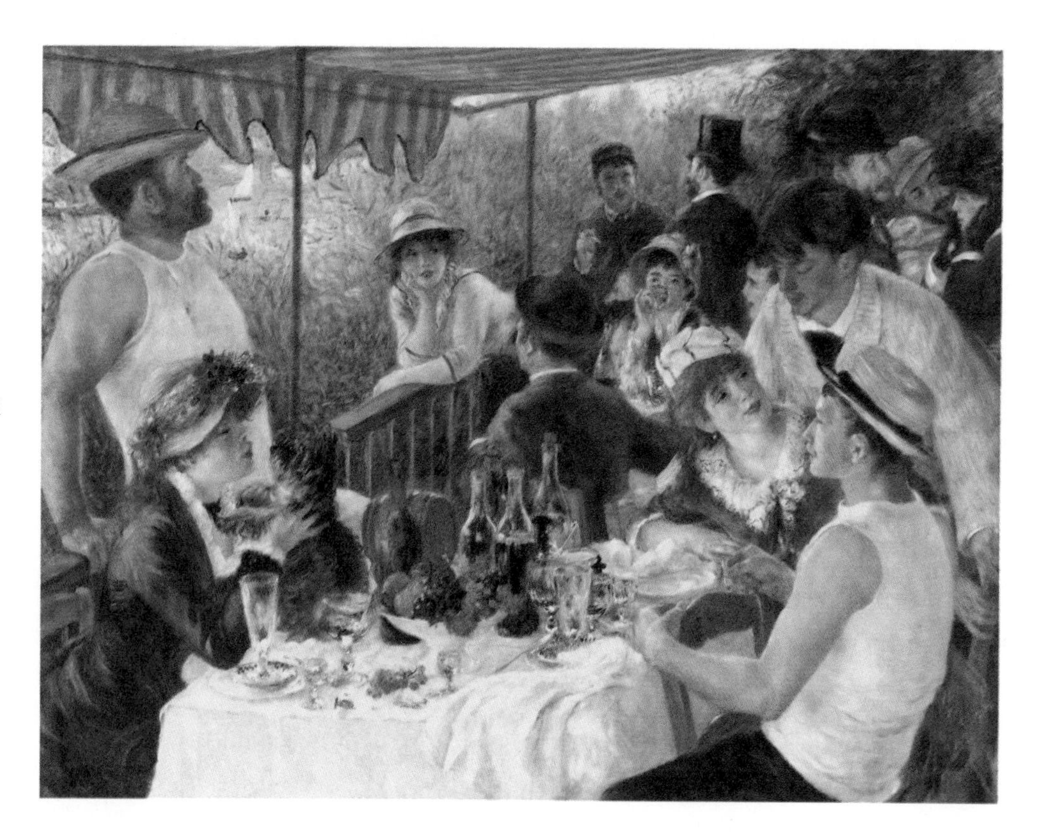

The Luncheon of the Boating Party by Pierre Auguste Renoir. The Phillips Collection, Washington, D.C.

Adulthood and the Later Years

This looks like a chapter about the later years, but it is relevant even if the reader is only 20. How you live life at 20 can profoundly affect the quality of your life at 60 or 80. What your later life will be like depends partly on your physical health and your financial security, but your expectations also play an important role. Most people, without realizing it, carry an unconscious stereotype, largely negative, of what it is like to be old—and they let themselves become that way. An old saying has it that "as the twig is bent, so grows the tree"—only, unlike a tree, you can bend your own twig.[1]

Before you will adopt nutrition behaviors that will enhance your health in old age, you must accept on a personal level that you, yourself, are aging. People who fear age try to deny that it is happening to them, and they distance themselves from old people, as if lack of association would keep them young. Everyone ages, though, and people who are prejudiced against older people are therefore prejudiced against *everyone,* including their own future selves. (Another form of prejudice is to view all old people as good, generous, and kind, when in fact bank robbers and crooks age, too.) To see what negative and positive views you hold about aging, try answering the following questions:

- In what ways do you expect your appearance to change as you grow older?
- What physical activities do you see yourself doing at 70?
- What will be your financial status? Will you be independent or dependent?
- What will your sex life be like? Will others see you as sexy?
- How many friends will you have? What will you do together?
- Will you be happy? Cheerful? Curious? Depressed? Uninterested in life or new things?

Your answers reveal not only what you think of other people now, but also what will probably become of you. You may wish to review some of the reasons for your answers, and if they are not supported by science, to change your beliefs.

Older people are an incredibly diverse group, and for the most part they are self-sufficient, socially sophisticated, mentally lucid, fully participating members of society who report themselves to be happy and healthy.[2] Most live in their own or relatives' homes, and only 5 percent live in nursing homes.[3] Three-fifths of the elderly are women.[4] Most have planned ahead financially, and about half need no financial assistance from the government.[5] Planning ahead is important, for the average income of older men in the United States is about $10,000 per year, and for women it is only half that amount.[6] Of aged black women, nearly half have yearly incomes of under $1000.

Figure 13–1
The Aging of the Population.
In 1900, 4 percent of the U.S. population were over 65; 11 percent are over 65 today; 12.5 percent (30,500,000 people) will be over 65 in the year 2000.

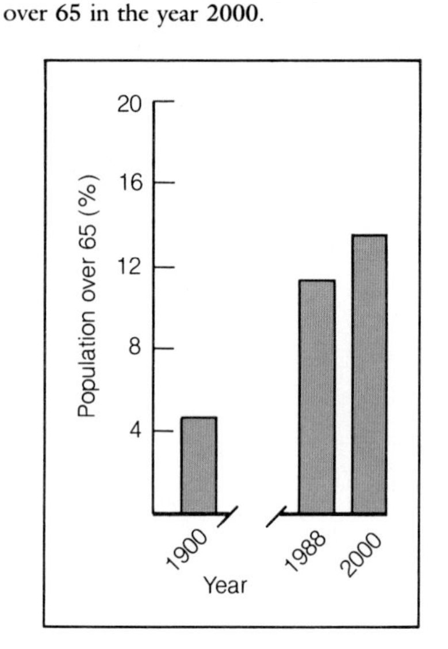

The bulk of the U.S. population is not yet old but aging, and the ratio of old people to young grows steadily larger (see Figure 13–1). In fact, the fastest growing age group is people over 85.

As people age, a lifetime of nutrition choices incurs consequences for the better or for the worse. While each day's intakes of nutrients may have only a minute effect on body organs and their functions, over years and decades their repeated effects accumulate to have major impacts. One writer has put it this way: "By age 65, the average American will have consumed 100,000 pounds of food, give or take a few tons. . . . Neglect will almost certainly be reflected in the state of his or her health by age 65, if not long before."[7] This being the case, it is of great importance for everyone to pay close attention now to nutrition. The young of today have benefits of science never afforded to the young of many years ago. It is likely that today's younger generations will reach even older ages and be healthier when they get there because of health habits they were taught to employ when they were young, including nutrition. And that is what this chapter is about.

The quality of the later years of life depends partly on health and financial status, and partly on expectations. Nutrition preparation has an impact on later health.

Nutrition and Disease Prevention

Nutrition alone cannot ensure a long and robust life. To think it can leads people to wrongly lay blame on those who get sick. Of a man suffering from cancer, for example, some may think, "A sedentary life with the wrong food is the cause." The man himself may waste his precious energy feeling guilty. But while some cancers are affected by the choices one makes (see Controversy 5), many individual cases are not—their causes are unknown, and they occur regardless of diet. Still, many diseases are nutrition sensitive, even if also responsive to other factors, a point made in Figure 1–5, p. 14. At one extreme are nutrient-deficiency diseases that can be completely cured by supplying the missing nutrients, and at the other extreme are certain genetic or inherited diseases that are completely unaltered by nutrition. Most fall in between, being influenced by each individual's inherited susceptibility, but responsive also to dietary manipulations that help to normalize metabolism and counteract the disease process. The potential influence of nutrition is well known in some instances, but in others it remains to be defined.

Among the better-known relationships between nutrition and disease are the following:

- Appropriate energy intake, abundant carbohydrate, adequate protein, and little fat help prevent *diabetes, obesity,* and related *cardiovascular diseases* such as atherosclerosis and hypertension (Chapter 3, Chapter 8, and Controversy 7), and may influence the development of some forms of *cancer* (Controversy 5).
- Adequate intakes of essential nutrients prevent *deficiency diseases* such as scurvy, goiter, anemia, and the like (Chapters 6 and 7).

- Variety in foods, as well as certain vegetables, may be protective against certain types of cancer (Controversy 5).
- Moderation in sugar intake helps prevent *dental caries* (Controversy 3 and Chapter 12).
- Appropriate fiber intakes help prevent malfunctions of the digestive tract such as *constipation, diverticulosis,* and possibly *colon cancer* (Chapter 3).
- Moderate sodium intake and adequate intakes of potassium, calcium, and other minerals help prevent *hypertension,* at least in people who are genetically predisposed to it (Controversy 7).
- Minimizing alcohol intake helps prevent cirrhosis of the liver, brain disease, and many other forms of damage to the body (Controversy 12).

Alzheimer's disease: a relentless, irreversible brain disease that attacks some people as they age; the final stage is complete helplessness and death.

cataracts (CAT-uh-racts): thickenings of the lens of the eye that can lead to blindness. Cataracts can be caused by injury, viral infection, toxic substances, genetic disorders—and possibly by some nutrient deficiencies or imbalances. A link exists between cataract formation and lactose intolerance or diabetes; its significance is not yet clear.

Three other examples of relationships between nutrition and disease should be added here. They are brain abnormalities, eyesight loss from cataracts, and arthritis. The relationships of nutrition to these three conditions are not as well known as those in the list above, but they are worth notice. One caution: be on the lookout for quacks selling nutritional "remedies" for these and other conditions of aging. Legitimate practitioners agree that the links to nutrition deserve more study, but do not warrant buying and taking supplements of nutrients. In fact, it is also possible that over a lifetime, supplements can build up in the body and cause toxicities, even if the amounts taken seem reasonable.

A group of conditions that affect the brain with aging progress slowly over a lifetime. Recent evidence suggests that some brain aging may actually be the result of gradual, insidious nutrient deficits. One study revealed that older people whose diets were lower in vitamin C or vitamin B_{12} were less able to think clearly, while those whose diets were poorer in riboflavin and folacin had poor memories. The researchers concluded that "subclinical malnutrition may play a small role in the depression of cognitive function in the elderly."[8]

Other studies have implicated other nutrient deficiencies in the aging of the brain. Deficiencies of the vitamins thiamin and niacin are well known to be partly responsible for degenerative changes in the mental function of alcohol abusers. Structural alterations in brain cells accompany the degenerative changes, even without alcohol abuse. Deficiencies of two other nutrients, copper and vitamin B_6, while not yet demonstrated to alter brain cell structures in people, do alter them in animals, and the deficiencies accelerate the aging of the nerve cells.[9]

A devastating brain disease is **Alzheimer's disease.** Its effects begin to be felt in people in their mid-60s as memory loss; it progresses over a period of months or years to the inability to perform everyday functions, and finally to the total inability to care for oneself. In the brain, the nerve pathways become progressively tangled and blocked. The mineral aluminum is found in higher than normal levels in diseased brain cells, but so far this seems to result from, rather than cause, the condition. Many nutrient supplements have been tried and for the most part, found ineffective in lessening the severity of the disease.[10] About 7 percent of the population will eventually suffer from Alzheimer's, and it usually runs in families.

Another age-related change is seen in the lens of the eye: **cataracts,** thickenings of the lenses that impair vision and ultimately lead to blindness. Cataracts occur even in well-nourished individuals due to injury, viral infections, toxic substances, and genetic disorders, but most cataracts are vaguely called senile

arthritis: a usually painful inflammation of a joint caused by many conditions, including infections, metabolic disturbances, or injury; joint structure is usually altered, with loss of function.

cataracts—meaning "caused by aging." Thoughtful scientists have wondered just what this really means, and have searched for a possible role of nutrient deficiencies, excesses, and imbalances in cataract causation. They have observed several possible (and, it should be emphasized, highly tentative) links: to protein, fat, or sugar (fructose derived from sucrose) excess, to excess energy intake (in people with diabetes), to deficiencies of the vitamins riboflavin or vitamin E, and to deficiencies of the minerals selenium or zinc. A link between lactose intolerance and cataracts is gaining strength, and researchers are trying to determine whether the presence of the milk sugar itself, or the dehydration caused by diarrhea in lactose-intolerant people, is the associated factor.[11]

Another major disease that disables the elderly is **arthritis,** a painful swelling of the joints that troubles many people as they grow older. During movement, the normal ends of bones are protected from wear by cartilage and by small sacs of fluid that act as a lubricant; with age, however, the protective padding materials disintegrate, and then joints wear, become malformed, and become painful to move. The cause of arthritis is unknown, but it afflicts millions around the world and is a major problem of the elderly.

Not effective against arthritis:

- Watercress.
- Burdock root.
- Vitamin D.
- Celery juice.
- Calcium.
- Megadoses of vitamins.
- Fasting.
- Fresh fruit.
- Honey.
- Lecithin.
- Yeast.
- Kelp.
- Raw liver.
- Fish liver oil.
- Alfalfa tea.
- *Aloe vera* liquid.
- Superoxide dismutase (SOD).
- 100 others.

Arthritis has for centuries been ascribed to poor diet, oftentimes in the form of quack remedies, including many bizarre diets advertised as arthritis cures. Two or three new popular books on diet for arthritis come out every year, urging people to eat no meat, or drink no milk, or eat all their food raw, or eat only "natural" food, or avoid all additives, or—who knows what will be next. Actually no known diet prevents, relieves, or cures arthritis,[12] but as long as people keep buying the books that make these claims, the law of supply and demand dictates that they will keep coming out.

One possible true link between arthritis and diet is through the immune system. It could be that in some cases of arthritis, the immune system has become defective and attacks the tissues of the bone coverings as it normally would an invader. The integrity of the immune system depends on adequate nutrition, and a poor diet probably worsens the condition. It is also possible that certain foods may stimulate the immune system to attack[13] (this fact is often exploited by faddists selling anti-arthritis diets). Another nutrient link that may prove significant in the future is the now-famous fatty acid found in fish oil, EPA. Chapter 4 told about EPA and heart health; research is beginning to show that the same diet recommended there, one low in saturated fat from red meats and dairy products and high in the fish oil EPA, might have potential to reduce the suffering of people with arthritis. Researchers theorize that EPA could interfere with the action of prostaglandins, chemicals involved in the inflammatory response that causes pain in arthritis.[14]

Weight loss is important for overweight persons with arthritis, because the joints affected are often weight-bearing joints that are stressed and irritated by having to carry excess poundage. Weight-loss diets alone often relieve the worst of the pain in arthritis clients, even that of arthritis in the hands (not weight bearing). Perhaps the drastic reduction in fat intake that accompanies the adoption of a calorie-restricted diet is beneficial for arthritis relief, with or without EPA added. Important to note: jogging and other weight-bearing exercise is not related to the development of arthritis—even in marathon runners.[15]

These brief discussions of brain disease, cataracts, and arthritis could be multiplied many-fold, both to provide further details and to add other diseases, but they have sufficed to show that nutrition can provide at least some protection against certain diseases commonly associated with aging. In fact, in general, it is beginning to look as if nutrition through the prime years may play a greater role than has been realized in preventing many changes once thought to be inevitable consequences of growing older.

A nutrition lifestyle that combines moderation with adequate intakes of all essential nutrients can forestall certain diseases and improve the quality of life into the later years.

life span: the maximum number of years of life attainable by a member of a species.

life expectancy: the average number of years lived by people in a given society.

The Aging Process

People today have longer life expectancies than any generation of the past. This truth is worth a moment's thought, and the meanings of two terms help to clarify it. One is **life span,** and the other is **life expectancy.** Life span is the documented maximum length of life possible for a species; the life span of human beings is about 115 years. Life expectancy is a more useful term—it is the average number of years people actually live in the conditions of their society. In 1983 in the United States, the life expectancy for women was 78 years and for men was 71 years, up from about 45 years in 1900. Some believe that life expectancies will continue rising.[16]

Advances in medical science—antibiotics and other treatments—are largely responsible for almost doubling the life expectancy in this century. Far fewer young people are dying from infections, and infant deaths are no longer common. Even deaths from cardiovascular disease are coming later in life, partly due to improvements in treatment, but also partly because people are taking seriously the advice to cut down on fat in the diet and take up exercising. Still, a biological schedule is built into the human organism (we call it aging) that cuts off life at a genetically fixed point in time.

Why we age as we do, and why we die, no one knows, although many researchers are trying to find out. Among the questions they are asking are:

- To what extent is aging inevitable? Can we retard it through changes in lifestyle and environment?
- What roles does nutrition play in aging, and what roles can it play in retarding aging?

With respect to the first question, it seems that aging is an inevitable, natural process, programmed into the genes at conception, but that people can adopt lifestyle habits such as exercising and attention to work and recreational environments that will slow the process within the natural limits set by heredity. And with respect to the second question, clearly, good nutrition can retard and ease the process in many significant ways. Table 13–1, which appears later in this chapter, proposes some changes with age that clearly respond to lifestyle choices. The next sections describe the natural aging of cells, organs, and the skeleton; then the roles of nutrition.

lipofuscin (lip-oh-FEW-sin): the aging pigment (*lipo* means "lipid"; *fuscus* means "brownish gray").

For more about evolution and natural selection, turn to Chapter 1.

Aging of Cells

Cells seem to age in response to outside (environmental) forces and also to undergo a built-in (genetic) aging process. Environmental stresses that promote aging include extremes of heat and cold, disease, lack of nutrients, lack of exercise, and the total lack of stimulation caused by disuse (for example, of the muscle cells in the legs of a person who can't walk). But even in the most pleasant and supportive of environments, inevitable changes take place in the structure and function of the body's cells.

All theories of aging agree that at some point the cells become incapable of replenishing their constituents. Take the muscles and nerves, for example. As muscles age, the vessels that deliver their blood supply atrophy, and some nerve cells that stimulate them to contract die off. With less blood and little stimulation, some muscle cells die and the muscles atrophy. Some of the active muscle cells are gradually replaced by inert connective tissue.

Theories of aging also agree that cells are programmed to stop reproducing after a certain number of cell divisions. Red blood cells undergo few divisions—they multiply only as long as they are in the marrow of the bones. When they move into the blood, they no longer reproduce; they work for four months and then die. Brain cells all stop reproducing before a baby is born.[17] Thus a newborn has all the brain cells he or she will ever have and has already lost a few. Thereafter, although a few cells may die each day of life, the losses are not noticeable because so many remain intact. After about age 65, though, the rate of cell death accelerates, and the losses are felt as slowed reflexes and impaired visual memory.* It seems strange that the human species should have evolved such a magnificent instrument for receiving, storing, interpreting, and retrieving information and yet not have evolved a method of repairing it, but it is not so strange in view of the theory of evolution, because evolution has only provided that people live long enough to reproduce the species. Our Stone-Age ancestors died at 20 or 30 years of age, passing on genes to their offspring that would enable them in turn to live to reproductive age. Natural selection did not mold the characteristics of human organisms beyond that age.

The aging process is a happenstance, then, and we must live with it as best we can. Fortunately, however, we have inherited magnificent equipment for learning and coping—our brains. Even though brains themselves age, the majority of older people retain excellent functioning, and further, possess wisdom attainable in only one way—by learning over a lifetime.

A third factor in the aging process seems to be that with the passage of time, cells become cluttered with debris—partially completed proteins and oxidized lipids that are never totally dismantled. This intracellular "sludge" interferes with the efficiency of operations within the cells. The lipid material that accumulates in the cells is known as **lipofuscin,** the pigment of old age.

Another factor may be that cells lose their ability to interpret the DNA genetic code words and so make their proteins incorrectly. As reduced amounts of protein or wrong proteins are produced, cell and organ functions that depend

*An older theory stated that brain cells died at a steady rate throughout life, but recent evidence disputes it. See D. Sinclair, *Human Growth after Birth* (New York: Oxford University Press, 1985), for a full discussion of the brain and aging.

on those proteins falter. Environmental stresses, such as radiation, may alter the DNA code itself. This, too, leads to the production of wrong proteins.

If wrong proteins are produced for any reason, another theory states, the body's immune system will react to them as if they were foreign proteins from outside and will produce antibodies to counteract them. Complexes then form between the antibodies and these proteins and accumulate in and among cells as useless debris. The **autoimmune theory** may account in part for the accumulation, in joints, of deposits that cause arthritis, as described earlier.

Finally, another theory of aging suggests that radiation from the earth (partly from nuclear weapons testing and partly from natural sources) and from outer space bombards molecules in the cells and splits them into highly reactive compounds known as **free radicals.** These free radicals then bind rigidly to other cellular molecules. This disrupts the informational content of important molecules, so the cells die. (Some investigators have suggested that the formation of free radicals might be retarded by the taking of vitamin E supplements.) None of these ideas about cellular aging are more than theories, but they suggest explanations for the aging of systems described in the next section.

autoimmune theory: the theory that aging occurs as the body fails to recognize its own protein compounds and creates antibodies against them.

free radicals: unstable molecular intermediates that arise during oxidation reactions. They are highly reactive and readily oxidize other molecules with which they come in contact.

Life expectancy has increased dramatically in this century because of advances in medicine and improved health habits. Each of the body's cells ages at an internally regulated rate, hastened or retarded by the environment. Theories of aging include gradual death of organ systems, genetically determined life span, intracellular debris, autoimmunity, and damage from free radicals.

Aging of Systems

The most visible physical changes of aging take place in the skin. As people age, the skin loses its elasticity and the layer of fat beneath it, so wrinkles increase. Many of the wrinkles follow the lines of muscles that are often flexed—hence the development of "character lines." You can almost tell someone's nature by their wrinkles—smilers develop facial lines different from those of frowners. Exposures to sun, wind, and cold hasten wrinkling. Muscles change, too, gradually diminishing and making thin people look angular. (Fat tissue may take the place of the lean in a plump person, and so this change may not show.) Body composition usually shifts away from the lean as people age, but it doesn't have to change much—regular exercise can prevent much muscle degeneration and prevent fat accumulation. Exercise, coupled with a high carbohydrate diet that provides just the right amounts of energy and protein, can help the body composition of an older person remain lean.

Body composition and exercise are discussed in Chapter 9.

Less visible but also important to nutrition are the changes that take place in the digestive system. The gums that hold the teeth in place are sensitive, and if not cared for properly throughout life, they may deteriorate, causing loss of teeth. Today, gum disease afflicts 90 percent of the population by age 65 to 74, and 45 percent of people over age 65 have no teeth at all.[18] Brushing, flossing, regular visits to the dentist, and avoidance of sticky sweet snacks help people hold onto their teeth throughout life. The senses of taste and smell diminish, changing the way people perceive food. Stronger seasonings may be required to make food taste good. The stomach's secretions of hydrochloric acid and enzymes decrease, as do the secretions of digestive juices by the pancreas and small intestine. The colon may, but doesn't necessarily, lose function, causing increased constipation and associated ills. A diet that contains fibrous fruits, vegetables, and grains, and plenty of fluid combined with exercise can help the bowels perform well throughout life.

The liver is somewhat different. Liver cells regenerate themselves throughout life, although fat may gradually infiltrate the liver, reducing its work output. The pancreas cells may become less responsive to high blood glucose levels, while the body's cells may become resistant to insulin, so that diabetes may develop. Although sometimes these conditions are genetically destined to occur, those that develop in later life are often a result of poor diet and lack of exercise, and are especially related to too much body fatness—obesity.

Fiber and colon functioning, and nutrition and diabetes are topics of—Chapter 3; the diet deemed advantageous to prevent heart disease is described in Controversy 4.

The heart and blood vessels also age. All organs and tissues depend on the circulation of nutrients and oxygen, so degenerative changes in the cardiovascular system critically affect all other systems. The decrease in blood flow through the kidneys makes them gradually less efficient at removing wastes and maintaining the blood's normal composition. As the heart pumps blood less forcefully, the capillary trees of the kidneys diminish in size; some kidney cells die. In this case, too, some heart and artery disease is genetically determined to occur, but often the team of proper diet and regular aerobic exercise can retard these degenerative processes. An adequate diet that is low in fat works to keep the passageways clear of plaques, and regular exercising ensures that an ample volume of blood is pumped into the kidneys, keeping the capillaries open. Should capillaries become blocked, exercise encourages the creation of new ones that bypass the damage.

Osteoporosis and its relation to diet are discussed in Chapter 7.

The lungs' capacity to inhale and exhale air may decrease by 50 percent. Maximum breathing capacity, maximum work rate, and maximum oxygen uptake can fall by 60 to 70 percent.[19] Here, exercise alone is the key to prevention. It has been shown that people need not lose their capacity to breathe deeply, as long as sufficient aerobic exercise is part of their regular routine.

Like the body's organ systems, the skeletal system is subject to change with the passage of time. Bone-building and bone-dismantling cells are constantly remodeling this structure, but with age, bone-building cells are lost, and so bone dismantling becomes more rapid than bone building. The result is osteoporosis—a disease that today afflicts close to half of all people over 65. The bones of a person with osteoporosis may become so fragile that simply tossing in bed at night can cause a break. In older people without frank osteoporosis, the reduced number of bone-building cells means that breaks do not heal as well or as rapidly as they once did. It is not yet known for sure the extent to which osteoporosis can be prevented, but it is clear that a lifetime of poor calcium intake, as well as inactivity, is strongly associated with its occurrence.

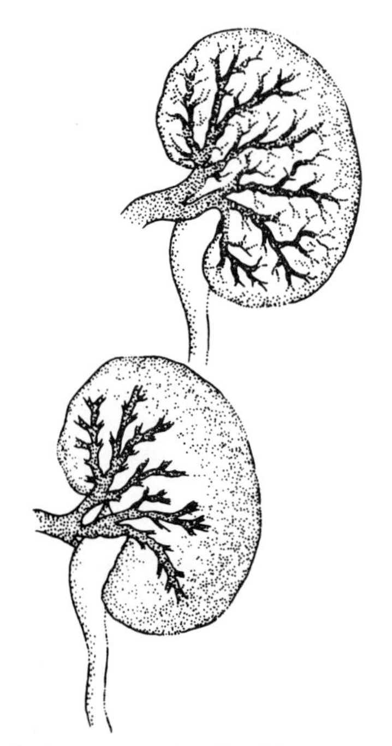

As the heart pumps less blood into an organ, the capillary trees within that organ recede, leaving some of the cells without nourishment. Exercise promotes maintenance and even growth of capillaries.

It is lucky for young people today that so much is known about the effects of diet and other health habits on aging. You would do well to take a course on health, to learn other measures beyond the scope of nutrition. Earlier, we promised you a table that would show some of the changes with age that a person with advance know-how can avoid, and some that are inevitable. Here it is—Table 13–1.

Aging affects every body tissue and organ: the brain, the digestive tract, the bones. Some of the changes are inevitable, but others are for the most part preventable through healthy habits that include proper diet and exercise.

Table 13–1

Changes with Age: Inevitable vs Preventable

Changes with Age	You Probably Cannot Change These	You Probably Can Slow or Prevent These Changes by Exercising, Eating an Adequate Diet, and Planning Ahead
Appearance		
Graying of hair	√	
Balding	√	
Drying and wrinkling of skin	√	
Nervous System		
Impairment of near vision	√	
Some loss of hearing	√	
Reduced taste and smell sensitivity	√	
Reduced touch sensitivity	√	
Slowed reactions (reflexes)	√	
Slowed mental function	√	
Mental confusion		√
Diminished visual memory	√	
Heart, Circulatory System, and Lungs		
Increased blood pressure		√
Increased resting heart rate		√
Decreased breathing capacity and oxygen uptake		√
Body Composition/Metabolism		
Increased body fatness		√
Raised blood cholesterol		√
Slowed energy metabolism		√
Other Physical Characteristics		
Decreased maximum work rate		√
Menopause (women)	√	
Loss of fertility (men)	√	
Loss of sexual functioning		√
Joints: loss of elasticity	√	
Joints: loss of flexibility		√
Oral health: loss of teeth, gum disease		√
Bone loss		√
Digestive problems, constipation		√

Source: Adapted from F. S. Sizer and E. N. Whitney, *Life Choices: Health Concepts and Strategies* (St. Paul: West, 1988), p. 398.

superoxide dismutase (SOD): an antioxidant enzyme found in animal tissues. Although widely advertised and sold as preventive medicine against aging, this enzyme, taken orally or injected, is ineffective.

Can Aging Be Prevented?

It is clear that health habits affect *health,* and good habits make aging more pleasant, but the question remains, Can people avoid growing old altogether? Can they take pills or potions, or is there anything else they can do to prolong life, and particularly, youth?

Although the search has gone on since the dawn of human history, the fountain of youth has yet to be located. Nonetheless, quacks who claim to have found it have been selling its waters for centuries. Products that claim antiaging effects are too numerous to list, but among them are such products as Gerovital H-3, a potion made of a painkiller, a preservative, and an antioxidant, none of which is of value in retarding aging or in the treatment or prevention of illness.[20] (Chapter 10 discussed the effects of antioxidants.)

One more such "treatment" is **superoxide dismutase (SOD).** SOD is an enzyme that occurs naturally in the cells of animals, including human beings. It acts as an antioxidant, as do vitamin C, vitamin E, and selenium. Animal species that live the longest, such as human beings, have the highest concentrations of SOD in their tissues, and it has been hoped that if the concentration of this enzyme in the human body could be raised, aging would slow, and life would be prolonged. It doesn't work.[21] Like other enzymes taken orally, SOD is digested in the stomach and intestine to fragments that the body uses to make its own proteins. If it were injected, it would still be external to cells and could cause irritation and allergic reactions, but could not prolong life. The trick would have to be to induce the cells to make more of it themselves (genetic engineering)—and even then, who is to say that higher levels would prolong life? The body tends to make the right amount of what it needs, as this book has shown in countless examples, and more SOD would probably not be better. Still, many health-food stores and other establishments are doing a brisk business selling it.

A different approach to the prevention of aging has been to study other cultures in the hope of finding an extremely long-lived race of people and then learning from them the secrets of long life. One scientist traveled far and wide in search of such people and found some, in two different geographical areas, who claimed to have lived for over 100 years. Further study revealed, however, that some of these people only claimed to be 100 or older, because in their societies age was venerated. Still, though, some did prove to be not only remarkably old, but also remarkably healthy and justifiably proud of it. The credit did not go to nutrition, these people did not eat according to any particular formula. One group ate a lot of meats and sweets; another used large amounts of alcohol and sugar. The secret—the one thing they all seemed to have in common—was that they lived physically active lives, and they remained active into old age. A recent study on longevity bears this out in this society, too; vigorous exercise and long life seem to go together.[22]

Still another approach has been drastic manipulation of the diet in animals, which has given rise to some interesting and suggestive findings. Rats live longer when their food intake is restricted, either in the early weeks of their lives, or even during adulthood. The restriction has to be severe, though—to 60 percent of the normal energy intake or even less. The life spans of rats were lengthened by such drastic restrictions of their food intakes, and especially their fat intakes, during the growth period. In one experiment, for example, animals allowed to eat freely lived to an average 656 days, while those whose feed was restricted lived to an average 949 days. The experiments were interesting because it was possible to study growth retardation of various organ systems and to speculate on the cause of the increased length of life of some of the animals—a delay in the onset of certain diseases, for example. The experiments did *not* suggest any direct applications to human nutrition, though, and there were distinct disadvantages to the animals given restricted feedings.

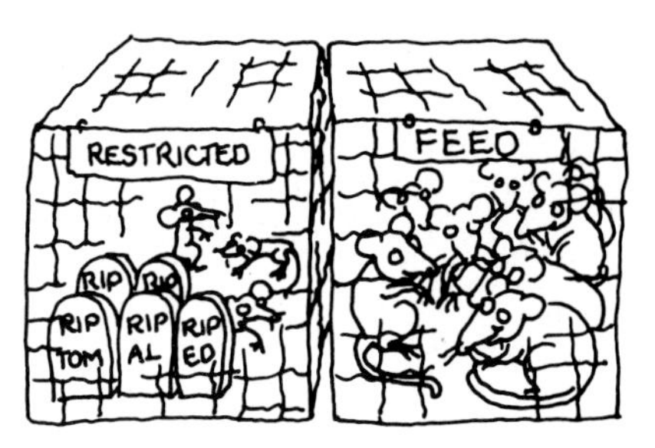

Some survive—but is it worth it?

For example, half of the restricted animals died *very* early (before 300 days). The average length of life was long because the few survivors lived a very long time. Also, the restriction retarded growth: "even the shortest period of food restriction in this study was comparable to restriction of the food intake of a human infant kept in an isolated environment for 20 to 25 years to an amount that would permit the infant to grow during that time to about the size of a one-year-old child."[23] Furthermore, the restricted animals that survived were malformed in a number of ways. It seems that extreme starvation to extend life, like any extreme, is hardly worth the price.

The views of the experts on food restriction can best be summed up by saying that disease can *shorten* people's lives, and that poor nutrition practices make diseases more likely and more severe. Adequate nutrition, then, by postponing and slowing disease processes, can help an individual reach the maximum life span—but cannot extend it further.[24] This brings us to a consideration of what exactly constitutes "good" nutrition for the aging.

Since time's beginning, people have sought to slow or reverse aging. No potion, pill, or powder is effective against aging.

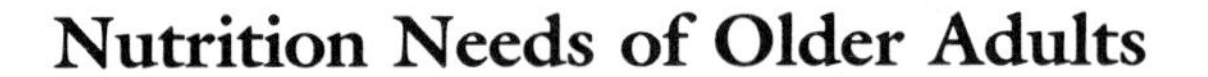

Nutrition Needs of Older Adults

Old age is a relatively new phenomenon—in the Stone Age, people's lives ended shortly after they had reproduced. Only recently has there been a population of senior citizens, and today, its numbers are growing larger. Scientists are working to find out how nutrient needs change as advancing age changes the body. So far, there is no RDA for older age groups—everyone over 50 is grouped together, even though needs change as aging progresses. No standard exists to which older people can compare their dietary intakes to be sure of meeting nutrient needs. Nor can health care professionals, such as dietitians, confidently state that food provided in care facilities for elderly clients is truly adequate. Clearly, the need for such standards is urgent now, and will become more so as the bulk of the population ages.

Some roadblocks stand in the way of researchers' determining RDA for the elderly. For one thing, aging changes different people in different ways, especially in their biochemistry, upon which nutrient needs are based. Members of other age groups bear much more resemblance to one another in this regard—you can count on all children to need extra energy for growth, on all pregnant women to need extra folacin for the making of blood, and so on. But as people age, their individual histories determine which nutrients they need more of, depending on diseases they have suffered and on their genetic predispositions to develop faulty nutrient absorption. For example, while one person may secrete less stomach acid at a certain age, and so absorb less iron, another person who maintains acid production may produce less of the intrinsic factor necessary to absorb vitamin B_{12}.

As a start toward developing RDA for older adults, researchers have come up with a list of factors to be considered.[25] The RDA should:

- Be aimed at the maintenance of *optimal* functioning of body systems, and at levels that may prevent age-related diseases, such as osteoporosis.
- Possibly be individualized according to health and history, rather than generalized to an age range.
- Take into account how nutrients are affected by other food components, such as fiber, and how they are affected by drugs that older people are likely to take.
- Take into account toxic effects of nutrient supplements that may build up over long-term use and become apparent in older people.

In addition, clear age divisions should be established for people aged 50 and older.

Right now, researchers possess insufficient information on which to establish a meaningful RDA for nutrients other than energy for older adults. Until an improved version of the RDA exists, the present RDA for adults will have to serve. The next sections give special attention to a few nutrients of concern.

Energy

Energy needs decrease with advancing age. For one thing, the number of active cells in each organ decreases, bringing about a reduction in the body's overall metabolic rate, although this is not inevitable. For another, older people usually reduce their physical activity (although they need not do so). The RDA for energy intakes for older people reflect an estimated reduction of about 5 percent per decade in energy output. The variation is great, so the ranges are wide (see the inside front cover), but average figures for people 75 and older are 2050 calories per day for men and 1600 for women.

PEM is protein-energy malnutrition; the symptoms are in Chapter 5.

Table 13–2

Eating Patterns for Older People

	Number of Exchanges	
Exchange List	*Woman (1500 cal)*	*Man (2000 cal)*
Milk (nonfat)	4	4
Vegetable	2	3
Fruit	4	6
Bread	5	9
Meat (lean)	6	7
Fat	6	8

Note: These patterns supply the food energy amounts recommended by the RDA for people over 50.

Table 13–2 shows food patterns that would supply amounts of calories a little lower than the RDA. On such a limited energy allowance, all foods must be nutrient dense. There is little leeway for such low-nutrient-density foods as sugar, sweets, fats, oils, or alcohol. Because obesity is well recognized as a shortener of the life span, these seem to be life-sustaining recommendations.

Energy intake should be adequate, however. Deficiency can cause protein-energy malnutrition (PEM), which is common in older people and often goes unnoticed. An observer, seeing the wasted muscle, weakness, and swelling of protein deficiency, may think "That person looks old," when in fact the symptoms are those of PEM. Older people who have been trying to lose weight or eating monotonous or bizarre diets are most likely to be affected.[26]

Activities of all kinds are recommended for maintenance of good health. Ideally, exercise should be part of each day's schedule, intense enough to increase the heartbeat and respiration rate for at least 20 minutes, and to prevent muscle atrophy. Many older persons believe that they can't participate in strenuous exercise, but studies have shown that they can do more than they think they can. Any exercise—even a ten-minute walk a day—is better than none, and with persistence, great improvement can be achieved at any age. Training not only improves muscles, but also increases the blood flow to the brain. Another reason to exercise: a person spending energy in physical activity can afford to eat more food, and with it, more nutrients.

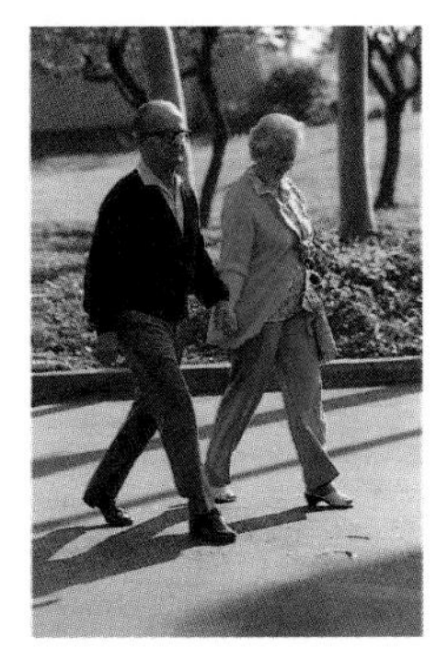

A person spending energy in physical activity can afford to eat more food.

Nutrients

The RDA committee assumes at present, based on the small amount of research available, that the need for ***protein*** is the same for older adults as it is for younger adults. However, as you grow older, you have to get this protein from less food, so you must seek out low-calorie sources of high-quality protein. To protect the protein from being used for energy, you have to include ample complex carbohydrates in your diet along with it.

Low hemoglobin levels have been shown to correlate with the protein (as well as the iron) content of the diet and may be the cause of the fatigue and apathy so often mentioned as a problem by older persons. The National Academy of Sciences recommends that older persons consume 12 percent of their calories as protein, which works out to an amount slightly above the RDA for most people. Too much protein may be as damaging as too little—excess protein causes the excretion of precious calcium, needed to protect the bones from osteoporosis. Food patterns that restrict fat and offer abundant carbohydrate typically supply up to 20 percent of the calories as protein, and this may be an ideal intake, especially for people whose protein needs are increased by illness.

Fat should be limited in the older person's diet, for many reasons. Cutting fat helps cut calories (recall that fat delivers two and a half times as many calories per unit of weight as the other energy nutrients) and may also help retard the development of atherosclerosis, cancer, arthritis, and other degenerative diseases. An appropriate intake might be 20 percent of the calories from fat. Of those, most should perhaps be from polyunsaturated and monounsaturated fat to contribute the essential fatty acids and to displace the saturated fat thought to contribute to high blood cholesterol. The polyunsaturated oils should be balanced between vegetable and fish sources.

Complex carbohydrate foods in great varieties should be emphasized in the older person's diet. Any educational campaign conducted to improve the diets of the elderly should make clear that where complex carbohydrates are found in food, a generous array of vitamins, minerals, and fiber follows.

The ***fiber*** recommendations for the general population should be stressed as well: increase the use of fruits, vegetables, and whole-grain cereals. The fiber in these foods is important to prevent constipation and to lower blood cholesterol. Cooking destroys some fiber in foods, but it also renders them easier to eat, so a person who has trouble chewing may prefer them. Such a person might then need to make a special effort to identify easy-to-eat foods such as cooked cereals, fruits, and vegetables that will be good sources of fiber.

The RDA for ***vitamins*** for the elderly are currently under study and probably will change. It seems likely that the RDA for some vitamins will decrease, while the RDA for others will increase. Among those that decrease may be vitamin A and folacin; among those that increase may be vitamin B_6, vitamin B_{12}, and

Supplements for the Elderly

Throughout this book, boxes such as these have brought to light many kinds of supplements and many of the claims that lure people to take them. Advertisers target older people for supplements and "health foods," by claiming their products prevent diseases, a claim to which elderly people attend. Even so, the elderly are, for the most part, reasonable in their approach—most avoid health-food stores, or they buy less there than others.[27] Do older people need supplements? If so, which?

To determine if a supplement is needed, consider first the needs of the people involved. Energy needs usually decrease with age due to a decline in basal metabolic rate and activity. This means older adults need to consume a more nutrient-dense diet; they need more nutrients per calorie from their food than when they were younger. Unfortunately, many older adults do just the opposite: they consume nutrient-poor diets. Compound the reduced energy needs with the increased needs for some nutrients (such as vitamin B_6, vitamin B_{12}, and vitamin D), and you can see that the nutrient density of the foods chosen must be extraordinarily high. Many older people take prescription drugs or have other conditions that push their nutrient needs up even further. Moreover, those who have had *slightly* inadequate diets throughout their lives may have developed considerable deficits by the time they are old—they may already be malnourished.

Can a supplement meet their needs? Sometimes, depending on the nutrient being supplemented. In most cases, though, the money people spend on nutrient supplements would be much better spent on nutritious foods. Even more important, self-prescribed vitamin-mineral supplements are sometimes taken in amounts so high as to be toxic. Even physicians do not always recommend the appropriate supplement or recognize that one is needed. Their clients may end up with the *wrong* vitamins and minerals prescribed or have none prescribed when supplements are needed. Surveys designed to find out what kinds of nutrient supplements older people are using tend to support the view that in many cases they are wasting their money. A study in a Southern California retirement community, for example, showed that 72 percent of the subjects were taking nutrient supplements—mostly of vitamins C and E—but that these choices were not related to the users' dietary intakes—that is, these were not the vitamins the subjects needed.[28]

In view of what is known about their nutrient needs, older people should first be encouraged to eat a balanced diet that is low in fat, high in fiber, and rich in vitamins and minerals. However, it may be appropriate to supplement the diet with a balanced, once-daily multivitamin-mineral preparation. Controversy 6, "Vitamin Supplements," identified some people who might need supplements. Many of these people could be elderly people—among them, habitual dieters, malnourished elderly people, people who eat bizarre or monotonous diets, people with illnesses that take away the appetite, people taking medications that interfere with the body's use of nutrients, people with diseases or other conditions that increase their metabolic needs, and strict vegetarians.

In addition, researchers specializing in the nutrition of the elderly have suggested a need for a vitamin D supplement (10 micrograms a day, or, in the old terminology, 400 IU).[29] As people age, they absorb less vitamin D from food, and they may make less when sunlight hits their skin.[30] Some authorities suggest that the RDA for vitamin D for older people should be set at 15 to 20 micrograms per day, rather than the 10 micrograms suggested for younger adults.[31] Evidence is accumulating that vitamin D therapy is important in the fight against osteoporosis, along with calcium, exercise, and for women, hormone therapy.[32]

Also, calcium supplements may be a wise addition—these were discussed in full in Chapter 7. Equally important is eliminating dietary factors that cause calcium excretion, such as caffeine overuse, unwarranted use of medication, or use of other drugs, including alcohol.

On the other hand, toxic overdoses must be avoided. The toxicity of vitamin D is particularly frightening (see Chapter 6)—so those using vitamin D supplements should be careful to take the recommended dose, not more, not less. Also, vitamin A is toxic, and the absorption of vitamin A increases with aging. Care must be taken to prevent vitamin A toxicity from even ordinary-dose supplements in the elderly.[33]

The older person would probably be wise to follow the rule of thumb that if the energy intake is below about 1500 calories, then a vitamin-mineral supplement is recommended—not a megavitamin, but just a once-daily type supplement. This means that many older persons, all except those who are so active that their energy allowances have remained high, should take this precaution. (Controversy 6 offered hints on how to choose a supplement, and Appendix D provides a comparison of those available.) Further, if the person cannot drink milk, calcium and vitamin D supplements may be of value. For anyone truly motivated to obtain the best possible health, however, it is never too late to learn to eat well, exercise regularly, and adopt whatever other lifestyle changes may be indicated to achieve that goal.

vitamin D; vitamin C and E requirements may remain the same.[34] While work progresses, it still seems likely that adequate vitamin intakes can, in general, best be ensured by improving the diet; the accompanying box examines the advisability of older people's using supplements.

Studies have shown that the one food group omitted most often by the elderly is the vegetable group. About 18 percent of older people are reported to eat no vegetables at all. Fruit is lacking in many diets, and up to one of every three older people report never eating fruit. Some men and women do not eat whole-grain breads and cereals, and so lose a significant source of many B vitamins and several minerals. The destruction of vitamin E by heat processing and oxidation is well known, and the processed and convenience foods so often used by the elderly and by nursing homes are thought to contribute to a vitamin E deficiency if their use continues over several years. Many, especially those who eat according to traditional ethnic foodways, do not drink milk and so risk vitamin D, as well as calcium, deficiency. The risk is greatest if they do not get much sun—for example, if they are homebound in nursing homes, or live in the North or in smoggy cities.[35] Each person whose diet is inadequate in any of these respects could alter it, using foods acceptable to that person, given the knowledge and motivation to do so. People who need more sun could arrange to get outdoors more, or to sit by an open sunny window some of the time.

Among the *minerals,* iron deserves first mention. Iron-deficiency anemia is not as common in older adults as in the past, but it still occurs in some, especially in those with low food energy intakes.[36] Low hemoglobin can result from a diet low in protein, as already mentioned; but diets low in iron are the usual cause. Heavy reliance on a "tea and toast" diet is cited as a double risk in this connection; what little iron the toast provides is poorly absorbable, while the tannins in tea inhibit iron absorption. (A similar substance in coffee inhibits iron absorption, too.[37]) The best insurance of an adequate iron intake is a colorful selection of foods that includes iron-containing red meats, as well as fruits and vegetables rich in vitamin C to aid in iron absorption.

Aside from diet, other factors in many older people's lives increase the likelihood of iron deficiency:

- Chronic blood loss from ulcers, hemorrhoids, or other disease conditions.
- Poor iron absorption due to reduced stomach acid secretion.
- Antacid use, which interferes with iron absorption.
- Use of medicines that cause blood loss, including anticoagulants, aspirin, and other arthritis medicines.

Anyone concerned with the nutrition status of an older person should not forget these possibilities.

Zinc deficiencies are common in older people; as many as 95 percent of old people may not get the zinc they need, and many miss the mark by more than half.[38] Increasing their meat intakes would be the simplest way to remedy this problem. Symptoms most often associated with zinc deficiencies are loss of taste and slowed wound healing. Loss of taste, however, may not respond to zinc supplementation, so it may often arise from some other factor associated with aging.

Another mineral often lacking in older people's diets is calcium, the need for which increases with advancing age. Bone loss occurs insidiously, and may be alarmingly extensive and severe before a person realizes there is any problem at all. The recommendation of 4 cups of milk a day for older adults is difficult to meet, especially for the person who is unaccustomed to using much milk at all, and some sources recommend even more.[39] However, there are many alternative foods for obtaining the needed calcium. If fresh milk causes gas, as some older people report, then low-fat cheese should be included. Dry nonfat milk can be incorporated into many foods. Soup stock made from bones can be used daily, and the bones of canned fish can be eaten with the fish as a calcium source.

Some authorities hold that all older people should limit their salt intakes. This is hard for people who rely on convenience foods and processed foods extensively, but it is suggested that they should eat fresh foods instead, whenever they can.

To obtain the needed minerals, the older person should follow the same recommendation as for vitamins. The basics of nutrition, first described in Chapter 2, still apply: adequacy, balance, calorie control, moderation, and variety.

The most important nutrient of all is *water.* The elderly need to be reminded to drink fluids, because they are likely to be somewhat insensitive to their own thirst signals. They should drink six to eight glasses a day, enough to bring their urine output to about 6 cups per day. A large percentage of foster home operators note that one of the biggest problems with their elderly clients is getting them to use more water and fruit juices.

You can tell from the color of your urine if you're getting enough water. Bright or dark yellow urine is too concentrated; you need more water. Pale yellow, almost colorless urine is dilute enough; your water intake is ample.

Older people need fewer calories but just as many or more nutrients as when they were younger. To continue meeting their nutrient needs, they have to place increased emphasis on foods of high nutrient density. It is important not to omit any classes of foods, but to consume members of every food group daily. Fiber and water are important, and the basic principles of nutrition still apply. Exercise can increase the daily energy output, so the person can afford to eat more food.

The Effects of Drugs on Nutrients

As people get older, illnesses tend to set in, and they use more medicines—from over-the-counter (OTC) types such as aspirins and laxatives to prescription drugs of all kinds. Most drugs interact with one or more nutrients in several ways, usually resulting in greater-than-normal needs for these nutrients. Drugs may:

- Change the person's eating habits, thereby reducing nutrient intakes (example: a drug that upsets the stomach depresses food intake).
- Reduce the absorption of nutrients from the food eaten (example: oil laxatives dissolve the fat-soluble vitamins and carry them out of the digestive tract).
- Change nutrient metabolism, so that the nutrients cannot perform their biological functions (example: certain cancer drugs mimic vitamins and take their places in key enzymes, rendering those enzymes ineffective).
- Hasten nutrient excretion (example: alcohol dislodges nutrients from their storage places, allowing them to circulate and be excreted by the kidneys).

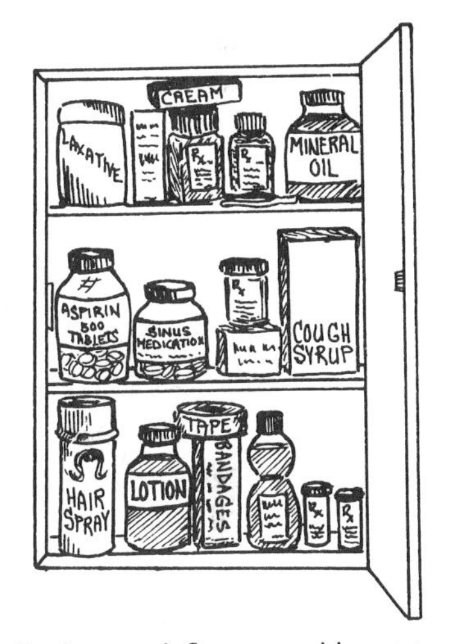

Medications can influence nutrition status.

Foods and nutrients can interfere with the actions of drugs, too. Prescription instructions take this into account and should be strictly followed.

The most common drug that can affect nutrition in old people is alcohol. A recent estimate sets the incidence of alcoholism in people over 60 in our society at 2 to 10 percent. Alcohol abuse has its most damaging impact on the vitamins thiamin and folacin and on the minerals calcium, magnesium, and zinc, but it affects nearly every nutrient to some extent. The substance itself provides only empty calories—no significant nutrients. Where it is a problem in elderly people, it must be recognized and dealt with. The effects of alcohol on a person of any age are explained in Controversy 12.

Of course, not everyone abuses alcohol, and for those who do not, it is relatively harmless to nutrition. In fact, a glass of wine, taken with food, relaxes, aids digestion, and adds to the enjoyment of meals. Used appropriately, wine and other alcoholic beverages can enhance health and enjoyment of life.

Over-the-counter drugs are freely available and useful for self-treatment, but are not harmless to nutrition. Mentioned in the list above, oil laxatives can carry nutrients, including bone-strengthening calcium and vitamin D, out of the body. In addition, a person who uses laxatives of any sort daily for a long time may find that the intestines can no longer function without them. Daily laxative use speeds up food transit time through the intestine so that many vitamins do not have time to be absorbed. Some laxatives contain fiber that lowers blood cholesterol, and could significantly alter blood lipids with long-term use.

Antacids also have nutrition effects. A person who takes Alka-Seltzer may not realize it, but it is loaded with sodium—a single 2-tablet dose exceeds some people's safe sodium intake for a whole day. It also neutralizes stomach acid, on which the absorption of many nutrients depends. Taking antacids regularly will cause the body to excrete many nutrients as wastes, rather than absorb them.

Like the effects of illnesses, the effects of drugs are cumulative over time. As one example, arthritis sufferers are often heavy users of aspirin, a superb painkiller and anti-inflammatory agent, but also an agent that prevents the passage of vitamin C from the plasma to the tissues. If plasma vitamin C levels are measured in these clients, then, no deficit is seen, and yet the tissues may be experiencing a deficit. A clinician, observing this effect, recommends "energetic vitamin C therapy" for clients taking large amounts of aspirin—not megadoses, to be sure, but doses of up to 200 milligrams, four times the RDA.[40] Another example: antibiotics kill intestinal bacteria that produce vitamin K, and many drugs produce a folacin deficiency. Anyone who finds it necessary to take one or several medications for more than just a few weeks should make special efforts to obtain amounts of nutrients greater than those recommended for other people. This goes for oral-contraceptive users, too (see box in Chapter 12).

Many more drugs than can be named here affect nutrition; the drugs mentioned in the next few paragraphs have been chosen because they are commonly used, or because they are particularly damaging to nutrition status. A common drug is the nicotine from tobacco; it is an appetite suppressant. One of the biggest problems people face upon quitting tobacco use is regulating food intake so as not to gain weight. Of course, the link between tobacco use and the development of cancer is strong, and people who continue to use it face much bigger problems than overweight. Smoking alters the metabolism of vitamin C; excretion of the vitamin is hastened in smokers, who may need more than other people to normalize blood levels.[41] The blood lipids are changed by smoking to favor cholesterol buildup, increasing the likelihood of heart disease.[42] The toxic minerals lead and cadmium are absorbed from cigarette smoke in the lungs.[43] Smoking affects nutrition, but correcting these nutrient effects will not prevent damage to the body caused by tobacco. Smoking has so many deleterious effects on health that it has been called the number one preventable health problem in the developed world.

Drugs that produce a feeling of pleasure, euphoria, are often abused; people who abuse them may stop eating and incur severe malnutrition. Such drugs are thought to stimulate pleasure centers in the brain in the same way that the brain's naturally occurring opiates do. In a normal person, eating triggers the endogenous opiates to stimulate the brain's pleasure centers; in the drug-addicted person, the brain's opiate production is suppressed and does not respond to eating—the person craves more drug instead of food. Animal studies show clearly that drugs suppress desire for food: animals, when given equal access to food and cocaine will ignore the food and choose the cocaine until they eventually starve.[44] Some prescription drugs—amphetamines, for example—can produce an addiction that has that effect on people, too.

Although not physically addicting, a marijuana cigarette has characteristic effects on sensory perception, including hearing, touch, taste, and smell and on perceptions of time, space, and the body. Among the taste changes apparently induced is a great enjoyment of eating, especially of sweets, but it is not known how this effect occurs; the drug apparently does not change the blood glucose level. The active ingredient in marijuana has been used successfully to alleviate the nausea caused by chemotherapy treatment of cancer, and to allow people who receive the treatment to eat.

hepatitis: inflammation of the liver caused by one of several types of viruses, transmitted by infected hypodermic needles (drug abuse, tattoos, blood transfusions), by eating infected seafood, or by contact with secretions of a person who has the disease; it often causes chronic liver disease.

Abusers of all drugs face multiple nutrition problems:

- They spend their money on drugs, not on food.
- They lose interest in food and seek drugs.
- They may use drugs that directly suppress the appetite.
- Their lifestyle is not conducive to good eating habits.
- They may contract wasting diseases, such as **hepatitis** or acquired immune deficiency syndrome (AIDS), from contaminated needles.
- They may abuse alcohol during withdrawal from the drug.

You might think that many years of living and experience would lend a person immunity to the lure of drug abuse, but drug use by the elderly is not confined to medicinal treatments. Old people are susceptible to alcohol and prescription drug addictions. Obtaining prescription drugs is no problem, for the elderly are rarely denied drug prescriptions when they request them. Under the drive of an addiction, they may go from physician to physician, garnishing from each the right to a vial of painkillers or tranquilizers, and ultimately fill each prescription and take all the pills. It is important to withhold judgment on an individual with a drug problem. Drug addiction is not a sign of weakness or of personality disorder; sufficient exposure to an addictive chemical is all that is required for dependence to develop. No one is exempt. One of the most important aspects of recovery from addiction is to identify and correct nutrition problems, possibly caused by the drug, while teaching and supporting adaptive eating habits.

COFFEE

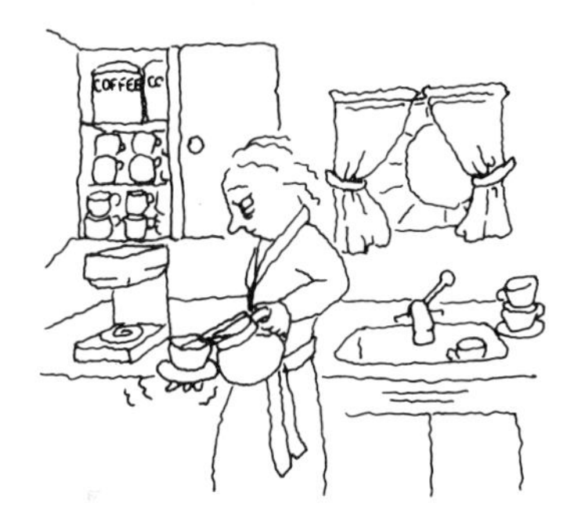

Caffeine has the distinction of being the drug most widely used by the human race. It is neither a medicine nor a euphoria-producing drug, but it is a mild stimulant of the central nervous system. Caffeine increases the respiration rate, heart rate, blood pressure, and secretion of the stress and other hormones, and it reduces blood flow to the brain by causing the brain's blood vessels to constrict. Its "wake-up" effect is maximal within an hour after the dose. In moderate amounts (50 to 200 milligrams a day), caffeine seems to be relatively harmless, although older people often find they cannot tolerate as much caffeine as they could when they were younger. Table 13–3 (p. 518) shows where caffeine is found, and in what quantities.

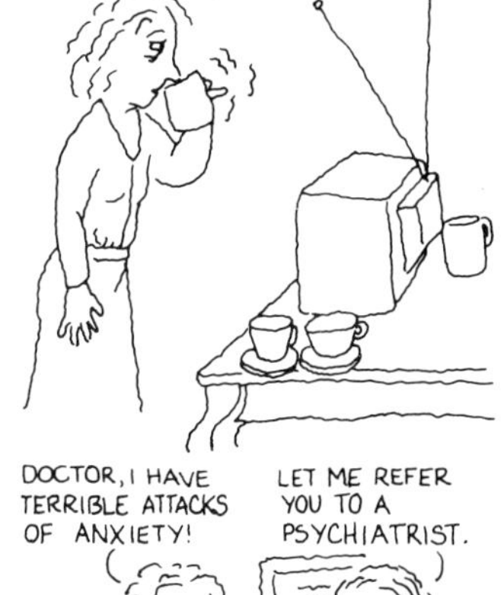

Caffeine is addictive, in that the body adapts to its presence. Sudden abstinence after long use, even if use has been moderate, or cutting back from a high to a low dose causes a characteristic withdrawal headache, curable only by taking more caffeine. This kind of headache is so common that many pain relievers include caffeine in their formulas, even though caffeine is ineffective for relieving other types of pain.

An overdose of caffeine produces a reaction indistinguishable from an anxiety attack. People who drink between 8 and 15 cups of coffee a day, for example, have been known to seek help from health care providers for complaints such as dizziness, agitation, restlessness, recurring headaches, intestinal discomfort, and sleep difficulties. Before prescribing a tranquilizer, the physician would do well to inquire about the caffeine consumption of such clients.

DOCTOR, I HAVE TERRIBLE ATTACKS OF ANXIETY!
LET ME REFER YOU TO A PSYCHIATRIST.

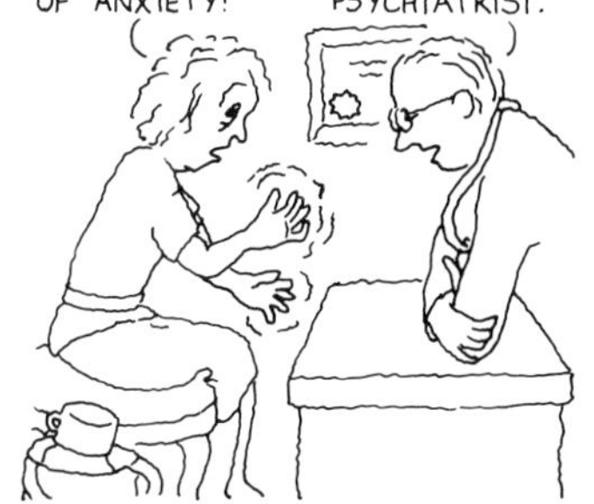

Anxiety may not be a "mental" symptom.

Table 13–3

Caffeine Content of Beverages, Foods, and OTC Drugs

Drinks and Foods	Average (mg)	Range (mg)
Coffee (5-oz cup)		
Brewed, drip method	130	110–150
Brewed, percolator	94	64–124
Instant	74	40–108
Decaffeinated, brewed or instant	3	1–5
Tea (5-oz cup)		
Brewed, major U.S. brands	40	20–90
Brewed, imported brands	60	25–110
Instant	30	25–50
Iced (12-oz glass)	70	67–76
Soft drinks (12-oz can)		
Dr. Pepper		40
Colas and cherry colas:		
regular		30–46
diet		2–58
caffeine free		0–trace
Jolt		72
Mountain Dew, Mello Yello		52
Big Red		38
Fresca, Hires Root Beer, 7–Up, Sprite,		0
Squirt, Sunkist Orange		0
Cocoa beverage (5-oz cup)	4	2–20
Chocolate milk beverage (8 oz)	5	2–7
Milk chocolate candy (1 oz)	6	1–15
Dark chocolate, semisweet (1 oz)	20	5–35
Baker's chocolate (1 oz)	26	26
Chocolate-flavored syrup (1 oz)	4	4
Drugs[a]		
Cold remedies (standard dose)		
Dristan		0
Coryban-D, Triaminicin		30
Diuretics (standard dose)		
Aqua-ban, Permathene H_2Off		200
Pre-Mens Forte		100
Pain relievers (standard dose)		
Excedrin		130
Midol, Anacin		65
Aspirin, plain (any brand)		0
Stimulants		
Caffedrin, NoDoz,Vivarin		200
Weight-control aids (daily dose)		
Prolamine		280
Dexatrim, Dietac		200

[a]Because products change, contact the manufacturer for an update on products you use regularly.

Source: Data from C. Lecos, The latest caffeine scoreboard, *FDA Consumer,* March 1984, p. 14; Measuring your life with coffee spoons. *Tufts University Diet and Nutrition Letter,* April 1984, pp. 3–6; Institute of Food Technologists, Expert Panel on Food Safety and Nutrition, *Evaluation of Caffeine Safety,* a publication (1986) available from the Institute of Food Technologists, 221 N. LaSalle St., Chicago, IL 60601.

Large doses of caffeine can also cause abnormal heartbeats, hypertension, and increased blood cholesterol and are believed to have caused heart attacks in people whose hearts were already damaged by degenerative disease. Caffeine is not considered a risk factor for the development of atherosclerosis. However, its vehicle coffee has been associated, together with other risk factors, with increased incidence of heart disease.[45] Coffee drinking seems to be part of a lifestyle in which something promotes heart disease, though it may not be the coffee itself.

Coffee has other nonnutrient effects—see Controversy 10.

Caffeine has effects on nutrition, too. The caffeine in just a few cups of coffee can double the excretion of calcium and magnesium; the amounts lost in one day are still small, but over years, they become significant. Caffeine also may induce benign (not cancerous) breast disease and may worsen premenstrual symptoms, especially in women who overuse it. Moderation in the use of caffeine-containing foods and beverages is advisable for all ages, and older people should be alert to the need to reduce their customary doses.

Age brings illness, and with it, increased use of medicines that can affect a person's nutrition. Older people can suffer from alcoholism as well as from other addictions. Caffeine is widely used, is habit-forming, and causes many changes in the body, including nutrient excretion.

Sources of Assistance

As mentioned at the start of this chapter, many elderly must live on little money in an expensive world. This has a direct effect on their nutrition, because food is among the few flexible items in the budget, and food money may be nibbled away by increases in the costs of rent, medical care, and the like. To economize, people may choose to do without nutritious foods, especially fruits, vegetables, and milk products.[46] Some older people have so little money to buy food that they resort to eating canned pet food instead of meat—a practice that can be dangerous. Pet foods may contain high levels of lead, insects, animal glands, and other contamination; they are not held to the same standards as are foods produced for people.

Poor dental health can contribute to malnutrition; if chewing causes pain, people naturally avoid such chewy (and nutritious) foods as meats and fresh fruits. Canned soups and syrupy fruits require little chewing, and so may be overused by some. In choosing such low-nutrient-density foods on a regular basis, people deny themselves the nutrients in fresh foods, and make malnutrition likely. In light of these and other problems and of the increasing numbers of people in the older age group, it is not surprising that individuals and agencies try to help.

Public Programs

In recent years, we have come to recognize that the responsibility for support in old age cannot be left entirely to the individual. Three major federal programs can help older persons with money problems, at least a little. Under Social Security, employees and employers pay into a fund from which the employee collects benefits at retirement. The Food Stamp program enables people who qualify to obtain stamps with which to buy food. The Supplemental Security Income program is aimed at directly improving the financial plight of the very poor, by increasing a person's or a family's income to the defined poverty level. This sometimes helps older people retain their independence.

Sources of support for the elderly:

- Social Security
- Food Stamps
- Supplemental Security Income

Another program to benefit the elderly is the Older Americans Act of 1965. Title IIIC (formerly Title VII) of this act is the "Nutrition Program for the Elderly." The major goals of this program are to provide:

Title IIIC of the Older Americans Act

- Low-cost nutritious meals.
- Opportunity for social interaction.
- Homemaker education and shopping assistance.
- Counseling and referral to other social services.
- Transportation services.

The program is intended to improve older people's nutrition status and enable them to avoid medical problems, continue living in communities of their own choice, and stay out of institutions.

Meals on Wheels

Sites chosen for congregate meals under this program must be accessible to most of the target population. Volunteers may also deliver meals to those who are homebound either permanently or temporarily; these efforts are known as Meals on Wheels. The program ensures nutrition, but its recipients miss out on the social benefit of the congregate meal sites; every effort is made to persuade them to come to the shared meals, if they can. Despite these programs, many eligible people are still missing meals and are malnourished simply because they don't know of the programs available.[47] Identification of such people should become a higher priority.

Food banks have been established in several areas to help older people stretch their food dollars. A food bank project buys industry's "irregulars"—products that have been mislabeled, underweighted, redesigned, or mispackaged and would ordinarily therefore be thrown away. Nothing is wrong with this food, and the industry can credit it as a donation. As government money dwindles, the nutrition status of low-income people of all ages depends more and more on private efforts such as food banking.

Food assistance programs serve the needs of the body, but many times the very best gift for elderly citizens is overlooked—it is a change of attitude. Our culture values the doers, those concerned with action and achievement. The Spanish mother may enjoy her child because he is sitting in her lap and laughing in her face; however, the Anglo-American mother is more likely preoccupied with how well her child is preparing for tomorrow. The elderly are aware of the status given those who are "doing something" and of the disrespect given those who lead a contemplative life in retirement.

It would take a near miracle to change the attitude of a nation, but individual persons can change their attitudes toward themselves as they age. Preparation for this period should include financial planning and developing of social skills to avert loneliness. It helps, too, to give of one's talents in volunteer or paid work; some think that being needed and contributing to humanity are keys to happiness in the later years. Intellectual pursuits can give meaning to the days.

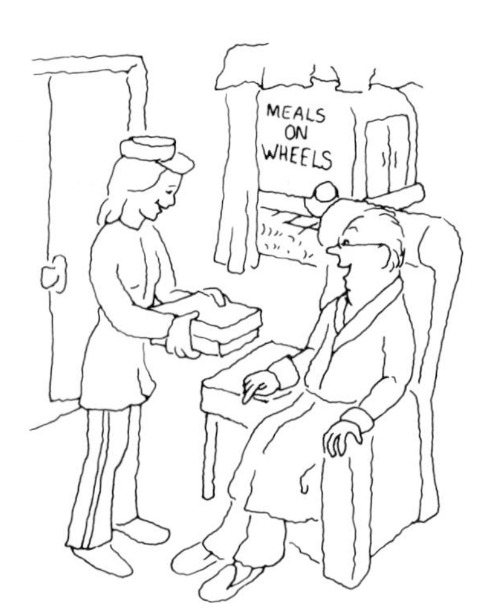

Stay-at-homes can get nourishing meals this way.

Each person must practice adjusting to change, especially when it comes without consent, to allow continued control over life. The goal is to enjoy life fully, with optimal health of mind and body.

Financial planning is needed to ensure support in the later years. Assistance programs are available for older people. Many programs directly improve nutrition status; some are aimed at helping to relieve financial problems. Wise adults will plan ahead to maximize their enjoyment of the later years.

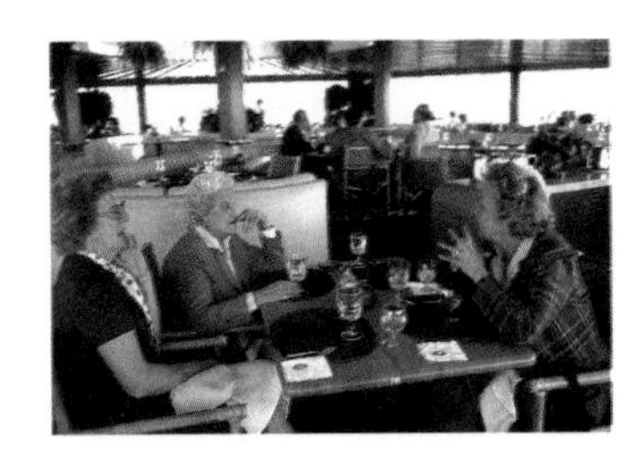

Social skills bring friends, friends bring happiness, and happiness is good for the appetite.

Nursing Homes and Day Care

When the care needs of an elderly person, say someone with Alzheimer's disease, make staying at home impossible, professional facilities can provide medical and other care. A variety of options exist; for example, some facilities provide assistance and limited medical care during the day while other family members attend to their own daytime needs. These facilities can provide day care, along with activities and a peer group for friendships. All these factors work together to give the elderly stimulating experiences; in such a setting, mealtimes are often a highlight. Another familiar alternative is the nursing home. A nursing home serves people who need constant medical care.

When inquiring into nursing homes or day care centers, a person should find out some things about the food service;

- Can the people choose their own food?
- How often are the menus repeated (is the cycle monotonous)?
- How often are fresh fruits and vegetables served? Is the food kept appropriately hot and cold until serving?
- Is a plate check conducted regularly, at least once a week, to discover what the resident is consuming?
- Does the staff keep track of each person's weight?
- Is there good communication between the nursing staff and the dietitian so that the dietitian will know if someone is not eating?
- Is the elderly person encouraged and helped to go to the dining room to eat in order to enjoy other people's company?
- Is the dining room attractive?
- Does someone help those who can't manage feeding themselves?
- Are minced meats offered to those who have problems with their dentures?
- Are religious and ethnic dietary requests honored?
- How high a proportion of the foods are prepackaged? (No guide can be given for what proportion is desirable, but it should be remembered that processed foods are low in vitamin content and high in salt.)

Other questions that the investigator will want to ask have to do with the general atmosphere of the facility, in recognition of the effect of social climate on a person's appetite. A nursing home or center that views participants as persons, not as patients, gets a mark in its favor.

Opinions differ on the philosophy to adopt for institutional menus. Managing a multitude of different special diets is difficult and expensive, and one authority recommends a "liberalized geriatric diet" for most cases, rather than diets tailored specifically for specific diseases. Based on the assumption that older people "should have the right to choose the food they eat," this general, liberal approach provides in one package the key characteristics of several special diets:

- 1500 to 2000 calories per day, mostly from nutrient-dense foods, with simple desserts.
- Minimal salt used in preparation.
- 50 to 60 grams protein per day from 2 cups milk and 4 to 6 ounces meat or alternate.
- At least 6 milligrams iron per day (the RDA for older people is 10 milligrams per day).
- Generous amounts of natural fiber.
- Fluid intake of 64 ounces per day.[48]

Further modifications are essential for people with severe disease conditions.

Nursing homes and adult day care facilities should be judged partly by the food they provide and partly by the attitudes they project.

Food Feature

Single Survival

Singles of all ages face problems concerning food purchasing, storing, and preparing. Large packages of meat and vegetables are often suitable for a family of four or more, and even a head of lettuce can spoil before one person can use it all. Many singles live in small dwellings, some without kitchens and freezers—for them, purchasing and storage problems are compounded. Following is a collection of ideas gathered from single people who have devised answers to these problems.

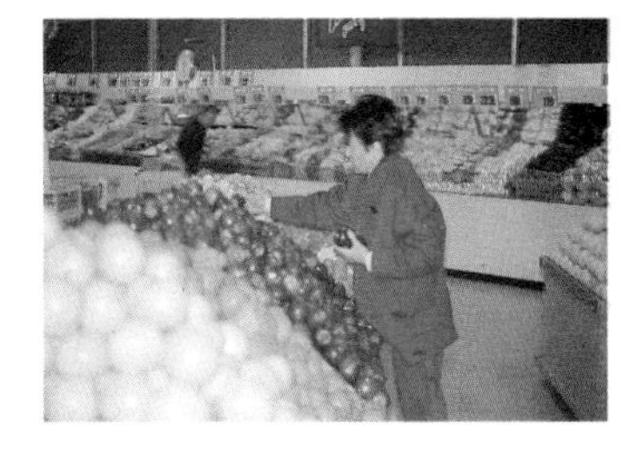

Buy only the amount you need.

Buy only what you will use: the small-size containers of food may be expensive, but it is also expensive to let the unused portion of a large-size container spoil before using. Buy only three pieces of each kind of fresh fruit: a ripe one, a medium-ripe one, and a green one. Eat the first right away and the second soon, and let the last one ripen to eat days later. Don't be timid about asking the grocer to break open a family-sized package of wrapped meat or fresh vegetables.

Think up a variety of ways to use a vegetable when you must buy it in large quantity. For example, you can divide a head of cauliflower into thirds. Cook one third and eat it as a hot vegetable. Put another third into a salad dressing marinade for use as an appetizer, and save the rest to use raw in salad. Make mixtures, using what you have on hand. A thick stew prepared from any leftover vegetables and bits of meat, with some added onion, pepper, celery, and potatoes, makes a complete and balanced meal—except for milk. But if you like creamed gravy, you can add dry nonfat milk to your stew.

Buy fresh milk in the sizes best suited for you. If your grocer doesn't carry pints or quarts of milk, try a nearby service station or convenience store.

Set aside a place for rows of glass jars containing shelf staple items that you can't buy in single-serving quantities—rice, tapioca, lentils and other dry beans, flour, cornmeal, dry nonfat milk, and cereal, to name only a few possibilities. Place each jar, tightly sealed, in the freezer for one night to kill any eggs or organisms before storing it on the shelf. Then the jars will keep bugs out of the foods indefinitely. The jars make an attractive display and will remind you of possibilities for variety in your menus. Cut the directions-for-use label from the package and store it in the jar.

Remember, light destroys riboflavin, so use opaque jars for enriched pasta and dry milk.

Cook for several meals at a time. For example, boil three potatoes with skins. Eat one hot, mashed with chives. When the others have cooled, use one to make a potato-cheese casserole ready to be put into the oven for the next evening's meal. Slice the third one into a covered bowl, and pour over it the juice from pickles, The pickled potato will keep several days in the refrigerator and can be used in a salad.

Experiment with stir-fried foods. Use a frying pan if you don't have a wok. A variety of vegetables and meats can be enjoyed this way; inexpensive vegetables such as cabbage and celery are delicious when crisp cooked in a little oil with soy sauce or lemon added. Cooked, leftover vegetables can be dropped in at the last minute. Frozen mixtures of Chinese or Polynesian vegetables are available in the larger grocery stores. Bonus: only one pan to wash. If you can afford a microwave oven, buy one; it will eliminate the need for most pots and pans,

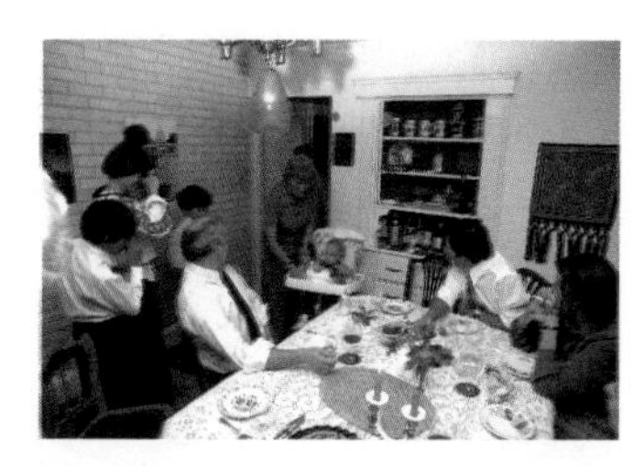

When shared with others, simple food is festive.

because you can assemble all your foods on your plate and cook them right there.

Depending on your freezer space, make double or even six times as much as you need of a dish that takes time to prepare: a casserole, vegetable pie, or meat loaf. Freeze individual portions in containers that can be microwaved or oven heated for serving later. Be sure to date these so you will use the oldest first.

Buy a loaf of bread and immediately store half, well wrapped, in the freezer (not the refrigerator, which will make it stale). Buy frozen vegetables in large bags rather than in small cartons. You can take out the exact amount you need and close the bag tightly with a rubber band or spring clothes pin. Season the bag of vegetables by adding some fresh herbs. Buy bunches of parsley, dill, and oregano or basil, keep just a few sprigs out for use during the next few days, and chop up the rest to add to the frozen vegetable bags, for low-cost elegance. Wrap individual portions of meat you wish to bake or broil (purchased in bulk) in thick aluminum foil: the foil can become the liner for the pan in which you bake or broil the meat, thus saving cleanup work. For meat to be microwaved, use sturdy plastic wrap to freeze each portion, and re-use the wrap to cover the cooking dish in the microwave. Put the portion in a brown bag marked "hamburger" or "chicken thighs". The bag is easy to locate in the freezer, and you'll know when your supply is running low.

Although the suggestions here will help the single person with the mechanics of food chores, they meet only a part of the need. Dr. Jack Weinberg, professor of psychiatry at the University of Illinois, wrote perceptively:

> It is not *what* the older person eats but *with whom* that will be the deciding factor in proper care for him. The oft-repeated complaint of the older patient that he has little incentive to prepare food for only himself is not merely a statement of fact but also a rebuke to the questioner for failing to perceive his isolation and aloneness and to realize that food . . . for one's self lacks the condiment of another's presence which can transform the simplest fare to the ceremonial act with all its shared meaning.[49]

Even for nutrition's sake, it is important to attend to loneliness at mealtimes; the person who is living alone must learn to connect food with socializing. Cook for yourself with the idea that you are also preparing for guests you might want to invite. Or invite guests and make enough food so that you will have some left for a later meal. With leftovers on hand, you can invite a single friend on the spur of the moment to "come over and share my frozen dinners with me tonight." Most elderly people, and in fact most people of any age, respond best not when they are made to feel dependent, such as when they are cared for in nursing homes, but when they share close proximity with others and interact with them.[50] So, go ahead and invite an older person in for a meal, but ask that person to bring the bread or otherwise include them in the planning.

When you are alone at mealtime, make it a special occasion; it is a good way to take care of yourself. For example, try this: set the table with tablecloth, napkin, a full complement of utensils, and a wildflower if you can. Set a pot of stew with vegetables and fresh herbs on low heat to cook, and make a salad. Go settle in a stuffed chair and enjoy a book, some soothing music, and a crackling cold glass of lemoned sparkling water, until the rich aroma of stew calls you to dinner. After serving your plate, light a candle, dim the lights, savor the food, and relish some of the best company you will ever have—your own.

shopping list:

- dry skim milk, pints of milk
- storage jars with tight-sealing lids
- fresh herbs
- bags of frozen fruits and vegetables
- clothespins for closing food bags
- small cans of fruits and vegetables
- freezer wrap, heavy aluminum foil
- small servings of lean meats
- 3 pieces of each kind of fruit: green, medium ripe, and ripe
- 3 potatoes
- a prepackaged bag of salad greens
- 1/2 dozen eggs

Notes

1. The discussion of ageism was adapted from F. S. Sizer and E. N. Whitney, *Life Choices: Health Concepts and Strategies* (St. Paul: West, 1988).
2. S. M. Golant, *A Place to Grow Old: The Meaning of Environment in Old Age* (New York: Columbia University Press, 1984), pp. 137, 316.
3. M. Chou, Selling to older Americans, *Cereal Foods World* 26 (1981): 633.
4. Senate Special Committee on Aging, American Association of Retired Persons, National Center for Health Statistics, Bureau of Labor Statistics, and the Population Reference Bureau as cited in Numbers show aging of America, *Tallahassee Democrat,* 17 February 1985.
5. Senate Special Committee on Aging, 1985.
6. Senate Special Committee on Aging, 1985.
7. L. Hofmann, ed., *The Great American Nutrition Hassle* (Palo Alto, Calif.: Mayfield, 1978), p. 89.
8. J. S. Goodwin, J. M. Goodwin, and P. J. Garry, Association between nutritional status and cognitive functioning in a healthy elderly population, *Journal of the American Medical Association* 249 (1983): 2917–2921.
9. E. J. Root and J. B. Longenecker, Brain cell alterations suggesting premature aging induced by dietary deficiency of vitamin B_6 and/or copper, *American Journal of Clinical Nutrition* 37 (1983): 540–552.
10. Alzheimer's disease: An aluminum connection? *Nutrition and the MD,* August 1985, p. 1.
11. The nutritional origin of cataracts, *Nutrition Reviews* 42 (1984): 377–379; F. Rosales and coauthors, Lactose digestion and milk consumption pattern in Guatemalan cataract patients (abstract), *American Journal of Clinical Nutrition* 43 (1986): 700.
12. The items shown in the margin were listed by K. A. Meister, Can diet cure arthritis? *ACSH News and Views,* September/October 1980, p. 10; and in Morsels and tidbits, *Nutrition and the MD,* January 1982.
13. L. G. Darlington, N. W. Ramsey, and J. R. Mansfield, Placebo-controlled, blind study of dietary manipulation therapy in rheumatoid arthritis, *Lancet* 1 (1986): 236–238.
14. J. M. Kremer and coauthors, Fish-oil fatty acid supplementation in active rheumatoid arthritis: A double-blinded, controlled crossover study, *Annuals of Internal Medicine* 106 (1987): 497–503.
15. N. E. Lane, D. A. Block, and H. H. Jones, Long distance running, bone density, and osteoarthritis, *Journal of the American Medical Association* 255 (1986): 1147–1151.
16. E. L. Schneider and J. D. Reed, Life extension, *New England Journal of Medicine* 312 (1985): 1159–1168.
17. D. Sinclair, *Human Growth after Birth* (New York: Oxford University Press, 1985), p. 217.
18. M. Allukian, Dentistry at the crossroads: The future is uncertain; the challenges are many (editorial), *American Journal of Public Health* 72 (1982): 653–654.
19. D. M. Watkin, The physiology of aging, *American Journal of Clinical Nutrition* 36 (supplement, October 1982): 750–758.
20. M. A. Dubick, Dietary supplements and health aids—a critical evaluation: 3. Natural and miscellaneous products, *Journal of Nutrition Education* 15 (1983): 123–128.
21. Life extension with SOD and other dietary antioxidants, *Nutrition and the MD,* December 1985, p. 3.
22. R. S. Paffenbarger and coauthors, Physical activity, all-cause mortality, and longevity of college alumni, *New England Journal of Medicine* 314 (1986): 605–613.
23. A. E. Harper, Nutrition, aging, and longevity, *American Journal of Clinical Nutrition* 36 (supplement, October 1982): 737–749.
24. Harper, 1982.
25. E. L. Schneider and coauthors, Recommended Dietary Allowances and the health of the elderly, *New England Journal of Medicine* 314 (1986): 157–160.
26. S. R. Gambert and A. R. Guansing, Protein-calorie malnutrition in the elderly, *Journal of the American Geriatrics Society* 28 (1980): 272–275.
27. L. Yung, I. Contento, and J. D. Gussow, Use of health foods by the elderly, *Journal of Nutrition Education* 3 (1984): 127–131.
28. G. E. Gray, A. Paganini-Hill, and R. K. Ross, Dietary intake and nutrient supplement use in a southern California retirement community, *American Journal of Clinical Nutrition* 38 (1983): 122–128.
29. Suter and Russell, 1987.
30. Schneider and coauthors, 1986.
31. A. M. Parfitt and coauthors, Vitamin D and bone health in the elderly, *American Journal of Clinical Nutrition* 36 (supplement, November 1982): 1014–1031.
32. B. E. Nordin and coauthors, A prospective trial of the effect of vitamin D supplementation on metacarpal bone loss in elderly women, *The American Journal of Clinical Nutrition* 42 (1985): 470–474; Y. Weisman, R. J. Schen, and Z. Eisenberg, Single oral high-dose vitamin D_3 prophylaxis in the elderly, *Journal of the American Geriatric Society* 34 (1986): 515–518, as reported in *Modern Medicine,* November 1986, p. 162.
33. J. B. Blumberg, Nutrient requirements for the healthy elderly, *Contemporary Nutrition* 6 (1986), a publication available from General Mills, Inc., P.O. Box 1172, Minneapolis, MN 55440.
34. P. M. Suter and R. M. Russell Vitamin requirements of the elderly, *American Journal of Clinical Nutrition* 45 (1987): 501–512.
35. Vitamin D status of the elderly: Contributions of sunlight exposure and diet, *Nutrition Reviews* 43 (1985): 78–80.
36. S. R. Lynch and coauthors, Iron status of elderly Americans, *American Journal of Clinical Nutrition* 36 (supplement, November 1982): 1032–1045.
37. T. A. Morck, S. R. Lynch, and J. D. Cook, Inhibition of food iron absorption by coffee, *American Journal of Clinical Nutrition* 37 (1983): 416–420.
38. H. N. Munro, P. M. Suter, and R. M. Russell, Nutrition requirements of the elderly, *Annual Review of Nutrition* 7 (1987): 23–49.
39. Munro, Suter, and Russell, 1987.
40. M. D. Altschule, *Nutritional Factors in General Medicine: Effects of Stress and Distorted Diets* (Springfield, Ill.: Charles C. Thomas, 1978), pp. 140–141.
41. A. B. Kallner, D. Hartmann, and D. H. Hornig, On the requirements of ascorbic acid in man: Steady-state turnover and body pool in smokers, *American Journal of Clinical Nutrition* 34 (1981): 1347–1355.
42. E. Koop, *The Health Consequences of Smoking,* a report (1983) of the surgeon general available from the Superintendent of Documents, U.S. Government Printing Office, Washington, D.C. 20402.
43. V. W. Bunker and coauthors, The intake and excretion of lead and cadmium by the elderly, *American Journal of Clinical Nutrition* 39 (1984): 803–808.
44. T. G. Aigner and R. L. Balster, Choice behavior in rhesus monkeys: Cocaine versus food, *Science* 201 (1978): 534–535.
45. A. Z. LaCroix and coauthors, Coffee consumption and the incidence of coronary heart disease, *New England Journal of Medicine* 315 (1986): 977–982, as described in *Modern Medicine,* February 1987, pp. 93–94.
46. N. M. Betts and V. M. Vivian, Factors related to the dietary ade-

quacy of noninstitutionalized elderly, *Journal of Nutrition for the Elderly* 4 (1985): 3–14.
47. Many frail elderly get inadequate food, according to Cornell study, *Journal of the American Dietetic Association* 86 (1986): 647.
48. E. Luros, A rational approach to geriatric nutrition, *Dietetic Currents, Ross Timesaver* 8 (November/December 1981).
49. J. Weinberg, Psychologic implications of the nutritional needs of the elderly, *Journal of the American Dietetic Association* 60 (1972): 293–296.
50. W. A. McIntosh and P. A. Shifflet, Influence of social support systems on dietary intake of the elderly, *Journal of Nutrition for the Elderly* 4 (1984): 5–18.

Food, Mood, and Time of Day

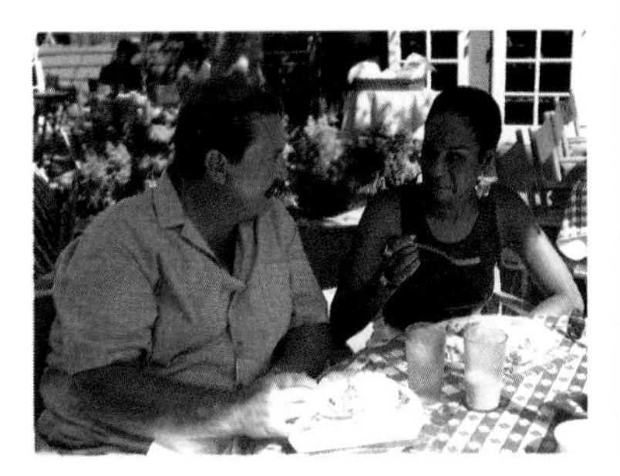

What you eat for breakfast may determine how you feel after lunch.

Why do you feel like eating a steak at one meal and a doughnut at another? Why do you feel sleepy after lunch and not after dinner? Why does depression cause some people to eat more, and others less, than they usually do? Or, putting these questions in general terms, does what you eat affect your mood? Does your mood affect what you eat? Researchers no longer doubt that food affects mood and the reverse, and they are beginning to understand how and why. Investigations into the effects have been more and more intense recently, and their focus is, of course, the brain.

The brain has its own survival at stake in directing the body when and what to eat. It is encased in the skull—a hard, inelastic helmet—for its own protection, and so cannot expand and contract as can, say, the liver or adipose tissue. It cannot store its own reserve energy supply in glycogen, fat, or other molecules, because those molecules take up space, and it cannot store oxygen with which to oxidize those fuels. Therefore, the brain must depend on the passing blood supply for its oxygen and fuels. Furthermore, its needs for those substances are extraordinary. The brain makes up only 2 percent of the adult's body weight, but at any given time it contains 15 percent of the body's blood, and it devours 20 to 30 percent of the fuels that support the basal metabolism. Its rapid metabolism makes its temperature a degree higher than that of the rest of the body. Should the blood deliver too little oxygen or glucose, coma would occur within minutes; should the blood supply be interrupted altogether, coma would ensue within 10 seconds and death within 5 minutes.[1] The brain also depends on the blood supply for amino acids, from which it makes its messenger molecules; for electrolytes, which it uses to transmit its electrical impulses; for other minerals and vitamins to facilitate these processes; for lipids to repair its cell membranes; and for water. Figure C13–1 shows how one cell within the brain communicates with another.

The brain is also extremely sensitive to fluctuations in its internal chemical composition. To protect itself from them, it has its own molecular sieve through which the blood must pass. The blood vessels that feed the brain differ from those that feed other organs in being lined with highly selective cells, known as the **blood-brain barrier,** that allow only desired constituents to enter the brain tissue. Whereas the environment outside the body may fluctuate widely in temperature, humidity, and chemical composition, the blood changes only a little, and the brain's internal milieu hardly fluctuates at all.

Because of its dependence on the blood supply, the brain continuously monitors it and sends messages to other organs when it needs their help in regulating it. At one time, the brain may need glucose; at another, protein. Should body stores be inadequate to supply the amounts needed, indications are that the brain may be able to direct eating to obtain carbohydrate at one time and protein at another, depending on what it needs. It is known that animals regulate the proportions of protein and carbohydrate that they consume. A possible explanation of how people may do so comes largely from research using animals, and it is presented here as an example of research into the connections between brain chemistry and food choices.

One of the ways the brain may be able to tell whether it needs carbohydrate or protein is by the amounts of **monoamines**—a type of **neurotransmitter**—available for its use. The monoamines are made in the nerve cells from single amino acids, by modifying them slightly.

The monoamines are an exception to the rule that the brain's internal chemistry hardly fluctuates at all. The amino acid building blocks (precursors) from which monoamines are made, unlike most molecules, are able to penetrate the blood-brain barrier, and do so in quantities that depend on their concentrations in the bloodstream. Thus the food a person eats can influence the brain chemistry by producing high or low concentrations of the precursor nutrients in an available form. Furthermore, once in the brain, these precursor nutrients exert **precursor control;** that is, the nerve cells respond to a larger or smaller supply of building blocks by making larger or smaller amounts of monoamines from them. These facts

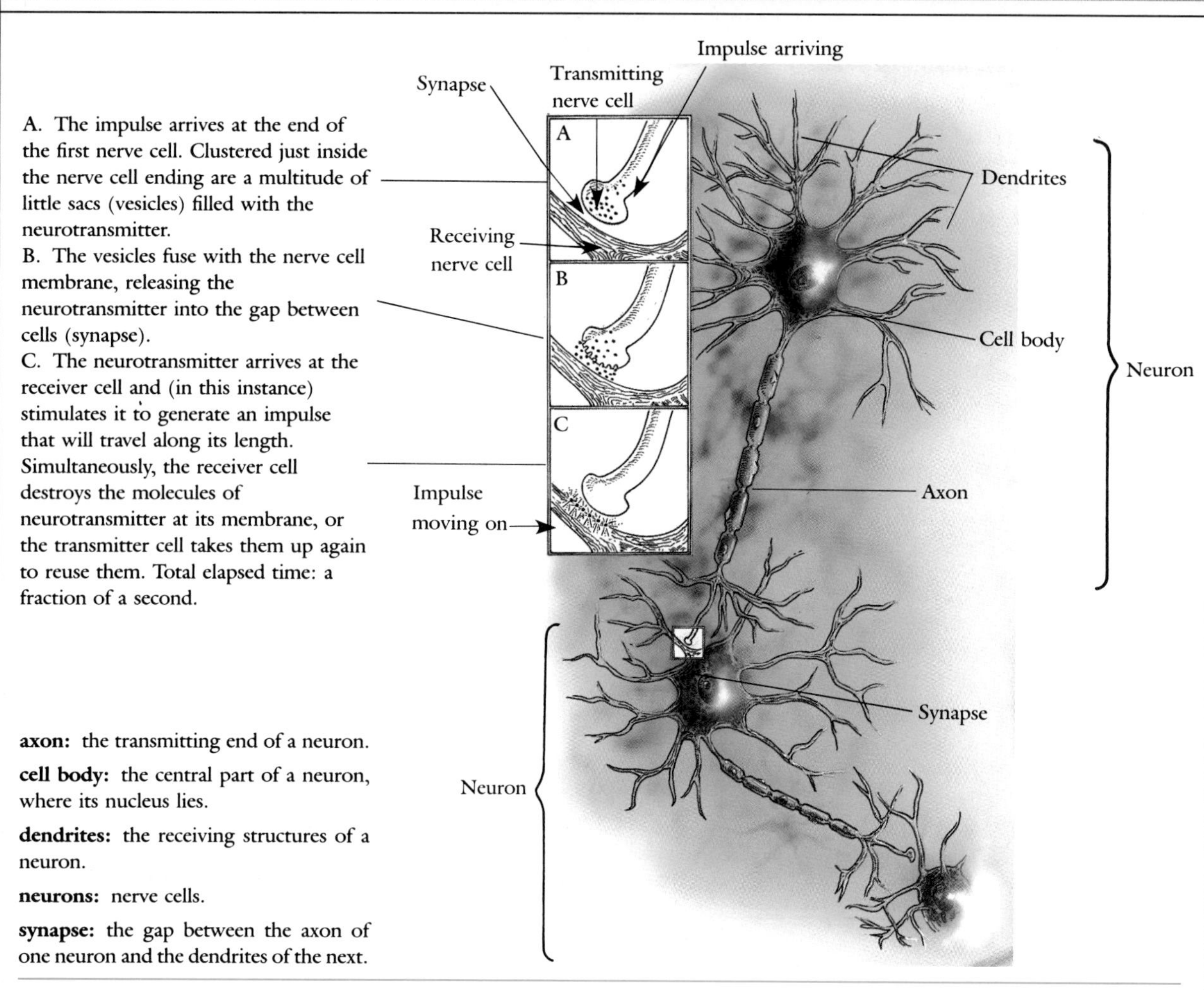

axon: the transmitting end of a neuron.

cell body: the central part of a neuron, where its nucleus lies.

dendrites: the receiving structures of a neuron.

neurons: nerve cells.

synapse: the gap between the axon of one neuron and the dendrites of the next.

Figure C13–1
Communication within the brain.
The mature human brain is composed of about 10 billion nerve cells, or **neurons,** which communicate with one another using a combination of electrical and chemical signals.[a] Each neuron is a long, slim cell with receiving structures **(dendrites)** at one end; a transmitting structure (the **axon**) at the other; and a bulge, the **cell body,** between. Electric impulses arise in the dendrites, pass through the cell body, and continue down the axon to its terminal. At the point where the terminal makes contact with the next nerve, it bulges slightly; two such bulges are shown in this figure and one is enlarged.

The electrical impulses that travel along nerve cells can, in some cases, jump unaided across the gap (called a **synapse**) from one cell to the next, but in most cases the gap between cells prevents electrical transmission. Communication across synapses usually requires the release of a chemical substance, or neurotransmitter, which flows across the gap. The first nerve cell (the one sending the impulse) releases a quantity of these molecules, and they diffuse across the synapse to reach the second (receiving) nerve cell. On arrival, they may make the receiving nerve cell either *more* or *less* likely to fire. Thus a neurotransmitter can either *stimulate* or *inhibit* the postsynaptic nerve. If it stimulates it, and the nerve fires, then an electrical impulse starts up and travels along the nerve to the other end, the next synapse. Thus messages are carried along nerves by electrical impulses and from one nerve to the next by chemical compounds, until they result in action (storage or integration of information, or contraction of a muscle) or die away.

A nerve cell "decides" to fire based on inputs from all the other cells in contact with it. If the amount of stimulation relative to the amount of inhibition is great enough to initiate an impulse, then the nerve cell will fire.

[a]The brain's 10 billion neurons are surrounded by 10 billion supporting cells, known as *glial cells,* not involved in nerve transmission.

link eating directly to brain chemistry and, as you will see in a moment, to mood and other sensations.

One monoamine whose brain concentration is especially sensitive to changes in precursor supply has been studied in depth: **serotonin,** made from its precursor, the amino acid tryptophan (see Figure C13–2). Ordinary meals, such as people eat every day, raise or lower the concentration of serotonin in the brain, depending on the meals' protein and carbohydrate content. Serotonin concentration in turn affects sensations and mood—so the composition of the meals people eat has real effects on how they feel afterward. A lack of tryptophan flowing into the brain can manifest itself in wakefulness and enhanced sensitivity to pain. An animal that has been made tryptophan deficient has a lowered threshold for pain; when it is given a single injection of tryptophan, its pain threshold becomes normal as its brain serotonin level is restored.[2]

The amount of tryptophan that enters the brain depends not only on the amount the person eats, but also on the total amounts of protein *and carbohydrate* the person eats. If tryptophan is eaten by itself, as a single amino acid, then its concentration in the blood rises, it flows into the brain, and brain serotonin increases proportionately. But normally, whole proteins containing tryptophan are eaten. In this case, some of the other large amino acids in the proteins compete with tryptophan for entry into the brain, because they use the same transport mechanism to get across the blood-brain barrier.* In this situation, tryptophan fails to enter the brain in increased quantities and so does not effectively enhance brain serotonin synthesis. If carbohydrate is fed along with the protein, however, it can "help" the protein deliver tryptophan to the brain, because it elicits the secretion of the hormone insulin. Insulin drives the other amino acids, but not tryptophan, into body cells, leaving the tryptophan free to enter the brain without competition. Thus, paradoxically, a meal high in carbohydrate, but not one high in protein, increases tryptophan's ease of transport into the brain and so promotes serotonin synthesis. It is not the total amount of tryptophan, then, but the amount relative to the competing amino acids, that affects the brain's serotonin level.

These facts may help explain how animals and human beings may know which kind of diet they have eaten last and what to eat next time. According to one theory, a high-carbohydrate meal raises their brain serotonin, makes them feel good, and so reduces their need for carbohydrate. They therefore eat more protein at the next meal. A high-protein

*The amino acids that share this transport system are tyrosine, phenylalanine, leucine, isoleucine, and valine. These amino acids also compete for absorption in the digestive tract.

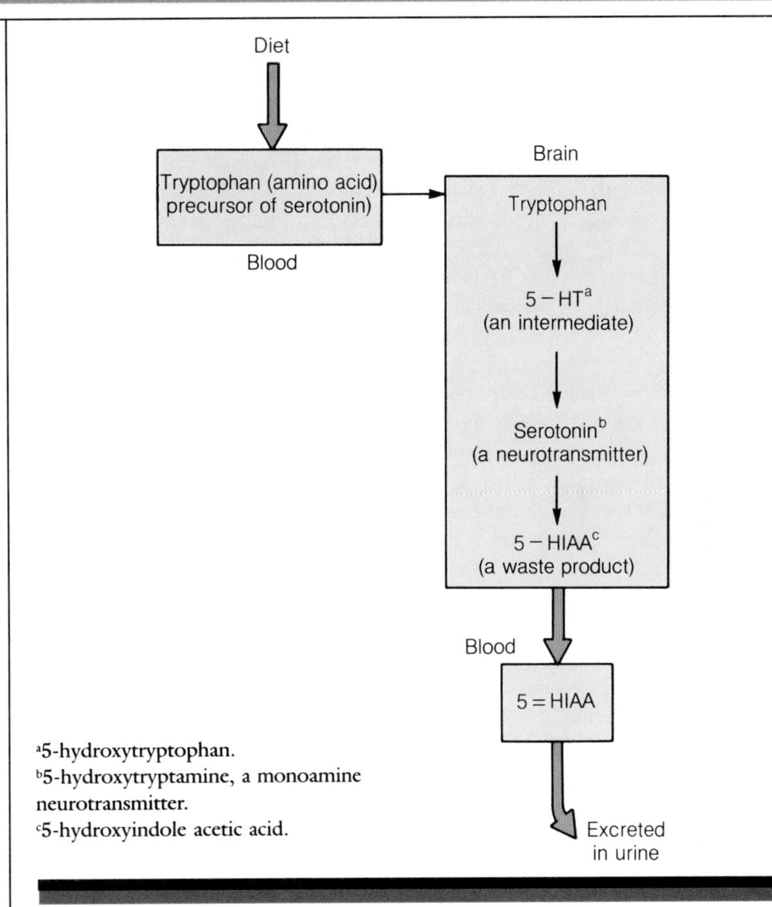

[a]5-hydroxytryptophan.
[b]5-hydroxytryptamine, a monoamine neurotransmitter.
[c]5-hydroxyindole acetic acid.

Figure C13–2
Serotonin synthesis in the brain.

meal creates a serotonin deficit, a loss of the good feeling, and therefore a craving for carbohydrate.[3]

One of the chief appeals of this theory is that it seems to account for what is observed to happen often with weight-control diets. The harder dieters try to restrict carbohydrate, the more they seem to crave it. The effect is accentuated if they are insulin resistant, as is likely if they are obese. When an insulin-resistant person eats carbohydrate, insulin's normal actions do not follow. The person's cells continue to be hungry for glucose; furthermore, brain serotonin does not rise, and so the carbohydrate craving is intensified.

The theory also helps explain why some people describe themselves as anxious, tense, and depressed before eating carbohydrate, and peaceful or relaxed afterward. The amino acid tryptophan given by itself has similar effects, consistent with the notion that it is the agent of carbohydrate's effect. (This doesn't mean people should dose themselves with tryptophan, of course. Tryptophan occurs in virtually all proteins—see p. 146 for specifics—and so all they need is a balanced assortment of amino acids, from protein, for an excess of any one could cause deficiencies of others, with consequent upsets of mood, and who knows what else? The box on p. 162 gave many reasons why amino acid supplements are a poor choice.)

Not all the evidence supports the theory that links serotonin to the appetite for carbohydrate. For example, under some circumstances, when animals eat tryptophan, they then eat *less* protein. This cannot be explained by changes in blood tryptophan, brain tryptophan, or brain serotonin levels.[4] Ongoing research should ultimately help to untangle this problem, but chances are that it will become more knotty before it becomes less so. Other hormones are probably involved. For example, carbohydrate and protein intakes affect not only insulin secretion, but also the secretion of insulin's opposing hormone, glucagon—and glucagon influences the synthesis of neurotransmitters, too.[5] Other hormones that affect the brain—or even that are synthesized inside the brain—after eating are cholecystokinin (the messenger that, outside the brain, communicates the arrival of fat to the gallbladder and pancreas) and calcitonin (a hormone that responds to the blood calcium level).

Carbohydrate or tryptophan can also induce fatigue or sleepiness. The effect of tryptophan in inducing sleep is particularly well known; 43 studies have now demonstrated it in people and animals.[6] Carbohydrate or tryptophan can also reduce sensitivity to mild pain and (in people over 40) increase the error rate in performance tests.[7] Brain serotonin may reduce aggression, too.[8]

Other avenues of investigation into such effects are also interesting, although many are just opening up and offer no more than tantalizing bits of information. For example, men and women may react differently to carbohydrates. A high-carbohydrate meal makes women sleepier and men calmer. Perhaps this is because women secrete more estrogen hormones than men. Estrogens can reduce serotonin synthesis in the brain, may favor a higher ratio of blood tryptophan to its competing amino acids, and may increase the number of serotonin receptors in the brain.[9] The monthly fluctuation of estrogen secretion may make women react differently to carbohydrate at different times of the month; as mentioned earlier (Chapter 12), women's appetites for carbohydrate are keener during the ten days prior to menstruation than during the ten days after.

The time of day also modulates these reactions: a high-starch breakfast has less effect than the same foods eaten at lunch.[10] Time-of-day effects like this influence both mood and eating behavior in many ways, as the next section shows.

Time of Day, Mood, and Eating Behavior

Whenever researchers have tried to study the effects of meals on how people feel, they have had to contend with a multitude of complications. How a meal affects a person seems to depend not only on the time of day, the composition of the meal, and the sex of the person, but also on the time of the *year,* the composition of the *last* meal, and on other aspects of the nature of the person.[11] What all this means, practically speaking, is that when a person claims that particular kinds of meals typically affect him or her in particular ways, even if the effects claimed are quite unlike the listener's experience, they may well be valid.

Time-of-day effects seem to have a lot to do with our evolutionary history. The postlunch slump that many people experience, for example, seems to be a consequence of the need our ancestors had to rest during the hot African noontime. It happens when the temperature is high and rising, and it happens regardless of exactly what time a person eats lunch, though the effect is greater the more carbohydrate the person eats.[12]

Many other things vary with a daily rhythm:

- Sleep and wakefulness.
- Cognitive and motor performance.
- Body temperature.
- Blood hormone (including sex hormone) levels.

■ Volume and composition of urine excreted.
■ Susceptibility to medicines, other drugs, and toxic agents.
■ Many nerve activities—photoreception, excitability, receptor sensitivities.[13]

The question of how these daily rhythms work has fascinated researchers for years, and their investigations have led to the conclusions reported here.

Naturally, because we live in a world in which day and night alternate on a regular 24-hour cycle, human beings do many things at intervals timed accordingly—a person typically sleeps at night, wakes in the morning, eats, performs tasks efficiently until after lunch, becomes sleepy and perhaps naps, performs efficiently again late in the day, eats again, and later sleeps. It used to be thought that sunlight and darkness were responsible for our cyclic behaviors, but it has now been found that the brain operates on such a cycle anyway. Kept in isolation, away from the light-dark cycle for weeks, both human beings and animals continue to perform these activities with a periodicity of about 25 (not 24) hours. The cycle, called **circadian rhythm** (*circa die* means "about a day"), is thus built in, and its basis in the brain is a sort of timer device that has been named the **biological clock.** The location of the clock has even been pinpointed. It is in a part of the hypothalamus connected to the retina of the eye. This location permits the eye to synchronize the internal clock with the day-night cycle. Since the earth's clock is faster, it normally overrides the person's clock, but if for any reason the person does not perceive the external day, the approximate rhythm will still be maintained. Influences other than light can also change the internal clock's setting, particularly temperature and, in human beings, social cues.[14]

The nerves of the clock manufacture a monoamine, **norepinephrine,** in small quantities during the day and in large quantities at night. One of the centers with which these nerves communicate is the **pineal gland,** a small gland in the brain that resembles the retina of the eye. (The Greeks named it the "third eye" when they first discovered it, and they thought it to be the seat of the soul.) When the pineal gland experiences the surge in norepinephrine level that occurs at night, it responds by intensifying its secretion of a hormone of its own, **melatonin,** which it makes from serotonin—almost all of it at night.[15] Melatonin, in turn, affects (among many things) the synthesis of a neurotransmitter, **dopamine,** that regulates (among many things) the ability to pay attention.

The chemistry and behavior of the brain at night are therefore different from its chemistry and behavior by day. Normally, people sleep at night. If they are awake, they are sleepy and subdued. If deprived of sleep for long (**insomnia**), they may become emotionally disturbed. Should the biological clock itself be abnormal, as it is in some people, sleep disorders, many abnormalities of hormone synthesis, and mental disorders are manifested.[16]

The body's chemistry is also different at different times of day, as is evident from its responses to drugs. For example, tumors are much more sensitive to anticancer drugs at certain times of day than at others, so the schedules on which the drugs are administered are adjusted accordingly.[17]

A familiar phenomenon related to daily rhythms is **jet lag.** It occurs when rapid travel across time zones suddenly forces people to reset their biological clocks by more than an hour or two. In reaction, people may feel dazed, become unable to concentrate, have trouble sleeping, and feel depressed.

People who must travel frequently can learn some tricks to help reset their bodies' clocks and prevent the worst of the jet lag effect. For example, a businessman who must fly from New York to California can make the day of arrival much more pleasant if he forces himself, a few days before the trip, to start staying up late, getting up late, and eating late according to New York standards. Then by the time he gets to California, he'll be adjusted to the new schedule. Of course, he goes through the same amount of disruption whether he makes the adjustment before or during his trip, but the preplanned change makes the first and succeeding days of the trip itself much more pleasant, and allows him to think and work much more efficiently than he would if he were suffering from jet lag. Alternatively, such a traveler can plan to arrive a day in advance, and use that day to adjust without work pressure. These steps are effective in averting much of the discomfort attributed to jet lag.

Depressed mood is linked in many other ways to eating behavior and time of day. In general, mood is depressed when people are hungry, as it is when they lack sleep or have to work too hard for too long. People's performance under such conditions deteriorates.[18] Many more specific connections also exist between depression, nutrition, and time. For example, some people have an abnormal way of sleeping, awaken several times a night—and invariably go and eat.[19] In other people, when severe depression occurs, it disturbs both their diets and their sleep patterns.[20]

Psychiatrists studying such connections describe the relationship between depression and eating behavior as "robust."[21] It is particularly strongly manifested in connection with the eating disorders—anorexia nervosa, bulimia, and obesity. Again, there are connections to the mood-regulating neurotransmitter serotonin. Even after recovery, people with bulimia have lower-than-normal levels of the serotonin product 5-HIAA (see Figure C13–2) in their brains. Certain subgroups of depressed people also have low 5-HIAA levels. It is believed that this may impair the ability of people with bulimia to experience satiety after eating a reasonable amount of food. Depression, in fact, is an invariable accompaniment to bulimia, and altered serotonin synthesis "may be of major significance in mediating the prominent clinical symptoms in bulimia."[22]

Another type of depression, known as major depression, affects the appetite in the opposite way and causes weight loss. Still another connection of eating behavior with depression is seasonal; it is sometimes called winter depression. Most people who have it have increased appetites, mostly for carbohydrate.[23]

Trace Elements and the Brain

The discussion thus far has shown how the energy-yielding nutrients, particularly carbohydrate and protein, affect neurotransmitter synthesis and mood. However, in the synthesis of neurotransmitters—whether norepinephrine, dopamine, or serotonin—other nutrients, of course, are involved. Iron is needed in one of the first steps. Vitamin B_6 and riboflavin are needed in later steps. These nutrients are but three among many, and deficiencies of them are reflected in depressed or otherwise disturbed mood.[24] Many of them cause anemia, which produces mental symptoms of its own (see Table C13–1):

- Protein-energy deficiency causes apathy, fretfulness, lack of energy, and lack of interest in food.
- Thiamin deficiency causes confusion, uncoordinated movements, depressed appetite, irritability, insomnia, fatigue, personality changes, and depression.[25]
- Riboflavin deficiency causes depression, hysteria, psychopathic behavior, lethargy, and hypochondria evident before clinical deficiency is detected.[26]
- Niacin deficiency causes irritability, agitated depression, headaches, sleeplessness, memory loss, emotional instability (early signs of pellagra onset), and mental confusion progressing to psychosis or delirium.
- Vitamin B_6 deficiency causes irritability, insomnia, weakness, depression, abnormal brainwave patterns, convulsions, the mental symptoms of anemia (Table C13–1), fatigue, and headaches.[27]
- Folacin deficiency causes the mental symptoms of anemia (Table C13–1), tiredness, apathy, weakness, forgetfulness, mild depression, abnormal nerve function, irritability, headache, disorientation, confusion, and inability to perform simple calculations.[28]
- Vitamin B_{12} deficiency causes degeneration of the peripheral nervous system and anemia.
- Vitamin C deficiency causes hysteria, depression, listlessness, lassitude, weakness, an aversion to work, hypochondria, social introversion, possible anemia, and fatigue.
- Vitamin A deficiency causes anemia.

Table C13–1

The Mental Symptoms of Anemia[a]
Lack of appetite
Apathy, listlessness
Clumsiness
Conduct disturbances
Shortened attention span
Hyperactivity
Irritability
Learning disorders (vocabulary, perception)
Lowered IQ
Low scores on latency and associative reactions
Reduced physical work capacity
Repetitive hand and foot movements

[a]These symptoms are not caused by anemia itself, but by iron deficiency in the brain. Children with much more severe anemias from other causes, such as sickle-cell anemia and thalassemia, show no reduction in IQ when compared with children without anemia.

Source: E. N. Whitney and L. K. DeBruyne, *Nutrition and Behavior,* a monograph (1987) available from Stickley Publishing Company, 210 W. Washington Sq., Philadelphia, PA 19106, with permission.

■ Iron deficiency causes fatigue, weakness, headaches, pallor, listlessness, irritability, and the mental symptoms of anemia (Table C13–1).
■ Magnesium deficiency causes apathy, personality changes, and hyperirritability.
■ Copper deficiency causes iron-deficiency anemia.
■ Zinc deficiency causes poor appetite, failure to grow, iron-deficiency anemia, irritability, emotional disorders, and mental lethargy.[29]

Trace elements affect brain function in many other ways, but this list should suffice to show how dramatically the way people eat can affect how they feel. Apparently, the saying "You are what you eat" is true not only physically, but also emotionally.

Food and Learning

One of the most important things the brain does is learn. Until recently, it was not known that food had anything to do with learning other than the obvious things—that nutrient deficiencies or low blood glucose levels impair the brain's function in general, including its ability to learn. Now, however, some specific connections are appearing between eating and remembering. For example, hungry mice, fed immediately after learning a task, later remember how to perform that task better than do mice fed before the learning session, or after a lag time. In terms of evolution, this makes sense: if an animal learns a new trick and it leads to food, the trick is worth remembering; it has survival value.[30]

How does food facilitate remembering? The details are not yet known, but it is known that the hormone cholecystokinin is involved. The hormone apparently activates memory by stimulating nerve fibers that lead from the stomach to the brain.[31] It is also known that polyunsaturated fat enables animals to learn better than does saturated fat.[32] On the other hand, neither the now-familiar neurotransmitter precursor tryptophan nor sugar seems to affect factors associated with learning, such as vigilance or memory.[33]

Another factor that does affect vigilance, of course, is caffeine. Students know that they have to stay awake to study, and they often use coffee, cola beverages, or wake-up pills to prolong their attention spans. What they may not have thought to ask is how the wake-up effect works; probably it works through prolonging the action of the neurotransmitter epinephrine.[34]

Research into the roles of nutrients in the brain is relatively new,

Miniglossary

biological clock: the structure within the hypothalamus that governs an organism's circadian rhythm.

blood-brain barrier: a barrier composed of the cells lining the blood vessels in the brain, which are so tightly glued to one another that substances can only get through the lining by crossing the cell bodies themselves. Thus the cells can use all their sophisticated equipment and be highly selective in permitting entry.

circadian rhythm: the cyclic rhythm of about 24 to 25 hours in duration that many body functions (such as temperature and blood pressure) follow.

dopamine: a neurotransmitter derived from melatonin that (among other things) regulates the ability to pay attention.

insomnia: inability to sleep, sleep disruption.

jet lag: disruption of a person's normal circadian rhythm, caused by rapid (jet) travel from one time zone to another.

melatonin: a hormone derived from serotonin, produced by the pineal gland, mostly at night.

monoamines: derivatives of single amino acids that, in the brain, serve as neurotransmitters.

neurotransmitter: a substance that is released at the end of one nerve cell when a nerve impulse arrives there, diffuses across the gap to the next nerve cell, and alters the membrane of that cell in such a way that it becomes either less or more likely to fire (or does fire).

norepinephrine: a compound related in structure to (and made from) the amino acid tyrosine. When secreted by the adrenal gland, it acts as a hormone; when secreted at the ends of nerve cells, it acts as a neurotransmitter.

pineal (pine-EE-ul) **gland:** a small gland within the brain that produces melatonin.

precursor control: control of a compound's synthesis by the availability of that compound's precursor. (The more precursor there is, the more of the compound is made.)

serotonin: A compound related in structure to (and made from) the amino acid tryptophan; it serves as one of the brain's principal neurotransmitters.

but has branched out into many lines of investigation. The more investigators learn, the more they want to find out, because so much territory remains to be explored. It is hoped that research into these areas will continue to be supported, not only because they are of interest, but also because they have great potential for enhancing human life.

Notes

1. M. B. Krassner, Diet and brain function, *Nutrition Reviews* (supplement), May 1986, pp. 12–15.
2. J. D. Fernstrom, Effects of the diet on brain neurotransmitters, *Metabolism* 26 (1977): 207–223; S. H. Zeisel and J. H. Growdon, Diet and brain neurotransmitters, *Nutrition and the MD,* April 1980.
3. J. D. Fernstrom, Acute and chronic effects of protein and carbohydrate ingestion on brain tryptophan levels and serotonin synthesis, *Nutrition Reviews* (supplement), May 1986, pp. 25–36.
4. Fernstrom, 1986.
5. W. M. Lovenberg, Biochemical regulation of brain function, *Nutrition Reviews* (supplement), May 1986, pp. 6–11.
6. E. L. Hartmann, Effect of L-tryptophan and other amino acids on sleep, *Nutrition Reviews* (supplement), May 1986, pp. 70–73.
7. R. J. Wurtman, Ways that foods can affect the brain, *Nutrition Reviews* (supplement), May 1986, pp. 2–6.
8. S. N. Young, The effect on aggression and mood of altering tryptophan levels, *Nutrition Reviews* (supplement), May 1986, pp. 112–122.
9. B. J. Spring and coauthors, Effects of carbohydrates on mood and behavior, *Nutrition Reviews* (supplement), May 1986, pp. 51–60.
10. Spring and coauthors, 1986.
11. A. Craig, Acute effects of meals on perceptual and cognitive efficiency, *Nutrition Reviews* (supplement), May 1986, pp. 163–171.
12. M. J. Thompson and D. W. Harsha, Our rhythms still follow the African sun, *Psychology Today,* January 1984, pp. 50–54.
13. J. S. Takahashi and M. Zatz, Regulation of circadian rhythmicity, *Science* 217 (1982): 1104–1110.
14. Takahashi and Zatz, 1982.
15. Takahashi and Zatz, 1982.
16. M. C. Moore-Ede, C. A. Czeisler, and G. S. Richardson, Circadian timekeeping in health and disease, *New England Journal of Medicine* 309 (1983): 469–476, 530–536.
17. W. Hrushesky, physician, University of Minnesota, as cited in Chemotherapy goes circadian, *American Health,* June 1986, pp. 10, 12.
18. Spring and coauthors, 1986.
19. I. Oswald and K. Adam, Rhythmic raiding of refrigerator related to rapid eye movement sleep, *British Medical Journal* 292 (1986): 589.
20. P. E. Mullen, C. R. Linsell, and D. Parker, Influence of sleep disruption and calorie restriction on biological markers for depression, *Lancet,* 8 November 1986, pp. 1051–1055.
21. T. D. Brewerton, M. M. Heffernan, and N. E. Rosenthal, Psychiatric aspects of the relationship between eating and mood, *Nutrition Reviews* (supplement), May 1986, pp. 78–88.
22. Brewerton, Heffernan, and Rosenthal, 1986.
23. Brewerton, Heffernan, and Rosenthal, 1986.
24. Unless otherwise cited, all of the listed symptoms can be found in R. S. Goodhart and M. E. Shils, eds., *Modern Nutrition in Health and Disease,* 6th ed. (Philadelphia: Lea and Febiger, 1980).
25. Marginal vitamin deficiency, *Nutrition and the MD,* July 1983, p. 3; D. Lonsdale and R. J. Shamberger, Red cell transketolase as an indicator of nutritional deficiency, *American Journal of Clinical Nutrition* 33 (1980): 205–211.
26. R. Sterner and W. Price, Restricted riboflavin: With subject behavioral effects in humans, *American Journal of Clinical Nutrition* 26 (1973): 150–160.
27. Marginal vitamin deficiency, 1983.
28. J. H. Pincus, E. H. Reynolds, and G. H. Glaser, Subacute combined system degeneration with folate deficiency, *Journal of the American Medical Association* 221 (1972): 496–497; Neurological disease in folic acid deficiency, *Nutrition Reviews* 39 (1981): 337–338.
29. A. S. Prasad, Clinical, biochemical and nutritional spectrum of zinc deficiency in human subjects: An update, *Nutrition Reviews* 7 (1983): 197–206.
30. S. Weisburd, Eat to remember, *Science News,* 23 May 1987, p. 327.
31. Weisburd, 1987.
32. Brain food, *Science News,* 11 January 1986, p. 24.
33. Spring and coauthors, 1986.
34. H. R. Lieberman, B. J. Spring, and G. S. Garfield, The behavioral effects of food constituents: Strategies used in studies of amino acids, protein, carbohydrate and caffeine, *Nutrition Reviews* (supplement), May 1986, pp. 61–70.

Chapter Fourteen

Contents

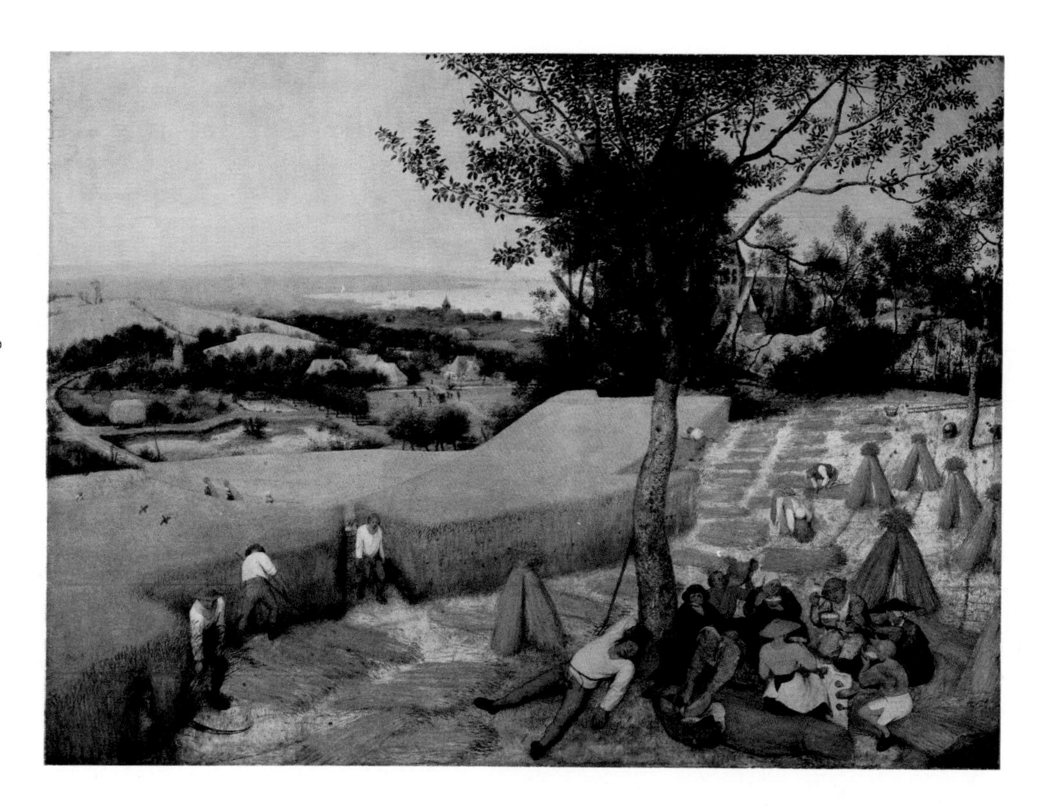

Detail of *The Harvesters* by Pieter Bruegel, the Elder. © Metropolitan Museum of Art, Rogers Fund, 1919. (19.164) Photograph by Eric Pollitzer.

Nutrition Status: Domestic and World

Throughout this book, the problems of overnutrition—obesity, heart disease, diabetes, and others—have been pressing concerns, for these are the diseases of the economically developed nations. Not everyone shares these problems, though. People in less-developed nations, and people in the less-privileged parts of our own nation, suffer the opposite problems—diseases caused by chronic, debilitating **hunger** and **malnutrition**.

What is hunger? How can it be permanently eradicated throughout the world? It is now generally agreed that emergency food relief is only a short-term solution at best. The real solutions lie in the development of self-sufficiency within each country.

This chapter begins with a discussion of some basic concepts—hunger and malnutrition, and their prevalence in the world. Next, it provides perspectives—first, on hunger in the United States, and then, on the causes and dimensions of world hunger. The chapter concludes with suggestions for personal involvement with the issues presented, including changes in lifestyle through voluntary simplicity. As you read, you are encouraged to challenge yourself with the answers to the following questions: What problems would you attack first in solving the problem of hunger and malnutrition? To what extent should the Western world get involved in tackling problems related to global hunger? Should we solve our own problems first? Remember too, as you read, that these issues are complex and often overwhelming from an individual's standpoint; however, it is usually better to light one small candle than to curse the darkness.

hunger: used in this chapter to describe the domestic and world food problem—a continuous lack of the nutrients necessary to achieve and maintain optimum health, well-being, and protection from disease. This type of hunger is also called **chronic undernutrition** and is the most basic and widespread form of hunger. **Famine** is the most visible form of hunger. Famine is a widespread lack of access to food due to natural disasters or war that causes a collapse in the food consumption in a society of chronically undernourished people.

malnutrition: impairment of health resulting from a relative deficiency or excess of specific nutrients necessary for health. (see also Chapter 1).

poverty: the state of having too little money to meet minimum needs for food, clothing, and shelter. As of the mid-1980s, the U.S. Department of Health and Human Services defines a poverty-level income as $10,650 annually for a family of four.

The Basics

Hunger and malnutrition have been with us throughout history and despite numerous development programs, they are not disappearing; the number of hungry and malnourished people continues to grow. Once viewed as a problem of overpopulation and inadequate food production, the major cause of hunger is now recognized to be the gap depicted in Figure 14–1 between the rich and the poor, both within and between countries. Other causes exist, but **poverty** is the main cause of hunger; malnutrition is primarily a problem of those who live in poverty. And why are people poor? For many reasons, including the greed of others; the lack of productive resources such as land, tools, and credit; unemployment; and a host of other factors.

There is a world of luxury foods, and another where food is the only luxury known. . . . There are those who live for the end of the working week and those who live in hopes of one beginning.[1]

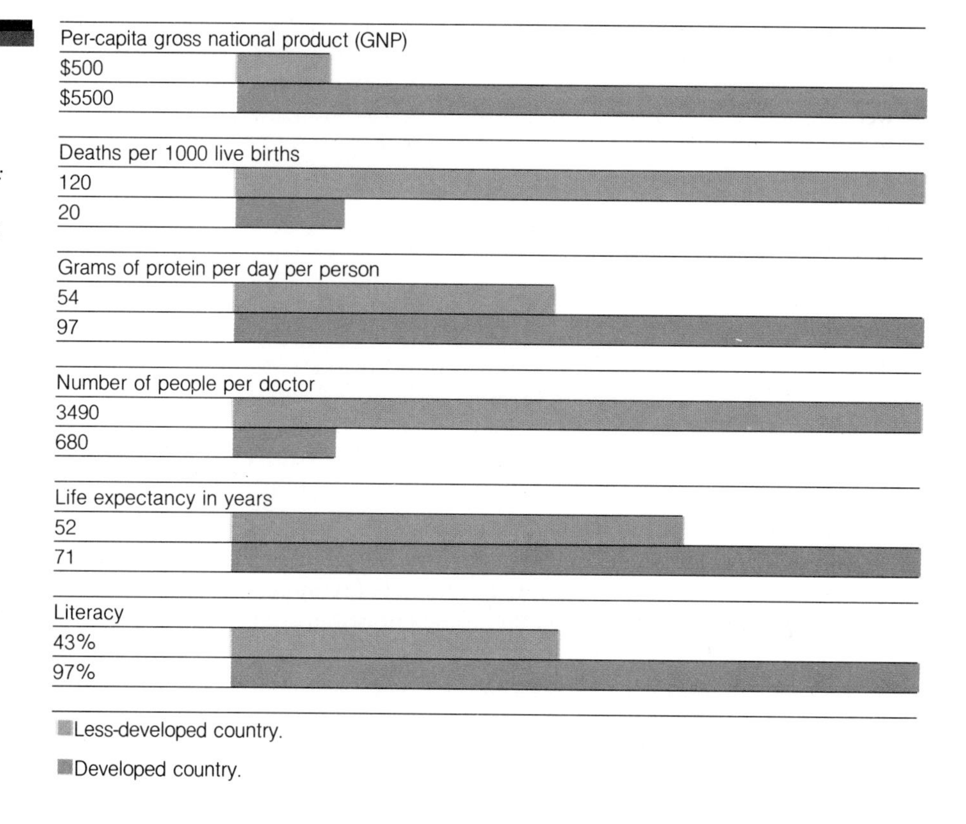

Figure 14–1
The Gap Between Developed and Less Developed Countries.
Source: U.S. Presidential Commission on World Hunger, *Overcoming World Hunger: The Challenge Ahead,* abridged ed. (Washington, D.C.: Government Printing Office, June 1980), p. 4.

How can hunger be controlled? To answer that question, other questions must be asked and answered first. What is restricting the poor's access to food? How can these restrictions be removed? Adequate nutrition can be achieved only when the economic, political, and social structures that hinder food consumption become the targets of change—both at home and abroad.

What Is Hunger?

Everyone knows the feeling of hunger as the urge to eat that signals the time for the next meal. But many know hunger as a constant companion, because that meal does not follow. Then hunger is ceaseless discomfort, weakness, and pain. The term as used here means a continuous lack of the nutrients necessary to achieve and maintain optimum health, well-being, and protection from disease. People who live with hunger may simply have too little food to eat, or may not choose enough nutritious foods from those available. To say this, though, is to fail to describe the depth of the experience of living without food. The following excerpt from a writer in India describes hunger in more personal terms:

> For hunger is a curious thing: at first it is with you all the time, waking and sleeping and in your dreams, and your belly cries out insistently, and there is a gnawing and a pain as if your very vitals were being devoured, and you must stop it at any cost, and you buy a moment's respite even while you know and fear the sequel. Then the pain is no longer sharp but dull, and this too is with you always, so that you think

> of food many times a day and each time a terrible sickness assails you, and because you know this you try to avoid the thought, but you cannot, it is with you. Then that too is gone, all pain, all desire, only a great emptiness is left, like the sky, like a well in drought, and it is now that the strength drains from your limbs, and you try to rise and you cannot, or to swallow and your throat is powerless, and both the swallow and the effort of retaining the liquid tax you to the uttermost.[2]

This excerpt from the statement of a woman from Boston describes hunger the same way:

> I've had no income and I've paid no rent for many months. My landlord let me stay. He felt sorry for me because I had no money. The Friday before Christmas he gave me ten dollars. For days I had had nothing but water. I knew I needed food; I tried to go out but I was too weak to walk to the store. I felt as if I were dying. I saw the mailman and told him I thought I was starving. He brought me food and then he made some phone calls and that's when they began delivering these lunches. But I had already lost so much weight that five meals a week are not enough to keep me going.
>
> I just pray to God I can survive. I keep praying I can have the will to save some of my food so I can divide it up and make it last. It's hard to save because I am so hungry that I want to eat it right away. On Friday, I held over two peas from the lunch. I ate one pea on Saturday morning. Then I got into bed with the taste of food in my mouth and I waited as long as I could. Later on in the day I ate the other pea.
>
> Today I saved the container that the mashed potatoes were in and tonight, before bed, I'll lick the sides of the container.
>
> When there are bones I keep them. I know this is going to be hard for you to believe and I am almost ashamed to tell you, but these days I boil the bones till they're soft and then I eat them. Today, there were no bones.[3]

All people need food. Regardless of race, religion, sex, or nationality, our bodies experience similarly the effects of hunger and malnutrition—listlessness, failure to thrive, stunted growth, mental retardation, muscle wastage, scurvy, pellagra, beriberi, anemia, rickets, osteoporosis, goiter, tooth decay, blindness, and a host of other effects, including death. Apathy and shortened attention span are two of a number of behavioral symptoms that are often mistaken for laziness, lack of intelligence, or mental illness in hungry or malnourished people.

Prevalence of Malnutrition

The United Nations Food and Agriculture Organization (FAO) estimates that of the world's 5-billion-plus people, at least half a billion suffer from some form of malnutrition.About 250 million are children of preschool age, and 10 million of these weigh less than 60 percent of the standard weight for their age. About 40,000 to 50,000 people die each day as a result of malnutrition. Millions of children die each year from the diseases of poverty: parasites and infectious diseases, such as whooping cough, measles, tuberculosis, and malaria, with accompanying diarrhea, which interact with poor nutrition in a vicious cycle. It is estimated that one child dies of these causes every two seconds[4]—15 have died in the 30 seconds it took you to read this paragraph. Four groups most often suffer the effects of hunger and malnutrition due to high nutrient needs or low tissue reserves: children, pregnant women, those who are ill, and the elderly.

acute PEM: acute protein-energy malnutrition, caused by recent severe food restriction, characterized by thinness for height.

chronic PEM: chronic protein-energy malnutrition, caused by long-term food deprivation, characterized in children by short height for age. For *PEM*, see p. 159.

low-birthweight (LBW) baby: a baby that weighs less than 5½ lb (2500 g) at birth. Such a baby is likely to get sick and be unable to do its job of obtaining nourishment by sucking and unable to win its mother's attention by energetic, vigorous cries and other healthy behavior. It can therefore become an apathetic, neglected baby, and this compounds the original malnutrition problems.

Marasmus and kwashiorkor: see Chapter 5.

The most widespread form of malnutrition among children in the developing world today is protein-energy malnutrition, or PEM (see p. 159). PEM takes two forms. Children who are thin for their height may be suffering from **acute PEM** or recent severe food restriction, whereas children who are short for their age have experienced **chronic PEM** or long-term food restriction. Stunted growth due to PEM, rather than symptoms of vitamin- and mineral-deficiency diseases, may be the most common sign of malnutrition in developing countries.[5] Breast-feeding permits infants in many developing countries to achieve weight and height gains equal to those of children in developed countries until about six months of age, but then the majority of these children fall behind in weight and height. Visitors to developing countries often overlook the PEM of children because they do not realize that the three- and four-year-old children they think they see are actually eight- or nine-years-old. Failure of children to grow is a warning that one of the extreme forms of PEM, marasmus or kwashiorkor, may soon follow.

Pregnant or lactating women, together with their young children, have a greater need for nutrients than other groups because these are supposed to be times of rapid growth (see Chapters 11 and 12). When family food is limited, these women and their children are the first to show the signs of undernutrition.

Women must gain weight during pregnancy to support normal fetal growth and development. Most women in developed countries gain an average of 12.5 kilograms (about 27 pounds). Studies among poor women show a weight gain often limited to 5 to 7 kilograms (11 to 15 pounds).[6] Birthweight is a potent indicator of the infant's future health status. The delivery of a **low-birthweight (LBW) baby** is more likely to be complicated by problems than that of a normal baby, and the LBW baby has a statistically greater chance of having birth defects, of contracting diseases, and of dying early in life. Low birthweight contributes to more than half of the deaths of children under five years of age. Many women

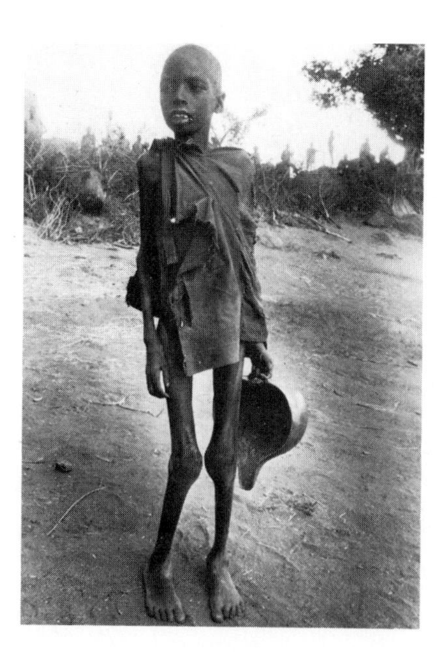

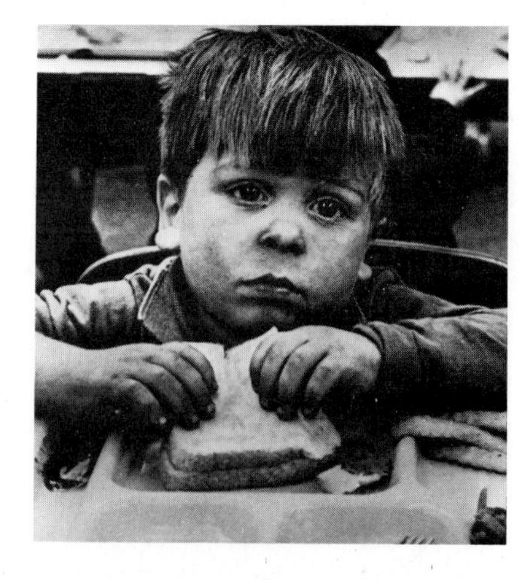

Malnutrition is widespread in developing nations but occurs in developed countries, too. Some children have food, but not the food they need.

in developing countries are responsible, even during their pregnancies, for most of the physical labor required to procure food for their families. The poor nutrition of some women results not only from their families' lack of access to food, but also to unequal distribution of the inadequate food supply within their own families. A mother will feed her husband, children, and other family members first, eating only whatever is left.

Cultural and social beliefs also limit food intake. In the Indian Punjab, the director of a program aimed at reducing malnutrition in local villages found that a malnutrition rate of 10 to 15 percent persisted even after a major effort to provide supplementary foods. The majority of those affected were very young girls, least able to demand their share and least recognized by other family members as deserving a fair share. In other areas of India, a child may be forbidden to eat curds and fruit because they are "cold," and bananas because they "cause convulsions."[7]

Other instances of malnutrition can be traced to inappropriate "modernization," such as replacing breast milk with formula feeding in environments and economic circumstances that make it impossible to feed formula safely. Breast milk, the recommended food for infants, is sterile and contains antibodies that enhance an infant's resistance to disease. Formula in bottles, however, in the absence of sterilization and refrigeration, is an ideal breeding ground for bacteria. More than 1.3 billion people in developing countries do not have access to safe drinking water.[8] Mixing contaminated water with milk powder and feeding this to infants often causes infections that lead to diarrhea, dehydration, and failure to absorb nutrients from the foods the children are given. Malnourished children cannot fight these infections effectively, and many die.

Even if children in developing countries are protected by breastfeeding at first, they must be weaned. The **weaning period** is one of the most dangerous periods for children. Infection often appears inevitable after weaning, caused by infected water, gruel, or other materials. The hazards to infants and children are reflected in mortality statistics. The **infant mortality rate** ranges from about 50 (Sri Lanka) to over 200 (Afghanistan) in the poorest of the developing countries as compared with an average of 13 to 20 in the developed countries. The death rate for children from one to four years old is no more favorable; it ranges from 20 to 30 times higher in developing countries than in developed countries.[9]

In the **third world,** the diet's basis is formed by bulky grains such as wheat, rice, millet, sorghum, and corn, and by starchy root crops such as cassava, sweet potatoes, plantain, and bananas. These may be supplemented with legumes (peas or beans) and, rarely, with animal proteins. Infants have small stomachs and most cannot eat enough of these staples (grains or root crops) to meet their daily energy and protein requirements. The infant needs to be fed more nutrient-dense foods during the weaning period. A great need exists to develop more adequate and inexpensive weaning foods in the developing countries. The most promising weaning foods are usually concentrated mixtures of grain and locally available **pulses**—that is, peas or beans.[10] Mothers are advised to continue breastfeeding while they introduce weaning foods.

Hunger and malnutrition are widespread in the world. Their main cause is poverty. Their chief victims are children, pregnant women, the ill and the elderly.

weaning period: the time during which an infant's diet is changed from breast milk to other nourishment.

infant mortality rate: the number of deaths during the first year of life per thousand live births.

third world: the underdeveloped nations of the world that are aligned with neither the communist nor the noncommunist blocs.

pulses: a term used for legumes, especially with reference to legumes that serve as staples in the diet of third world countries.

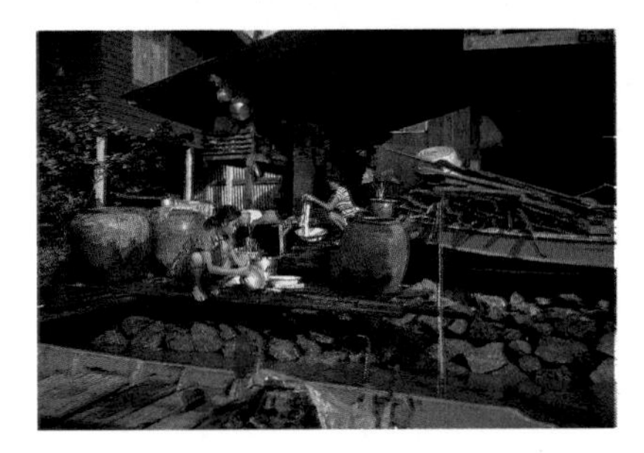

Women wash dishes, clothes, and children in the rivers along which their homes are built. The jugs are used to collect and store both rain water and river water.

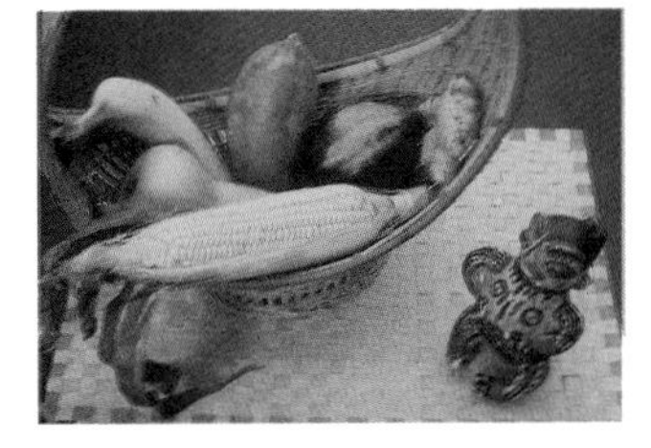

A child can't eat enough of these bulky foods to obtain adequate nourishment.

Hunger in the United States

A way of delineating developed versus developing countries is by the terms "first world," "second world," "third world" and "fourth world." "First world" refers to the developed market economy nations (Western Europe, North America, Japan, Australia, and New Zealand). "Second world" refers to developed nations with centrally planned economies (Eastern Europe and the USSR). "Third world" is used for the developing countries. "Fourth world" refers to the poorest of the third world countries.

The specter of hunger in a land of plenty is sobering. How could the wealthiest nation in the world, consumer of 40 percent of the world's resources but having only 6 percent of the world's population, not be able to meet the food needs of its poor?

Almost without exception, findings cite increased poverty as the single most important cause of American hunger. The 1985 Physician's Task Force on Hunger in America found that, in the United States alone, "at least 20 million citizens suffer from hunger at least some days each month."[11] Despite economic gains over the last few years, millions of Americans experience this dehumanizing and debilitating specter of hunger—especially infants, low-income women, the elderly, ethnic minorities, dislocated farm families, and former blue-collar workers, who have been forced out of manufacturing (oil, natural gas, steel, and mining) into the service sector.

The Past

During the 1930s, Congress was concerned about the plight of farmers in this country who were losing their farms and the economic depression facing U.S. families. It was then that Congress established the authority to buy and distribute excess food commodities. A few years later, Congress created the Food Stamp program to enable people to buy food. Then, in 1946, it passed the National School Lunch Act as a response to testimony from the surgeon general that 70 percent of the boys who had had poor nutrition 10 to 12 years before had been rejected by the draft. Still, in the 1960s, it was evident that large numbers of people were going hungry in the United States, and, as a result, some of them suffered seriously from malnutrition.

Nutrition surveys taken at intervals ever since the 1940s to investigate people's nutritional health in the United States have demonstrated a consistent relationship between family income and nutrition status—the lower the income, the less adequate the nutrition status. The Preschool Nutrition Survey (1968 to 1970) showed that low-income preschoolers were of smaller physical size and had lower blood hemoglobin concentrations than higher-income children. The Ten-State Nutrition Survey (1968 to 1970) also showed that low-income children were more frequently of smaller physical size. The Health and Nutrition Examination Survey (HANES, 1971 to 1974) showed a relationship between family income and the intake of energy, protein, and calcium; the lower the income, the less adequate the intake of these nutrients.

According to the U.S. Department of Agriculture's 1977 to 1978 Nationwide Food Consumption Survey, only 12 percent of low-income households spending at the Thrifty Food Plan level (the amount allotted to food stamp households whose incomes are below 130 percent of the poverty level) obtained 100 percent of the RDA, and only 34 percent obtained 80 percent of the RDA for selected indicator nutrients. The same survey shows that the "food shopping expertise of households with low food costs, with low income, and receiving food stamps was as good or better than that of other households." It appears that poor families have difficulty nourishing themselves, despite their generally good shopping habits because they are unable to buy sufficient amounts of food.

According to the same 1977–1978 survey, the percentage of households that met or exceeded the RDA rose and fell with income. Thus it appears that income confers the ability to obtain a nutritionally adequate diet. Table 14–1 shows the results for six nutrients. People with lower incomes had lower intakes of five of them.

The surveys reveal the reality that people can and do suffer from many kinds of malnutrition on the domestic scene. Few severe deficiencies are apparent, but subclinical iron deficiency and some overt anemia are widespread. Protein deficiencies are seen among poor pregnant and lactating women. Intakes of many nutrients have been impossible to study in depth to date, due to lack of knowledge about their presence in foods or lack of techniques for accurately assessing their presence in the body, but problems are suspected with respect to folacin, vitamin B_6, magnesium, and zinc.

As a result of the evidence accumulated during the 1960s and 1970s showing that hunger was a problem in the United States, this country took on the problems of poverty and hunger as national priorities. Programs were developed in hopes of preventing malnutrition in those people found to be at risk. The Food Stamp program was expanded to serve more people. School lunch and breakfast programs were enlarged so that children could have adequate nutrition while they learned. Feeding programs were started to reach senior citizens. The supplemental food program was established for low-income pregnant women, infants, and children (WIC) to supply food and nutrition counseling during the years when nutrition makes the most crucial difference of all.

The result of these efforts was that hunger diminished as a serious problem for this country. That the food assistance programs made a difference was doc-

Table 14–1

Nationwide Food Consumption Survey Findings

	Percentage of Persons with Nutrient Intakes at or below 70% of RDA[a]			
Nutrient	*Income to $6,000*	*Income $6,000–$9,999*	*Income $10,000–$15,999*	*Income $16,000 and Over*
Vitamin A	36%	33%	32%	29%
Vitamin B_6[b]	59%	51%	49%	48%
Vitamin C	30%	29%	27%	23%
Calcium	49%	43%	39%	39%
Iron	29%	31%	33%	33%
Magnesium	48%	40%	36%	35%

[a]Data represent percentage of persons in each income group with intakes at or below 70% of RDA. Example: 36% of all those surveyed whose incomes were at or below $6000 per year had vitamin A intakes below 70% of the RDA.

[b]Vitamin B_6 intakes may not be as deficient as they appear. People who get along on minimal protein intakes need less than the RDA of vitamin B_6 to handle the amount of protein they consume.

umented in several studies, including comparative observations made in 1967 and 1977. In 1967 a Field Foundation report stated:

> Wherever we went and wherever we looked we saw children in significant numbers who were hungry and sick, children for whom hunger is a daily fact of life, and sickness in many forms, an inevitability. The children we saw were more than malnourished. They were hungry, weak, apathetic. Their lives were being shortened. They are visibly and predictably losing their health, their energy, their spirits. They are suffering from hunger and disease, and directly or indirectly, they are dying from them—which is exactly what starvation means.

In 1977 a report by the same group stated:

> Our first and overwhelming impression is that there are far fewer grossly malnourished people in this country today than there were ten years ago. . . . This change does not appear to be due to an overall improvement in living standards or to a decrease in joblessness in those areas. In fact, the facts of life for Americans living in poverty remain as dark or darker than they were ten years ago. But in the area of food there is a difference. The Food Stamp program, school lunch and breakfast programs, and the Women-Infant-Children programs have made the difference.[12]

If this is true, why are numerous groups today reporting that hunger in America is on the rise? The next section addresses this question.

The Present

Once again in the 1980s, the problem of hunger has returned to America. Of the "new poor" who are taking advantage of the various types of emergency food assistance are many families with children. Many are two-parent families experiencing the effects of long-term unemployment, or single women with children who receive no support from absent fathers. Many are poor families receiving food stamps that run out before the end of the month. Through the late 1960s and 1970s, hunger was often associated with the chronic poor, including the homeless, street people, and the long-term unemployed. Now, this pattern is changing. These groups are still hungry, but hunger is appearing among more segments of the population, including infants, small children, local families with residences, bankrupt farm families, single mothers, young adults, married couples, the newly unemployed, and the working poor.

Why is there now a resurgence of the hunger problem in the United States? Nationally, most studies conducted since 1980 have attributed the increases in hunger throughout the country to worsening economic conditions among the poor. Table 14–2 depicts increases in poverty between 1980 and 1984 among a number of population groups.

Major reductions in federal spending for antipoverty programs have taken place throughout the 1980s. Federal expenditures for human services programs were cut by $110 billion to reduce the national debt during the period from 1982 to 1985. Programs were eliminated, eligibility requirements were tightened, no adjustments were allowed for inflation, and budgets for the remaining programs were slashed. Some of the most severe reductions came in programs directly affecting those deepest in poverty, including Aid to Families with Dependent Children (AFDC), food stamps, low-income housing assistance, and child nutrition. Funding for the school lunch programs was cut by one-third.[13]

Table 14–2

Increases in U.S. Poverty, 1980-1984

Category	National Rate of Poverty Increases
Infants and Children Under the Age of Six	+63%
The "Working Poor"(Families who Receive 75% of Their Income from Jobs as Opposed to Public Assistance Benefits)	+56%
Poor Married Couples (Two Parent Families)	+47%
Young Adults Living Independently (Their Own Households)	+13%
Single Parent Families, (Usually Headed by Women)	+10%
The Elderly	A decline, −3%

Source: The United States Bureau of Census, *Statistical Updates,* Washington, D.C., 1985.

Cuts in college financial aid effectively blocked a pathway out of poverty taken by many in the past.

Studies have been conducted by various groups: the U.S. Conference of Mayors, the National Council of Churches, the Citizen's Commission on Hunger in New England, Bread for the World, the President's Task Force on Food Assistance, the Physician's Task Force on Hunger, and the Food Research and Action Center. Numerous states have conducted local surveys as well. All have reached the conclusion that hunger is again a serious problem in the United States. As one indicator, more soup kitchens are serving more meals to more people than at any other time since the Great Depression.[14]

The U.S. Conference of Mayors, in its survey of food assistance in 25 major cities, found that the need for emergency food had increased by 28 percent between 1984 and 1985, and then by another 25 percent in 1986. The report also noted that 17 percent of emergency food needs were going unmet in the cities surveyed. Why?

Causes of Hunger in the United States

Most experts agree that poverty is the major cause of hunger in the United States, but other causes also contribute, including:

- Excessive consumption of nutrient-poor "junk food" by people of all income groups, resulting in nutrient deficiencies.
- Alcoholism and chronic substance abuse, often contributing to increased poverty and malnutrition among not only the afflicted individuals, but their families as well.
- Mental illness, loneliness, isolation, depression, and despair resulting in people's loss of concern for their own physical well-being.
- The reluctance of people, particularly the elderly, to accept what is perceived as welfare or charity.
- Delays in receiving requested food stamps and other public assistance benefits.
- An increase in the number of single mothers without the means to care for their children.

- Poor management of limited family financial resources.
- Health problems of old age, precipitating an inability to purchase and prepare food.
- Lack of proper nutritional balance in the food available to hungry persons through emergency feeding programs and food assistance organizations; programs must take what they can get and pass it on to hungry persons.
- Lack of access to assistance programs because of intimidation, ineligibility, and other reasons.
- Insufficient community food resources to feed the hungry.
- Insufficient community transportation systems to deliver food to hungry persons who have no transportation.[15]

Toward a Solution

Solutions are available to the problems of hunger and inadequate nutrition. What is required is individuals willing to take action and to work together. Regardless of the type and level of involvement a person chooses, each person can make a difference. The government programs described in this chapter need people's support in a number of ways. Individual people can:

- Assist in these programs themselves as volunteers.
- Help develop means of informing low-income persons of food-related services and programs for which they are eligible.
- Help increase the accessibility of existing programs and services to those who need them.
- Document the needs that exist in their own communities. Refer to the Food and Research Action Center's booklet, entitled *How to Document Hunger in Your Community* or Bread for the World's *Hunger Watch USA* handbook (addresses provided at the end of this chapter).
- Join with others in the community who have similar interests; support groups that speak for the poor.

Besides individual actions, any person who is concerned about the problems of poverty and malnutrition in the United States can exercise the right to express political views. Develop and express your own convictions on how to improve food assistance programs to better meet our people's nutrition needs. Decide what local, state, and national governments should do to help, and communicate your decisions to your elected officials for needed legislative changes.

In the United States, family income correlates with nutrition status. Government efforts between the 1940s and the 1970s improved U.S. nutrition status. In the 1980s increasing poverty has worsened the U.S. hunger problem. Other causes also contribute to it. Political action is needed to improve it.

World Hunger

According to the *1986 World Population Data Sheet,* life expectancy at birth in the United States is now 75 years. In Japan, Iceland, and Sweden it is 77 years. Worldwide, life expectancy averages 62 years, but in Africa it is 50, and in Sierra

Leone it is only 34. Many factors relate to this, but nutrition is one of the major ones. The phenomenon of world hunger is different from that of domestic hunger as portrayed by these statistics. In fact, most people would find it hard to imagine the severity of third world poverty:

> Many hundreds of millions of people in the poorest countries are preoccupied solely with survival and elementary needs. For them, work is frequently not available, or pay is low, and conditions barely tolerable. Homes are constructed of impermanent materials and have neither piped water nor sanitation. Electricity is a luxury. Health services are thinly spread, and in rural areas only rarely within walking distance. Permanent insecurity is the condition of the poor. There are no public systems of social security in the event of unemployment, sickness, or death of a wage earner in the family. Flood, drought, or disease affecting people or livestock can destroy livelihood without hope of compensation. In the wealthy countries, ordinary men and women face genuine economic problems—uncertainty, inflation, the fear if not the reality of unemployment. But they rarely face anything resembling the total deprivation found in the poor countries.[16]

Strangely, although hunger exists because people do not have enough to eat, it is also true that the world already produces enough food to provide the basics of nutrition to all human beings. The next section examines some of the conditions that account for the widespread hunger and poverty seen in this world of abundance.

Causes and Dimensions

Table 14–3 reveals the human dimensions of the world hunger problem; Table 14–4 shows that it has many causes. It is a problem of supply and demand, of inappropriate technology, of environmental abuse, of demographic distribution, of unequal access to resources, of extremes of dietary patterns, and of unjust economic systems. Two generalizations and an important question are suggested by these tables.

1. The underlying causes of global hunger and poverty are complex and interrelated.
2. Hunger is a product of poverty resulting from the ways in which governments and businesses manage national and international economies.
3. The question "Why are people hungry?" has been answered: "Because they are poor." The question that remains to be answered is "Why are people poor?"

A diagram of poverty-hunger relationships is presented in Figure 14–2.

Colonialism

The colonial era caused hunger and malnutrition for millions of people in developing countries, and even today colonial-type practices are followed. The current problems arose as consequences of human and natural factors related to colonialism. Look at Africa, for example.

The African continent was originally colonized so that it could be used as a source of raw materials for Western industrialized nations. Agricultural production for local consumption was neglected. There were few opportunities for education. Traditional family structure and community organization were dis-

Table 14–3

The Realities of Hunger

The United Nations reports that there are 520 million malnourished people in the world.
Each year, 15 to 20 million people die of hunger-related causes, including diseases brought on by lowered resistance due to malnutrition. Of every four of these, three are children.
Over 40% of all deaths in poor countries occur among children under five years old.
The United Nations (UNICEF) states that 17 million children died last year from preventable diseases—one every two seconds, 40,000 a day. (A vaccination immunizing one child against a major disease costs 7 cents.) At least 50 million children are permanently blinded each year simply through lack of vitamin A.
More than 500 million people in poor countries suffer from chronic anemia due to inadequate diet.
Every day, the world produces 2 lb of grain for every man, woman, and child on earth. This is enough to provide everyone with 3000 kcal day, well above the average need of 2300 kcal.
A person born in the rich world will consume 30 times as much food as a person born in the poor world.
The poor countries have nearly 75% of the world's population, but consume only about 15% of the world's available energy.
Almost half the world's people earn less than $200 a year—many use 80 to 90% of that income to obtain food.
Of the nearly 5 billion people on earth, more than 1 billion drink contaminated water.
Water-related disease claims 25 million lives a year. Of these, 15 million are under five years of age.
There are 800 million illiterates. In many countries, half of the population over 15 is illiterate. Two-thirds of these are women.

Sources: *World Hunger: Facts,* available from Oxfam America, 115 Broadway, Boston, MA 02116; Office on Global Education, Church World Service, 2115 N Charles St., Baltimore, MD 21218.

rupted. The infrastructure was designed merely to move Africa's minerals, metals, cash crops, and wealth to Europe. Much of this same activity continues today but it is not called colonialism.

By the time the African nations were beginning to achieve their independence from colonial rule, many of their forests had already been timbered to meet needs abroad. Deforestation continued, both in order to provide farmland for the growing population and to make way for large commercial farms to grow foods and commodities for export. Treeless slopes undergo rapid topsoil erosion. When no more trees are available to be chopped for firewood, people use animal dung as fuel instead of as fertilizer. To meet the growing demands for food, they farm the land intensively, and leave it fallow for too short a time to permit it to recover its fertility. All these factors make the land less productive and more vulnerable to drought.

As more and more land is used for commercial farming, the rural poor are moved onto marginal lands unsuited for adequate food production. Such lands require irrigation and fertilizer beyond the means of the poor. Throughout much of Africa, land that first grew forests and then grew beans, grains, or vegetables

Table 14–4

Causes of the World Food Problem

Worldwide Problems

1. Natural catastrophes—drought, heavy rains and flooding, crop failures.
2. Environmental degradation—soil erosion and inadequate water resources.
3. Food supply-and-demand imbalances.
4. Inadequate food reserves.
5. Warfare and civil disturbances.
6. Migration—refugees.
7. Culturally based food prejudices.
8. Declining ecological conditions in agricultural regions.

Problems of the Developing World	Problems of the Industrialized World
1. Underdevelopment.	1. Excessive use of natural resources.
2. Excessive population growth.	2. Pollution.
3. Lack of economic incentives—farmers using inappropriate methods and laboring on land they may lose or can never hope to own.	3. Inefficient, animal-protein diets.
4. Parents lacking knowledge of basic nutrition for their children.	4. Inadequate research in science and technology.
5. Insufficient government attention to the rural sector.	5. Excessive government bureaucracy.
	6. Loss of farmland to competing uses.

Problems Linking Industrial and Developing Worlds

1. Unequal access to resources.
2. Inadequate transfer of research and technology.
3. Lack of development planning.
4. Insufficient food aid.
5. Excessive food aid.
6. Politics of food aid and nutrition education.
7. Inappropriate technological research.
8. Inappropriate role of multinational corporations.
9. Insufficient emphasis on agricultural development for self-sufficiency.

Source: Adapted from C. G. Knight and R. P. Wilcox, *Triumph of Triage? The World Food Problem in Geographical Perspective,* resource paper no. 75–3 (Washington, D.C.: Association of American Geographers, 1976), p. 4.

for local people's use now grows foods for export. This may be called "economic colonialism." Wealthy Africans and foreign investors use the more fertile lands for cotton, sesame, sugar, cocoa, coffee, tea, tobacco, and livestock. Production of food grains per capita has declined for the last 20 years in Africa while sugarcane production has doubled and tea quadrupled. Chad recently had a record cotton crop simultaneously with famine at epidemic levels. Sixty percent of national earnings for Ghana, the Sudan, Somalia, Ethiopia, Zambia, and Malawi are derived from cash crops that finance both luxury imported goods for the minority and international debts. Imagine what happens when the international market prices for these commodities fall.

Figure 14–2
Behind Hunger Stands Poverty.

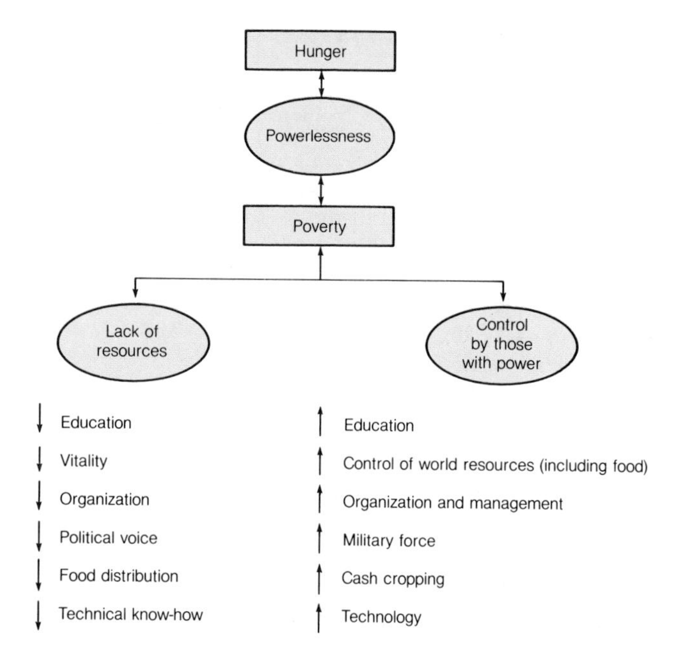

Overpopulation

Fernando is a child of 5 in Bolivia. His father, a hardworking copper miner, and his mother care for him and his six brothers and sisters. Fernando has rickets, is anemic, is small in stature and weak in body. Because of the lack of clean water in his village, he and other members of his family suffer from continual diarrhea. If Fernando is lucky enough to become an adult, he will remain small in stature and weak in body. If Fernando dies soon, his parents will feel impelled to bring another child into the world in the hope that a new child will live to adulthood and be able to care for the parents in old age.

The transition of population growth rates from a slow-growth stage (with high birth and death rates), through a rapid-growth stage (in which birth rates are high and death rates are low), to a low-growth stage (with low birth and death rates) is known as the **demographic transition.**

The current world population is approximately 5 billion, and for the year 2000 the projected United Nations figure is 6 billion. These facts justify concern over the world's capacity to produce adequate food in the future. It does not necessarily follow, however, that "too many people" is the cause of the world food problem. Actually, poverty seems to be at the root of the problem, and both hunger and overpopulation are caused by poverty. Three major factors affect third world population growth: birth rates, death rates, and standards of living. Low-income countries have high birth and death rates and a low standard of living. When a people's standard of living rises, giving them better access to health care, family planning, and education, the death rate falls first, but then the birth rate also falls. As the standard of living continues to improve, the family earns sufficient income to risk having smaller numbers of children. A family depends on its children to cultivate the land, to secure food and water, and to make the adults secure in their old age. If a family is confronted with ongoing poverty, parents will choose to have many children to ensure that some will survive to adulthood. Children represent the "social security" of the poor. The improvement of poor people's economic status helps relieve the need for this "insurance," and so helps reduce the birth rate. Table 14–5 shows the relationships between the infant mortality rate and the population growth rate, and reveals that hunger and poverty in a nation reflect not only the level of national development, but also the people's sense of security.[17]

In many countries where economic growth has occurred and resources have been distributed relatively equally among all groups, the rates of population growth have decreased. Examples include parts of Costa Rica, Sri Lanka, Taiwan, and West Malaysia. In countries where economic growth has occurred but the resources have been unevenly distributed, population growth has remained high.

arable: capable of being plowed. (*arare* means "to plow").

Table 14–5
Effect of Hunger on Population Growth Rate

	Hungry Countries	Nonhungry Countries
Average infant mortality rate	113 per 1000	35 per 1000
Total infant deaths per year	10.6 million	1.4 million
Size of population	2.3 billion	2.3 billion
Average rate of population increase	2.4% per year	1.0% per year
Total births per year	86.4 million	38.6 million

Source: Adapted from *The Ending Hunger Briefing Workbook,* 1982, available from The Hunger Project, 2015 Steiner Street, San Francisco, CA 94115, pp. 26, 30.

Examples are Brazil, Mexico, the Philippines, and Thailand, where a large family continues to be a major economic asset for the poor.[18]

Distribution of Resources/Land Reform

Land reform—giving people a more meaningful stake in food production, development, and the benefits of society—can combine with population control to increase everyone's assets. To introduce this section, a few facts must be presented:[19]

- Much of the world's agriculture is primitive. More than 50 percent of all food consumed in the world is still hand produced.
- In many countries, up to 90 percent of the population lives on rural land.
- Of the more than 150 nations of the world, fewer than 24 are democracies. Most governments dictate the day-to-day lives of their people and their policies may not be equitable.
- Securing enough food on a day-to-day basis is a problem for as many as a billion human beings.
- The land in many parts of the world does not support the growing of food, even by the wealthy. Furthermore, the poor are often crowded onto mountainous slopes that are even less **arable.**

The problem of unequal distribution of resources exists not only between rich and poor nations but also between rich and poor people within nations. The FAO estimates that world food production averages about 3000 calories per person per day, but food is distributed unequally. Huge amounts of soybeans and grains are fed to livestock to produce protein foods the poor cannot afford to purchase. Also, by some estimates, at least 20 percent or more of the total food produced is lost to pests and spoilage.[20]

Again, the problem is poverty; the symptom is inability to purchase basic food for sustenance. But the wealthy nations cannot simply give to the poor; this only weakens them further; self-reliance is the goal. The question of policymakers and nutrition planners is, how do we increase the productivity of the

Green Revolution: the development and widespread adoption of high-yielding strains of wheat, corn, and rice in developing countries. "Green Revolution" is a popular term also used to describe almost any package of modern agriculture technology delivered to developing countries.

appropriate technology: a technology that utilizes locally abundant resources in preference to locally scarce resources. Developing countries usually have a large labor force and little capital; the appropriate technology would therefore be labor-intensive.

If you give a man a fish, he will eat for a day. If you teach him to fish, he will eat for a lifetime.

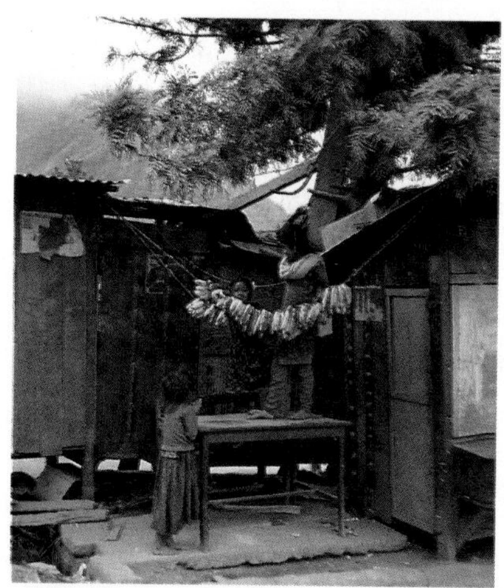

Children help to string up bananas that the family hopes to sell.

rural poor in a way that supports self-reliance? Much is involved, but four things are basic and are required simultaneously. The poor must have greater access to land, capital, technology, and knowledge.[21] Some international food aid may also be required during the development period. Despite all development efforts, however, a country's own political desire must be to improve the conditions of all its people.

Governments can learn from recent history the importance of developing local agricultural technology. A major effort made in the 1960s—the **Green Revolution**—had only minimal success because it was not in harmony with local realities. It was an effort to bring the genetic-engineered, petroleum-demanding agricultural technology of the industrial world to the developing countries, but the high-yielding strains of wheat and rice that were selected required irrigation, chemical fertilizers, and pesticides—all costly, and beyond the economic means of too many of the farmers in the developing world.

Instead of transplanting industrial technology into the developing countries, there is a need to develop small, efficient farms and local structures for marketing, credit, transportation, food storage, and agricultural education. International research centers need to examine the conditions of tropical countries and orient their research toward **appropriate technology**—labor-intensive rather than energy-intensive agricultural methods.

Environmental concerns must be taken more seriously as well. As important as the amount of land available for crop production is the condition of the soil and the availability of water. Soil erosion is now accelerating on every continent, at a rate that threatens the world's ability to continue feeding itself. Erosion of soil has always occurred; it is a natural process, but in the past it has been compensated for by processes that build the soil up. Farmers should alternate soil-building crops with soil-devouring crops, a practice known as crop rotation. An acre of soil planted one year in corn, the next in wheat, and the next in clover loses 2.7 tons of topsoil each year, but if it is planted only in corn three years in a row, it will lose 19.7 tons a year.[22] When farmers must choose whether

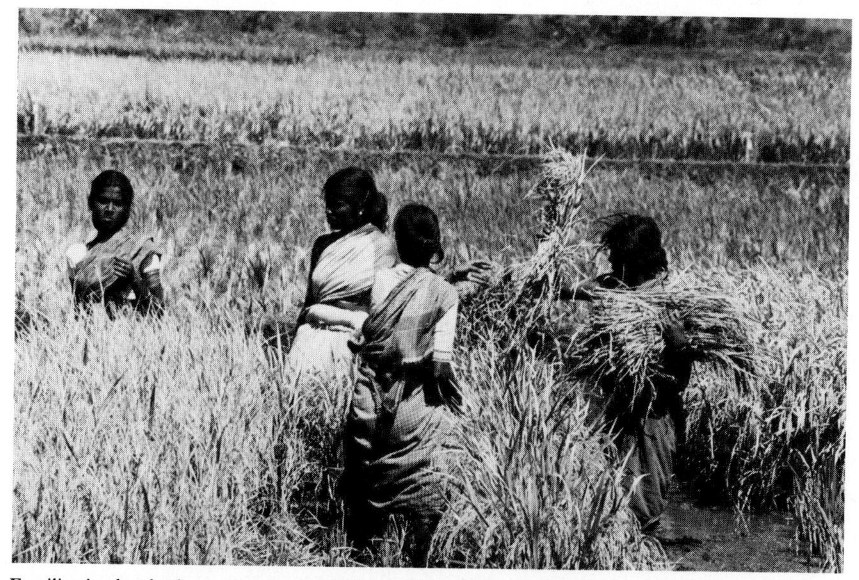

Families in developing countries depend on their children to help provide for daily needs.

to make three times as much money planting corn year after year or rotate crops and go bankrupt, naturally they choose the profits. Ruin may not follow immediately, but it will follow.[23]

multinational corporations: international organizations with direct investments and/or operative facilities in more than one country. Examples are U.S. oil and food companies.

Food for Profit

Businesspeople, economists, and some development specialists often extol the benefits to third world countries deemed to result from the investments of **multinational corporations,** especially in fostering economic growth. Other observers, however, are convinced that the multinationals have done more harm than good. Because the negative effects have included malnutrition, the topic of this chapter, they are emphasized here.[24]

A multinational corporation's primary concern is profit, and it supports political and economic systems that exploit the poor:

> Agribusiness is now buying or renting more and more arable land. Decisions on what to plant and where to distribute the harvest are made with the balance sheet in mind. Thus it is profitable in poor countries to use land for exportable luxuries even while the people are suffering severe malnutrition because not enough grain is grown for local consumption.[25]

The classic example of the subtle exploitation of the poor, related to nutrition, is the competition for farmland between cash crops and food crops. The tragic scenario unfolds this way: Large landowners and multinational corporations control the best farmlands and use them mainly to grow crops that can be exported for profit. Indigenous persons work for below-subsistence wages and are forced onto marginal lands to do their own farming. The poor work hard, but they are cultivating crops for other people, rather than for themselves. The money they earn is not enough even to buy the products they help produce. The poor never acquire their share of the profits realized from the marketing of their products. The results: imported foods—bananas, beef, cocoa, coconut, coffee, pineapple, sugar, tea, winter tomatoes, and others—fill *our* grocery stores, while the poor who grow these foods have even less food and resources than before. Additional cropland is diverted for nonfood cash crops—tobacco, rubber, cotton, and other agricultural products. These practices also contribute to the bankruptcy experienced by American farmers; cash crops often undersell American-grown produce because they have been produced with government supported financial aid.

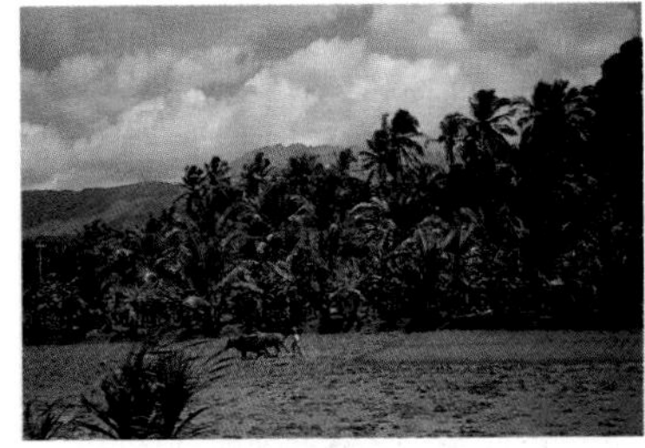

Man and oxen ploughing a field in rural India.

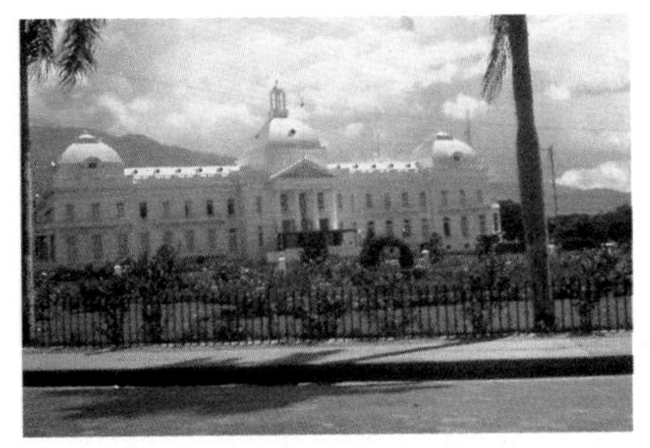

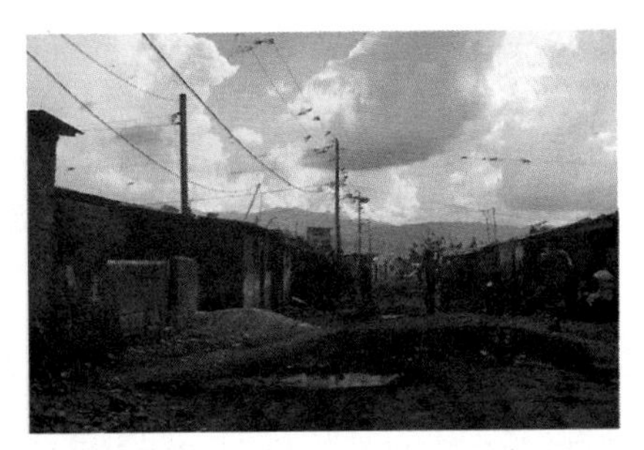

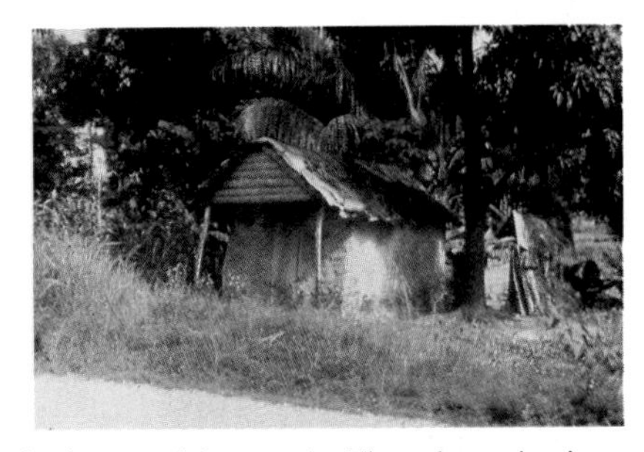

The stark contrasts between rich and poor within a single developing country are depicted here in the homes of the people. The ruler maintains a palace while the majority of the population live in city tenements or rural huts.

Export-oriented agriculture thus uses the labor, land, capital, and technology that is needed to help local families produce their own food. For example, the effort required to produce bananas for export could be reallocated to provide food for the local people. It has been suggested that one solution to the world food problem is not that the developed countries should *give* more food aid, but that they should *take* less food away from the poor countries.[26] Truly, imported foods raised on land from which thousands of small farmers have been displaced symbolizes the exploitation of the poor as vividly as does a bottle of contaminated formula in the mouth of a dying infant.

Countless examples can be cited to illustrate how natural resources are diverted from producing food for domestic consumption to producing luxury crops for those who can afford them. A few such examples are included here:[27]

- Africa is a net *exporter* of barley, beans, peanuts, fresh vegetables, and cattle (not to mention luxury crop exports such as coffee and cocoa), yet it has a higher incidence of PEM among young children than any other continent.
- Mexico now supplies the United States with over half its supply of several winter and early spring vegetables, while infant deaths associated with poor nutrition are common.
- Half of Central America's agricultural land produces food for export, while in several of its countries the poorest 50 percent of the population eat only half the protein they need. (The richest 5 percent, on the other hand, consume two to three times more than they need.)

Besides diverting acreage away from the traditional staples of the diet, multinationals may also contribute to hunger by way of their marketing techniques. Their advertisements lead many consumers with limited incomes to associate products like cola beverages, cigarettes, infant formula, and snack foods with good health and prosperity. These promotions are tragically inappropriate for these people. A poor family's nutrition status suffers when its tight budget is pinched further by purchase of such goods.

The United Nations has commissioned several studies in the hopes of establishing an international code of conduct for the multinational corporations.[28] These powerful organizations could have an immense impact on national economies for good, rather than for ill. Remember, too, that we, directly or indirectly (as shareholders) are the multinationals. We could, therefore, if we chose, increase the credit and capital available to the developing world; and these resources, if properly used, could help to eliminate hunger. The multinationals also possess the scientific knowledge and organizational skills needed to help develop improved food and agricultural systems. However, experience reveals that wise control of these corporations is necessary to ensure that human needs do not become subordinate to political and financial gains.

Contributors to the world hunger problem have been colonialism, overpopulation, maldistribution of land, and use of third world countries' resources to produce cash crops for export when those countries' people need those resources themselves.

Toward a Solution

Although the problem of world hunger is overwhelming, it can be broken down into many small, local problems. Significant strides can then be made toward solving them at the local level. Even if the problem of poverty itself is not immediately or fully solved, progress is possible. For example, infants and children need not be raised in middle-class homes to be protected from malnutrition. Slight modifications of the children's own diets can be immensely beneficial. Encouraging examples are provided by recent experiences in Sierra Leone, Nepal, and Southeast Asia.

In Sierra Leone, Bennimix was developed from subsistence crops and introduced as a supplement to infants' diets. Rice, sesame (benniseed), and peanuts were hand pounded to make a flour meal and then cooked. The local children found it tasty—and, whereas they had been malnourished before, they thrived when Bennimix was added to their diets. The village women formed a cooperative to reduce the household drudgery of preparation, and they rotated the work on a weekly or monthly basis.[29] The government also established a manufacturing plant to produce and market the mixture at subsidized prices. The success of the venture appeared to lie in involving the local people in the process of identifying the problem and devising its solution. It was not considered enough only to accomplish the goals of an agency; the needs of the people were remembered.

A similar success was achieved in Nepal by maximizing use of local resources and facilities to prepare a supplementary food. Ingredients for the food were soybeans, corn, and wheat, mixed in a 2:1:1 proportion, and yielding a concentrated "superflour" of high biological value suitable for infants and children. A Nutrition Rehabilitation Center tested this superflour by giving the undernourished children and their mothers two cereal-based meals a day, and giving the children three additional small meals of superflour porridge daily. Within ten days the undernourished children had gained weight, lost their edema, and recovered their appetites and social alertness. The mothers, who saw with their own eyes the remarkable recoveries of their children, were motivated to learn how to make the tasty supplementary food and incorporate it into their local foodstuffs and customs.[30]

Another success story is the research surrounding the winged bean plant, cultivated in Southeast Asia for years, but only recently studied by the National Academy of Sciences. The plant is easily cultivated, even in sandy soil and tropical climates, needs no fertilizer, and is completely edible. The winged bean is similar to the soybean, but is much easier to grow. Complemented with corn, it can be made into a weaning food with the protein quality of milk and a high vitamin A content.[31]

These three examples offer little hope that the world food situation can be improved by simple means, because the real issue of poverty remains to be addressed. One-shot intervention programs—offering nutrition education, food distribution, food fortification, and the like—are not enough. It is difficult to describe the misery a mother feels when she has received education about nutrition but is unable to purchase the foods her family needs. She now knows *why* her child is sick and dying but is helpless in *applying* her new knowledge.

Focus on Children. There is hopeful news for children in underdeveloped countries and in neglected parts of the United States. **GOBI** is a plan set forth by **UNICEF** that can cut the number of hunger-related child deaths from 40,000 to 20,000 a day. GOBI is an acronym for four simple, but profoundly important, elements of UNICEF's "Child Survival" campaign: Growth charts, oral rehydration therapy, breast milk, and immunization.

The use of growth charts requires a worldwide education campaign. A mother can learn to weigh her child every month and chart the child's growth on a

GOBI: an acronym for the elements of UNICEF's child survival campaign: growth charts, oral rehydration therapy, breast milk, and immunization.

UNICEF: the United Nations Children's Fund, formerly the United Nations International Children's Emergency Fund.

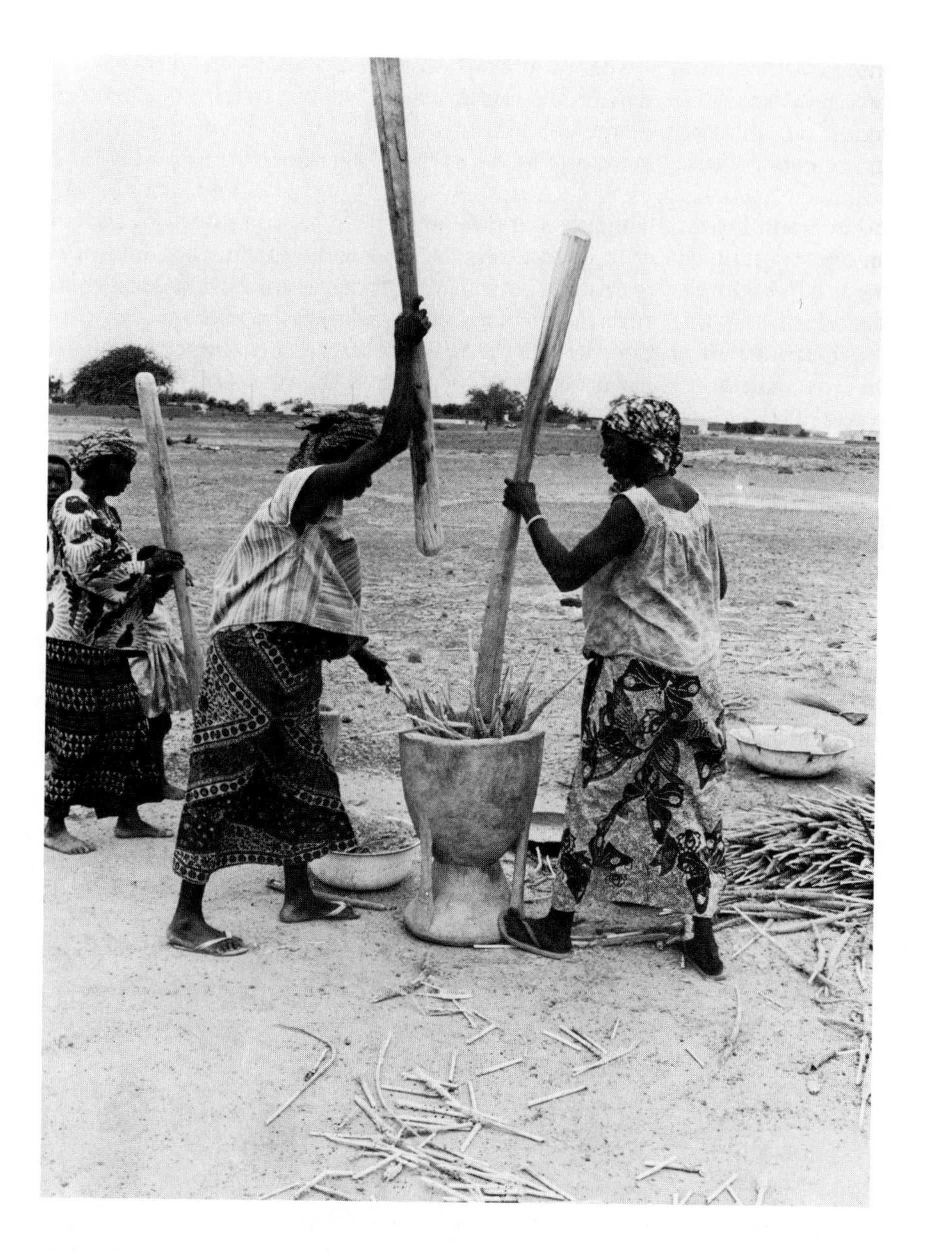

In Nepal, the women worked together in a first step toward self-sufficiency.

specially designed paper growth chart. She can learn to detect for herself the early stages of "hidden malnutrition" that can leave a child irreparably retarded in mind and body. Then at least she can know she needs to take steps to remedy the malnutrition—if she can.

The importance of oral rehydration therapy (ORT) is that most children who die of malnutrition don't starve to death—they die because their health has been compromised by bacteria and infections causing diarrhea. Until recently, there was no easy way of stopping the infection-diarrhea cycle and saving their lives. Oral rehydration therapy is the administration of a simple solution of sugar, salt, and water to treat dehydration caused by diarrhea.* The solution

*Only in the event of an emergency, when medical help is not otherwise available: mix one level teaspoon (5 milliliters) of salt with 8 level teaspoons (40 milliliters) of sugar in a quart (1 liter) of drinking water.

increases the body's ability to absorb fluids by 2500 percent.[32] Mothers can make up the ORT solution themselves using locally available ingredients. International development groups also provide packets of these salts to mothers in rural and urban areas.

The promotion of breastfeeding among mothers in developing countries has many benefits. Breast milk is hygienic, is readily available, is nutritionally sound, and provides infants with immunological protection specific for their environments. In the developing world, its advantages over formula feeding can mean the difference between life and death.

As for immunizations, they could prevent most of the 5 million deaths each year from measles, diphtheria, tetanus, whooping cough, poliomyelitis, and tuberculosis. However, adequate protein nutrition is necessary in order for vaccinations to be useful. UNICEF's goal is to immunize all of the world's children by 1990. It used to be difficult to keep vaccines stable in their long journeys from laboratory to remote villages. However, a new measles vaccine has been discovered that does not require refrigeration. The result: universal measles immunization for young children is now possible.

Focus on Women. Women make up 50 percent of the world's population. Any solution to the problems of poverty and hunger is incomplete and even hopeless if it fails to address the role of women in developing countries. We have noted that the main cause of hunger is poverty. Women and children represent the majority of those living in poverty.

In many countries, over 90 percent of the population lives in rural areas. The lot of a woman living in rural poverty is often an oppressive one. Not only is she dealing with the impoverishment of rural life in an underdeveloped nation, but she must also cope with life in a male-dominated society. Her needs are rarely met, yet she is expected to carry the burden of her family's survival alone. Women are oftentimes overworked and underfed. In many cultures, they are the last to get food, despite the fact that they spend hours each day procuring water and firewood, and pounding grains by hand. In many countries, women in the rural areas are not only the primary food producers, but also are responsible for child care and food preparation. Often they have to work as harvesters on other people's lands as well. Husbands are frequently absent, having gone to live in the cities in search of work or having found employment on distant commercial farms—growing export crops.

Development projects are often large in scale and highly technological, and they overlook women's needs. Yet women play a vital role in the nutrition of their nations' people. Their nutrition during pregnancy and lactation determines the future health of their children. They are almost always the ones who feed their families, and if they are weakened by malnutrition themselves, or ignorant as to how to feed others, the consequences ripple outward to affect many other individuals. In recent years, the importance of the role women play in these countries has begun to be understood. Various countries now offer development programs with women in mind.

Six basic strategies are at the heart of women's programs:

- Removing barriers to financial credit—so that women can obtain loans for raw materials and equipment to enhance their role in food production..
- Providing access to time-saving technologies—seed grinders, for example.
- Providing appropriate training—for the purpose of self-reliance.

- Teaching management and marketing skills—to avoid exploitation.
- Making health and day-care services available—to provide a healthy environment for these women's children.
- Forming of women's support groups—to foster strength by means of cooperative efforts.[33]

The recognition of women's needs by some development organizations is an encouraging trend in the efforts to contend with the world hunger crisis.

Progress toward solutions of individual nations' hunger problems can be made via appropriate local efforts. Effective programs focus on children and women and train women to better support their own and their families' economic and nutritional well-being.

Personal Action

To summarize what is known about the world food situation, let us examine the conclusions of the Presidential Commission on World Hunger. The members of the commission are convinced that worldwide efforts to overcome hunger and malnutrition and to foster self-reliant development must be intensive. Their major conclusions are listed in Table 14–6.

Now is an opportune time to exercise our global citizenship on behalf of the poor. One of the most important steps individuals can take is to urge government and corporate policymakers to make hunger a priority item, just as the issues of energy, inflation, and ecology are. Three of the most powerful social movements of recent history began with moral outrage against dehumanizing situations—sex discrimination, slavery, and the war in Vietnam. Vigorous voices

Table 14–6

Presidential Commission on World Hunger: Conclusions

- The major world hunger problem today is the prevalence of chronic undernutrition—which calls for a political, as well as a technical, solution.
- The world hunger problem is getting worse rather than better.
- A major crisis of global food supply—of even more serious dimensions than the present energy crisis—appears likely by the year 2000, unless steps are taken now to facilitate a significant increase in food production in the developing nations.
- Rising global demand for food must be met within resource limits—of land, water, energy, and agricultural inputs.
- There is no ideal food, no perfect diet, no universally acceptable agricultural system waiting to be transplanted from one geographic, climatic, or cultural setting to another. Assistance programs must focus on self-reliance and respond to the needs of each country. Needs and requirements cannot be generalized.
- In addition to action by the industrialized nations, decisive steps to build more effective national food systems must be taken by the developing countries.
- The outcome of the war on hunger, by the year 2000 and beyond, will be determined not by forces beyond human control, but by decisions and actions well within the capability of nations and people working individually and together.

Source: Adapted from Presidential Commission on World Hunger, *Overcoming World Hunger: The Challenge Ahead* (Washington, D.C.: Government Printing Office, 1980), pp. 180–185.

are needed to influence the policies of our governments and corporations, since their present policies of food trade, aid, and investment appear to be keeping the third world *underdeveloped*. To remain silent is to render support to the status quo. To urge change is to make it known that the way to achieve food adequacy for everyone in a sensible time span is with a detailed, monitored, aggressive policy of redistribution, both at the international and national levels.

Among the possibilities for personal action are these:

Hunger exists not because we can't end it, but simply because we haven't.—World Runners

- Read more about national and international development issues. Discuss these issues with a group of friends or co-workers. Be able to articulate them to others. Be open to new ideas and solutions.
- Help raise money for volunteer agencies working abroad. Their projects directly affect some portion of the poor at the grassroots level, and are more likely to get food and funds into the hands of the poor than are those of top-heavy bureaucracies. A guide to world hunger organizations is available from *Seeds* (see p. 565).
- Learn about agribusiness. Huge food-producing corporations can make a major difference to people's and the earth's future. Your knowledge of how they operate can enable you to influence them to make a difference in the right direction. These corporations are responsive to the consumers to whom they sell, so what you demand from them influences what they produce. If consumers will pay for exotic fruits to be flown in from half a world away, then the industry will produce them. You communicate your wishes to those food companies whenever you buy, or don't buy, their products. Consider boycotting products imported from developing countries as cash crops or products of companies that market goods inappropriately in the third world. What we choose to eat affects not only our lives, but also the lives of those who produce it.
- Attend or organize an event to raise your community's awareness of world food issues. World Food Day occurs annually on October 16, commemorating the founding of FAO, the United Nations agency responsible for improving global access to food. Oxfam America sponsors the Fast for a World Harvest each year in November.
- Support local groups such as food banks and soup kitchens. Donate time, funding, or food.
- Write letters, as often as possible. Ask your government legislators what they are doing to end world hunger. Share your knowledge with them. Write to local newspapers—provide them with information on hunger issues to be shared with their readers. Oxfam America and Bread for the World have guidelines to help you write effectively to these people.

It follows, of course, that careful planning is required so that the poor themselves realize the potential benefits being suggested here. Guidelines must be developed, to divert to needy markets the resources this country would make available, and these guidelines must be reflected in the policies of our government. In the words of an author who has devoted intensive study to world hunger:

> Doing good for the sake of doing good is self-interest. To most people, ethical concerns are of value. Compassion and human decency may not lend themselves neatly to cost-benefit analysis, but the desire for sound moral values is a legitimate rationale for

government action. Somehow, affluent societies must learn to accept this kind of self-interest as a basis for public policy.[34]

Meanwhile, what can we do in a personal way, to improve the chances of the future well-being of the world and its people? The problems may appear so great that they seem approachable only by way of worldwide political decisions. But consider this: you can also help change the world through the personal choices you make each day.[35] To describe some ways in which an individual can accomplish this, especially through daily food choices, is perhaps the most fitting way to conclude this book.

Individuals can help the world's hungry by speaking up, by raising money, by supporting local food distribution efforts, and by supporting enlightened legislation.

Food Feature

Voluntary Simplicity

The Food Features throughout this book have been filled with practical suggestions for attaining the ideals of personal nutrition presented in the chapters. It turns out that many of those suggestions that best support personal health also support the health of the whole earth as well.

How we choose to live our individual lives is ultimately a personal matter; however, our choices have an impact on the way the rest of the world's people live and die. Our nation, with 6 percent of the world's population, consumes about 40 percent of the world's food and energy resources. The food problem depends partly on the demands we place on the world's finite natural resources. In a sense, therefore, we contribute to the world food problem. People in affluent nations have the freedom and means to choose their lifestyles; people in poor nations do not. We can find ways to reduce our consumption of the world's nonrenewable resources; we can use only what is absolutely required. The admonition, so familiar in childhood, to "clean your plate," as if that would alleviate the suffering of some starving stranger, could well be replaced with the mandate simply to "consume less food." It is ironic that whereas other societies cannot secure enough clean water for people to drink, our society produces bottles of pop that contain 1 calorie of artificial sweetener in 12 ounces of water, and that cost 800 calories of energy, each, to produce. Choosing a diet at the level of necessity, rather than excess, would reduce the resource demands made by our industrial agriculture. It would also produce humanitarian and economic benefits.

One major way to reduce the demands we make on world resources is to depend less on animal-based proteins and to use more plant-based proteins. Even one meal a week per person would make a difference. Meat does not necessarily have to be eliminated totally from the diet, because ruminants (cattle, sheep, and goats) can use forage crops and crop residues produced on land not suitable to other crops.[36] In so doing, these animals convert plants indigestible by humans into high-quality animal protein. Today, however, much rich cropland is used to grow animal feed instead of foods for humans. The animals are then fed these grain and protein feeds in feedlots, where they are fattened much faster than if they had grazed on pastureland. Figure 14–3 shows the different rates at which animals convert feed to edible animal protein. As shown, chickens require about 3 pounds of grain to produce 1 pound of meat, whereas cattle require 16 pounds of grain to do the same.

Cattle are also grown on land cleared for that purpose from irreplaceable tropical rainforests—an ongoing process that is wiping out one of the world's last great natural resources (see Controversy 14). By simply cutting back on our beef consumption and substituting less land-costly plant-protein sources, we could perhaps rescue some of the last of those forests and certainly could help make large amounts of land available for human food production. We would also realize other ecological benefits, including decreased water and fertilizer requirements. Irrigation for raising food for beef cattle forage crops alone requires 4 to 45 times more water than for other field crops.[37]

Figure 14–3
A Protein Factory in Reverse.

[a]Soy constitutes only 12% of steer feed and 20 to 25% of poultry feed.
Source: F. M. Lappe, *Diet for a Small Planet* (New York: Ballentine Books, 1975), p. 11. Institute for Food and Development Policy, 1885 Mission St., San Francisco, CA 94103. Reprinted with permission of the Institute for Food and Development Policy.

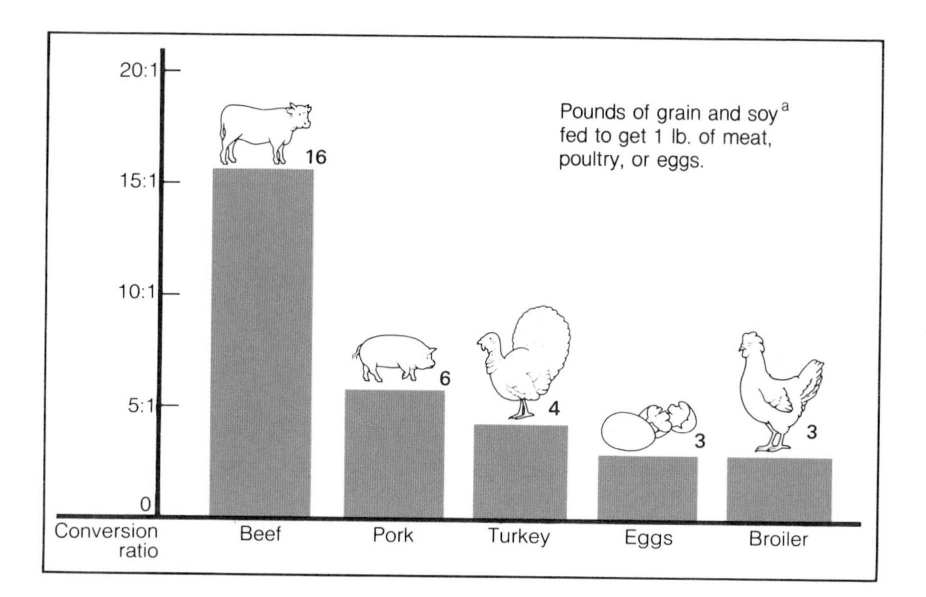

A second way in which the developed world can better the quality of life in the developing countries is to shift to a less energy-dependent lifestyle. The primary reason to alter our food and energy consumption patterns is not to redistribute our food to developing countries, but to reduce the demand we make on their resources. This would make those resources available to them for their own self-development.

Every personal choice that every person makes affects the well-being of everyone else, whether the person is aware of it or not. Some hold, therefore, that all people have the responsibility to make sure they can answer yes to the question, If everyone lived as I do, would the children of today grow up in a better world? Those who study the future are convinced that the hope of the world lies in everyone's adopting a simple lifestyle. As one such person put it, "the widespread simplification of life is vital to the well-being of the entire human family."[38]

This is not to suggest that people should adopt a life of poverty—emphatically not. It is said that "poverty is repressive, simplicity is liberating. Poverty generates a sense of helplessness . . . simplicity fosters creativity. Poverty is mean and degrading . . . simplicity is enabling."[39] In other words, to become poor would solve nothing—poverty obstructs personal growth; simplicity opens the way to it. What *is* advocated has nothing to do with wealth. It is a lifestyle, a commitment to live more simply in view of the world's limited resources.[40]

Voluntary simplicity involves a thousand small decisions relating to food choices and other choices—of which we will offer 15. Before reading them, be sure to understand that they are not "the" rules, but only a sampling deemed appropriate by one school of thought. *Voluntary* is a key word, just as *simplicity* is. Each individual must look within to discover a personal sense of what is appropriate. Each person needs to find a balance, personally suitable, that leads him or her between the extremes of poverty and self-indulgence.

Many organizations concerned with the world's future have set themselves the task of identifying ways for individuals to simplify their lives for the benefit of all. A sampling of the ideas they have generated is presented in Table 14–7.

Table 14–7

Foodways to Simplify Life

1. Select nutrient-dense foods most often.
2. Select unprocessed foods, grown locally.
3. Buy staple foods in bulk containers.
4. Buy fresh foods in season.
5. Learn to preserve foods.
6. Conserve food, and conserve its nutritional value. Buy all foods in recyclable containers.
7. Eat lower on the food chain—more plant foods, less meat.
8. If you eat beef, look for forage-fed or grass-fed beef.
9. If you eat beef, choose domestic, not foreign-grown beef. Don't feed beef to pets.
10. Reduce your intakes of refined sugar and other nonnutritive products.
11. Grow your own fruits and vegetables, whenever possible. Use organic fertilizer and biological pesticides. Eat wild foods.
13. Organize a food co-op.
14. Bake bread, home-prepare other foods.
15. Drink homemade beverages.

Sources: Ideas from Center for Science in the Public Interest, Simple Lifestyle Team, *99 Ways to a Simple Lifestyle* (Garden City, N.Y.: Anchor Books, 1977), and D. Katz and M. T. Goodwin, *Food: Where Nutrition, Politics, and Culture Meet* (Washington, D.C.: Center for Science in the Public Interest, 1976), p. 155.

Interestingly, the suggestions seem to address two problems that, on the face of them, might seem to require different solutions. The first is to bring about the greatest possible improvement in one's own nutrition; the second is to take all possible dietary steps for the well-being of the earth and its people.

The first item on the list, "Select nutrient-dense foods most often," captures in a sentence possibly the most important personal nutrition advice in this book. For the earth, too, it is vitally important. The concept of nutrient density was introduced in Chapter 2, and the tables of nutrients per hundred calories in Chapters 6 and 7 showed that, most often, vegetables are richest in nutrients. If people use more vegetables to attain nutrient adequacy each day, they eat less meat; and as this chapter has made clear, vegetables demand far fewer of the earth's limited resources, measured in calories, than do meats. Fats and sugars *lower* the nutrient density of foods, and are also costly to the earth to produce.

The second item on the list, "Select unprocessed foods, grown locally," is equally applicable to self and world. Unprocessed, in this sense, means with the nutrients left in, sugar and fat left out. You already know why you should select unprocessed, or whole, foods for personal nutrition. To appreciate why they are also good for the earth, and why the local varieties are preferred, consider how potatoes grown far away might become a processed food, say potato chips, in your grocery store. To make the chips, the whole potatoes are transported on fuel-burning trucks from the farm to the factory, where power-driven machines strip them of some of their parts (and some of their nutrients); other machines alter their shape and consistency; others add sugar, salt, and fat (each additive produced at its own factory); the mixture is cooked and dried in electrical equipment; and still more machines portion out the finished potato chips into plastic or cellophane containers (all produced with many other fuel-gobbling machines at many other factories and trucked in). Then the chips are shipped: the containers are boxed together and hauled by still other fuel-burning trucks to the distribution center, from which they will be delivered to the air-conditioned or heated grocery store and stacked in brightly lighted cases for the consumer to purchase. Now compare: a consumer stops at a roadside stand to buy potatoes, within viewing distance of the farm. Not only is the person's nutrition best served, but the cost of potato nutrition per calorie of the earth's resources is immeasurably lower. Even if the potatoes are brought in from the next county and sold in the grocery store, they are far preferable, in terms of their energy cost, to the potato chips.

The same considerations apply to item 3—"Buy staple foods in bulk or recyclable containers." Bulk containers involve much less energy consumption at the manufacturing end; you can use your own small jars or canisters over and over again, at home. Recyclable containers require replacement infrequently. As for item 4, "Buy fresh foods in season," such a choice saves all the costs, not only of packing, but also of cold storage, that otherwise would be incurred. "Learn to preserve foods" is item 5. When local produce is in season, it is least expensive. If you buy more than you need and quick-cook and freeze some, you can then eat that food later for a price no higher, except for what it has cost you to store it.

Item 6 on the list is "Conserve food, and conserve its nutritional value." Once you have purchased the food, whatever the cost to the earth in producing it, be sure to obtain the full nutrient contribution it can make to your health. Prepare no more than you will serve; serve no more than you will eat. And cook it with care: the plant captured sunlight and used fertilizer to synthesize and store its nutrients. The animal consumed plants to do the same thing. The Food Feature of Chapter 6 showed ways of conserving those nutrients to make a difference to people's nutritional health. Here too, what is good for you is good for the earth.

Items 7 through 10 say to eat less meat, particularly less beef, and less sugar (and to this we would add, less fat). Implicit in this is the admonition to eat more vegetables, legumes, and whole foods of all sorts, and to appreciate the natural flavors of foods without sugar and fat. The costs of meat have been previously delineated; fats and sugars cost as much energy to produce as any processed food, and often more. The land on which sugarcane and oil seeds grow yields products devoid of nutrients and rich in energy, excesses of which are linked to obesity and associated ills. That same land could be used instead to produce vitamin-rich carrots, or broccoli, or simply not farmed at all, but allowed to support the natural environment upon which all life depends.

Item 11 suggests that you grow your own fruits and vegetables, whenever possible. To do so promotes your health in a non-energy-consuming way—you expend your own energy, outdoors, in a healthful environment instead of in an air-conditioned spa or a heated ice-skating rink. Then you eat the food you've produced—requiring less to be produced for you by others.

Item 12 recommends that you "Organize a food co-op"—that is, a grocery store or buying club that you and your neighbors or friends run for yourselves. The theory is that cooperatives generate self-reliance and expand the human potential of their participants. Their members, who pay minimal dues, can save money on food and other basic items, and more money by volunteering their labor.

Routes to Involvement

You may want to learn more about organizations dealing with food policy issues. Agencies willing to help you get the facts include:

- Bread for the World
  6411 Chillum Pl. NW
  Washington, D.C. 20012
- Oxfam America
  115 Broadway
  Boston, MA 02116
- Seeds
  222 East Lake Drive
  Decatur, GA 30030
- Food Research and Action Center
  1319 F St. N.W. Suite 500
  Washington, D.C. 20004
- The Hunger Project
  2015 Steiner St.
  San Francisco, CA 94115
- Institute for Food and Development Policy
  1885 Mission St.
  San Francisco, CA 94103
- Interreligious Taskforce on U.S. Food Policy
  110 Maryland Ave. NE
  Washington, D.C. 20002

Most supermarkets' first objective is to make money. Highly processed impulse items increase their profit margin: supermarkets make more money from sugared cereals, sodas, candy, and other end-of-aisle displays than from nutritious foods. In contrast, cooperative stores are more responsive to their customers—they are owned by the consumers, so there is no conflict of interest. They can offer bulk quantities of unprocessed foods for very little above wholesale prices and resist low-quality, jazzily packaged foods. If they produce profits, they return them to their members, or reinvest them in a way the members approve. Many communities already have food cooperatives operating; for those that do not, resources are available to show how to start them.*

Items 13 and 14 recommend that you prepare your own bread, other food products, and beverages. Some may think they don't have the time or the will to bake bread, but there is much to be said for considering it. Home-baked bread can be more delicious than any bread bought from the store. The time

*Examples: G. Stern, *How to Start Your Own Food Co-op: A Guide to Wholesale Buying* (New York: Walker and Company, 1974); T. Vellela, *Food Coops for Small Groups* (New York: Workman Publishing, 1975).

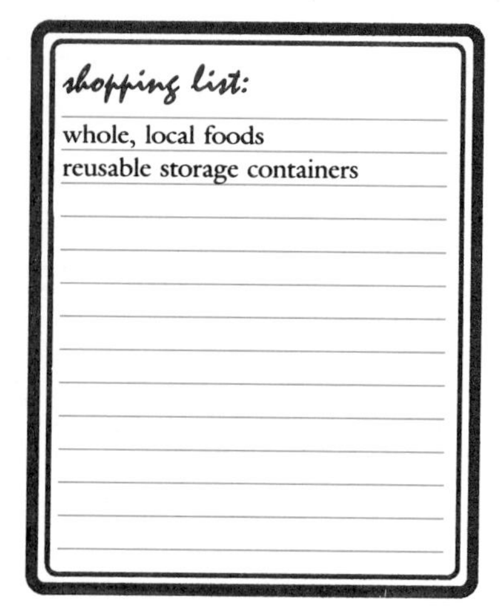

and energy spent baking it are time and energy not spent doing something else (driving a car, consuming luxury goods and services). The choice is a possible one to make—provided that you are willing to exchange some other activity for it. People who learn to enjoy producing their own food obtain a satisfaction from it that may make it less necessary for them to consume items that are more costly in terms of land, resources, and other people's energy.

The last suggestion is to "Eat wild foods." For many people, this is not a possibility, but for some, it is. The same philosophy applies: it is the simplest and most cost-free possible way of obtaining nourishment. Many people are not aware of foods that grow in wild places near their homes—or even as weeds in nearby public parks. Local botanical societies can inform you about these plants—and also about the importance of harvesting conservatively and replacing the seeds so that they will be there again next year.

No doubt, everyone can make some of these choices; a lucky few can make them all. Personal lifestyles do matter, for a society is nothing more than the sum of its individuals. As we go, so goes our world.

Notes

1. A. H. Boerma, Keynote address, Second World Food Congress, The Hague, June 1970, in *FAO Studies in Food and Population,* FAO Economic and Social Development Series, no. 1, p. 129, Rome, 1976.
2. K. Markandaya, *Nectar in a Sieve,* 2d American ed. (New York: John Day Company, 1955), pp. 121–122. Reprinted in *Ending Hunger.* © 1985 The Hunger Project.
3. L. Schwartz-Nobel, *Starving in the Shadow of Plenty* (New York: Putnam, 1981), pp. 35–36. © 1981 by G. Putnam Co.
4. D. R. Gwatkin, How many die? A set of demographic estimates of the annual number of infant and child deaths in the world, *American Journal of Public Health* 70 (1980): 1286–1289.
5. S. N. Gershoff, Science—Neglected ingredient of nutrition policy, *Journal of the American Dietetic Association* 70 (1977): 471.
6. M. Cameron and Y. Hofvander, *Manual on Feeding Infants and Young Children,* 2d ed. (New York: Protein Advisory Board of the United Nations, 1976), p. 1.
7. Dr. Carol Dyer's findings related to social and cultural beliefs about food in India, from A. Berg, *The Nutrition Factor* (Washington, D.C.: Brookings Institute, 1973), p. 46.
8. I. Rozov, The decade: Not just pumps and pipes, *World Health,* April/May 1983, p. 29.
9. World Bank, *World Development Report 1981,* Table 21.
10. P. Pellet, The role of food mixtures in combating childhood malnutrition, in *Nutrition in the Community,* ed. D. McLaren (New York: Wiley, 1978), pp. 185–202.
11. Harvard University School of Public Health, *Physician's Task Force on Hunger in America* (Cambridge, Mass.: Harvard University School of Public Health, 1986).
12. N. Kotz, *Hunger in America: The Federal Response* (New York: The Field Foundation, 1979), p. 17.
13. Harvard University School of Public Health, 1986.
14. J. Lelyveld, Hunger in America, *Seeds,* December 1985, pp. 6–11.
15. Florida Department of Health and Rehabilitative Services and the Florida Task Force on Hunger, *Hunger in Florida: A Report to the Legislature,* April 1986, pp. 32–33.
16. Independent Commission on International Issues, *North-South: A Program for Survival* (Cambridge, Mass.: MIT Press, 1980), pp. 49–50. © 1980 MIT Press.
17. The story of Fernando told in the margin is from: D. Burgess, The future of hungry children abroad, *Journal of Current Social Issues,* Summer 1975, p. 36.
18. J. Kocher, Not too many but too little, in J. D. Gussow, *The Feeding Web: Issues in Nutritional Ecology* (Palo Alto, Calif.: Bull Publishing, 1978), pp. 81–83.
19. R. R. Spitzer, *No Need for Hunger* (Danville, Ill.: Interstate Printers and Publishers, 1981), pp. 20–23.
20. *Nutrition Week* 13 (1983): pp. 4–5.
21. M. R. Langham, L. Polopolus, and M. L. Upchurch, *World Food Issues* (Gainesville, Fla.: University of Florida Press, 1982), pp. 18–20.
22. National Agricultural Lands Study, *Soil Degradation: Effects on Agricultural Productivity, Interim Report No. 4* (Washington, D.C.: USDA, November 1980), as cited by L. R. Brown, World population growth, soil erosion, and food security, *Science* 214 (1981): 995–1002.
23. Brown, 1981.
24. For the other side of the argument—offering multinationals as part of the solution rather than the problem—see M. L. Kastens, Harvest of hunger: How government meddling threatens the world's food supply, *Futurist* 15, no. 5 (1981): 5–10.
25. R. J. Barnet, Multinationals: A dissenting view, *Saturday Review* 3 (1976): 11, 58.
26. G. Kent, Food trade: The poor feed the rich, *Food and Nutrition Bulletin* 4 (1982): 25–33.
27. F. M. Lappe and J. Collins, *Food First: Beyond the Myth of Scarcity* (Boston: Houghton Mifflin, 1978), p. 15.
28. Interreligious Taskforce on U.S. Food Policy, *Identifying a Food*

Policy Agenda for the 1980s: A Working Paper (Washington, D.C.: January 1980), p. 30.
29. J. M. Steckle, Improving food utilization in developing countries, *Canadian Home Economics Journal* 27 (1977): 34–39.
30. *National Conference on Primary Health Care* (Kathmandu: Ministry of Health, Health Services Coordination Committee, WHO, UNICEF, 1977), pp. 9, 25, as cited by M. E. Frantz, Nutrition problems and programs in Nepal, *Hunger Notes* 2 (1980): 5–8.
31. The Hunger Project, *A Shift in the Wind* 13 (1982): 3.
32. Oral rehydration therapy, *World Health* (Geneva: WHO), June 1985.
33. Oxfam America, *Facts for Action: Women Creating a New World,* Number 3, 1986, p. 3.
34. A. Berg, The trouble with triage, *New York Times Magazine,* 15 June 1975, p. 26.
35. The case for optimism, in E. Cornish and members and staff of the World Future Society, *The Study of the Future: An Introduction to the Art and Science of Understanding and Shaping Tomorrow's World* (Washington, D.C.: World Future Society, 1977), pp. 34–37.
36. The argument in favor of maintaining animal agriculture is discussed in Spitzer, 1981, pp. 183–202.
37. C. G. Knight and R. P. Wilcox, *Triumph or Triage? The World Food Problem in Geographical Perspective,* resource paper no. 75–3 (Washington, D.C.: Association of American Geographers, 1976), p. 53.
38. D. Elgin, *Voluntary Simplicity: Toward a Way of Life That Is Outwardly Simple, Inwardly Rich* (New York: Morrow, 1981), p. 25.
39. Elgin, 1981, pp. 32–34.
40. R. E. Pestle, T. A. Cornille, and K. Solomon, Lifestyle alternatives: Development and evaluation of an attitude scale, *Home Economics Research Journal,* December 1982, pp. 175–182.

Must the Rainforest Die for Fast Food?

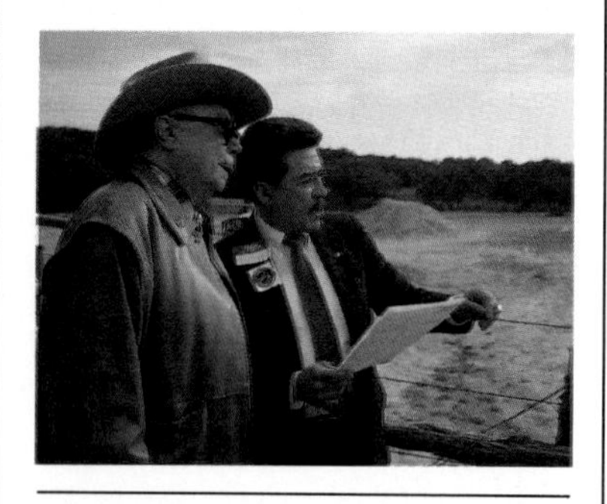

Do we inherit the land from our parents, or do we borrow it from our children?

On a mountainous slope in Central America, a person walks a narrow trail, the Trail of the Giants, within a towering forest. Alongside the trail, and for miles on each side of it, huge trees loom more than a hundred feet tall, and measure 20 feet across at the base. Heavy vines bedeck their trunks, ferns and mosses grow among them, orchids blaze brilliantly in patches of sunlight at intervals along their height. Huge iridescent moths flutter from light to shade to light; vivid hummingbirds dart from branch to branch; birds call. High in the canopy, monkeys chatter, and flocks of parrots gab and squawk in noisy confabulations. Rain falls frequently in drenching torrents; between times, the forest's own water falls in constant drips from the tip of every leaf to the leaf below, to feed a diverse garden of vegetation on the forest floor. The forest's soil is thin, less than an inch deep, for although tons of leaf litter, bark, branches, and animal droppings fall from the trees, uncountable quantities of molds, fungi, and bacteria break them down as fast as they fall. Below the thin soil lies impermeable clay.

The forest has been here for millions of years. It is vast, mysterious, and welcoming. It is three-dimensional—miles wide, miles long, and over a hundred feet deep. Millions on millions of species of animals and plants not yet known to science thrive in its honeycomb of multitudinous spaces. Within 1 acre of this forest dwell 800,000 pounds of living things.[1]

When that acre is cleared to plant grass and grow beef, it will be useful for that purpose for about eight years. Then the soil's fertility will be used up. The last of the soil will wash away, leaving bare clay. When the whole region's forest is gone, there will no longer be trees to draw moisture from underground and release it into the air. The whole region will become dryer, rain will cease to fall, and the land will become uninhabitable, not only for cattle, but for all other life, including human beings. It will require vast applications of fertilizer, pesticides, and irrigation to make it "useful" for any purpose whatever.

Eight years—a short time for a million-year-old acre of forest to die. And within that time span, the acre will produce 50 pounds of cattle per year—400 pounds in all. Of that, 200 pounds is usable meat, enough to yield 800 four-ounce hamburgers. The trade-off: 55 square feet of forest, representing half a ton of forest life, lost permanently for each hamburger.[2]

Why is this happening? Is there no other land left on which hamburger meat can be grown? It turns out that is not the problem. All over Latin America, and in fact all over the world, the same process is taking place. The case of Central America is used here to illustrate what is happening, how it has come about, and what, perhaps, can be done about it.

Central America's Rainforests

The land on which the forest lies is considered arable land, although poor for the purpose. Like nearly all such land in Central America, it is privately owned or owned by the government. In Latin America generally, 7 percent of the landowners control 93 percent of the arable land,[3] and fewer than half of all rural families own enough to support a family; many own none at all. The population is growing; in 1980, rural Mexico and Central America contained 35 million people; it is projected that 20 years later there will be 22 million more, and that 90 percent of them will occupy land formerly covered by tropical rainforest.

The pathway to destruction often begins when logging trucks move in, to extract the most valuable woods for use in the building industries. The logging teams take down many of the towering giants of the forest—mahoganies, cedars, and other valued trees, together with a tangle of vines, ferns, nests, and associated wildlife. They destroy about half of the forest's canopy, but more significantly, they leave behind roads.

When the loggers leave, settlers enter—landless families fleeing inequitable land distribution and population pressure elsewhere in the country, searching for homes and means of livelihood. They slash away the remaining forest, burning it as they go, and overrun the indigenous people to establish little settlements from our innumerable fast-food hamburger establishments. Consumers buy the beef, and the trees continue to fall. Meanwhile, ironically, our domestic beef farmers are going broke. Their beef costs more to produce (because land, supplies, and labor cost more), and consumers are less willing to pay for it.

The money to convert Central America's rainforests to grasslands comes largely from international banks, which have supplied billions of dollars to finance cattle ranching in Central and South America since 1970. The money goes not only for land purchases, but for roads, fences, packing plants, pest control, and new ports for export. The banks claim that they are helping to close Central America's "nutrition gap," but in reality, they are doing nothing of the kind. They prefer to finance the production of a resource that will be paid for by the U.S. market for cheap imported beef rather than to finance an effort to improve the native people's malnutrition problems with no sure return in sight.

Some argue that the process benefits the country as a whole. It is, after all, a form of economic development. It brings money in; it encourages international trade. So it does, but this ignores the question of to whom, within the country, the money is going. As beef production in Central America has increased, the people there have eaten less and less beef, for two reasons. First, foreign companies are willing to pay higher prices than the people can pay, so the people can't afford to buy the beef. Second, the population has increased, so more people are competing for the beef that remains within the country. Honduras, which produces the least food per person of any country in Latin America, sells half its beef to the United States. Even an American house cat eats more beef than the average Central American.[9]

How Can the Process Be Stopped?

People concerned with the destruction of tropical rainforests to grow beef ask the questions, Why can't we produce our own beef? Why can't we import beef from elsewhere? In fact, we do both. The average American's beef consumption is 105 pounds per person per year, and we do produce most of this ourselves. The beef we import comes mostly from Australia, New Zealand, Brazil, Argentina, Ireland, the Dominican Republic, and Haiti. Only 13.5 percent of imported beef is from Central America, representing only 2 percent of the total we consume, or about 2 pounds per person (220 square feet of rainforest per person per year). Why can't we simply exclude that 2 pounds from our imports, and shop for it elsewhere?

If we did so, it is true that Central Americans who depend on the American market for income from this source would suffer. Although the amount is small to us, it is large to them. Costa Rica, for example, sells up to two-thirds of its total beef to the United States. Belize is just beginning to clear its forests to sell us beef, but it has high hopes for the future. In El Salvador, where no rainforests remain, beef sales to the United States amount to 9 million pounds a year. Panama sells less that is directly imported into the United States, but sells to ships passing through the Canal. Honduras has already been mentioned. Of Latin American countries outside Central America, only Mexico and Brazil sell relatively small amounts of their beef to the United States—Mexico, due to domestic need; and Brazil, because imports of its beef are restricted. Its cattle are subject to a disease that would endanger U.S. cattle, should it get a foothold here. (Still, the United States does import 46 million pounds of beef from Brazil each year.)[10]

Table C14–1

Rainforests and Their Rate of Destruction—Central America

Country	Rainforest Remaining[a]	Rate of Loss per Year
Costa Rica	28,000 km²	1000 km²
Guatemala	26,000 km²	600 km²
Panama	22,000 km²	500 km²
Honduras	20,000 km²	700 km²
Costa Rica	16,000 km²	600 km²
Belize	9,800 km²	32 km²
Mexico	8,000 km²	600 km²
El Salvador	0 km²	—km²
Total	130,000 km²	4,032 km²

[a]1982 statistics.

Source: J. D. Nations and D. I. Komer, Rainforests and the hamburger society, *Environment*, April 1983, pp. 12–20, Table 1, p. 14. Reprinted with permission of the Helen Dwight Reid Educational Foundation. Published by Heldref Publications, 4000 Albemarle St., N.W., Washington, D.C. 20016. Copyright © 1988.

and build their homes. They hope to stay all their lives, but they cannot survive for long, for the crops they plan drain the soil of its nutrients in only a year or two, and then begin to fail. Weeds and insect pests overwhelm them, and soon they are forced to sell out to moneyed speculators who are gathering up cleared land with a view to development. The settlers move on, to slash and burn other areas of forest. The government tolerates their doing so, because otherwise it would have to face the pressure to redistribute to the landless the large estates and company holdings owned by the few. "Thus, the pioneer families receive a few years of crops in exchange for converting the rainforest to grassland for the benefit of someone else."[4]

In many instances, the land-occupying, crop-growing step is skipped. The government or a large landowner, supported by national development loans, will simply pay people to ready the land for use by removing its trees and vegetation. A family can move onto a piece of land, clear it, and then sell it for $80 a **hectare** (2½ acres) to a weekend rancher from the United States. Eighty dollars is a lot of money to a landless family; land-clearing can become a way of life.

The larger landowners plan to use the land for cattle industry development, and they are influential enough to obtain support for the purpose from an international bank. Beef production begins. Initially, they stock the land with 1 head of cattle per hectare, which is all it will support. By the fifth to the tenth year, however, they can only grow one head of cattle per 5 to 7 hectares. From such a herd density they will obtain, at best, about 22 pounds of beef per hectare each year, or less than 10 pounds per acre.[5]

The contrast with the original forest yield could hardly be greater. The natives in such an area, living on small, cleared patches beneath the undisturbed forest canopy, were able to grow 13,000 pounds of shelled corn *and* 10,000 pounds of root and vegetable crops on each hectare of plots for five to seven years. Then they would allow the plots to return to forest and clear others. They rotated their crops of citrus, rubber, cacao, avocado, and papaya in a system known as **agroforestry**, which could be continued indefinitely. If the government of the country wanted to solve its people's hunger problem, it could do no better than to encourage an agricultural method like this one. "Food production systems practiced by traditional rainforest Indians are, without exception, more productive than the pasturelands that are replacing these systems."[6]

Anyway, on the land we are speaking of, the forest and its people are gone, and the land has been cleared. Beef production continues on this cleared land for a few years, but it becomes less successful each year. The cattle trample the hillsides and loosen the soil; torrential rains wash it away. Within seven to ten years, the land is eroded beyond repair—useless, now, for forest, families' crops, *or* beef production. It is a wasteland. The whole process takes less than ten years. In the next ten years, a *larger* area of forest will suffer the same fate, for the population has grown, and the number of landless, needy people has grown greater.

By way of this process, between 1950 and 1980, nearly two-thirds of Central America's lowland and mountainside rainforests were cleared or severely degraded.[7] Within 20 more years, the process will be over, for no more forest will be left (see Figure C14–1 and Table C14–1). In El Salvador, the forest has been totally destroyed already.

The United States creates much of the demand for beef that provides the driving force for the entire process. U.S. companies annually purchase more than 330 million pounds of beef from Central American countries alone—an amount that represents 90 percent of that region's beef exports.[8] The demand comes largely

Figure C14–1
Deforestation in Central America, 1950 to 1985.

Source: USAID and IIED, Earthscan, as adapted by T. Peterson, Hunger and the environment, *Seeds,* October 1987, Figure, p. 7.

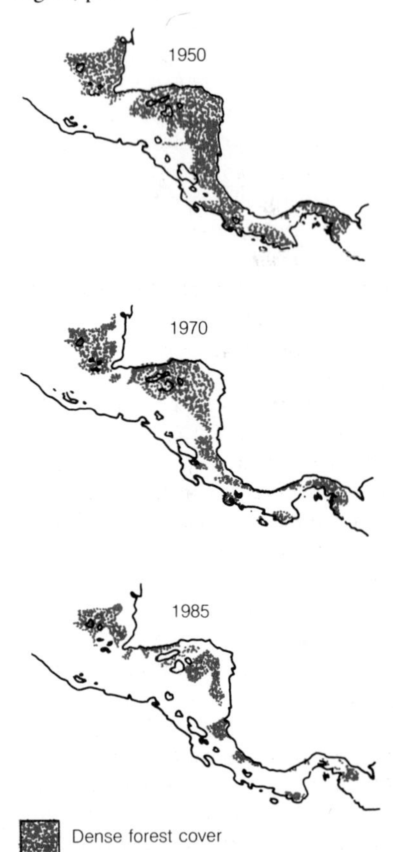

So the Central American beef exporters would suffer, but only the wealthy ones. Few of their profits filter down to the peasants, and the loss of those profits therefore would not hurt the peasants. The export of beef makes the country's gross national product look better, and puts more wealth in the hands of the already-wealthy. Unfortunately for the poor, it is those wealthy who have the loudest voice to influence policies made by U.S. companies and government. If beef production were to cease, even the wealthy would not suffer for long; they would simply have to turn to other means of making money. Growing other cash crops—sugarcane, oil palm, coffee, bananas, pineapples—would be less destructive than growing beef, but beef dominates the Central American export crops, because it brings quicker profits to the wealthy.

In theory, it would be perfectly possible to exclude Central American beef from domestic consumption. Even if the U.S. government were reluctant to go along, individual consumers could boycott the product, or could boycott fast-food companies that use it—but for one problem. There is no way of knowing which beef comes from where.

The beef slaughtered in Central America is looked over at packing sites in the countries of origin, by U.S. Department of Agriculture (USDA) officials. Then it is packed into 60-pound boxes of deboned cuts, frozen, and transported by refrigerator ships to port cities in Florida and California, where it again passes through the hands of USDA officials. Thereafter, it carries no identifying marks. After it gets into the country, it is all "domestic," and it may change hands several more times, passing through customhouse brokers and meat packers, before it finds its way into fast food hamburgers, lunch meats, sausages, hotdogs, chili, soups, stews, hash, TV dinners, pot pies, baby foods, pet foods, and (in the port of origin, Miami) restaurant fare for customers who prefer lean beef. The ultimate packers do not know where it comes from. A fast food franchise may claim that it uses only domestic beef, without being aware that such is not the case.

The problem is solvable. In fact, it has been called *simple* to arrive at a solution. For maximum speed and effectiveness, it requires the participation of four sets of people:

1. Knowledgeable U.S. biologists and others in a position to influence Central American policy must encourage recognition of the fact that clearing for beef production is a destructive and economically wasteful use of the rainforests.
2. U.S. legislators must pass laws phasing out beef imports from rainforest regions, in recognition of the fact that, although such imports may have helped hold down the price of beef by 5 cents a pound, the costs in other than mercenary terms are unbearable (see Figure C14–2).
3. The international banks must redirect their loans from supporting the beef industry to supporting systems of food production that will not destroy the environment and the people's hopes for a future livelihood.
4. American consumers must put pressure on the international banks and on their legislators to take these actions. Until they do, consumers should refuse to buy any beef products except where positive proof exists that the beef was produced on U.S. farmland, or at least not produced on cleared rainforest land. (This could be achieved by legislating an improved system of labeling beef from its point of origin and tracking it thereafter.)

High-yield, intensive agricultural systems [such as] agroforestry [and] terracing . . . have already been tested and found viable by U.S. and Latin American scientists. These systems can simultaneously produce food for local populations and crops for export, all on land that has already been cleared. What the systems presently lack is political and financial support. By expanding these sustained-yield agricultural practices, the Central American countries could increase their populations' food production while at the same time conserving their nations' remaining forest resources.

—James D. Nations and Daniel I. Komer

Should additional reasons be needed to persuade people not to use beef of unknown origin, some are available. Central American beef is more and more contaminated with unacceptably high concentrations of toxic pesticides not allowed on U.S. crops. Rejections of imported beef by the USDA because of such residues have doubled in recent years, and sometimes, shipments have had to be cut off altogether. DDT, which is still produced in the United States although it cannot be used here, is exported, sprayed on crops in Latin America, eaten by the cattle, and returned to us in the beef.[11]

If we fail to save the rainforests, it will not be the earth's first such loss. Countless times in human history, the same story has been repeated in other environments: people have multiplied, and in the effort to obtain enough food to survive, they have destroyed the environments on which they depended. The Mayan people, who vanished and left behind the famous temples tourists marvel at, are now thought to have died out because they destroyed the forest they lived in as their population grew. (Forests surround the temples once again, although they are not as rich in species as the original ones were, and it has taken hundreds of years to restore them.) The mountains of China are now bare over thousands of square miles because people of earlier times, living in primitive conditions, burned all the trees for firewood. Now, erosion has worn the mountains to bare rock and the land is uninhabitable. The cedars of Lebanon were wiped out the same way, beginning in biblical times, and even the Sahara Desert is a desert partly because of human misuse of once-fertile land.[12]

The vast wastelands of China, Lebanon, and the Sahara, as well as the deserts of Afghanistan, New Mexico, Easter Island, and others, were created by people living primitively, knocking down trees one by one, cutting them up by hand, and burning them stick by stick. Developers financed by international banks can devour the land much faster. They can be stopped, if at all, only by the new awareness, described in the next section, that all people's interests will ultimately be served by the same policies.

Hunger and the Environment

Once upon a time there were four groups of people who disagreed. The conservationists wanted to save the environment, whatever it might cost in terms of money or people's hardship. The population-control advocates felt it was more urgent by far to slow down the world's increasing birth rate. The world hunger people argued that the world's highest priority should be to feed the world's already-existing hungry people. The international development people believed that the hope of the future lay in amplifying each country's gross national product. These groups are now discovering that they cannot achieve a stable improvement in any of these areas without tackling them all simultaneously. They admit that hunger and development issues cannot be separated from environmental issues. They see that only an international attack on the root causes of poverty will save the natural environment, and that only a massive effort to save and protect the world's natural resources will solve the problems of poverty and hunger.[13] Formerly adversaries, these groups are now joining together and sharing their goals. In place of the old views that *national* economies must be bettered, and that people must be fed, they are now realizing that "it is not enough to achieve the end of hunger. We must do it in a way that can be sustained."[14]

Central to the new awareness is the realization that the crucial factors, everywhere, are *soil, trees,* and *water*. Without the preservation of trees, soil is lost. Tree loss exposes the soil to wind erosion, rain erosion, and drying. The land crusts over, and then even when the rain falls, it washes off. Without the soil, the earth, which brings forth our food, can no longer support human life.

Soil loss worldwide, due to deforestation, is horrendous, and is increasing every year. At present, it amounts to 25 billion tons a year, enough to fill Yankee Stadium 175,000 times.[15] Where there are trees, nature creates new soil at the rate of a centimeter every 80 to 280 years, but soil loss due to human misuse of the land today is taking place at a much greater rate, such that a quarter of the world's arable land is destined to become permanent wasteland.

Development as traditionally practiced by the wealthy for their own profit cannot permanently achieve

Figure C14–2

Development Costs with Environment Reckoned In

BALANCE SHEET	
Income from beef	$10,000,000
Cost of producing beef (land, labor, technology, etc.)	−4,000,000
PROFIT	$6,000,000

Old way of doing a balance book (example)

BALANCE SHEET	
Income from beef	$10,000,000
Cost of producing beef (land, labor, technology, etc.)	−4,000,000
Loss of irreplaceable forest land for all future	−100,000,000
LOSS	−94,000,000

New way of doing a balance book (example)

solutions to any of the world's problems. Developers operating this way forget to evaluate the environment as productive capital even though they use it as such. To make clear what they are doing, we need new bookkeeping systems, with columns reckoning the real costs of environmental degradation, as illustrated in Figure C14–2.[16]

The new concept is that of **sustainable development**. It is:

- Stable—it does not disrupt the ecology or culture of the land in which it takes place.
- Nonexploitative—it involves the rational use of renewable resources; it does not plunder and leave desolation behind.
- Resilient—it is adaptable to changes, whether in the weather or in governments.
- User friendly—its methods are easy for the people who are to use them to understand.
- Productive—it creates surpluses above people's minimum needs for survival.
- Self-reliant—it helps people become free of dependence on handouts and assistance from outside.
- Complicated and challenging—it requires much more intimate knowledge of individual locales and situations than does, say, one massive technology (such as beef production) applied all over an area.[17]

The differences between the development practiced by the banks and governments promoting beef production in Central America and that advocated here are illustrated in Figure C14–3.

Figure C14–3
Traditional Versus Sustainable Development.

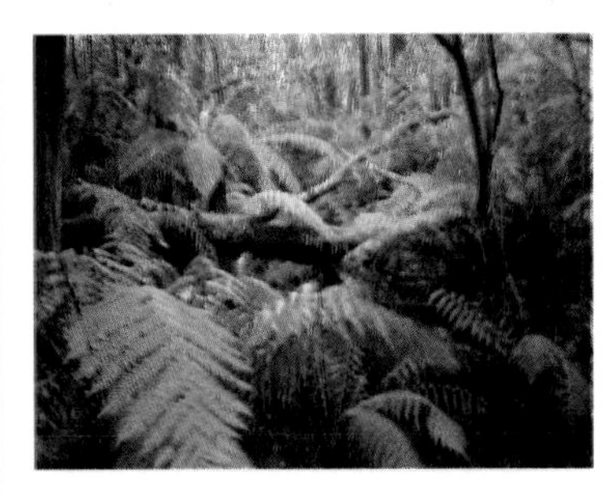

Sustainable development. People must support the earth if the earth is to support them.

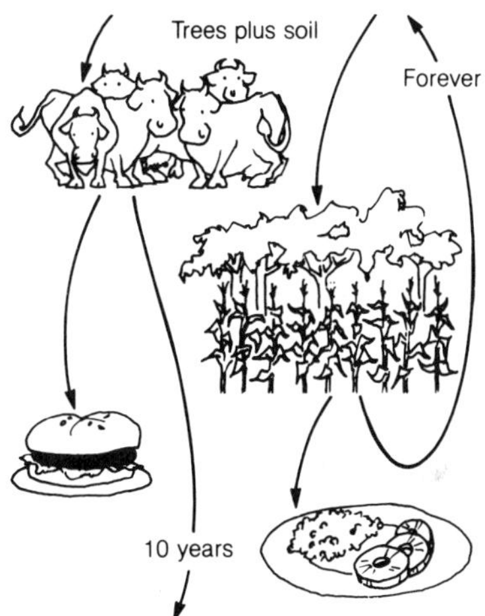

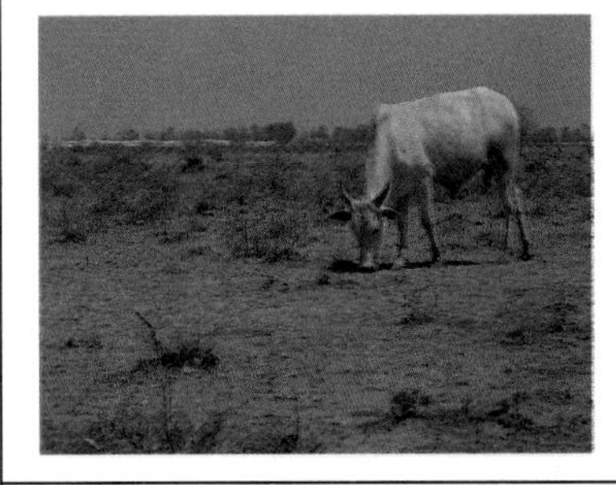

Traditional development. People drain the earth's resources, and the earth ceases to support them.

Hope for the Future

Possibly, awareness of these facts will dawn among those who have the power to change things, but it will have to come fast. By the year 2000, the fate of the remaining rainforest will have been decided. Some hopeful signs have appeared recently. The World Bank, for example, has changed its policies somewhat. In 1982, it lent Brazil half a billion dollars to move 200,000 landless people to the northwest region to clear forestlands and try to start farms, although it was warned by biologists that the soil, without trees, would not support agriculture. Now, ac-

Miniglossary

agroforestry: agriculture within a tropical rainforest, as practiced by the indigenous people, notable for not destroying the forest.

hectare: a measure of land area, 2½ acres.

sustainable development: development that betters people's economic well-being not only in the short term, but also in the long term.

cording to reports, the World Bank may be becoming more sensitive to environmental concerns.[18]

Another hopeful sign is the concept of "Debt for Nature," applied recently in Bolivia. Bolivia owed a debt of $650,000 to a U.S. bank, which it could not repay. The bank devalued the loan to $100,000, and a conservation group, Conservation International, paid it off. In return, Bolivia agreed to preserve 3.7 million acres for endangered species at the headwaters of the Amazon River, and set up an endowment to manage the land. Thus the bank got some of its money back, Bolivia retired its debt, and some forestland was saved.

Many more such signs are needed. The earth will take care of us only if we take care of it. This is something the Indians have always known. In words spoken by one of their chiefs:

> This we know. The Earth does not belong to man; man belongs to the earth. This we know. All things are connected like the blood which unites one family. All things are connected.
>
> Whatever befalls the earth befalls the sons of the earth. Man did not weave the web of life, he is merely a strand in it. Whatever he does to the web, he does to himself.
>
> —Chief Seattle, 1854

We do not inherit land from our parents, we borrow it from our children.

A person walks the Trail of the Giants in a forest in Central America. The person is filled with wonder and fear. How long will the forest remain? Let us hope—forever.

Notes

1. C. Uhl and G. Parker, Viewpoint: Our steak in the jungle, *BioScience* 36 (1986): 642.
2. Uhl and Parker, 1986.
3. J. D. Nations and D. I. Komer, Rainforests and the hamburger society, *Environment,* April 1983, pp. 12–20.
4. Nations and Komer, 1983.
5. Nations and Komer, 1983.
6. Nations and Komer, 1983.
7. U.S. Department of Agriculture statistics, cited by Nations and Komer, 1983.
8. Nations and Komer, 1983.
9. Nations and Komer, 1983.
10. Nations and Komer, 1983.
11. Nations and Komer, 1983.
12. M. W. Mikewell, The deforestation of Mount Lebanon, *Geographical Review* 59 (1969): 1–28; J. J. Cloudsley-Thompson, Recent expansion of the Sahara, in the Introduction to *Key Environments: Sahara Desert,* ed. J. J. Cloudsley-Thompson (Oxford: Pergamon Press, 1984), pp. 8–14.
13. T. Peterson, Hunger and the environment, *Seeds,* October 1987, pp. 6–13.
14. Peterson, 1987.
15. Peterson, 1987.
16. G. H. Brundtland, in the Foreword to L. Timberlake, *Only One Earth: Living for the Future* (New York: Sterling, 1987), p. 8. The idea for Figure C14–2 was inspired by an idea presented in the Foreword, p. 8, by Gro Harlem Brundtland, Prime Minister of Norway and Chairman of the World Commission on Environment and Development.
17. Timberlake, 1987, pp. 21–22.
18. Peterson, 1987.

Appendixes

A
B
C
D
E
F
G
H
I

Appendix A

Table of Food Composition

A

This table of food composition is not the standard table found in most nutrition textbooks. The list of foods chosen is an expanded version of that presented in the 1985 edition of the USDA *Home and Garden Bulletin Number 72, Nutritive Value of Foods*. The *Bulletin,* however, does not contain all the foods listed here nor the values for dietary fiber, vitamin B_6, folacin, magnesium, or zinc.

To achieve a complete and reliable listing of nutrients for all the foods, many sources of information had to be researched. Government sources of information are the primary base for all the data: USDA *Handbooks 8–1* through *8–16* and the 1986 release of the USDA's *Home and Garden Bulletin Number 72, Nutritive Value of Foods*. In addition, provisional USDA information of nutrient values—both published and unpublished—and many conversations with the staff members at the USDA Human Nutrition Information Service in Hyattsville, Maryland, have provided professional assistance to refine the data.

Even with all the government sources available, there are still many missing nutrient values, and as the various government data are updated, conflicting values are reported from the USDA for the same items. To fill in the missing values and resolve discrepancies, other sources of information were used. These reliable sources include refereed journal articles, food composition tables from Canada and England, information from other nutrient data banks and publications, unpublished scientific data, and manufacturers' data.

Estimates of nutrient amounts for foods and nutrients include all possible adjustments in the interest of accuracy. When multiple values were reported for a nutrient, the numbers were averaged and weighted with consideration of the original number of samples in the separate sources. Whenever water percentages were available, estimates of nutrient amounts were adjusted for water content. When no water percentage was given, it was assumed to be that shown in the table. Whenever a reported weight appeared inconsistent (cooked eggplant and collards), many kitchen tests were made, and the average weight of the typical product was given as tested.

When estimates of nutrient amounts in cooked foods were derived from reported amounts in raw foods, published retention factors were applied. Some reported data for combination foods were modified in this table to include newer data available for major ingredients. For example, since the "pies" were analyzed and reported, newer data on fruits have been published. Older reported data on certain bakery items were updated for the new enrichment levels for certain nutrients.

At the end of this table is a list of food items from major fast food chains. Major nutrients are from available information from manufacturers, and other nutrients are estimates calculated from known values of major ingredients. These values are representative of the products offered at this time, but may change as manufacturers modify the recipes, modify the amount of sodium, change suppliers, and so forth.

Considerable effort has been made to report the most accurate data available and to eliminate missing values. There will always be changes in the future, and the authors* welcome any suggestions or comments.

It Is Important to Know

that there can be many different nutrient values reported for foods. Many factors influence the amounts of nutrients in foods, including the mineral content of the soil, the method of processing, genetics, diet of the animal or fertilizer of the plant, season of the year, methods of analysis, difference in moisture content of the samples analyzed, length and method of storage, and methods of cooking the food.

As a result, different nutrient values for the same food item are reported, even by reliable sources. Although each nutrient from USDA government data is presented as a single number in some USDA publications, it is actually an average of a range of data. In the more detailed reports

*This table has been prepared for West Publishing Company and is copyrighted by ESHA Research in Salem, Oregon—the developer and publisher of "The Food Processor®" computerized nutrition systems. The major sources for the data from the U.S. Department of Agriculture are supplemented by over 350 additional sources of information. Because the list of references is so extensive, it is not provided here, but it is available from the publisher.

(Handbook 8 series), the number of samples is identified, and the standard deviation of the data is also noted. USDA data will have different reported values for foods as well, as older information is replaced with newer data in the more recent publications. Therefore, nutrient data should be viewed and used only as a guide, a close approximation of nutrient content.

Dietary fiber deserves a special word. Estimates of dietary fiber are included for all the foods in this table. The sources of this information are primarily from Southgate (England), many journal articles, some of the latest published data from the USDA, and extensive unpublished information from the USDA Human Nutrition Information Service in Hyattsville, Maryland.

It is important to know that this is emerging data, and to expect additional research and refinement of analytical techniques to modify the data in the future. Dietary fiber is composed of cellulose, hemicellulose, lignin, pectin, gums, and mucilages. Very little data is yet available on the gum and mucilage components in foods, but there is considerable data on the other components.

Many different analytical techniques are used to measure various components of fiber, and these methods are undergoing their own review of accuracy in the scientific community. In this table, either an estimate of the total dietary fiber (a specific analytical technique) or a combination of measures for the insoluble components and pectin, when available, is used.

Vitamin A is reported in retinol equivalents. The amount of this vitamin can vary by the season of the year. Reported values in both dairy products and plants are higher in summer and early fall than in winter. The values reported here represent year-round averages. In the organ meats of all animal products (liver especially) there is a large amount of vitamin A, and these amounts vary widely, depending on the background of the animal. The vitamin is present in very small amounts in regular meat and is often reported as a trace.

Newer reported vitamin A values for some plant foods have increased significantly due to additional information and sometimes to newer plant genetics. New vitamin A values for canned pumpkin are 3.5 times greater than the previously reported values. This information was used to modify the vitamin A value of pumpkin pie, which was not yet updated.

The energy and nutrients in recipes and combination foods vary widely, depending on the ingredients. The various fatty acids and cholesterol are influenced by the type of fat used (the specific type of oil, vegetable shortening, butter, margarine, etc.).

Total fats, as well as the breakdown of total fats to saturated, monounsaturated, and polyunsaturated fats, are listed in the table. The fatty acids seldom add up exactly to the total. This is due to rounding and to the existence of small amounts of other fatty acid components that are not included in the basic three categories.

Niacin values are for preformed niacin and do not include additional niacin that may form in the body from the conversion of tryptophan.

Table A–1

Food Composition

Grp	Ref	Food Description	Measure	Wt (g)	H_2O (%)	Ener (cal)	Prot (g)	Carb (g)	Dietary Fiber (g)	Fat (g)	Fat Breakdown (g)		
											Sat	Mono	Poly
		BEVERAGES											
		Alcoholic:											
		Beer:											
1	1	Regular (12 fl oz)	1½ c	356	92	146	1	13	1	0	0	0	0
1	2	Light (12 fl oz)	1½ c	354	95	100[1]	1	5	<1	0	0	0	0
		Gin, rum, vodka, whiskey:											
1	3	80 proof	1½ fl oz	42	67	97	0	<.1	0	0	0	0	0
1	4	86 proof	1½ fl oz	42	64	105	0	<.1	0	0	0	0	0
1	5	90 proof	1½ fl oz	42	62	110	0	<.1	0	0	0	0	0
		Wine:											
1	6	Dessert (4 fl oz)	½ c	118	72	181[2]	<1	14[2]	0	0	0	0	0
1	7	Red	3½ fl oz	103	88	74	<1	2	0	0	0	0	0
1	8	Rosé	3½ fl oz	103	89	73	<1	2	0	0	0	0	0
1	9	White medium	3½ fl oz	103	90	70	<1	1	0	0	0	0	0
		Carbonated:[3]											
1	10	Club soda (12 fl oz)	1½ c	355	100	0	0	0	0	0	0	0	0
1	11	Cola beverage (12 fl oz)	1½ c	370	89	151	<1	39	0	0	0	0	0
1	12	Diet cola (12 fl oz)	1½ c	355	100	2	<1	<1	0	0	0	0	0
1	13	Diet soda pop–average (12 fl oz)	1½ c	355	100	2	<1	<1	0	0	0	0	0
1	14	Ginger ale (12 fl oz)	1½ c	366	91	124	<1	32	0	0	0	0	0
1	15	Grape soda (12 fl oz)	1½ c	372	89	161	0	42	0	0	0	0	0
1	16	Lemon-lime (12 fl oz)	1½ c	368	90	149	0	38	0	0	0	0	0
1	17	Orange (12 fl oz)	1½ c	372	88	177	0	46	0	0	0	0	0
1	18	Pepper-type soda (12 fl oz)	1½ c	368	89	151	0	38	0	0	0	0	0
1	19	Root beer (12 fl oz)	1½ c	370	89	152	<1	39	0	0	0	0	0
		Coffee:[3]											
1	20	Brewed	1 c	240	99	2[5]	<1	1	<1	0	0	0	0
1	21	Prepared from instant	1 c	240	99	2[5]	<1	1	0	0	0	0	0
		Fruit drinks, noncarbonated:[6]											
1	22	Fruit punch drink, canned	1 c	253	88	118	<1	30	0	<1	t	t	t
1	23	Grape drink, canned	1 c	250	88	112	0	35	<1	<1	t	t	t
		Lemonade, frozen:											
1	26	Concentrate (6-oz can)	¾ c	219	52	397	1	103	1	<1	.1	t	.1
1	27	Lemonade prepared from frozen concentrate	1 c	248	89	100	<1	26	<1	<1	t	t	t
		Limeade, frozen:											
1	28	Concentrate (6-oz can)	¾ c	218	50	408	<1	108	1[8]	<1	t	t	.1
1	29	Limeade prepared from frozen concentrate	1 c	247	89	102	<1	27	<1[8]	<1	t	t	t
1	24	Pineapple grapefruit, canned	1 c	250	88	117	1	29	0	<1	t	t	.1
1	25	Pineapple orange, canned	1 c	250	87	125	3	29	0	<1	t	t	.1
		Fruit and vegetable juices: see Fruit and Vegetable sections											

(1)Calories can vary from 78 to 131 for 12 fl oz.

(2)Values for sweet dessert wine. Dry dessert wines contain 149 cal and 5 g of carbohydrate.

(5)Calorie values from USDA vary from 1 to 4 calories per cup.

(6)Usually less than 10% fruit juice.

(8)Dietary fiber values are estimated from values for lemonade.

KEY: 1 = BEV 2 = DAIRY 3 = EGGS 4 = FAT/OIL 5 = FRUIT 6 = BAKERY 7 = GRAIN 8 = FISH 9 = BEEF 10 = POULTRY 11 = SAUSAGE 12 = MIXED/FAST 13 = NUTS/SEEDS 14 = SWEETS 15 = VEG/LEG 16 = MISC 22 = SOUP/SAUCE

Chol (mg)	Calc (mg)	Iron (mg)	Magn (mg)	Phos (mg)	Pota (mg)	Sodi (mg)	Zinc (mg)	VT-A (RE)	Thia (mg)	Ribo (mg)	Niac (mg)	V-B6 (mg)	Fola (µg)	VT-C (mg)
0	18	.11	23	44	89	19	.07	0	.02	.09	1.61	.18	21	0
0	18	.14	18	43	64	10	.11	0	.03	.11	1.39	.12	15	0
0	0	.02	0	2	1	<1	.02	0	<.01	<.01	<.01	t	0	0
0	0	.02	0	2	1	<1	.02	0	<.01	<.01	<.01	0	0	0
0	0	.02	0	2	1	<1	.02	0	<.01	<.01	<.01	0	0	0
0	9	.28	11	11	109	11	.08	0	.02	.02	.25	0	<1	0
0	8	.44	13	14	115	6	.09	0	<.01	.03	.08	.04	2	0
0	9	.39	10	15	102	5	.06	0	<.01	.02	.08	.03	1	0
0	9	.33	11	14	82	5	.07	0	<.01	<.01	.07	.01	<1	0
0	17	.15	4	0	6	75	.36	0	0	0	0	0	0	0
0	9	.13	3	46	4	14	.05	0	0	0	0	0	0	0
0	12	.11	4	30	0	21[4]	.28	0	.02	.08	0	0	0	0
0	14	.14	3	38	7	21[4]	.18	0	0	0	0	0	0	0
0	12	.66	3	1	5	25	.18	0	0	0	0	0	0	0
0	12	.31	4	0	3	57	.26	0	0	0	0	0	0	0
0	9	.25	2	1	4	41	.18	0	0	0	.06	0	0	0
0	19	.23	4	4	9	46	.38	0	0	0	0	0	0	0
0	12	.14	1	41	2	38	.15	0	0	0	0	0	0	0
0	19	.18	4	2	3	49	.26	0	0	0	0	0	0	0
0	4	.96	14	2	130	5	.04	0	0	0	.53	0	<1	0
0	8	.12	11	8	87	8	.07	0	0	<.01	.69	0	0	0
0	19	.52	5	2	64	56	.31	4	.06	.06	.05	0	3	75
0	3	.41	5	3	13	16	.28	t	.08	.01	.07	.01	<1	85
0	15	1.58	11	19	148	8	.17	21	.06	.21	.16	.06	22	39[7]
0	8	.41	5	5	38	8	.09	5	.01	.05	.04	.01	6	10[7]
0	11	.22	60	13	129	<.01	.11	t	.02	.02	.22	.11	24	26
0	7	.06	2	3	33	6	.05	t	<.01	<.01	.05	.03	7	7
0	18	.77	15	14	154	34	.15	9	.07	.04	.67	.10	26	115
0	13	.67	14	10	116	9	.14	133	.07	.05	.52	.12	27	56

(4)Value for product sweetened with aspartame only; sodium is 32 mg if a blend of aspartame and sodium saccharin is used; 75 mg if just sodium saccharin is used.

(7)Vitamin C can range from 5 to 72 mg in a small can of frozen concentrate, and from 1 to 18 mg in 1 c lemonade.

(For purposes of calculations, use "0" for t, <1, <.1, <.01, etc.)

A

Table A–1

Food Composition

Grp	Ref	Food Description	Measure	Wt (g)	H_2O (%)	Ener (cal)	Prot (g)	Carb (g)	Dietary Fiber (g)	Fat (g)	Fat Breakdown (g)		
											Sat	Mono	Poly
BEVERAGES—Con.													
		Tea:[3]											
1	30	Brewed	1 c	240	100	2	<.01	<1	0	0	0	0	0
1	31	From instant, unsweetened	1 c	237	100	2	<1	<1	0	0	0	0	0
1	32	From instant, sweetened	1 c	262	91	86	<.01	22	0	0	0	0	0
DAIRY													
		Butter: see Fats and Oils, #158, 159, 160											
		Cheese, natural:											
2	33	Blue	1 oz	28	42	100	6	1	0	8	5.3	2.2	.2
2	34	Brick	1 oz	28	41	105	6	1	0	8	5.3	2.4	.2
2	35	Brie	1 oz	28	48	95	6	<1	0	8	5.0	2.3	.3
2	36	Camembert	1 oz	28	52	85	6	<1	0	7	4.3	2.0	.2
		Cheddar:											
2	37	Cut pieces	1 oz	28	37	114	7	<1	0	9	6.0	2.7	.3
2	38	1″ cube	1 ea	17	37	69	4	<1	0	6	3.6	1.6	.2
2	39	Shredded	1 c	113	37	455	28	1	0	37	24	11	1
		Cottage:											
2	40	Creamed, large curd	1 c	225	79	235	28	6	0	10	6.4	3.0	.3
2	41	Creamed, small curd	1 c	210	79	215	26	6	0	9	6.0	2.7	.3
2	42	With fruit	1 c	226	72	279	22	30	0	8	4.9	2.2	.3
2	43	Low fat 2%	1 c	226	79	205	31	8	0	4	2.8	1.2	.1
2	44	Low fat 1%	1 c	226	82	164	28	6	0	2	1.5	.7	<.1
2	45	Dry curd	1 c	145	80	123	25	3	0	1	.4	.2	<.1
2	46	Cream	1 oz	28	54	99	2	1	0	10	6.2	2.8	.4
2	47	Edam	1 oz	28	42	101	7	<1	0	8	5.0	2.3	.2
2	48	Feta	1 oz	28	55	75	5	1	0	6	4.2	1.3	.2
2	49	Gouda	1 oz	28	42	101	7	1	0	8	5.0	2.2	.2
2	50	Gruyère	1 oz	28	33	117	8	<1	0	9	5.4	2.9	.5
2	51	Gorgonzola	1 oz	28	39	111	7	0	0	9	5.5	2.4	.5
2	52	Liederkranz	1 oz	28	53	87	5	0	0	8	5.3	2.2	.2
2	53	Monterey jack	1 oz	28	41	106	7	<1	0	9	5.4	2.4	.2
		Mozzarella, made with:											
2	54	Whole milk	1 oz	28	54	80	5	1	0	6	3.7	1.9	.2
2	55	Park skim milk, low moisture	1 oz	28	49	80	8	1	0	5	3.1	1.4	.1
2	56	Muenster	1 oz	28	42	104	6	<1	0	8	5.4	2.5	.2
		Parmesan, grated:											
2	57	Cup, not pressed down	1 c	100	18	455	42	4	0	30	19	8.7	.7
2	58	Tablespoon	1 tbsp	5	18	23	2	<1	0	2	1	.4	<.1
2	59	Ounce	1 oz	28	18	129	12	1	0	9	5.4	3.0	.2
2	60	Provolone	1 oz	28	41	100	7	1	0	8	4.8	2.1	.2
		Ricotta, made with:											
2	61	Whole milk	1 c	246	72	428	28	8	0	32	20	8.9	1
2	62	Part skim milk	1 c	246	74	340	28	13	0	19	12	5.7	.6
2	63	Romano	1 oz	28	31	110	9	1	0	8	4.9	2.2	.2
2	64	Swiss	1 oz	28	37	107	8	1	0	8	5.0	2.1	.3

(3) Mineral content varies depending on water source.

KEY: 1 = BEV 2 = DAIRY 3 = EGGS 4 = FAT/OIL 5 = FRUIT 6 = BAKERY 7 = GRAIN 8 = FISH 9 = BEEF 10 = POULTRY 11 = SAUSAGE 12 = MIXED/FAST 13 = NUTS/SEEDS 14 = SWEETS 15 = VEG/LEG 16 = MISC 22 = SOUP/SAUCE

Chol (mg)	Calc (mg)	Iron (mg)	Magn (mg)	Phos (mg)	Pota (mg)	Sodi (mg)	Zinc (mg)	VT-A (RE)	Thia (mg)	Ribo (mg)	Niac (mg)	V-B6 (mg)	Fola (μg)	VT-C (mg)
0	0	.05	7	1	89	7	.05	0	0	.03	.1	0	12	0
0	5	.05	5	3	47	8	.07	0	0	<.01	<.01	<.09	<1	0
0	1	.04	3	3	49	t	.02	0	0	.04	.09	0	5	0
21	150	.09	7	110	73	396	.75	65	<.01	.11	.29	.05	10	0
27	191	.13	7	128	38	159	.73	86	<.01	.1	.03	.02	6	0
28	52	.14	6	53	43	178	.7	57	.02	.15	.11	.07	18	0
20	110	.09	6	98	53	236	.68	71	<.01	.14	.18	.06	18	0
30	204	.20	8	146	28	176	.92	86	<.01	.11	.02	.02	5	0
18	124	.12	5	88	17	107	.54	52	<.01	.07	.01	.01	3	0
119	815	.77	31	579	111	701	3.51	342	.03	.42	.09	.08	21	0
34	135	.26	11	297	190	911	.8	108	.05	.37	.30	.14	27	t
31	126	.29	11	277	177	850	.8	101	.04	.34	.27	.14	26	t
25	108	.25	9	236	151	915	.66	81	.04	.29	.23	.12	22	t
19	155	.36	14	340	217	918	.95	45	.05	.42	.33	.17	30	0
10	138	.32	12	302	193	918	.86	25	.05	.37	.29	.15	28	t
10	46	.33	6	151	47	19	.68	12	.04	.21	.23	.12	21	0
31	23	.34	2	30	34	84	.33	124	<.01	.06	.03	.01	4	0
25	207	.12	8	152	53	274	1.06	72	.01	.11	.02	.02	5	0
25	140	.18	5	96	18	316	.81	36	.04	.23	.29	.02	3	0
32	198	.07	8	155	34	232	1.1	49	<.01	.10	.02	.02	6	0
31	287	.06	4	172	23	95	1	98	.02	.08	.03	.02	3	0
25	149	.12	8	121	26	513	.57	103	.01	.09	.2	.04	9	0
21	110	.12	7	100	68	390	.7	91	.01	.18	.1	.04	34	0
26	212	.2	8	126	23	152	.85	81	<.01	.11	.02	.02	3	0
22	147	.05	5	105	19	106	.7	68	<.01	.07	.02	.02	2	0
15	207	.08	8	149	27	150	.82	54	<.01	.1	.03	.02	3	0
27	203	.12	8	133	38	178	.84	90	<.01	.09	.03	.02	3	0
79	1376	.95	51	807	107	1862	3.19	173	.04	.39	.32	.1	8	0
4	69	.05	3	40	5	93	.16	9	<.01	.02	.02	<.01	<1	0
22	390	.27	14	229	30	528	1	49	.01	.11	.09	.03	2	0
20	214	.15	8	141	39	248	.89	75	<.01	.09	.04	.02	3	0
124	509	.94	28	389	257	207	2.85	330	.03	.48	.26	.11	14	0
76	669	1.09	4	449	307	307	3.29	278	.05	.46	.19	.05	14	0
29	302	.23	12	215	26	340	1	40	.01	.1	.02	.03	2	0
26	272	.05	10	171	31	74	1.1	72	<.01	.1	.03	.02	2	0

(For purposes of calculations, use "0" for t, <1, <.1, <.01, etc.)

Table A–1

Food Composition

Grp	Ref	Food Description	Measure	Wt (g)	H_2O (%)	Ener (cal)	Prot (g)	Carb (g)	Dietary Fiber (g)	Fat (g)	Fat Breakdown (g) Sat	Mono	Poly
DAIRY—Con.													
		Pasteurized processed cheese products:											
2	65	American	1 oz	28	39	106	6	1	0	9	5.6	2.5	.3
2	66	Swiss	1 oz	28	42	95	7	1	0	7	4.6	2.0	.2
2	67	American cheese food	1 oz	28	44	93	6	2	0	7	4.4	2.0	.2
2	68	American cheese spread	1 oz	28	48	82	5	2	0	6	3.8	1.8	.2
		Cream, sweet:											
		Half and half (cream and milk):											
2	69	Cup	1 c	242	81	315	7	10	0	28	17	8	1
2	70	Tablespoon	1 tbsp	15	81	20	<1	1	0	2	1.1	.5	.1
		Light, coffee or table:											
2	71	Cup	1 c	240	74	469	6	9	0	46	29	13	1.7
2	72	Tablespoon	1 tbsp	15	74	30	<1	1	0	3	1.8	.8	.1
		Light whipping cream, liquid:											
2	73	Cup	1 c	239	64	699	5	7	0	74	46	22	2.1
2	74	Tablespoon	1 tbsp	15	64	44	<1	<1	0	5	2.9	1.4	.1
		Heavy whipping cream, liquid:											
2	75	Cup	1 c	238	58	821	5	7	0	88	55	25	3.3
2	76	Tablespoon	1 tbsp	15	58	51	<1	<1	0	6	3.5	1.6	.2
		Whipped cream, pressurized:											
2	77	Cup	1 c	60	61	154	2	8	0	13	8.3	3.9	.5
2	78	Tablespoon	1 tbsp	4	61	10	<1	1	0	1	.5	.2	<.1
		Cream, sour, cultured:											
2	79	Cup	1 c	230	71	493	7	10	0	48	30	14	1.8
2	80	Tablespoon	1 tbsp	14	71	30	<1	1	0	3	1.8	.9	.1
		Cream products—imitation and part dairy:											
		Coffee whitener:											
2	81	Frozen or liquid	1 tbsp	15	77	20	<1	2	0	2	1.4	t	t
2	82	Powdered	1 tsp	2	2	11	<.1	1	0	1	.6	t	t
		Dessert topping, frozen:											
2	83	Cup	1 c	75	50	239	1	17	0	19	16	1.2	.4
2	84	Tablespoon	1 tbsp	5	50	15	<.1	1	0	1	1.0	.1	t
		Dessert topping from mix:											
2	85	Cup	1 c	80	67	151	3	13	0	10	8.6	.7	.2
2	86	Tablespoon	1 tbsp	5	67	9	<1	1	0	1	.5	<.1	t
		Dessert topping, pressurized:											
2	87	Cup	1 c	70	60	185	1	11	0	16	13	1.4	.2
2	88	Tablespoon	1 tbsp	4	60	11	<.1	1	0	1	.8	.1	t
		Sour dressing, part dairy:											
2	89	Cup	1 c	235	75	416	8	11	0	39	31	4.6	1.1
2	90	Tablespoon	1 tbsp	15	75	25	1	1	0	2	2.0	.3	.1
		Imitation sour cream:											
2	91	Cup	1 c	230	71	479	5	15	0	45	41	1.4	.1
2	92	Tablespoon	1 tbsp	14	71	29	<1	1	0	3	2.5	.1	t
		Milk fluid:											
2	93	Whole Milk	1 c	244	88	150	8	11	0	8	5.1	2.4	.3
2	94	2% low-fat milk	1 c	244	89	121	8	12	0	5	2.9	1.4	.2
2	95	2% milk solids added[10]	1 c	245	89	125	9	12	0	5	2.9	1.4	.2

(10)Milk solids added, label claims less than 10 g protein per cup.

KEY: 1 = BEV 2 = DAIRY 3 = EGGS 4 = FAT/OIL 5 = FRUIT 6 = BAKERY 7 = GRAIN 8 = FISH 9 = BEEF 10 = POULTRY
11 = SAUSAGE 12 = MIXED/FAST 13 = NUTS/SEEDS 14 = SWEETS 15 = VEG/LEG 16 = MISC 22 = SOUP/SAUCE

Chol (mg)	Calc (mg)	Iron (mg)	Magn (mg)	Phos (mg)	Pota (mg)	Sodi (mg)	Zinc (mg)	VT-A (RE)	Thia (mg)	Ribo (mg)	Niac (mg)	V-B6 (mg)	Fola (μg)	VT-C (mg)
27	174	.11	6	211	46	406	.93	82	<.01	.1	.02	.02	2	0
24	219	.17	8	216	61	388	1.02	65	<.01	.08	.01	.01	2	0
18	163	.24	9	130	79	337	.85	62	<.01	.12	.04	.02	2	0
16	159	.09	8	201	69	381	.78	54	.01	.12	.04	.03	2	0
89	254	.17	25	230	314	98	1.23	259	.09	.36	.19	.09	6	2
6	16	.01	2	14	20	6	.08	16	<.01	.02	.01	<.01	<1	t
159	231	.1	21	192	292	95	.65	437	.08	.35	.14	.08	6	2
10	14	<.01	1	12	18	6	.04	27	<.01	.02	<.01	<.01	<1	t
265	166	.07	17	146	231	82	.60	705	.06	.30	.1	.07	9	1
17	10	<.01	1	9	15	5	.04	44	<.01	.02	<.01	<.01	<1	t
326	154	.07	17	149	179	89	.55	1002	.05	.26	.09	.06	10	1
20	10	<.01	1	9	11	6	.03	63	<.01	.02	<.01	<.01	<1	t
46	61	.03	6	54	88	78	.22	124	.02	.04	.04	.03	1	0
3	4	<.01	<1	3	5	5	.01	8	<.01	<.01	<.01	<.01	<1	0
102	268	.14	26	195	331	123	.69	448	.08	.34	.15	.04	25	2
6	16	<.01	2	12	20	7	.04	27	<.01	.02	<.01	<.01	2	t
0	1	<.01	<1	10	29	12	<.01	1[9]	0	0	0	0	0	0
0	<1	.02	<1	8	16	4	.01	<1[9]	0	<.01	0	0	0	0
0	5	.09	1	6	14	19	.03	65[9]	0	0	0	0	0	0
0	<1	<.01	<1	<1	1	1	<.01	4[9]	0	0	0	0	0	0
8	72	.03	8	69	121	53	.22	39[9]	.02	.09	.05	.02	3	<1
.5	4	<.01	<1	4	8	3	.14	2[9]	<.01	<.01	<.01	<.01	<1	t
0	4	.01	1	13	13	43	.01	33[9]	0	0	0	0	0	0
0	<1	<.01	<1	1	1	3	<.01	2[9]	0	0	0	0	0	0
13	266	.07	23	205	381	113	.87	5[9]	.09	.38	.17	.04	28	2
1	17	<.01	2	13	24	7	.05	<1[9]	<.01	.02	.01	<.01	2	t
0	6	.01	—	102	369	235	0	0	0	0	0	0	0	0
0	<1	<.01	—	6	22	14	0	0	0	0	0	0	0	0
33	291	.12	33	228	370	120	.94	76	.09	.4	.2	.1	12	2
22	297	.12	33	232	377	122	.96	140	.1	.4	.21	.1	12	2
18	314	.12	35	245	397	128	.98	140	.1	.42	.22	.11	12	2

[9]Vitamin A value is largely from beta-carotene used for coloring.

(For purposes of calculations, use "0" for t, <1, <.1, <.01, etc.)

Table A–1

Food Composition

Grp	Ref	Food Description	Measure	Wt (g)	H_2O (%)	Ener (cal)	Prot (g)	Carb (g)	Dietary Fiber (g)	Fat (g)	Fat Breakdown (g) Sat	Mono	Poly
DAIRY—Con.													
		Milk, Fluid—con.											
2	96	1% low-fat milk	1 c	244	90	102	8	12	0	3	1.6	.8	.1
2	97	1% milk solids added[10]	1 c	245	90	105	9	12	0	2	1.5	.7	.1
2	98	Skim milk	1 c	245	91	86	8	12	0	<1	.3	.1	t
2	99	Skim milk solids added[10]	1 c	245	90	91	9	12	0	1	.4	.2	t
2	100	Buttermilk	1 c	245	90	99	8	12	0	2	1.3	.6	.1
		Milk, canned:											
2	101	Sweetened condensed	1 c	306	27	982	24	166	0	27	17	7.4	1
2	102	Evaporated, whole	1 c	252	74	340	17	25	0	20	12	5.9	.6
2	103	Evaporated, skim	1 c	255	79	200	19	29	0	<1	.3	.2	t
		Milk, dried:											
2	104	Buttermilk	1 c	120	3	464	41	59	0	7	4.3	2.0	.3
		Instant, nonfat:											
2	105	Envelope[11]	1 ea	91	4	326	32	48	0	1	.4	.2	t
2	106	Cup	1 c	68	4	244	24	36	0	<1	.3	.1	t
2	107	Goat milk	1 c	244	87	168	9	11	0	10	6.5	2.7	.4
2	108	Kefir[13]	1 c	233	82	160	9	9	0	4	2.9	1.2	.1
		Milk beverages and powdered mixes:											
		Chocolate:											
2	109	Whole	1 c	250	82	210	8	26	<1	8	5.3	2.5	.3
2	110	2% fat	1 c	250	84	180	8	26	<1	5	3.1	1.5	.2
2	111	1% fat	1 c	250	84	160	8	26	<1	2	1.5	.7	.1
		Chocolate-flavored beverages:											
2	112	Powder containing nonfat dry milk	1 oz	28	1	100	4	23	<1	1	.7	.4	t
2	113	Choc drink prepared with water	¾ c	206	86	100	4	23	<1	1	.7	.4	t
2	114	Powder without nonfat dry milk	¾ oz	22	<1	75	1	20	<1	<1	.4	.2	t
2	115	Choc drink prepared with whole milk	1 c	266	81	226	9	31	<1	9	5.5	2.6	.3
2	116	Eggnog, commercial	1 c	254	74	342	10	34	0	19	11	5.7	.9
		Malted milk, chocolate flavor:											
2	117	Powder[14], 3 heaping tsp	¾ oz	21	1	79	1	18	<1	1	.5	.2	.1
2	118	Malted milk prepared with whole milk	1 c	265	81	229	9	30	<1	9	5.2	2.6	.4
		Malted milk, natural flavor:											
2	119	Powder[14], 3 heaping tsp	¾ oz	21	2	87	2	16	0	2	.9	.4	.3
2	120	Malted milk prepared with whole milk	1 c	265	81	237	10	27	0	10	6.0	2.8	.6
		Milk shakes:											
2	121	Chocolate (10 fl oz)	1¼ c	283	72	360	10	58	<1	10	6.6	3.0	.4
2	122	Vanilla (10 fl oz)	1¼ c	283	75	314	10	51	<1	8	5.3	2.4	.3

(10) Milk solids added, label claims less than 10 g protein per cup.
(11) Yields 1 qt fluid milk when reconstituted according to package directions.
(13) Most values provided by product labeling.
(14) The latest USDA data from *Handbook 8–14* on beverages updates previous USDA data.

KEY: 1 = BEV 2 = DAIRY 3 = EGGS 4 = FAT/OIL 5 = FRUIT 6 = BAKERY 7 = GRAIN 8 = FISH 9 = BEEF 10 = POULTRY 11 = SAUSAGE 12 = MIXED/FAST 13 = NUTS/SEEDS 14 = SWEETS 15 = VEG/LEG 16 = MISC 22 = SOUP/SAUCE

Chol (mg)	Calc (mg)	Iron (mg)	Magn (mg)	Phos (mg)	Pota (mg)	Sodi (mg)	Zinc (mg)	VT-A (RE)	Thia (mg)	Ribo (mg)	Niac (mg)	V-B6 (mg)	Fola (μg)	VT-C (mg)
10	300	.12	34	235	381	123	.96	145	.1	.41	.21	.1	12	2
10	314	.12	35	245	397	128	.98	145	.1	.42	.22	.11	12	2
4	302	.1	28	247	406	126	.92	149	.09	.34	.22	.1	14	2
5	316	.12	37	255	419	130	1	149	.1	.43	.22	.11	12	2
9	285	.12	26	219	371	257	1.03	20	.08	.38	.14	.08	12	2
104	868	.58	78	775	1136	389	2.88	248	.28	1.27	.64	.16	34	8
74	657	.48	60	510	764	267	1.94	136	.12	.8	.49	.13	18	5
10	738	.7	68	497	845	293	2.18	300	.11	.8	.4	.14	22	3
83	1421	.36	131	1119	1910	621	4.82	65	.47	1.9	1.05	.41	57	7
16	1120	.28	107	896	1552	500	4.01	646[12]	.38	1.59	.81	.31	45	5
12	837	.21	80	670	1160	373	3.06	483[12]	.28	1.19	.61	.23	34	4
28	326	.12	34	270	499	122	.73	137	.12	.34	.68	.11	2	3
10	350	.5	28	319	205	50	.9	155	.45	.44	.3	.09	20	6
31	280	.6	33	251	417	149	1.02	73	.09	.41	.31	.1	12	2
17	284	.6	33	254	422	151	.91	143	.09	.41	.32	.1	12	2
7	287	.6	33	256	425	152	1.02	148	.1	.41	.32	.1	12	2
1	89	.29	23	88	223	139	.46	<1	.03	.17	.18	.04	3	1
1	89	.29	23	88	223	139	.46	<1	.03	.17	.18	.04	3	1
0	8	.68	21	28	128	45	.33	<1	<.01	.03	.11	<.01	4	t
33	300	.8	54	256	498	165	1.26	76	.1	.43	.32	.1	12	3
149	330	.51	47	278	420	138	1.17	203	.09	.48	.27	.13	2	4
1	13	.48	15	37	130	53	.17	4	.04	.04	.42	.04	4	t
34	304	.6	47	265	499	172	1.09	80	.13	.44	.62	.14	16	3
4	63	.15	20	75	159	103	.21	19	.11	.19	1.1	.08	10	1
37	354	.27	52	303	529	223	1.14	94	.2	.59	1.31	.19	22	3
37	319	.88	47	288	567	273	1.15	64	.16	.69	.46	.14	10	1
32	344	.26	35	289	492	232	1.01	90	.13	.52	.52	.15	9	2

[12]With added vitamin A.

(For purposes of calculations, use "0" for t, <1, <.1, <.01, etc.)

A

Table A–1

Food Composition

Grp	Ref	Food Description	Measure	Wt (g)	H_2O (%)	Ener (cal)	Prot (g)	Carb (g)	Dietary Fiber (g)	Fat (g)	Fat Breakdown (g) Sat	Mono	Poly
DAIRY–Con.													
		Milk desserts, frozen:											
		Ice cream, regular vanilla (about 11% fat):											
		Hardened:											
2	123	½ gallon	½ gal	1064	61	2153	38	254	0	115	71	33	4
2	124	Cup	1 c	133	61	269	5	32	0	14	8.3	4.1	.5
2	125	Fluid ounces	3 oz	50	61	101	2	12	0	5	3.3	1.6	.2
2	126	Soft serve	1 c	173	60	377	7	38	0	22	14	6.7	1.0
		Ice cream, rich vanilla (about 16% fat), hardened:											
2	127	½ gallon	½ gal	1188	59	2805	33	256	0	190	118	55	7
2	128	Cup	1 c	148	59	349	4	32	0	24	15	6.8	.9
		Ice milk, vanilla (about 4% fat):											
		Hardened:											
2	129	½ gallon	½ gal	1048	69	1467	41	232	0	45	28	13	1.7
2	130	Cup	1 c	131	69	184	5	29	0	6	3.5	1.6	.2
2	131	Soft serve (about 3% fat)	1 c	175	70	223	8	38	0	5	2.9	1.3	.2
		Sherbet (2% fat):											
2	132	½ gallon	½ gal	1542	66	2158	17	469	0	30	19	8.8	1.1
2	133	Cup	1 c	193	66	270	2	59	0	4	2.4	1.1	.1
		Milk desserts, other:											
2	134	Custard, baked	1 c	265	77	305	14	29	0	15	6.8	5.4	.7
		Pudding, canned:											
2	135	Chocolate	5 oz	142	68	205	3	30	<1	11	9.5	.5	.1
2	136	Tapioca	5 oz	142	74	160	3	28	0	5	4.8	t	t
2	137	Vanilla	5 oz	142	69	220	2	33	0	10	9.5	.3	.1
		Puddings, prepared from dry mix with whole milk:											
2	138	Chocolate, instant	1 c	260	71	310	8	54	<1	7	4.6	2.2	.4
2	139	Chocolate, regular, cooked	½ c	130	73	150	4	25	<1	4	2.4	1.1	.1
2	140	Rice	½ c	132	73	155	4	27	<1	4	2.3	1.1	.1
2	141	Tapioca	½ c	130	75	145	4	25	0	4	2.3	1.1	.1
2	142	Vanilla, instant	½ c	130	73	150	4	27	0	4	2.2	1.1	.2
2	143	Vanilla, regular, cooked	½ c	130	74	145	4	25	0	4	2.3	1	.1
2	144	Soybean milk	1 c	263	92	87	9	6	0	4	.5	.7	2.1
		Yogurt, low fat:											
2	145	Fruit added[15]	1 c	227	74	231	10	43	<1	2	1.6	.7	.1
2	146	Plain	1 c	227	85	144	12	16	0	3	2.3	1.0	.1
2	147	Vanilla or coffee flavor	1 c	227	79	193	11	31	0	3	1.8	.8	.1
2	148	Yogurt, made with nonfat milk	1 c	227	85	127	13	17	0	<1	.3	.1	t
2	149	Yogurt, made with whole milk	1 c	227	88	138	8	11	0	7	4.8	2.0	.2
EGGS													
		Raw, large:											
3	150	Whole, without shell	1 ea	50	75	79	6	1	0	6	1.7	2.2	.7
3	151	White	1 ea	33	88	16	3	<1	0	<.1	0	0	0
3	152	Yolk	1 ea	17	49	63	3	<.1	0	6	1.7	2.2	.7

(15)Carbohydrate and calories vary widely—consult label if more precise values are needed.

KEY: 1 = BEV 2 = DAIRY 3 = EGGS 4 = FAT/OIL 5 = FRUIT 6 = BAKERY 7 = GRAIN 8 = FISH 9 = BEEF 10 = POULTRY 11 = SAUSAGE 12 = MIXED/FAST 13 = NUTS/SEEDS 14 = SWEETS 15 = VEG/LEG 16 = MISC 22 = SOUP/SAUCE

Chol (mg)	Calc (mg)	Iron (mg)	Magn (mg)	Phos (mg)	Pota (mg)	Sodi (mg)	Zinc (mg)	VT-A (RE)	Thia (mg)	Ribo (mg)	Niac (mg)	V-B6 (mg)	Fola (µg)	VT-C (mg)
478	1405	.96	149	1075	2053	926	11.3	1064	.41	2.63	1.08	.49	22	6
59	176	.12	18	134	257	116	1.41	133	.05	.33	.13	.06	3	1
22	66	.04	7	50	97	44	.53	50	.02	.12	.05	.02	1	t
153	236	.43	25	199	338	153	1.99	199	.08	.45	.18	.1	9	1
701	1212	.83	131	927	1770	867	9.74	1758	.36	2.27	.93	.43	23	5
88	151	.1	16	115	221	108	1.21	219	.04	.28	.12	.05	2	1
146	1404	1.47	147	1035	2117	838	4.40	419	.61	2.78	.94	.68	21	6
18	176	.18	19	129	265	105	.55	52	.08	.35	.12	.09	3	1
13	274	.28	29	202	412	163	.86	44	.12	.54	.18	.13	5	1
113	827	2.47	124	594	1588	709	10.6	308	.26	.71	1.05	.2	108	31
14	103	.31	15	74	198	88	1.33	39	.03	.09	.13	.03	14	4
278	297	1.1	37	310	387	209	1.53	146	.11	.5	.3	.13	24	1
1	74	1.2	24	117	254	285	.70	31	.04	.17	.6	.03	3	t
1	119	.3	24	113	212	252	.70	t	.03	.14	.4	.03	3	t
1	79	.2	24	94	155	305	.70	t	.03	.12	.6	.03	3	t
28	260	.6	48	658	352	880	1.18	66	.08	.36	.22	.13	10	2
15	146	.4	24	120	190	167	.59	34	.05	.2	.1	.06	5	1
15	133	.5	16	110	165	140	.60	33	.10	.18	.6	.05	6	1
15	131	.1	16	103	167	152	.50	34	.04	.18	.1	.05	6	1
15	129	.1	16	273	164	375	.50	33	.04	.17	.1	.05	6	1
15	132	.1	16	102	166	178	.50	34	.04	.18	.1	.05	6	1
0	55	.8	57	126	340	55	.40	10	.02	.08	.5	.28	28	0
10	345	.16	33	271	442	133	1.68	25	.08	.4	.22	.09	21	2
14	415	.18	40	326	531	159	2.02	36	.10	.49	.26	.11	25	2
11	388	.16	36	306	497	150	1.88	30	.10	.46	.24	.1	23	2
4	452	.2	43	354	579	173	2.20	5	.11	.53	.28	.12	28	2
29	275	.11	27	216	352	104	1.34	68	.07	.32	.17	.07	16	1
274	28	1.04	6	90	65	69	.61	78	.04	.15	.03	.06	32	0
0	4	.01	3	4	45	50	.06	0	<.01	.09	.03	<.01	5	0
272	26	.95	3	86	15	8	.55	94	.04	.07	.01	.05	26	0

(For purposes of calculations, use "0" for t, <1, <.1, <.01, etc.)

A

Table A–1

Food Composition

Grp	Ref	Food Description	Measure	Wt (g)	H_2O (%)	Ener (cal)	Prot (g)	Carb (g)	Dietary Fiber (g)	Fat (g)	Fat Breakdown (g)		
											Sat	Mono	Poly
EGGS—Con.													
		Cooked:											
3	153	Fried in butter	1 ea	46	72	95	5	1	0	6	2.4	2.4	.7
3	154	Hard-cooked, shell removed	1 ea	50	75	79	6	1	0	6	1.7	2.2	.7
3	155	Hard-cooked, chopped	1 c	136	75	215	17	2	0	15	4.6	6.1	2.0
3	156	Poached	1 ea	50	74	79	6	1	0	5	1.7	2.2	.7
3	157	Scrambled with milk and butter (also omelet)	1 ea	64	73	95	6	1	0	7	3.0	2.8	.8
FATS and OILS													
		Butter:											
4	158	Stick	½ c	113	16	813	1	<.1	0	92	57	27	3.4
4	159	Tablespoon	1 tbsp	14	16	100	<1	<.1	0	11	7.2	3.3	.4
4	160	Pat (about 1 tsp)[18]	1 ea	5	16	34	<.1	<.1	0	4	2.5	1.2	.2
		Fats, cooking (vegetable shortening):											
4	161	Cup	1 c	205	0	1812	0	0	0	205	51	91	54
4	162	Tablespoon	1 tbsp	13	0	15	0	0	0	13	3.3	5.8	3.4
		Lard:											
4	163	Cup	1 c	205	0	1849	0	0	0	205	80	93	23
4	164	Tablespoon	1 tbsp	13	0	115	0	0	0	13	5.1	5.9	1.5
		Margarine:											
		Imitation (about 40% fat), soft:											
4	165	8-oz container	8 oz	227	58	785	1	1	0	88	18	36	31
4	166	Tablespoon	1 tbsp	14	58	50	<.1	<.1	0	5	1.1	2.2	2.0
		Regular, hard (about 80% fat):											
4	167	Cup	½ c	113	16	812	1	1	0	91	18	41	29
4	168	Tablespoon	1 tbsp	14	16	100	<1	<1	0	11	2.3	5.1	3.6
4	169	Pat[18]	1 ea	5	16	36	<.1	<.1	0	4	.8	1.8	1.3
		Regular, soft (about 80% fat):											
4	170	8-oz container	8 oz	227	16	1626	2	1	0	183	31	65	79
4	171	Tablespoon	1 tbsp	14	16	100	1	<.1	0	11	2.0	4.0	4.9
		Spread (about 60% fat), hard:											
4	172	Cup	½ c	113	37	610	1	0	0	69	16	29	20
4	173	Tablespoon	1 tbsp	14	37	75	<.1	0	0	8	2.0	3.6	2.5
4	174	Pat[18]	1 ea	5	37	25	<.1	0	0	3	.7	1.3	.9
		Spread (about 60% fat), soft:											
4	175	8 oz container	8 oz	227	37	1225	1	0	0	138	29	72	31
4	176	Tablespoon	1 tbsp	14	37	75	<.1	0	0	8	1.8	4.4	1.9
		Oils:											
		Corn:											
4	177	Cup	1 c	218	0	1927	0	0	0	218	28	53	128
4	178	Tablespoon	1 tbsp	14	0	125	0	0	0	14	1.8	3.4	8.2

(18)Pat is 1″ square, ⅓″ high; 90 per lb.

KEY: 1 = BEV 2 = DAIRY 3 = EGGS 4 = FAT/OIL 5 = FRUIT 6 = BAKERY 7 = GRAIN 8 = FISH 9 = BEEF 10 = POULTRY 11 = SAUSAGE 12 = MIXED/FAST 13 = NUTS/SEEDS 14 = SWEETS 15 = VEG/LEG 16 = MISC 22 = SOUP/SAUCE

Chol (mg)	Calc (mg)	Iron (mg)	Magn (mg)	Phos (mg)	Pota (mg)	Sodi (mg)	Zinc (mg)	VT-A (RE)	Thia (mg)	Ribo (mg)	Niac (mg)	V-B6 (mg)	Fola (μg)	VT-C (mg)
278	28	.92	5	90	58	162	.64	94	.04	.13	.03	.05	22	0
274	28	1.04	6	90	65	69	.72	78	.04	.14	.03	.06	24	0
745	76	2.84	17	245	177	188	1.96	212	.10	.39	.08	.15	67	0
273	28	1.04	6	90	65	146	.72	78	.04	.13	.03	.05	24	0
282	54	.93	109	109	97	176	.7	102	.04	.18	.04	.06	22	t
247	27	.18	2	26	29	933[16]	.06	852[17]	<.01	.04	.05	<.01	3	0
31	3	.02	<1	3	4	116[16]	<.01	106[17]	<.01	<.01	<.01	t	<1	0
11	1	<.01	<1	1	1	41[16]	<.01	38[17]	t	<.01	<.01	t	<1	0
0	0	0	0	0	0	0	.1	0	0	0	0	0	0	0
0	0	0	0	0	0	0	0	0	0	0	0	0	0	0
195	t	0	<1	6	t	t	.23	0	0	0	0	0	0	0
12	t	0	<1	<1	t	t	.01	0	0	0	0	0	0	0
0	40	0	2	31	57	2178[19]	.23	2254[20]	.01	.05	.03	.01	2	t
0	2	0	<1	2	4	136[19]	.03	141[20]	<.01	<.01	<.01	<.01	<1	t
0	34	.07	3	26	48	1066[19]	.23	1122[20]	.01	.04	.03	.01	1	t
0	4	<.01	<1	3	6	133[19]	.03	139[20]	<.01	<.01	<.01	<.01	<1	t
0	1	<.01	<1	1	2	47[19]	.01	50[20]	t	<.01	<.01	t	<1	t
0	60	0	5	46	86	2448[19]	.46	2254[20]	.02	.07	.04	.02	2	t
0	4	0	<1	3	5	153[19]	.03	140[20]	<.01	<.01	<.01	<.01	<1	t
0	24	0	2	18	34	1123[19]	.17	1122[20]	<.01	.03	.02	<.01	<1	t
0	3	0	<1	2	4	139[19]	.02	139[20]	<.01	<.01	<.01	<.01	<1	t
0	1	0	<1	1	1	50[20]	<.01	50[20]	t	<.01	<.01	t	<1	t
0	47	0	4	37	68	2256[19]	.34	2254[20]	.16	.06	.04	.01	2	t
0	3	0	<1	2	4	139[19]	.02	139[20]	.01	<.01	<.01	<.01	<1	t
0	0	0	—	0	0	0	.4	0	0	0	0	0	<1	0
0	0	0	—	0	0	0	.03	0	0	0	0	0	0	0

(16)For salted butter; unsalted butter contains 12 mg sodium per stick, or 1/2 c, 1.5 mg/tbsp, or .5 mg/pat.

(17)Values for vitamin A are a year-round average.

(19)For salted margarine.

(20)Based on average vitamin A content of fortified margarine. Federal specifications require a minimum of 15,000 IU/lb.

(For purposes of calculations, use "0" for t, <1, <.1, <.01, etc.)

A

Table A–1

Food Composition

Grp	Ref	Food Description	Measure	Wt (g)	H_2O (%)	Ener (cal)	Prot (g)	Carb (g)	Dietary Fiber (g)	Fat (g)	Fat Breakdown (g) Sat	Mono	Poly
		FATS and OILS—Con.											
		Olive:											
4	179	Cup	1 c	216	0	1909	0	0	0	216	29	159	18
4	180	Tablespoon	1 tbsp	14	0	125	0	0	0	14	1.9	10	1.2
		Peanut:											
4	181	Cup	1 c	216	0	1909	0	0	0	216	36	100	69
4	182	Tablespoon	1 tbsp	14	0	125	0	0	0	14	2.4	6.5	4.5
		Safflower:											
4	183	Cup	1 c	218	0	1927	0	0	0	218	20	26	162
4	184	Tablespoon	1 tbsp	14	0	125	0	0	0	14	1.3	1.7	10
		Soybean:											
4	185	Cup	1 c	218	0	1927	0	0	0	218	33	94	82
4	186	Tablespoon	1 tbsp	14	0	125	0	0	0	14	2	6	5
		Soybean/cottonseed:											
4	187	Cup	1 c	218	0	1927	0	0	0	218	39	64	105
4	188	Tablespoon	1 tbsp	14	0	125	0	0	0	14	3	4	7
		Sunflower:											
4	189	Cup	1 c	218	0	1927	0	0	0	218	23	43	143
4	190	Tablespoon	1 tbsp	14	0	125	0	0	0	14	1.4	2.7	9.2
		Salad dressings/ sandwich spreads:											
4	191	Blue cheese:	1 tbsp	15	32	75	1	1	<1	8	1.5	1.9	4.3
		French:											
4	192	Regular	1 tbsp	16	35	85	<.1	1	<1	9	1.4	4	3.5
4	193	Low calorie	1 tbsp	16	75	24	<.1	2	<1	2	.2	.3	1
		Italian:											
4	194	Regular	1 tbsp	14	34	80	<1	1	<1	9	1.3	3.7	3.2
4	195	Low calorie	1 tbsp	15	86	5	<.1	1	<1	t	t	t	t
		Mayonnaise:											
4	196	Regular	1 tbsp	14	15	100	<1	<1	0	11	1.7	3.2	5.8
4	197	Imitation	1 tbsp	15	63	35	0	2	0	3	.5	.7	1.6
4	198	Ranch style	½ c	119	35	435	4	6	0	45	6.7	19	17
4	199	Salad dressing—mayo type	1 tbsp	15	40	58	<1	4	0	5	.7	1.4	2.7
4	200	Tartar sauce	1 tbsp	14	34	74	<1	1	<1	8	1.2	2.6	3.9
		Thousand Island:											
4	201	Regular	1 tbsp	16	46	60	<1	2	<1	6	1.0	1.3	3.2
4	202	Low calorie	1 tbsp	15	69	25	<1	2	<1	2	.2	.4	.9
		Salad dressings, prepared from home recipe:											
4	203	Cooked type[21]	1 tbsp	16	69	25	1	2	0	2	.5	.6	.3
4	204	Vinegar and oil	1 tbsp	16	47	70	0	0	0	8	1.5	2.4	3.9
		FRUITS and FRUIT JUICES											
		Apples:											
		Raw, with peel:											
5	205	2¾″ diam (about 3 per lb with cores)	1 ea	138	84	80	<1	21	4	<1	.1	t	.1
5	206	3¼″ diam (about 2 per lb with cores)	1 ea	212	84	125	<1	32	7	1	.1	t	.2

(21) Fatty acid values apply to product made with regular margarine.

Key: 1 = BEV 2 = DAIRY 3 = EGGS 4 = FAT/OIL 5 = FRUIT 6 = BAKERY 7 = GRAIN 8 = FISH 9 = BEEF 10 = POULTRY 11 = SAUSAGE 12 = MIXED/FAST 13 = NUTS/SEEDS 14 = SWEETS 15 = VEG/LEG 16 = MISC 22 = SOUP/SAUCE

Chol (mg)	Calc (mg)	Iron (mg)	Magn (mg)	Phos (mg)	Pota (mg)	Sodi (mg)	Zinc (mg)	VT-A (RE)	Thia (mg)	Ribo (mg)	Niac (mg)	V-B6 (mg)	Fola (μg)	VT-C (mg)
0	<1	.83	<1	3	0	0	.13	0	0	0	0	0	<1	0
0	t	.05	<1	t	0	0	<.01	0	0	0	0	0	0	0
0	t	.06	<1	0	0	0	.02	t	0	0	0	0	<1	0
0	t	<.01	<1	0	0	0	<.01	t	0	0	0	0	0	0
0	0	0	—	0	0	0	.41	0	0	0	0	0	0	0
0	0	0	—	0	0	0	.03	0	0	0	0	0	0	0
0	<1	.05	<1	1	0	0	.4	0	0	0	0	0	<1	0
0	t	0	<1	t	0	0	.03	0	0	0	0	0	t	0
0	0	0	—	0	0	0	.4	0	0	0	0	0	<1	0
0	0	0	—	0	0	0	.03	0	0	0	0	0	0	0
0	0	0	0	0	0	0	—	0	0	0	0	0	0	0
0	0	0	0	0	0	0	—	0	0	0	0	0	0	0
3	12	.03	<1	11	6	<1	.28	10	<.01	.02	.01	<.01	8	t
0	2	.06	<1	1	2	188	.01	t	t	t	t	<.01	0	t
0	6	.07	—	5	3	306	.03	t	t	t	t	0	t	t
0	1	.03	<1	1	5	162	.02	3	t	t	t	.03	0	t
0	1	.03	<1	1	4	136	0	t	t	t	t	0	t	t
8	2	.07	<1	4	5	80	.02	12	<.01	<.01	<.01	<.01	<1	0
4	0	0	—	0	2	75	—	0	0	0	0	0	t	0
47	119	.31	12	100	158	522	.43	86	.04	.17	.08	.05	6	1
4	2	.03	<1	4	1	105	0	13	<.01	<.01	t	<.01	t	0
4	3	.1	<1	4	11	182	.02	9	<.01	<.01	<.01	<.01	<1	t
4	2	.09	<1	3	18	110	.03	15	<.01	<.01	.03	<.01	6	t
2	2	.09	<1	3	17	153	0	14	<.01	<.01	.03	<.01	<1	t
9	13	.08	—	14	19	117	0	20	.01	.02	.04	0	<1	t
0	0	0	—	0	1	0	—	0	0	0	0	0	—	0
0	10	.25	6	10	159	1	.05	7	.02	.02	.11	.07	4	8
0	15	.38	9	23	244	1	.08	11	.04	.03	.16	.1	6	12

(For purposes of calculations, use "0" for t, <1, <.1, <.01, etc.)

A

Table A–1

Food Composition

Grp	Ref	Food Description	Measure	Wt (g)	H_2O (%)	Ener (cal)	Prot (g)	Carb (g)	Dietary Fiber (g)	Fat (g)	Fat Breakdown (g) Sat	Mono	Poly
		FRUITS and JUICES—Con.											
		Apples—con.											
5	207	Raw, peeled slices	1 c	110	84	65	<1	16	3	<1	.1	t	.1
5	208	Dried, sulfured	10 ea	64	32	155	1	42	9	<1	t	t	.1
5	209	Apple juice, bottled or canned[23]	1 c	248	88	116	<1	29	1	<1	.1	t	.1
		Applesauce:											
5	210	Sweetened	1 c	255	80	195	1	51	4	<1	.1	t	.1
5	211	Unsweetened	1 c	244	88	106	<1	28	5	<1	t	t	t
		Apricots:											
5	212	Raw, without pits (about 12 per lb with pits)	3 ea	106	86	51	2	12	2	<1	t	.2	.1
		Canned (fruit and liquid):											
5	213	Heavy syrup	1 c	258	78	214	1	55	4	<1	t	.1	t
5	214	Halves	3 ea	85	78	70	<1	18	1	<.1	t	t	t
5	215	Juice pack	1 c	248	87	119	2	31	4	<.1	t	t	t
5	216	Halves	3 ea	84	87	40	<1	10	1	<.1	t	t	t
		Dried:											
5	217	Dried halves	10 ea	35	31	83	1	22	3	<1	t	.1	t
5	218	Cooked, unsweetened, with liquid	1 c	250	75	210	3	55	7	<1	t	.2	.1
5	219	Apricot nectar, canned	1 c	251	85	141	1	36	2	<1	t	.1	t
		Avocados, raw, edible part only:											
5	220	California (½ lb with refuse)	1 ea	173	73	305	4	12	5	30	4.5	19	3.5
5	221	Florida (1 lb with refuse)	1 ea	304	80	340	5	27	9	27	5	15	5
5	222	Mashed, fresh, average	1 c	230	74	370	5	17	6	35	6	22	5
		Bananas, raw, without peel:											
5	223	Whole, 8¾″ long (weighs 175 g with peel)	1 ea	114	74	105	1	27	3	<1	.2	.1	.1
5	224	Slices	1 c	150	74	138	2	35	4	1	.3	.1	.1
5	225	Blackberries, raw	1 c	144	86	74	1	18	10	1	.3	.1	.1
		Blueberries:											
5	226	Raw	1 c	145	85	82	1	21	5	1	<.1	.2	.3
		Frozen, sweetened:											
5	227	10-oz container	10 oz	284	77	230	1	62	9	<1	.1	.1	.2
5	228	Cup	1 c	230	77	185	1	51	7	<1	.1	.1	.2
		Cherries:											
5	229	Sour, red pitted, canned water pack	1 c	244	90	90	2	22	3	<1	.1	.1	.1
5	230	Sweet, raw, without pits	10 ea	68	81	49	1	11	1	1	.1	.2	.2
		Cranberry juices:											
5	231	Cranberry juice cocktail[26]	1 c	253	85	145	<.1[27]	37	1	<1	t	t	.1
5	232	Cranberry-apple juice	1 c	253	86	169	<1	43	1	1[29]	.2	.1	.4
5	233	Cranberry sauce, canned, strained	1 c	277	61	419	1	108	2	<1	.1	.1	.2

(23)Also applies to pasteurized apple cider.

(26)Data here are from the newest USDA *Handbook 8–14* on beverages. These data are somewhat different from that presented in *Handbook 8–9* on fruits and fruit juices.

(27)The newest USDA *Handbook 8–14* data on beverages indicates "0" for protein.

(29)The newest USDA *Handbook 8–14* data on beverages indicates "0" for fat.

Key: 1 = BEV 2 = DAIRY 3 = EGGS 4 = FAT/OIL 5 = FRUIT 6 = BAKERY 7 = GRAIN 8 = FISH 9 = BEEF 10 = POULTRY 11 = SAUSAGE 12 = MIXED/FAST 13 = NUTS/SEEDS 14 = SWEETS 15 = VEG/LEG 16 = MISC 22 = SOUP/SAUCE

Chol (mg)	Calc (mg)	Iron (mg)	Magn (mg)	Phos (mg)	Pota (mg)	Sodi (mg)	Zinc (mg)	VT-A (RE)	Thia (mg)	Ribo (mg)	Niac (mg)	V-B6 (mg)	Fola (μg)	VT-C (mg)
0	4	.1	3	8	124	1	.04	5	.02	.01	.1	.05	<1	4
0	9	.9	10	24	288	56[22]	.13	0	0	.1	.59	.08	<1	3
0	17	.92	8	17	295	7	.07	t	.05	.04	.25	.07	<1	2[24]
0	10	1	7	18	156	8	.1	3	.03	.07	.50	.07	2	4[24]
0	7	.29	7	18	183	5	.06	7	.03	.06	.46	.06	2	3[24]
0	15	.58	8	21	313	1	.28	277	.03	.04	.64	.06	9	11
0	23	.77	18	33	361	10	.27	317	.05	.06	.97	.14	4	8
0	7	.26	6	10	119	3	.09	105	.02	.02	.32	.05	1	3
0	30	.74	24	50	409	9	.27	419	.04	.05	.85	.18	5	12
0	10	.25	8	17	139	3	.1	142	.01	.02	.29	.06	2	4
0	16	1.65	16	41	482	3	.26	253	<.01	.05	1.05	.06	4	1
0	40	4.2	42	103	1222	8	.66	591	.01	.07	2.36	.28	0	4
0	18	.96	13	23	286	8	.23	330	.02	.04	.65	.16	3	2[25]
0	19	2.04	70	73	1097	21	.73	106	.19	.21	3.32	.48	113	14
0	33	1.6	104	119	1484	14	1.28	186	.33	.37	5.84	.85	162	24
0	25	2.3	90	95	1378	24	.97	141	.25	.28	4.42	.64	142	18
0	7	.35	32	22	451	1	.19	9	.05	.11	.62	.66	24	10
0	9	.46	43	29	593	1	.25	12	.07	.15	.81	.87	31	13
0	46	.8	29	30	282	0	.39	24	.04	.06	.58	.08	49	30
0	9	.24	7	15	129	9	.16	15	.07	.07	.7	.05	9	20
0	16	1.11	7	20	169	4	.14	12	.06	.15	.72	.17	19	3
0	13	.9	6	16	138	3	.14	10	.05	.12	.58	.14	16	2
0	27	3.34	15	25	240	17	.17	184	.04	.1	.43	.11	20	5
0	10	.3	8	13	152	0	.04	15	.03	.04	.3	.02	3	5
0	8	.38	5	5	45	5	.18	1	.02	.02	.09	.05	<1	90[28]
0	18	.15	5	7	68	5	.1	t	.01	.05	.15	.06	<1	81[28]
0	11	.61	8	17	72	80	.09	6	.04	.06	.28	.05	2	6

(22)Sodium bisulfite used to preserve color; unsulfured product would contain lower levels of sodium.

(24)Value based on products without added ascorbic acid. Bottled apple juice with added ascorbic acid usually contains 41.6 mg/100 g, or 103 mg per cup. Check label for specific vitamin C values.

(25)Without added ascorbic acid. Products with added ascorbic acid contain 136 mg per cup. Check label.

(28)Nutrient added.

(For purposes of calculations, use "0" for t, <1, <.1, <.01, etc.)

Table A–1

Food Composition

Grp	Ref	Food Description	Measure	Wt (g)	H_2O (%)	Ener (cal)	Prot (g)	Carb (g)	Dietary Fiber (g)	Fat (g)	Fat Breakdown (g) Sat	Mono	Poly
		FRUITS and FRUIT JUICES—Con.											
		Dates:											
5	234	Whole, without pits	10 ea	83	22	228	2	61	7	<1	.2	.1	t
5	235	Chopped	1 c	178	22	489	4	131	16	1	.4	.2	.1
5	236	Figs, dried	10 ea	187	28	477	6	122	24	2	.4	.5	1.1
		Fruit cocktail, canned, fruit and liquid:											
5	237	Heavy syrup pack	1 c	255	80	185	1	48	3	1	<.1	<.1	.1
5	238	Juice pack	1 c	248	87	115	1	29	3	<.1	t	t	t
		Grapefruit:											
		Raw 3¾″ diam, whole fruit weighs 1 lb 1 oz with refuse (peel membrane, seeds):											
5	239	Pink/red, half fruit, edible part	1 half	123	91	37	1	9	2	<1	t	t	<.1
5	240	White, half fruit, edible part[30]	1 half	118	90	39	1	10	1	<1	t	t	<.1
5	241	Canned sections with liquid	1 c	254	84	152	1	39	2	<1	<.1	<.1	.1
		Grapefruit juice:											
5	242	Raw	1 c	247	90	96	1	23	<1	<1	<.1	<.1	.1
		Canned:											
5	243	Unsweetened	1 c	247	90	93	1	22	<1	<1	<.1	<.1	.1
5	244	Sweetened	1 c	250	87	115	1	28	<1	<1	<.1	<.1	.1
		Frozen concentrate, unsweetened											
5	245	Undiluted, 6-fl-oz can	¾ c	207	62	300	4	72	1	1	.2	.2	.3
5	246	Diluted with 3 cans water	1 c	247	89	102	1	24	<1	<1	.1	<.1	.1
		Grapes, raw, European type (adherent skin):											
5	247	Thompson seedless	10 ea	50	81	35	<1	9	1	<1	.1	t	.1
5	248	Tokay/Emperor, seeded types	10 ea	57	81	40	<1	10	1	<1	.1	t	.1
		Grape juice:											
5	249	Bottled or canned	1 c	253	84	155	1	38	1	<1	.1	t	.1
		Frozen concentrate, sweetened:											
5	250	Undiluted, 6-fl-oz can	¾ c	216	54	385	1	96	4	1	.2	<.1	.2
5	251	Diluted with 3 cans water	1 c	250	87	128	<1	32	1	<1	.1	t	.1
5	252	Kiwi fruit, raw, peeled (about 5 per lb with skin)	1 ea	76	83	46	1	11	1	<1	t	.2	.2
5	253	Lemons, raw, without peel and seeds (about 4 per lb whole)	1 ea	58	89	17	1	5	1	<1	t	t	.1
		Lemon juice											
		Fresh:											
5	254	Cup	1 c	244	91	60	1	21	1	0	0	0	0
5	255	Tablespoon	1 tbsp	15	91	4	<.1	1	<1	0	0	0	0
		Canned or bottled, unsweetened:											
5	256	Cup	1 c	244	92	52	1	16	1	1	.1	<.1	.2
5	257	Tablespoon	1 tbsp	15	92	5	<.1	1	<1	<.1	t	t	t
		Frozen, single strength, unsweetened:											
5	258	Cup	1 c	244	92	54	1	16	1	1	.1	<.1	.3
5	259	Tablespoon	1 tbsp	15	92	3	<.1	1	<1	<.1	t	t	t

(30) Weight is for edible portion. Weight with rind is 241 g for one-half.

A

Key: 1 = BEV 2 = DAIRY 3 = EGGS 4 = FAT/OIL 5 = FRUIT 6 = BAKERY 7 = GRAIN 8 = FISH 9 = BEEF 10 = POULTRY 11 = SAUSAGE 12 = MIXED/FAST 13 = NUTS/SEEDS 14 = SWEETS 15 = VEG/LEG 16 = MISC 22 = SOUP/SAUCE

Chol (mg)	Calc (mg)	Iron (mg)	Magn (mg)	Phos (mg)	Pota (mg)	Sodi (mg)	Zinc (mg)	VT-A (RE)	Thia (mg)	Ribo (mg)	Niac (mg)	V-B6 (mg)	Fola (μg)	VT-C (mg)
0	27	1	29	33	541	2	.24	4	.07	.08	1.83	.16	14	0
0	58	2.14	63	70	1161	5	.52	9	.16	.18	3.92	.34	29	0
0	269	4.18	111	128	1331	21	.94	25	.13	.17	1.3	.42	16	1
0	16	.73	14	28	224	15	.21	52	.05	.05	.95	.11	1	5
0	20	.53	17	34	235	10	.21	76	.03	.04	1	.13	2	7
0	13	.15	10	11	158	0	.09	32[31]	.04	.03	.23	.05	15	47
0	14	.07	11	9	175	0	.08	1	.04	.02	.32	.05	12	39
0	36	1.02	25	25	328	4	.21	0	.1	.05	.62	.05	22	54
0	22	.49	30	37	400	2	.13	2[32]	.1	.05	.49	.11	52	94
0	17	.49	24	27	378	2	.22	2	.1	.05	.57	.05	26	72
0	20	.9	24	28	405	5	.15	2	.1	.06	.8	.05	26	67
0	56	1.02	78	101	1002	6	.38	6	.3	.16	1.6	.32	26	248
0	20	.34	26	34	337	2	.12	2	.1	.05	.54	.11	52	83
0	5	.13	3	7	92	1	.03	4	.05	.03	.15	.06	4	5
0	6	.15	4	8	105	1	.03	4	.05	.03	.17	.06	4	6
0	22	.61	24	27	334	8	.13	2	.07	.09	.66	.16	6	t[33]
0	28	.78	32	32	160	15	.28	6	.11	.2	.93	.32	9	179[34]
0	10	.26	11	11	53	5	.10	2	.04	.07	.31	.1	4	60[34]
0	20	.3	23	30	252	4	.08[32]	13	.02	.04	.4	.04[35]	17[35]	74
0	15	.35	2	9	80	1	.06	2	.02	.01	.06	.05	7	31
0	18	.08	16	14	303	2	.12	5	.07	.02	.24	.12	32	112
0	1	<.01	1	1	19	<1	<.01	t	<.01	<.01	.01	<.01	2	7
0	26	.31	22	21	248	50[36]	.15	4	.10	.02	.48	.1	25	61
0	2	.02	1	1	15	3[36]	.01	t	<.01	<.01	.03	<.01	2	4
0	19	.30	20	20	218	4	.12	3	.14	.03	.33	.15	23	77
0	1	.02	1	1	14	<1	<.01	t	<.01	<.01	.02	<.01	1	5

(31)Vitamin A in Texas red grapefruit would be 74 RE.
(32)Vitamin A for white grapefruit juice; pink or red grapefruit juice = 109 RE per cup.
(33)Without added ascorbic acid.
(34)With added ascorbic acid.
(35)Data are estimated from other fruit data.
(36)Sodium benzoate and sodium bisulfite added as preservatives.

(For purposes of calculations, use "0" for t, <1, <.1, <.01, etc.)

Table A–1

Food Composition

Grp	Ref	Food Description	Measure	Wt (g)	H_2O (%)	Ener (cal)	Prot (g)	Carb (g)	Dietary Fiber (g)	Fat (g)	Fat Breakdown (g) Sat	Mono	Poly
FRUITS and FRUIT JUICES—Con.													
		Lime juice:											
		Fresh:											
5	260	Cup	1 c	246	90	65	1	22	1	<1	<.1	<.1	.1
5	261	Tablespoon	1 tbsp	15	90	4	<.1	1	<1	<.1	t	t	t
5	262	Canned or bottled, unsweetened	1 c	246	92	50	1	16	1	1	.1	.1	.2
5	263	Mangos, raw, edible part (weighs 300 g with skin and seeds)	1 ea	207	82	135	1	35	3	1	.1	.2	.1
		Melons, raw, without rind and cavity contents:											
5	264	Cantaloupe, 5″ diam (2⅓ lb whole (with refuse), orange flesh	½ ea	267	90	94	2	22	3	1	.1	.1	.2
5	265	Honeydew, 6½″ diam (5¼ lb whole with refuse), slice = ⅒ melon	1 slice	129	90	45	1	12	1	<1	t	t	<.1
5	266	Nectarines, raw, without pits, 2½″ diam	1 ea	136	86	67	1	16	3	1	.1	.2	.3
		Oranges, raw:											
5	267	Whole without peel and seeds 2⅝″ diam (weighs about 180 g with peel and seeds)	1 ea	131	87	60	1	15	3	<1	t	<.1	<.1
5	268	Sections, without membranes	1 c	180	87	85	2	21	4	<1	<.1	<.1	<.1
		Orange juice:											
5	269	Fresh, all varieties	1 c	248	88	111	2	26	<1	<1	.1	.1	.1
5	270	Canned, unsweetened	1 c	249	89	105	2	25	<1	<1	<.1	.1	.1
5	271	Chilled	1 c	249	88	110	2	25	1	1	.1	.1	.2
		Frozen concentrate:											
5	272	Undiluted (6-oz can)	¾ c	213	58	339	5	81	3	<1	.1	.1	.1
5	273	Diluted with 3 parts water by volume	1 c	249	88	110	2	27	1	<1	t	<.1	<.1
5	274	Orange and grapefruit juice, canned	1 c	247	89	105	2	25	<1	<1	<.1	<.1	.1
		Papayas, raw:											
5	275	½″ slices	1 c	140	89	60	1	14	2	<1	.1	.1	<.1
5	276	Whole fruit, cubes, 3½″ diam by 5⅛″, without seeds and skin (1 lb with refuse)	1 ea	304	89	117	2	30	5	<1	.1	.1	.1
		Peaches:											
		Raw:											
5	277	Whole, 2½″ diam, peeled, pitted (about 4 per lb with peels and pits)	1 ea	87	88	37	1	10	2	<.1	t	<.1	<.1
5	278	Sliced	1 c	170	88	73	1	19	4	<1	t	.1	.1
		Canned, fruit and liquid:											
		Heavy syrup pack											
5	279	Cup	1 c	256	79	190	1	51	4	<1	<.1	.1	.1
5	280	Half	1 ea	81	79	60	<1	16	1	<.1	t	<.1	<.1
		Juice pack											
5	281	Cup	1 c	248	88	109	2	29	4	<.1	t	<.1	<.1
5	282	Half	1 ea	77	88	34	<1	9	1	<.1	t	t	t

Key: 1 = BEV 2 = DAIRY 3 = EGGS 4 = FAT/OIL 5 = FRUIT 6 = BAKERY 7 = GRAIN 8 = FISH 9 = BEEF 10 = POULTRY 11 = SAUSAGE 12 = MIXED/FAST 13 = NUTS/SEEDS 14 = SWEETS 15 = VEG/LEG 16 = MISC 22 = SOUP/SAUCE

Chol (mg)	Calc (mg)	Iron (mg)	Magn (mg)	Phos (mg)	Pota (mg)	Sodi (mg)	Zinc (mg)	VT-A (RE)	Thia (mg)	Ribo (mg)	Niac (mg)	V-B6 (mg)	Fola (μg)	VT-C (mg)
0	22	.08	14	18	268	2	.15	3	.05	.03	.25	.11	21	72
0	1	<.01	1	1	17	<1	.01	t	<.01	<.01	.01	.08	1	4
0	30	.6	16	25	185	39[36]	.15	4	.08	.01	.4	.07	20	16
0	21	.26	18	22	323	4	.07	806	.12	.12	1.21	.28	39	57
0	29	.56	19	45	825	24	.43	861	.1	.06	1.53	.31	80	113
0	8	.09	9	13	350	13	.11	5	.1	.02	.77	.08	39	32
0	6	.21	11	22	288	0	.12	100	.02	.06	1.35	.03	5	7
0	52	.14	13	18	237	t	.09	27	.11	.05	.37	.08	40	70
0	72	.19	18	25	326	t	.4	37	.16	.07	.51	.11	83	96
0	27	.50	27	42	496	2	.12	50	.22	.07	.99	.1	109	124
0	20	1.1	27	35	436	5	.17	44	.15	.07	.78	.22	15	86
0	25	.42	28	27	473	2	.11	19[37]	.28	.05	.7	.13	45[37]	82[37]
0	68	.75	73	121	1436	6	.38	59	.6	.14	1.53	.33	331	294
0	22	.27	24	40	474	2	.13	19	.2	.04	.5	.11	109	97
0	20	1.1	24	35	390	7	.18	29	.14	.07	.83	.06	20	72
0	33	.3	14	12	247	9	.10	282	.04	.04	.47	.03	26	92
0	72	.3	31	16	780	8	.22	612	.08	.10	1.03	.06	48	188
0	4	.1	6	10	171	0	.12	47	.01	.04	.86	.02	3	6
0	9	.19	11	20	335	1	.18	91	.03	.07	1.68	.03	6	11
0	8	.69	13	29	235	16	.22	85	.03	.06	1.57	.05	8	7
0	2	.22	4	9	75	5	.07	27	<.01	.02	.5	.01	3	2
0	15	.72	18	43	317	11	.26	94	.02	.04	1.44	.05	8	9
0	5	.21	6	13	98	3	.09	29	<.01	.01	.45	.01	3	3

(37)Values for juice from California oranges indicate the following values for 1 c: 36 RE of vitamin A, 72μg of folacin, and 106 mg of vitamin C.

(For purposes of calculations, use "0" for t, <1, <.1, <.01, etc.)

Table A–1

Food Composition

Grp	Ref	Food Description	Measure	Wt (g)	H_2O (%)	Ener (cal)	Prot (g)	Carb (g)	Dietary Fiber (g)	Fat (g)	Fat Breakdown (g) Sat	Mono	Poly
		FRUITS and FRUIT JUICES—Con.											
		Peaches—con.											
		Dried:											
5	283	Uncooked	10 ea	130	32	311	5	80	10	1	.1	.4	.5
5	284	Cooked, fruit and liquid	1 c	258	78	200	3	51	5	1	.1	.2	.3
		Frozen, sliced, sweetened:											
5	285	10-oz package	1 ea	284	75	267	2	68	6	<1	<.1	.1	.2
5	286	Cup, thawed measure	1 c	250	75	235	2	60	5	<1	<.1	.1	.2
		Pears:											
		Raw, with skin, cored:											
5	287	Bartlett, 2½″ diam (about 2½ per lb, whole)	1 ea	166	84	98	<1	25	5[39]	1	<.1	.1	.2
		Pears, raw, with skin, cored—con.											
5	288	Bosc, 2½″ diam (about 3 per lb, whole)	1 ea	141	84	85	1	21	4[39]	<1	.1	.1	.1
5	289	D'Anjou, 3″ diam (about ½ per lb, whole)	1 ea	200	84	120	1	30	6[39]	1	.1	.2	.2
		Canned, fruit and liquid:											
		Heavy syrup pack:											
5	290	Cup	1 c	255	80	188	1	49	5[39]	<1	t	.1	.1
5	291	Half	1 ea	79	80	59	<1	15	2[39]	<1	t	t	t
		Juice pack:											
5	292	Cup	1 c	248	86	123	1	32	5[39]	<1	t	<.1	<.1
5	293	Half	1 ea	77	86	38	<1	10	2[39]	<.1	t	t	t
5	294	Dried halves	10 ea	175	27	459	3	122	19	1	.1	.2	.3
		Pineapple:											
5	295	Raw chunks, diced	1 c	155	86	76	1	19	3	1	.1	.1	.2
		Canned, fruit and liquid:											
		Heavy syrup pack:											
5	296	Crushed, chunks, tidbits	1 c	255	79	199	1	52	2	<1	t	<.1	.1
5	297	Slices	1 ea	58	79	45	<1	12	1	<.1	t	t	<.1
		Juice Pack:											
5	298	Crushed, chunks, tidbits	1 c	250	84	150	1	39	2	<1	t	<.1	.1
5	299	Slices	1 ea	58	84	35	<1	9	1	<.1	t	t	t
5	300	Pineapple juice, canned, unsweetened	1 c	250	86	140	1	34	1	<1	t	t	.1
		Plantains, without peel:											
5	301	Raw slices (one whole plantain weights 179 g without peel)	1 c	148	65	181	2	47	4[41]	1	.3	.1	.1
5	302	Cooked, boiled, sliced	1 c	154	67	179	1	48	4	<1	.1	<.1	.1
		Plums, without pits:											
		Raw											
5	303	Medium 2⅛″ diam	1 ea	66	85	36	1	9	1	<1	<.1	.3	.1
5	304	Small, 1½″ diam	1 ea	28	85	15	<1	4	1	<1	t	.1	<.1
		Canned, purple, with liquid:											
		Heavy Syrup pack:											
5	305	Cup	1 c	258	76	230	1	60	4	<1	t	.2	.1
5	306	Plums	3 ea	110	76	98	<1	25	2	<1	t	.1	t

[39] Dietary fiber data vary 2.4 to 3.4 g/100 g for fresh pears; 1.6 to 2.6 g/100 g for canned pears.

[41] Dietary fiber value partially derived from data for bananas.

Key: 1 = BEV 2 = DAIRY 3 = EGGS 4 = FAT/OIL 5 = FRUIT 6 = BAKERY 7 = GRAIN 8 = FISH 9 = BEEF 10 = POULTRY 11 = SAUSAGE 12 = MIXED/FAST 13 = NUTS/SEEDS 14 = SWEETS 15 = VEG/LEG 16 = MISC 22 = SOUP/SAUCE

Chol (mg)	Calc (mg)	Iron (mg)	Magn (mg)	Phos (mg)	Pota (mg)	Sodi (mg)	Zinc (mg)	VT-A (RE)	Thia (mg)	Ribo (mg)	Niac (mg)	V-B6 (mg)	Fola (μg)	VT-C (mg)
0	37	5.28	54	155	1295	9	.74	281	<.01	.28	5.69	.09	6	6
0	23	3.37	35	99	825	6	.46	51	.01	.05	3.92	.1	<1	10
0	9	1.05	14	31	369	17	.14	81	.04	.10	1.9	.05	9	268[38]
0	8	.93	12	28	325	16	.13	71	.03	.09	1.63	.04	8	236[38]
0	19	.41	9	18	208	1	.20	3	.03	.07	.17	.03	12	7
0	16	.40	8	16	176	t	.17	3	.03	.06	.1	.03	10	6
0	22	.50	11	22	250	t	.24	4	.04	.08	.2	.04	14	8
0	13	.56	11	18	166	13	.21	1	.03	.06	.62	.04	3	3
0	4	.17	3	5	51	4	.06	t	.01	.02	.19	.01	<1	1
0	22	.71	17	29	238	10	.22	1	.03	.03	.5	.04	5	4
0	7	.22	5	9	74	3	.07	t	<.01	<.01	.15	.01	2	1
0	59	3.68	58	103	932	10	.68	t	.01	.25	2.4	.01	21	12
0	11	.57	21	11	175	2	.12	4	.14	.06	.65	.14	16	24
0	36	.97	40	18	265	3	.31	4	.23	.06	.73	.19	12	19
0	8	.22	9	4	60	1	.70	1	.05	.01	.17	.04	3	4
0	35	.70	35	15	305	3	.25	10	.24	.05	.71	.19	12	24
0	8	.16	8	4	71	1	.06	2	.06	.01	.17	.04	3	6
0	43	.65	34	20	335	3	.28	1	.14	.06	.64	.24	58	27[40]
0	4	.89	55	50	739	6	.21	167[42]	.08	.08	1.02	.44	33	27
0	3	.89	49	43	716	8	.2	140	.07	.08	1.16	.37	40	17
0	3	.07	4	7	114	<1	.07	21	.03	.06	.33	.05	3	6
0	1	.03	2	3	48	<1	.03	9	.01	.03	.14	.02	<1	3
0	23	2.17	13	34	235	49	.18	67	.04	.1	.75	.07	6	1
0	10	.92	6	14	100	21	.08	29	.02	.04	.32	.03	3	<1

(38)With added ascorbic acid.

(40)Without added ascorbic acid. If added, contains 96 mg per cup.

(42)Vitamin A values range from 1.5 RE for white-fleshed varieties to 178 RE for yellow-fleshed varieties.

(For purposes of calculations, use "0" for t, <1, <.1, <.01, etc.)

A

Table A–1

Food Composition

Grp	Ref	Food Description	Measure	Wt (g)	H_2O (%)	Ener (cal)	Prot (g)	Carb (g)	Dietary Fiber (g)	Fat (g)	Fat Breakdown (g) Sat	Mono	Poly
		FRUITS and FRUIT JUICES—Con.											
		Plums, without pits—con.											
		Juice pack:											
5	307	Cup	1 c	252	84	146	1	38	6	<.1	t	<.1	t
5	308	Plums	3 ea	95	84	55	<1	14	2	<.1	t	t	t
		Prunes, dried, pitted:											
5	309	Uncooked (10 prunes with pits weigh 97 g):	10 ea	84	32	201	2	53	13[43]	<1	<.1	.3	.1
5	310	Cooked, unsweetened, fruit and liquid (250 g with pits)	1 c	212	70	227	3	60	17	<1	<.1	.3	.1
5	311	Prune juice, bottled or canned	1 c	256	81	181	2	45	3	<.1	t	<.1	t
		Raisins, seedless:											
5	312	Cup, not pressed down	1 c	145	15	435	5	115	10	1	.2	<.1	.2
5	313	One packet, ½ oz	½ oz	14	15	41	1	11	1	<.1	t	t	t
		Raspberries:											
5	314	Raw	1 c	123	87	60	1	14	9	1	t	.1	.4
		Frozen, sweetened											
5	315	10-oz container	10 oz	284	73	293	2	74	15	<1	t	<.1	.3
5	316	Cup, thawed measure	1 c	250	73	255	2	65	14	<1	t	<.1	.2
5	317	Rhubarb, cooked, added sugar	1 c	240	68	279	1	75	5	<1	t	t	.1
		Strawberries:											
5	318	Raw, whole, capped	1 c	149	92	45	1	10	3	1	<.1	.1	.3
		Frozen, sliced, sweetened:											
5	319	10-oz container	10 oz	284	73	273	2	74	6	<1	t	.1	.2
5	320	Cup, thawed measure	1 c	255	73	245	1	66	6	<1	t	.1	.2
		Tangerines, without peel and seeds:											
5	321	Raw (2⅜″ whole)	1 ea	84	88	37	<1	9	2	<1	t	<.1	<.1
5	322	Canned, light syrup, fruit and liquid	1 c	252	83	154	1	41	4	<1	<.1	<.1	.1
5	323	Tangerine juice, canned, sweetened	1 c	249	87	125	1	30	1	<1	<.1	<.1	.1
		Watermelon, raw, without rind and seeds											
5	324	Piece, 1″ thick by 10″ diam (weighs 2 lb with refuse)	1 pce	482[44]	92	152	3	35	2	2	.3	.2	1
5	325	Diced	1 c	160	92	50	1	11	1	1	.1	.1	.4
		BAKED GOODS: BREADS, CAKES, COOKIES, CRACKERS, PIES, PANCAKES, TORTILLAS											
6	326	Bagels, plain, enriched, 3½″ diam	1 ea	68	29	200	7	38	1	2	.3	.5	.7
		Biscuits:											
6	327	From home receipe	1 ea	28	28	100	2	13	1	5	1.2	2	1.3
6	328	From mix	1 ea	28	29	94	2	14	1	3	.8	1.4	.9
6	329	From refrigerated dough	1 ea	20	30	65	1	10	1	2	.6	.9	.6
6	330	Bread crumbs, dry grated (see 364, 365 for soft crumbs)	1 c	100	7	390	13	73	4	5	1.5	1.6	1

(43) Dietary fiber data can vary to a lower value of approximately 8.1g for 10 prunes.
(44) 926 g with rind and seeds.

Key: 1 = BEV 2 = DAIRY 3 = EGGS 4 = FAT/OIL 5 = FRUIT 6 = BAKERY 7 = GRAIN 8 = FISH 9 = BEEF 10 = POULTRY 11 = SAUSAGE 12 = MIXED/FAST 13 = NUTS/SEEDS 14 = SWEETS 15 = VEG/LEG 16 = MISC 22 = SOUP/SAUCE

Chol (mg)	Calc (mg)	Iron (mg)	Magn (mg)	Phos (mg)	Pota (mg)	Sodi (mg)	Zinc (mg)	VT-A (RE)	Thia (mg)	Ribo (mg)	Niac (mg)	V-B6 (mg)	Fola (μg)	VT-C (mg)
0	25	.86	20	38	388	3	.28	254	.06	.15	1.19	.1	8	7
0	10	.32	8	15	147	1	.1	96	.02	.06	.45	.04	3	3
0	43	2.08	38	66	626	3	.45	167	.07	.14	1.65	.22	3	3
0	49	2.35	43	74	708	4	.51	65	.05	.21	1.53	.46	<1	6
0	31	3.02	36	64	707	10	.54	t	.04	.18	2.01	.56	1	11
0	71	3.02	48	140	1089	17	.46	1	.23	.13	1.19	.36	5	5
0	7	.29	5	14	105	2	.04	t	.02	.01	.12	.04	<1	<1
0	27	.7	22	15	187	0	.57	16	.04	.11	1.11	.07	32	31
0	43	1.85	37	48	324	3	.51	17	.05	.13	.65	.1	74	47
0	38	1.62	32	43	285	3	.45	15	.05	.11	1.5	.09	65	41
0	348	.5	30	19	230	2	.19	17	.04	.06	.48	.05	13	8
0	21	.57	16	28	247	2	.19	4	.03	.1	.34	.09	28	85
0	31	1.7	20	37	278	9	.17	7	.05	.14	1.1	.09	47	118
0	28	1.5	18	33	250	8	.15	6	.04	.13	1.02	.08	42	106
0	12	.08	10	8	132	1	.38	77	.09	.02	.13	.06	17	26
0	18	.93	19	25	197	15	.60	212	.13	.11	1.1	.11	34	50
0	45	.5	20	35	443	2	.07	105	.15	.05	.25	.08	8	55
0	38	.82	52	41	560	10	.34	176	.39	.1	.96	.69	10	47
0	13	.27	17	14	186	3	.11	59	.13	.03	.32	.23	3	15
0	29	1.8	14	46	50	245	.35	0	.26	.20	2.4	.03	16	0
t	47	.7	7	36	32	195	.20	3	.08	.08	.8	.01	2	t
t	59	.58	7	129	57	265	.18	4	.12	.11	.85	.01	2	t
1	4	.47	3	79	18	249	.08	0	.08	.05	.67	<.01	1	0
5	122	4.1	31	141	152	736	.50	0	.35	.35	4.8	.02	28	0

(For purposes of calculations, use "0" for t, <1, <.1, <.01, etc.)

A

Table A–1

Food Composition

Grp	Ref	Food Description	Measure	Wt (g)	H_2O (%)	Ener (cal)	Prot (g)	Carb (g)	Dietary Fiber (g)	Fat (g)	Fat Breakdown (g) Sat	Mono	Poly
		BAKED GOODS—Con.											
		Breads:											
6	331	Boston brown bread, canned, 3¼″ slice	1 pce	45	45	95	2	21	2	1	.26	.13	.14
		Cracked wheat bread (¼ cracked-wheat flour, ¾ enr wheat flour):											
6	332	1-lb loaf	1 ea	454	35	1190	42	227	23	16	3.1	4.3	5.7
6	333	Slice (18 per loaf)	1 pce	25	35	65	2	12	1	1	.2	.2	.3
6	334	Slice, toasted	1 pce	21	26	65	2	12	1	1	.2	.2	.3
		French/Vienna bread, enriched:											
6	335	1-lb loaf	1 ea	454	34	1270	43	230	8	18	4	6	6
6	336	French, slice, 5 × 2½ × 1″	1 pce	35	34	100	3	18	1	1	.3	.4	.5
6	337	Vienna, slice 4¾ × 4 × ½″	1 pce	25	34	70	2	13	<1	1	.2	.3	.3
		French toast: see Mixed Dishes, and Fast Foods, 691											
		Italian bread, enriched:											
6	338	1-lb loaf	1 ea	454	32	1255	41	256	5	4	.6	.3	1.6
6	339	Slice, 4½ × 3¼ × ¾″	1 pce	30	32	83	3	17	<1	<1	<.1	t	.1
		Mixed grain bread, enriched:											
6	340	1-lb loaf	1 ea	454	37	1165	45	212	18	17	3	4	7
6	341	Slice (18 per loaf)	1 pce	25	37	65	2	12	1	1	.2	.2	.4
6	342	Slice, toasted	1 pce	23	27	65	2	12	1	1	.2	.2	.4
		Oatmeal bread, enriched:											
6	343	1-lb loaf	1 ea	454	37	1145	38	212	16	20	4	7	8
6	344	Slice (18 per loaf)	1 pce	25	37	65	2	12	1	1	.2	.4	.5
6	345	Slice, toasted	1 pce	23	30	65	2	12	1	1	.2	.4	.5
6	346	Pita pocket bread, enr, 6½″ round	1 ea	60	31	165	6	33	1	1	.1	.1	.4
		Pumpernickel bread (⅔ rye flour, ⅓ enr wheat flour):											
6	347	1-lb loaf	1 ea	454	37	1160	42	218	19	16	3	4	6
6	348	Slice, 5 × 4 × ⅜″	1 pce	32	37	80	3	15	1	1	.2	.3	.5
6	349	Slice, toasted	1 pce	29	28	80	3	15	1	1	.2	.3	.5
		Raisin bread, enriched:											
6	350	1-lb loaf	1 ea	454	33	1260	38	239	12	18	4	7	7
6	351	Slice (18 per loaf)	1 pce	25	33	68	2	13	1	1	.2	.4	.4
6	352	Slice, toasted	1 pce	21	24	68	2	13	1	1	.2	.4	.4
		Rye bread, light (⅓ rye flour, ⅔ enr wheat flour):											
6	353	1-lb loaf	1 ea	454	37	1190	38	218	30	17	3.3	5.2	5.5
6	354	Slice, 4¾ × 3¾ × 7/16″	1 pce	25	37	65	2	12	2	1	.2	.3	.3
6	355	Slice, toasted	1 pce	22	28	65	2	12	2	1	.2	.3	.3
		Wheat bread (blend of enr wheat flour and whole-wheat flour):[45]											
6	356	1-lb loaf	1 ea	454	37	1160	43	213	25	19	3.9	7.3	4.5
6	357	Slice (18 per loaf)	1 pce	25	37	65	2	12	1	1	.2	.4	.3
6	358	Slice, toasted	1 pce	23	28	65	3	12	1	1	.2	.4	.3

[45] A blend of white and whole-wheat flour—no official ratio specified.

A

KEY: 1 = BEV 2 = DAIRY 3 = EGGS 4 = FAT/OIL 5 = FRUIT 6 = BAKERY 7 = GRAIN 8 = FISH 9 = BEEF 10 = POULTRY 11 = SAUSAGE 12 = MIXED/FAST 13 = NUTS/SEEDS 14 = SWEETS 15 = VEG/LEG 16 = MISC 22 = SOUP/SAUCE

Chol (mg)	Calc (mg)	Iron (mg)	Magn (mg)	Phos (mg)	Pota (mg)	Sodi (mg)	Zinc (mg)	VT-A (RE)	Thia (mg)	Ribo (mg)	Niac (mg)	V-B6 (mg)	Fola (µg)	VT-C (mg)
3	41	.90	40	72	131	113	.35	0	.06	.04	.7	.06	8	0
0	295	12.1	218	581	608	1966	6.36	0	1.73	1.73	15.3	.42	218	t
0	16	.67	12	32	34	106	.35	0	.1	.1	.84	.02	12	t
0	16	.67	12	32	34	106	.35	0	.07	.1	.84	.02	9	t
0	499	14	91	386	409	2633	2.9	0	2.09	1.59	18.2	.24	168	t
0	39	1.08	7	30	32	203	.22	0	.16	.12	1.4	.02	13	t
0	28	.77	5	21	23	145	.16	0	.12	.09	1	.01	9	t
							3.1							
0	77	12.7	106	350	336	2656	.2	0	1.86	1.06	15.1	.24	160	0
0	5	.8	7	23	22	176		0	.12	.07	1	.02	11	0
0	472	14.8	222	962	990	1870	5.45	t	1.77	1.73	18.9	.47	295	t
0	27	.8	12	55	56	106	.3	t	.1	.1	1.1	.03	16	t
0	27	.8	12	55	56	106	t	t	.08	.1	1.1	.02	12	t
0	267	12	154	563	707	2231	4.45	0	2.09	1.2	15.4	.07	15	0
0	15	.7	8	31	39	124	.24	0	.12	.07	.85	<.01	<1	0
0	15	.7	8	31	39	124	.24	0	.09	.07	.85	<.01	<1	0
0	49	1.45	16	60	71	339	.47	0	.27	.12	2.21	.02	23	0
0	322	12.4	309	990	1966	2461	5.18	0	1.54	2.36	15	.72	222	0
0	23	.88	22	71	141	177	.4	0	.11	.17	1.06	.05	16	0
0	23	.88	22	71	141	177	.4	0	.09	.17	1.06	.05	12	0
0	463	14.1	114	395	1058	1657	2.81	1	1.5	2.81	18.6	.15	159	t
0	25	.78	6	22	59	92	.15	t	.08	.15	1.02	<.01	9	t
0	25	.80	6	22	59	92	.15	t	.06	.15	1.02	<.01	8	t
0	363	12.3	109	658	926	3164	5.77	0	1.86	1.45	15	.43	177	0
0	20	.68	6	36	51	175	.38	0	.1	.08	.83	.02	10	0
0	20	.68	6	36	51	175	.38	0	.08	.08	.83	.02	8	0
0	572	15.8	209	835	627	2447	4.77	t	2.09	1.45	20.5	.49	204	t
0	32	.87	12	47	35	135	.26	t	.12	.08	1.13	.03	11	t
0	32	.9	12	47	35	135	.26	t	.10	.08	1.2	.02	8	t

(For purposes of calculations, use "0" for t, <1, <.1, <.01, etc.)

A

Table A–1

Food Composition

Grp	Ref	Food Description	Measure	Wt (g)	H_2O (%)	Ener (cal)	Prot (g)	Carb (g)	Dietary Fiber (g)	Fat (g)	Fat Breakdown (g) Sat	Mono	Poly
		BAKED GOODS—Con.											
		Bread—con.											
		White bread, enriched:											
6	359	1-lb loaf	1 ea	454	37	1210	38	222	12	18	5.6	6.5	4.2
6	360	Slice (18 per loaf)	1 pce	25	37	65	2	12	1	1	.3	.4	.2
6	361	Slice, toasted	1 pce	22	28	65	2	12	1	1	.3	.4	.2
6	362	Slice (22 per loaf)	1 pce	20	37	55	2	10	1	1	.3	.3	.2
6	363	Slice, toasted	1 pce	17	28	55	2	10	1	1	.3	.3	.2
		White bread cubes, crumbs:											
6	364	Cubes, soft	1 c	30	37	80	3	15	1	1	.4	.4	.3
6	365	Crumbs, soft	1 c	45	37	120	4	22	1	2	.6	.6	.4
		Whole-wheat bread:											
6	366	1-lb loaf	1 ea	454	38	1110	44	206	51	20	6	7	5
6	367	Slice (16 per loaf)	1 pce	28	38	70	3	13	3	1	.4	.4	.3
6	368	Slice, toasted	1 pce	25	29	70	3	13	3	1	.4	.4	.3
		Bread stuffing, prepared from mix:											
6	369	Dry type	1 c	140	33	500	9	50	1	31	6	13	10
6	370	Moist type, with egg	1 c	203	61	420	9	40	1	26	5	11	8
		Cakes, prepared from mixes:[46]											
		Angel food cake:											
6	371	Whole cake, 9 3/4" diam tube	1 ea	635	38	1510	38	342	3	2	.4	.2	1
6	372	Piece, 1/12 of cake	1 pce	53	38	125	3	29	<1	<1	t	t	.1
6	373	Boston cream pie, 1/8 of cake	1 pce	120	35	260	3	44	<1	8	2.8	3.1	1.5
		Coffee cake:											
6	374	Whole cake, 7 3/4 × 5 1/8 × 1 1/4"	1 ea	430	30	1385	27	225	3	41	12	17	10
6	375	Piece, 1/6 of cake	1 pce	72	30	230	5	38	1	7	2.0	2.8	1.6
		Devil's food with chocolate frosting:											
6	376	Whole cake, 2 layer, 8 or 9" diam	1 ea	1107	24	3755	49	645	5	136	56	51	20
6	377	Piece, 1/16 of cake	1 pce	69	24	235	3	40	<1	8	3.5	3.2	1.2
6	378	Cupcakes, 2 1/2" diam	1 ea	35	24	120	2	20	<1	4	1.8	1.6	.6
		Gingerbread:											
6	379	Whole cake, 8" square	1 ea	570	37	1575	18	291	3	39	10	16	11
6	380	Piece, 1/9 of cake	1 pce	63	37	174	2	32	<1	4	1.1	1.8	1.2
		Yellow, with chocolate frosting, 2 layer:											
6	381	Whole cake, 8 or 9" diam	1 ea	1108	26	3735	45	638	5	125	48	49	22
6	382	Piece, 1/16 of cake	1 pce	69	26	235	3	40	<1	8	3	3.1	1.4
		Cakes from home recipes with enriched flour:											
		Carrot cake, cream cheese frosting:[47]											
6	383	Whole, 9 × 13" cake	1 ea	1536	23	6175	63	775	11	328	66	135	108
6	384	Piece, 1/16 of 9 × 13" sheet cake 2 1/4 × 3 1/4"	1 pce	96	23	385	4	48	1	21	4	8	7
		Fruitcake, dark, 7 1/2" diam tube, 2 1/4" high:[47]											
6	385	Whole cake	1 ea	1361	18	5185	74	783	38	228	48	113	52
6	386	Piece, 1/32 of cake, 2/3" arc	1 pce	43	18	165	2	25	1	7	1.5	3.6	1.6

(46) Excepting angel food cake, cakes were made from mixes containing vegetable shortening, and frostings were made with margarine. All mixes use enriched flour.

(47) Made with vegetable oil.

KEY: 1 = BEV 2 = DAIRY 3 = EGGS 4 = FAT/OIL 5 = FRUIT 6 = BAKERY 7 = GRAIN 8 = FISH 9 = BEEF 10 = POULTRY 11 = SAUSAGE 12 = MIXED/FAST 13 = NUTS/SEEDS 14 = SWEETS 15 = VEG/LEG 16 = MISC 22 = SOUP/SAUCE

Chol (mg)	Calc (mg)	Iron (mg)	Magn (mg)	Phos (mg)	Pota (mg)	Sodi (mg)	Zinc (mg)	VT-A (RE)	Thia (mg)	Ribo (mg)	Niac (mg)	V-B6 (mg)	Fola (µg)	VT-C (mg)
0	572	12.9	95	490	508	2334	2.81	t	2.13	1.41	17	.15	159	t
0	32	.71	5	27	28	129	.15	t	.12	.08	.94	<.01	9	t
0	32	.71	5	27	28	129	.15	t	.09	.08	.94	<.01	9	t
0	25	.57	4	22	22	103	.12	t	.09	.06	.75	<.01	7	t
0	25	.6	4	21	22	103	.12	t	.07	.06	.75	<.01	7	t
0	38	.85	6	32	34	154	.19	t	.14	.09	1.13	.01	10	t
0	57	1.28	9	49	50	231	.28	t	.21	.14	1.69	.01	16	t
0	327	15.5	422	1180	799	2887	7.63	t	1.59	.95	17.4	.85	250	t
0	20	.96	26	74	50	180	.5	t	.1	.06	1.07	.05	16	t
0	20	.96	26	74	50	180	.5	t	.08	.06	1.07	.05	12	t
0	92	2.2	30	136	126	1254	.55	273	.17	.2	2.5	.02	14	0
67	81	2.03	45	134	118	1023	.78	256	.1	.18	1.62	.04	20	t
0	527	2.73	51	1086	845	3226	.81	0	.32	1.27	1.6	.08	51	0
0	44	.23	4	91	71	269	.07	0	.03	.11	.13	<.01	4	0
20	26	.6	11	70	40	225	.23	70	.01	.18	.7	.05	7	0
279	262	7.3	27	748	469	1853	3.7	194	.82	.9	7.7	.12	30	1
47	44	1.22	4	125	78	310	.62	32	.14	.15	1.29	.02	5	t
598	653	22.1	200	1162	1439	2900	7.95	498	1.11	1.66	10	.32	82	1
37	41	1.4	12	72	90	181	.5	31	.07	.1	.6	.02	<1	t
19	21	.7	6	37	46	92	.25	16	.04	.05	.32	.01	3	t
6	513	10.8	41	570	1562	1733	5.52	0	.86	1.03	7.4	.07	36	1
1	57	1.2	4	63	173	192	.61	0	.1	.11	.82	<.01	4	t
576	1008	15.5	72	2017	1208	2515	3.31	465	1.22	1.66	11.1	.45	80	1
36	63	.96	4	126	75	157	.21	29	.08	.1	.69	.03	5	t
1183	707	21	197	998	1720	4470	8.15	246	1.83	1.97	14.7	1.38	243	23
74	44	1.3	12	62	108	279	.51	15	.11	.12	.9	.86	15	1
640	1293	37.6	340	1592	6138	2123	6.8	422	2.41	2.55	17	1.72	54	504
20	41	1.2	11	50	194	67	.21	13	.08	.08	.5	.05	2	16

(For purposes of calculations, use "0" for t, <1, <.1, <.01, etc.)

Table A–1

Food Composition

Grp	Ref	Food Description	Measure	Wt (g)	H_2O (%)	Ener (cal)	Prot (g)	Carb (g)	Dietary Fiber (g)	Fat (g)	Fat Breakdown (g) Sat	Mono	Poly
		BAKED GOODS—Con.											
		Cakes—con.											
		Sheet cake, plain, no frosting:[48]											
6	387	Whole cake, 9″ square	1 ea	777	25	2830	35	434	3	108	30	45	26
6	388	Piece, 1/9 of cake	1 pce	86	25	315	4	48	<1	12	3.3	5	2.8
		Sheet cake, plain, unckd white frosting:[48]											
6	389	Whole cake, 9″ square	1 ea	1096	21	4020	37	694	3	129	42	50	26
6	390	Piece, 1/9 of cake	1 pce	121	21	445	4	77	<1	14	5	6	3
		Pound cake:[49]											
6	391	Loaf, 8 1/2 × 3 1/2 × 3 1/4″	1 ea	514	22	2025	33	265	4	94	21	41	27
6	392	Piece, 1/17 of loaf, 1/2″ slice	1 pce	30	22	120	2	15	<1	5	1.2	2.4	1.6
		Cakes, commercial:											
		Pound cake:											
6	393	Loaf, 8 1/2 × 3 1/2 × 3″	1 ea	500	24	1935	26	257	4	94	52	30	4
6	394	Slice, 1/17 of loaf, 1/2″ slice	1 pce	29	24	110	2	15	<1	5	3.0	1.7	.2
		Snack cakes:											
6	395	Chocolate w/creme filling, 2 small cakes per package	1 ea	28	20	105	1	17	<1	4	1.7	1.5	.6
6	396	Sponge cake w/creme filling, 2 small cakes per package	1 ea	42	19	155	1	27	<1	5	2.3	2.1	.5
		White cake with white frosting, 2-layer cake:											
6	397	Whole cake, 8 or 9″ diam	1 ea	1140	24	4170	43	670	5	148	33	62	42
6	398	Piece, 1/16 of cake	1 pce	71	24	260	3	42	<1	9	2.1	3.8	2.6
		Yellow cake with chocolate frosting, 2-layer:											
6	399	Whole cake, 8 or 9″ diam	1 ea	1108	23	3895	40	620	5	175	92	59	10
6	400	Piece, 1/16 of cake	1 pce	69	23	245	2	39	<1	11	5.7	3.7	.6
		Cheesecake:											
6	401	Whole cake, 9″ diam	1 ea	1110	46	3350	60	317	5	213	120	66	15
6	402	Piece, 1/12 of cake	1 pce	92	46	278	5	26	<1	18	9.9	5.4	1.2
		Cookies made with enriched flour:											
		Brownies with nuts:											
6	403	Commercial with frosting, 1 1/2 × 1 3/4 × 7/8	1 ea	25	13	100	1	16	<1	4	1.6	2	.6
6	404	Home recipe, 1 3/4 × 1 3/4 × 7/8″[47]	1 ea	20	10	95	1	11	<1	6	1.4	2.8	1.2
		Chocolate chip cookies:											
6	405	Commercial, 2 1/4″ diam	4 ea	42	4	180	2	28	<1	9	2.9	3.1	2.6
6	406	Home recipe, 2 1/3″ diam[50]	4 ea	40	3	185	2	26	1	11	3.9	4.3	2
6	407	From refrigerated dough, 2 1/4″ diam	4 ea	48	5	225	2	32	<1	11	4	4.4	2

(47)Made with vegetable oil.
(48)Cakes made with vegetable shortening; frosting with margarine.
(49)Made with margarine.
(50)Made with vegetable shortening.

KEY: 1 = BEV 2 = DAIRY 3 = EGGS 4 = FAT/OIL 5 = FRUIT 6 = BAKERY 7 = GRAIN 8 = FISH 9 = BEEF 10 = POULTRY
11 = SAUSAGE 12 = MIXED/FAST 13 = NUTS/SEEDS 14 = SWEETS 15 = VEG/LEG 16 = MISC 22 = SOUP/SAUCE

Chol (mg)	Calc (mg)	Iron (mg)	Magn (mg)	Phos (mg)	Pota (mg)	Sodi (mg)	Zinc (mg)	VT-A (RE)	Thia (mg)	Ribo (mg)	Niac (mg)	V-B6 (mg)	Fola (μg)	VT-C (mg)
552	497	11.7	56	793	614	2331	2.75	373	1.24	1.4	10.1	.26	54	2
61	55	1.3	6	88	68	258	.31	41	.14	.15	1.1	.03	15	t
636	548	11	56	822	669	2488	2.90	647	1.21	1.42	9.9	.27	110	2
70	61	1.2	6	91	74	275	.32	71	.13	.16	1.1	.03	12	t
555	339	9.3	48	473	483	1645	2.69	1033	.93	1.08	7.8	.39	55	1
32	20	.5	3	28	28	97	.16	60	.05	.06	.5	.02	3	t
1100	146	9.3	48	517	443	1857	1.95	715	.96	1.12	8.1	.38	55	1
64	8	.5	3	30	26	108	.11	41	.06	.06	.5	.02	3	t
15	21	1	2	26	34	105	.17	4	.06	.09	.7	.01	3	0
7	14	.6	3	44	37	155	.21	9	.07	.06	.6	.02	4	0
46	536	15.5	60	1585	832	2827	1.77	194	3.19	2.05	27.6	.16	64	0
3	33	1	4	99	52	176	.11	12	.2	.13	1.7	.01	4	0
609	366	19.9	72	1884	1972	3080	3.3	488	.78	2.22	10	.45	80	0
38	23	1.24	4	117	123	192	.21	30	.05	.14	.62	.03	5	0
2053	622	5.33	111	977	1088	2464	4.66	833	.33	1.44	5.11	.71	200	56
170	52	.44	9	81	90	204	.39	69	.03	.12	.42	.06	17	5
14	13	.6	14	26	50	59	.36	18	.08	.07	.33	.04	5	t
18	9	.4	11	26	35	51	.31	6	.05	.05	.3	.04	4	t
5	16	.8	9	41	56	140	.3	15	.1	.23	.9	.02	4	t
18	13	1	14	34	82	82	.22	5	.06	.06	.58	.03	4	0
22	13	1.04	10	34	62	173	.24	8	.06	.1	.89	<.01	4	0

(For purposes of calculations, use "0" for t, <1, <.1, <.01, etc.)

A

Table A–1

Food Composition

Grp	Ref	Food Description	Measure	Wt (g)	H_2O (%)	Ener (cal)	Prot (g)	Carb (g)	Dietary Fiber (g)	Fat (g)	Fat Breakdown (g) Sat	Mono	Poly
BAKED GOODS—Con.													
		Cookies—con.											
6	408	Fig bars	4 ea	56	12	210	2	42	1	4	1	1.5	1
6	409	Oatmeal raisin cookies, 2 5/8" diam	4 ea	52	4	245	3	36	<1	10	2.5	4.5	2.8
6	410	Peanut butter cookies, home recipe, 2 5/8" diam[50]	4 ea	48	3	245	4	28	1	14	4	5.8	2.8
6	411	Sandwich-type cookies, all	4 ea	40	2	195	2	29	<1	8	2	3.6	2.2
		Shortbread cookies:											
6	412	Commercial, small	4 ea	32	6	155	2	20	<1	8	2.9	3	1.1
6	413	From home recipe, large[49]	2 ea	28	3	145	2	17	<1	8	1.3	2.7	3.4
6	414	Sugar cookies from refrigerated dough, 2 1/2" diam	4 ea	48	4	235	2	31	<1	12	2.3	5	3.6
6	415	Vanilla wafers	10 ea	40	4	185	2	29	<1	7	1.8	3	1.8
6	416	Corn chips	1 oz	28	1	155	2	16	<1	9	1.4	2.4	3.7
		Crackers:[53]											
6	417	Cheese crackers	10 ea	10	4	50	1	6	<1	3	.9	1.2	.3
6	418	Cheese crackers with peanut butter	4 ea	30	3	150	4	19	<1	7	1.6	3.2	1.2
6	419	Graham crackers	2 ea	14	4	60	1	11	1	2	.4	.6	.4
6	420	Melba toast, plain	1 pce	5	4	20	1	4	<1	<1	.1	.1	.1
6	421	Rye wafers, whole grain	2 ea	14	5	55	1	10	1	1	.3	.4	.3
6	422	Saltine crackers[54]	4 ea	12	4	50	1	9	<1	1	.5	.4	.2
6	423	Snack-type crackers, round	3 ea	9	3	45	1	6	<1	3	.6	1.2	.3
6	424	Wheat crackers, thin	4 ea	8	3	35	1	5	<1	1	.5	.5	.4
6	425	Whole-wheat wafers	2 ea	8	4	35	1	5	<1	2	.5	.6	.4
6	426	Croissants, 4 1/2 × 4 × 1 3/4"	1 ea	57	22	235	5	27	<1	12	3.5	6.7	1.4
		Danish pastry:											
6	427	Packaged ring, plain, 12 oz	1 ea	340	27	1305	21	152	3	71	22	29	16
6	428	Round piece, plain, 4 1/4" diam 1" high	1 ea	57	27	220	4	26	<1	12	3.6	4.8	2.6
6	429	Ounce, plain	1 oz	28	28	110	2	13	<1	6	1.8	2.4	1.3
6	430	Round piece with fruit	1 pce	65	30	235	4	28	1	13	3.9	5.2	2.9
		Doughnuts:											
6	431	Cake type, plain, 3 1/4" diam	1 ea	50	21	210	3	24	<1	12	2.8	5	3
6	432	Yeast-leavened, glazed, 3 3/4" diam	1 ea	60	27	235	4	26	<1	13	5.2	5.5	.9
		English muffins:											
6	433	Plain, enriched	1 ea	57	42	140	4	26	2	1	.3	.2	.3
6	434	Toasted	1 ea	50	29	140	4	26	2	1	.3	.2	.3
		Muffins, 2 1/2" diam, 1 1/2" high											
		From home recipe:											
6	435	Blueberry[50]	1 ea	45	37	135	3	20	1	5	1.5	2.1	1.2
6	436	Bran[47]	1 ea	45	35	125	3	19	2	6	1.4	1.6	2.3
6	437	Cornmeal	1 ea	45	33	145	3	21	2	5	1.5	2.2	1.4
		From commercial mix:											
6	438	Blueberry	1 ea	45	33	140	3	22	1	5	1.4	2	1.2
6	439	Bran	1 ea	45	28	140	3	24	2	4	1.3	1.6	1
6	440	Cornmeal	1 ea	45	30	145	3	22	2	6	1.7	2.3	1.4

(47)Made with vegetable oil.

(49)Made with margarine.

(50)Made with vegetable shortening.

(53)Crackers made with enriched flour except for rye wafers and whole-wheat wafers.

(54)Made with lard.

KEY: 1 = BEV 2 = DAIRY 3 = EGGS 4 = FAT/ OIL 5 = FRUIT 6 = BAKERY 7 = GRAIN 8 = FISH 9 = BEEF 10 = POULTRY 11 = SAUSAGE 12 = MIXED/FAST 13 = NUTS/SEEDS 14 = SWEETS 15 = VEG/LEG 16 = MISC 22 = SOUP/SAUCE

Chol (mg)	Calc (mg)	Iron (mg)	Magn (mg)	Phos (mg)	Pota (mg)	Sodi (mg)	Zinc (mg)	VT-A (RE)	Thia (mg)	Ribo (mg)	Niac (mg)	V-B6 (mg)	Fola (μg)	VT-C (mg)
27	40	1.36	15	34	162	180	.36	6	.08	.07	.73	.07	4	t
2	18	1.1	26	58	90	148	.53	12	.09	.08	1	.03	6	0
22	21	1.1	19	60	110	142	.36	5	.07	.07	1.9	.04	12	0
0	12	1.4	20	40	66	189	.12	0	.09	.07	.8	.01	1	0
27	13	.8	4	39	38	123	.15	8	.1	.09	.9	.01	3	0
0	6	.55	4	31	18	125	.13	89	.08	.06	.71	<.01	2	t
29	50	.9	8	91	33	261	.24	11	.09	.06	1.1	.02	4	0
25	16	.8	6	36	50	150	.12	14	.07	.1	1	.01	4	0
0	35	.5	19	52	52	233	.42	11	.04	.05	.4	.04[51]	3[52]	1
6	11	.3	2	17	17	112	.1	5	.05	.04	.4	.01	—	0
4	26	1.2	2	94	64	338	.06	2	.16	.12	2.4	.03	—	0
0	6	.37	5	20	36	86	.11	0	.02	.03	.6	.01	2	0
0	6	.1	—	10	11	44	—	0	.01	.01	.1	.01	—	0
0	7	.5	16	44	65	115	1.6	0	.06	.03	.5	.03	10	0
4	3	.5	3	12	17	165	.07	0	.06	.05	.6	<.01	2	0
0	9	.3	2	18	12	90	.05	t	.03	.03	.3	<.01	1	0
0	3	.3	7[55]	15	17	69	.24[55]	t	.04	.03	.4	.01	3[55]	0
0	3	.2	7[55]	22	31	59	.24	0	.02	.03	.4	.01	3[55]	0
13	20	2.1	6	64	68	452	.32	13	.17	.13	1.3	.03	18	0
292	360	6.5	68	347	316	1302	2.86	99	.95	1.02	8.5	.12	84	t
49	60	1.1	11	58	53	218	.48	17	.16	.17	1.4	.02	14	t
24	30	.55	6	29	27	109	.24	8	.08	.09	.7	.01	7	t
56	17	1.3	13	80	57	233	.55	11	.16	.14	1.4	.02	16	t
20	22	.8	12	111	58	192	.25	5	.12	.12	1.1	.02	4	t
21	17	1.4	12	55	64	222	.3	t	.28	.12	1.8	.28	13	0
0	96	1.7	11	67	331	378	.41	0	.26	.18	2.14	.02	18	0
0	96	1.7	11	67	331	378	.41	0	.23	.18	2.14	.02	15	0
19	54	.9	11	46	47	198	.29	9	.1	.11	.9	<.01	12	1
24	60	1.4	11	125	99	189	.37	30	.11	.13	1.3	.01	9	3
23	66	.9	13	59	57	169	.34	15	.11	.11	.9	.04	5	t
45	15	.9	5	90	54	225	.23	11	.11	.13	1.17	<.01	14	<1
28	27	1.7	4	182	50	385	.95	14	.08	.12	1.9	.12	19	0
42	30	1.3	13	128	31	291	.34	16	.09	.09	.8	.04	5	t

(51) B_6 values vary from 0 to .04 g between various brands—check label.

(52) Folacin values estimated and derived from values for cornmeal and corn tortillas.

(55) Values derived from whole-wheat recipes and retention values.

(For purposes of calculations, use "0" for t, <1, <.1, <.01, etc.)

A

Table A–1

Food Composition

Grp	Ref	Food Description	Measure	Wt (g)	H_2O (%)	Ener (cal)	Prot (g)	Carb (g)	Dietary Fiber (g)	Fat (g)	Fat Breakdown (g) Sat	Mono	Poly
		BAKED GOODS—Con.											
		Pancakes, 4″ diam:											
6	441	Buckwheat, from mix; egg and milk added	1 ea	27	58	55	2	6	1	2	.9	.9	.5
6	442	Plain, from home recipe	1 ea	27	50	60	2	9	1	2	.5	.8	.5
6	443	Plain, from mix; egg, milk, oil added	1 ea	27	54	60	2	8	1	2	.5	.9	.5
		Piecrust, with enriched flour, baked:[50]											
6	444	Home recipe, 9″ shell	1 ea	180	15	900	11	79	4	60	15	26	16
		From mix:											
6	445	Piecrust for 2-crust pie	1 ea	320	19	1485	20	141	6	93	23	41	25
6	446	1 pie shell	1 ea	180	19	835	11	79	4	52	13	23	14
		Pies, 9″ diam; pie crust made with veg shortening, enriched flour:											
		Apple pie:[56]											
6	447	Whole pie	1 ea	945	48	2420	22	360	19	105	25	46	29
6	448	Piece, 1/6 of pie	1 pce	158	48	405	4	60	3	18	4.1	7.6	4.9
		Banana cream pie:[57]											
6	449	Whole pie	1 ea	1190	66	1917	38	283	10	77	27	29	15
6	450	1/6 of pie	1 pce	198	66	320	6	47	2	13	4.5	4.9	2.5
		Blueberry pie:[56]											
6	451	Whole pie	1 ea	945	51	2285	23	330	22	102	24	45	28
6	452	Piece, 1/6 of pie	1 pce	158	51	380	4	55	4	17	4.0	7.5	4.7
		Cherry pie:[56]											
6	453	Whole pie	1 ea	945	47	2465	26	363	15	107	25	47	30
6	454	Piece, 1/6 of pie	1 pce	158	47	410	4	61	2	18	4.2	7.8	4.9
		Chocolate cream pie:[58]											
6	455	Whole pie	1 ea	1051	63	1864	42	255	4	76	27	30	15
6	456	Piece, 1/6 of pie	1 pce	175	63	311	7	43	1	13	4.5	5.0	2.5
		Custard pie:											
6	457	Whole pie	1 ea	910	58	1760	46	204	4	85	28	35	17
6	458	Piece, 1/6 of pie	1 pce	152	58	293	8	34	1	14	.9	5.8	2.8
		Lemon meringue pie:[56]											
6	459	Whole Pie	1 ea	840	47	2140	31	317	5	86	21	37	22
6	460	Piece, 1/6 of pie	1 pce	140	47	355	5	53	1	14	3.5	6.2	3.7
		Peach pie:[56]											
6	461	Whole pie	1 ea	945	48	2410	24	361	17	105	25	46	29
6	462	Piece, 1/6 of pie	1 pce	158	48	405	4	61	3	17	4.1	7.7	4.8
		Pecan pie:[56]											
6	463	Whole pie	1 ea	825	20	3500	38	551	10	142	24	75	34
6	464	Piece, 1/6 of pie	1 pce	138	20	583	6	92	2	24	3.9	13	5.7
		Pumpkin pie:[56]											
6	465	Whole Pie	1 ea	910	59	2250	54	308	15	94	34	37	17
6	466	Piece, 1/6 of pie	1 pce	152	59	375	9	51	3	16	5.7	6.1	2.8

(50)Made with vegetable shortening.

(56)Recipes updated for latest USDA values for fruits/nuts/fruit juice.

(57)Recipe based on pie crust, cooked vanilla pudding, 2 bananas.

(58)Based on value for pie crust, cooked chocolate pudding with meringue.

KEY: 1 = BEV 2 = DAIRY 3 = EGGS 4 = FAT/OIL 5 = FRUIT 6 = BAKERY 7 = GRAIN 8 = FISH 9 = BEEF 10 = POULTRY 11 = SAUSAGE 12 = MIXED/FAST 13 = NUTS/SEEDS 14 = SWEETS 15 = VEG/LEG 16 = MISC 22 = SOUP/SAUCE

Chol (mg)	Calc (mg)	Iron (mg)	Magn (mg)	Phos (mg)	Pota (mg)	Sodi (mg)	Zinc (mg)	VT-A (RE)	Thia (mg)	Ribo (mg)	Niac (mg)	V-B6 (mg)	Fola (µg)	VT-C (mg)
20	59	.4	18	91	66	125	.5	17	.04	.05	.2	.06	6	t
16	27	.5	4	38	33	115	.21	10	.06	.07	.5	.02	4	t
16	36	.7	4	71	43	160	.22	7	.09	.12	.8	.01	3	t
0	25	4.5	31	90	90	1100	1.5	0	.54	.4	5	.17	32	0
0	131	9.3	44	272	179	2600	1.19	0	1.07	.79	9.89	.27	57	0
0	74	5.23	25	153	101	1462	.79	0	.6	.44	5.57	.15	32	0
0	170	10	61	300	600	2844	1.6	177	1.04	.76	9.5	.5	48	2
0	28	1.67	10	50	100	476	.27	30	.17	.13	1.6	.08	8	t
90	880	6.54	186	810	2006	2532	4.05	222	.9	1.75	7.41	1.61	104	20
15	147	1.09	31	135	334	422	.68	37	.15	.29	1.24	.27	17	3
0	155	12.3	60	274	756	2533	1.68	188	1.04	.85	10.4	.43	84	36
0	26	2.1	10	46	126	423	.28	31	.17	.14	1.73	.07	14	6
0	220	19	91	350	920	2873	1.87	685	1.13	.85	9.5	.5	93	5
0	37	3.17	15	58	153	480	.31	114	.19	.14	1.58	.08	16	1
90	958	7.66	176	881	1332	2565	4.34	204	.81	1.83	6.22	.48	73	3
15	160	1.28	29	147	222	428	.72	34	.14	.3	1.04	.08	12	<1
888	742	8.64	110	880	1040	2000	4.75	386	.82	1.6	5.5	.51	91	1
148	124	1.44	18	147	173	333	.79	64	.14	.27	.92	.08	15	t
822	150	8.4	54	412	420	2369	3.06	438	.59	.84	5	.3	78	25
137	25	1.4	9	69	70	395	.51	73	.1	.14	.83	.05	13	4
0	160	11.3	98	332	1408	2533	2.11	555	1.04	.93	13.9	.39	72	28
0	27	1.9	16	55	235	423	.35	93	.17	.15	2.30	.07	12	5
822	210	12	192	777	781	1823	8.8	250	1.63	.99	6.6	.51	110	0
137	35	2	32	130	130	304	1.47	42	.27	.17	1.1	.09	18	0
655	1200	15	220	1260	2400	1947	5.75	11169[59]	.82	1.76	7.3	.68	117	6
109	200	2.5	37	210	400	325	.96	1861[59]	.14	.29	1.22	.11	20	1

(59)Latest USDA values of Vitamin A for canned pumpkin are almost 3.5 times greater than previously published values. Canned pumpkin is usually a blend of pumpkin and winter squash.

(For purposes of calculations, use "0" for t, <1, <.1, <.01, etc.)

Table A–1

Food Composition

Grp	Ref	Food Description	Measure	Wt (g)	H_2O (%)	Ener (cal)	Prot (g)	Carb (g)	Dietary Fiber (g)	Fat (g)	Fat Breakdown (g) Sat	Mono	Poly
		BAKED GOODS—Con.											
		Pies, fried, commercial:											
6	467	Apple	1 ea	85	43	255	2	32	2	14	5.8	6.6	.6
6	468	Cherry	1 ea	85	43	250	2	32	1	14	5.8	6.7	.6
		Pretzels, made with enriched flour:											
6	469	Thin sticks, 2¼″ long	10 ea	3	2	10	<1	2	<1	<1	t	<.1	<.1
6	470	Dutch twists, 2¾ × 2⅝″	1 ea	16	2	65	2	13	<1	1	.1	.2	.2
6	471	Thin twists, 3¼ × 2¼ × ¼″	10 ea	60	3	240	6	48	1	2	.4	.8	.6
		Rolls and buns, enriched:											
		Commercial:											
6	472	Cloverleaf rolls, 2½″ diam, 2″ high	1 ea	28	32	85	2	14	1	2	.5	.8	.6
6	473	Hotdog buns	1 ea	40	34	115	3	20	1	2	.5	.8	.6
6	474	Hamburger buns	1 ea	45	34	129	4	23	1	2	.6	.9	.7
6	475	Hard rolls, white, 3¾″ diam, 2″ high	1 ea	50	25	155	5	30	1	2	.4	.5	.6
6	476	Submarine rolls or hoagies, 11½ × 3 × 2½	1 ea	135	31	400	11	72	2	8	1.8	3	2.2
		From home recipe:											
6	477	Dinner rolls 2½″ diam, 2″ high	1 ea	35	26	120	3	20	1	3	.8	1.2	.9
6	478	Toaster pastries, fortified	1 ea	54	13	210	2	38	1	6	1.7	3.6	.4
		Tortillas:											
6	479	Corn, enriched, 6″ diam	1 ea	30	45	65	2	13	1	1	.1	.3	.6
6	480	Flour, 8″ diam	1 ea	35	27	105	3	19	1	3	.4	1.2	1.0
6	481	Taco shells	1 ea	11	4	48	1	8	1	2	.2	.6	1.2
		Waffles, 7″ diam:											
6	482	From home recipe	1 ea	75	37	245	7	26	2	13	4	4.9	2.6
6	483	From mix, egg/milk added	1 ea	75	42	205	7	27	2	8	2.7	2.9	1.5
		GRAIN PRODUCTS: CEREALS, FLOUR, GRAINS, PASTA and NOODLES, POPCORN											
		Barley, pearled:											
7	484	Dry, uncooked	1 c	200	11	700	16	158	16	2	.3	.2	.9
7	485	Cooked	1 c	200	72	196	5	44	4	1	.1	.1	.3
		Breakfast cereals, hot, cooked:											
		Corn grits (hominy) cooked:											
7	486	Yellow, enriched, regular and quick prepared	1 c	242	85	146	3	31	1	<1	t	.1	.2
7	487	White, instant, prepared from packet	1 ea	137	85	80	2	18	<1	<1	t	.1	.1
		Cream of Wheat®, cooked:											
7	488	Regular, quick, instant	1 c	244	86	140	4	29	1	1	.1	.1	.2
7	489	Mix and eat, plain, packet	1 ea	142	82	100	3	21	<1	<1	.1	.1	.1
7	490	Malt-O-Meal® cereal, cooked	1 c	240	88	122	4	26	1	<1	t	t	.1

KEY: 1 = BEV 2 = DAIRY 3 = EGGS 4 = FAT/OIL 5 = FRUIT 6 = BAKERY 7 = GRAIN 8 = FISH 9 = BEEF 10 = POULTRY 11 = SAUSAGE 12 = MIXED/FAST 13 = NUTS/SEEDS 14 = SWEETS 15 = VEG/LEG 16 = MISC 22 = SOUP/SAUCE

Chol (mg)	Calc (mg)	Iron (mg)	Magn (mg)	Phos (mg)	Pota (mg)	Sodi (mg)	Zinc (mg)	VT-A (RE)	Thia (mg)	Ribo (mg)	Niac (mg)	V-B6 (mg)	Fola (μg)	VT-C (mg)
14	12	.94	6	34	42	326	.14	3	.09	.06	1	.03	4	1
13	11	.7	7	41	61	371	.15	19	.06	.06	.6	.04	8	1
0	1	.06	<1	3	3	48	.03	0	<.01	<.01	.13	<.01	<1	0
0	4	.32	4	15	16	258	.17	0	.05	.04	.7	<.01	3	0
0	16	1.2	15	55	61	966	.42	0	.19	.15	2.6	.01	10	0
t	33	.81	6	44	36	155	.22	t	.14	.09	1.1	.01	11	t
0	54	1.19	8	44	56	241	.36	t	.2	.13	1.58	.01	15	t
0	61	1.34	9	49	63	271	.41	t	.22	.15	1.78	.02	17	t
0	24	1.4	14	46	49	313	.44	0	.2	.12	1.7	.02	17	0
0	100	3.8	31	115	128	683	1.17	0	.54	.33	4.5	.09	49	0
12	16	1.1	10	36	41	98	.32	8	.12	.12	1.2	.01	12	0
0	104	2.16	10	104	91	248	.31	100[60]	.17	.18	2.27	.2	43	4
0	42	.6	18	55	43	1	.36	8	.05	.03	.4	.09	6	0
0	21	.55	13	59	35	134	.27	0	.13	.08	1.2	.01	16	0
0	21	.21	9	27	20	50	.17	4	<.01	.01	.2	.02	2	0
102	154	1.5	11	135	129	445	.61	39	.18	.24	1.5	.03	13	t
59	179	1.2	11	257	146	515	.52	49	.14	.23	.9	.03	4	t
0	32	4.2	51	378	320	6	4.47	0	.24	.1	7.9	.45	40	0
0	6	1.17	12	112	72	2	1.15	0	.05	.02	1.7	.09	10	0
0	1	1.55[61]	11	29	54	0[62]	.17	15[63]	.24[61]	.15[61]	1.96[61]	.06	2	0
0	7	1[61]	5	16	29	343	.08	0	.18[61]	.08[61]	1.3[61]	.03	1	0
0	54[64]	10.9[64]	12	43[65]	46	5[65 66]	.35	0	.24[64]	.07[64]	1.5[64]	.02	9	0
0	20[64]	8.10[64]	7	20[64]	38	241	.20	376[64]	.43[64]	.28[64]	5[64]	.01	5	0
0	5	9.6[64]	14	24[64]	31	2[66]	.17	0	.48[64]	.24[64]	5.8[64]	.02	5	0

(60)Vitamin A values from label declaration varies from 100 to 150 RE for major brands.

(61)Nutrient added.

(62)Cooked without salt. If salt is added according to label recommendation, sodium content is 540 mg.

(63)Value for yellow corn grits; cooked white corn grits contain 0 RE of Vitamin A.

(64)Nutrient added–value based on label declaration.

(65)For regular and instant cereal. For quick cereal, phosphorus is 102 mg, and sodium is 142 mg.

(66)Cooked without salt. If added according to label recommendations, sodium content is 390 mg for Cream of Wheat; 324 mg for Malt-O-Meal; 374 mg for oatmeal.

(For purposes of calculations, use "0" for t, <1, <.1, <.01, etc.)

Table A–1

Food Composition

Grp	Ref	Food Description	Measure	Wt (g)	H_2O (%)	Ener (cal)	Prot (g)	Carb (g)	Dietary Fiber (g)	Fat (g)	Fat Breakdown (g) Sat	Mono	Poly
GRAIN PRODUCTS—Con.													
		Oatmeal or rolled oats, cooked:											
7	491	Regular, quick, instant, nonfortified	1 c	234	85	145	6	25	9	2	.4	.8	1
		Instant, fortified:											
7	492	Plain, from packet	¾ c	177	86	104	4	18	7	2	.3	.6	.7
7	493	Flavored, from packet	¾ c	164	76	160	5	31	6	2	.3	.7	.8
7	494	Whole-wheat cereal, cooked	1 c	245	88	110	4	23	6	1	.1	.1	.3
		Breakfast cereals, ready to eat:											
7	495	All-Bran®	⅓ c	28	3	70	4	21	8	<1	.1	.1	.3
7	496	Cap'n Crunch®	1 c	37	2	156	2	30	1	3	2.2	.4	.5
7	497	Cheerios®	1 c	23	5	89	3	16	1	1	.3	.5	.6
7	498	Corn Flakes, Kellogg's®	1¼ c	28	3	110	2	24	<1	<.1	t	t	.1
7	499	Corn Flakes, Post Toasties®	1¼ c	28	3	110	2	24	<1	<.1	t	t	.1
7	500	40% Bran Flakes, Kellogg's®	1 c	39	3	125	5	30	6	1	.14	.14	.4
7	501	40% Bran Flakes, Post®	1 c	47	3	152	5	37	6	1	.2	.2	.3
7	502	Froot Loops®	1 c	28	2	111	2	25	<1	1	.2	.1	.1
7	503	Golden Grahams®	1 c	39	2	150	2	33	1	1	1.0	.1	.2
7	504	Granola, homemade	1 c	122	3	595	15	67	8	33	5.8	9.4	17
7	505	Grape Nuts®	½ c	57	3	202	7	26	3	<1	t	t	.2
7	506	Honey Nut Cheerios®	1 c	33	3	125	4	26	1	1	.1	.3	.3
7	507	Lucky Charms®	1 c	32	3	125	3	26	1	1	.2	.4	.5
7	508	Nature Valley® Granola	1 c	113	4	503	12	76	7	20	13	2.8	2.8
7	509	100% Natural® cereal, plain	¼ c	28	2	135	3	18	2	6	4.1	1.2	.5
7	510	Product 19®	1 c	33	3	126	3	27	<1	<1	t	t	.1
7	511	Raisin Bran, Kellogg's®	1 c	49	8	211	5	53	6	2	.2	.2	.5
7	512	Raisin Bran, Post®	1 c	56	9	174	5	43	6	1	.2	.2	.4
7	513	Rice Krispies, Kellogg's®	1 c	29	2	112	2	25	<1	<1	t	t	.1
7	514	Puffed Rice®	1 c	14	3	56	1	13	<1	<1	t	t	<.1
7	515	Shredded Wheat®	¾ c	32	5	115	3	25	4	1	.1	.1	.3
7	516	Special K®	1½ c	32	2	125	6	24	<1	<1	t	t	t
7	517	Super Sugar Crisp®	1 c	33	2	123	2	30	1	<1	t	t	.1
7	518	Sugar Frosted Flakes ®	1 c	35	3	133	2	32	<1	<1	t	t	t
7	519	Sugar Smacks®	¾ c	28	3	106	2	25	<1	<1	.1	.1	.2
7	520	Total®	1 c	33	4	116	3	26	2	1	.1	.1	.4
7	521	Trix®	1 c	28	2	108	2	25	<1	<1	.2	.1	.1
7	522	Wheaties®	1 c	29	5	101	3	23	3	<1	.1	.1	.2
		Buckwheat:											
		Flour:											
7	523	Dark	1 c	98	12	338	11	71	8	3	.5	.8	.9
7	524	Light	1 c	98	12	340	6	78	6	1	.2	.4	.4
7	525	Whole grain, dry	1 c	175	11	586	20	128	16	4	.8	1.4	1.5
		Bulgar:											
7	526	Dry, uncooked	1 c	170	10	600	19	129	16	3	1.2	.3	1.2
7	527	Cooked	1 c	135	56	246	10	44	7	1	.4	.1	.4

A

KEY: 1 = BEV 2 = DAIRY 3 = EGGS 4 = FAT/OIL 5 = FRUIT 6 = BAKERY 7 = GRAIN 8 = FISH 9 = BEEF 10 = POULTRY 11 = SAUSAGE 12 = MIXED/FAST 13 = NUTS/SEEDS 14 = SWEETS 15 = VEG/LEG 16 = MISC 22 = SOUP/SAUCE

Chol (mg)	Calc (mg)	Iron (mg)	Magn (mg)	Phos (mg)	Pota (mg)	Sodi (mg)	Zinc (mg)	VT-A (RE)	Thia (mg)	Ribo (mg)	Niac (mg)	V-B6 (mg)	Fola (µg)	VT-C (mg)
0	20	1.59	56	178	132	1[66]	1.15	4	.26	.05	.3	.05	10	0
0	163[61]	6.32[61]	51	133	99	285[61]	1	453[61]	.53[61]	.29[61]	5.49[61]	.74	150	0
0	168[61]	6.7[61]	51	148	137	254[61]	1	460[61]	.53[61]	.38[61]	5.9[61]	.77	150	t
0	17	1.2	33	127	118	3	1.23	0	.15	.05	1.5	.14	25	0
0	23	4.5[61]	106	264	350	320	3.7	375[61]	.37[61]	.43[61]	5[61]	.5	100	15[61]
0	6	9.83[64]	15	47	48	278	4.01	5[61]	.66[64]	.71[64]	8.64[64]	1	238	0
0	38	3.6[61]	31	109	82	246	.63	304[61]	.32[61]	.32[61]	4[61]	.4	5	12[61]
0	1	1.8[61]	3	18	26	351	.08	375[61]	.37[61]	.42[61]	5[61]	.51	100	15[61]
0	1	.7[61]	3	12	33	297	.08	375[61]	.37[61]	.42[61]	5[61]	.51	100	0
0	19	11.2[61]	71	192	248	363	5.15	522[61]	.51[61]	.59[61]	6.86[61]	.7	138	0
0	21	7.47[61]	102	296	251	431	2.5	629[61]	.62[61]	.72[61]	8.3[61]	.85	166	0
0	3	4.5[61]	7	24	26	145	3.7	375[61]	.4[61]	.4[61]	5[61]	.5	100	15[61]
0	24	6.2[61]	16	56	86	476	.34	516[61]	.5[61]	.6[61]	6.9[61]	.7	—	21[61]
0	76	4.84	141	494	612	12	4.47	4	.73	.31	2.14	.43	99	1
0	22	2.46	38	142	190	394	1.24	753[61]	.8[61]	.8[61]	10[61]	1	200	0
0	23	5.2[61]	39	122	115	299	.87	437[61]	.4[61]	.5[61]	5.8[61]	.6	4	17[61]
0	36	5.1[61]	27	88	66	227	.56	424[61]	.4[61]	.5[61]	5.6[61]	.6	—	17[61]
0	71	3.78	116	354	389	232	2.19	8	.39	.19	.83	.32	85	0
0	49	.83	34	104	138	12	.63	2	.09	.15	.6	.64	8	0
0	4	21[61]	12	47	51	378	.5	1769[61]	1.7[61]	2[61]	23.3[61]	2.3	466	70[61]
0	33	31.6[61]	96	263	404	386	6.6	500[61]	.66[61]	.76[61]	8.78[61]	.87	140	0
0	27	9.01[61]	96	237	349	370	3.01	750[61]	.74[61]	.85[61]	10[61]	1.02	200	0
0	4	1.8[61]	10	34	30	340	.48	388[61]	.4[61]	.4[61]	5[61]	.5	100	15[61]
0	1	.15[61]	4	14	16	<1	.14	0	.01[61]	.01[61]	.42[61]	.01	3	0
0	12	1.35	42	112	115	3	1.05	0	.08	.09	1.67	.08	16	0
0	9	5.06[61]	18	62	55	298	4.16	429[61]	.45[61]	.45[61]	5.63[61]	.56	112	17[61]
0	7	2.1[61]	20	60	123	29	1.7	437[61]	.4[61]	.5[61]	5.8[61]	.6	116	0
0	1	2.2[61]	3	26	22	284	.05	463[61]	.5[61]	.5[61]	6.2[61]	.6	124	19[61]
0	3	1.8[61]	13	31	42	75	.28	375[61]	.37[61]	.43[61]	5[61]	.5	100	15[61]
0	56	21[61]	37	137	123	409	.78	1769[61]	1.7[61]	2[61]	23.3[61]	2.3	466	70[61]
0	6	4.5[61]	6	19	26	179	.13	375[61]	.4[61]	.4[61]	4.9[61]	.5	—	15[61]
0	44	4.6[61]	32	100	108	363	.65	388[61]	.4[61]	.4[61]	5.1[61]	.5	9	15[61]
0	32	2.5	135	298	490	1	2.65	0	.58	.15	2.75	.41	125	0
0	11	1	47	86	314	1	2.56	0	.09	.05	.47	.09	100	0
0	200	6.7	315	494	784	4	4.4	0	1.05	.26	7.7	.37	52	0
0	49	9.5	130	575	389	7	3.2	0	.48	.24	7.7	.38	80	0
0	27	2.87	57	263	151	3	2.81	0	.08	.05	4.1	.07	18	0

(61)Nutrient added.

(64)Nutrient added–value based on label declaration.

(66)Cooked without salt. If added according to label recommendations, sodium content is 390 mg for Cream of Wheat; 324 mg for Malt-O-Meal; 374 mg for oatmeal.

(For purposes of calculations, use "0" for t, <1, <.1, <.01, etc.)

Table A–1

Food Composition

Grp	Ref	Food Description	Measure	Wt (g)	H_2O (%)	Ener (cal)	Prot (g)	Carb (g)	Dietary Fiber (g)	Fat (g)	Fat Breakdown (g) Sat	Mono	Poly
		GRAIN PRODUCTS—Con.											
		Cornmeal:											
7	528	Whole-ground, unbolted, dry	1 c	122	12	435	11	90	9	5	.5	1.1	2.5
7	529	Bolted, nearly whole, dry	1 c	122	12	440	11	91	7	4	.5	1.1	2.5
7	530	Degermed, enriched, dry	1 c	138	12	502	11	108	4	2	.2	.4	.9
7	531	Degermed, enriched, cooked	1 c	240	88	120	3	26	1	<1	.1	.1	.3
		Macaroni, cooked:											
7	532	Firm stage, hot	1 c	130	64	190	6	39	1	1	.1	.1	.3
7	533	Tender stage, cold	1 c	105	72	115	4	24	1	<1	.1	.1	.2
7	534	Tender stage, hot	1 c	140	72	155	5	32	1	1	.1	.1	.2
7	535	Millet, cooked	½ c	95	86	54	1	11	1	<1	.1	.1	.2
		Noodles:											
7	536	Egg noodles, cooked	1 c	160	70	200	7	37	<1	2	.5	.6	.6
7	537	Chow mein, dry	1 c	45	11	220	6	26	<1	11	2.1	7.3	.4
7	538	Spinach noodles, dry	3½ oz	100	10	380	14	71	1	4	1.0	1.1	1.1
		Popcorn:											
7	539	Air popped, plain	1 c	8	4	30	1	6	1	<1	t	.1	.2
7	540	Popped in veg oil/salted	1 c	11	3	55	1	6	1	3	.5	1.4	1.2
7	541	Sugar-syrup coated	1 c	35	4	135	2	30	<1	1	.1	.3	.6
		Rice:											
7	542	Brown rice, cooked	1 c	195	70	232	5	50	4	1	.3	.3	.4
		White, enriched, all types:											
7	543	Raw, dry	1 c	185	12	670	12	149	3	1	.2	.2	.3
7	544	Cooked without salt	1 c	205	73	223	4	50	1	<1	.1	.1	.1
7	545	Instant, prepared without salt	1 c	165	73	180	4	40	<1	<1	.1	.1	.1
		White, parboiled/converted rice:											
7	546	Raw, dry	1 c	185	10	683	14	150	3	1	.2	.2	.4
7	547	Cooked, hot	1 c	175	73	186	4	41	1	<1	t	t	<.1
7	548	Wild rice, cooked	½ c	100	76	92	4	19	3	<1	.1	.1	.1
7	549	Rye flour medium	1 c	115	11	392	13	85	9	2	.4	.5	.9
		Spaghetti, cooked:											
7	550	Firm stage, hot	1 c	130	64	190	6	39	1	1	.1	.1	.3
7	551	Tender stage, hot	1 c	140	72	155	5	32	1	1	.1	.1	.2
7	552	Whole-wheat spaghetti, cooked	1 c	123	67	151	7	32	4	<1	.1	.1	.2
7	553	Wheat bran	½ c	18	12	38	3	11	8	1	.1	.1	.4
		Wheat germ:											
7	554	Raw	1 c	75	12	272	20	35	2	8	1.4	1.2	4.9
7	555	Toasted	1 c	113	4	431	33	56	3	12	2.1	1.8	7.3
7	556	Rolled wheat, cooked	1 c	240	80	142	4	32	5	1	.1	.1	.3
7	557	Whole-grain wheat, cooked	⅓ c	50	86	28	1	6	1	<1	<.1	<.1	.1
		Wheat flour (unbleached):											
		All-purpose white flour, enriched:											
7	558	Sifted	1 c	115	12	419	12	88	3	1	.2	.1	.5
7	559	Unsifted	1 c	125	12	455	13	95	3	1	.2	.1	.6
7	560	Cake or pastry flour, enriched, sifted	1 c	96	12	349	7	76	2	1	.2	.1	.4
7	561	Self-rising, enriched, unsifted	1 c	125	12	440	12	93	3	1	.2	.1	.6
7	562	Whole wheat, from hard wheats	1 c	120	12	400	16	85	15	2	.3	.3	1.1

KEY: 1 = BEV 2 = DAIRY 3 = EGGS 4 = FAT/OIL 5 = FRUIT 6 = BAKERY 7 = GRAIN 8 = FISH 9 = BEEF 10 = POULTRY
11 = SAUSAGE 12 = MIXED/FAST 13 = NUTS/SEEDS 14 = SWEETS 15 = VEG/LEG 16 = MISC 22 = SOUP/SAUCE

A

Chol (mg)	Calc (mg)	Iron (mg)	Magn (mg)	Phos (mg)	Pota (mg)	Sodi (mg)	Zinc (mg)	VT-A (RE)	Thia (mg)	Ribo (mg)	Niac (mg)	V-B6 (mg)	Fola (μg)	VT-C (mg)
0	24	2.2	130	312	346	1	2.15	62	.46	.13	2.4	.57	33	0
0	21	2.2	129	272	303	1	2.15	62	.37	.1	2.3	.56	29	0
0	8	5.93	65	137	166	1	1.15	61	.61	.36	4.8	.34	29	0
0	2	1.48	17	34	38	1	.23	14	.14	.1	1.2	.06	6	0
0	14	2.1	17	85	103	1	.61	0	.23	.13	1.82	.1	4	0
0	8	1.31	12	53	64	1	.39	0	.15	.08	1.13	.07	3	0
0	11	1.74	15	70	85	1	.52	0	.2	.11	1.5	.09	4	0
0	3	1.1	38	47	64	1	.42	0	.1	.06	.4	.03	10	0
50	16	2.6	28	94	70	3	.2	34	.22	.13	1.9	.01	7	0
5	14	.4	—	41	33	450	.1	0	.05	.03	.6	.03	10	0
0	41	4.54	38	154	460	35	2.2	18	.98	.47	6.89	.27	73	0
0	1	.2	23	22	20	<1	.22	1	.03	.01	.2	.02	3	0
0	3	.27	25	31	19	86	.28	2	.01	.02	.1	.02	3	0
0	2	.5	29	47	90	<1	.29	3	.13	.02	.4	.03	3	0
0	23	1.17	72	142	137	0	1.05	0	.18	.04	2.73	.29	10	0
0	44	5.4	63	174	170	9	2.41	0	.81	.06	6.48	.3	18	0
0	21	2.87	23	57	57	0	.84	0	.22	.02	2.05	.1	4	0
0	5	1.32	16	31	0	0[67]	.64	0	.21	.02	1.65	.02	7	0
0	111	5.4	34	370	278	17	2.03	0	.81	.07	6.5	.48	22	0
0	33	1.4	11	100	75	9	.56	0	.19	.02	2.1	.17	7	0
0	5	1.1	33	85	55	2	1.17	0	.11	.16	1.6	1.31	35	0
0	36	2.72	90	340	304	1	1.67	0	.36	.15	2.45	.25	91	0
0	14	2.08	17	85	103	1	.61	0	.23	.13	1.82	.1	9	0
0	11	1.74	15	70	85	1	.52	0	.2	.11	1.5	.09	8	0
0	19	1.06	43	106	200	16	.91	0	.21	.09	1.54	.87	25	0
0	21	1.95	91	223	205	3	2.34	0	.14	.06	4.86	.25	46	0
0	54	4.5	252	838	620	2	11	0	1.51	.51	3.15	.69	246	0
0	50	8.71	362	1294	1070	4	18.9	0	1.89	.93	6.32	1.13	474	0
0	19	1.7	58	182	202	2	1.96	0	.17	.07	2.2	.08	27	0
0	3	.3	12	30	29	1	.44	0	.04	.01	.4	.35	6	0
0	18	5.06	24	100	109	2	.76	0	.73	.46	6.08	.05	18	0
0	20	5.5	26	109	119	3	.82	0	.8	.5	6.61	.05	20	0
0	16	4.22	20	70	91	2	.63	0	.6	.38	5.08	.04	15	0
0	331	5.5	26	583	113	1349	.83	0	.8	.5	6.61	.05	20	0
0	49	5.16	168	446	444	4	2.96	0	.66	.14	5.16	.4	58	0

(67)If prepared with salt according to label recommendation, sodium would be 608 mg.

(For purposes of calculations, use "0" for t, <1, <.1, <.01, etc.)

Table A–1

Food Composition

Grp	Ref	Food Description	Measure	Wt (g)	H_2O (%)	Ener (cal)	Prot (g)	Carb (g)	Dietary Fiber (g)	Fat (g)	Fat Breakdown (g) Sat	Mono	Poly
		MEATS: FISH and SHELLFISH											
		Clams:											
8	563	Raw meat only	3 oz	85	82	63	11	2	t	1	.1	.1	.2
8	564	Canned, drained	3 oz	85	77	126	22	4	t	2	.2	.2	.5
		Cod:											
8	565	Baked with butter	3½ oz	100	75	114	23	0	0	6	3.2	1.5	.5
8	566	Batter fried	3½ oz	100	61	199	20	7	0	10	2.6	4.4	2.9
8	567	Poached, no added fat	3½ oz	100	76	94	21	0	0	1	.2	.1	.6
8	568	Crab meat, canned	1 c	135	76	133	28	1	0	2	.3	.3	.6
8	569	Fish sticks, breaded pollock	2 ea	57	46	155	9	14	t	7	1.8	2.9	1.8
		Flounder/sole, baked with lemon juice:											
8	570	With butter	3 oz	85	73	140	20	t	0	6	3.2	1.5	.5
8	571	With margarine	3 oz	85	73	140	20	t	0	6	1.2	2.3	1.9
8	572	Without added fat	3 oz	85	78	99	21	0	0	1	.3	.3	.4
8	573	Haddock, breaded/fried[68]	3 oz	85	61	175	17	7	<1	9	2.4	3.9	2.4
8	574	Halibut, broiled with butter and lemon juice	3 oz	85	72	140	22	0	0	6	3.3	1.6	.7
8	575	Herring, pickled	3 oz	85	55	223	12	8	0	15	2.0	10	1.4
8	576	Ocean perch, breaded/fried	3 oz	85	59	185	16	7	<1	11	3	5	3
		Oysters:											
		Raw:											
8	577	Eastern	1 c	248	85	170	18	10	0	6	1.6	.6	1.8
8	578	Pacific	1 c	248	82	200	23	12	0	6	1.3	.9	2.2
		Cooked:											
8	579	Eastern, breaded, fried	1 ea	45	65	90	5	5	0	5	1.4	2.1	1.4
8	580	Western, simmered	3½ oz	100	71	135	14	7	0	4	.8	.7	1.5
8	581	Pollock, cooked, dry heat	3 oz	85	74	96	20	0	0	1	.2	.2	.5
		Salmon:											
8	582	Canned pink, solids and liquid	3 oz	85	69	118	17	0	0	5	1.3	1.5	1.7
8	583	Broiled or baked	3 oz	85	62	183	23	0	0	9	1.6	4.5	2.1
8	584	Smoked	3 oz	85	72	100	16	0	0	4	.8	1.7	.9
8	585	Atlantic sardines, canned, drained	3 oz	85	60	177	21	0	0	10	1.3	3.3	4.4
8	586	Scallops, breaded, from frozen	6 ea	93	59	200	17	10	<1	10	2.5	4.2	2.7
		Shrimp:											
8	587	Cooked, boiled, 18 large shrimp	3½ oz	100	77	99	21	0	0	1	.3	.2	.4
8	588	Canned, drained	⅔ c	85	73	102	20	1	0	2	.3	.3	.6
8	589	Fried, 7 medium[71]	3 oz	85	53	206	18	10	<1	10	1.8	3.3	4.3
8	590	Trout, cooked, dry heat	3 oz	85	63	129	22	<1	0	4	.7	1.1	1.3
		Tuna, light, canned, drained solids:											
8	591	Oil pack	3 oz	85	60	169	25	0	0	7	1.3	2.5	2.5
8	592	Water pack	3 oz	85	71	111	25	0	0	<1	.1	.1	.1

(68) Dipped in egg, milk and bread crumbs; fried in vegetable shortening.

(71) Dipped in egg, bread crumbs, and flour; fried in vegetable shortening.

KEY: 1 = BEV 2 = DAIRY 3 = EGGS 4 = FAT/OIL 5 = FRUIT 6 = BAKERY 7 = GRAIN 8 = FISH 9 = BEEF 10 = POULTRY 11 = SAUSAGE 12 = MIXED/FAST 13 = NUTS/SEEDS 14 = SWEETS 15 = VEG/LEG 16 = MISC 22 = SOUP/SAUCE

Chol (mg)	Calc (mg)	Iron (mg)	Magn (mg)	Phos (mg)	Pota (mg)	Sodi (mg)	Zinc (mg)	VT-A (RE)	Thia (mg)	Ribo (mg)	Niac (mg)	V-B6 (mg)	Fola (µg)	VT-C (mg)
29	39	11.9	8	144	267	47	1.16	77	.09	.18	1.5	.07	13	9
57	78	23.8	16	287	534	95	2.32	145	.01	.36	2.85	.07	4	3
60	24	.6	42	140	245	224	.58	20	.09	.08	2.5	.28	11	1
55	80	.5	24	200	370	100	1	t	.02	.02	1.8	.09	3	t
60	29	.5	42	140	245	110	.58	14	.09	.08	2.5	.28	14	t
120	137	1.13	52	351	505	450	5.42	14	.11	.11	1.85	.41	22	0
64	11	.42	14	103	149	332	.38	18	.07	.1	1.2	.03	10	0
68	16	.28	50	187	272	145	.53	54	.07	.1	1.9	.20	10	1
55	16	.28	50	187	273	151	.53	69	.07	.1	1.9	.20	10	1
58	16	.28	50	246	292	89	.53	10	.07	.1	1.9	.20	10	1
75	34	1	26	183	270	123	.85	20	.06	.1	2.9	.13	14	0
45	51	.91	91	242	490	100	.5	150	.06	.08	6.1	.34	6	1
11	65	1.04	8	76	59	740	.45	219	.03	.12	2.8	.11	2	0
66	94	1.2	26	191	241	138	.42	20	.10	.11	2	.22	7	0
136	111	16.6	135	344	568	277	226[69]	223	.34	.41	3.3	.12	25	24
136	20	12.7	55	402	417	263	41.2[69]	223	.17	.58	5	.12	25	72
35	49	3	14	73	64	70	9[69]	44	.07	.1	1.3	.02	2	4
77	75	8.57	31	234	312	165	48[69]	97	.15	.29	2.1	.07	11	15
82	5	.24	31	250	329	98	.51	19	.06	.07	1.4	.06	4	t
37	181[70]	.72	29	279	277	471	.78	14	.02	.16	5.6	.10	13	0
74	6	.47	26	234	319	56	.43	53	2.0	.15	5.7	.19	14	0
20	9	.72	15	139	149	666	.26	22	.02	.09	4.0	.24	2	0
121	325[70]	2.5	33	417	337	429	1.11	57	.07	.19	4.5	.14	10	0
57	39	.76	55	219	310	431	.99	21	.04	.10	1.4	.18	11	0
195	39	3.1	34	137	182	224	1.56	18	.03	.03	2.59	.13	4	t
147	50	2.3	35	198	179	143	1.07	15	.02	.03	2.34	.09	2	0
150	57	1.1	34	185	191	292	1.17	26	.11	.12	2.61	.08	7	0
62	73	2.1	33	272	539	29	1.18	19	.07	.19	2.3	.41	6	3
15	11	1.2	26	265	176	301	.77	20	.03	.09	10.1	.32	5	0
15	10	2.7	26	158	267	303	.77	20	.03	.10	13.2	.32	5	0

[69] Value varies widely.

[70] If bones are discarded, calcium value is greatly reduced.

(For purposes of calculations, use "0" for t, <1, <.1, <.01, etc.)

A

Table A–1

Food Composition

Grp	Ref	Food Description	Measure	Wt (g)	H_2O (%)	Ener (cal)	Prot (g)	Carb (g)	Dietary Fiber (g)	Fat (g)	Fat Breakdown (g) Sat	Mono	Poly
		MEAT and MEAT PRODUCTS											
		Beef, cooked[72]											
		Braised, simmered, pot roasted:											
		Relatively fat, like chuck blade:											
9	593	Lean and fat, piece 2½ × 2½ × ¾″	3 oz	85	43	325	22	0	0	26	11	12	1
9	594	Lean only from #593	2.2 oz	62	53	167	19	0	0	9	3.9	4.2	.3
		Relatively lean, like round:											
9	595	Lean and fat, piece 4⅛ × 2¼ × ¾″	3 oz	85	54	222	25	0	0	13	5	6	1
9	596	Lean only from #595	2.8 oz	78	57	173	25	0	0	8	2.7	3.4	.3
		Ground beef, broiled, patty 3 × ⅝″:											
9	597	Lean	3 oz	85	56	231	21	0	0	16	6	7	1
9	598	Regular	3 oz	85	54	246	20	0	0	18	7	8	1
9	599	Heart, simmered	3 oz	85	64	148	24	<1	0	5	1.4	1.1	1.2
9	600	Liver, fried	3 oz	85	56	185	23	7	0	7	2.4	1.5	1.5
		Roasts, oven cooked, no added liquid:											
		Relatively fat, rib:											
9	601	Lean and fat, piece 4⅛ × 2¼ × ½″	3 oz	85	46	324	19	0	0	27	11	12	1
9	602	Lean only	3 oz	61	58	204	23	0	0	12	5	5	.4
		Relatively lean, round:											
9	603	Lean and fat, piece 2½ × 2½ × ¾″	3 oz	85	57	213	23	0	0	13	5	6	1
9	604	Lean only	3 oz	75	63	162	24	0	0	6	2.3	2.6	.3
		Steak, broiled, sirloin:											
9	605	Lean and fat, piece 2 ½ × 2½ × ¾″	3 oz	85	54	238	22	0	0	16	6.6	7.0	.6
9	606	Lean only	3 oz	72	60	172	24	0	0	8	3.0	3.2	.3
9	607	Beef, canned, corned	3 oz	85	58	213	23	0	0	13	5	5	1
9	608	Beef, dried, cured	2.5 oz	72	57	120	21	0	0	3	1.1	1.2	.2
		Lamb, cooked:											
		Chops (3 per lb with bone):											
		Arm chops, braised:											
9	609	Lean and fat	2.2 oz	63	44	220	20	0	0	15	7	6	1
9	610	Lean part of #609	1.7 oz	48	49	135	17	0	0	7	3	3	.4
		Loin chops, broiled:											
9	611	Lean and fat	2.8 oz	80	54	235	22	0	0	16	7	6	1
9	612	Lean part of #611	2.3 oz	64	61	140	19	0	0	6	2.6	2.4	.4
		Leg, roasted											
9	613	Lean and fat, piece 4⅛ × 2¼ × ½″	3 oz	85	59	205	22	0	0	13	6	5	.8
9	614	Lean only from #613	3 oz	85	64	163	23	0	0	7	2.8	2.6	.5
		Rib, roasted:											
9	615	Lean and fat, piece 2½ × 2½ × ¾″	3 oz	85	47	315	18	0	0	26	12	11	1.5
9	616	Lean only from #615	2 oz	57	60	130	15	0	0	7	3.2	3	5
		Pork, cured, cooked (see also #669–672):											
9	617	Bacon, medium slices	3 pce	19	13	109	6	<1	0	9	3.3	4.5	1.1
9	618	Canadian-style bacon	2 pce	47	62	86	11	1	0	4	1.3	1.9	.4
		Ham, roasted											
9	619	Lean and fat, 2 pieces 4⅛ × 2¼ × ¼″	3 oz	85	58	207	18	0	0	14	5	7	2
9	620	Lean only	3 oz	85	66	133	21	0	0	5	1.6	2.2	.5
9	621	Ham, canned, roasted	3 oz	85	66	140	18	<1	0	7	2.4	3.5	.8

[72] Outer layer of fat removed to about 1/2" of the lean. Deposits of fat within the cut remain.

KEY: 1 = BEV 2 = DAIRY 3 = EGGS 4 = FAT/OIL 5 = FRUIT 6 = BAKERY 7 = GRAIN 8 = FISH 9 = BEEF 10 = POULTRY
11 = SAUSAGE 12 = MIXED/FAST 13 = NUTS/SEEDS 14 = SWEETS 15 = VEG/LEG 16 = MISC 22 = SOUP/SAUCE

Chol (mg)	Calc (mg)	Iron (mg)	Magn (mg)	Phos (mg)	Pota (mg)	Sodi (mg)	Zinc (mg)	VT-A (RE)	Thia (mg)	Ribo (mg)	Niac (mg)	V-B6 (mg)	Fola (μg)	VT-C (mg)
87	11	2.5	15	162	190	53	6.66	t	.06	.20	2.0	.21	5	0
66	8	2.3	14	146	163	44	6.37	t	.05	.18	1.7	.18	4	0
81	5	2.8	20	217	248	43	4.36	t	.06	.21	3.3	.29	9	0
75	4	2.7	20	212	240	40	4.27	t	.06	.20	3.2	.28	6	0
74	9	1.8	18	134	256	65	4.56	t	.04	.18	4.4	.22	8	0
76	9	2.1	17	144	248	70	4.40	t	.03	.16	4.9	.23	8	0
164	5	6.4	22	213	198	54	2.66	0	.12	1.31	3.5	.18	2	1
410	9	5.3	20	392	309	90	4.63	9120[69]	.18	3.52	12.3	1.22	187	19
72	10	1.8	16	145	250	54	4.40	t	.06	.15	2.8	.21	6	0
68	10	2.2	21	181	320	63	5.90	t	.07	.18	3.5	.26	7	0
70	6	2.3	21	188	300	53	5.41	t	.08	.21	2.95	.31	6	0
69	5	2.5	23	205	328	55	6.01	t	.08	.23	3.18	.34	7	0
67	7	1.9	20	166	299	54	3.91	t	.07	.15	4.0	.32	6	0
64	7	2.1	23	185	336	57	4.44	t	.08	.17	4.54	.36	7	0
73	17	1.8	12	94	116	855	3.03	0	.02	.13	2.07	.11	5	1
46	4	3.2	23	125	320	2500	3.77	0	.05	.23	2.7	.14	4	0
77	16	1.5	11	132	195	46	2.9	t	.04	.16	4.4	.11	2	0
59	12	1.3	11	111	162	36	2.26	t	.03	.13	3	.11	2	0
78	16	1.4	21	162	272	62	3.11	t	.09	.21	5.5	.12	18	0
60	12	1.3	18	145	241	54	2.69	t	.08	.18	4.4	.1	16	0
78	8	1.73	20	162	273	57	3.79	t	.09	.25	5.5	.17	3	0
76	7	1.75	20	175	288	58	3.89	t	.09	.23	5.36	.19	3	0
77	19	1.4	15	139	224	60	4	t	.08	.18	5.5	.14	3	0
50	12	1	13	111	179	46	2.26	t	.05	.13	3.50	.09	2	0
16	2	.32	5	64	92	303	.62	0	.13	.05	1.39	.05	1	6[73]
27	5	.38	10	138	181	719	.79	0	.38	.09	3.22	.21	2	10[73]
53	6	.74	16	182	243	1009	1.97	0	.51	.19	3.8	.32	3	0
47	6	.8	19	193	269	1128	2.19	0	.58	.22	4.27	.4	3	0
35	6	.91	16	188	298	908	1.97	0	.82	.21	4.27	.33	4	19[73]

[69]Value varies widely.

[73]Values based on products containing added ascorbic acid or sodium ascorbate. If none added, ascorbic acid content would be negligible.

(For purposes of calculations, use "0" for t, <1, <.1, <.01, etc.)

Table A–1

Food Composition

Grp	Ref	Food Description	Measure	Wt (g)	H_2O (%)	Ener (cal)	Prot (g)	Carb (g)	Dietary Fiber (g)	Fat (g)	Fat Breakdown (g) Sat	Mono	Poly
		MEATS: POULTRY and POULTRY PRODUCTS											
		Pork, fresh, cooked:											
		Chops, loin (cut 3 per lb with bone):											
		Broiled:											
9	622	Lean and fat	3.1 oz	87	50	275	24	0	0	19	7	9	2
9	623	Lean only from #622	2.5 oz	72	57	166	23	0	0	8	2.6	3.4	.9
		Pan fried:											
9	624	Lean and fat	3.1 oz	89	45	334	21	0	0	27	10	13	3
9	625	Lean only for #624	2.4 oz	67	54	178	19	0	0	11	3.7	4.8	1.3
		Leg, roasted:											
9	626	Lean and fat, piece 2½ × 2½ × ¾"	3 oz	85	53	250	21	0	0	18	6	8	2
9	627	Lean only from #626	3 oz	85	60	187	24	0	0	9	3.2	4.2	1.1
		Rib, roasted:											
9	628	Lean and fat, piece 2½ × 2½ × ¾"	3 oz	85	51	270	21	0	0	20	7	9	2
9	629	Lean only from #628	2½ oz	71	57	175	20	0	0	10	3.4	4.4	1.2
		Shoulder, braised:											
9	630	Lean and fat, 3 pieces 2½ × 2½ × ¼"	3 oz	85	47	295	23	0	0	22	8	10	2
9	631	Lean only from #630	2.4 oz	67	54	165	22	0	0	8	3	4	1
		Veal, medium fat, cooked:											
9	632	Veal cutlet, braised or broiled, 4⅛ × 2¼ × ½"	3 oz	85	60	185	23	0	0	9	4	4	1
9	633	Veal rib roasted, 2 pieces 4⅛ × 2¼ × ¼"	3 oz	85	55	230	23	0	0	14	6	6	1
9	634	Veal liver, simmered	3 oz	85	53	222	25	3	0	11	5	3	4
		Chicken, cooked:											
		Fried, batter dipped:[74]											
10	635	Breasts (5.6 oz with bones)	1 ea	140	52	364	35	13	<1	18	5	8	4
10	636	Drumsticks (3.4 oz with bones)	1 ea	72	53	193	16	6	<1	11	3	5	3
10	637	Thighs	1 ea	86	52	238	19	8	<1	14	4	6	3
10	638	Wings	1 ea	49	46	159	10	5	<1	11	3	4	3
		Fried, flour coated:[74]											
10	639	Breasts (4.2 oz with bones)	1 ea	98	57	218	31	2	<1	9	2.4	3.4	1.9
10	640	Drumsticks (2.6 oz with bones)	1 ea	49	57	120	13	1	<1	7	1.8	2.7	1.6
10	641	Thighs	1 ea	62	54	162	17	2	<1	9	2.5	3.6	2.1
10	642	Wings	1 ea	32	49	103	8	1	<1	7	1.9	2.8	1.6
		Roasted:											
10	643	All types of meat	1 c	140	64	266	40	0	0	10	2.9	3.7	2.4
10	644	Dark meat	1 c	140	63	286	38	0	0	14	3.7	5.0	3.2
10	645	Light meat	1 c	140	65	242	43	0	0	6	1.8	2.2	1.4
10	646	Breasts, without skin	½ ea	86	65	142	27	0	0	3	.9	1.1	.7
10	647	Drumsticks	1 ea	44	67	76	12	0	0	2	.7	.8	.6
10	648	Thighs	1 ea	62	59	153	16	0	0	10	2.9	3.8	2.1
10	649	Chicken meat, stewed, all types	1 c	140	67	248	38	0	0	9	2.6	3.3	2.2
10	650	Chicken liver, simmered	1 ea	20	68	30	5	2	0	1	.4	.3	.2
10	651	Duck, roasted, meat only	½ duck	221	64	445	52	0	0	25	9.2	8.2	3.2

(74)Fried in vegetable shortening.

A

KEY: 1 = BEV 2 = DAIRY 3 = EGGS 4 = FAT/OIL 5 = FRUIT 6 = BAKERY 7 = GRAIN 8 = FISH 9 = BEEF 10 = POULTRY
11 = SAUSAGE 12 = MIXED/FAST 13 = NUTS/SEEDS 14 = SWEETS 15 = VEG/LEG 16 = MISC 22 = SOUP/SAUCE

Chol (mg)	Calc (mg)	Iron (mg)	Magn (mg)	Phos (mg)	Pota (mg)	Sodi (mg)	Zinc (mg)	VT-A (RE)	Thia (mg)	Ribo (mg)	Niac (mg)	V-B6 (mg)	Fola (µg)	VT-C (mg)
84	4	.7	22	184	312	61	1.68	3	.87	.24	4.35	.35	4	<1
71	4	.66	22	176	302	56	1.61	2	.83	.22	3.99	.34	4	<1
92	4	.75	23	190	323	64	1.74	3	.91	.24	4.58	.35	4	<1
71	3	.67	21	178	305	57	1.61	2	.84	.22	4.03	.34	4	<1
79	5	.85	18	210	280	50	2.43	2	.54	.27	3.89	.33	8	<1
80	6	.95	21	239	317	54	2.77	2	.59	.3	4.2	.38	10	<1
69	9	.76	16	190	313	37	1.67	3	.5	.24	4.17	.3	7	<1
56	8	.71	15	182	300	33	1.58	2	.45	.22	3.8	.28	6	<1
93	6	1.4	12	162	286	75	3.23	3	.46	.26	4.4	.31	4	0
76	5	1.3	15	235	151	68	3.87	2	.4	.24	4	.31	4	0
109	9	.8	15	196	258	56	3.48	t	.06	.21	4.6	.27	3	0
109	10	.7	20	211	259	57	3.48	t	.11	.26	6.6	.27	3	0
280	11	12.1	22	456	385	100	5.23	6464[69]	.21	3.56	14	.62	272	31
119	28	1.75	34	258	282	385	1.33	28	.16	.2	14.7	.6	8	0
62	12	.97	14	106	134	194	1.67	19	.08	.15	3.67	.2	6	0
80	16	1.24	18	134	165	248	1.75	25	.1	.2	4.92	.23	8	0
39	10	.63	8	59	68	157	.67	17	.05	.07	2.58	.15	3	0
88	16	1.17	29	228	253	74	1.07	15	.08	.13	13.5	.57	4	0
44	6	.66	11	86	112	44	1.42	12	.04	.11	2.96	.17	4	0
60	8	.93	15	116	147	55	1.56	18	.06	.15	4.31	.21	5	0
26	5	.4	6	48	57	25	.56	12	.02	.04	2.14	.13	1	0
125	21	1.69	35	273	340	120	2.94	22	.1	.25	12.8	.65	8	0
130	21	1.86	33	250	336	130	3.92	30	.1	.32	9.17	.5	11	0
118	21	1.49	38	302	345	108	1.73	12	.09	.16	17.4	.84	5	0
73	13	.89	25	196	220	64	.86	5	.06	.1	11.8	.52	3	0
41	5	.57	11	81	108	42	1.4	8	.03	.1	2.67	.17	4	0
58	8	.83	14	108	137	52	1.46	30	.04	.13	3.95	.19	4	0
116	20	1.63	29	210	252	98	2.79	21	.07	.23	8.56	.37	8	0
126	3	1.7	2	62	28	10	.87	983	.03	.35	.89	.12	154	3
198	27	5.97	44	449	557	143	5.75	51	.57	1.04	11.3	.55	22	0

(69)Value varies widely.

(For purposes of calculations, use "0" for t, <1, <.1, <.01, etc.)

A

Table A–1

Food Composition

Grp	Ref	Food Description	Measure	Wt (g)	H_2O (%)	Ener (cal)	Prot (g)	Carb (g)	Dietary Fiber (g)	Fat (g)	Fat Breakdown (g) Sat	Mono	Poly
MEATS: POULTRY and POULTRY PRODUCTS—Con.													
		Turkey, roasted, meat only:											
10	652	Dark meat	3 oz	85	63	159	24	0	0	6	2.1	1.4	1.8
10	653	Light meat	3 oz	85	66	133	25	0	0	3	.9	.5	.7
10	654	All types, chopped or diced	1 c	140	65	240	41	0	0	7	2.3	1.5	2.0
10	655	All types, slices	3 oz	85	65	145	25	0	0	4	1.4	.9	1.2
		Poultry food products (see also #664, 668, 673, 676):											
10	656	Canned, boneless chicken	5 oz	142	69	235	31	0	0	11	3.1	4.5	2.5
10	657	Chicken frankfurters	1 ea	45	58	115	6	3	0	9	2.5	3.8	1.8
10	658	Chicken roll, light meat	2 pce	57	69	90	11	1	0	4	1.2	1.7	.9
10	659	Gravy and turkey, frozen package	5 oz	142	85	95	8	7	<1	4	1.2	1.4	.7
10	660	Turkey loaf, breast meat	2 pce	42	72	46	10	0	0	1	.2	.2	.1
10	661	Turkey patties, breaded, fried	1 ea	64	50	181	9	10	<1	12	3	5	3
10	662	Turkey, frozen, roasted, seasoned	3 oz	85	68	130	18	3	0	5	1.6	1	1.4
MEATS: SAUSAGES and LUNCHMEATS													
		Bologna:											
11	663	Beef and pork	1 pce	28	54	89	3	1	0	8	3.0	3.8	.7
11	664	Turkey	2 pce	57	66	113	8	1	0	9	3.0	3.7	2.5
11	665	Braunschweiger sausage	2 pce	57	48	205	8	2	0	18	6.2	8.5	2.1
11	666	Brown-and-serve sausage links, cooked	1 ea	13	45	50	2	<1	0	5	1.7	2.2	.5
		Frankfurters (see also #657)											
11	667	Beef and pork	1 ea	45	54	145	5	1	0	13	4.8	6.2	1.2
11	668	Turkey	1 ea	45	63	102	6	1	0	8	2.4	2.7	2.1
		Ham:											
11	669	Ham lunchmeat, canned, 3 x 2 x ½″	1 pce	21	52	70	3	<1	0	6	2.3	3.0	.8
11	670	Chopped ham, packaged	2 pce	22	61	98	7	<1	0	8	2.6	3.9	.9
11	671	Ham lunchmeat, regular	2 pce	57	65	103	10	2	0	6	1.9	2.8	.7
11	672	Ham lunchmeat, extra lean	2 pce	57	70	75	11	1	0	3	.9	1.3	.3
11	673	Turkey ham	2 pce	57	71	75	11	<1	0	3	1.0	.8	.8
11	674	Pork sausage link, cooked[76]	1 ea	13	45	50	3	<1	0	4	1.4	1.8	.5
		Salami:											
11	675	Pork and beef	2 pce	57	60	145	8	1	0	11	4.6	5.2	1.1
11	676	Turkey	2 pce	57	66	111	9	<1	0	8	2.3	2.6	2.0
11	677	Dry, beef and pork	2 pce	20	35	85	5	<1	0	7	2.4	3.4	.6
11	678	Sandwich spreads, pork and beef	1 tbsp	15	60	35	1	2	0	3	.9	1.1	.4
11	679	Vienna sausage, canned	1 ea	16	60	45	2	<1	0	4	1.5	2.0	.3
MIXED DISHES and FAST FOODS													
12	680	Beef and vegetable stew, homemade	1 c	245	82	220	16	15	3	11	4.4	4.5	.5
12	681	Beef pot pie, homemade[77]	1 pce	210	55	515	21	39	1	30	8	13	7
12	682	Chicken à la king, home recipe	1 c	245	68	470	27	12	1	34	13	13	6
12	683	Chicken and noodles, home recipe	1 c	240	71	365	22	26	1	18	5	7	4
12	684	Chicken chow mein, canned	1 c	250	89	95	7	18	5	1	.1	.1	.8

(76)One patty (8 per pound) of bulk sausage is equivalent to 2 links.
(77)Crust made with vegetable shortening and enriched flour.

KEY: 1 = BEV 2 = DAIRY 3 = EGGS 4 = FAT/OIL 5 = FRUIT 6 = BAKERY 7 = GRAIN 8 = FISH 9 = BEEF 10 = POULTRY 11 = SAUSAGE 12 = MIXED/FAST 13 = NUTS/SEEDS 14 = SWEETS 15 = VEG/LEG 16 = MISC 22 = SOUP/SAUCE

Chol (mg)	Calc (mg)	Iron (mg)	Magn (mg)	Phos (mg)	Pota (mg)	Sodi (mg)	Zinc (mg)	VT-A (RE)	Thia (mg)	Ribo (mg)	Niac (mg)	V-B6 (mg)	Fola (µg)	VT-C (mg)
72	27	1.99	21	174	247	67	3.8	0	.05	.21	3.1	.3	8	0
59	16	1.14	24	186	259	54	1.73	0	.05	.11	5.81	.46	5	0
106	35	2.49	37	298	418	99	4.34	0	.09	.26	7.62	.64	10	0
64	21	1.51	22	181	254	60	2.64	0	.05	.15	4.63	.39	6	0
88	20	2.2	17	158	196	714	2.13	48	.02	.18	8.99	.5	4	3
45	43	.9	8	48	38	616	1	17	.03	.05	1.39	.09	2	0
28	24	.55	10	89	129	331	.41	14	.04	.07	3	.31	2	0
26	20	1.32	11	115	87	787	.99	18	.03	.18	2.55	.14	2	0
17	3	.17	8	97	118	608	.48	0	.02	.04	3.54	.15	2	0[75]
40	9	1.41	12	173	176	512	1.5	7	.06	.12	1.47	.13	2	0
45	4	1.4	20	207	253	578	2.37	0	.04	.14	5.3	.24	5	0
16	3	.43	3	26	51	289	.55	0	.05	.04	.73	.05	1	6[73]
56	47	.87	8	74	113	498	.99	0	.03	.09	2.1	.1	3	t
89	6	5.32	6	96	113	652	1.62	2406	.14	.87	4.78	.19	57	5[73]
9	1	.1	2	14	25	105	.15	0	.05	.02	.40	.03	<1	0
23	5	.52	5	39	75	504	.83	0	.09	.05	1.18	.06	2	12[73]
44	53	.77	8	71	84	550	1	17	.11	.12	1.77	.09	2	t
13	1	.15	2	17	45	271	.31	0	.08	.04	.66	.04	1	t
21	3	.4	5	58	119	573	.77	0	.23	.07	1.4	.13	2	1[73]
32	4	.56	11	140	188	746	1.21	0	.49	.14	2.98	.19	2	16[73]
27	4	.43	10	124	198	810	1.09	0	.53	.13	2.74	.26	2	15[73]
32	6	1.56	12	108	184	565	1.56	0	.04	.15	2.72	.16	4	0
11	4	.16	2	24	47	168	.33	0	.1	.03	.59	.04	<1	t
37	7	1.5	7/	66	113	607	1.22	0	.14	.2	2.02	.12	0	7[73]
46	11	.93	9	73	125	535	1.25	0	.06	.15	2.23	.14	5	t
16	2	.3	4	28	76	372	.64	0	.12	.06	.97	.1	0	6[73]
6	2	.12	1	9	16	152	.15	1	.03	.02	.26	.02	<1	0
8	2	.14	1	8	16	152	.26	0	.01	.02	.26	.02	<1	0
71	29	2.9	41	184	613	292	3.9	568	.15	.17	4.7	.28	37	17
42	29	3.8	6	149	334	596	3.17	517	.29	.29	4.8	.24	29	6
221	127	2.5	20	358	404	760	1.8	272	.1	.42	5.4	.23	11	12
103	26	2.2	34	247	149	600	2.07	130	.05	.17	4.3	.16	9	1
8	45	1.3	14	85	418	725	1.3	28	.05	.1	1	.09	12	13

(73)Values based on products containing added ascorbic acid or sodium ascorbate. If none added, ascorbic acid content would be negligible.

(75)If sodium ascorbate is added, product contains 11 mg ascorbic acid.

(For purposes of calculations, use "0" for t, <1, <.1, <.01, etc.)

Table A–1

Food Composition

Grp	Ref	Name / Food Description	Measure	Wt (g)	H_2O (%)	Ener (cal)	Prot (g)	Carb (g)	Dietary Fiber (g)	Fat (g)	Fat Breakdown (g) Sat	Mono	Poly
MIXED DISHES and FAST FOODS—Con.													
12	685	Chicken chow mein, home recipe	1 c	250	78	255	23	10	4	11	4	4	3
12	686	Chicken pot pie, home recipe[77]	1 pce	232	57	545	23	42	2	31	10	16	7
12	687	Chili with beans, canned	1 c	255	76	286	15	31	6	14	6	6	1
12	688	Chop suey with beef and pork	1 c	250	75	300	26	13	2	17	4	7	4
12	689	Corn pudding[78]	1 c	250	76	271	11	32	9	13	6.3	4.3	1.7
12	690	Cole slaw[79]	1 c	120	82	84	2	15	2	3	.5	.9	1.6
12	691	French toast, home recipe[81]	1 pce	65	53	156	6	15	1	8	2.4	3.1	1.6
		Macaroni and cheese:											
12	692	Canned[82]	1 c	240	80	230	9	26	1	10	5	3	1
12	693	Home recipe[49]	1 c	200	58	430	17	40	1	22	10	7	4
12	694	Quiche lorraine, ⅛ of 8″ quiche[77]	1 pce	176	47	600	13	29	<1	48	23	18	4
		Spaghetti (enriched) in tomato sauce:											
		With cheese:											
12	695	Canned	1 c	250	80	190	6	39	2	2	.4	.4	.5
12	696	Home recipe	1 c	250	77	260	9	37	2	9	3	3.6	1.2
		With meatballs:											
12	697	Canned	1 c	250	78	260	12	29	3	10	2	4	3
12	698	Home recipe	1 c	248	70	330	19	39	3	12	4	4	2
		Burritos:[83]											
12	699	Beef and bean	1 ea	175	54	390	21	40	5	17	7	7	2
12	700	Bean	1 ea	174	55	322	13	47	8	10	4	3	2
		Cheeseburgers:											
12	701	Regular	1 ea	112	46	300	15	28	1	15	7	6	1
12	702	4-oz patty	1 ea	194	46	524	30	40	2	31	15	12	1
12	703	Chicken patty sandwiches	1 ea	157	52	436	25	34	1	22	6	10	5
12	704	Corn dogs	1 ea	111	45	330	10	27	<1	20	8	10	1
12	705	Enchiladas[84]	1 ea	230	72	235	20	24	2	16	8	7	.6
12	706	English muffins with egg, cheese, bacon	1 ea	138	49	360	18	31	2	18	8	8	.7
		Fish sandwiches:											
12	707	Regular, with cheese	1 ea	140	43	420	16	39	1	23	6	7	8
12	708	Large, without cheese	1 ea	170	48	470	18	41	1	27	6	9	10
		Hamburgers with buns:											
12	709	Regular	1 ea	98	46	245	12	28	1	11	4	5	1
12	710	4-oz patty	1 ea	174	50	445	25	38	1	21	7	12	1
12	711	Hotdogs/frankfurters and buns	1 ea	85	53	260	8	21	1	15	5	7	2
12	712	Cheese pizza, ⅛ of 15″ round[77]	1 pce	120	46	290	15	39	2	9	4	3	1
12	713	Roast beef sandwiches	1 ea	150	52	345	22	34	1	13	4	7	2
12	714	Beef tacos	1 ea	81	55	195	9	15	1	11	4	6	1

(49)Made with margarine.

(77)Crust made with vegetable shortening and enriched flour.

(78)Recipe: 55% yellow corn, 23% whole milk, 14% egg, 4% sugar, 3% salt, and 1% pepper.

(79)Recipe: 41% cabbage; 12% celery; 12% table cream; 12% sugar; 7% green pepper; 6% lemon juice; 4% onion; 3% pimento; 3% vinegar; 2% each for salt, dry mustard, and white pepper.

(81)Recipe: 35% whole milk, 32% white bread, 29% egg, and cooked in 4% margarine.

(82)Made with corn oil.

(83)Made with a 10½″-diameter flour tortilla.

(84)USDA data were unspecified for type of enchilada.

A

Key: 1 = BEV 2 = DAIRY 3 = EGGS 4 = FAT/OIL 5 = FRUIT 6 = BAKERY 7 = GRAIN 8 = FISH 9 = BEEF 10 = POULTRY 11 = SAUSAGE 12 = MIXED/FAST 13 = NUTS/SEEDS 14 = SWEETS 15 = VEG/LEG 16 = MISC 22 = SOUP/SAUCE

Chol (mg)	Calc (mg)	Iron (mg)	Magn (mg)	Phos (mg)	Pota (mg)	Sodi (mg)	Zinc (mg)	VT-A (RE)	Thia (mg)	Ribo (mg)	Niac (mg)	V-B6 (mg)	Fola (μg)	VT-C (mg)
75	58	2.5	28	293	473	718	2.12	50	.08	.23	4.3	.41	19	10
56	70	3	25	232	343	594	2	735	.32	.32	4.9	.46	29	5
43	119	8.75	115	393	932	1330	5.10	86	.12	.27	.91	.34	41	4
68	60	4.8	32	248	425	1053	3.58	60	.28	.38	5	.32	22	33
230	100	1.4	38	143	402	138	1.26	89	1.03	.32	2.47	.29	63	7
10[80]	54	.7	12	38	218	28	.24	98	.08	.07	.33	.17	32	39
140	87	1.34	13	105	112	257	.66	80	.12	.16	1.05	.05	18	t
24	199	1	31	182	139	730	1.34	72	.12	.24	1	.02	8	t
44	362	1.8	37	322	240	1086	1.35	232	.2	.4	1.8	.05	10	1
285	211	1	23	276	283	653	1.95	454	.11	.32	1.2	.15	17	t
3	40	2.8	16	88	303	955	1.12	120	.35	.28	4.5	.13	6	10
8	80	2.3	26	135	408	955	1.3	140	.25	.18	2.3	.2	8	13
23	53	3.3	20	113	245	1220	2.39	100	.15	.18	2.3	.12	5	5
89	124	3.7	40	236	665	1009	2.45	159	.25	.3	.4	.19	7	22
52	165	2.7	61	274	388	516	3.30	58	.26	.29	4.36	.73	48	5
15	181	2.53	76	243	427	1030	2.37	58	.26	.23	2.4	1.01	55	5
44	135	2.3	22	174	219	672	2.53	65	.26	.24	3.7	.11	20	1
104	236	4.45	43	320	407	1224	5.27	128	.33	.48	7.37	.23	23	3
68	44	1.87	30	173	194	2732	1	16	.29	.26	9.21	.37	18	4
37	34	1.94	22	303	164	1252	1.44	t	.28	.17	3.27	.11	2	3
19	322	3.29	76	198	653	1332	1.2	352	.18	.26	t	.25	19	t
213	197	3.1	28	290	201	832	1.86	160	.46	.5	3.71	.15	35	1
56	132	1.85	29	223	274	667	.95	25	.32	.27	3.3	.1	24	3
90	61	2.23	34	246	375	621	.88	15	.35	.24	3.52	.12	42	1
32	56	2.2	19	107	202	463	2	14	.23	.24	3.8	.12	16	1
71	75	4.84	40	225	404	763	5.01	28	.38	.38	7.85	.28	24	2
23	59	1.71	13	83	113	745	1.19	t	.29	.19	2.48	.07	17	12
56	220	1.6	40	216	230	699	1.73	106	.34	.29	4.2	.04	40	2
55	60	4.04	38	222	338	757	3.66	32	.39	.33	6.02	.28	42	2
21	109	1.15	36	134	263	456	1.56	57	.09	.07	1.41	.12	14	1

(80)From dairy cream in recipe.

(For purposes of calculations, use "0" for t, <1, <.1, <.01, etc.)

Table A–1

Food Composition

Grp	Ref	Food Description	Measure	Wt (g)	H_2O (%)	Ener (cal)	Prot (g)	Carb (g)	Dietary Fiber (g)	Fat (g)	Fat Breakdown (g) Sat	Mono	Poly
		MIXED DISHES and FAST FOODS—Con.											
12	715	Potato salad with mayonnaise and egg[85]	1 c	250	76	358	7	28	4	21	4	6	9
12	716	Spinach soufflé[86]	1 c	136	74	218	11	3	4	18	7	7	3
12	717	Tuna salad[87]	1 c	205	63	375	33	19	2	19	3	5	9
		Additional Fast Foods at the end of this appendix.											
		NUTS, SEEDS and PRODUCTS											
		Almonds:											
13	718	Slivered, packed	1 c	135	4	795	27	28	14[88]	70	7	46	15
		Whole, dried:											
13	719	Cup	1 c	142	4	837	28	29	15[88]	74	7	48	16
13	720	Ounce	1 oz	28	4	167	6	6	3[88]	15	1	10	3
13	721	Almond butter	1 tbsp	16	1	101	2	3	1	9	1	6	2
13	722	Brazil nuts, dry (about 7)	1 oz	28	3	186	4	4	2	19	5	7	7
		Cashew nuts:											
		Dry roasted, salted:											
13	723	Cup	1 c	137	2	787	21	45	8	63	13	37	11
13	724	Ounce	1 oz	28	2	163	4	9	2	13	3	8	2
		Oil roasted, salted:											
13	725	Cup	1 c	130	4	748	21	37	8	63	12	37	11
13	726	Ounce	1 oz	28	4	163	5	8	2	14	3	8	2
13	727	Cashew butter	1 tbsp	16	3	94	3	4	1	8	2	5	1
13	728	European chestnuts, roasted, 1 c = approx 17 kernels	1 c	143	40	350	5	76	19	3	.6	1.1	1.2
		Coconut:											
		Raw											
13	729	Piece 2 × 2 × 1/2″	1 pce	45	47	159	2	7	6	15	13	.6	.2
13	730	Shredded/grated[94]	1 c	80	47	283	3	12	11	27	24	1	.3
		Dried, shredded/grated:											
13	731	Unsweetened	1 c	78	3	515	5	19	19	50	45	2	.6
13	732	Sweetened	1 c	93	16	466	3	44	19	33	29	1	.4
		Filberts (hazelnuts), chopped:											
13	733	Cup	1 c	115	5	727	15	18	8	72	5	57	7
13	734	Ounce	1 oz	28	5	179	4	4	2	18	1	14	2
		Macadamia nuts, oil roasted, salted:											
13	735	Cup	1 c	134	2	962	10	17	5	103	15	81	2
13	736	Ounce	1 oz	28	2	204	2	4	1	22	3	17	.4
		Mixed nuts, salted:											
13	737	Dry roasted	1 c	137	2	814	24	35	11	70	10	43	15
13	738	Roasted in oil	1 c	142	2	876	24	30	11	80	12	45	19

(85)Recipe: 62% potatoes; 12% egg; 8% mayonnaise; 7% celery; 6% sweet pickle relish; 2% onion; 1% each for green pepper, pimiento, salt, and dry mustard.

(86)Recipe: 29% whole milk, 26% spinach, 13% egg white, 13% cheddar cheese, 7% egg yolk, 7% butter, 4% flour, 1% salt and pepper.

(87)Made with drained chunk light tuna, celery, onion, pickle relish, and mayonnaise-type salad dressing.

(88)Values reported for dietary fiber in almonds vary from 7.0 to 14.3g/100 g

(94)1 c packed = 130 g.

Key: 1 = BEV 2 = DAIRY 3 = EGGS 4 = FAT/OIL 5 = FRUIT 6 = BAKERY 7 = GRAIN 8 = FISH 9 = BEEF 10 = POULTRY 11 = SAUSAGE 12 = MIXED/FAST 13 = NUTS/SEEDS 14 = SWEETS 15 = VEG/LEG 16 = MISC 22 = SOUP/SAUCE

Chol (mg)	Calc (mg)	Iron (mg)	Magn (mg)	Phos (mg)	Pota (mg)	Sodi (mg)	Zinc (mg)	VT-A (RE)	Thia (mg)	Ribo (mg)	Niac (mg)	V-B6 (mg)	Fola (µg)	VT-C (mg)
170	48	1.63	39	130	635	1323	.78	82	.19	.15	2.23	.35	17	25
184	230	1.34	37	231	202	763	1.29	675	.09	.3	.48	.12	62	3
80	31	2.5	42	281	531	877	1.16	53	.06	.14	13.3	.49	41	6
0	359	4.94	400	702	988	15	3.94	0	.28	1.05	4.54	.15	79	1
0	378	5.2	420	738	1034	15[89]	4.15	0	.3	1.11	4.77	.16	83	1
0	75	1.04	84	147	208	3[89]	.83	0	.06	.22	.95	.03	17	t
0	43	.59	48	84	121	2[90]	.49	0	.02	.1	.46	.01	0	t
0	50	.96	64	170	170	0	1.3	t	.28	.04	.46	.07	1	t
0	62	8.22	356	671	774	877[91]	7.67	0	.27	.27	1.92	.35	95	0
0	13	1.7	74	139	160	181[91]	1.59	0	.06	.06	.4	.07	20	0
0	53	5.33	332	554	689	814[92]	6.18	0	.55	.23	2.34	.33	88	0
0	12	1.16	72	121	151	177[92]	1.35	0	.12	.05	.51	.07	19	0
0	7	.09	41	73	87	2[93]	.83	0	.05	.03	.26	.04	11	0
0	42	1.3	47	153	846	3	.81	3	.35	.25	1.92	.71	100	37
0	6	1.09	14	51	160	9	.49	0	.03	<.01	.24	.02	12	1
0	12	1.94	26	90	285	16	.88	0	.05	.02	.43	.04	21	3
0	20	2.59	70	161	423	29	1.57	0	.05	.08	.47	2.34	7	1
0	14	1.79	47	100	313	244	1.69	0	.03	.02	.44	.29	9	1
0	216	3.76	328	359	512	3	2.76	8	.57	.13	1.31	.7	83	1
0	53	.93	81	89	126	1	.68	2	.14	.03	.32	.17	20	t
0	60	2.41	157	268	441	348[95]	1.47	1	.28	.15	2.71	.33	79	0
0	13	.51	33	57	94	74[95]	.31	3	.06	.03	.57	.07	17	0
0	96	5.07	308	596	817	917[96]	5.21	2	.27	.27	6.44	.41	69	1
0	153	4.56	334	659	825	926[96]	7.22	3	.71	.32	7.19	.34	118	1

(89)Salted almonds contain 1108 mg sodium per cup, 221 mg/oz.
(90)Salted almond butter contains 72 mg sodium per tablespoon.
(91)Dry-roasted cashews without salt contain 21 mg sodium per cup, or 4 mg/oz.
(92)Oil-roasted cashews without salt contain 22 mg sodium per cup, or 5 mg/oz.
(93)Salted cashew butter contains 98 mg sodium per tablespoon.
(95)Macadamia nuts without salt contain 9 mg sodium per cup, or 2 mg/oz.
(96)Mixed nuts without salt contain about 15 mg sodium per cup.

(For purposes of calculations, use "0" for t, <1, <.1, <.01, etc.)

Table A–1

Food Composition

Grp	Ref	Food Description	Measure	Wt (g)	H_2O (%)	Ener (cal)	Prot (g)	Carb (g)	Dietary Fiber (g)	Fat (g)	Fat Breakdown (g) Sat	Mono	Poly
		NUTS, SEEDS and PRODUCTS—Con.											
		Peanuts:											
		Oil roasted, salted:											
13	739	Cup	1 c	145	2	837	39	27	12	71	10	36	23
13	740	Ounce	1 oz	28	2	163	8	5	2	14	2	7	4
		Dried, unsalted:											
13	741	Cup	1 c	146	7	827	37	24	14	72	10	36	23
13	742	Ounce	1 oz	28	7	161	7	5	3	14	2	7	4
13	743	Peanut butter	1 tbsp	16	2	94	4	3	1	8	1.5	3.8	2.3
		Pecans, halves, dried:											
13	744	Cup	1 c	108	5	720	8	20	7[99]	73	6	46	18
13	745	Ounce	1 oz	28	5	190	2	5	2[99]	19	1.5	12	5
13	746	Pine nuts/piñons, dried	1 oz	28	6	161	3	5	2	17	3	7	7
13	747	Pistachio nuts, dried, shelled	1 oz	28	4	164	6	7	1	14	2	9	2
13	748	Pumpkin kernels, dried, unsalted	1 oz	28	7	154	7	5	2	13	2	4	6
13	749	Sesame seeds, hulled, dried	¼ c	38	5	221	10	4	6	21	3	8	9
		Sunflower seed kernels:											
13	750	Dry	¼ c	36	5	205	8	7	2	18	2	3	12
13	751	Oil roasted	¼ c	34	3	208	7	5	2	19	2	4	13
13	752	Tahini (sesame butter)	1 tbsp	15	3	91	3	3	2	8	1	3	4
		Black walnuts, chopped:											
13	753	Cup	1 c	125	4	759	30	15	11	71	5	16	47
13	754	Ounce	1 oz	28	4	172	7	3	2	16	1	4	11
		English walnuts, chopped:											
13	755	Cup	1 c	120	4	770	17	22	8	74	7	17	47
13	756	Ounce	1 oz	28	4	182	4	5	2	18	2	4	11
		SWEETENERS and SWEETS: see also Dairy (milk desserts) and Baked Goods											
14	757	Apple butter	2 tbsp	35	52	66	<1	16	<1	<1	.1	t	.1
14	758	Caramel, plain or chocolate	1 oz	28	8	115	1	22	<1	3	2.2	.3	.1
		Chocolate (see also, #784, 785, 971):											
		Milk chocolate:											
14	759	Plain	1 oz	28	1	145	2	16	<1	9	5.4	3	.3
14	760	With almonds	1 oz	28	2	150	3	15	1	10	4.4	4.7	1.0
14	761	With peanuts	1 oz	28	1	155	5	10	2	12	3.5	5.2	2.7
14	762	With rice cereal	1 oz	28	2	140	2	18	1	7	4.4	2.5	.2
14	763	Semisweet chocolate chips	1 c	170	1	860	7	97	5	61	36	20	2
14	764	Sweet dark chocolate	1 oz	28	1	150	1	16	1	10	5.9	3.3	.3
14	765	Fondant candy, uncoated(mints, candy corn, other)	1 oz	28	3	105	0	27	0	0	0	0	0
14	766	Fudge, chocolate	1 oz	28	8	115	<1	21	<1	3	2.1	1	.1
14	767	Gum drops	1 oz	28	12	98	0	25	0	<1	t	t	.1
14	768	Hard candy, all flavors	1 oz	28	1	109	0	28	0	0	0	0	0

(99)Dietary fiber data calculated/derived from data on other nuts.

Key: 1 = BEV 2 = DAIRY 3 = EGGS 4 = FAT/OIL 5 = FRUIT 6 = BAKERY 7 = GRAIN 8 = FISH 9 = BEEF 10 = POULTRY
11 = SAUSAGE 12 = MIXED/FAST 13 = NUTS/SEEDS 14 = SWEETS 15 = VEG/LEG 16 = MISC 22 = SOUP/SAUCE

Chol (mg)	Calc (mg)	Iron (mg)	Magn (mg)	Phos (mg)	Pota (mg)	Sodi (mg)	Zinc (mg)	VT-A (RE)	Thia (mg)	Ribo (mg)	Niac (mg)	V-B6 (mg)	Fola (μg)	VT-C (mg)
0	125	2.78	273	734	982	626[97]	9.6	0	.38	.16	20.5	.45	181	0
0	24	.54	53	144	200	123[97]	1.88	0	.07	.03	4.20	.09	36	0
0	85	4.72	263	559	1047	23	4.78	0	.97	.19	20.7	.43	153	0
0	17	.92	51	109	204	5	.93	0	.19	.04	4.02	.08	30	0
0	5	.29	25	52	116	75[98]	.40	0	.02	.02	2.15	.06	13	0
0	39	2.3	138	314	423	1[100]	5.91	14	.92	.14	.96	.2	42	2
0	10	.6	36	83	111	3[100]	1.55	4	.24	.04	.25	.05	11	1
0	2	.87	67	10	178	20	1.22	1	.35	.06	1.24	.08	19	1
0	38	1.93	45	143	310	2[101]	.38	7	.22	.05	.31	.06	16	t
0	12	4.25	152	333	229	5[102]	2.12	11	.06	.09	.50	.03	26	t
0	49	2.93	130	291	153	15	2.23	t	.27	.03	1.76	.29	38	0
0	42	2.44	128	254	248	1	1.82	2	.82	.09	1.62	.46	85	t
0	19	2.26	43	385	163	205[103]	1.76	2	.11	.1	1.4	.4	79	<1
0	21	.95	53	119	69	5	1.57	1	.24	.02	.85	.06	15	1
0	73	3.84	253	580	655	1	4.28	37	.27	.14	.86	.7	82	1
0	16	.87	57	132	149	0	.97	8	.06	.03	.2	.16	19	t
0	113	2.93	203	380	602	12	3.28	15	.46	.18	1.25	.67	79	4
0	27	.69	48	90	142	3	.78	4	.11	.04	.3	.16	19	1
0	5	.25	2	13	89	1	.01	0	<.01	<.01	.07	<.01	<1	1
1	42	.4	2	35	54	64	.1	t	.01	.05	.1	<.01	0	t
6	50	.4	16	61	96	23	.37	10	.02	.1	.1	.02	<1	t
5	61	.56	33	77	125	23	.48	7	.03	.13	.31	.02	4	t
3	32	.68	35	87	155	19	.68	5	.11	.07	2.2	.05	16	t
6	48	.2	13	57	100	46	.29	8	.01	.08	.1	.01	<1	t
0	51	5.8	230	178	593	24	2.39	3	.1	.14	.9	.04	22	t
0	7	.6	32	41	86	5	.42	1	.01	.04	.1	<.01	4	t
0	2	.1	—	2	1	57	.1	0	<.01	<.01	.01	<.01	0	0
1	22	.3	7	24	42	54	.15	t	.01	.03	.1	<.01	2	t
0	2	.1	—	—	1	10	0	0	0	<.01	.01	0	0	0
0	6	.1	<1	2	1	7	0	0	0	0	0	0	0	0

(97)Peanuts without salt contain 22 mg sodium per cup, or 4 mg/oz.
(98)Peanut butter without added salt contains 3 mg sodium per tablespoon.
(100)Salted pecans contain 816 mg sodium per cup, or 214 mg/oz.
(101)Salted pistachios contain approx 221 mg sodium per ounce.
(102)Salted pumpkin/squash kernels contain approximately 163 mg sodium per ounce.
(103)Unsalted sunflower seeds contain 1 mg sodium per 1/4 cup.

(For purposes of calculations, use "0" for t, <1, <.1, <.01, etc.)

Table A–1

Food Composition

Grp	Ref	Food Description	Measure	Wt (g)	H_2O (%)	Ener (cal)	Prot (g)	Carb (g)	Dietary Fiber (g)	Fat (g)	Fat Breakdown (g)		
											Sat	Mono	Poly
		SWEETENERS and SWEETS—Con.											
14	769	Jelly beans	1 oz	28	6	104	<.01	26	0	<.01	t	t	.1
14	770	Marshmallows	4 ea	28	17	90	<1	23	0	0	0	0	0
14	771	Gelatin salads/desserts	½ c	120	84	70	2	17	<1	0	0	0	0
		Honey:											
14	772	Cup	1 c	339	17	1030	1	279	0	0	0	0	0
14	773	Tablespoon	1 tbsp	21	17	65	<.1	17	0	0	0	0	0
		Jams or preserves:											
14	774	Tablespoon	1 tbsp	20	29	54	<1	14	<1	<.1	0	t	t
14	775	Packet	1 ea	14	29	38	<.1	9	<1	<.1	0	t	t
		Jellies:											
14	776	Tablespoon	1 tbsp	18	28	49	<.1	13	0	<.1	t	t	t
14	777	Packet	1 ea	14	28	39	<.1	10	0	<.1	t	t	t
14	778	Popsicles, 3 oz when fluid	1 ea	95	80	70	0	18	0	0	0	0	0
		Sugars:											
14	779	Brown sugar	1 c	220	2	820	0	212	0	0	0	0	0
		White sugar, granulated											
14	780	Cup	1 c	200	1	770	0	199	0	0	0	0	0
14	781	Tablespoon	1 tbsp	12	1	45	0	12	0	0	0	0	0
14	782	Packet	1 ea	6	1	25	0	6	0	0	0	0	0
14	783	White sugar, powdered, sifted	1 c	100	<1	385	0	99	0	0	0	0	0
		Syrups:											
		Chocolate:											
14	784	Thin type	2 tbsp	38	37	85	1	22	1	<1	.2	.1	.1
14	785	Fudge type	2 tbsp	38	25	125	2	21	1	5	3	2	.2
14	786	Molasses, blackstrap [104]	2 tbsp	40	24	85	0	22	0	0	0	0	0
14	787	Pancake table syrup (corn and maple)	¼ c	84	25	244	0	64	0	0	0	0	0
		VEGETABLES AND LEGUMES											
15	788	Alfalfa seeds, sprouted	1 c	33	91	10	1	1	1	<1	t	t	.1
15	789	Artichokes, cooked globe (300 g with refuse)	1 ea	120	86	53	3	12	4	<1	.1	t	.1
		Asparagus, green, cooked:											
		From raw:											
15	790	Cuts and tips	½ c	90	92	22	2	4	2	<1	.1	t	.1
15	791	Spears, ½″ diam at base	4 spears	60	92	15	2	3	1	<1	<.1	t	.1
		From frozen:											
15	792	Cuts and tips	1 c	180	91	50	5	9	3	1	.2	t	.3
15	793	Spears, ½″ diam at base	4 spears	60	91	17	2	3	1	<1	.1	t	.1
15	794	Canned, spears, ½″ diam at base	4 spears	80	95	11	2	2	1	<1	.1	t	.2
15	795	Bamboo shoots, canned, drained slices	1 c	131	94	25	2	4	3	<1	.1	t	.2

(104)Light molasses would contain about 66 mg calcium, 2.1 mg iron, 18 mg magnesium, and 366 mg potassium for 2 tbsp.

Key: 1 = BEV 2 = DAIRY 3 = EGGS 4 = FAT/OIL 5 = FRUIT 6 = BAKERY 7 = GRAIN 8 = FISH 9 = BEEF 10 = POULTRY
11 = SAUSAGE 12 = MIXED/FAST 13 = NUTS/SEEDS 14 = SWEETS 15 = VEG/LEG 16 = MISC 22 = SOUP/SAUCE

Chol (mg)	Calc (mg)	Iron (mg)	Magn (mg)	Phos (mg)	Pota (mg)	Sodi (mg)	Zinc (mg)	VT-A (RE)	Thia (mg)	Ribo (mg)	Niac (mg)	V-B6 (mg)	Fola (μg)	VT-C (mg)
0	1	.3	—	1	11	7	0	0	0	<.01	.01	—	0	0
0	1	.45	1	2	2	25	<.01	0	0	<.01	.01	<.01	0	0
0	2	.1	<1	23	91	55	.05	0	.01	.01	.2	<.01	0	0
0	17	1.7	8	20	173	17	.27	0	.02	.14	1	.06	<1	3
0	1	.11	<1	1	11	1	.02	0	<.01	<.01	.06	<.01	2	t
0	4	.2	1	2	18	2	<.01	t	<.01	.01	.04	<.01	2	<1
0	3	.14	<1	1	13	1	<.01	t	<.01	<.01	.03	<.01	1	t
0	2	.12	<1	1	16	4	0	t	<.01	<.01	.04	<.01	2	1
0	1	.09	<1	1	12	3	0	t	<.01	<.01	.03	<.01	2	1
0	0	.01	—	0	4	11	0	0	0	0	0	0	0	0
0	187	4.8	135	56	757	97	.08	0	.02	.07	.20	0	0	0
0	3	.1	<1	.1	7	5	.08	0	0	0	0	0	0	0
0	<1	<.01	<1	t	t	t	<.01	0	0	0	0	0	0	0
0	t	<.01	<1	t	t	t	<.01	0	0	0	0	0	0	0
0	0	.08	<1	0	4	2	<.01	0	0	0	0	0	0	0
0	6	.75	26	49	85	36	.39	1	<.01	.02	.11	<.01	3	0
0	38	.5	18	60	82	42	.39	13	.02	.08	.07	<.01	3	0
0	274[104]	10.1[104]	103[104]	34	1171[104]	38	0	0	.04	.08	.8	.11	6	0
0	2	.06	<.01	8	14	38	0	0	0	0	0	t	t	0
0	11	.32	9	23	26	2	.30	5	.03	.04	.16	.01	12	3
0	47	1.62	47	72	316	79	.43	17	.07	.06	.71	.1	53	9
0	22	.59	17	55	279	4	.43	75	.09	.11	.95	.13	88	25
0	14	.4	11	37	186	2	.29	50	.06	.07	.63	.09	59	16
0	41	1.15	23	99	392	7	1.01	147	.12	.18	1.87	.16	176	44
0	14	.38	8	33	131	2	.34	49	.04	.06	.62	.06	59	15
0	11	.5	8	30	122	278[105]	.32	38	.05	.07	.7	.04	69	13
0	10	.42	6	33	105	9	.30	1	.03	.03	.18	—	40	1

(105)Special dietary pack contains 3 mg sodium

(For purposes of calculations, use "0" for t, <1, <.1, <.01, etc.)

Table A–1

Food Composition

Grp	Ref	Food Description	Measure	Wt (g)	H_2O (%)	Ener (cal)	Prot (g)	Carb (g)	Dietary Fiber (g)	Fat (g)	Fat Breakdown (g) Sat	Mono	Poly
		VEGETABLES and LEGUMES—Con.											
		Beans (see also Great northern, #855; Kidney beans, #860; Navy beans, #876; Pinto beans, #898; Refried beans, #921; Soybeans, #925):											
15	796	Black beans, cooked	1 c	172	66	227	15	41	15	1	.2	.1	.4
		Lima beans:											
15	797	Thick seeded (Fordhooks), cooked from frozen	½ c	85	74	85	5	16	5	<1	.1	t	.1
15	798	Thin seeded (baby), cooked from frozen	½ c	90	72	94	6	17	5	<1	.1	t	.1
15	799	Cooked from dry, drained	1 c	182	67	230	15	42	10	1	.2	.1	.3
		Snap beans/green beans, cuts and french style:											
15	800	Cooked from raw	1 c	125	89	44	2	10	3	<1	.1	t	.2
15	801	Cooked from frozen	1 c	135	92	36	2	8	3	<1	<.1	t	.1
15	802	Canned, drained	1 c	136	93	26	2	6	2	<1	<.1	t	.1
		Navy beans, canned:											
15	803	Beans w/pork and tomato sauce	1 c	253	73	247	13	49	19	3	1.0	1.1	.3
15	804	Beans w/pork and sweet sauce	1 c	253	71	282	13	53	18	4	1.4	1.6	.5
15	805	Beans with frankfurters	1 c	257	70	365	17	40	17	17	6	7	2
		Bean sprouts (mung):											
15	806	Raw	1 c	104	90	32	3	6	2	<1	.1	t	.1
15	807	Cooked, stir fried	1 c	124	84	62	5	13	3	<1	.1	.1	.1
15	808	Cooked, boiled, drained	1 c	124	93	26	3	5	2	<1	<.1	t	<.1
		Beets:											
		Cooked from fresh:											
15	809	Sliced or diced	½ c	85	91	26	1	6	2	<.1	t	t	t
15	810	Whole beets, 2″ diam	2 beets	100	91	31	1	7	2	<.1	t	t	t
		Canned:											
15	811	Sliced or diced	½ c	85	91	27	1	6	2	<1	t	t	<.1
15	812	Pickled slices	½ c	114	82	74	1	19	2	<1	t	t	<.1
15	813	Beet greens, cooked, drained	1 c	144	89	40	4	8	3	<1	<.1	.1	.1
		Black-eyed peas, cooked:											
15	814	From dry, drained	1 c	171	70	198	13	36	11	1	.2	.1	.4
15	815	From fresh, drained	1 c	171	70	198	13	36	7	1	.2	.1	.4
15	816	From frozen, drained	1 c	170	66	224	14	40	7	1	.3	.1	.5
		Broccoli:											
		Raw:											
15	817	Chopped	1 c	88	91	24	3	5	3	<1	.1	t	.2
15	818	Spears	1 spear	151	91	42	4	8	6	<1	.1	<.1	.3

Key: 1 = BEV 2 = DAIRY 3 = EGGS 4 = FAT/OIL 5 = FRUIT 6 = BAKERY 7 = GRAIN 8 = FISH 9 = BEEF 10 = POULTRY 11 = SAUSAGE 12 = MIXED/FAST 13 = NUTS/SEEDS 14 = SWEETS 15 = VEG/LEG 16 = MISC 22 = SOUP/SAUCE

Chol (mg)	Calc (mg)	Iron (mg)	Magn (mg)	Phos (mg)	Pota (mg)	Sodi (mg)	Zinc (mg)	VT-A (RE)	Thia (mg)	Ribo (mg)	Niac (mg)	V-B6 (mg)	Fola (µg)	VT-C (mg)
0	47	3.6	121	241	611	1	1.9	1	.42	.10	.87	.12	256	0
0	19	1.16	29	54	347	45	.37	16	.06	.05	.91	.1	55	11
0	25	1.76	50	101	370	26	.5	15	.06	.05	.69	.1	58	5
0	52	4.36	97	231	1817	5	1.87	0	.29	.10	1.2	.14	273	0
0	58	1.6	32	48	373	4	.45	83[106]	.09	.12	.77	.07	42	12
0	61	1.11	29	33	151	17	.84	71[107]	.07	.1	.56	.08	42	11
0	36	1.22	18	26	148	340[108]	.39	47[109]	.02	.08	.27	.05	40	6
17	141	4.6	88	297	759	1113	2.6	31	.13	.12	1.3	.20	57	8
17	155	4.2	87	266	673	849	3.8	29	.12	.15	.89	.22	95	8
15	123	4.5	71	267	604	1105	4.8	40	.15	.14	2.3	.12	77	6
0	14	.95	22	56	154	6	.43	2	.09	.13	.78	.09	63	14
0	16	2.4	38	70	200	14	1.12	3	.17	.22	1.49	.1	72	20
0	15	.81	18	34	125	12	.58	2	.06	.13	1.01	.05	35	14
0	9	.53	31	26	266	42	.21	1	.03	.01	.23	.03	49	5
0	11	.62	37	31	312	49	.25	1	.03	.01	.27	.03	86	6
0	13	1.55	13	15	126	233[110]	.18	1	.01	.04	.15	.04	27	4
0	13	.47	17	19	169	301	.3	1	.03	.06	.29	.03	35	3
0	165	2.74	97	58	1308	346	.72	734	.17	.42	.72	.19	47	36
0	42	4.3	91	266	476	6	2.2	3	.35	.1	.85	.17	356	<1
0	46	3.3	91	266	476	6	2.2	3	.35	.09	.85	.17	355	<1
0	40	3.6	85	208	638	9	2.42	13	.42	.11	1.24	.16	240	4
0	42	.78	22	58	286	24	.36	136[111]	.06	.1	.56	.14	62	82
0	72	1.33	38	99	490	41	.6	233[111]	.1	.18	.96	.24	107	141

(106)For green varieties; yellow beans contain 10 RE/cup.
(107)For green varieties; yellow beans contain 15 RE.
(108)Dietary pack contains 3 mg sodium.
(109)For green varieties; yellow beans contain 14 RE.
(110)Dietary pack contains 39 mg sodium.
(111)Vitamin A for whole plant: leaves are 1600 RE/100 g raw; flower clusters are 300/100 g raw; stalks are 40 RE/100 g raw.

(For purposes of calculations, use "0" for t, <1, <.1, <.01, etc.)

Table A–1

Food Composition

Grp	Ref	Food Description	Measure	Wt (g)	H_2O (%)	Ener (cal)	Prot (g)	Carb (g)	Dietary Fiber (g)	Fat (g)	Fat Breakdown (g)		
											Sat	Mono	Poly
		VEGETABLES and LEGUMES—Con.											
		Broccoli—con.											
		Cooked from raw:											
15	819	Spears	1 spear	180	90	53	5	10	7	<1	.1	<.1	.2
15	820	Chopped	1 c	156	90	46	5	9	6	<1	.1	<.1	.2
		Cooked from frozen:											
15	821	Spear, small piece	1 spear	30	91	8	1	2	1	<.1	t	t	t
15	822	Chopped	1 c	184	91	51	6	10	6	<1	<.1	t	.1
		Brussels sprouts:											
15	823	Cooked from raw	1 c	156	87	60	6	13	6	1	.2	.1	.4
15	824	Cooked from frozen	1 c	155	87	65	6	13	5	1	.1	.1	.3
		Cabbage, common varieties:											
15	825	Raw, shredded or chopped	1 c	70	92	16	1	4	2	<1	t	t	.1
15	826	Cooked, drained	1 c	150	94	32	1	7	4	<1	.1	<.1	.2
		Chinese cabbage:											
15	827	Bok choy or Pak-choi, cooked, drained	1 c	170	96	20	3	3	3	<1	<.1	t	.1
15	828	Pe-Tsai, raw, chopped	1 c	76	94	11	1	3	2	<1	<.1	t	.1
		Cabbage, red, coarsely chopped:											
15	829	Raw	1 c	70	92	19	1	4	2	<1	t	t	.1
15	830	Cooked	½ c	75	94	16	1	3	4	<1	t	t	.1
15	831	Savoy cabbage, coarsely chopped, raw	1 c	70	91	20	1	4	2	<.1	t	t	<.1
		Carrots:											
		Raw:											
15	832	Whole, 7½ × 1⅛″	1 carrot	72	88	31	1	7	2	<1	t	t	.1
15	833	Grated	½ c	55	88	24	1	6	2	<1	t	t	<.1
		Cooked, sliced, drained:											
15	834	Cooked from raw	½ c	78	87	35	1	8	3	<1	<.1	t	.1
15	835	Cooked from frozen	½ c	73	90	26	1	6	3	<.1	t	t	<.1
15	836	Canned, sliced, drained	½ c	73	93	17	1	4	2	<1	<.1	t	.1
15	837	Carrot juice	¾ c	184	89	73	2	17	2	<1	.1	t	.1
		Cauliflower:											
15	838	Raw, flowerets	½ c	50	92	12	1	3	1	<.1	t	t	<.1
		Cooked, drained, flowerets:											
15	839	From raw	½ c	62	92	15	1	3	2	<1	t	t	.1
15	840	From frozen	1 c	180	94	34	3	7	4	<1	.1	<.1	.2
		Celery, pascal type, raw:											
15	841	Large outer stalk, 8 × 1½″ (at root end)	1 stalk	40	95	6	<1	1	1	<.1	t	t	t
15	842	Diced	½ c	60	95	10	<1	2	1	<.1	t	t	<.1
		Chick-peas (see Garbanzo, #854)											
		Collards, cooked, drained:											
15	843	From raw	1 c	145	96	20	2	4	4	<1	.1	<.1	.1
15	844	From frozen	1 c	170	88	61	5	12	5	1	.1	.1	.4
		Corn:											
		Cooked, drained:											
15	845	From raw, on cob, 5″ long	1 ear	77	70	83	3	19	4	1	.2	.3	.5
15	846	From frozen, on cob, 3½″ long	1 ear	63	73	59	2	14	3	<1	.1	.1	.2
15	847	Kernels, cooked from frozen	½ c	82	76	67	3	17	4	<.1	t	t	<.1

Key: 1 = BEV 2 = DAIRY 3 = EGGS 4 = FAT/OIL 5 = FRUIT 6 = BAKERY 7 = GRAIN 8 = FISH 9 = BEEF 10 = POULTRY 11 = SAUSAGE 12 = MIXED/FAST 13 = NUTS/SEEDS 14 = SWEETS 15 = VEG/LEG 16 = MISC 22 = SOUP/SAUCE

Chol (mg)	Calc (mg)	Iron (mg)	Magn (mg)	Phos (mg)	Pota (mg)	Sodi (mg)	Zinc (mg)	VT-A (RE)	Thia (mg)	Ribo (mg)	Niac (mg)	V-B6 (mg)	Fola (μg)	VT-C (mg)
0	205	2.16	106	86	293	20	.55	254[111]	.15	.37	1.36	.36	123	113
0	178	1.78	94	74	254	16	.48	220[111]	.13	.32	1.18	.31	107	98
0	15	.18	6	17	54	7	.09	57[111]	.02	.02	.14	.04	26	12
0	94	1.13	37	101	331	44	.56	348[111]	.1	.15	.84	.24	104	74
0	56	1.88	32	87	491	17	.5	112	.17	.12	.95	.31	94	97
0	38	1.15	37	84	504	36	.55	91	.16	.17	.83	.27	157	71
0	32	.4	10	16	172	12	.12	9	.04	.02	.21	.07	40	33
0	50	.58	22	38	308	29	.24	13	.09	.08	.34	.1	31	36
0	158	1.77	18	49	630	57	.43	437	.05	.11	.73	.3	32	44
0	59	.23	10	22	181	7	.17	91	.03	.04	.3	.18	60	21
0	36	.35	11	29	144	8	.15	3	.04	.02	.21	.15	19	40
0	28	.27	8	21	105	6	.11	2	.03	.01	.15	.1	9	26
0	25	.28	20	29	161	20	.26	70	.05	.02	.21	.13	32	22
0	19	.36	11	32	233	25	.14	2025	.07	.04	.67	.11	10	7
0	15	.28	8	24	178	19	.11	1547	.05	.03	.51	.08	8	5
0	24	.48	10	24	177	52	.23	1915	.03	.04	.4	.19	11	2
0	21	.35	7	19	115	43	.17	1292	.02	.03	.32	.09	8	2
0	19	.47	6	17	131	176[112]	.19	1006	.01	.02	.4	.08	7	2
0	44	.57	26	77	538	54	.33	3167	.17	.1	.71	.4	7	11
0	14	.29	7	23	178	7	.09	t	.04	.03	.32	.12	33	36
0	17	.26	7	22	200	4	.15	t	.04	.04	.34	.12	32	34
0	31	.74	16	43	250	33	.23	4	.07	.1	.56	.16	74	56
0	14	.19	5	10	114	35	.07	5	.01	.01	.12	.01	4	3
0	22	.29	7	16	170	53	.1	8	.02	.02	.18	.02	5	4
0	113	.59	16	15	135	27	.93	322	.03	.06	.34	.06	55	14
0	357	1.9	52	46	427	85	.46	1017	.08	.2	1.08	.19	129	45
0	2	.47	25	79	192	13	.37	17[113]	.17	.06	1.24	.18	36	5
0	2	.38	18	47	158	3	.4	13[113]	.11	.04	.96	.14	19	3
0	2	.25	15	39	114	4	.29	20[113]	.06	.06	1.05	.18	19	2

(111)Vitamin A for whole plant: leaves are 1600 RE/100 g raw; flower clusters are 300/100 g raw; stalks are 40 RE/100 g raw.

(112)Dietary pack contains 31 mg sodium.

(113)For yellow varieties; white varieties contain only a trace of vitamin A.

(For purposes of calculations, use "0" for t, <1, <.1, <.01, etc.)

Table A–1

Food Composition

Grp	Ref	Food Description	Measure	Wt (g)	H_2O (%)	Ener (cal)	Prot (g)	Carb (g)	Dietary Fiber (g)	Fat (g)	Fat Breakdown (g) Sat	Mono	Poly
		VEGETABLES and LEGUMES—Con.											
		Corn—con.											
		Canned:											
15	848	Cream style	½ c	128	79	93	2	23	6	<1	.1	.2	.3
15	849	Whole kernel, vacuum pack	1 c	210	77	166	5	41	10	1	.2	.3	.5
		Cowpeas; (see Black-eyed peas, #814–816)											
15	850	Cucumbers with peel, ⅛″ thick, 2⅛″ diam	6 slices	28	96	4	<1	1	<1	<.1	t	t	t
		Dandelion greens:											
15	851	Raw	1 c	55	86	25	1	5	1	<1	.1	<.1	.2
15	852	Chopped, cooked, drained	1 c	105	90	35	2	7	1	1	.2	<.1	.4
15	853	Eggplant, cooked	1 c	160	92	45	1	11	6	<1	.1	<.1	.2
15	854	Garbanzo beans (chick-peas), cooked	1 c	164	60	269	15	45	9	4	.4	1.0	2.0
15	855	Great northern beans, cooked	1 c	177	69	210	15	38	12	1	.3	<.1	.3
15	856	Escarole/curly endive, chopped	1 c	50	94	8	1	2	1	<1	t	t	<.1
15	857	Jerusalem artichokes, raw slices	1 c	150	78	114	3	26	2	<.1	—	t	t
		Kale, cooked, drained:											
15	858	From raw	1 c	130	91	42	4	7	4	1	.1	<.1	.3
15	859	From frozen	1 c	130	90	39	4	7	3	1	.1	.1	.3
15	860	Kidney beans, canned	1 c	256	78	208	13	38	20	1	.1	.1	.4
15	861	Kohlrabi slices, cooked from raw	1 c	165	90	48	3	11	2	<1	t	t	.1
15	862	Lentils, cooked from dry	1 c	198	70	231	18	40	10	1	.1	.1	.4
		Lettuce:											
		Butterhead/Boston types:											
15	863	Head, 5″ diam	1 head	163	96	21	2	4	3	<1	.1	t	.2
15	864	Leaves, 2 inner or outer	2 leaves	15	96	2	<1	<1	<1	<.1	t	t	t
		Iceberg/crisphead:											
15	865	Head, 6″ diam	1 head	539	96	70	5	11	9	1	.1	<.1	.5
15	866	Wedge, ¼ of head	1 wedge	135	96	18	1	3	2	<1	<.1	t	.1
15	867	Chopped or shredded	1 c	56	96	7	1	1	1	<1	t	t	.1
15	868	Loose leaf, chopped	1 c	56	94	10	1	2	1	<1	t	t	.1
		Romaine:											
15	869	Chopped	1 c	56	95	9	1	1	1	<1	t	t	.1
15	870	Inner leaf	1 leaf	10	95	2	<1	<1	<1	<.1	t	t	t
		Mushrooms:											
15	871	Raw, sliced	½ c	35	92	9	1	2	1	<1	t	t	.1
15	872	Cooked from raw, pieces	½ c	78	91	21	2	4	2	<1	.1	t	.1
15	873	Canned, drained	½ c	78	91	19	2	4	2	<1	<.1	t	.1
		Mustard greens:											
15	874	Cooked from raw	1 c	140	94	21	3	3	3	<1	t	.2	.1
15	875	Cooked from frozen	1 c	150	94	28	3	5	4	<1	t	.2	.1
15	876	Navy beans, cooked from dry	1 c	182	63	259	16	48	16	1	.3	.1	.5
		Okra, cooked:											
15	877	From fresh pods	8 pods	85	90	27	2	6	3	<1	<.1	t	<.1
15	878	From frozen slices	½ c	92	91	34	2	7	3	<1	.1	.1	.1

Key: 1 = BEV 2 = DAIRY 3 = EGGS 4 = FAT/OIL 5 = FRUIT 6 = BAKERY 7 = GRAIN 8 = FISH 9 = BEEF 10 = POULTRY 11 = SAUSAGE 12 = MIXED/FAST 13 = NUTS/SEEDS 14 = SWEETS 15 = VEG/LEG 16 = MISC 22 = SOUP/SAUCE

Chol (mg)	Calc (mg)	Iron (mg)	Magn (mg)	Phos (mg)	Pota (mg)	Sodi (mg)	Zinc (mg)	VT-A (RE)	Thia (mg)	Ribo (mg)	Niac (mg)	V-B6 (mg)	Fola (μg)	VT-C (mg)
0	4	.49	22	65	172	365[114]	.68	12[113]	.03	.07	1.23	.08	57	6
0	11	.88	48	134	390	572[115]	.97	51[113]	.09	.15	2.46	.12	104	17
0	4	.08	3	5	42	1	.07	1	<.01	<.01	.09	.01	4	1
0	103	1.71	20	36	218	42	.62	770	.1	.14	.39	.04	64	19
0	147	1.89	26	44	244	46	.8	1229	.14	.18	.5	.04	82	19
0	10	.56	21	35	397	5	.24	10	.12	.03	.96	.14	23	2
0	80	4.7	78	275	477	11	2.51	4	.19	.1	.86	.23	282	2
0	121	3.8	88	293	692	4	1.55	<1	.28	.11	1.2	.21	181	2
0	26	.41	8	14	157	11	.40	103	.04	.04	.2	.01	71	3
0	21	5.1	26	117	644	6	.10	3	.3	.09	1.95	.11	15	6
0	94	1.17	23	36	296	30	.31	962	.07	.09	.70	.18	30	53
0	179	1.22	23	36	417	20	.23	826	.06	.15	.87	.11	31	33
0	69	3.1	79	269	658	889	1.4	0	.28	.18	1.3	.18	126	3
0	41	.66	31	74	561	34	.32	6	.07	.03	.64	.14	13	89
0	37	6.6	71	356	731	4	2.5	2	.34	.15	2.1	.35	358	3
0	52	.49	18	38	419	8	.42	158	.1	.1	.49	.11	119	13
0	5	.04	2	3	39	t	.04	15	<.01	<.01	.04	.01	11	1
0	102	2.7	48	108	852	48	1.19	178	.25	.16	1.01	.22	302	21
0	26	.68	12	27	213	12	.3	45	.06	.04	.25	.05	76	5
0	11	.28	5	11	89	5	.12	19	.03	.02	.1	.02	31	2
0	38	.78	6	14	148	5	.18	106	.03	.04	.22	.03	60	10
0	20	.62	3	25	162	4	.18	146	.06	.06	.28	.03	76	13
0	4	.11	<1	5	29	t	.03	26	.01	.01	.05	.06	14	2
0	2	.43	4	36	130	1	.3	0	.04	.16	1.44	.03	7	1
0	5	1.36	9	68	278	2	.68	0	.06	.23	3.48	.07	14	3
0	9	.62	6	52	101	332	.56	0	.05	.17	1.25	.06	10	0
0	104	1.56	21	57	283	22	.3	424	.06	.09	.61	.18	20	35
0	152	1.68	20	36	209	38	.3	671	.06	.08	.39	.16	20	21
0	128	4.5	107	285	670	2	1.93	<1	.37	.11	.97	.30	255	1
0	54	.38	48	48	274	4	.47	49	.11	.05	.74	.16	39	14
0	88	.62	47	42	215	3	.57	47	.09	.11	.72	.04	134	11

(113)For yellow varieties; white varieties contain only a trace of vitamin A.

(114)Dietary pack contains 4 mg sodium per ½ cup.

(115)Dietary pack contains 6 mg sodium per cup.

(For purposes of calculations, use "0" for t, <1, <.1, <.01, etc.)

Table A–1

Food Composition

Grp	Ref	Food Description	Measure	Wt (g)	H_2O (%)	Ener (cal)	Prot (g)	Carb (g)	Dietary Fiber (g)	Fat (g)	Fat Breakdown (g) Sat	Mono	Poly
		VEGETABLES and LEGUMES—Con.											
		Onions:											
		Raw:											
15	879	Chopped	1 c	160	91	54	2	12	3	<1	.1	.1	.2
15	880	Sliced	1 c	115	91	39	1	8	2	<1	.1	<.1	.1
15	881	Cooked, drained, chopped	½ c	105	92	30	1	7	2	<1	<.1	t	.1
15	882	Dehydrated flakes	¼ c	14	4	45	1	12	1	<.1	t	t	<.1
15	883	Onions, spring, chopped, bulb and top	½ c	50	91	13	1	3	2	<.1	t	t	<.1
15	884	Onion rings, breaded, prepared from frozen	2 rings	20	29	80	1	8	<1	5	1.7	2.2	1
		Parsley:											
		Raw											
15	885	Chopped	½ c	30	88	10	1	2	2	<.1	t	t	<.1
15	886	Sprigs	10 sprigs	10	88	3	<1	1	1	<.1	t	t	t
15	887	Freeze dried	¼ c	1	2	4	<1	1	1	<.1	t	t	<.1
15	888	Parsnips, sliced, cooked	1 c	156	78	125	2	30	4	1	.1	.2	.1
		Peas:											
		Black-eyed (see Black-eyed peas, #814–816)											
15	889	Edible pods, cooked	1 c	160	89	67	5	11	5	<1	.1	<.1	.2
		Green:											
15	890	Canned, drained	½ c	85	82	59	4	11	5	<1	.1	<.1	.1
15	891	Cooked from frozen	½ c	80	80	63	4	11	8	<1	<.1	t	.1
15	892	Split, green, cooked from dry	1 c	196	69	231	16	41	10	1	.1	.2	.3
		Peppers, hot:											
		Hot green chili:											
15	893	Canned	½ c	68	92	17	1	4	1	<.1	t	t	<.1
15	894	Raw	1 pepper	45	88	18	1	4	1	<.1	t	t	.1
15	895	Jalapenos, chopped, canned	½ c	68	90	17	1	3	2	<1	.4	t	.2
		Peppers, sweet, green:											
15	896	Whole pod (90 g with refuse), raw	1 pod	74	93	18	1	4	1	<1	.1	t	.2
15	897	Cooked, chopped (1 pod cooked = 73 g)	½ c	68	95	12	<1	3	1	<1	<.1	t	.1
15	898	Pinto beans, cooked from dry	1 c	171	64	235	14	44	19	1	.2	.2	.3
		Potatoes:[122]											
		Baked in oven, 4¾ × 2⅓″ diam											
15	899	With skin	1 potato	202	71	220	5	51	4	<1	.1	t	.1
15	900	Flesh only	1 potato	156	75	145	3	34	4	<1	<.1	t	.1
15	901	Skin	1 ea	58	47	115	2	27	1	<.1	t	t	<.1
		Baked in microwave, 4¾ × 2⅓″ diam:											
15	902	With skin	1 potato	202	72	212	5	49	4	<1	.1	t	.1
15	903	Flesh only	1 potato	156	74	156	3	36	4	<1	<.1	t	.1
15	904	Skin	1 ea	58	64	77	2	17	1	<.1	t	t	<.1

(122)Vitamin C varies with length of storage. After 3 months of storage approximately two-thirds of the ascorbic acid remains; after 6 to 7 months, about one-third remains.

A

Key: 1 = BEV 2 = DAIRY 3 = EGGS 4 = FAT/OIL 5 = FRUIT 6 = BAKERY 7 = GRAIN 8 = FISH 9 = BEEF 10 = POULTRY 11 = SAUSAGE 12 = MIXED/FAST 13 = NUTS/SEEDS 14 = SWEETS 15 = VEG/LEG 16 = MISC 22 = SOUP/SAUCE

Chol (mg)	Calc (mg)	Iron (mg)	Magn (mg)	Phos (mg)	Pota (mg)	Sodi (mg)	Zinc (mg)	VT-A (RE)	Thia (mg)	Ribo (mg)	Niac (mg)	V-B6 (mg)	Fola (µg)	VT-C (mg)
0	40	.59	16	46	248	3	.29	0	.1	.02	.16	.25	32	13
0	29	.43	12	33	178	2	.21	0	.07	.01	.12	.18	23	10
0	29	.21	11	24	159	8	.19	0	.04	<.01	.08	.19	13	6
0	36	.22	13	42	227	3	.26	0	.11	<.01	<.01	.22	23	11
0	30	.94	10	16	128	2	.22	250	.04	.07	.1	.03	8	23
0	6	.3	1	16	26	75	.07	5	.06	.03	.7	.02	1	t
0	39	1.86	13	12	161	12	.22	156	.02	.03	.21	.05	55	27
0	13	.62	4	4	54	4	.07	52	<.01	.01	.07	.02	18	9
0	2	.75	5	8	88	5	.09	89	.01	.03	.15	.02	22	2
0	58	.9	46	108	573	16	.4	0	.13	.08	1.1	.15	91	20[116]
0	67	3.15	42	89	383	6	.6	21	.2	.12	.86	.23	48	77
0	17	.81	15	57	.147	186[117]	.6	65	.1	.07	.62	.05	38	8
0	19	1.25	23	72	134	70	.75	53	.23	.14	1.18	.09	47	8
0	26	2.52	71	195	710	4	1.96	1	.37	.11	1.7	.09	127	1
0	5	.34	8	12	143	10	.02	42[118]	.01	.03	.54	.08	35	46
0	8	.54	11	21	153	3	.14	35[119]	.04	.04	.43	.12	10	109
0	18	1.9	8	12	92	995	.13	116	.02	.03	.34	.08	35	9
0	4	.94	10	16	144	2	.13	39[120]	.06	.04	.41	.12	12	95[120]
0	3	.6	7	10	88	1	.08	26[121]	.04	.02	.25	.07	10	76[121]
0	82	4.5	95	273	800	3	1.85	<1	.32	.16	.68	.27	294	3
0	20	2.75	55	115	844	16	.65	0	.22	.07	3.32	.7	22	26
0	8	.55	39	78	610	8	.45	0	.16	.03	2.18	.47	14	20
0	20	2.2	25	59	332	12	.28	0	.07	.07	1.78	.35	12	8
0	22	2.5	54	212	903	16	.73	0	.24	.07	3.46	.69	24	31
0	8	.64	39	170	641	11	.51	0	.2	.04	2.54	.5	19	24
0	27	3.44	22	48	377	9	.3	0	.04	.04	1.29	.28	10	9

(116)Value for Vitamin C is highest right after harvest and drops after that.

(117)Dietary pack contains 1.7 mg sodium.

(118)For green chili peppers; red varieties contain 809 RE vitamin A.

(119)For green chili peppers; red varieties contain 484 RE vitamin A.

(120)For green sweet peppers; red varieties contain 570 RE vitamin A and 141 mg ascorbic acid.

(121)For green sweet peppers; red varieties contain 256 RE vitamin A and 113 mg ascorbic acid.

(For purposes of calculations, use "0" for t, <1, <.1, <.01, etc.)

Table A–1

Food Composition

Grp	Ref	Food Description	Measure	Wt (g)	H_2O (%)	Ener (cal)	Prot (g)	Carb (g)	Dietary Fiber (g)	Fat (g)	Fat Breakdown (g) Sat	Mono	Poly
		VEGETABLES and LEGUMES—Con.											
		Potatoes—con.											
		Boiled, about 2½" diam:											
15	905	Peeled after boiling	1 potato	136	77	119	2	27	3	<1	<.1	t	.1
15	906	Peeled before boiling	1 ea	135	78	116	2	27	2	<1	<.1	t	.1
		French fried, strips 2-3½" long, frozen											
15	907	Oven heated	10 strips	50	53	111	2	17	2	4	2.1	1.8	.3
15	908	Fried in veg oil	10 strips	50	38	158	2	20	2	8	2.5	1.6	3.8
15	909	Hashed brown, from frozen	1 c	156	56	340	5	44	2	18	7	8	2
		Mashed:											
15	910	Home recipe with milk[123]	1 c	210	78	162	4	37	1	1	.7	.3	.1
15	911	Home recipe with milk and margarine	1 c	210	76	222	4	35	1	9	2.2	3.7	2.5
15	912	Prepared from flakes; water, milk, butter, salt added	1 c	210	76	237	4	32	1	12	7.2	3.3	.5
		Potato products, prepared:											
		Au gratin:											
15	913	From dry mix	1 c	245	79	228	6	31	4	10	6.3	3	.3
15	914	From home recipe[125]	1 c	245	74	322	12	28	4	19	12	5	1
		Potato salad (see Mixed Dishes #715)											
		Scalloped:											
15	915	From dry mix	1 c	245	79	228	5	31	5	11	6.5	3.0	.5
15	916	Home recipe[127]	1 c	245	81	210	7	26	5	9	5.5	2.6	.4
15	917	Potato chips	14 chips	28	2	148	2	15	<1	10	2.6	1.8	5.2
		Pumpkin:											
15	918	Cooked from raw, mashed	1 c	245	94	50	2	12	4	<1	.1	t	t
15	919	Canned	1 c	245	90	83	3	20	5	1	.4	.1	<.1
15	920	Red radishes	10 radishes	45	95	7	<1	2	1	<1	t	t	t
15	921	Refried beans, canned	1 c	253	72	270	16	47	22	3	1	1.2	.4
15	922	Sauerkraut, canned with liquid	1 c	236	92	44	2	10	4	<1	.1	<.1	.1
		Seaweed:											
15	923	Kelp, raw	1 oz	28	82	12	1	3	1	<1	.1	<.1	t
15	924	Spirulina, dried	1 oz	28	5	82	16	7	1	2	.8	.2	.6
15	925	Soybeans, cooked from dry	1 c	172	63	298	29	17	5	15	2.2	3.4	8.7
		Soybean products:											
15	926	Miso	½ c	138	42	284	16	39	4[130]	8	1.2	1.9	4.7
15	927	Tofu	½ c	124	85	94	10	2	2[130]	6	.9	1.3	3.4
		Spinach:											
15	928	Raw, chopped	1 c	56	92	12	2	2	2	<1	<.1	t	.1
		Cooked, drained:											
15	929	From raw	1 c	180	91	41	5	7	6	<1	.1	t	.2
15	930	From frozen (leaf)	1 c	190	90	53	6	10	6	<1	.1	t	.2
15	931	Canned, drained solids	1 c	214	92	50	6	7	8	1	.2	<.1	.5

(123)Recipe: 84% potatoes, 15% whole milk, 1% salt.
(125)Recipe: 55% potatoes, 30% whole milk, 9% cheddar cheese, 3% butter, 2% flour, 1% salt.
(127)Recipe: 59% potatoes, 36% whole milk, 2% butter, 2% flour, 1% salt.
(130)Estimate based on cooked soybeans.

Key: 1 = BEV 2 = DAIRY 3 = EGGS 4 = FAT/OIL 5 = FRUIT 6 = BAKERY 7 = GRAIN 8 = FISH 9 = BEEF 10 = POULTRY 11 = SAUSAGE 12 = MIXED/FAST 13 = NUTS/SEEDS 14 = SWEETS 15 = VEG/LEG 16 = MISC 22 = SOUP/SAUCE

Chol (mg)	Calc (mg)	Iron (mg)	Magn (mg)	Phos (mg)	Pota (mg)	Sodi (mg)	Zinc (mg)	VT-A (RE)	Thia (mg)	Ribo (mg)	Niac (mg)	V-B6 (mg)	Fola (µg)	VT-C (mg)
0	7	.42	30	60	515	6	.41	0	.14	.03	1.96	.41	14	18
0	10	.42	26	54	443	7	.37	0	.13	.03	.18	.36	12	10
0	4	.67	11	43	229	15	.21	0	.06	.01	1.15	.12	8	6
0	10	.38	17	47	366	108	.19	0	.09	.01	1.63	.12	14	5
0	24	2.36	26	112	680	53	.5	0	.17	.03	3.78	.2	26	10
4	55	.57	39	100	628	636	.6	12	.18	.08	2.35	.49	17	14
4[124]	54	.55	37	97	607	619	.58	41	.18	.11	2.2	.47	17	13
4[124]	103	.46	37	118	490	697	.37	44	.23	.08	1.41	.02	16	20
12	203	.78	37	233	537	1076	.59	76	.05	.2	2.3	.1	3	8
56[126]	292	1.56	48	277	970	1064	1.69	93	.16	.28	2.43	.43	20	24
27	88	.93	34	137	497	835	.61	51	.05	.14	2.52	.1	3	8
29[128]	140	1.41	46	154	926	821	.98	46	.17	.23	2.58	.44	21	26
0	7	.34	17	43	369	133[129]	.3	0	.04	<.01	1.19	.14	13	12
0	37	1.4	22	74	564	3	.45	265	.08	.19	1.01	.16	33	12
0	64	3.41	56	85	504	12	.42	5404	.06	.13	.9	.14	30	10
0	9	.13	4	8	104	11	.13	t	<.01	.02	.14	.03	12	10
0	118	4.5	99	214	994	1071	3.45	0	.12	.14	1.2	.28	150	15
0	72	3.47	31	46	401	1561	.44	4	.05	.05	.34	.31	4	35
0	48	.81	34	12	25	66	.35	3	.01	.04	.13	—	51	—
0	34	8.08	55	33	386	297	—	16	.68	1.04	3.63	.1	—	3
0	175	8.84	148	421	886	1	2.0	2	.27	.49	.69	.4	93	3
0	92	3.78	58	211	226	5032	4.58	12	.13	.35	1.19	.3	46	0
0	130	6.65	127	120	150	9	1.0	11	1.0	.06	.24	.06	19	.1
0	55	1.52	44	27	312	44	.3	376	.04	.11	.41	.11	109	16
0	244	6.42	157	100	838	126	1.37	1474	.17	.42	.88	.44	262	40
0	277	2.89	131	91	566	163	1.33	1479	.11	.32	.8	.28	204	23
0	271	4.92	162	94	740	683[131]	.99	1878	.03	.29	.83	.21	209	31

(124)For margarine; if butter is used, cholesterol = 25 mg for 29 total mg.
(126)For butter; if margarine is used, cholesterol = 37 mg.
(128)For butter; if margarine is used cholesterol = 15 mg.
(129)If no salt is added, sodium = 2 mg.
(131)Dietary pack contains 58 mg sodium.

(For purposes of calculations, use "0" for t, <1, <.1, <.01, etc.)

Table A–1

Food Composition

Grp	Ref	Food Description	Measure	Wt (g)	H_2O (%)	Ener (cal)	Prot (g)	Carb (g)	Dietary Fiber (g)	Fat (g)	Fat Breakdown (g) Sat	Mono	Poly
		VEGETABLES and LEGUMES—Con.											
		Spinach soufflé (see Mixed Dishes)											
		Squash, summer varieties, cooked slices:											
15	932	Varieties averaged	1 c	180	94	36	2	8	3	1	.1	<.1	.2
15	933	Crookneck	1 c	180	94	36	2	8	3	1	.1	<.1	.2
15	934	Zucchini	1 c	180	95	29	1	7	3	<.1	t	t	<.1
		Squash, winter varieties, cooked:											
		Varieties averaged, baked:											
15	935	Mashed	1 c	245	89	96	2	21	6	1	.3	.1	.7
15	936	Baked cubes	1 c	205	89	79	2	18	5	1	.3	.1	.5
15	937	Acorn, baked, mashed	1 c	245	90	83	2	22	6	<1	<.1	t	.1
15	938	Butternut, baked cubes	1 c	205	88	83	2	21	5	<1	<.1	t	.1
		Sweet potatoes:											
		Cooked, 5 × 2″ diam:											
15	939	Baked in skin, peeled	1 potato	114	73	118	2	28	3	<1	<.1	t	.1
15	940	Boiled without skin	1 potato	151	73	160	2	37	4	<1	.1	t	.2
15	941	Candied, 2½ × 2″	1 pce	105	67	144	1	29	2	3	1.4	.7	.2
		Canned:											
15	942	Solid pack, mashed	1 c	265	74	258	5	59	6	<1	.1	t	.2
15	943	Vacuum pack, mashed	1 c	255	76	233	4	54	6	<1	.1	t	.2
15	944	Vacuum pack, 2¾ × 1″	1 pce	40	76	36	1	8	1	<.1	t	t	<.1
		Tomatoes:											
		Raw:											
15	945	Whole, 2⅗″ diam	1 tomato	123	94	24	1	5	2	<1	<.1	<.1	.1
15	946	Chopped	1 c	180	94	35	2	8	3	<1	.1	.1	.2
15	947	Cooked from raw	1 c	240	92	60	3	14	5	1	.1	.1	.3
15	948	Canned, solids and liquid	1 c	240	94	47	2	10	2	1	.1	.1	.2
15	949	Tomato juice, canned	1 c	244	94	42	2	10	2	<1	t	t	.1
		Tomato products, canned:											
15	950	Paste	1 c	262	74	220	10	49	6	2	.3	.4	1.0
15	951	Puree	1 c	250	87	102	4	25	4	<1	<.1	<.1	.1
15	952	Sauce	1 c	245	89	74	3	18	3	<1	.1	.1	.2
15	953	Turnips, cubes, cooked from raw	½ c	78	94	14	1	4	1	<.1	t	t	<.1
		Turnip greens, cooked:											
15	954	From raw (leaves and stems)	1 c	144	94	29	2	6	4	<1	.1	t	.1
15	955	From frozen (chopped)	½ c	82	90	24	3	4	2	<1	.1	t	.1
15	956	Vegetable juice cocktail, canned	1 c	242	94	46	2	11	1	<1	<.1	<.1	.1
		Vegetables, mixed:											
15	957	Canned, drained	1 c	163	87	77	4	15	7	<1	.1	<.1	.2
15	958	Frozen, cooked, drained	1 c	182	83	107	5	24	7	<1	.1	t	.1

Key: 1 = BEV 2 = DAIRY 3 = EGGS 4 = FAT/OIL 5 = FRUIT 6 = BAKERY 7 = GRAIN 8 = FISH 9 = BEEF 10 = POULTRY 11 = SAUSAGE 12 = MIXED/FAST 13 = NUTS/SEEDS 14 = SWEETS 15 = VEG/LEG 16 = MISC 22 = SOUP/SAUCE

Chol (mg)	Calc (mg)	Iron (mg)	Magn (mg)	Phos (mg)	Pota (mg)	Sodi (mg)	Zinc (mg)	VT-A (RE)	Thia (mg)	Ribo (mg)	Niac (mg)	V-B6 (mg)	Fola (μg)	VT-C (mg)
0	48	.64	44	69	346	2	.71	52[132]	.08	.07	.92	.12	36	9
0	48	.64	44	69	346	2	.71	52[132]	.09	.09	.92	.17	36	10
0	23	.63	40	72	455	5	.32	43[132]	.07	.07	.77	.14	30	8
0	34	.81	20	49	1071	2	.64	872	.21	.06	1.72	.18	69	24
0	28	.67	16	41	895	3	.54	730	.17	.05	1.43	.15	57	20
0	65	1.37	63	67	645	6	.27	63	.24	.02	1.30	.29	28	16
0	84	1.23	59	55	583	7	.27	1435	.15	.04	1.99	.25	39	31
0	32	.52	23	63	397	12	.33	2488	.08	.14	.7	.28	26	28
0	32	.8	15	41	278	20	.4	2575	.08	.21	1	.36	22	26
0[133]	27	1.2	12	27	198	74	.16	440	.02	.04	.41	.17	12	7
0	77	3.4	61	133	536	191	.54	3857	.07	.23	2.4	.48	42	13
0	56	2.27	57	125	796	136	.46	2036	.09	.14	1.89	.48	42	67
0	9	.36	9	20	125	21	.07	319	.01	.02	.3	.08	7	11
0	9	.59	14	28	255	10	.13	139	.07	.06	.74	.09	12	22[134]
0	12	.86	20	42	372	15	.19	204	.11	.09	1.08	.14	17	32[134]
0	20	1.44	33	70	624	25	.32	325	.17	.14	1.72	.15	23	50
0	63[135]	1.45	29	46	529	390[136]	.38	145	.11	.07	1.76	.22	35	36
0	22	1.41	27	47	537	881[137]	.34	136	.12	.08	1.64	.27	49	45
0	92	7.84	134	207	2442	170[138]	2.1	647	.41	.5	8.44	1	40	111
0	37	2.32	60	99	1051	49[139]	.54	340	.18	.14	4.29	.38	39	88
0	34	1.88	46	78	908	1481[140]	.6	240	.16	.14	2.82	.33	39	32
0	18	.17	6	15	106	39	.08	0	.02	.02	.23	.05	7	9
0	198	1.15	32	41	293	41	.29	792	.07	.1	.59	.26	171	40
0	125	1.59	21	27	184	12	.34	654	.04	.06	.38	.06	32	18
0	27	1.02	27	41	467	883	.48	283	.1	.07	1.76	.34	38	67
0	44	1.71	26	68	474	243	.67	1899	.07	.08	.94	.13	38	8
0	46	1.49	40	93	308	64	.89	779	.13	.22	1.55	.14	35	6

(132)Applies to squash including skin; flesh has no appreciable vitamin A value.
(133)For recipe using margarine; if butter is used, cholesterol = 8 mg.
(134)Year-round average. From June through October, ascorbic acid is approximately 32 mg and 47 mg, respectively, for one tomato and 1 c chopped tomato. From November through May, market samples average around 12 and 18 mg, respectively.
(135)Calcium is added as a firming agent.
(136)Dietary pack contains 31 mg sodium.
(137)If no salt is added, sodium content is 24 mg.
(138)If salt is added, sodium content is 2070 mg.
(139)If salt is added, sodium content is 998 mg.
(140)With salt added.

(For purposes of calculations, use "0" for t, <1, <.1, <.01, etc.)

A

Table A–1

Food Composition

Grp	Ref	Food Description	Measure	Wt (g)	H_2O (%)	Ener (cal)	Prot (g)	Carb (g)	Dietary Fiber (g)	Fat (g)	Fat Breakdown (g) Sat	Mono	Poly
		VEGETABLES and LEGUMES—Con.											
		Water chestnuts, canned:											
15	959	Slices	½ c	70	86	35	1	9	1	<.1	t	t	t
15	960	Whole	4 ea	28	86	14	<1	3	<1	<1	t	t	t
		MISCELLANEOUS											
16	961	Carob flour	1 c	103	3	185	5	92	12	1	.1	.2	.2
		Baking powders for home use:											
		Sodium aluminum sulfate:											
16	962	With monocalcium phosphate monohydrate	1 tsp	3	2	5	t	1	0	0	0	0	0
16	963	With monocalcium phosphate monohydrate, calcium sulfate	1 tsp	3	1	5	t	1	0	0	0	0	0
16	964	Straight phosphate	1 tsp	4	2	5	t	1	0	0	0	0	0
16	965	Low sodium	1 tsp	4	1	5	t	1	0	0	0	0	0
16	966	Basil, ground	1 tbsp	5	6	11	1	3	1	<1	—	—	—
		Catsup:											
16	967	Cup	1 c	273	69	290	5	69	1	1	.2	.2	.4
16	968	Tablespoon	1 tbsp	17	69	18	<1	4	<1	<.1	t	t	<.1
16	969	Celery seed	1 tsp	2	6	8	<1	1	<1	<1	.1	.3	.1
16	970	Chili powder	1 tsp	3	8	8	<1	1	1	<1	.1	.1	.2
		Chocolate											
16	971	Baking	1 oz	28	2	145	4	8	2	15	9	5	.5
		Semi-sweet, milk, and dark chocolates (see Sweeteners and Sweets, #759, 763, 764)											
16	972	Coriander, fresh	¼ c	4	93	<1	<.1	<1	<1	<.1	—	—	—
16	973	Cinnamon	1 tsp	2	10	5	<.1	2	1	<.1	t	t	t
16	974	Curry powder	1 tsp	2	10	5	<1	1	<1	<1	—	—	—
		Garlic:											
16	975	Cloves	4 cloves	12	59	18	1	4	<1	<.1	t	t	<.1
16	976	Powder	1 tsp	3	6	9	<1	2	<1	<.1	t	t	t
16	977	Gelatin, dry, plain	1 envelope	7	13	25	6	0	1	t	t	t	t
16	978	Ginger root, raw, sliced	5 slices	11	87	8	<1	2	<1	<.1	t	t	t
16	979	Mustard, prepared, (1 packet = 1 tsp)	1 tsp	5	80	4	<1	.3	<1	<1	t	.2	t
		Miso (see #926 under Vegetables and Legumes, Soybean products):											
		Olives:											
16	980	Green	10 olives	39	78	45	<1	<1	2	4.5	.6	3.6	.3
16	981	Ripe, pitted[141]	10 olives	47	81	50	<1	3	1	4.5	.8	3.4	.3
16	982	Onion powder	1 tsp	2	5	5	<1	2	<1	<.1	t	t	t
16	983	Oregano, ground	1 tsp	2	7	5	<1	1	<1	<1	t	t	.1
16	984	Paprika	1 tsp	2	10	6	<1	1	<1	<1	t	t	.2
16	985	Pepper, black	1 tsp	2	11	5	<1	1	<1	<.1	<.1	<.1	<.1
		Pickles:											
16	986	Dill, medium, 3¾ × 1¼″ diam	1 pickle	65	93	5	<1	1	1	<1	<.1	t	<.1
16	987	Fresh pack, slices, 1½″ diam × ¼″ thick	4 slices	30	79	20	<1	5	<1	<.1	t	t	t
16	988	Sweet, small, about 2½ × ¾″ diam	1 pickle	15	61	20	<.1	5	<1	<.1	t	t	t
16	989	Pickle relish, sweet	1 tbsp	15	63	20	<.1	5	<1	<.1	t	t	<.1

[141] This is the most recent tested data from the California Olive Industry, October 1986.

Key: 1 = BEV 2 = DAIRY 3 = EGGS 4 = FAT/OIL 5 = FRUIT 6 = BAKERY 7 = GRAIN 8 = FISH 9 = BEEF 10 = POULTRY 11 = SAUSAGE 12 = MIXED/FAST 13 = NUTS/SEEDS 14 = SWEETS 15 = VEG/LEG 16 = MISC 22 = SOUP/SAUCE

Chol (mg)	Calc (mg)	Iron (mg)	Magn (mg)	Phos (mg)	Pota (mg)	Sodi (mg)	Zinc (mg)	VT-A (RE)	Thia (mg)	Ribo (mg)	Niac (mg)	V-B6 (mg)	Fola (μg)	VT-C (mg)
0	3	.61	3	14	82	6	.27	t	<.01	.02	.25	—	8	1
0	1	.25	1	5	33	2	.11	t	<.01	<.01	.1	—	3	<1
0	359	3.0	56	81	852	36	.94	1	.06	.48	2.0	.38	30	<1
0	58	0	t	87	5	329	0	0	0	0	0	0	0	0
0	183	0	—	45	4	290	0	0	0	0	0	0	0	0
0	239	0	—	359	6	312	0	0	0	0	0	0	0	0
0	207	0	—	314	891	t	0	0	0	0	0	0	0	0
0	95	1.89	18	22	154	2	.26	42	<.01	.01	.31	—	—	3
0	60	2.2	57	137	991	2845	.64	382	.25	.19	4.4	.29	14	41
0	4	.14	4	9	54	156	.04	24	.02	.01	.27	.02	<1	3
0	38	.97	10	11	30	4	.15	t	.01	.01	.1	—	—	<1
0	7	.37	4	8	50	26	.07	91	<.01	.02	.2	—	1	2
0	22	1.9	82	109	235	1	1.01	1	.01	.1	.38	.01	18	0
0	4	.08	1	1	22	1	—	11	<.01	<.01	.03	—	—	<1
0	28	.87	1	1	12	1	.04	1	<.01	<.01	.03	.02	—	1
0	10	.62	5	7	31	1	.09	2	<.01	<.01	.07	—	—	<1
0	22	.2	3	18	48	2	1.06	0	.02	.01	.08	.40	<1	4
0	2	.08	2	12	31	1	.07	0	.01	<.01	.02	—	2	t
0	1	0	2	0	2	6	0	0	0	0	0	<.01	0	0
0	2	.05	5	3	46	1	.22	0	<.01	<.01	.08	.02	2	1
0	4	.1	2	4	7	63	.03	0	<.01	.01	.07	<.01	0	t
0	24	.6	9	6	21	936	.03	12	<.01	<.01	.01	<.01	<1	t
0	42	1.5	10	10	4	410	.14	18	<.01	<.01	0.2	<.01	<1	<1
0	8	.06	3	7	20	1	.05	0	<.01	<.01	.01	.03	3	t
0	24	.66	4	3	25	t	.07	10	<.01	t	.09	—	—	1
0	4	.54	4	7	49	1	.1	127	.01	.04	.35	—	—	1
0	9	.49	4	4	27	1	.03	t	<.01	<.01	.02	0	—	0
0	17	.7	8	14	130	928	.18	7	<.01	.01	.01	<.01	<1	4
0	10	.55	2	8	60	201	0	4	t	<.01	<.01	<.01	0	2
0	2	.25	2	2	30	107	<.01	1	<.01	<.01	<.01	<.01	0	1
0	3	.12	<1	2	30	107	.01	2	t	t	<.01	0	0	1

(For purposes of calculations, use "0" for t, <1, <.1, <.01, etc.)

Table A–1

Food Composition

Grp	Ref	Food Description	Measure	Wt (g)	H_2O (%)	Ener (cal)	Prot (g)	Carb (g)	Dietary Fiber (g)	Fat (g)	Fat Breakdown (g)		
											Sat	Mono	Poly
MISCELLANEOUS—Con.													
		Popcorn (see Grain Products, #539-541)											
16	990	Salt	1 tsp	6	0	0	0	0	0	0	0	0	0
16	991	Vinegar, cider	1 tbsp	15	94	2	0	1	0	0	0	0	0
		Yeast:											
16	992	Baker's, dry, active, package	1 package	7	5	20	3	3	<.01	<1	t	.1	t
16	993	Brewer's, dry	1 tbsp	8	5	25	3	3	<1	<.1	t	t	0
SOUPS, SAUCES, AND GRAVIES													
		Soups, canned, condensed:											
		Prepared with equal volume of whole milk:											
22	994	Clam chowder, New England	1 c	248	85	163	10	17	2	7	3.0	2.3	1.1
22	995	Cream of chicken	1 c	248	85	191	8	15	<1	11	5	4	2
22	996	Cream of mushroom	1 c	248	85	205	6	15	<1	14	5	3	5
22	997	Tomato	1 c	248	85	160	6	22	<1	6	2.9	1.6	1.1
		Prepared with equal volume of water:											
22	998	Bean with bacon	1 c	253	84	173	8	23	3	6	1.5	2.2	1.8
22	999	Beef broth, bouillon, consommé	1 c	240	98	16	3	1	0	<1	.3	.2	t
22	1000	Beef noodle	1 c	244	92	84	5	9	<1	3	1.2	1.2	.5
22	1001	Chicken noodle	1 c	241	92	75	4	9	<1	2	.7	1.1	.6
22	1002	Chicken rice	1 c	241	94	60	4	7	1	2	.5	.9	.4
22	1003	Clam chowder, Manhatten	1 c	244	90	78	4	12	1	2	.4	.4	1.3
22	1004	Cream of chicken	1 c	244	91	115	3	9	1	7	2.1	3.3	1.5
22	1005	Cream of mushroom	1 c	244	90	130	2	9	1	9	2.4	1.7	4.2
22	1006	Minestrone	1 c	241	91	80	4	11	1	2	.5	.7	1.1
22	1007	Split pea with ham	1 c	253	82	189	10	28	1	4	1.8	1.8	.6
22	1008	Tomato	1 c	244	90	86	2	17	<1	2	.4	.4	1.0
22	1009	Vegetable beef	1 c	244	92	79	6	10	1	2	.9	.8	.1
22	1010	Vegetarian vegetable	1 c	241	92	70	2	12	1	2	.3	.8	.7
		Soups, dehydrated:											
		Unprepared, dry products:											
22	1011	Bouillon	1 packet	6	3	15	1	1	0	1	.3	.2	t
22	1012	Onion	1 packet	7	4	20	1	4	<1	<1	.1	.2	.1
		Prepared with water:											
22	1013	Chicken noodle	¾ c	188	94	40	2	6	<1	1	.2	.4	.3
22	1014	Onion	¾ c	184	96	20	1	4	<1	<1	.1	.3	.1
22	1015	Tomato vegetable	¾ c	189	94	41	1	8	<1	1	.3	.3	.1
		Sauces:											
		From dry mixes:											
22	1016	Cheese sauce, prepared with milk	1 c	279	77	305	16	23	<1	17	9	5	2
22	1017	Hollandaise, prepared with milk	1 c	259	84	240	5	14	—	20	12	6	1
22	1018	White sauce, prepared with milk	1 c	264	81	240	10	21	<1	13	6	5	2
		From home recipe:											
22	1019	White sauce, medium[143]	1 c	250	73	395	10	24	<1	30	9	12	7

[143] Made with enriched flour, margarine, and whole milk.

A

Key: 1 = BEV 2 = DAIRY 3 = EGGS 4 = FAT/OIL 5 = FRUIT 6 = BAKERY 7 = GRAIN 8 = FISH 9 = BEEF 10 = POULTRY 11 = SAUSAGE 12 = MIXED/FAST 13 = NUTS/SEEDS 14 = SWEETS 15 = VEG/LEG 16 = MISC 22 = SOUP/SAUCE

Chol (mg)	Calc (mg)	Iron (mg)	Magn (mg)	Phos (mg)	Pota (mg)	Sodi (mg)	Zinc (mg)	VT-A (RE)	Thia (mg)	Ribo (mg)	Niac (mg)	V-B6 (mg)	Fola (μg)	VT-C (mg)
0	14	<.01	0	3	.3	2132	0	0	0	0	0	0	0	0
0	1	.09	<1	1	15	t	.02	0	0	0	0	0	0	0
0	4	1.1	16	90	140	4	.42	t	.17	.38	2.7	.14	266	t
0	17[142]	1.39	18	140	152	10	.63	t	1.25	.34	3.16	.4	313	t
22	187	1.48	23	157	300	992	1.3	40	.07	.24	1.03	.13	12	3
27	180	.67	18	152	273	1046	.68	94	.07	.26	.92	.07	8	1
20	178	.59	20	156	270	1076	.64	38	.08	.28	.81	.06	15	2
17	159	1.82	23	148	450	932	.29	109	.13	.25	1.52	.16	21	68
3	81	2.05	44	132	403	952	1.03	89	.09	.03	.57	.04	32	2
1	15	.41	9	31	130	782	.6	0	<.01	.05	1.87	.07	2	0
5	15	1.1	6	46	100	952	1.54	63	.07	.06	1.07	.04	4	<1
7	17	.78	5	36	55	1106	.4	71	.05	.06	1.39	<.01	2	t
7	17	.75	1	22	101	815	.26	66	.02	.02	1.13	.02	1	t
2	34	1.89	10	58	261	1808	.93	92	.06	.05	1.34	.08	10	3
10	34	.61	3	37	88	986	.63	56	.03	.06	.82	.02	2	t
2	46	.5	5	49	100	1032	.59	0	.05	.09	.7	.01	3	1
2	34	.92	7	56	312	911	.73	234	.05	.04	.94	.10	16	1
0	22	2.3	48	213	399	1008	1.32	44	.15	.08	1.5	.07	2	1
0	13	1.76	8	34	263	872	.24	69	.09	.05	1.42	.11	15	67
5	17	1.11	6	41	173	956	2	189	.04	.05	1.03	.08	11	2
0	21	1.08	7	35	209	823	.46	301	.05	.05	.92	.06	11	1
1	4	.1	4	19	27	1019	.01	t	t	.01	.3	.01	—	0
t	10	.14	3	23	47	627	.06	t	.02	.04	.4	<.01	2	t
2	24	.37	5	24	23	957	.15	5	.05	.04	.66	<.01	1	<1
0	9	.14	6	22	48	635	.06	t	.02	.04	.36	<.01	2	<1
0	6	.47	15	23	78	856	.12	14	.04	.03	.59	.04	2	5
53	569	.3	32	438	552	1565	.95	117	.15	.56	.3	.1	12	2
52	124	.9	—	127	124	1564	—	220	.05	.18	.1	.5	—	t
34	425	.3	35	256	444	797	1.15	92	.08	.45	.5	.08	14	3
32	292	.9	35	238	381	888	1.05	340	.15	.43	.8	.1	12	2

(142)Value varies from 6 to 60 mg.

(For purposes of calculations, use "0" for t, <1, <.1, <.01, etc.)

Table A–1

Food Composition

Grp	Ref	Food Description	Measure	Wt (g)	H_2O (%)	Ener (cal)	Prot (g)	Carb (g)	Dietary Fiber (g)	Fat (g)	Fat Breakdown (g)		
											Sat	Mono	Poly
		SOUPS, SAUCES, AND GRAVIES—Con.											
		Sauces—con.											
		Ready to serve:											
22	1020	Barbeque sauce	1 tbsp	16	81	10	<1	2	<1	<1	<.1	.1	.1
22	1021	Soy sauce	1 tbsp	18	71	9	1	2	0	0	0	0	0
		Gravies:											
		Canned:											
22	1022	Beef	1 c	233	88	124	9	11	<1	5	2.8	2.3	.2
22	1023	Chicken	1 c	238	85	189	5	13	<1	14	3.4	6.1	3.6
22	1024	Mushroom	1 c	238	89	120	3	13	<1	6	1	3	2.4
		From dry mix:											
22	1025	Brown	1 c	261	91	80	3	14	<1	2	.9	.8	.1
22	1026	Chicken	1 c	260	91	85	3	14	<1	2	.5	.9	.4

A

Key: 1 = BEV 2 = DAIRY 3 = EGGS 4 = FAT/OIL 5 = FRUIT 6 = BAKERY 7 = GRAIN 8 = FISH 9 = BEEF 10 = POULTRY 11 = SAUSAGE 12 = MIXED/FAST 13 = NUTS/SEEDS 14 = SWEETS 15 = VEG/LEG 16 = MISC 22 = SOUP/SAUCE

Chol (mg)	Calc (mg)	Iron (mg)	Magn (mg)	Phos (mg)	Pota (mg)	Sodi (mg)	Zinc (mg)	VT-A (RE)	Thia (mg)	Ribo (mg)	Niac (mg)	V-B6 (mg)	Fola (μg)	VT-C (mg)
0	3	.12	<1	3	27	128	.03	14	<.01	<.01	.06	.01	<1	t
0	3	.4	6	20	32	10[illegible]9	.07	0	.01	.02	.61	.03	3	0
7	14	1.63	3	70	189	117	2.33	0	.07	.08	1.54	.02	7	0
5	48	1.1	5	69	260	1375	1.91	264	.04	.1	1.06	.02	3	0
0	17	1.6	—	36	252	1357	1.66	0	.08	.15	1.6	.05	0	0
2	66	.2	t	47	61	1147	.01	0	.04	.09	.9	<.01	—	0
3	39	.3	—	47	62	1134	.32	0	.05	.15	.8	.03	—	3

(For purposes of calculations, use "0" for t, <1, <.1, <.01, etc.)

A

Table A–1

Food Composition

Grp	Ref	Food Description	Measure	Wt (g)	H_2O (%)	Ener (cal)	Prot (g)	Carb (g)	Dietary Fiber (g)	Fat (g)	Fat Breakdown (g) Sat	Mono	Poly
ARBY'S													
12	1402	Bac'n Cheddar, deluxe	1 ea	226	56	526	27	33	<1	37	10	16	11
		Roast beef sandwiches:											
12	1403	Regular	1 ea	147	51	353	22	32	<1	15	7	5	2
12	1404	Junior	1 ea	86	48	218	12	22	<1	9	4	3	2
12	1405	Super	1 ea	234	58	501	25	50	<1	22	9	8	5
12	1406	Deluxe	1 ea	247	62	486	26	43	<1	23	9	8	5
12	1407	Beef 'n Cheddar	1 ea	197	57	455	26	28	<1	27	8	12	7
		Chicken Sandwiches:											
12	1408	Chicken breast sandwich	1 ea	195	52	509	26	36	<1	29	6	11	12
12	1409	Chicken salad sandwich	1 ea	156	53	386	18	33	<1	20	–	–	–
12	1410	Chicken salad & croissant	1 ea	150	50	472	22	16	<1	36	–	–	–
12	1411	Chicken club sandwich	1 ea	210	44	621	26	57	<1	32	–	–	–
12	1412	Hot ham and cheese sandwich	1 ea	156	62	292	23	19	<1	14	5	6	3
12	1413	Turkey deluxe sandwich	1 ea	197	61	375	24	33	<1	17	4	5	8
		Baked Potatoes											
12	1414	Plain	1 ea	312	75	290	8	66	6	<1	t	t	t
12	1415	Deluxe, w/butter & sour cream	1 ea	340	74	648	18	59	6	38	22	10	2
12	1416	W/broccoli & cheese	1 ea	340	70	541	13	72	6	22	10	7	3
12	1417	W/mushrooms & cheese	1 ea	321	70	506	16	61	6	22	10	7	3
12	1418	Taco	1 ea	425	70	619	23	73	6	27	11	9	3
		Milkshakes											
12	1419	Chocolate	1 ea	340	74	451	10	77	<1	12	3	7	2
12	1420	Jamocha	1 ea	326	75	368	9	59	0	11	3	6	2
12	1421	Vanilla	1 ea	312	75	330	11	46	0	12	4	5	2
Source: Arby's Inc, Atlanta Georgia for the basic nutrients. Values for dietary fiber, magnesium, phosphorus, potassium, zinc, vitamin A (in RE's), B6, folacin, some of the fatty acids, and percent water, are estimates calculated from known values for major ingredients.													
BURGER KING													
		Croissant Sandwiches											
12	1422	With egg, bacon & cheese	1 ea	119	49	335	15	20	<1	24	13	8	2
12	1423	With egg, sausage & cheese	1 ea	163	49	538	19	20	<1	41	20	12	3
12	1424	With egg, ham & cheese	1 ea	145	58	335	18	20	<1	20	12	7	1
		Whopper Sandwiches											
12	1425	Whopper	1 ea	265	57	640	27	42	<1	41	16	19	4
12	1426	Whopper w/ cheese	1 ea	289	57	723	31	43	<1	48	20	20	3
12	1427	Double beef	1 ea	351	56	850	46	52	<1	52	20	24	5
12	1428	Double w/cheese	1 ea	374	55	950	51	54	<1	60	24	28	4
12	1429	Whopper, Junior	1 ea	136	52	370	15	31	<1	17	6	8	1
12	1430	Whopper, Junior w/cheese	1 ea	158	55	420	17	32	<1	20	9	8	1
12	1431	Hamburger	1 ea	109	46	275	15	29	<1	12	5	6	<1
12	1432	Cheeseburger	1 ea	120	45	317	17	30	<1	15	7	6	1
12	1433	Bacon double cheeseburger	1 ea	159	41	510	33	27	<1	31	14	15	2
12	1434	Chicken sandwich	1 ea	230	46	688	26	56	<1	40	11	17	10
12	1435	Chicken tenders	1 ea	95	50	204	20	10	0	10	3	4	2
12	1436	Ham & cheese sandwich	1 ea	230	59	471	24	44	<1	23	10	8	4
12	1437	Whaler fish sandwich	1 ea	189	45	488	19	45	<1	27	6	9	10

KEY: 1 = BEV 2 = DAIRY 3 = EGGS 4 = FAT/OIL 5 = FRUIT 6 = BAKERY 7 = GRAIN 8 = FISH 9 = BEEF 10 = POULTRY
11 = SAUSAGE 12 = MIXED/FAST 13 = NUTS/SEEDS 14 = SWEETS 15 = VEG/LEG 16 = MISC 22 = SOUP/SAUCE

Chol (mg)	Calc (mg)	Iron (mg)	Magn (mg)	Phos (mg)	Pota (mg)	Sodi (mg)	Zinc (mg)	VT-A (RE)	Thia (mg)	Ribo (mg)	Niac (mg)	V-B6 (mg)	Fola (μg)	VT-C (mg)
83	100	2.70	—	—	422	1672	—	85	.15	.26	6	—	—	4
39	80	3.60	16	120	200	588	2.4	t	.23	.43	7.6	.20	14	<1
20	40	1.80	8	60	197	345	1.2	t	.15	.26	4	.10	7	t
40	100	4.50	25	190	500	798	3.8	225	.38	.60	9	.30	21	36
59	100	6.30	25	190	500	1288	3.8	10	.30	.34	5	.30	22	t
63	80	5.40	24	260	335	955	3.3	86	.12	.34	5	.22	19	<1
83	100	3.60	30	180	390	1082	1.0	17	.23	.26	10	.38	18	<1
30	–	–	–	–	–	630	–	–	–	–	–	–	–	–
12	–	–	–	–	–	725	–	–	–	–	–	–	–	–
108	–	–	–	–	–	1300	–	–	–	–	–	–	–	–
45	200	1.80	31	405	312	1350	2.4	60	.98	.51	6	.31	26	24
39	80	2.70	30	250	346	1047	2.3	30	.23	.43	12	.52	20	5
0	20	1.80	80	175	1300	12	1.0	0	.30	.14	5	1.08	30	63
72	300	2.70	83	200	1340	475	1.1	300	.23	.43	6	1.10	33	63
24	150	2.70	97	400	1400	475	2.0	200	.30	.34	6	1.15	60	63
21	300	2.70	91	440	1345	635	2.1	250	.23	.43	7	1.25	36	63
145	450	3.60	105	530	1425	1065	4.7	860	.38	.26	8	1.40	38	63
36	300	1.10	48	350	410	341	1.2	85	.12	.60	.4	.14	14	2
35	300	1.10	36	350	525	262	1.1	85	.09	.51	3	.14	14	t
32	300	.70	36	350	686	281	1.1	85	.12	.60	t	.14	37	2

Chol (mg)	Calc (mg)	Iron (mg)	Magn (mg)	Phos (mg)	Pota (mg)	Sodi (mg)	Zinc (mg)	VT-A (RE)	Thia (mg)	Ribo (mg)	Niac (mg)	V-B6 (mg)	Fola (μg)	VT-C (mg)
249	136	2.00	20	249	182	762	1.5	150	.32	.30	2	.06	24	t
293	145	2.90	19	292	284	1042	2.4	150	.36	.32	4	.06	24	t
262	136	2.20	24	317	256	987	1.9	150	.49	.32	3	.06	24	t
94	80	4.90	43	237	547	842	4.5	60	.33	.41	7	.40	35	14
117	210	4.90	47	360	570	1126	5.1	85	.34	.48	7	.40	35	14
188	91	7.30	60	387	760	1080	8.5	60	.34	.56	10	.50	45	14
211	222	7.30	65	510	730	1535	9.1	85	.35	.63	10	.50	45	14
41	40	2.80	24	127	275	486	2.3	30	.23	.25	4	.20	17	6
52	105	2.80	27	189	287	628	2.6	85	.23	.29	4	.20	17	6
37	37	2.70	23	124	235	509	2.4	15	.23	.25	4	.12	18	3
48	102	3.80	26	186	247	651	2.6	70	.23	.29	4	.13	24	3
104	168	3.80	37	328	363	728	5.1	85	.31	.42	6	.30	30	t
82	79	3.30	54	274	375	1423	1.2	13	.45	.31	10	.40	18	t
47	18	.70	24	236	200	636	.6	5	.08	.08	7	.34	10	t
70	195	3.20	42	384	419	1534	2.4	85	.87	.42	6	.31	25	7
84	t	2.20	40	249	366	592	.1	20	.28	.21	4	.13	3	t

Table A–1

Food Composition

Grp	Ref	Food Description	Measure	Wt (g)	H_2O (%)	Ener (cal)	Prot (g)	Carb (g)	Dietary Fiber (g)	Fat (g)	Fat Breakdown (g) Sat	Mono	Poly
		BURGER KING—Con.											
12	1438	Whaler sandwich w/cheese	1 ea	201	45	530	21	46	<1	30	7	9	10
12	1439	French fries, regular	1 svg	74	37	227	3	24	<1	13	5	4	1
12	1440	Onion rings, regular	1 svg	79	37	274	4	28	<1	16	5	7	4
		Milkshakes											
12	1441	Chocolate, medium	1 ea	273	76	320	8	46	<1	12	–	–	–
12	1442	Vanilla, medium	1 ea	273	74	321	9	49	<1	10	–	–	–
		Pies											
12	1443	Apple pie	1 ea	125	51	305	3	44	<1	12	–	–	–
12	1444	Cherry pie	1 ea	128	42	357	4	55	<1	13	–	–	–
12	1445	Pecan pie	1 ea	113	20	459	5	64	1	20	3	11	5
		Source: Burger King Corporation for basic nutrients. Values for fatty acids, dietary fiber, vitamin A (RE's), folacin and percent water, calculated from known values for major ingredients.											
		DAIRY QUEEN											
		Ice cream cones											
12	1446	Small	1 ea	85	65	140	3	22	0	4	2	1	<1
12	1447	Regular	1 ea	142	65	240	6	38	0	7	–	–	–
12	1448	Large	1 ea	213	65	340	9	57	0	10	–	–	–
		Dipped ice cream cones											
12	1449	Small	1 ea	92	58	190	3	25	<1	9	–	–	–
12	1450	Regular	1 ea	156	58	340	6	42	<1	16	–	–	–
12	1451	Large	1 ea	234	58	510	9	64	<1	24	–	–	–
		Sundaes											
12	1452	Small	1 ea	106	60	190	3	33	<1	4	–	–	–
12	1453	Regular	1 ea	177	60	310	5	56	<1	8	–	–	–
12	1454	Large	1 ea	248	60	440	8	78	<1	10	–	–	–
12	1455	Banana Split	1 ea	383	67	540	9	103	<1	11	–	–	–
12	1456	Peanut buster parfait	1 ea	305	52	740	16	94	<1	34	–	–	–
12	1457	Hot fudge brownie delight	1 ea	266	55	600	9	85	<1	25	–	–	–
12	1458	Strawberry shortcake	1 ea	312	61	540	10	100	<1	11	–	–	–
12	1459	Buster bar	1 ea	149	45	460	10	41	<1	29	–	–	–
12	1460	Dilly bar	1 ea	85	55	210	3	21	<1	13	–	–	–
12	1461	DQ ice cream sandwich	1 ea	60	47	140	3	24	<1	4	–	–	–
		Milkshakes:											
12	1462	Small	1 ea	291	63	490	10	82	<1	13	–	–	–
12	1463	Regular	1 ea	418	63	710	14	120	<1	19	–	–	–
12	1464	Large	1 ea	588	63	990	19	168	<1	26	–	–	–
		Malted milkshakes:											
12	1465	Small	1 ea	291	60	520	10	91	<1	13	–	–	–
12	1466	Regular	1 ea	418	60	760	14	134	<1	18	–	–	–
12	1467	Large	1 ea	588	60	1060	20	187	<1	25	–	–	–
12	1468	Float	1 ea	397	76	410	5	82	0	7	–	–	–
12	1469	Freeze	1 ea	397	72	500	9	89	0	12	–	–	–
		Mr. Misty											
12	1470	Regular	1 ea	330	81	250	0	63	0	0	0	0	0
12	1471	Kiss	1 ea	89	81	70	0	17	0	0	0	0	0
12	1472	Freeze	1 ea	411	72	500	9	91	0	12	–	–	–
12	1473	Float	1 ea	411	78	390	5	74	0	7	–	–	–
12	1474	Chicken sandwich	1 ea	220	46	670	29	46	<1	41	8	15	17

A

KEY: 1 = BEV 2 = DAIRY 3 = EGGS 4 = FAT/OIL 5 = FRUIT 6 = BAKERY 7 = GRAIN 8 = FISH 9 = BEEF 10 = POULTRY 11 = SAUSAGE 12 = MIXED/FAST 13 = NUTS/SEEDS 14 = SWEETS 15 = VEG/LEG 16 = MISC 22 = SOUP/SAUCE

Chol (mg)	Calc (mg)	Iron (mg)	Magn (mg)	Phos (mg)	Pota (mg)	Sodi (mg)	Zinc (mg)	VT-A (RE)	Thia (mg)	Ribo (mg)	Niac (mg)	V-B6 (mg)	Fola (μg)	VT-C (mg)
95	112	2.20	43	311	378	734	1.1	40	.27	.24	4	.13	3	t
14	t	.50	21	114	360	160	.3	0	.10	.30	7.5	.23	20	t
0	124	.80	18	195	173	665	.4	–	t	t	t	.07	8	t
–	260	1.60	46	262	567	202	1.0	–	.13	.55	t	–	–	t
–	295	t	32	284	505	205	1.0	–	.11	.57	t	–	–	t
4	t	1.20	t	31	122	412	.2	4	.27	.16	.6	.03	7	5
6	t	1.10	12	37	166	204	.2	15	.24	.16	.5	.03	4	8
4	24	1.10	16	84	204	374	<1	16	.28	.18	.6	.06	15	t

Chol (mg)	Calc (mg)	Iron (mg)	Magn (mg)	Phos (mg)	Pota (mg)	Sodi (mg)	Zinc (mg)	VT-A (RE)	Thia (mg)	Ribo (mg)	Niac (mg)	V-B6 (mg)	Fola (μg)	VT-C (mg)
10	100	.40	13	100	134	45	.47	30	.03	.17	t	.04	2	t
15	150	.70	20	200	220	80	.70	60	.06	.34	t	.06	3	t
25	250	1.40	30	300	330	115	1.0	90	.12	.51	t	.09	4	t
10	100	.40	13	100	134	55	.47	30	.03	.17	t	.04	2	t
20	150	.70	20	200	220	100	.70	60	.06	.34	t	.06	3	t
30	250	1.40	30	300	330	145	1.0	90	.12	.51	t	.09	4	t
10	100	.40	13	150	145	75	.45	30	.03	.17	.17	.03	2	t
20	200	1.10	26	200	290	120	.90	60	.06	.34	.3	.06	4	t
30	250	1.40	40	300	435	165	1.35	120	.12	.43	.4	.09	6	t
30	250	1.80	60	350	670	150	2.1	225	.15	.51	.4	.80	9	15
30	250	1.80	50	450	500	250	1.5	90	.15	.43	2	.10	7	t
20	200	1.80	30	300	300	225	.90	90	.12	.34	.3	.06	4	t
25	250	1.80	–	300	–	215	–	–	.23	.51	t	–	–	12
10	100	1.10	–	250	–	175	–	–	.12	.17	2	–	–	t
10	100	.40	–	100	–	50	–	–	.03	.17	t	–	–	t
5	60	.04	–	60	–	40	–	–	.03	.07	.4	–	–	t
35	350	1.80	30	400	480	180	.10	75	.15	.60	.3	.14	3	t
50	450	2.70	43	500	690	260	.14	105	.23	.77	.4	.20	4	t
70	700	3.60	60	800	960	360	.20	150	.30	1.2	.8	.28	6	t
35	350	2.70	30	400	480	180	.10	75	.15	.60	.4	.14	3	t
50	450	4.50	43	600	690	260	.14	105	.30	.85	.8	.20	4	t
70	700	5.40	60	800	960	360	.20	150	.38	1.2	1.20	.28	6	t
20	200	1.10	–	200	–	85	–	60	.06	.26	t	–	–	t
30	300	1.80	–	350	–	180	–	120	.15	.51	t	–	–	t
0	t	t	–	t	–	10	–	0	t	t	t	–	–	t
0	t	t	–	t	–	10	–	–	t	t	t	–	–	t
30	300	1.40	–	200	–	140	–	–	.12	.51	t	–	–	t
20	200	.70	–	200	–	95	–	–	.06	.26	t	–	–	t
75	t	.40	15	60	200	870	.5	8	.06	t	.1	.16	9	9

Table A–1

Food Composition

Grp	Ref	Food Description	Measure	Wt (g)	H_2O (%)	Ener (cal)	Prot (g)	Carb (g)	Dietary Fiber (g)	Fat (g)	Fat Breakdown (g) Sat	Mono	Poly
		DAIRY QUEEN-Con.											
12	1475	Fish filet sandwich	1 ea	170	52	400	20	41	<1	16	4	6	6
12	1476	Fish filet sandwich w/cheese	1 ea	177	51	440	24	39	<1	21	7	7	6
		Hamburgers											
12	1477	Single	1 ea	148	51	360	21	33	<1	16	6	7	1
12	1478	Double	1 ea	210	52	530	36	33	<1	28	10	13	2
12	1479	Triple	1 ea	272	52	710	51	33	<1	45	17	21	4
		Cheeseburgers											
12	1480	Single	1 ea	162	51	410	24	33	<1	20	8	8	1
12	1481	Double	1 ea	239	51	650	43	34	<1	37	15	14	2
12	1482	Triple	1 ea	301	52	820	58	34	<1	50	20	20	3
		Hotdogs											
12	1483	Regular	1 ea	100	50	280	11	21	<1	16	6	7	2
12	1484	With cheese	1 ea	114	49	330	15	21	<1	21	8	8	2
12	1485	With chili	1 ea	128	55	320	13	23	2	20	8	8	2
		Super Hotdogs											
12	1486	Regular	1 ea	175	48	520	17	44	<1	27	9	12	3
12	1487	With cheese	1 ea	196	48	580	22	45	<1	34	11	13	3
12	1488	With chili	1 ea	218	53	570	21	47	2	32	11	13	3
12	1489	French fries, small	1 svg	71	47	200	2	25	<1	10	4	3	<1
12	1490	French fries, large	1 svg	113	47	320	3	40	<1	16	7	5	1
12	1491	Onion Rings	1 svg	85	28	280	4	31	<1	16	5	7	4
		Source: International Dairy Queen Inc., Minneapolis, MN for basic nutrients. Values for dietary fiber, magnesium, potassium, zinc, fatty acids, vitamin A (RE's), B6, folacin and percent water, calculated from known values for the major ingredients.											
		JACK IN THE BOX											
12	1492	Breakfast Jack sandwich	1 ea	126	49	307	18	30	<1	13	–	–	–
12	1493	Canadian crescent	1 ea	134	42	472	19	25	<1	31	–	–	–
12	1494	Sausage crescent	1 ea	156	38	584	22	28	<1	43	–	–	–
12	1495	Supreme crescent	1 ea	146	38	547	20	27	<1	40	–	–	–
12	1496	Pancakes breakfast	1 ea	232	45	626	16	79	<1	27	–	–	–
12	1497	Scrambled egg breakfast	1 ea	267	51	719	26	55	<1	44	–	–	–
12	1498	Hamburger	1 ea	98	44	276	13	30	<1	12	–	–	–
12	1499	Cheeseburger	1 ea	113	44	323	16	32	<1	15	–	–	–
12	1500	Jumbo Jack	1 ea	205	57	485	26	38	<1	26	–	–	–
12	1501	Jumbo Jack w/cheese	1 ea	246	56	630	32	45	<1	35	–	–	–
12	1502	Bacon cheeseburger supreme	1 ea	231	45	724	34	44	<1	46	–	–	–
12	1503	Swiss & baconburger	1 ea	231	52	643	33	31	<1	43	–	–	–
12	1504	Ham & swiss burger	1 ea	203	44	638	36	37	<1	39	–	–	–
12	1505	Chicken supreme	1 ea	228	52	601	31	39	<1	36	–	–	–
12	1506	Moby Jack sandwich	1 ea	137	40	444	16	39	<1	25	–	–	–
12	1507	Club Pita	1 ea	177	64	284	22	30	<1	8	–	–	–
		Tacos											
12	1508	Regular	1 ea	81	57	191	8	16	<1	11	–	–	–
12	1509	Super	1 ea	135	63	288	12	21	<1	17	–	–	–
12	1510	Chicken strips dinner	1 ea	180	23	689	40	65	–	30	–	–	–
12	1511	Shrimp dinner	1 ea	165	16	731	22	77	<1	37	–	–	–
12	1512	Pasta seafood salad	1 ea	150	52	394	15	32	2	22	–	–	–

KEY: 1 = BEV 2 = DAIRY 3 = EGGS 4 = FAT/OIL 5 = FRUIT 6 = BAKERY 7 = GRAIN 8 = FISH 9 = BEEF 10 = POULTRY
11 = SAUSAGE 12 = MIXED/FAST 13 = NUTS/SEEDS 14 = SWEETS 15 = VEG/LEG 16 = MISC 22 = SOUP/SAUCE

Chol (mg)	Calc (mg)	Iron (mg)	Magn (mg)	Phos (mg)	Pota (mg)	Sodi (mg)	Zinc (mg)	VT-A (RE)	Thia (mg)	Ribo (mg)	Niac (mg)	V-B6 (mg)	Fola (μg)	VT-C (mg)
50	60	.70	20	200	370	875	.3	<1	.15	.26	3	.16	40	<1
60	150	.40	22	250	370	1035	.3	30	.15	.26	3	.16	20	<1
45	100	3.60	33	150	290	630	4.5	10	.30	.17	5	.18	16	t
85	100	6.30	45	300	410	660	6.4	20	.45	.34	9	.28	23	t
135	100	9.00	60	450	532	690	8.2	28	.60	.51	14	.33	29	t
50	200	3.60	35	250	300	790	5.0	110	.30	.17	5	.20	20	t
95	350	6.30	50	500	443	980	7.3	160	.45	.43	9	.30	30	t
145	350	9.00	65	700	550	1010	9.2	200	.60	.60	14	.55	37	t
45	80	1.40	21	100	130	830	1.4	t	.12	.14	3	.08	20	<1
55	150	1.40	24	200	140	990	1.9	85	.12	.17	3	.08	24	<1
55	80	1.80	38	150	170	985	1.8	60	.15	.26	4	.17	30	<1
80	150	2.70	24	150	210	1365	2.8	t	.23	.26	5	.14	35	<1
100	250	1.40	38	300	220	1605	2.5	100	.23	.26	5	.16	39	<1
100	150	2.70	48	250	250	1595	2.5	60	.23	.43	6	.25	45	<1
10	t	.34	16	60	450	115	t	0	.06	t	.8	.16	15	9
15	t	1.08	24	100	700	185	.3	0	.09	.03	1.2	.30	25	15
15	20	.72	16	60	110	140	.3	15	.09	t	.4	.08	10	2

Chol (mg)	Calc (mg)	Iron (mg)	Magn (mg)	Phos (mg)	Pota (mg)	Sodi (mg)	Zinc (mg)	VT-A (RE)	Thia (mg)	Ribo (mg)	Niac (mg)	V-B6 (mg)	Fola (μg)	VT-C (mg)
203	170	3.10	24	310	190	871	1.8	–	.47	.41	3	.11	–	<1
226	125	3.40	–	–	–	851	–	–	.50	.40	3.6	–	–	3
187	170	2.90	–	–	–	1012	–	–	.60	.51	4.6	–	–	t
178	150	2.70	–	–	–	1053	–	–	.64	.54	4.2	–	–	t
85	100	2.70	36	633	237	1670	1.9	–	.60	.43	5	.19	3	27
260	250	2.40	55	483	635	1110	3.0	–	.68	.59	5	.34	1	12
29	70	2.70	20	115	165	521	1.8	9	.36	.24	3.2	.10	–	1
42	160	2.70	22	194	177	749	2.3	57	.36	.27	3.3	.10	–	1
64	97	6.90	35	208	390	905	3.7	–	.51	.21	7	.25	–	5
110	250	4.50	49	411	499	1665	4.8	–	.53	.34	12	.31	–	5
70	310	4.90	–	–	–	1307	–	–	.56	.51	8.8	–	–	3
99	230	4.70	–	–	–	1354	–	–	.45	.41	6.8	–	–	3
117	268	6.10	–	–	–	1330	–	–	.76	.48	7.6	–	–	10
60	240	3.00	–	–	–	1582	–	–	.52	.37	10.6	–	–	4
47	160	2.20	30	263	246	820	1.1	–	.40	.25	2.8	.08	–	<1
43	80	–	–	–	–	953	–	–	.78	.29	5.9	–	–	4
21	100	1.10	35	146	257	460	1.2	–	.07	.17	1.0	.13	–	<1
37	150	1.60	45	198	347	765	1.8	–	.12	.08	1.4	.18	–	2
100	110	4.00	–	–	–	1213	–	–	.45	.29	18.6	–	–	12
157	370	4.90	–	–	–	1510	–	–	.39	.17	7	–	–	12
48	208	5.90	–	–	–	1570	–	–	.38	.23	1.8	–	–	21

A

Table A–1

Food Composition

Grp	Ref	Food Description	Measure	Wt (g)	H_2O (%)	Ener (cal)	Prot (g)	Carb (g)	Dietary Fiber (g)	Fat (g)	Fat Breakdown (g) Sat	Mono	Poly
		JACK IN THE BOX—Con.											
12	1513	Taco salad	1 ea	358	81	377	31	10	1	24	–	–	–
		Nachos											
12	1514	Cheese	1 svg	155	36	571	15	49	–	35	–	–	–
12	1515	Supreme	1 svg	340	70	718	23	66	–	40	–	–	–
12	1516	French fries	1 svg	68	40	221	2	27	<1	12	–	–	–
12	1517	Hash brown potatoes	1 svg	90	60	68	2	15	<1	12	–	–	–
12	1518	Onion rings	1 svg	108	28	382	5	39	<1	23	–	–	–
		Milkshakes											
12	1519	Chocolate	1 ea	322	77	330	11	55	0	7	–	–	–
12	1520	Strawberry	1 ea	328	77	320	10	55	0	7	–	–	–
12	1521	Vanilla	1 ea	317	76	320	10	57	0	6	–	–	–
12	1522	Apple turnover	1 ea	119	38	410	4	45	<1	24	–	–	–

Source: Jack in the Box Restaurants, Foodmaker, Inc., San Diego, CA for basic nutrients. Some values for dietary fiber, magnesium, phosphorus, potassium, zinc, vitamin A (RE's), B6, folacin, and fatty acids, calculated from known values for major ingredients.

Grp	Ref	Food Description	Measure	Wt (g)	H_2O (%)	Ener (cal)	Prot (g)	Carb (g)	Dietary Fiber (g)	Fat (g)	Fat Breakdown (g) Sat	Mono	Poly
		KENTUCKY FRIED CHICKEN											
		Original Recipe:											
12	1253	Center breast	1 ea	95	52	236	24	7	<1	14	4	7	2
12	1251	Side breast	1 ea	69	39	199	16	7	<1	12	3	5	3
12	1250	Drumstick	1 ea	47	53	117	12	3	<1	7	2	3	2
12	1252	Thigh	1 ea	88	49	257	18	7	<1	18	4	7	4
12	1249	Wing	1 ea	42	44	136	10	4	<1	9	2	4	2
		Dinners:											
12	1254	2 pce dinner, white	1 ea	322	64	604	30	48	1	32	7	12	10
12	1255	2 pce dinner, dark	1 ea	346	65	643	35	46	1	35	8	13	11
12	1256	2 pce dinner, combination	1 ea	341	63	661	33	48	1	38	8	14	11
		Extra crispy recipe:											
12	1261	Center breast	1 ea	104	39	297	24	14	<1	16	4	7	4
12	1259	Side breast	1 ea	84	39	286	17	14	<1	18	5	7	4
12	1258	Drumstick	1 ea	58	51	155	13	5	<1	9	2	4	2
12	1260	Thigh	1 ea	107	45	343	20	13	<1	23	6	10	6
12	1257	Wing	1 ea	53	36	201	11	9	<1	14	4	6	3
		Dinners:											
12	1262	2 pce dinner, white	1 ea	348	60	755	33	60	1	43	10	16	12
12	1263	2 pce dinner, dark	1 ea	375	62	765	38	55	1	54	11	16	13
12	1264	2 pce dinner, combination	1 ea	371	60	902	36	58	1	48	12	18	14
12	1265	Mashed potatoes	⅓ c	80	81	60	2	12	<1	1	<1	<1	<1
12	1266	Chicken gravy	⅓ c	78	76	59	2	4	<1	4	1	2	<1
12	1267	Dinner roll	1 ea	21	31	61	2	11	<1	1	<1	<1	<1
12	1268	Corn on the cob	1 ea	143	70	176	5	32	2	3	<1	1	1
12	1269	Coleslaw	⅓ c	79	76	103	1	12	<1	6	1	2	3
12	1381	Kentucky nuggets	1 ea	16	44	46	3	2	<1	3	1	2	<1
		Kentucky nugget sauces											
12	1382	Barbeque	2 tbsp	30	51	35	<1	7	–	1	<1	<1	<1
12	1383	Sweet & sour	2 tbsp	30	50	58	<1	13	–	1	<1	<1	<1
12	1384	Honey sauce	1 tbsp	15	50	49	0	12	–	<1	–	–	–
12	1385	Mustard sauce	2 tbsp	30	52	36	1	6	–	1	–	–	–
12	1386	Kentucky fries	1 svg	119	45	268	5	33	<1	13	3	8	1
12	1387	Mashed potatoes & gravy	⅓ c	86	80	62	2	10	<1	1	<1	<1	<1
12	1388	Buttermilk biscuit	1 ea	75	27	269	5	32	<1	14	4	8	1

KEY: 1 = BEV 2 = DAIRY 3 = EGGS 4 = FAT/OIL 5 = FRUIT 6 = BAKERY 7 = GRAIN 8 = FISH 9 = BEEF 10 = POULTRY 11 = SAUSAGE 12 = MIXED/FAST 13 = NUTS/SEEDS 14 = SWEETS 15 = VEG/LEG 16 = MISC 22 = SOUP/SAUCE

Chol (mg)	Calc (mg)	Iron (mg)	Magn (mg)	Phos (mg)	Pota (mg)	Sodi (mg)	Zinc (mg)	VT-A (RE)	Thia (mg)	Ribo (mg)	Niac (mg)	V-B6 (mg)	Fola (μg)	VT-C (mg)
102	280	4.30	–	–	–	1436	–	–	.18	.53	6	–	–	7
37	370	1.40	–	–	–	1154	–	–	.11	.19	1	–	–	3
65	410	3.20	–	–	–	1782	–	–	.15	.26	3.2	–	–	8
8	10	.50	23	75	360	164	.26	<1	.07	.03	1.20	.18	–	3
0	t	.70	–	–	–	15	–	<1	.03	t	.08	–	–	4
27	30	1.40	16	69	109	407	.40	<1	.21	.12	1.80	.06	–	3
25	350	.70	55	330	650	270	1.20	–	.15	.59	.60	.18	–	3
25	350	.40	40	328	613	240	1.10	–	.15	.43	.40	.16	–	3
25	350	.30	38	312	599	230	1.00	<1	.15	.34	.40	.20	–	<1
15	11	1.40	10	33	69	350	.20	–	.23	.12	2.50	.03	–	<1

Chol (mg)	Calc (mg)	Iron (mg)	Magn (mg)	Phos (mg)	Pota (mg)	Sodi (mg)	Zinc (mg)	VT-A (RE)	Thia (mg)	Ribo (mg)	Niac (mg)	V-B6 (mg)	Fola (μg)	VT-C (mg)
87	30	1.17	28	205	267	631	.72	6	.08	.11	7.57	.31	8	2
70	50	.98	19	151	176	558	.77	4	.06	.08	5.66	.20	6	1
63	12	.80	13	95	122	207	1.29	3	.04	.09	2.38	.09	4	1
109	34	1.45	22	169	217	566	1.65	5	.08	.16	4.03	.17	9	2
55	22	.68	10	76	86	302	.58	3	.03	.04	2.28	.10	4	1
133	142	3.31	61	326	643	1528	1.88	77	.22	.19	10.0	.50	39	37
180	116	3.90	66	363	720	1441	3.47	77	.25	.32	8.46	.46	42	37
172	126	3.78	64	344	684	1536	2.76	77	.24	.27	8.36	.47	41	37
79	62	1.29	29	218	244	584	.77	6	.11	.11	7.89	.30	11	2
65	57	1.12	21	157	188	564	.88	5	.12	.13	5.37	.24	9	2
66	11	.95	14	100	147	263	1.32	4	.07	.11	3.07	.16	6	1
109	49	1.49	24	185	228	549	1.73	7	.12	.19	5.35	.17	11	2
59	16	.65	12	77	100	312	.67	3	.06	.09	2.94	.11	5	1
132	143	6.03	65	333	689	1544	2.08	77	.31	.29	10.4	.56	43	37
183	130	4.09	70	383	776	1480	3.58	77	.32	.38	10.4	.54	46	37
176	135	6.40	68	361	729	1529	2.93	77	.31	.35	10.3	.49	45	37
<1	21	.28	14	41	218	228	.16	5	.01	.04	.96	.11	7	5
2	9	.48	2	10	21	398	.04	1	.01	.03	.47	<.01	2	<1
1	21	.53	6	28	29	118	.20	1	.10	.04	.98	.01	7	<1
<1	7	.79	53	134	323	12	.99	27	.14	.11	1.80	.22	71	2
4	29	.19	9	20	115	171	.13	28	.03	.03	.20	.07	10	19
12	2	.13	4	29	33	140	.22	30	.02	.03	1.00	.04	1	2
1	6	.24	5	10	75	450	.05	37	.01	.01	.19	.02	3	<1
1	5	.16	2	5	39	148	.02	6	.01	.02	.04	.01	1	<1
t	1	.11	<1	<1	6	10	<.01	0	.01	<.01	.04	t	1	3
1	10	.26	6	15	23	346	.09	1	.02	.01	.16	.02	3	1
1	24	.94	28	78	606	81	.31	0	.17	.06	2.70	.18	20	3
1	19	.35	9	28	137	297	.11	5	.01	.04	1.00	.08	8	1
1	77	1.22	9	264	95	521	.29	30	.28	.13	1.80	.03	8	<1

Table A–1

Food Composition

Grp	Ref	Food Description	Measure	Wt (g)	H_2O (%)	Ener (cal)	Prot (g)	Carb (g)	Dietary Fiber (g)	Fat (g)	Fat Breakdown (g) Sat	Mono	Poly
		KENTUCKY FRIED CHICKEN—Con.											
12	1389	Potato salad	⅓ c	90	76	141	2	13	1	9	1	3	5
12	1390	Baked beans	⅓ c	89	71	105	5	18	6	1	<1	<1	<1
12	1391	Chicken Little sandwich	1 ea	57	52	177	6	17	1	9	2	3	3
		Source: Kentucky Fried Chicken Corporation											
		LONG JOHN SILVER'S											
		Fish, batter fried											
12	1523	Fish & fryes, 3 pce	1 ea	350	55	853	43	64	<1	48	–	–	–
12	1524	Fish & fryes, 2 pce	1 ea	260	53	651	30	53	<1	36	–	–	–
12	1525	Fish dinner, 3 pce	1 ea	540	60	1180	47	93	<1	70	–	–	–
		Fish, breaded & fried											
12	1526	Fish dinner, 3 pce	1 ea	450	60	940	35	84	<1	52	–	–	–
12	1527	Fish dinner, 2 pce	1 ea	400	60	818	26	76	<1	46	–	–	–
		Chicken											
12	1528	Chicken plank dinner, 3 pce	1 ea	370	60	885	32	72	<1	51	–	–	–
12	1529	Chicken plank dinner, 4 pce	1 ea	440	60	1037	41	82	<1	59	–	–	–
12	1530	Chicken nugget dinner, 6 pce	1 ea	300	60	699	23	54	<1	45	–	–	–
12	1531	Clam chowder	1 svg	185	85	128	7	15	<1	5	–	–	–
12	1532	Clam dinner	1 ea	460	60	955	22	100	<1	58	–	–	–
12	1533	Fish & chicken dinner	1 ea	460	60	935	36	73	<1	55	–	–	–
12	1534	Oyster dinner	1 ea	360	60	789	17	78	<1	45	–	–	–
12	1535	Scallop dinner	1 ea	320	60	747	17	66	<1	45	–	–	–
12	1536	Seafood platter	1 ea	410	60	976	29	85	<1	58	–	–	–
12	1537	Batter fried shrimp dinner	1 ea	300	60	711	17	60	<1	45	–	–	–
12	1538	Fish sandwich platter	1 ea	400	60	835	30	84	<1	42	–	–	–
		Salads											
12	1539	Ocean chef	1 ea	320	85	229	27	13	2	8	–	–	–
12	1540	Seafood	1 ea	480	85	426	19	22	2	30	–	–	–
12	1541	Cole slaw	1 svg	98	70	182	1	11	<1	15	–	–	–
12	1542	Fries	1 svg	85	42	247	4	31	<1	12	–	–	–
12	1543	Hush puppies	1 ea	47	37	145	3	18	<1	7	–	–	–
		Source: Long John Silver's Inc., Lexington, KY.											
		McDONALD'S											
		Sandwiches											
12	1221	Big Mac	1 ea	200	48	570	25	39	1	35	12	13	8
12	1222	Quarter Pounder	1 ea	160	49	427	25	29	1	24	9	11	2
12	1223	Quarter Pounder w/cheese	1 ea	186	48	525	30	31	1	32	13	12	2
12	1224	Filet-O-Fish sandwich	1 ea	143	44	435	15	36	<1	26	6	9	9
12	1225	Hamburger	1 ea	100	46	263	12	28	<1	11	4	5	1
12	1226	Cheeseburger	1 ea	114	45	318	15	29	<1	16	7	6	1
12	1227	French fries	1 svg	68	37	220	3	26	<1	12	5	4	1
12	1228	Chicken McNuggets	6 ea	109	49	323	19	15	<1	20	5	11	2
		Sauces											
12	1229	Mustard Sauce	1 ea	30	53	63	1	11	<1	2	<1	1	1
12	1230	Barbecue	1 ea	32	51	60	<1	14	<1	<1	<1	<1	<1
12	1231	Sweet & sour	1 ea	32	50	64	<1	15	<1	<1	<1	<1	<1

KEY: 1 = BEV 2 = DAIRY 3 = EGGS 4 = FAT/OIL 5 = FRUIT 6 = BAKERY 7 = GRAIN 8 = FISH 9 = BEEF 10 = POULTRY 11 = SAUSAGE 12 = MIXED/FAST 13 = NUTS/SEEDS 14 = SWEETS 15 = VEG/LEG 16 = MISC 22 = SOUP/SAUCE

Chol (mg)	Calc (mg)	Iron (mg)	Magn (mg)	Phos (mg)	Pota (mg)	Sodi (mg)	Zinc (mg)	VT-A (RE)	Thia (mg)	Ribo (mg)	Niac (mg)	V-B6 (mg)	Fola (μg)	VT-C (mg)
11	10	.32	15	32	256	396	.29	27	.07	.02	.60	.19	7	3
1	54	1.43	29	90	229	387	1.29	10	.06	.04	.50	.07	32	2
20	39	1.40	10	105	114	398	.93	6	.15	.14	1.65	.07	11	<1
17	–	–	–	–	–	611	–	–	–	–	–	–	–	–
27	–	–	–	–	–	1543	–	–	–	–	–	–	–	–
56	–	–	–	–	–	2076	–	–	–	–	–	–	–	–
55	–	–	–	–	–	763	–	–	–	–	–	–	–	–
37	–	–	–	–	–	1579	–	–	–	–	–	–	–	–
95	–	–	–	–	–	2161	–	–	–	–	–	–	–	–
127	–	–	–	–	–	1297	–	–	–	–	–	–	–	–
75	–	–	–	–	–	1402	–	–	–	–	–	–	–	–
64	–	–	–	–	–	986	–	–	–	–	–	–	–	–
113	–	–	–	–	–	1086	–	–	–	–	–	–	–	–
12	–	–	–	–	–	367	–	–	–	–	–	–	–	–
13	–	–	–	–	–	1	–	–	–	–	–	–	–	–
1	–	–	–	–	–	405	–	–	–	–	–	–	–	–
106	–	–	–	–	–	2025	–	–	–	–	–	–	–	–
75	–	–	–	–	–	1352	–	–	–	–	–	–	–	–
119	–	–	–	–	–	2797	–	–	–	–	–	–	–	–
101	–	–	–	–	–	1900	–	–	–	–	–	–	–	–
76	–	–	–	–	–	1526	–	–	–	–	–	–	–	–
25	–	–	–	–	–	1918	–	–	–	–	–	–	–	–
25	–	–	–	–	–	2433	–	–	–	–	–	–	–	–
25	–	–	–	–	–	853	–	–	–	–	–	–	–	–
83	203	4.90	38	314	249	979	4.69	38	.48	.38	7.20	.27	21	3
80	98	4.30	37	249	322	718	5.11	23	.35	.32	7.20	.27	23	3
107	255	4.84	41	382	341	1195	5.70	128	.37	.41	7.07	.23	23	3
47	133	2.47	27	229	150	800	.89	28	.36	.23	3.00	.10	20	2
29	84	2.85	19	126	142	506	2.09	14	.31	.22	4.08	.12	17	2
40	169	2.84	23	205	157	730	2.60	67	.30	.24	4.33	.12	21	2
9	9	.61	27	101	564	109	.32	5	.12	.02	2.26	.22	19	13
63	11	1.25	26	283	302	512	.89	27	.16	.14	7.52	.38	11	2
3	8	.17	6	15	23	259	.09	1	.01	<.01	.08	.01	3	<1
<1	4	.12	5	10	75	309	.05	5	.01	.01	.08	.02	3	1
<1	2	.08	2	5	39	186	.02	20	.01	.01	.07	.01	1	<1

A

Table A–1

Food Composition

Grp	Ref	Food Description	Measure	Wt (g)	H_2O (%)	Ener (cal)	Prot (g)	Carb (g)	Dietary Fiber (g)	Fat (g)	Fat Breakdown (g) Sat	Mono	Poly
McDONALD'S—Con.													
		Milkshakes											
12	1232	Chocolate	10 fl oz	291	70	383	10	66	<1	9	4	2	<1
12	1233	Strawberry	10 fl oz	290	72	362	9	62	<1	9	4	3	<1
12	1234	Vanilla	10 fl oz	291	73	352	10	60	<1	8	4	3	<1
		Sundaes											
12	1235	Hot fudge	1 ea	164	60	357	7	58	<1	11	5	3	1
12	1236	Strawberry	1 ea	164	62	320	6	54	<1	9	3	3	1
12	1237	Caramel	1 ea	165	57	361	7	61	<1	10	3	3	1
12	1238	Soft ice cream cone	1 ea	115	65	189	4	31	<1	5	2	1	<1
		Pies											
12	1239	Fried Apple	1 ea	85	45	253	2	29	<1	14	5	7	1
12	1240	Fried Cherry	1 ea	88	44	260	2	32	<1	14	5	7	1
		Cookies, package											
12	1241	McDonaldland cookies	1 pkg	67	3	308	4	49	<1	10	4	5	1
12	1242	Chocolate chip cookies	1 pkg	69	3	342	4	45	<1	16	8	6	1
		Breakfast items:											
12	1243	English muffin, w/butter	1 ea	63	42	186	5	30	<1	5	2	2	1
12	1244	Egg McMuffin	1 ea	138	51	340	19	31	<1	16	6	5	2
12	1245	Hot Cakes w/butter & syrup	1 ea	214	46	500	8	94	<1	10	4	4	1
12	1246	Scrambled eggs	1 ea	98	70	180	13	3	<1	13	5	5	2
12	1247	Sausage	1 svg.	53	43	210	10	1	<1	19	7	9	2
12	1248	Hash brown potato patty	1 ea	55	56	144	1	15	<1	9	3	5	1
12	1392	Sausage McMuffin	1 ea	115	38	427	18	30	<1	26	10	11	3
12	1393	Sausage McMuffin w/egg	1 ea	165	47	517	23	32	<1	33	13	14	4
12	1394	Biscuit, plain	1 ea	85	27	330	5	37	<1	18	8	7	2
12	1395	Biscuit w/sausage	1 ea	121	32	467	12	35	<1	31	12	14	4
12	1396	Biscuit w/sausage & egg	1 ea	175	43	585	20	36	<1	40	15	17	5
12	1397	Biscuit w/bacon, egg & cheese	1 ea	145	41	483	17	33	<1	32	10	14	3
		Salads											
12	1398	Chef salad	1 ea	273	84	226	21	6	2	13	6	4	1
12	1399	Shrimp salad	1 ea	264	88	99	14	5	2	3	1	1	<1
12	1400	Garden salad	1 ea	204	91	91	6	4	2	6	3	2	<1
12	1401	Chicken salad oriental	1 ea	280	88	146	23	5	2	4	1	1	1

Source: McDonald's Corporation, Oak Brook, Illinois. Some values for Salads estimated from known values for major ingredients.

Grp	Ref	Food Description	Measure	Wt (g)	H_2O (%)	Ener (cal)	Prot (g)	Carb (g)	Dietary Fiber (g)	Fat (g)	Sat	Mono	Poly
TACO BELL													
		Burritos:											
12	1544	Bean	1 ea	191	58	360	13	54	8	11	5	5	1
12	1545	Beef	1 ea	191	58	402	22	38	2	17	8	7	1
12	1546	Bean & beef	1 ea	191	58	381	17	46	5	14	7	6	1
12	1547	Burrito supreme	1 ea	248	66	422	17	46	5	19	9	8	1
12	1548	Double beef supreme	1 ea	262	66	465	23	41	2	23	11	10	1
12	1549	Enchirito	1 ea	213	66	382	20	30	5	20	10	8	1
12	1550	Fajita (steak taco)	1 ea	142	65	235	15	20	2	11	5	4	1

A

KEY: 1 = BEV 2 = DAIRY 3 = EGGS 4 = FAT/OIL 5 = FRUIT 6 = BAKERY 7 = GRAIN 8 = FISH 9 = BEEF 10 = POULTRY 11 = SAUSAGE 12 = MIXED/FAST 13 = NUTS/SEEDS 14 = SWEETS 15 = VEG/LEG 16 = MISC 22 = SOUP/SAUCE

Chol (mg)	Calc (mg)	Iron (mg)	Magn (mg)	Phos (mg)	Pota (mg)	Sodi (mg)	Zinc (mg)	VT-A (RE)	Thia (mg)	Ribo (mg)	Niac (mg)	V-B6 (mg)	Fola (μg)	VT-C (mg)
30	320	.84	45	306	533	300	1.16	72	.13	.44	.50	.14	14	3
32	322	.17	34	289	487	207	1.02	86	.12	.44	.35	.14	11	4
31	329	.18	34	326	500	200	1.05	79	.12	.70	.35	.14	35	3
27	215	.61	35	236	410	170	.98	58	.07	.31	1.12	.13	11	2
25	174	.38	28	180	290	90	.80	58	.07	.30	1.03	.05	20	3
31	200	.23	30	230	338	145	.87	70	.07	.31	1.01	.05	13	4
24	183	.12	17	160	182	109	.64	55	.06	.36	.44	.06	3	1
7	14	.62	6	27	39	398	.16	3	.02	.02	.19	.02	5	1
8	12	.59	7	27	39	427	.15	11	.03	.02	.25	.02	3	1
10	12	1.47	11	74	52	358	.34	8	.23	.23	2.85	.03	6	1
18	29	1.56	29	108	170	313	.50	23	.12	.21	1.70	.03	6	1
15	117	1.51	13	74	71	310	.50	42	.28	.49	2.61	.04	17	1
259	226	2.93	26	322	168	885	1.92	145	.47	.44	3.77	.21	30	1
47	3	2.23	28	501	187	1070	.69	64	.26	.36	2.27	.12	9	5
514	61	2.53	13	264	135	205	1.66	187	.08	.47	.20	.20	65	1
39	16	.82	9	95	127	423	1.47	9	.27	.11	2.07	.18	1	1
4	5	.40	13	67	247	325	.17	1	.06	.01	.82	.13	6	4
59	168	2.25	24	186	215	942	1.68	114	.70	.25	4.14	.15	23	1
287	196	3.47	30	288	294	1044	2.36	198	.84	.50	4.46	.20	33	<1
9	74	1.30	10	299	108	786	.33	54	.21	.15	1.70	.03	9	<1
48	82	2.05	17	353	231	1147	1.31	18	.56	.22	3.39	.12	12	1
285	119	3.43	24	476	312	1301	2.10	126	.53	.49	3.85	.19	35	1
263	2	2.57	20	461	232	1269	1.55	196	.30	.43	2.32	.10	44	2
125	222	1.30	25	200	400	850	1.40	125	.35	.33	5.20	.04	60	20
187	64	.87	60	180	420	570	1.90	71	.13	.13	1.70	.06	60	10
110	104	.63	18	80	280	100	.40	65	.08	.16	.94	.06	60	10
92	47	1.40	20	140	350	270	.66	120	.14	.17	7.60	.34	61	22

Chol (mg)	Calc (mg)	Iron (mg)	Magn (mg)	Phos (mg)	Pota (mg)	Sodi (mg)	Zinc (mg)	VT-A (RE)	Thia (mg)	Ribo (mg)	Niac (mg)	V-B6 (mg)	Fola (μg)	VT-C (mg)
14	120	2.19	65	210	427	921	2.05	65	.66	.39	2.74	1.00	55	2
59	103	2.11	35	225	313	994	4.00	100	.31	.44	3.44	.23	27	2
36	111	2.15	50	220	370	958	2.67	80	.49	.42	3.09	.59	38	2
35	142	2.21	50	227	437	952	3.00	185	.45	.45	3.14	.52	40	9
59	140	2.45	52	230	434	1054	4.00	200	.34	.49	3.68	.30	30	9
56	260	2.10	61	263	423	1260	3.51	157	.39	.41	2.12	.61	29	3
14	119	3.03	24	150	207	507	3.18	133	.41	.34	2.74	.17	15	3

Table A–1

Food Composition

Grp	Ref	Food Description	Measure	Wt (g)	H_2O (%)	Ener (cal)	Prot (g)	Carb (g)	Dietary Fiber (g)	Fat (g)	Fat Breakdown (g) Sat	Mono	Poly
		TACO BELL—Con.											
		Tacos:											
12	1551	Regular	1 ea	78	55	184	10	11	1	11	6	3	1
12	1552	Taco bellgrande	1 ea	170	63	351	18	20	2	22	13	6	1
12	1553	Taco light	1 ea	170	59	411	19	18	2	29	18	8	1
12	1554	Soft taco	1 ea	92	52	228	12	18	2	12	5	4	1
		Tostadas:											
12	1555	Regular	1 ea	156	67	243	10	28	7	11	5	4	1
12	1556	Beefy tostada	1 ea	198	69	322	15	22	4	20	10	8	1
12	1557	Bellbeefer	1 ea	177	63	312	17	32	<1	13	6	4	2
12	1558	Mexican pizza	1 ea	269	55	714	28	43	5	48	31	14	2
12	1559	Taco salad with salsa	1 ea	601	73	949	36	63	5	62	40	18	3
		Nachos:											
12	1560	Regular	1 ea	106	40	356	7	38	<1	19	12	5	1
12	1561	Bellgrande	1 ea	333	58	719	23	65	6	49	23	20	2
12	1562	Pintos & cheese	1 ea	128	69	194	9	19	7	10	5	4	<1
12	1563	Taco sauce	1 ea	3.7	96	2	<1	<1	<1	<1	<1	<1	<1
12	1564	Salsa	1 ea	90.7	95	18	1	4	1	<1	<1	<1	<1
12	1565	Cinnamon Crispas	1 ea	47.3	1	266	3	27	<1	16	13	2	1

Source: Taco Bell Corporation, California for most nutrient values. Values for Dietary fiber, mono-unsaturated fat, magnesium, phosphorus, zinc, folacin, Vitamin B6, Vitamin A in REs, and percentage water are estimates calculated from known values of major ingredients.

Grp	Ref	Food Description	Measure	Wt (g)	H_2O (%)	Ener (cal)	Prot (g)	Carb (g)	Dietary Fiber (g)	Fat (g)	Sat	Mono	Poly
		WENDY's											
		Hamburgers:											
12	1566	Single, on white bun, no toppings	1 ea	117	41	350	21	27	<1	18	7	9	1
12	1567	Single, on multigrain bun, no toppings	1 ea	211	45	527	30	28	2	33	12	13	2
12	1568	Double, on white bun, no toppings	1 ea	197	44	560	41	32	<1	34	7	13	8
12	1569	Big classic	1 ea	241	63	470	26	36	2	25	7	10	5
		Cheeseburgers:											
12	1570	Bacon cheeseburger	1 ea	147	46	460	29	23	<1	28	13	13	2
12	1571	Single, w/all toppings	1 ea	215	50	548	30	32	2	33	13	12	5
12	1572	Double, w/all toppings	1 ea	291	50	735	48	27	2	48	18	18	6
		Baked Potatoes:											
12	1573	Plain	1 ea	250	75	249	6	52	5	<1	<1	<1	<1
12	1574	W/bacon & cheese	1 ea	372	71	610	16	55	5	31	17	11	3
12	1575	W/broccoli & cheese	1 ea	377	74	502	13	56	5	25	11	8	4
12	1576	W/cheese	1 ea	404	71	727	17	56	5	32	20	10	2
12	1577	W/chili & cheese	1 ea	453	72	653	21	64	8	28	14	12	1
12	1578	W/sour cream & chives	1 ea	280	71	405	7	54	5	18	11	5	1
12	1579	Chili	1 c	256	77	260	21	26	5	8	3	4	<1
12	1580	French fries	1 svg	106	43	306	4	38	<1	15	7	5	2
12	1581	Frosty dairy dessert	1 c	216	35	354	7	53	0	13	5	3	2
12	1582	Chocolate chip cookie	1 ea	64	5	320	3	40	1	17	6	6	5

Source: Wendy's International, for most nutrient values. Some of the values for Dietary fiber, the types of fatty acids, magnesium, phosphorus, zinc, folacin, Vitamin B6, Vitamin A in REs, and percentage water are estimates calculated from known values of major ingredients.

KEY: 1 = BEV 2 = DAIRY 3 = EGGS 4 = FAT/OIL 5 = FRUIT 6 = BAKERY 7 = GRAIN 8 = FISH 9 = BEEF 10 = POULTRY
11 = SAUSAGE 12 = MIXED/FAST 13 = NUTS/SEEDS 14 = SWEETS 15 = VEG/LEG 16 = MISC 22 = SOUP/SAUCE

Chol (mg)	Calc (mg)	Iron (mg)	Magn (mg)	Phos (mg)	Pota (mg)	Sodi (mg)	Zinc (mg)	VT-A (RE)	Thia (mg)	Ribo (mg)	Niac (mg)	V-B6 (mg)	Fola (μg)	VT-C (mg)
32	78	1.10	16	100	159	274	2.12	42	.07	.14	1.07	.12	10	1
55	165	1.91	18	100	334	470	2.12	132	.13	.28	1.91	.12	13	5
57	156	2.07	18	100	316	575	2.12	128	.10	.28	1.78	.12	13	5
32	116	2.27	18	100	178	516	2.12	42	.39	.22	2.74	.12	10	1
18	161	1.81	62	195	401	670	1.55	84	.40	.22	1.15	1.01	47	3
40	185	1.96	43	206	408	764	2.97	152	.24	.29	1.61	.56	31	6
39	174	2.36	22	125	299	855	2.10	121	.16	.30	1.73	.12	<1	5
81	453	3.08	80	400	449	1364	5.40	355	.36	.39	2.00	1.11	60	7
85	393	5.92	130	460	1222	1763	5.59	450	.69	.78	4.00	1.30	140	25
9	178	.99	40	200	158	423	.80	27	.03	.16	.09	.14	4	2
43	323	4.19	100	400	763	1312	4.30	280	.52	.47	2.36	.98	33	12
19	139	1.75	110	156	384	733	2.17	87	.43	.21	1.15	.21	68	1
0	2	.07	–	–	13	126	–	19	<.01	<.01	.06	–	–	<1
0	36	.60	–	–	163	376	–	112	.02	.14	–	–	–	2
2	25	.71	–	–	36	122	–	<1	.03	.02	.18	–	–	<1

Chol (mg)	Calc (mg)	Iron (mg)	Magn (mg)	Phos (mg)	Pota (mg)	Sodi (mg)	Zinc (mg)	VT-A (RE)	Thia (mg)	Ribo (mg)	Niac (mg)	V-B6 (mg)	Fola (μg)	VT-C (mg)
65	32	4.50	20	118	220	410	2.10	–	.22	.25	5.00	.12	<1	<1
86	167	4.01	46	368	464	814	4.65	–	.35	.31	5.55	.28	36	6
125	48	6.30	42	339	431	575	8.35	–	.22	.43	9.00	.47	29	<1
81	43	4.55	34	200	468	901	5.11	31	.26	.24	4.80	.25	30	12
65	136	3.60	33	296	332	860	5.14	82	.27	.28	5.70	.24	25	1
84	177	4.00	33	339	430	864	4.41	111	.34	.35	5.29	.25	28	6
165	180	5.40	50	470	620	883	8.80	112	.36	.53	10.0	.46	31	6
0	34	2.82	67	169	1362	58	.65	0	.28	.11	3.82	.70	68	10
36	207	3.94	79	657	1602	1560	2.81	250	.52	.39	7.68	.82	68	13
20	226	3.44	76	449	1478	435	.76	370	.31	.27	4.06	.77	95	33
27	742	3.04	67	423	1472	1371	.65	240	.28	.21	3.84	.70	68	7
18	686	4.58	85	354	1682	1538	2.07	220	.32	.23	5.07	.80	83	9
5	45	2.82	68	177	1376	171	.68	15	.28	.13	3.82	.70	69	7
30	64	4.50	60	320	594	1070	3.78	300	.15	.17	3.00	.26	40	6
15	13	1.02	45	197	689	105	.51	0	.15	.04	2.96	.27	33	12
45	257	.86	43	238	518	194	.92	143	.11	.45	.31	.12	17	<1
7	10	1.09	15	62	102	237	.46	0	.05	.08	.58	.03	6	0

Appendix B

Recommended Nutrient Intakes for Canadians

Table B–1

Average Energy Requirements

Age	Sex	Average Height (cm)	Average Weight (kg)	Requirements[a]					
				Cal/Kg	*MJ/Kg*	*Cal/Day*	*MJ/Day*	*Cal/Cm*	*MJ/Cm*
Months									
0–2	Both	55	4.5	120–100[b]	0.50–0.42[b]	500	2.0	9.0	0.04
3–5	Both	63	7.0	100– 95[b]	0.42–0.40[b]	700	2.8	11.0	0.05
6–8	Both	69	8.5	95– 97[b]	0.40–0.41[b]	800	3.4	11.5	0.05
9–11	Both	73	9.5	97– 99[b]	0.41	950	3.8	12.5	0.05
Years									
1	Both	82	11	101	0.42	1100	4.8	13.5	0.06
2–3	Both	95	14	94	0.39	1300	5.6	13.5	0.06
4–6	Both	107	18	100	0.42	1800	7.6	17.0	0.07
7–9	M	126	25	88	0.37	2200	9.2	17.5	0.07
	F	125	25	76	0.32	1900	8.0	15.0	0.06
10–12	M	141	34	73	0.30	2500	10.4	17.5	0.07
	F	143	36	61	0.25	2200	9.2	15.5	0.06
13–15	M	159	50	57	0.24	2800	12.0	17.5	0.07
	F	157	48	46	0.19	2200	9.2	14.0	0.06
16–18	M	172	62	51	0.21	3200	13.2	18.5	0.08
	F	160	53	40	0.17	2100	8.8	13.0	0.05
19–24	M	175	71	42	0.18	3000	12.4		
	F	160	58	36	0.15	2100	8.8		
25–49	M	172	74	36	0.15	2700	11.2		
	F	160	59	32	0.13	1900	8.0		
50–74	M	170	73	31	0.13	2300	9.6		
	F	158	63	29	0.12	1800	7.6		
75+	M	168	69	29	0.12	2000	8.4		
	F	155	64	23	0.10	1500	6.0		

[a]Requirements can be expected to vary within a range of ± 30%.
[b]First and last figures are averages at the beginning and at the end of the three-month period.
Source: Health and Welfare Canada, *Recommended Nutrient Intakes for Canadians* (Ottawa: Canadian Government Publishing Centre, 1983), Table II.1, pp. 22–23, as revised in the second printing.

B

Table B–2

Recommended Nutrient Intakes

Age	Sex	Weight (kg)	Protein (g/day)[a]	Fat-Soluble Vitamins: *Vitamin A (RE/day)*[b]	*Vitamin D (μg/day)*[c]	*Vitamin E (mg/day)*[d]
Months						
0–2	Both	4.5	11[f]	400	10	3
3–5	Both	7.0	14[f]	400	10	3
6–8	Both	8.5	17[f]	400	10	3
9–11	Both	9.5	18	400	10	3
Years						
1	Both	11	19	400	10	3
2–3	Both	14	22	400	5	4
4–6	Both	18	26	500	5	5
7–9	M	25	30	700	2.5	7
	F	25	30	700	2.5	6
10–12	M	34	38	800	2.5	8
	F	36	40	800	2.5	7
13–15	M	50	50	900	2.5	9
	F	48	42	800	2.5	7
16–18	M	62	55	1000	2.5	10
	F	53	43	800	2.5	7
19–24	M	71	58	1000	2.5	10
	F	58	43	800	2.5	7
25–49	M	74	61	1000	2.5	9
	F	59	44	800	2.5	6
50–74	M	73	60	1000	2.5	7
	F	63	47	800	2.5	6
75 +	M	69	57	1000	2.5	6
	F	64	47	800	2.5	5
Pregnancy (additional)						
First trimester			15	100	2.5	2
Second trimester			20	100	2.5	2
Third trimester			25	100	2.5	2
Lactation (additional)			20	400	2.5	3

Note: Recommended intakes of energy and of certain nutrients are not listed in this table because of the nature of the variables upon which they are based. The figures for energy are estimates of average requirements for expected patterns of activity. For nutrients not shown, the following amounts are recommended: **thiamin,** 0.4 mg/1000 cal (0.48 mg/5000) kJ); **riboflavin,** 0.5 mg/1000 cal (0.6 mg/5000 kJ); **niacin,** 7.2 niacin equivalents/1000 cal (8.6 NE/5000 kJ); **vitamin B_6,** 15 μg (as pyridoxine)/g protein; **phosphorus,** same as calcium.

Recommended intakes during periods of growth are taken as appropriate for individuals representative of the midpoint in each age group. All recommended intakes are designed to cover individual variations in essentially all of a healthy population subsisting upon a variety of common foods available in Canada.

Table B–2 continued

Recommended Nutrient Intakes

Water-Soluble Vitamins			Minerals				
Vitamin C (mg/day)	*Folacin (μg/day)*[c]	*Vitamin B_{12} (μg/day)*	*Calcium (mg/day)*	*Magnesium (mg/day)*	*Iron (mg/day)*	*Iodine (μg/day)*	*Zinc (mg/day)*
20	50	0.3	350	30	0.4[g]	25	2[h]
20	50	0.3	350	40	5	35	3
20	50	0.3	400	45	7	40	3
20	55	0.3	400	50	7	45	3
20	65	0.3	500	55	6	55	4
20	80	0.4	500	65	6	65	4
25	90	0.5	600	90	6	85	5
35	125	0.8	700	110	7	110	6
30	125	0.8	700	110	7	95	6
40	170	1.0	900	150	10	125	7
40	170	1.0	1000	160	10	110	7
50	160	1.5	1100	220	12	160	9
45	160	1.5	800	190	13	160	8
55	190	1.9	900	240	10	160	9
45	160	1.9	700	220	14	160	8
60	210	2.0	800	240	8	160	9
45	165	2.0	700	190	14	160	8
60	210	2.0	800	240	8	160	9
45	165	2.0	700	190	14[i]	160	8
60	210	2.0	800	240	8	160	9
45	165	2.0	800	190	7	160	8
60	210	2.0	800	240	8	160	9
45	165	2.0	800	190	7	160	8
0	305	1.0	500	15	6	25	0
20	305	1.0	500	20	6	25	1
20	305	1.0	500	25	6	25	2
30	120	0.5	500	80	0	50	6

[a]The primary units are grams per kilogram of body weight. The figures shown here are examples.
[b]One retinol equivalent (RE) corresponds to the biological activity of 1 μg of retinol, 6 μg of β-carotene, or 12 μg of other carotenes.
[c]Expressed as cholecalciferol or ergocalciferol.
[d]Expressed as *d*-α-tocopherol equivalents, relative to which β- and γ-tocopherol and α-tocotrienol have activities of 0.5, 0.1, and 0.3, respectively.
[e]Expressed as total folate.
[f]The assumption is made that the protein is from breast milk or is of the same biological value as that of breast milk at first, and that between three and nine months the child is weaned. Adjustments for the changing quality of protein have been made accordingly.
[g]It is assumed that breast milk is the source of iron up to two months of age.
[h]Based on the assumption that breast milk is the source of zinc for the first two months.
[i]After menopause the recommended intake is 7 mg/day.

Source: Health and Welfare Canada, ***Recommended Nutrient Intakes for Canadians*** (Ottawa: Canadian Government Publishing Centre, 1983), Table X.1, pp. 179–180, as revised in the second printing.

B

Appendix C

Aids to Calculation

Many mathematical problems have been worked out for you as examples at appropriate places in the text. This appendix aims to help with the use of the metric system and with those problems not fully explained elsewhere.

Conversion Factors (see Inside Back Cover)

Conversion factors are useful mathematical tools in everyday calculations, like the ones encountered in the study of nutrition. Skill in the use of conversion factors is especially desirable as the United States and Canada "go metric."

A conversion factor is a fraction in which the numerator (top) and the denominator (bottom) express the same quantity in different units. For example, 2.2 pounds and 1 kilogram are equivalent; they express the same weight. The conversion factor used to change pounds to kilograms or vice versa is:

$$\frac{2.2 \text{ lb}}{1 \text{ kg}} \text{ or } \frac{1 \text{ kg}}{2.2 \text{ lb}}.$$

Because either of these factors equals 1, a measurement can be multiplied by the factor without changing the value of the measurement. Thus its units can be changed.

The correct factor to use in a problem is the one with the unit you are seeking in the numerator (top) of the fraction.

Following are three examples of problems commonly encountered in nutrition study; they illustrate the usefulness of conversion factors.

Example 1 Convert 1/4 cup to an approximate number of milliliters for use in a recipe.

1. The conversion factor is:

$$\frac{1 \text{ c}}{250 \text{ ml}} \text{ or } \frac{250 \text{ ml}}{1 \text{ c}}.$$

2. Multiply 1/4 cup by the factor:

$$\frac{1}{4} \not{c} \times \frac{250 \text{ ml}}{1 \not{c}} = 62.5 \text{ ml, or about } 60 \text{ ml.}$$

Example 2 Convert the weight of 130 pounds to kilograms.

1. Choose the conversion factor in which the unit you are seeking is on top:

$$\frac{1 \text{ kg}}{2.2 \text{ lb}}.$$

2. Multiply 130 pounds by the factor:

$$130 \not{lb} \times \frac{1 \text{ kg}}{2.2 \not{lb}} = \frac{130 \text{ kg}}{2.2} = \text{59 kg (rounded off to nearest whole number).}$$

Example 3 How many grams of saturated fat are contained in a 4-ounce hamburger? A 3-ounce hamburger contains 8 grams of saturated fat.

1. You are seeking grams of saturated fat; therefore, the conversion factor is:

$$\frac{8 \text{ g saturated fat}}{3 \text{ oz hamburger}}.$$

2. Multiply 4 ounces of hamburger by the conversion factor:

$$4 \not{oz} \text{ hamburger} \times \frac{8 \text{ g saturated fat}}{3 \not{oz} \text{ hamburger}} = \frac{4 \times 8 \text{ g}}{3}$$
$$= \text{11 g saturated fat (rounded off to nearest whole number).}$$

Percentages

A percentage is a comparison between a number of items (perhaps your intake of calories) and a standard number (perhaps the number of calories recommended for your age and sex—your energy RDA). The standard number is the number you divide by. The answer you get after the division must be multiplied by 100 to be stated as a percentage (*percent* means "per 100").

Example 4 What percentage of the RDA for calories is your calorie intake?

1. Find your energy RDA (inside front cover). We'll use 2100 calories to demonstrate.

2. Total your calorie intake for a day—for example, 1200 calories.

C

3. Divide your calorie intake by the RDA calories:

1200 cal (your intake) ÷ 2100 cal (RDA) = 0.573.

4. Multiply your answer by 100 to state it as a percentage:

0.573 × 100 = 57.3 = 57% (rounded off to the nearest whole number).

In some problems in nutrition, the percentage may be more than 100. For example, suppose your daily intake of vitamin A is 3200 RE and your RDA (male) is 1000 RE. Your intake as a percentage of the RDA is more than 100 percent (that is, you consume more than 100 percent of your vitamin A RDA). The following calculations show your vitamin A intake as a percentage of the RDA:

$$3200 \div 1000 = 3.2.$$
$$3.2 \times 100 = 320\% \text{ of RDA.}$$

Sometimes the comparison is between a part of a whole (for example, your calories from protein) and the total amount (your total calories). In this case, the total number is the one you divide by.

Example 5 What percentages of your total calories for the day come from protein, fat, and carbohydrate?

1. Using Appendix A and your diet record, find the total grams of protein, fat, and carbohydrate you consumed—for example, 60 grams protein, 80 grams fat, and 285 grams carbohydrate.

2. Multiply the number of grams by the number of calories from 1 gram of each energy nutrient (conversion factors):

$$60 \text{ g protein} \times \frac{4 \text{ cal}}{1 \text{ g protein}} = 240 \text{ cal.}$$

$$80 \text{ g fat} \times \frac{9 \text{ cal}}{1 \text{ g fat}} = 720 \text{ cal.}$$

$$285 \text{ g carbohydrate} \times \frac{4 \text{ cal}}{1 \text{ g carbohydrate}} = 1140 \text{ cal.}$$

$$240 + 720 + 1140 = 2100 \text{ cal.}$$

3. Find the percentage of total calories from each energy nutrient (see Example 4):

$$\text{Protein: } 240 \div 2100 = 0.114.$$
$$0.114 \times 100 = 11.4 = 11\% \text{ of calories.}$$

$$\text{Fat: } 720 \div 2100 = 0.342.$$
$$0.342 \times 100 = 34.2 = 34\% \text{ of calories.}$$

$$\text{Carbohydrate: } 1140 \div 2100 = 0.542.$$
$$0.542 \times 100 = 54.2$$
$$= 54\% \text{ of calories.}$$

$$11\% + 34\% + 54\% = 99\% \text{ of calories (total).}$$

The percentages total 99 percent rather than 100 percent because a little was lost from each number in rounding off. Either 99 or 101 is a reasonable total in problems like this.

Ratios

A ratio is a comparison of two or three values in which one of the values is reduced to 1. A ratio compares identical units and so is expressed without units. For example, the P:S ratio is a comparison of the grams of polyunsaturated fat to grams of saturated fat in the diet.

Example 6 Find the P:S ratio of your diet.

1. Using Appendix A and your diet record, find the grams of linoleic acid (polyunsaturated fat) and grams of saturated fat. Say they are 32 grams linoleic acid and 25 grams saturated fat.

2. Divide the larger of the amounts above by the smaller—divide linoleic acid grams by saturated fat grams:

$$\text{Linoleic acid (g)} \div \text{saturated fat (g)}.$$
$$32 \text{ g} \div 25 \text{ g} = 1.28$$

3. The P:S ratio is usually expressed as correct to one decimal place: 1.28 = 1.3. The P:S ratio of your diet is 1.3:1 (read as "one point three to one" or simply "one point three").

Appendix D

Vitamin/Mineral Supplements Compared

The following tables are useful for comparing the essential vitamin and mineral contents of supplements commonly available in the United States. Notice that blank columns have been provided for the addition of locally available products you may wish to compare with those shown here.*

Not all ingredients in vitamin/mineral preparations are of proven benefit. To facilitate meaningful comparison, the tables list only the nutrients known to be essential in human nutrition. Other nutrients and compounds found on the labels of these supplements are listed in the table notes.

When a supplement is needed that supplies certain nutrients, these tables will ease the task of selecting an appropriate one. Notice, for example, that some preparations marketed for the elderly are composed largely of alcohol, with few vitamins or minerals. These are "tonics," not vitamin/mineral supplements. A tonic may be useful if the only need is for comfort and the benefit of the placebo effect, but if an elderly person needs a balanced assortment of vitamins and minerals and cannot easily take pills, it may be advisable to suggest a liquid preparation designated for infants.

Notice the very low levels of calcium present in some of these preparations. A product that supplies 20 milligrams of calcium provides only 2 percent of an adult's RDA for calcium and would have no significant impact on a person's calcium nutrition.

*These tables are reprinted, with permission, from L. K. DeBruyne and S. R. Rolfes, *Selection of Supplements,* a 1986 monograph in the *Nutrition Clinics* series available from Stickley Publishing Co., 210 Washington Sq., Philadelphia, PA 19106.

Table D–1

Supplements for Infants and Children

Company	Lederle	Miles Laboratories	Mead-Johnson	Mead-Johnson	Radiance	Chocks
Product	Centrum Jr.	Flintstones with Iron	Poly-Vi-Sol	Poly-Vi-Sol Iron and Zinc	Chewable for Children	Bugs Bunny plus Iron
Age of Intended Users	*Children over 4*	*Children over 2*	*Infants*	*Children and Adults*	*Children 2 to 12*	*Children over 2*
Recommended Daily Dose	*1 Chewable*	*1 Chewable*	*1 ml Dropper*	*1 Chewable*	*1 Chewable*	*1 Chewable*
Vitamins						
Vitamin A (IU)	5000	2500	1500	2500	4000	2500
Vitamin D (IU)	400	400	400	400	400	400
Vitamin E (IU)	15	15	5	15	3.4	15
Vitamin C (mg)	60	60	35	60	60	60
Thiamin (B_1) (mg)	1.5	1.05	0.5	1.05	2	1.05
Riboflavin (B_2) (mg)	1.7	1.2	0.6	1.2	2.4	1.2
Vitamin B_6 (mg)	2	1.05	0.4	1.05	2	1.05
Vitamin B_{12} (μg)	6	4.5	2	4.5	10	4.5
Niacin (mg)	20	13.5	8	13.5	10	13.5
Folacin (mg)	0.4	0.3	—	0.3	—	0.3
Minerals						
Calcium (mg)	—	—	—	—	19	—
Phosphorus (mg)	—	—	—	—	—	—
Iron (mg)	18	15	—	12	12	15
Potassium (mg)	1.6	—	—	—	4	—
Mangnesium (mg)	25	—	—	—	22	—
Zinc (mg)	10	—	—	8	—	—
Copper (mg)	2	—	—	—	0.2	—
Iodine (μg)	—	—	—	—	—	—
Manganese (mg)	1	—	—	—	—	—
Cost per day[a]						

[a]Divide the total retail price for the container by the number of doses per container. For example, XYZ Vitamins are sold in bottles of 100 tablets, and the recommended dose is 2 tablets per day; there are 50 doses in the bottle. At $5.00 per bottle, XYZ Vitamins cost $.10 per day.

Table D–1

(continued)

Neolife	J. B. Williams	Upjohn	Amway	Shaklee	Richardson Vicks	Ross Labs	Miles Labs	Other
Vita Squares	Popeye with Mins/ Iron	Unicap	Nutrilite	Vita-Lea Children	Life-Stage Children	Vi-Daylin with Iron	Flintstones Complete	
Children over 2	*Children*	*Children*	*Children*	*Children over 4*	*Children 4 to 12*	*Children under 4*	*Children over 4*	
3 Chewables	*1 Chewable*	*1 Chewable*	*1 Chewable*	*2 Chewables*	*2 Chewables*	*1 Dropper*	*1 Chewable*	
3000	2500	5000	2500	2000	5000	1500	5000	
400	400	400	400	400	400	400	400	
9	15	15	10	10	30	5	30	
60	60	60	40	60	60	35	60	
1.5	1.05	1.5	0.7	1.1	1.5	0.5	1.5	
1.5	1.2	1.7	0.8	1.2	1.7	0.6	1.7	
1.2	1.05	2	0.7	1.5	2	0.4	2	
3	4.5	6	3	3	6	1.5	6	
10	13.5	20	9	14	20	8	20	
0.2	0.3	0.4	0.2	0.3	0.4	—	0.4	
—	—	—	—	130	—	—	100	
—	—	—	—	100	—	—	100	
3	15	—	5	10	9	10	18	
—	—	—	—	—	—	—	—	
—	40	—	—	60	—	—	20	
—	12	—	—	1.5	—	—	15	
0.002	1.5	—	—	0.2	—	—	—	
75	105	—	—	15	—	—	150	
1	—	—	—	—	—	—	2.5	

Note: Radiance chewables also contain 2 mg pantothenic acid, 10 mg biotin, 2 mg inositol, and 2 mg of a choline compound.
Neolife chewables also contain 10 mg pantothenic acid, 0.075 mg inositol, 0.05 mg of a choline compound, 15 mg biotin, and 15 mg PABA.
Williams chewables also contain 2.5 mg pantothenic acid and 37.5 mg biotin.
Amway chewables also contain 5 mg pantothenic acid.
Shaklee chewables also contain 4 mg pantothenic acid and 0.1 mg biotin.
Lederle chewables also contain 1.4 mg chlorine (recommended daily dose for children 2 to 4 is ½ tablet).
Richardson Vicks chewables also contain 10 mg pantothenic acid and 0.3 mg biotin.

D

Table D–2

Supplements for Adults

Company	**Lederle**	**Parke-Davis**	**Squibb**	**Miles Labs**	**Radiance**	**Neolife**	**Amway**
Product	**Centrum A to Zinc**	**Myadec**	**Theragran M**	**One-a-Day Plus Iron**	**Nutri-Mega**	**Formula IV**	**Nutrilite Double X**
Recommended Daily Dose	*1 Tablet*	*1 Tablet*	*1 Tablet*	*1 Tablet*	*2 Tablets*	*2 Capsules*	*9 Tablets*
Vitamins							
Vitamin A (IU)	5000	10,000	10,000	5000	10,000	4000	15,000
Vitamin D (IU)	400	400	400	400	400	400	400
Vitamin E (IU)	30	30	15	30	300	10	30
Vitamin C (mg)	90	250	200	60	300	90	500
Thiamin (B_1) (mg)	2.25	10	10.3	1.5	50	10	15
Riboflavin (B_2) (mg)	2.6	10	10	1.7	50	10	15
Vitamin B_6 (mg)	3	5	4.1	2	50	10	15
Vitamin B_{12} (g)	9	6	5	6	50	10	9
Niacin (mg)	20	100	100	20	50	50	35
Folacin (mg)	0.4	0.4	—	0.4	0.4	0.4	0.4
Minerals							
Calcium (mg)	162	—	—	—	200	—	900
Phosphorus (mg)	125	—	—	—	50	—	450
Iron (mg)	27	20	12	18	18	25	18
Potassium (mg)	7.7	—	—	—	30	10	—
Magnesium (mg)	100	100	65	—	50	35	300
Zinc (mg)	22.5	20	1.5	—	15	—	15
Copper (mg)	3	2	2	—	2	2	2
Iodine (μg)	150	150	150	—	150	100	150
Manganese (mg)	7.5	1.25	1	—	30	10	5
Cost per day [a]							

[a]Divide the total retail price for the container by the number of doses per container. For example, XYZ Vitamins are sold in bottles of 100 tablets, and the recommended dose is 2 tablets per day; there are 50 doses in the bottle. At $5.00 per bottle, XYZ Vitamins cost $.10 per day.

Table D–2

(continued)

J. B. Williams	Origin	Miles Labs	Mineralab	Richardson Vicks	Richardson Vicks	J. B. Williams	Upjohn	Squibb	Other
Vitabank	**Multi-vitamin**	**One-a-Day Plus Minerals**	**Added Pro-tection III**	**Lifestage–Women**	**Lifestage–Men**	**Femiron**	**Unicap Plus Iron**	**Theragran Z**	
1 Tablet	*1 Tablet*	*1 Tablet*	*6 Tablets*	*1 Tablet*	*1 Tablet*	*1 Tablet*	*1 Tablet*	*1 Tablet*	
5000	10,000	5000	10,000	5000	10,000	5000	5000	10,000	
400	400	400	200	400	400	400	400	400	
30	30	30	400	30	50	15	15	15	
90	250	60	1200	100	200	60	60	200	
2.25	20	1.5	100	3	10	1.5	1.5	10.3	
2.6	20	1.7	50	3.4	10	1.7	1.7	10	
3	5	2	100	4	5	2	2	4.1	
9	6	6	100	12	6	6	6	5	
20	150	20	40	40	100	20	20	100	
0.4	0.4	0.4	0.8	0.4	0.4	0.4	0.4	—	
170	100	129.6	500	—	—	10	—	—	
130	—	100	—	—	—	—	—	—	
18	30	18	20	27	18	20	18	12	
7.5	5	5	99	—	—	—	—	—	
100	50	100	500	100	100	—	—	—	
15	7.5	15	30	15	15	—	—	22.5	
2	1	2	2	2	2	—	—	2	
150	150	150	200	150	150	—	—	150	
2.5	1.5	2.5	20	—	1.25	—	—	1	

Note: Lederle Centrum A to Zinc also contains 10 mg pantothenic acid, 45 μg biotin, 25 μg selenium, 15 μg molybdenum, 15 μg chromium, and 7 mg chlorine.

Radiance Nutri-Mega also contains 50 mg pantothenic acid, 50 μg biotin, 50 mg inositol, 50 mg PABA, 50 mg of a choline compound, and 80 mg lecithin.

Neolife Formula IV also contains 12 mg pantothenic acid, 65 mg inositol, 30 mg PABA, 30 mg lecithin, 40 mg diastase, 45 mg lipase (pancreatin), 168 mg linoleic acid, 40 mg pancrein, and 10 mg betaine.

Origin Multivitamins also contains 20 mg pantothenic acid, 25 μg biotin, 10 mg inositol, and 20 mg of a choline compound.

Amway Nutrilite Double X also contains 10 mg panthothenic acid, 5 μg chromium, and 5 μg selenium.

J.B. Williams Vitabank also contains 18 mg pantothenic acid and 25 μg selenium.

Miles Labs One-a-Day plus Minerals also contains 10 mg pantothenic acid, 10 μg chromium, 10 μg selenium, and 10 μg molybdenum.

Miles Labs One-a-Day plus Iron also contains 30 μg biotin, 10 mg pantothenic acid, and 50 μg vitamin K.

Squibb Theragran Z and M also contain 18.4 mg pantothenic acid.

Parke-Davis Myadec also contains 20 mg pantothenic acid.

Mineral Lab Added Protection III also contains 500 mg pantothenic acid, 300 μg biotin, 150 mg of a choline compound, 100 mg inositol, 50 mg PABA, 100 mg citrus bioflavinoid complex, 200 μg chromium, 200 μg selenium, 100 μg molybdenum, 5000 IU beta-carotene, 150 mg niacinamide, and 100 μg trace elements.

Richardson Vicks Lifestage for Women and Men also contain 10 and 20 mg pantothenic acid, respectively.

Upjohn Unicap plus Iron also contains 10 mg pantothenic acid.

Table D–3

Supplements and Tonics for the Elderly

Company	Ross Labs	Lederle	J.B. Williams	J.B. Williams	Upjohn	Other
Product	Vi-Daylin Plus Iron	Gevrabon	Geritol	Geritol	Unicap Senior	
Recommended Daily Dose	*1 Tsp*	*1 Oz*	*1 Oz*	*1 Tablet*	*1 Tablet*	
Vitamins						
Vitamin A (IU)	2500	—	—	—	5000	
Vitamin D (IU)	400	—	—	—	—	
Vitamin E (IU)	15	—	—	—	15	
Vitamin C (mg)	60	—	—	75	60	
Thiamin (B_1) (mg)	1.05	5	5	5	1.2	
Riboflavin (B_2) (mg)	1.2	2.5	5	5	1.7	
Vitamin B_6 (mg)	1.05	1	1	0.5	2	
Vitamin B_{12} (μg)	4.5	1	1.5	3	6	
Niacin (mg)	13.5	50	100	30	14	
Folacin (mg)	—	—	—	—	0.4	
Minerals						
Calcium (mg)	—	—	—	2	—	
Phosphorus (mg)	—	—	—	—	—	
Iron (mg)	10	15	100	50	10	
Potassium (mg)	—	—	—	—	5	
Magnesium (mg)	—	2	—	—	—	
Zinc (mg)	—	2	—	—	15	
Copper (mg)	—	—	—	—	2	
Iodine (μg)	—	100	—	—	150	
Manganese (mg)	—	2	—	—	1	
Alcohol (%)	0.5	18	12	—	—	
Cost per day[a]						

[a]Divide the total retail price for the container by the number of doses per container. For example, XYZ Vitamins are sold in bottles of 100 tablets, and the recommended dose is 2 tablets per day; there are 50 doses in the bottle. At $5.00 per bottle, XYZ Vitamins cost $.10 per day.

Note: Lederle Gevrabon also contains 100 mg inositol and 100 mg of a choline compound.
J.B. Williams Geritol also contains 100 mg of a choline compound, 50 mg methionine, and 4 mg panthenol.
Upjohn Unicap Senior also contains 10 mg pantothenic acid.

Appendix E

Food Exchange Systems

For an introduction to the use of exchange systems, see Chapter 2. The U.S. and Canadian exchange systems are presented here.

The U.S. Exchange System

The U.S. system divides the foods suitable for use in planning a healthy diet into six lists—the starch/bread, meat, meat alternate, vegetable, fruit, milk, and fat lists.* These lists are shown in Tables E–1 through E–6. Following these lists are three other tables of foods: free foods, combination foods, and foods for occasional use.

Table E–1

Starch/Bread List (15 g carbohydrate, 3 g protein, 80 cal)
For starchy foods not on this list, the general rule is that ½ c of cereal grain or pasta is 1 serving; 1 oz of a bread product is 1 serving.

Amount	Food
Cereals/Grains/Pasta	
⅓ c	Bran cereals, concentrated[a]
½ c	Bran cereals, flaked[a]
½ c	Bulgur (cooked)
½ c	Cooked cereals
2½ tbsp	Cornmeal (dry)
3 tbsp	Grapenuts
½ c	Grits (cooked)
¾ c	Other ready-to-eat unsweetened cereals
½ c	Pasta (cooked)
1½ c	Puffed cereal
⅓ c	Rice, white or brown (cooked)
½ c	Shredded wheat
3 tbsp	Wheat germ[a]
Dried Beans/Peas/Lentils	
¼ c	Baked beans[a]
⅓ c	Beans and peas (cooked) such as black-eyed, kidney, white, split[a]
⅓ c	Lentils (cooked)[a]
Starchy Vegetables	
½ c	Corn[a]
1 cob	Corn on the cob, 6 inches long[a]
½ c	Lima beans[a]
½ c	Peas, green (canned or frozen)[a]
½ c	Plantains[a]
1 small (3 oz)	Potatoes, baked
½ c	Potatoes, mashed
¾ c	Squash, winter (acorn, butternut)
⅓ c	Yams, sweet potatoes, plain
Bread	
½ (1 oz)	Bagels
2 (⅔ oz)	Bread sticks, crisp, 4 × ½ inch
1 c	Croutons, low fat
½ muffin	English muffins
½ (1 oz)	Frankfurter or hamburger buns
½ loaf	Pita, 6 inches across
1 (1 oz)	Plain rolls, small
1 slice (1 oz)	Raisin bread, unfrosted
1 slice (1 oz)	Rye, pumpernickel[a]
1 tortilla	Tortillas, 6 inches across
1 slice (1 oz)	White (including French, Italian)
1 slice (1 oz)	Whole wheat
Crackers/Snacks	
8 crackers	Animal crackers
3 crackers	Graham crackers, 2½ inches square
¾ oz	Matzoth
5 slices	Melba toast
24 crackers	Oyster crackers
3 c	Popcorn (popped, no fat added)
¾ oz	Pretzels
4 crackers	Rye crisp, 2 × 3½ inches
6 crackers	Saltine-type crackers
2–4 slices (¾ oz)	Whole-wheat crackers, no fat added (crisp breads)

[a]3 g or more of dietary fiber per serving. Average fiber contents of whole-grain products is 2 g per serving.

(continued on following page)

*The U.S. exchange system presented here is based on material in *Exchange Lists for Meal Planning*, 1986, prepared by committees of the American Diabetes Association and the American Dietetic Association, with permission of both organizations.

Table E–1

(continued)

Amount	Food
Starchy Foods Prepared with Fat	
(Count as 1 starch/bread serving, plus 1 fat serving.)	
1 biscuit	Biscuits 2½ inches across
½ c	Chow mein noodles
1 (2 oz)	Corn bread, 2-inch cube
6 crackers	Crackers, round butter type
10 (1½ oz)	French fried potatoes, 2 inches to 3½ inches long
1 muffin	Muffins, plain, small
2 pancakes	Pancakes, 4 inches across
¼ c	Stuffing, bread (prepared)
2 taco shells	Taco shells, 6 inches across
1 waffle	Waffle, 4½ inches square
4–6 crackers (1 oz)	Whole-wheat crackers, fat added

E

Table E–2

Meat/Meat Alternate Lists (Lean meat = 7 g protein, 3 g fat, 55 cal. Medium-fat meat = 7 g protein, 5 g fat, 75 cal. High-fat meat = 7 g protein, 8 g fat, 100 cal.)

Lean Meat and Alternates		
Beef:	1 oz	USDA Good or Choice grades of lean beef, such as round, sirloin, and flank steak; tenderloin; and chipped beef[a]
Pork:	1 oz	Lean pork, such as fresh ham; canned, cured, or boiled ham[a]; Canadian bacon,[a] tenderloin.
Veal:	1 oz	All cuts are lean except for veal cutlets (ground or cubed); examples of lean veal are chops and roasts
Poultry:	1 oz	Chicken, turkey, Cornish hen (without skin)
Fish:	1 oz	All fresh and frozen fish
	2 oz	Crab, lobster, scallops, shrimp, clams (fresh or canned in water)[a]
	6 medium	Oysters
	¼ c	Tuna (canned in water)[a]
	1 oz	Herring (uncreamed or smoked)
	2 medium	Sardines (canned)
Wild Game:	1 oz	Venison, rabbit, squirrel
	1 oz	Pheasant, duck, goose (without skin)
Cheese:	¼ c	Any cottage cheese
	2 tbsp	Grated Parmesan
	1 oz	Diet cheeses (with less than 55 cal oz)[a]
Other:	1 oz	95% fat-free luncheon meat
	3 whites	Egg whites
	¼ c	Egg substitutes with less than 55 cal/¼ c
Medium-Fat Meat and Alternates		
Beef:	1 oz	Most beef products fall into this category; examples are all ground beef, roasts (rib, chuck, rump), steaks (cubed, porterhouse, T-bone), and meat loaf.
Pork:	1 oz	Most pork products fall into this category; examples are chops, loin roast, Boston butt, cutlets
Lamb:	1 oz	Most lamb products fall into this category; examples are chops, leg, and roast.
Veal:	1 oz	Cutlet (ground or cubed, unbreaded)
Poultry:	1 oz	Chicken (with skin), domestic duck or goose (well drained of fat), ground turkey
Fish:	¼ c	Tuna (canned in oil and drained)[a]
	¼ c	Salmon (canned)[a]
Cheese:		Skim or part-skim milk cheeses, such as:
	¼ c	Ricotta
	1 oz	Mozzarella
	1 oz	Diet cheeses (with 56 to 80 cal/oz)[a]
Other:	1 oz	86% fat-free luncheon meat[a]
	1	Eggs (high in cholesterol, limit to 3 per week)
	¼ c	Egg substitutes with 56 to 80 cal/¼ c
	4 oz	Tofu (2½ × 2¾ × 1 inch)
	1 oz	Liver, heart, kidney, sweetbreads (high in cholesterol)

[a]400 mg or more of sodium per exchange. Meats contribute no fiber to the diet.

Table E–2

(continued)

High-Fat Meat and Alternates		
Beef:	1 oz	Most USDA Prime cuts of beef, such as ribs, corned beef[a]
Pork:	1 oz	Spareribs, ground pork, pork sausage (patty or link)[a]
Lamb:	1 oz	Patties (ground lamb)
Fish:	1 oz	Any fried fish product
Cheese:	1 oz	All regular cheeses,[a] such as American, blue, cheddar, Monterey, Swiss
Other:	1 oz	Luncheon meat[a] such as bologna, salami, pimiento loaf
	1 oz	Sausage,[a] such as Polish, Italian[a]
	1 oz	Knockwurst, smoked
	1 oz	Bratwurst[a]
	1 frank (10/lb)	Frankfurters (turkey or chicken)[a]
	1 tbsp	Peanut butter (contains unsaturated fat)
Count as 1 high-fat meat plus 1 fat exchange:		
1 frank	(10/lb)	Frankfurters (beef, pork, or combination)[a]

[a]400 mg or more of sodium per exchange. Meats contribute no fiber to the diet.

Table E–3

Vegetable List

(5 g carbohydrate, 2 g protein, 25 cal) All portion sizes, except as otherwise noted, are ½ c of any cooked vegetable or vegetable juice, 1 c of any raw vegetable.

Artichokes (½ medium)	Mushrooms, cooked
Asparagus	Okra
Beans (green, wax, Italian)	Onions
Bean sprouts	Pea pods
Beets	Peppers (green)
Broccoli	Rutabagas
Brussels sprouts	Sauerkraut[a]
Cabbage, cooked	Spinach, cooked
Carrots	Summer squash (crookneck)
Cauliflower	Tomatoes (one large)
Eggplant	Tomato/vegetable juice[a]
Greens (collard, mustard, turnip)	Turnips
Kohlrabi	Water chestnuts
Leeks	Zucchini, cooked

[a]400 mg or more of sodium per serving. Most vegetable servings contain 2 to 3 g of dietary fiber.

Starchy vegetables such as corn, peas, and potatoes are found on the Starch/Bread List.
For free vegetables, see free food list.

Table E–4

Fruit List

(15 g carbohydrate, 60 cal) All portion sizes, unless otherwise noted, are ½ c of fresh fruit or fruit juice, ¼ c of dried fruit.

Amount	Food
Fresh, Frozen, and Unsweetened Canned Fruit	
1 apple	Apples (raw, 2 inches across)
½ c	Applesauce (unsweetened)
4 apricots	Apricots (medium, raw)
½ c or 4 halves	Apricots (canned)
½ banana	Bananas (9 inches long)
¾ c	Blackberries (raw)[a]
¾ c	Blueberries (raw)[a]
⅓ melon	Cantaloupe (5 inches across)
1 c	Cantaloupe (cubes)
12 cherries	Cherries (large, raw)
½ c	Cherries (canned)
2 figs	Figs (raw, 2 inches across)
½ c	Fruit cocktail (canned)
½ grapefruit	Grapefruit (medium)
¾ c	Grapefruit (segments)
15 grapes	Grapes (small)
⅛ melon	Honeydew melon (medium)
1 c	Honeydew melon (cubes)
1 kiwi	Kiwi fruit (large)
¾ c	Mandarin oranges
½ mango	Mangoes (small)
1 nectarine	Nectarine (1½ inches across)[a]
1 orange	Orange (2½ inches across)
1 c	Papayas
1 peach or ¾ c	Peach (2¾ inches across)
½ c or 2 halves	Peaches (canned)
½ large or 1 small	Pear
½ c or 2 halves	Pears (canned)
2 persimmons	Persimmons (medium, native)
¾ c	Pineapple (raw)
⅓ c	Pineapple (canned)
2 plums	Plums (raw, 2 inches across)
½ pomegranate	Pomegranate[a]
1 c	Raspberries (raw)[a]
1¼ c	Strawberries (raw, whole)[a]
2 tangerines	Tangerines (2½ inches across)
1¼ c	Watermelon (cubes)

[a]3 or more g of dietary fiber per serving. Average fiber contents of fresh, frozen, and dry fruits: 2 g per serving.

E

Table E–4

(continued)

Amount	Food
Dried Fruit	
4 rings	Apples[a]
7 halves	Apricots[a]
2½ medium	Dates
1½ figs	Figs[a]
3 medium	Prunes[a]
2 tbsp	Raisins
Fruit Juice	
½ c	Apple juice/cider
⅓ c	Cranberry juice cocktail
½ c	Grapefruit juice
⅓ c	Grape juice
½ c	Orange juice
½ c	Pineapple juice
⅓ c	Prune juice

[a]3 or more g of dietary fiber per serving. Average fiber contents of fresh, frozen, and dry fruits: 2 g per serving.

Table E–5

Milk List

Nonfat and very low-fat milk = 12 g carbohydrate, 8 g protein, trace fat, 90 cal.

Low-fat milk = 12 g carbohydrate, 8 g protein, 5 g fat, 120 cal.

Whole milk = 12 g carbohydrate, 8 g protein, 8 g fat, 150 cal.

Amount	Food
Nonfat and Very Low-Fat Milk	
1 c	Nonfat milk
1 c	½% milk
1 c	1% milk
1 c	Low-fat buttermilk
½ c	Evaporated nonfat milk
⅓ c	Dry nonfat milk
8 oz	Plain nonfat yogurt
Low-Fat Milk	
1 c fluid	2% milk
8 oz	Plain low-fat yogurt (with added nonfat milk solids)
Whole Milk	
1 c	Whole milk
½ c	Evaporated whole milk
8 oz	Whole plain yogurt

Table E–6

Fat List (5 g fat, 45 cal)

Amount	Food
Unsaturated Fats	
⅛ medium	Avocados
1 tsp	Margarine
1 tbsp	Margarine, diet[a]
1 tsp	Mayonnaise
1 tbsp	Mayonnaise, reduced calorie[a]
	Nuts and seeds:
6 whole	Almonds, dry roasted
1 tbsp	Cashews, dry roasted
20 small or 10 large	Peanuts
2 whole	Pecans
2 whole	Walnuts
1 tbsp	Other nuts
1 tbsp	Pine nuts, sunflower seeds (without shells)
	Pumpkin seeds
2 tsp	Oil (corn, cottonseed, safflower,
1 tsp	soybean, sunflower, olive, peanut)
10 small or 5 large	Olives[a]
1 tbsp	Salad dressing (all varieties)[a]
2 tsp	Salad dressing, mayonnaise type
1 tbsp	Salad dressing, mayonnaise type, reduced calorie
2 tbsp	Salad dressing, reduced calorie[b]
Saturated Fats	
1 slice	Bacon[a]
1 tsp	Butter
½ oz	Chitterlings
2 tbsp	Coconut, shredded
2 tbsp	Coffee whitener, liquid
4 tsp	Coffee whitener, powder
1 tbsp	Cream (heavy, whipping)
2 tbsp	Cream (light, coffee, table)
2 tbsp	Cream, sour
1 tbsp	Cream cheese
¼ oz	Salt pork[a]

Note: 2 tbsp low-calorie salad dressing is a free food.

[a]If more than one or two servings are eaten, these foods have 400 mg or more of sodium.

[b]400 mg or more of sodium per serving.

Table E–7

Free Foods

A free food is any food or drink that contains less than 20 cal/serving. People with diabetes are advised to eat as much as they want of those items that have no serving size specified. They may eat two or three servings per day of those items that have a specific serving size. It is suggested that they spread them out through the day.

Drinks	
	Bouillon[a] or broth without fat
	Bouillon, low sodium
	Carbonated drinks, sugar-free
	Carbonated water
	Club soda
1 tbsp	Cocoa powder, unsweetened
	Coffee/tea
	Drink mixes, sugar-free
	Tonic water, sugar-free
Nonstick Pan Spray	
Fruit	
½ c	Cranberries, unsweetened
½ c	Rhubarb, unsweetened
Vegetables (raw, 1 c)	
	Cabbage
	Celery
	Chinese cabbage[b]
	Cucumbers
	Green onions
	Hot peppers
	Mushrooms
	Radishes[b]
	Zucchini[b]
Salad Greens	
	Endive
	Escarole
	Iceberg lettuce
	Romaine
	Spinach
Sweet Substitutes	
	Candy, hard, sugar-free
	Gelatin, sugar-free
2 tsp	Jam/jelly, sugar-free
1–2 tbsp	Pancake syrup, sugar-free
	Sugar substitutes (saccharin, aspartame)
2 tbsp	Whipped topping
Condiments	
1 tbsp	Catsup
	Horseradish
	Mustard
	Pickles, dill, unsweetened[a]
2 tbsp	Salad dressing, low calorie
1 tbsp	Taco sauce
	Vinegar
Seasonings	
	Basil (fresh)
	Celery seeds
	Chili powder
	Chives
	Cinnamon
	Curry
	Dill
	Flavoring extracts (vanilla, almond, walnut, peppermint, butter, lemon, etc.)
	Garlic
	Garlic powder
	Herbs
	Hot pepper sauce
	Lemon
	Lemon juice
	Lemon pepper
	Lime
	Lime juice
	Mint
	Onion powder
	Oregano
	Paprika
	Pepper
	Pimiento
	Soy sauce[a]
	Soy sauce, low sodium ("lite")
	Spices
	Wine, used in cooking
	Worcestershire sauce

[a]400 mg or more of sodium per serving
[b]3 g or more of fiber per serving

[a]400 mg or more of sodium per serving
[b]3 g or more of fiber per serving

E

Table E–8

Combination foods

Much of the food we eat is mixed together in various combinations that do not fit into only one exchange list. This is a list of average values for some typical combination foods. It will help you fit these foods into your meal plan. Ask your dietitian for information about any other foods you'd like to eat. The *American Diabetes Association/American Dietetic Association Family Cookbook* and the *American Diabetes Association Holiday Cookbook* have many recipes and further information about many foods, including combination foods. Check your library or local bookstore.

Food	Amount	Exchanges
Casseroles	1 c (8 oz)	2 starch, 2 medium-fat meat, 1 fat
Cheese pizza, thin crust[a]	¼ of 15-oz, or ¼ of 10-inch, pizza	2 starch, 1 medium-fat meat, 1 fat
Chili with beans (commercial)[a,b]	1 c (8 oz)	2 starch, 2 medium-fat meat, 2 fat
Chow mein (without noodles or rice)[a,b]	2 c (16 oz)	1 starch, 2 vegetable, 2 lean meat
Macaroni and cheese[a]	1 c (8 oz)	2 starch, 1 medium-fat meat, 2 fat
Soup		
Bean[(a, b)]	1 c (8 oz)	1 starch, 1 vegetable, 1 lean meat
Chunky, all varieties[a]	10¾-oz can	1 starch, 1 vegetable, 1 medium-fat meat
Cream (made with water)[a]	1 c (8 oz)	1 starch, 1 fat
Vegetable[a] or broth[a]	1 c (8 oz)	1 starch
Spaghetti and meatballs (canned)[a]	1 c (8 oz)	2 starch, 1 medium-fat meat, 1 fat
Sugar-free pudding (made with nonfat milk)	½ c	1 starch
If beans are used as a meat substitute:		
Dried beans[b], peas,[b] lentils[b]	1 c (cooked)	2 starch, 1 lean meat

[a]400 mg or more of sodium per serving
[b]3 g or more of fiber per serving

Foods for Occasional Use

Food	Amount	Exchanges
Angel food cake	1/12 cake	2 starch
Cake, no icing	1/12 cake, or a 3-inch square	2 starch, 2 fat
Cookies	2 small (1¾ inches across)	1 starch, 1 fat
Frozen fruit yogurt	⅓ c	1 starch
Gingersnaps	3 cookies	1 starch
Granola	¼ c	1 starch, 1 fat
Granola bars	1 small	1 starch, 1 fat
Ice cream, any flavor	½ c	1 starch, 2 fat
Ice milk, any flavor	½ c	1 starch, 1 fat
Sherbet, any flavor	¼ c	1 starch
Snack chips, all varieties[a]	1 oz	1 starch, 2 fat
Vanilla wafers	6 small	1 starch, 1 fat

[a]If more than one serving is eaten, these foods have 400 mg or more of sodium.

The Canadian System

The Canadian system is similar to the U.S. exchange system, but the serving sizes and some of the foods listed are different. This system, as explained in the handbook *Good Health Eating Guide*, is a revision of the Canadian exchange system of meal planning.* Features of the Canadian system include the following:

- Foods are divided into six groups according to carbohydrate, protein, and fat content.
- Foods are interchangeable within a group.
- Most foods are eaten in measured amounts.

New features of the system include the following:

- An energy value is given for each food group.
- Protein foods low in fat are emphasized in the protein foods group. Protein foods containing extra fat are identified.
- The user is able to distinguish between complex and simple carbohydrates (starches and sugars).

*The tables for the Canadian system are taken from *Good Health Eating Guide* (Toronto: Canadian Diabetes Association, 1981), and are used with the association's permission.

Table E–9

Protein Foods Group (7 g protein, 3 g fat, 55 cal)

Food	Measure	Mass (weight), g
Cheese		
All types, made from partly skim milk (e.g., mozzarella, part skim)	1 piece, 5 × 2 × 2 cm (2 × 3/4 × 3/4 inch)	25
Cottage cheese, all types	50 ml (1/4 c)	55
Fish		
Anchovies (see extras)		
Canned, drained (e.g., chicken haddie, mackerel, salmon, tuna)	50 ml (1/4 c)	30
Cod tongues/cheeks	75 ml (1/3 c)	50
Fillet or steak (e.g., Boston blue, cod, flounder, haddock, halibut, perch, pickerel, pike, salmon, shad, sole, trout, whitefish)	1 piece, 6 × 2 × 2 cm (2½ × 3/4 × 3/4 inch)	30
Herring	1/3 fish	30
Octopus	50 ml (1/4 c)	40
Sardines	2 medium or 3 small	30
Seal, walrus	1 slice, 6 × 4 × 1 cm (2½ × 1½ × ½ inch)	25
Smelts	2 medium	30
Squid	50 ml (1/4 c)	40
Shellfish		
Clams, mussels, oysters, scallops, snails	3 medium	30
Crab, lobster, flaked	50 ml (1/4 c)	30
Shrimp, fresh	5 large	30
frozen	10 medium	30
canned	18 small	30
dry pack	50 ml (1/4 c)	30
Meat and Poultry (e.g., beef, chicken, ham, lamb, pork, turkey, veal, wild game)		
Back bacon	3 slices, thin	25
Chops	½ chop, with bone	35
Minced or ground, lean	30 ml (2 tbsp)	25
Sliced, lean	1 slice, 10 × 5 × 5 mm (4 × 2 × 1/4 inch)	25
Steak, lean	1 piece, 4 × 3 × 2 cm (1½ × 1¼ × 3/4 inch)	25
Organ Meats		
Heart, liver	1 slice, 5 × 5 × 1 cm (2 × 2 × ½) inch)	25
Kidney, sweetbreads, chopped	50 ml (1/4 c)	25
Tongue	1 slice, 8 × 6 × 5 mm (3¼ × 2½ × 1/4 inch)	25
Tripe, 1 piece = 4 cm × 4 cm × 8 mm (1½ × 1½ × 3/8 inch)	5 pieces	50
Soybean		
Bean curd or tofu, 1 block = 6 × 6 × 4 cm (2½ × 2½ × 1½ inches)	½ block	70
The following choices contain extra fat, so use them less often.		
Cheese		
Cheese, all types made from whole milk (e.g., brick, brie, camembert, cheddar, Edam, Tilsit)	1 piece, 5 × 2 × 2 cm (2 × 3/4 × 3/4 inch)	25
Cheese, coarsely grated (e.g., cheddar)	75 ml (1/3 c)	25
Cheese, dry, finely grated (e.g., Parmesan)	45 ml (3 tbsp)	15
Cheese, ricotta	50 ml (1/4 c)	55

E

Table E–9

(continued)

Food	Measure	Mass (weight), g
Eggs		
Eggs, scrambled	50 ml (1/4 c)	55
Eggs, in shell, raw or cooked	1 medium	50
Eggs, without shell, cooked or poached in water	1 medium	45
Fish		
Eel	5 cm, 4 cm diameter (2 inches, 1 1/2-inch diameter)	50
Meat		
Bologna	1 slice, 5mm, 10-cm diameter (1/4 inch, 4-diameter)	40
Canned luncheon meat	1 slice, 85 × 45 × 10 mm (3 1/2 × 1 3/4 × 1/2 inch)	40
Corned beef, fresh	1 slice, 10 × 5 × 5 mm (4 × 2 × 1/4 inch)	25
Corned beef, canned	1 slice, 75 × 55 × 5 mm (3 × 2 1/4 × 1/4 inch)	25
Ground beef, medium fat	30 ml (2 tbsp)	25
Meat spreads, canned	45 ml (3 tbsp)	35
Paté (see Fats and Oils group)		
Sausage, garlic, Polish, or knockwurst	1 slice, 1 cm, 5-cm diameter (1/2 inch, 2-inch diameter)	50
Sausage, pork, link	1 link	25
Spareribs or shortribs, with bone	10 × 6 cm (4 × 2 1/2 inches)	65
Summer sausage or salami	1 slice, 5 mm, 10-cm diameter (1/4 inch, 4-diameter)	40
Stewing beef	1 cube, 25 mm (1 inch)	25
Wieners	1/2 medium	25
Miscellaneous		
Blood pudding	1 slice, 5 × 1 cm (2 × 1/2 inch)	25
Peanut butter, all kinds	15 ml (1 tbsp)	15

Table E–10

Starchy Foods Group (15 g carbohydrate [starch], 2 g protein, 68 cal)

Food	Measure	Mass (weight), g
Breads		
Bagels	½	25
Bread crumbs	50 ml (¼ c)	25
Bread cubes	250 ml (1 c)	25
Bread sticks, 11 × 1 cm (4½ × ½ inches)	2	20
Brewis, cooked	50 ml (¼ c)	45
English muffins, crumpets	½	25
Flour	40 ml (2½ tbsp)	20
Hamburger buns	½	30
Hot dog buns	½	30
Kaiser rolls	½	25
Matzoth, 15-cm (6-inch square)	1	20
Melba toast, rectangular	4	15
Pita, 20-cm (8-inch) diameter	¼	25
Plain rolls	1 small	25
Raisin bread	1 slice	25
Rusks	2	20
Rye, coarse or pumpernickel, 10 cm × 10 cm × 8 mm (4 × 4 × ⅜ inch)	½ slice	25
Tortillas, 15 cm (6 inches)	1	20
White (French and Italian)	1 slice	25
Whole wheat, cracked wheat, rye, white enriched	1 slice	25
Cereals		
Bran flakes, 40% bran	125 ml (½ c)	20
Cooked cereals, cooked	125 ml (½ c)	125
dry	30 ml (2 tbsp)	20
Cornmeal, cooked	125 ml (½ c)	125
dry	30 ml (2 tbsp)	20
Ready-to-eat unsweetened cereals	250 ml (1 c)	20
Shredded wheat biscuit, rectangular or round	1	20
Shredded wheat, bite size	125 ml (½ c)	20
Wheat germ	75 ml (⅓ c)	30
Cookies and Biscuits		
See "Prepared Foods" (below)		
Grains		
Barley, cooked	125 ml (½ c)	120
dry	30 ml (2 tbsp)	20
Bulgar, kasha, cooked, moist	125 ml (½ c)	70
cooked, crumbly	75 ml (⅓ c)	40
dry	30 ml (2 tbsp)	20
Rice, cooked, loosely packed	125 ml (½ c)	105
cooked, tightly packed	75 ml (⅓ c)	70
Tapioca, pearl and granulated, quick cooking, dry	30 ml (2 tbsp)	15
Pasta		
Macaroni, cooked	125 ml (½ c)	70
Noodles, cooked	125 ml (½ c)	80
Spaghetti, cooked	125 ml (½ c)	70

Table E–10

(continued)

Food	Measure	Mass (weight), g
Starchy Vegetables		
Beans and peas, dried, cooked	125 ml (1/2 c)	80
Breadfruit	1 slice	75
Corn, canned, whole kernel	125 ml (1/2 c)	85
canned, creamed	75 ml (1/3 c)	60
Corn on the cob, 13 cm, 4-cm diameter (5 inches, 1 1/2-inch diameter)	1 small cob	140
Cornstarch	30 ml (2 tbsp)	15
Plantains	1/3 small	50
Popcorn, unbuttered, large kernel	750 ml (3 c)	20
Potatoes, whipped	125 ml (1/2 c)	105
Potatoes, whole, 13 cm, 5-cm diameter (5 inches, 2-inch diameter)	1/2	95
Yams, sweet potatoes, 13 cm, 5-cm diameter (5 inches, 2-inch diameter)	1/2	75
Prepared Foods (these have the equivalent of 1 tsp fat or 1 fat exchange in them)		
Baking powder biscuits, 5-cm (2-inch) diameter	1	30
Cookies, plain (e.g., digestive, oatmeal)	2	20
Cupcakes, uniced, 5-cm (2-inch) diameter	1 small	35
Doughnuts, cake type, plain, 7-cm (2 3/4-inch) diameter	1	30
Muffins, plain, 6-cm (2 1/2-inch) diameter	1 small	40
Pancakes, homemade using 50 ml (1/4 c) batter	1 small	50
Potatoes, french fried, 5 × 9 cm (2 × 3 1/2 inches)	10	65
Soup, canned (prepared with equal volume of water)	250 ml (1 c)	260
Waffles, homemade, using 50 ml (1/4 c) batter	1 small	35

E

Table E–11

Milk Group

Type of Milk	Carbohydrate	Protein	Fat	Energy
Nonfat	6 g	4 g	0 g	40 cal
2%	6 g	4 g	2 g	58 cal
Whole	6 g	4 g	4 g	76 cal

Food	Measure	Mass (weight), g
Milk	125 ml (1/2 c)	125
Buttermilk	125 ml (1/2 c)	125
Evaporated milk	50 ml (1/4 c)	50
Powdered milk, regular	30 ml (2 tbsp)	15
instant	50 ml (1/4 c)	15
Unflavoured yogurt	125 ml (1/2 c)	125

Table E–12

Fruits and Vegetables Group
(10 g carbohydrate [simple sugar], 1 g protein, 44 cal)

Food	Measure	Mass (weight), g
Fruits (fresh, frozen without sugar, canned in water)		
Apples, raw	½ medium	75
raw, without skin and core	½ medium	65
sauce	125 ml (½ c)	120
Apricots, raw	2 medium	115
canned, in water	4 halves, plus 30 ml (2 tbsp) liquid	110
Bake-apples (cloudberries), raw	125 ml (½ c)	120
Bananas, 15 cm (6 inches), with peel	½ small	75
peeled'	½ small	50
Blackberries, raw	125 ml (½ c)	70
canned, in water	125 ml (½ c), plus 30 ml (2 tbsp) liquid	100
Blueberries, raw	125 ml (½ c)	120
Boysenberries, raw	125 ml (½ c)	70
canned, in water	125 ml ½ c), plus 30 ml (2 tbsp) liquid	100
Cantaloupe, wedge with rind, 13-cm (5-inch) diameter	¼	240
cubed or diced	250 ml (1 c)	160
Cherries, raw, with pits	10	75
raw, without pits	10	70
canned, in water, with pits	75 ml (⅓ c) plus 30 ml (2 tbsp) liquid	90
canned, in water, without pits	75 ml (⅓ c), plus 30 ml (2 tbsp) liquid	85
Crabapples, raw	1 small	55
Cranberries, raw	250 ml (1 c)	100
Figs, raw	1 medium	50
canned, in water	3 medium, plus 30 ml (2 tbsp) liquid	100
Foxberries, raw	250 ml (1 c)	100
Fruit, mixed, cut up	125 ml (½ c)	120
Fruit cocktail, canned, in water	125 ml (½ c), plus 30 ml (2 tbsp) liquid)	120
Gooseberries, raw	250 ml (1 c)	150
canned, in water	250 ml (1 c), plus 30 ml (2 tbsp) liquid	230
Grapefruit, raw, with rind	½ small	185
raw, sectioned	125 ml (½ c)	100
canned, in water	125 ml (½ c), plus 30 ml (2 tbsp) liquid	120
Grapes, raw, slip skin	125 ml (½ c)	75
raw, seedless	125 ml (½ c)	75
canned, in water	75 ml (⅓ c), plus 30 ml (2 tbsp) liquid	115
Guavas, raw	½	50
Honeydew melon, raw, with rind	1/10	225
cubed or diced	250 ml (1 c)	170
Huckleberries, raw	125 ml (½ c)	70
Kiwi fruit, raw, with skin	2	155
Kumquats, raw	3	60
Litchi fruit, raw	8	120
Loganberries, raw	125 ml (½ c)	70
Loquats, raw	8	130
Mandarin oranges, raw, with rind	1	135
raw, sectioned	125 ml (½ c)	100
canned, in water	125 ml (½ c), plus 30 ml (2 tbsp) liquid	100
Mangoes, raw, without skin and seed	⅓	65
diced	75 ml (⅓ c)	65
Nectarines	½ medium	75

E

Table E–12

(continued)

Food	Measure	Mass (weight), g
Fruits, continued		
Oranges, raw, with rind	1 small	90
raw, sectioned	125 ml (½ c)	90
Papayas, raw, with skin and seeds	¼ medium	150
raw, without skin and seeds	¼ medium	100
cubed or diced	125 ml (½ c)	100
Peaches, raw, with seed and skin, 6-cm (2½-inch) diameter	1 large	130
raw, sliced, diced	125 ml (½ c)	100
canned, in water, halves or slices	125 ml (½ c), plus 30 ml (2 tbsp) liquid	120
Pears, raw, with skin and core	½	90
raw, without skin and core	½	85
canned, in water, halves	2 halves, plus 30 ml (2 tbsp) liquid	90
Persimmons, raw, native	1	30
raw, Japanese	¼	50
Pineapple, raw	1 slice, 8-cm diameter, 2 cm thick (3⅓-inch diameter, ¾ inch thick)	75
canned, in juice, diced	75 ml (⅓ c), plus 15 ml (1 tbsp) liquid	55
canned, in juice, sliced	1 slice, plus 15 ml (1 tbsp) liquid	55
canned, in water, diced	125 ml (½ c), plus 30 ml (2 tbsp) liquid	100
canned, in water, sliced	2 slices, plus 15 ml (1 tbsp) liquid	100
Plums, raw, prune type	2	60
damson	6	65
Japanese	1	70
canned, in apple juice	2, plus 30 ml (2 tbsp) liquid	70
canned, in water	3, plus 30 ml (2 tbsp) liquid	100
Pomegranates, raw	½	140
Raspberries, raw, black or red	125 ml (½ c)	65
canned, in water	125 ml (½ c), plus 30 ml (2 tbsp) liquid	100
Saskatoons (see *blueberries*)		
Strawberries, raw	250 ml (1 c)	150
canned, in water	250 ml (1 c), plus 30 ml (2 tbsp) liquid	240
Tangelos, raw	1	205
Tangerines, raw	1	115
raw, sectioned	125 ml (½ c)	100
Watermelon, raw, with rind	1 wedge, 125-mm triangle, 22 mm thick (5-inch triangle, 1 inch thick)	310
cubed or diced	250 ml (1 c)	160
Dried Fruit		
Apples	5 pieces	15
Apricots	4 halves	15
Banana flakes	30 ml (2 tbsp)	15
Currants	30 ml (2 tbsp)	15
Dates, without pits	2	15
Peaches	1 half	15
Pears	1 half	15
Prunes, raw, with pits	2	15
raw, without pits	2	10
stewed, no liquid	2	20
stewed, with liquid	2, plus 15 ml (1 tbsp) liquid	35
Raisins	30 ml (2 tbsp)	15

E

Table E–12

(continued)

Food	Measure	Mass (weight), g
Juices (no sugar added, or unsweetened)		
Apple, carrot, papaya, pear, pineapple, pomegranate	75 ml (1/3 c)	80
Apricot, grape, guava, mango, prune	50 ml (1/4 c)	55
Grapefruit, loganberry, orange, raspberry, tangelo, tangerine	125 ml (1/2 c)	130
Tomato, tomato-based mixed vegetable	250 ml (1 c)	255
Vegetables (fresh, frozen, or canned)		
Artichokes, Jerusalem, mature or late season[a]	2 small	50
Beets, diced or sliced	125 ml (1/2 c)	85
Carrots, diced	125 ml (1/2 c)	75
Parsnips, mashed	125 ml (1/2 c)	80
Peas, fresh or frozen	125 ml (1/2 c)	80
canned	75 ml (1/3 c)	55
Pumpkin, mashed	125 ml (1/2 c)	45
Rutabagas, mashed	125 ml (1/2 c)	85
Sauerkraut	250 ml (1 c)	235
Snowpeas	10 pods	100
Squash, yellow or winter, mashed	125 ml (1/2 c)	115
Succotash	75 ml (1/3 c)	55
Tomatoes, canned	250 ml (1 c)	240
Turnips, mashed	125 ml (1/2 c)	115
Vegetables, mixed	125 ml (1/2 c)	90
Water chestnuts	8 medium	50

[a]Jerusalem artichokes contain inulin, which converts to carbohydrate during storage, in or out of the ground. Jerusalem artichokes in early season (autumn) are low in carbohydrate, but in late season (winter/spring) they become a fruits and vegetables choice.

E

Table E–13

Extra Vegetables Group
(½ cup, 3.5 g carbohydrate, 14 cal)

Artichokes, globe or french	Celery	Okra
Artichokes, Jerusalem, early season[a]	Chard	Onions, green or mature
Asparagus	Cucumbers	Parsley
Bamboo shoots	Eggplant	Pepper, green or red
Beans, string, green or yellow	Endive	Radishes
Bean sprouts, mung or soy	Fiddleheads	Rhubarb
Bitter melon (balsam pear)	Greens (beet, collard, dandelion, mustard, turnip, etc.)	Shallots
Bok choy	Kale	Spinach
Broccoli	Kohlrabi	Sprouts (alfalfa, radish, etc.)
Brussels sprouts	Leeks	Tomatoes, raw
Cabbage	Lettuce	Vegetable marrow
Cauliflower	Mushrooms	Watercress
		Zucchini

If eaten in large amounts, the following foods must be counted as 1 fruits and vegetables choice:

Brussels sprouts, cooked, 250 ml (1 c)	155 g
Eggplant, cooked, diced, 250 ml (1 c)	200 g
Kohlrabi, cooked, diced, 250 ml (1 c)	140 g
Leeks, cooked, edible parts of 4 leeks	100 g
Okra, cooked, sliced, 250 ml (1 c)	160 g
Onions, mature, cooked, 250 ml (1 c)	210 g
Rhubarb, cooked, no sugar added, 250 ml (1 c)	244 g
Tomatoes, raw, 2 medium (6-cm or 2½-inch diameter) *or* 1 large (13-cm or 5-inch diameter)	270 g

[a]Jerusalem artichokes contain inulin, which converts to carbohydrate during storage, in or out of the ground. Jerusalem artichokes in early season (autumn) are low in carbohydrate, but in late season (winter/spring) they become a fruits and vegetables choice.

Table E–14

Fats and Oils Group (5 g fat, 45 cal)

Food	Measure	Mass (weight), g
Avocado pears	⅛	30
Bacon, side, crisp	1 slice	5
Butter	5 ml (1 tsp)	5
Cheese spreads	15 ml (1 tbsp)	15
Coconut, fresh	45 ml (3 tbsp)	15
dried	15 ml (1 tbsp)	10
Cream, half and half (cereal) 10%	30 ml (2 tbsp)	30
light (coffee), 20%	15 ml (1 tbsp)	15
whipping, 32 to 37%	15 ml (1 tbsp)	15
sour, 12 to 14%	45 ml (3 tbsp)	35
Cream cheese	15 ml (1 tbsp)	15
Gravy	30 ml (2 tbsp)	30
Lard	5 ml (1 tsp)	5
Margarine	5 ml (1 tsp)	5
Nuts, shelled:		
Almonds	8 nuts	20
Brazil nuts	2 nuts	5
Cashews	5 nuts	10
Filberts, hazelnuts	5 nuts	10
Macadamia nuts	3 nuts	5
Peanuts	10 nuts	10
Pecans	5 halves	5
Pignolias, pine nuts	25 ml (5 tsp)	10
Pistachios, shelled	20 nuts	10
in shell	20 nuts	20
Pumpkin and squash seeds	20 ml (4 tsp)	10
Sesame seeds	15 ml (1 tbsp)	10
Sunflower seeds, shelled	15 ml (1 tbsp)	10
in shell	45 ml (3 tbsp)	15
Walnuts	4 halves	10
Oil, cooking and salad	5 ml	5
Olives, green	10	45
ripe	7	40
Paté, liverwurst, meat spreads	15 ml (1 tbsp)	15
Salad dressings: blue, French, Italian, mayonnaise, thousand island	5 ml (1 tsp)	5
Salt pork, raw or cooked	5 ml	5
Sesame oil	5 ml	5

E

Table E–15

Extras (may be used without measuring)

Beverages
Bouillon or clear broth
Bouillon from cube, powder or liquid
Coffee, clear
Consommé
Herbal teas, unsweetened
Mineral water
Soda water, club soda
Sugar-free soft drinks
Tea, clear
Water

Condiments
Chowchow, unsweetened tomato pickles
Garlic
Gelatin, unsweetened
Ginger root
Horseradish, uncreamed
Lemon juice or lemon wedges
Lime juice or lime wedges
Mustard
Parsley
Pickles, unsweetened dill pickles or sour cucumber pickles
Pimientos
Soy sauce
Vinegar
Worcestershire sauce

Herbs and Spices
Salt, pepper, thyme, marjoram, cinnamon, etc.

Miscellaneous
Artificial sweeteners, such as cyclamate or saccharin
Baking powder, baking soda
Dulse
Flavorings and extracts (e.g., vanilla)
Rennet

Table E–16

Extras
(2.5 g carbohydrate, 15 cal, limited to amount indicated)

Anchovies	2 fillets
Barbecue sauce	15 ml (1 tbsp)
Bran, natural	30 ml (2 tbsp)
Brewer's yeast	5 ml (1 tsp)
Carob powder	5 ml (1 tsp)
Catsup	5 ml (1 tsp)
Chili sauce	5 ml (1 tsp)
Cocoa powder	5 ml (1 tsp)
Cranberry sauce, unsweetened	15 ml (1 tbsp)
Dietetic fruit spreads	5 ml (1 tsp)
Maraschino cherries	1 cherry
Nondairy coffee whitener	5 ml (1 tsp)
Nuts, chopped pieces	5 ml (1 tsp)
Relish	5 ml (1 tsp)
Sugar substitutes, granular	5 ml (1 tsp) (3 to 4 packages)
Whipped topping	15 ml (1 tbsp)
Yogurt, plain	30 ml (2 tbsp)

The Exchange Lists are the basis of a meal planning system designed by a committee of the American Diabetes Association and The American Dietetic Association. While designed primarily for people with diabetes and others who must follow special diets, the Exchange Lists are based on principles of good nutrition that apply to everyone.

Appendix F

Nutrition Resources

People interested in nutrition often want to know where, in their own town or county, they can find reliable nutrition information. One place you are not likely to find it is the local library, where fad diet books sit side by side on the shelf with books of facts. However, wherever you live, there are several sources you can turn to:

- The Department of Health may have a nutrition expert.
- The local extension agent is often an expert.
- The food editor of your local paper may be well informed.
- The dietitian at the local hospital had to fulfill a set of qualifications before he or she became an R.D. (see Controversy 2).
- There may be knowledgeable professors of nutrition or biochemistry at a nearby college or university.

The syndicated column on nutrition by J. Mayer and J. Goldberg, which appears in many newspapers, presents well-researched, reliable answers to current questions. The column by R. Alfin-Slater and D. B. Jelliffe is also accurate and trustworthy. In addition, you may be interested in building a nutrition library of your own. Books you can buy, journals you can subscribe to, and addresses you can write to for general information are given below.

Books

A 54-page list of references with critiques of each, *Nutrition References and Book Reviews,* is available for purchase from the Chicago Nutrition Association. (See "Addresses," below.)

The following 900-page paperback has a chapter on each of 58 topics, including energy, obesity, 32 nutrients, several diseases, malnutrition, growth and its assessment, immunity, alcohol, fiber, dental health, drugs, and toxins. The only major omissions seem to be nutrition and food intake and national nutrition status surveys. Watch for an update; these come out every several years:

- *Nutrition Reviews' Present Knowledge in Nutrition,* 5th ed. Washington, D.C.: Nutrition Foundation, 1984.

Another book that readers may wish to add to their libraries is the latest edition of *Recommended Dietary Allowances,* available from the National Academy of Sciences (see "Addresses," below). The Canadian equivalent is *Recommended Nutrient Intakes for Canadians,* available by mail from the Canadian Government Publishing Centre, Supply and Services Canada, Ottawa, Ontario K1A OS9 Canada.

We also recommend our own book, which explores current nutrition topics other than those treated here.

- Whitney, E. N., Hamilton, E. M. N., and Boyle, M. A. *Understanding Nutrition,* 4th ed. St. Paul, Minn.: West, 1987.

Two excellent cookbooks for families wishing to prepare truly healthful meals are:

- White, A., and the Society for Nutrition Education. *The Family Health Cookbook.* New York: McKay, 1980.
- *The American Heart Association Cookbook,* 4th ed. New York: David McKay, 1984.

F

Journals

Nutrition Today, the publication of the Nutrition Today Society, is an excellent magazine for the interested layperson. It makes a point of raising controversial issues and providing a forum for conflicting opinions. References are seldom printed in the magazine but are available on request. Six issues per year, from Director of Membership Services, Nutrition Today Society. (See "Addresses," below.)

The *Journal of the American Dietetic Association,* the official publication of the ADA, contains articles of interest to dietitians and nutritionists, news of legislative action on food and nutrition, and a very useful section of abstracts of articles from many other journals of nutrition and related areas. Twelve issues per year, from the American Dietetic Association. (See "Addresses," below.)

Nutrition Reviews, a publication of the Nutrition Foundation, Inc., does much of the work for the library researcher, compiling recent evidence on current topics and presenting extensive bibliographies. Twelve issues per year, from the Nutrition Foundation. (See "Addresses," below.)

Nutrition and the MD is a monthly newsletter that provides up-to-date, easy to read, and practical information on nutrition for health care providers. It is available from PM, Inc. (See "Addresses," below.)

Other journals that deserve mention here are the *Journal of Nutrition, Food Technology,* the *American Journal of Clinical Nutrition,* and the *Journal of Nutrition Education. FDA Consumer,* a government publication with many articles of interest to the consumer, is available from the Food and Drug Administration (see "Addresses," below). Many other journals of value are referred to throughout this book.

Some of this book's Controversies, as well as other articles of interest to consumers, are available as individual booklets called *Nutrition Clinics.* You can write for a free publication list from the George F. Stickley Company (address below). Many of the other organizations listed below will also provide publication lists free on request.

Addresses

U.S. government The U.S. Department of Agriculture (USDA) has several divisions. The USDA's Food Safety and Inspection Service (FSIS) inspects and analyzes domestic and imported meat, poultry, and meat and poultry food products; establishes standards and approves recipes and labels of processed meat and poultry products; and monitors the meat and poultry industries for violations of inspection laws. To obtain publications or ask questions, write or call:

- FSIS Consumer Inquiries
  USDA
  Washington, DC 20250
  (202) 472-4485

The USDA's Agricultural Research Service (ARS) conducts research to fulfill the diverse needs of agricultural users— from farmers to consumers—in the areas of crop and animal production, protection, processing, and distribution; food safety and quality; and natural resources conservation. Write to the Information Division, ARS, USDA (same address).

The USDA's Human Nutrition Information Service (HNIS) maintains the USDA's Nutrient Data Bank, conducts the Nationwide Food Consumption Survey, monitors nutrient content of the U.S. food supply, provides nutrition guidelines for education and action programs, collects and disseminates food and nutrition materials, and conducts nutrition education research. Write to:

- HNIS, USDA
  Federal Center Building
  Hyattsville, MD 20782

The USDA's Food and Nutrition Service (FNS) administers the food stamp program; the national school lunch and school breakfast programs; the special supplemental food program for women, infants, and children (WIC); and the food distribution, child care food, summer food service, and special milk programs. Write to:

- FNS, USDA
  500 12th Street SW
  Washington, DC 20250

The USDA's Agricultural Marketing Service (AMS) operates a variety of marketing programs and services—several of interest to consumers—that include developing grades and standards for the trading of food and other farm products and carrying out grading services on request from packers and processors; inspecting egg products for wholesomeness; administering marketing orders that aid in the marketing of milk, fruits, vegetables, and related specialty crops like nuts; and administering truth-in-seed labeling; and other regulatory programs. Write to:

- Information Division, AMS, USDA
  Washington, DC 20250

The USDA's *Food News for Consumers,* a quarterly newsletter, is available from the Government Printing Office. Other government addresses are:

- Food and Drug Administration (FDA)
  5600 Fishers Lane
  Rockville, MD 20852
- The Food and Nutrition Information Education Resources Center (FNIERC)
  National Agriculture Library
  10301 Baltimore Boulevard, Room 304
  Beltsville, MD 20705
  (301) 344-3719
- National Academy of Sciences/National Research Council (NAS/NRC)
  2101 Constitution Avenue NW
  Washington, DC 20418
- National Center for Health Statistics (NCHS)
  U.S. Department of Health and Human Services (USDHHS)
  Public Health Service
  3700 East-West Highway
  Hyattsville, MD 20782
- U.S. Government Printing Office
  The Superintendent of Documents
  Washington, DC 20402

Canadian government

- Department of Community Health
  1075 Ste-Foy Road, 7th Floor
  Quebec, Quebec G1S 2M1 Canada
- Home Economics Directorate
  880 Portage Avenue, 2nd Floor
  Winnipeg, Manitoba R3G OP1 Canada

- Nutrition Programs
  446 Jeanne Mance Building
  Tunney's Pasture
  Ottawa, Ontario K1A 1B4 Canada
- Nutrition Services
  Box 488
  Halifax, Nova Scotia B3J 3R8 Canada
- Nutrition Services
  P.O. Box 6000
  Fredericton, New Brunswick E3B 5H1 Canada
- Public Health Resource Service
  15 Overlea Boulevard, 5th Floor
  Toronto, Ontario M4H 1A9 Canada

Consumer and advocacy groups

- Action for Children's Television (ACT)
  46 Austin Street
  Newtonville, MA 02160
- Center for Science in the Public Interest (CSPI)
  1755 S Street NW
  Washington, DC 20009
- Children's Foundation
  1420 New York Avenue NW, Suite 800
  Washington, DC 20005
- Community Nutrition Institute
  1146 19th Street NW
  Washington, DC 20036
- The Consumer Information Center
  Department 609K
  Pueblo, Colorado 81009
- Food Research and Action Center (FRAC)
  2011 I Street NW
  Washington, DC 20006
- National Council against Health Fraud, Inc.
  PO Box 1276
  Loma Linda, CA 92354
- National Self-Help Clearinghouse
  33 West 42nd Street, Room 1227
  New York, NY 10036

Professional and service organizations

- Al-Anon Family Group Headquarters
  P.O. Box 182
  Madison Square Station
  New York, NY 10010
- Alcoholics Anonymous World Services
  P.O. Box 459
  Grand Central Station
  New York, NY 10017
- American Academy of Pediatrics
  PO Box 1034
  Evanston, IL 60204
- American College of Nutrition
  100 Manhattan Avenue, #1606
  Union City, NJ 07087
- American Dental Association
  211 East Chicago Avenue
  Chicago, IL 60611
- American Diabetes Association
  2 Park Avenue
  New York, NY 10016
- American Dietetic Association
  430 North Michigan Avenue
  Chicago, IL 60611
- American Heart Association
  7320 Greenville Avenue
  Dallas, TX 75231
- American Home Economics Association
  2010 Massachusetts Avenue NW
  Washington, DC 20036
- American Institute for Cancer Research
  803 West Broad Street
  Falls Church, VA 22046
- American Institute of Nutrition
  9650 Rockville Pike
  Bethesda, MD 20014
- American Medical Association
  Nutrition Information Section
  535 North Dearborn Street
  Chicago, IL 60610
- The American National Red Cross
  Food and Nutrition Consultant
  National Headquarters
  Washington, DC 20006
- American Public Health Association
  1015 Fifteenth Street NW
  Washington, DC 20005
- Amerian Society for Clinical Nutrition
  9650 Rockville Pike
  Bethesda, MD 20014
- The Canadian Diabetes Association
  123 Edward Street, Suite 601
  Toronto, Ontario M5G 1E2 Canada
- The Canadian Dietetic Association
  385 Yonge Street
  Toronto, Ontario M4T 1Z5 Canada
- The Chicago Nutrition Association
  8158 Kedzie Avenue
  Chicago, IL 60652
- George F. Stickley Company
  210 West Washington Square
  Philadelphia, PA 19106
- Institute of Food Technologists
  221 North La Salle Street
  Chicago, IL 60601

- La Leche League International, Inc.
  9616 Minneapolis Avenue
  Franklin Park, IL 60131
- March of Dimes Birth Defects Foundation (National Headquarters)
  1275 Mamaroneck Avenue
  White Plains, NY 10605
- National Clearinghouse for Alcohol Information
  Box 2345
  Rockville, MD 20850
- National Council on Alcoholism
  733 Third Avenue
  New York, NY 10017
- National Nutrition Consortium
  1635 P Street NW, Suite 1
  Washington, DC 20036
- Nutrition Foundation, Inc.
  1126 Sixteenth St. NW, Suite 111
  Washington, DC 20036
- Nutrition Today Society
  428 East Preston Street
  Baltimore, MD 21202
- Overeaters Anonymous (OA)
  2190 190th Street
  Torrance, CA 90504
  (213) 320-7941
- PM, Inc. (Publisher of *Nutrition and the MD)*
  14545 Friar, #106
  Van Nuys, CA 91411
- Society for Nutrition Education
  1736 Franklin Street
  Oakland, CA 94612
- Technical Information Center
  Office on Smoking and Health
  5600 Fishers Lane, Room 1–16
  Rockville, MD 20857

Trade organizations Trade organizations produce many excellent free materials on nutrition. Naturally, they also promote their own products. The student must learn to differentiate between slanted and valid information. We find the brief reviews in *Contemporary Nutrition* (General Mills), the *Dairy Council Digest,* Ross Laboratories' *Dietetic Currents,* and R. A. Seelig's reviews from the United Fresh Fruit and Vegetable Association to be generally useful and reliable.

- ABC Corporation
  1330 Avenue of the Americas
  New York, NY 10019
- American Egg Board
  1460 Renaissance Street
  Park Ridge, IL 60068
- American Meat Institute
  P.O. Box 3556
  Washington, DC 20007
- Best Foods
  Consumer Service Department
  Division of CPC International
  Internation Plaza
  Englewood Cliffs, NJ 07623
- Bordon Farm Products
  Borden Company, Consumer Affairs
  180 East Broad Street
  Columbus, OH 43215
- Campbell Soup Company
  Food Service Products Division
  375 Memorial Avenue
  Camden, NJ 08101
- Del Monte Teaching Aids
  PO Box 9075
  Clinton, IA 52736
- Fleischmann's Margarines
  Standard Brands, Inc.
  625 Madison Avenue
  New York, NY 10022
- General Foods Consumer Center
  250 North Street
  White Plains, NY 10625
- General Mills
  PO Box 113
  Minneapolis, MN 55440
- Gerber Products Company
  445 State Street
  Fremont, MI 49412
- H. J. Heinz
  Consumer Relations
  PO Box 57
  Pittsburgh, PA 15230
- Hunt-Wesson Foods
  Educational Services
  1645 West Valencia Drive
  Fullerton, CA 92634
- Kellogg Company
  Department of Home Economics Services
  Battle Creek, MI 49016
- McGraw-Hill Films
  Care of Association Films, Inc.
  600 Grand Avenue
  Ridgefield, NJ 07657
- Mead Johnson Nutritionals
  2404 Pennsylvania Avenue
  Evansville, IN 47721
- National Commission on Egg Nutrition
  205 Touvy Avenue
  Park Ridge, IL 60668

- National Dairy Council
  6300 North River Road
  Rosemont, IL 60018-4233
- Nestlé Company
  Home Economics Division
  100 Bloomingdale Road
  White Plains, NY 10605
- Oscar Mayer Company
  Consumer Service
  PO Box 1409
  Madison, WI 53701
- Pillsbury Company
  1177 Pillsbury Building
  608 Second Avenue South
  Minneapolis, MN 55402
- The Potato Board
  1385 South Colorado Boulevard, Suite 512
  Denver, CO 80222
- Rice Council
  PO Box 22802
  Houston, TX 77027
- Ross Laboratories
  Director of Professional Services
  625 Cleveland Avenue
  Columbus, OH 43216
- Sister Kenny Institute
  Chicago Avenue at 27th Street
  Minneapolis, MN 55407
- Soy Protein Council
  1800 M Steet NW
  Washington, DC 20036
- Sunkist Growers
  Consumer Service, Division BB
  Box 7888
  Valley Annex
  Van Nuys, CA 91409
- United Fresh Fruit and Vegetable Association
  727 N. Washington Street
  Alexandria, VA 22314
- Vitamin Information Bureau
  383 Madison Avenue
  New York, NY 10017
- Vitamin Nutrition Information Service (VNIS)
  Hoffmann-LaRoche
  340 Kingsland Avenue
  Nutley, NJ 07110
- Wheat Flour Institute
  600 Maryland Avenue
  Washington, DC 20024

Organizations concerned with world hunger

- Bread for the World
  802 Rhode Island Avenue NE
  Washington, DC 20018
- The Hunger Project
  2015 Steiner Street
  San Francisco, CA 94115
- Institute for Food and Development Policy
  1885 Mission Street
  San Francisco, CA 94103
- Interreligious Taskforce on U.S. Food Policy
  110 Maryland Avenue NE
  Washington, DC 20002
- Meals for Millions/Freedom from Hunger Foundation
  1800 Olympic Boulevard
  PO Drawer 680
  Santa Monica, CA 90406
- Oxfam America
  115 Broadway
  Boston, MA 02116
- Worldwatch Institute
  1776 Massachusetts Avenue NW
  Washington, DC 20036

United Nations

- Food and Agriculture Organization (FAO)
  North American Regional Office
  1325 C Street SW
  Washington, DC 20025
- World Health Organization (WHO)
  1211 Geneva 27
  Switzerland

Appendix G

Supplementary Glossary

For consumers who are interested in knowing the meanings of terms that appear in advertising or on labels, and that are not mentioned elsewhere in this book, this glossary offers a few. Some of these terms appear both in the main text and here. In those cases, the definition given in the text is that used in nutrition, and the definition given here is the meaning of the term when it appears on a label. A few other terms that are not used in this text appear here, just so that people looking for them in the index can find their definitions.

acetic acid: see *antimicrobial agents.*

agar: see *stabilizers (thickeners).*

aloe: a tropical plant of widely acclaimed, but unproven, medicinal value. The gel of the plant is often added to lotions and creams, and sometimes is included in preparations for internal use.

aluminum phosphate: see *anticaking agents.*

anticaking agents: substances added to keep products such as salts and powders free flowing. Examples are magnesium carbonate, calcium silicate, aluminum phosphate, or similar compounds.

antimicrobial agents: compounds added to products to prevent spoilage by bacteria or mold. Familiar among them are acetic acid (vinegar) and sodium chloride (salt). Others are benzoic, propionic, and sorbic acids; nitrites and nitrates; and sulfur dioxide.

antioxidant: a compound that protects others from oxidation by being oxidized itself. Oxidation is a chemical reaction in which oxygen or a similar reactant changes the nature of other chemicals, usually to the detriment of the product or the nutrients it contains. Examples are BHA, BHT, and propyl gallate.

arabic: see *stabilizers (thickeners).*

artificial colors: a type of food additive (see also Chapter 10). Vegetable dyes are extracted from vegetables such as beets and carrots. Food colors are a mix of vegetable dyes and synthetic dyes approved by the FDA for use in food.

aspartame: the generic name for an artificial sweetener (see page 95). Sold under the trade names Nutrasweet and Equal. See also *Nutrasweet* and *Equal.*

benzoic acid: see *antimicrobial agents.*

beta-carotene: an orange pigment found in plants. The food industry uses it to color foods; the body converts it to active vitamin A, so it is both a food additive and a nutrient. See also *artificial colors.*

BHA, BHT: see *antioxidant.*

bicarbonate: see *leavening agents.*

bioflavonoids: substances in foods that supply no nutritional need. Some are called "vitamin P" (erroneously) by faddists.

bleaching agents: substances used to whiten foods, such as flour and cheese, and to speed up the maturing of cheese. Peroxides are examples.

caffeine: a central nervous system stimulant that, when used as a food additive, lends a bitter flavor note. See also *flavoring agents.*

calcium carbonate: a calcium compound in frozen and canned goods that, along with many other such compounds, acts as a firming agent. See also *firming agents.*

calcium silicate: see *anticaking agents.*

carotene: see *beta-carotene.*

carrageenan: see *stabilizers (thickeners).*

cell salts: a mineral preparation sold in health-food stores supposed to have been prepared from living, healthy cells. It is not necessary to take such preparations, and it may be dangerous.

chelating agents: acids added to foods to prevent discoloration, flavor changes, and rancidity that might occur because of processing. Examples are citric acid, malic acid, and tartaric acid (cream of tartar). See also p. 387.

cholecalciferol (COAL-ee-cal-SIFF-er-ol)**:** the chemical name for vitamin D.

citric acid: see *chelating agents.*

cobalamin (co-BAL-uh-min)**:** an alternative name for vitamin B_{12} (*cobal* means "cobalt containing"; *amine* means "vitamin").

coloring agents: see *artificial colors.*

cream of tartar: see *chelating agents.*

dextrins: short chains of glucose formed by breaking down starch. The word sometimes appears on food labels, because dextrins can be used as thickening agents in foods.

diglycerides: see *emulsifiers.*

empty-calorie food: a popular term used to denote a food that contains no nutrients, only calories. Actually, almost all foods contain some nutrients. Therefore, most nutritionists prefer to say "food of low nutrient density."

G

emulsifiers: chemicals that attract both fats and water, and act to help the two to mix (see also Chapter 4). Examples of emulsifiers used in foods are lecithin, monoglycerides and diglycerides, and propylene glycol esters.
Equal: a household artificial sweetener, made from aspartame mixed in a lactose base. See also *aspartame*.
firming agents: substances added to processed fruits and vegetables to preserve a firm texture through the cooking or freezing treatments.
flavoring agents: Substances used to add or enhance flavor (see artificial flavors and flavor enhancers in Chapter 10).
gelatin: a soluble form of the protein collagen, used to thicken foods.
gliadin (GLIGH-uh-den)**:** a fraction of the gluten protein.
gluten (GLOOT-en)**:** a protein found in wheat, oats, rye, and barley.
guar: see *stabilizers (thickeners)*.
gums: see *stabilizers (thickeners)*.
humectants: substances used to retain moisture in foods, and to improve their texture.
hydrolyzed protein: an intact protein treated with acids or enzymes to yield a combination of free amino acids and short peptide chains.
leavening agents: substances added to create bubbles of carbon dioxide in grain products to make them light in texture. Examples are yeast, bicarbonates, and phosphates.
lecithin: a fatty compound made by the body (see Chapter 4); it is often added as an emulsifier in processed foods. See also *emulsifiers*.
locust bean gum: see *stabilizers (thickeners)*.
magnesium carbonate: see *anticaking agents*.
malic acid: see *chelating agents*.
meat replacements: textured vegetable protein products formulated to look and taste like meat, fish, or poultry. Many of these are designed to match the known nutrient contents of animal-protein foods, but sometimes they fall short. See also *textured vegetable protein*.
meat tenderizer: a preparation of enzymes (proteases) that can be applied to meat before cooking to break down its tough connective tissues, making them tender. The chief enzyme in a meat tenderizer is papain (PAP-ane).
monoglycerides: see *emulsifiers*.
Nutrasweet: the trade name given to a concentrated form of aspartame used by food manufacturing firms to sweeten their products. **Nutrasweet blend** is a combination sweetener that includes Nutrasweet and saccharin. See also *aspartame*.
papain: see *meat tenderizer*. Also called papaya enzyme.
para-aminobenzoic acid (PABA): a substance found in foods, probably not an essential nutrient for human beings.
peroxide: see *bleaching agents*.
phosphates: see *leavening agents*.
propionic acid: see *antimicrobial agents*.
propyl gallate: see *antioxidant*.
propylene glycol esters: see *emulsifiers*.
protein isolate: a protein with high biological value has been chemically separated from a source containing a variety of proteins; different from amino acids in that the protein is extracted whole.
rose hips: fruits of rose plants, high in vitamin C, used in herbal teas and other mixtures, and as a vitamin C source for the manufacture of supplements.
rutin: one of the bioflavonoids, not an essential nutrient in human nutrition. See also *bioflavonoids*.
sorbic acid: see *antimicrobial agents*.
stabilizers (thickeners): substances used to maintain foam, emulsions, or suspensions in products, or to thicken them. Examples are gums such as carrageenan, guar, locust bean, tragacanth, xanthan gum, gum arabic, agar (a seaweed extract), starch, and pectin.
sulfur dioxide: see *antimicrobial agents*.
tartaric acid: see *chelating agents*.
tartrazine: a food coloring agent, also known as yellow dye no. 5; its presence must be declared on labels, because some people are allergic to it.
textured vegetable protein (TVP): soybean protein processed for use in imitation meat products.
thickeners: see *stabilizers (thickeners)*.
tragacanth: see *stabilizers (thickeners)*.
TVP: see *textured vegetable protein*.
water-miscible (MISS-ih-bul)**:** a term used to describe fat-soluble compounds, such as some vitamins, that readily mix with water and can be absorbed without fat.
xanthan gum: see *stabilizers (thickeners)*.

Appendix H

Self-Study Forms

Form 1

Nutrient Intakes (use one form for each day)

Food Description	Approximate Measure or Weight	Ener[a] (cal)	Prot[b] (g)	Carb[b] (g)	Fiber[b] (g)	Fat[b] (g)	Fat Breakdown (g)[b]		
							Sat	*Mono*	*Poly*
Total									

[a]Compute these values to the nearest whole number.
[b]Compute these values to one decimal place.
[c]Compute these values to two decimal places.

Chol[a] (mg)	Calc[a] (mg)	Iron[c] (mg)	Magn[a] (mg)	Phos[a] (mg)	Pota[a] (mg)	Sodi[a] (mg)	Zinc[b] (mg)	Vit-A[a] (RE)	Thia[c] (mg)	Ribo[c] (mg)	Niac[b] (mg)	V-B6[b] (mg)	Fola[a] (mcg)	VitC[b] (mg)

H

Form 2

Average Daily Energy and Nutrient Intakes

Day	Date	Ener (cal)	Prot (g)	Carb (g)	Fiber (g)	Fat (g)	Fat Breakdown (g)		
							Sat	*Mono*	*Poly*
1									
2									
3									
4									
5									
6									
7[a]									
Total									
Average daily intake (divide total by 7[b])									

[a]Use fewer lines if you recorded fewer days.
[b]Divide by 3 if you recorded 3 days' intakes, etc.

Form 3

Comparison with a Standard Intake

	Ener (cal)	Prot (g)	Carb (g)	Fiber (g)	Fat (g)	Fat Breakdown (g)		
						Sat	*Mono*	*Poly*
Average daily intake (from Form 2)								
Standard[a]			X	25	X	X	X	X
Intake as percentage of standard[b]								

[a]Taken from RDA tables (inside front cover) or Recommended Nutrient Intakes for Canadians (Appendix B).
[b]For example, if your intake of protein was 50 g and the standard for a person of your age and sex was 46 g, then you consumed $(50 \div 46) \times 100$, or 109 percent of the standard.

Chol (mg)	Calc (mg)	Iron (mg)	Magn (mg)	Phos (mg)	Pota (mg)	Sodi (mg)	Zinc (mg)	Vit-A (RE)	Thia (mg)	Ribo (mg)	Niac (mg)	V-B6 (mg)	Fola (mcg)	Vit-C (mg)

Chol (mg)	Calc (mg)	Iron (mg)	Magn (mg)	Phos (mg)	Pota (mg)	Sodi (mg)	Zinc (mg)	Vit-A (RE)	Thia (mg)	Ribo (mg)	Niac (mg)	V-B6 (mg)	Fola (mcg)	Vit-C (mg)
<300														

Form 4

Percentage of Calories from Protein, Fat, and Carbohydrate

My intakes from Form 3:

Protein:	___ g/day × 4 cal/g = (P) ______	cal/day
Fat:	___ g/day × 9 cal/g = (F) ______	cal/day
Carbohydrate:	___ g/day × 4 cal/g = (C) ______	cal/day
	Total cal/day = (T) ______	cal/day[a]

Percentage of calories from protein:

$\frac{(P)}{(T)} \times 100 =$ ___ % of total calories

Percentage of calories from fat:

$\frac{(F)}{(T)} \times 100 =$ ___ % of total calories

Percentage of calories from carbohydrate:

$\frac{(C)}{(T)} \times 100 =$ ___ % of total calories[b]

[a] This total will not agree perfectly with the total calories recorded on Form 1, but should agree within 20%.

[b] The three percentages can total 99, 100, or 101, depending on the way in which figures were rounded off earlier. For recommended balance, see Self-Study 2.

H

Form 5

Food Selection Scorecard

Food Group and Recommended Intake	Your Intake from Group (specify food and amount)	Your Score
Fruits and vegetables—4 or more portions (½ cooked edible portion or 3 to 4 oz, 100 g, raw); at least 1 raw daily		
1 portion vitamin A–rich dark green or deep orange fruit or vegetable (any food with more than your RDA) = 10 points (no more than 10 points allowed)		
1 portion vitamin C–rich fruit or vegetable (any food with more than your RDA) = 10 points (no more than 10 points allowed)		
Other fruits and vegetables, including potatoes = 2.5 each		
Subtotal (no more than 25 points allowed)		
Breads and cereals—4 or more portions of whole-grain or enriched (1 oz dry-weight cereal or 1-oz slice bread or equivalent grain product)		
1 portion cereal or 2 bread equivalents = 10 points (no more than 10 points allowed)		
Other bread equivalents = 5 points each		
Subtotal (no more than 25 points allowed)		
Milk and milk products—2 or more portions (8 oz fluid milk; calcium equivalents are 1 ½ oz hard cheese. 2 c cottage cheese, 1 pint ice milk or ice cream)		
One portion = 12.5 points		
Subtotal (no more than 25 points allowed)		

H

Form 5

(continued)

Food Group and Recommended Intake	Your Intake from Group (specify food and amount)	Your Score
Meat and meat alternates—2 or more portions of meat (2 to 3 oz of cooked meat, fish, or poultry, 2 eggs, (¾ c cooked legumes, 4 tbsp peanut butter, 2 to 3 oz nuts).		
2 portions meat = 25 points		
Subtotal (no more than 25 points allowed)		
Grand total (no more than 100 points)		

The above are foundation foods. Additional foods are those that do not fit into the above groupings but add flavor, interest, variety, and (often) calories. List those eaten:

Form 6

Diet Planning by Exchange Groups

Exchange List	Number of Exchanges[b]	Amounts to Be Delivered[a]			
		Carbohydrate ____ *g*	*Protein* ____ *g*	*Fat* ____ *g*	*Energy*[c] ____ *cal*
Starch/bread					
Meat					
Vegetable					
Fruit					
Milk					
Fat					
	Total actually delivered				

[a]From step 2, p. 308 or 309.
[b]From steps 4, 5, 6.
[c]From step 7.

H

Form 7

Meal Patterns

Exchange List	Total Exchanges to Be Consumed Daily[a]	Exchanges Consumed at Each Meal				
		Breakfast	*Lunch*	*Snack*	*Dinner*	*Snack*
Starch/bread						
Meat						
Vegetable						
Fruit						
Milk						
Fat						

[a]From Form 6, column 2.

H

H

Form 8

Nutrient Density of Foods

Food Item	Size of Serving I Would Eat	A Amount of Nutrient #1 (________) That One Serving Would Supply (% of my RDA)	B Amount of Nutrient #2 (________) That One Serving Would Supply (% of my RDA)	C Amount of Nutrient #3 (________) That One Serving Would Supply (% of my RDA)	D Amount of Food Energy That One Serving Would Supply (% of my RDA)	E A/D	F B/D	G C/D	Nutrient Score E + F + G

Appendix I

Summary of Digestion and Absorption

Chapter 1 described the remarkable human body and briefly introduced the digestive system. Chapters 3, 4, and 5 showed how the digestion and absorption of carbohydrates, lipids, and protein proceed. This appendix puts the whole picture together.

The cells lining the intestinal tract secrete powerful juices and **enzymes** to disintegrate nutrients (especially carbohydrate and protein) into their component parts. Two organs outside the digestive tract—the liver with its associated gallbladder, and the pancreas—also contribute digestive juices through a common duct into the small intestine. The presence of these digestive juices and enzymes requires that still other cells specialize in protecting the digestive system cells of the **mucous membranes**. They secrete a thick, viscous substance known as **mucus,** which coats the intestinal tract lining and ensures that it will not itself be digested (see Figure I–1).

The cells of the intestinal lining can recognize the nutrients needed by the body and absorb enough of them to nourish all the body's cells. Every nutrient that enters the body fluids must traverse a cell of the intestinal lining. To work efficiently, each cell has a velvety covering of tiny hairs (**microvilli**), which can trap the nutrient particles. The intestinal tract lining is composed of a single sheet of these cells, and the sheet pokes out into millions of finger-shaped projections (**villi**). Each villus is lined with muscle, so it can actively wave about, stirring and making contact with the intestinal contents. Each villus also has its own capillary network and a lymph vessel so that nutrients transferred across its selective cells can immediately mingle into the body fluids.

The process of rendering foods into nutrients and absorbing these into the body fluids is remarkably efficient. In a healthy body, more than 90 percent of the carbohydrate, fat, and protein that pass through the intestinal tract are digested to glucose, glycerol and fatty acids, and amino acids in time to be absorbed. The small intestine with its villi, if spread out completely flat, would occupy a third of a football field in area. Its cells, weighing perhaps 4 to 5 pounds, absorb enough nutrients in a few hours a day to nourish the other 150 or so pounds of cells in the body.

The process of digestion is diagramed in full in Figure I–2. The first part, the mouth, is designed for physically breaking down foods. The teeth cut off a bite-size portion and then, aided by the tongue, grind it finely enough to be mixed with saliva and swallowed. The esophagus carries the mixture to the stomach. The stomach is supplied with several sets of muscles to mix and grind it further and

Figure I–1 The Digestive Tract Lining.

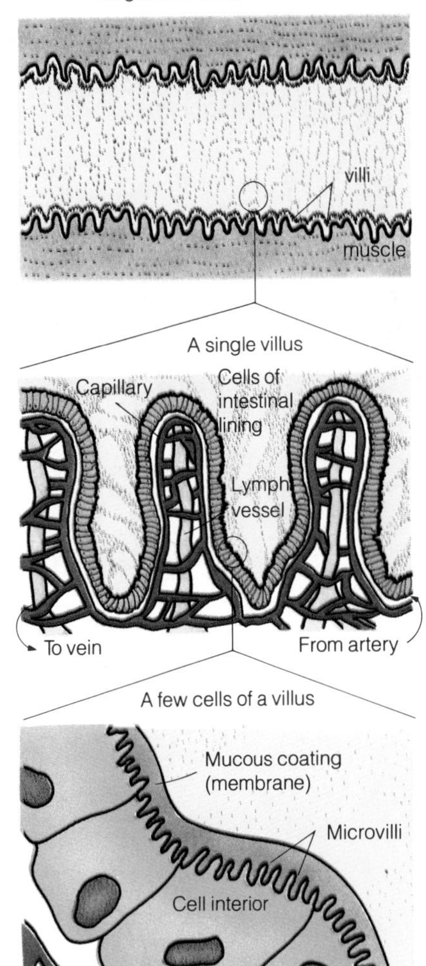

I

Figure I–2 The Digestive System.

Fiber	Starch
The mechanical action of the mouth crushes and tears fiber in food and mixes it with saliva to moisten it for swallowing.	The salivary glands secrete a watery fluid into the mouth to moisten the food. An enzyme begins digestion by splitting starch into smaller polysaccharides and maltose. This digestion continues after the food is swallowed until stomach acid and enzymes start to digest the salivary enzymes.
Most fiber passes intact through the digestive tract to the large intestine. Here, some types of fiber are digested to glucose by bacterial enzymes, and the free glucose molecules are absorbed into the body. Fiber in the large intestine holds water and regulates bowel activity. Some fiber binds cholesterol and certain minerals and carries them out in the feces.	The pancreas produces carbohydrate-digesting enzymes and releases them through the common bile duct into the small intestine. These enzymes split polysaccharides into disaccharides. Then enzymes on the surface of the small intestinal cells break these into simple sugars (monosaccharides). The cells absorb the monosaccharides as they are freed.

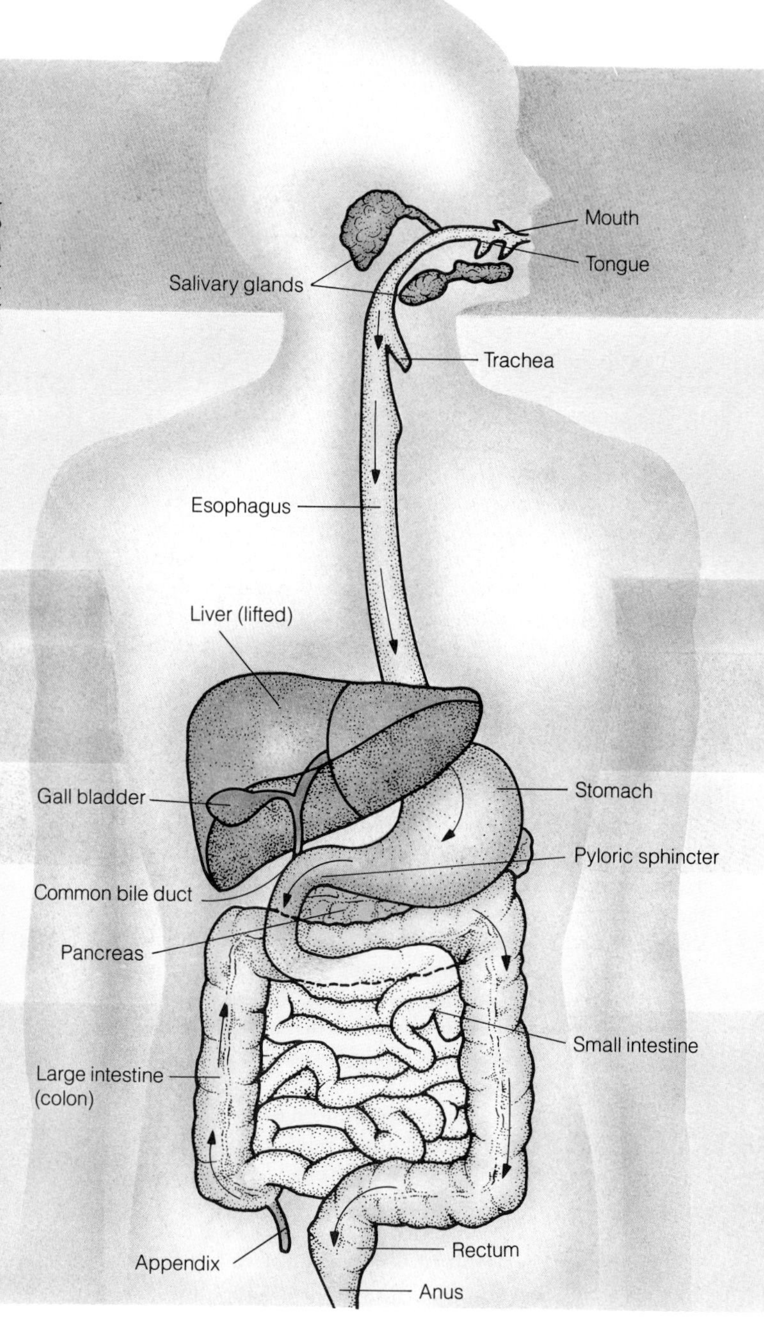

I

Protein

In the mouth, chewing crushes and softens protein-rich foods and mixes them with saliva to be swallowed.

Stomach acid works to uncoil protein strands and activate stomach enzymes. Then the enzymes break the strands into smaller fragments.

In the small intestine, the fragments of protein are split into free amino acids, dipeptides, and tripeptides with the help of enzymes from the pancreas and small intestine. Enzymes on the surface of the small intestinal cells break these peptides into amino acids, and they are absorbed through the cells into the blood. The large intestine carries any undigested protein residue out of the body. Normally, practically all the protein is digested and absorbed.

Fat

Fat floats up from the other foods in the watery stomach acid. The stomach digests a small percentage of fat. The liver secretes bile; the gallbladder stores it and releases it through the common bile duct into the small intestine when fat arrives there. The bile emulsifies the fat, making it ready for enzyme action.

The pancreas produces fat-digesting enzymes and releases them through the common bile duct into the small intestine. These enzymes split triglycerides into monoglycerides, free fatty acids, and glycerol, which are absorbed. Some fatty materials escape absorption and are carried out of the body via the large intestine.

Vitamins

Water-soluble vitamins need little action by the digestive organs except absorption in the small intestine. However, vitamin B_{12} requires "intrinsic factor" produced by the stomach in order to be absorbed.

Bile from the liver, stored in the gallbladder, is released through the common bile duct into the small intestine when fat is present there. The bile emulsifies fat-soluble vitamins and aids in their absorption with other fats. The bacteria in the large intestine releases vitamin K, which is absorbed there.

Minerals and Water

All digestive reactions take place in water secreted into the digestive tract by various organs. The salivary glands of the mouth are the first to contribute water.

The stomach secrets enough watery fluid to turn a moist, chewed mass of swallowed food into a liquid.

Stomach acid acts on iron to make it more absorbable. Vitamin C and a factor in meat also increases iron absorption. Binders in vegetables and grains "tie up" zinc and calcium, making them unavailable for absorption. If a person's body has plenty of a certain mineral like iron, zinc, or calcium, then the small intestine absorbs a smaller percentage of that mineral from food than it would if the person was deficient.

The small intestine, along with the pancreas and liver, secretes its own fluids for a total of about 2 gallons of water secreted into the digestive tract per day. This water is not lost, but is conserved by reabsorption in the large intestine.

Absorption of calcium depends on adequate vitamin D status. Other minerals, like sodium and potassium, are absorbed in the small and large intestines whether or not the person has sufficient amounts of the minerals in the body.

Table I–1

Digestive Tract Secretions

Digestive Tract Secretions
Salivary glands:
Saliva
Salivary amylase (enzyme that breaks down starch)
Stomach (gastric) glands:
Gastric juice
Hydrochloric acid (uncoils protein)
Gastric proteases (enzymes that break down protein)
Mucus (thick coating that protects the stomach wall from these secretions)
Intestinal cells:
Intestinal amylase and proteases (enzymes that break down carbohydrate and protein)
Mucus (thin coating that protects the intestinal wall)
Liver and gallbladder:
Bile (emulsifier that separates fat into small particles that enzymes can attack)
Pancreas:
Bicarbonate (neutralizes acid fluid from stomach so intestinal and pancreatic enzymes can work on its contents)
Pancreatic amylase, lipases, and proteases (enzymes that break down carbohydrate, fat, and protein)

secretes acid and enzymes that will begin to break it apart chemically. Table I–1 summarizes the secretions of the digestive organs.

During the preparatory stage, as the complex carbohydrate known as starch is released from a food (such as bread), an enzyme present in the saliva starts to break it down chemically to smaller units. But this action is stopped when the carbohydrate units reach the stomach, because glands in the stomach wall exude hydrochloric acid. The salivary enzyme that breaks up starch is digested in the stomach, together with other proteins. Further dismantling of carbohydrate occurs after it leaves the stomach.

Fats and oils, taken as part of such complex foods as meats or nuts or in relatively pure form as butter or oil, are not much affected until after leaving the stomach.

Proteins are eaten as part of such foods as meat, milk, and soybeans. Although no chemical action on them takes place in the mouth, chewing and mixing protein with saliva is an important part of preparing it for the chemical action that begins in the stomach. There, enzymes and hydrochloric acid break apart the large, complex protein molecules into smaller pieces known as peptides and finally into dipeptides, tripeptides, and amino acids.

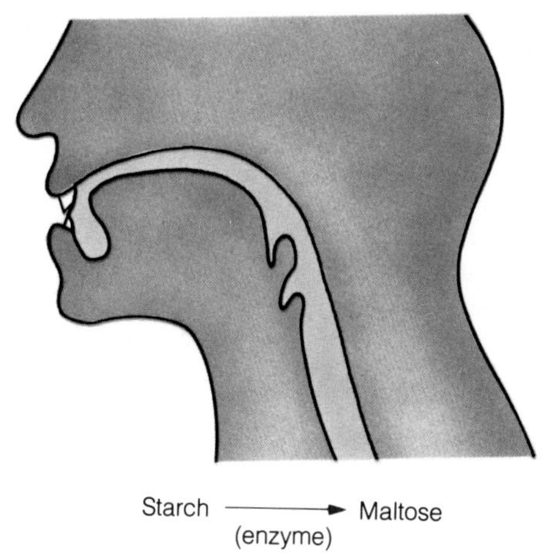

Digestion in the mouth.

Some of the early stages of digestion, such as chewing and swallowing, are under conscious control. Actions in the esophagus and in the stomach require no thought, although they do make us aware that things are happening there. After swallowing, the digestive apparatus works in a manner too complicated for the conscious brain (cortex) to be bothered with; at this juncture, you must relinquish all awareness and put your trust in the ability of each cell to perform its own specialized job.

The complicated chemical dismantling that takes place beyond the stomach requires that only small amounts be processed at one time. To accomplish this, the **pylorus**, a circular muscle surrounding the lower end of the stomach, controls the exit of the contents, allowing only a little at a time to be squirted forcefully into the small intestine.

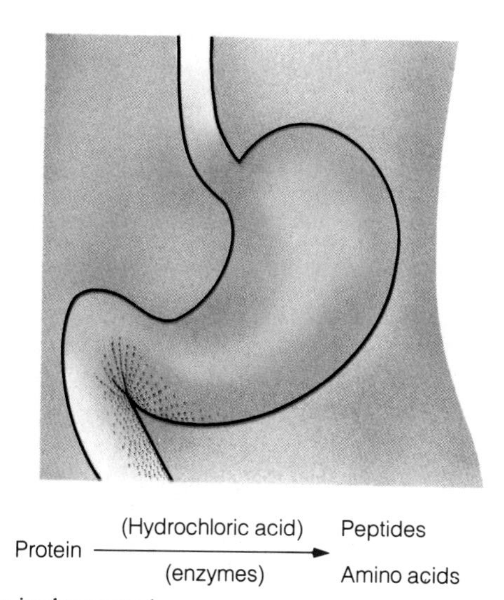

Digestion in the stomach.

Gradually the stomach empties itself by means of these powerful squirts.

The small intestine is "the" organ of digestion and absorption; it finishes the job the mouth and stomach have started. It is actually about 20 feet long, but it is called small because its diameter is small compared with that of the large intestine (colon). Its contents must touch its walls in order to make contact with the secretions and in order to be absorbed at the proper places. At the end of the small intestine, a circular muscle (similar in function to the pylorus at the end of the stomach) controls the flow of the contents going into the colon.

The small intestine works with the precision of a laboratory chemist. As the thoroughly liquefied and partially digested nutrient mixture arrives there, hormonal messages tell the gallbladder to send its emulsifier, bile, in amounts matched to the amount of fat present. Other hormones notify the pancreas to release **bicarbonate** in amounts precisely adjusted to neutralize the stomach acid, as well as to release enzymes of the appropriate kinds and quantities to continue dismantling whatever large molecules remain. Such messages also keep the strong muscles imbedded in the walls of the intestine contracting, in a squeezing activity called **peristalsis**, so that the contents will be pressed along to the next region. Peristalsis is stimulated by the presence of roughage or fiber and is quieted by the presence of fat, which requires a longer time for digestion.

Meanwhile, as the pancreatic and intestinal enzymes act on the bonds that hold the large nutrients together, smaller and smaller units make their appearance in the intestinal

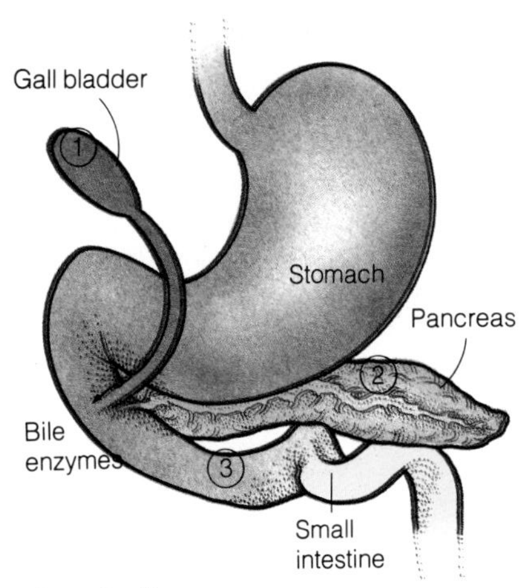

Small intestine—details.

1. The gallbladder sends bile into the small intestine by way of a duct.
2. The pancreas sends enzymes (and bicarbonate).
3. The small intestine also secretes enzymes.

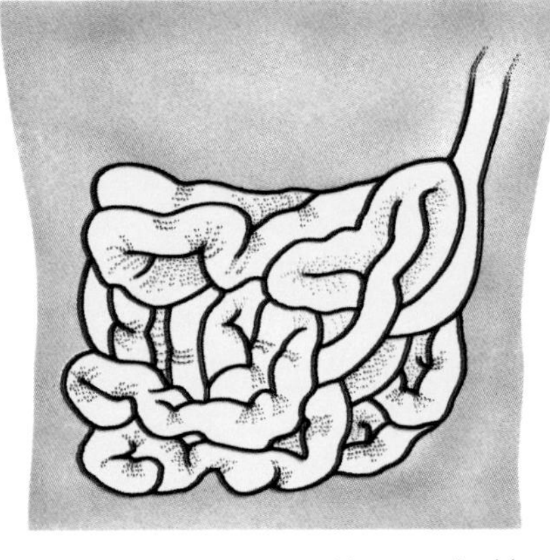

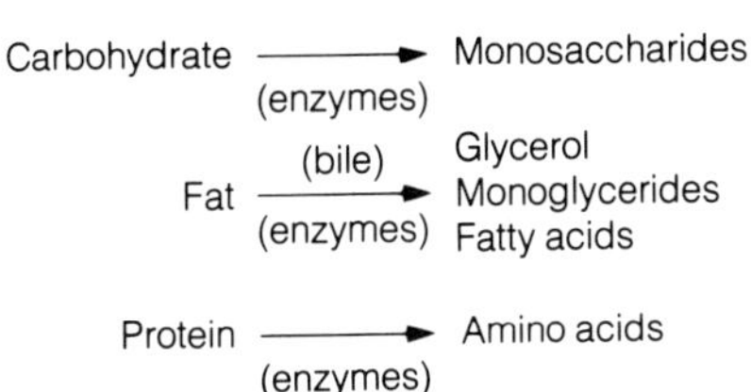

Digestion in the small intestine.

Miniglossary

bicarbonate: a commonly occurring chemical that neutralizes acid; a secretion of the pancreas.

enzymes: large protein molecules that facilitate specific chemical reactions. Enzymes often have chemical names ending in *-ase*, such as amylase (an enzyme that splits starch or amylose). The ending *-ase* indicates an enzyme; the root tells what it digests. Other examples: protease (an enzyme that splits protein) and lipase (an enzyme that splits fats).

microvilli (MY-croh-VILL-ee, MY-croh-VILL-eye): tiny hairlike projections on each cell of the intestinal tract lining that can trap nutrient particles and translocate them into the cells (singular: **microvillus**).

mucus (MYOO-cus): a thick, slippery coating of the intestinal tract lining (and other body linings) that protects the cells from exposure to digestive juices. The adjective form is *mucous*. The **mucous membrane** is the digestive tract lining.

peristalsis (perri-STALL-sis): the wavelike squeezing motions of the stomach and intestines that push their contents along.

pylorus (pye-LORE-us): the circular muscle that regulates the opening at the bottom of the stomach. See Figure I–2.

villi (VILL-ee, VILL-eye): poked-out parts of the sheet of cells that line the gastrointestinal tract; the villi make the surface area much greater than it would otherwise be (singular: **villus**).

fluids. Finally, units that the cells can use—glucose, glycerol, fatty acids, and amino acids, among others—are released. These are contacted and absorbed through the intestinal villi. Nutrients released early, such as simple sugars, and those requiring no special handling, such as the water-soluble vitamins, are absorbed high in the small intestine: nutrients that are released more slowly are absorbed further down. The lymphatic and circulatory systems then take over the job of transporting the nutrients to the cell consumers. The lymph at first carries most of the products of fat digestion and the fat-soluble vitamins, later delivering them to the blood. The blood carries the products of carbohydrate and protein digestion, the water-soluble vitamins, and the minerals. By the time the remaining mixture reaches the end of the small intestine, little is left but water, indigestible residue (mostly fiber), and dissolved minerals. The cells lining the colon are specialized for absorbing these minerals and retrieving the water for recycling. The final waste product, the feces, a smooth paste of a consistency suitable for excretion, is stored in the colon. Such a system can adjust to whatever mixture of foods is presented. Although a meal may be eaten in half an hour, the nutrients it provides reach the body fluids over a span of about four hours.

Index

U.S. RDA for Adults

Nutrient	RDA for an Adult Male (1968)	RDA for an Adult Female (1968)	U.S. RDA for Adults[a]
Nutrients that must *appear on the label:*[b]			
Protein (g), PER ≥ casein[c]	45	—	45
Protein (g) PER < casein	65	55	65
Vitamin A (RE)	1000[d]	800[d]	1000[d]
Vitamin C (ascorbic acid) (mg)	60	55	60
Thiamin (vitamin B_1) (mg)	1.4	1.0	1.5
Riboflavin (vitamin B_2) (mg)	1.7	1.5	1.7
Niacin (mg)	18	13	20
Calcium (g)	0.8	0.8	1.0
Iron (mg)	10	18	18
Nutrients that may *appear on the label:*			
Vitamin D (IU)	—	—	400[e]
Vitamin E (IU)	30[f]	25[f]	30[f]
Vitamin B_6 (mg)	2.0	2.0	2.0
Folic acid (folacin) (mg)	0.4	0.4	0.4
Vitamin B_{12} (μg)	6	6	6
Phosphorus (g)	0.8	0.8	1.0
Iodine (μg)	120	100	150
Magnesium (mg)	350	300	400
Zinc (mg)	—	—	15
Copper (mg)	—	—	2
Biotin (mg)	—	—	0.3
Pantothenic acid (mg)	—	—	10

[a]Separate tables of U.S. RDA are published for infants, children, and pregnant and lactating women.
[b]Must appear whenever nutrition labeling is required.
[c]PER is an index of protein quality explained in Chapter 5. Casein is milk protein.
[d]1000 RE was originally expressed as 5000 IU. 800 RE was originally expressed as 4000 IU.
[e]400 IU vitamin D is the same as 10 μg; see inside front cover.
[f]30 IU vitamin E is the same as 30 mg. 25 IU vitamin E is the same as 25 mg. The RDA for vitamin E has since been lowered.

Note: As of 1980, the U.S. RDA numbers used on labels were still those taken from the 1968 RDA. There was no great need to update them, because they still would be judged generous by any standard, and because the expense of converting labels to a different set of numbers would be too great to warrant the change. The circled numbers are those chosen for the U.S. RDA from the adult male and female recommendations. In each case, the higher number is chosen. In the cases of thiamin, niacin, iodine, and magnesium, the RDA for an adolescent boy are used, because these are even higher than the adult RDA. In the cases of calcium and phosphorus, 1 g/day is used, more than the adult RDA. Pregnant and lactating women and rapidly growing teenagers have RDA even higher than this, but 1 g was considered generous enough for use as a standard for labels.

In the cases of the last four nutrients—zinc, copper, biotin, and pantothenic acid—RDA had not been set as of 1968, but these nutrients were known to be essential. The agency set "guestimates" for these so that labels showing percentages of U.S. RDA could include them. As of 1980, all four of these nutrients were included in the RDA tables, but the U.S. RDA values were not changed to correspond; they were considered close enough already.

Source: Adapted from *Food Technology* 28, no. 7 (1974):5.